Clinical Scenarios in Surgery

Decision Making and Operative Technique

SECOND EDITION

Clinical Scenarios in Surgery

Decision Making and Operative Technique

SECOND EDITION

Justin B. Dimick, MD, MPH
George D. Zuidema Professor of Surgery
Chief, Division of Minimally Invasive
    Surgery
Department of Surgery
University of Michigan
Ann Arbor, Michigan

Gilbert R. Upchurch Jr., MD
Woodward Professor & Chair
Department of Surgery
University of Florida
Professor of Surgery
Vascular Surgery Division
UF Health Shands Hospital
Gainesville, Florida

Christopher J. Sonnenday, MD, MHS
Associate Professor of Surgery, Health
    Management & Policy
Department of Surgery
University of Michigan
Ann Arbor, Michigan

Lillian S. Kao, MD, MS
Professor
Department of Surgery
McGovern Medical School at the
    University of Texas Health Science
    Center at Houston
Houston, Texas

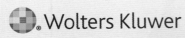 Wolters Kluwer

Philadelphia · Baltimore · New York · London
Buenos Aires · Hong Kong · Sydney · Tokyo

Senior Acquisitions Editor: Keith Donnellan
Editorial Coordinator: Lauren Pecarich
Marketing Managers: Rachel Mante Leung
Production Project Manager: Joan Sinclair
Design Coordinator: Stephen Druding
Manufacturing Coordinator: Beth Welsh
Prepress Vendor: SPi Global

Second Edition

9 8 7 6 5 4 3

Printed in China

Library of Congress Cataloging-in-Publication Data
Names: Dimick, Justin B., editor. | Upchurch, Gilbert R., editor. | Sonnenday, Christopher J., editor. | Kao, Lillian S., editor.
Title: Clinical scenarios in surgery : decision making and operative technique / [edited by] Justin B. Dimick, Gilbert R. Upchurch Jr., Christopher J. Sonnenday, Lillian S. Kao.
Other titles: Clinical scenarios in surgery.
Description: Second edition. | Philadelphia : Wolters Kluwer, [2019] | Preceded by Clinical scenarios in surgery / editors, Justin B. Dimick, Gilbert R. Upchurch Jr., Christophr J. Sonnenday. c2013. | Includes bibliographical references and index.
Identifiers: LCCN 2018036067 | ISBN 9781496349071 (hardback)
Subjects: | MESH: Surgical Procedures, Operative—methods | Decision Making | Case Reports
Classification: LCC RD34 | NLM WO 16.1 | DDC 617—dc23 LC record available at https://lccn.loc.gov/2018036067

shop.lww.com

To my wife, Anastasia, and our children, Mary and Paul, for their love and support. To the dedicated general surgery residents, who will use the contents of this book to heal and comfort our patients.

—Justin B. Dimick

To the faculty and residents at the University of Florida for accepting me as a Gator.

—Gilbert R. Upchurch Jr.

To the general surgery residents of the University of Michigan, for their constant inspiration and dedication to patient care.

—Christopher J. Sonnenday

To the general surgery faculty and residents at McGovern Medical School at the University of Texas Health Science Center at Houston and to the providers at Red Duke Trauma Institute and Memorial Hermann Hospital-Texas Medical Center for their dedication to high-quality, patient-centered surgical care.

—Lillian S. Kao

CONTRIBUTORS

Daniel Albo, MD, PhD
Chief, Division of Surgical Oncology
Department of Surgery
Baylor College of Medicine
Director, GI Oncology Program
Dan L. Duncan Cancer Center
Baylor College of Medicine
Houston, Texas

Christina V. Angeles, MD
Assistant Professor of Surgery
Division of Surgical Oncology
Geisel School of Medicine
Attending Surgeon
Dartmouth-Hitchcock Medical Center
Lebanon, New Hampshire

Stanley W. Ashley, MD
Instructor of Surgery
Department of Surgery
Harvard Medical School
Brigham and Women's Hospital
Boston, Massachusetts

Naira Baregamian, MD
Assistant Professor of Surgery
Division of Surgical Oncology & Endocrine Surgery
Vanderbilt University Medical Center
Nashville, Tennessee

Carlton C. Barnett Jr., MD
Professor of Surgery
Department of Surgery
University of Colorado
Position Chief, Surgical Oncology VAMC
Rocky Mountain Regional VA Medical Center
Denver, Colorado

Douglas C. Barnhart, MD, MSPH
Professor, Division of Pediatric Surgery
University of Utah School of Medicine
Program Director, Pediatric Surgery Fellowship
Medical Director for Surgical Patient Safety and Quality
Primary Children's Hospital
Salt Lake City, Utah

Meredith Barrett, MD
General Surgery House Officer
University of Michigan
Ann Arbor, Michigan

Jessica M. Bensenhaver, MD, MS, FACS
Director of Breast Oncology
Research Director, International Center for the Study of Breast
 Cancer Subtypes
Department of Surgery
Henry Ford Health System
Detroit, Michigan

Noelle L. Bertelson, MD, FACS, FASCRS
Attending Surgeon
Colon and Rectal Surgery
Colon and Rectal Clinic of Colorado
St. Joseph Hospital
Denver, Colorado

Kunjan S. Bhakta, MD
Clinical Lecturer of Surgery
Department of Surgery
University of Michigan
Ann Arbor, Michigan

James H. Black III, MD, FACS
The David Goldfarb, MD Associate Professor of Surgery
Director, Division of Vascular Surgery and
 Endovascular Therapy
Johns Hopkins Hospital
Baltimore, Maryland

Jeffrey A. Blatnik, MD
Assistant Professor
Department of Surgery
Washington University in St. Louis
Barnes-Jewish Hospital
St. Louis, Missouri

Melissa M. Boltz, DO, MBA
Assistant Professor of Surgery
Penn State Milton S. Hershey Medical Center
Hershey, Pennsylvania

Judy C. Boughey, MD
Vice Chair for Research
Department of Surgery
Professor of Surgery
Mayo Clinic
Mayo Clinic Hospital, Methodist Campus
Rochester, Minnesota

Brooke C. Bredbeck, MD
Department of Surgery
University of Michigan
Ann Arbor, Michigan

Steven W. Bruch, MD, MSc
Clinical Associate Professor
Department of Surgery
University of Michigan
CS Mott Children's Hospital Pediatric Surgery
Ann Arbor, Michigan

Terry Lynn Buchmiller, MD
Associate Professor
Harvard Medical School and Boston
 Children's Hospital
Boston, Massachusetts

Richard A. Burkhart, MD
Assistant Professor
Department of Surgery and Oncology,
Johns Hopkins University & Hospital
Baltimore, Maryland

Clay Cothren Burlew, MD, FACS
Professor of Surgery
Department of Surgery
University of Colorado
Director, Surgical Intensive Care Unit
Denver Health Medical Center
Denver, Colorado

Richard E. Burney, MD
Professor Emeritus of Surgery
Department of Surgery
Michigan Medicine
University of Michigan Hospitals
Ann Arbor, Michigan

William R. Burns, MD
Assistant Professor
Department of Surgery
University of Michigan
Surgeon, Michigan Medicine
Ann Arbor, Michigan

John C. Byrn, MD
Clinical Associate Professor of Surgery
Division of Colorectal Surgery
Department of Surgery
University of Michigan Health System
Ann Arbor, Michigan

Jeremy Cannon, MD, FACS
Associate Professor of Surgery
Division of Trauma, Critical Care and Emergency Surgery
Department of Surgery
Perelman School of Medicine, University of Pennsylvania
Philadelphia, Pennsylvania

Benjamin David Carr, MD
House Officer
Department of Surgery
University of Michigan, Michigan Medicine
Ann Arbor, Michigan

Stacey A. Carter, MD
Assistant Professor
Michael E. DeBakey Department of Surgery
Baylor College of Medicine
Houston, Texas

Eugene P. Ceppa, MD
Associate Professor of Surgery
Indiana University School of Medicine
Indianapolis, Indiana

William Z. Chancellor, MD
Resident
Department of Surgery
University of Virginia School of Medicine
Charlottesville, Virginia

Andrew C. Chang, MD
Associate Professor and Head
Section of Thoracic Surgery
University of Michigan, Michigan Medicine
Ann Arbor, Michigan

Alfred E. Chang, MD
Hugh Cabot Professor of Surgery
Division of Surgical Oncology, Department of Surgery
University of Michigan Health Systems
Ann Arbor, Michigan

Anthony Charles, MD, MPH, FACS
Associate Professor of Surgery
School of Medicine
Director, UNC-ECMO Program
University of North Carolina
Chapel Hill, North Carolina

Herbert Chen, MD, FACS
Fay Fletcher Kerner Endowed Chair and Professor
Chairman and Surgeon-in-Chief
Department of Surgery
University of Alabama at Birmingham Health
University of Alabama at Birmingham
Birmingham, Alabama

Sonia Cohen, MD, PhD
Surgery Resident
Department of Surgery
Masachusetts General Hospital
Boston, Masachusetts

Bryan A. Cotton, MD, MPH
John B. Holmes Professor in Clinical Sciences
McGovern Medical School at the University of Texas Health
Trauma Surgeon
Red Duke Trauma Institute at Memorial Hermann Hospital-TMC
Houston, Texas

Robert A. Cowles, MD
Associate Professor of Surgery
Yale School of Medicine
New Haven, Connecticut

Christopher J. Crellin, MD
Resident Physician
Obstetrics and Gynecology
Tripler Army Medical Center
Honolulu, Hawaii

Michael W. Cripps, MD, MSCS, FACS
Assistant Professor
Division of General and Acute Care Surgery
Department of Surgery
University of Texas Southwestern Medical Center at Dallas
Medical Director, Surgical Intensive Care Unit
Parkland Memorial Hospital
Dallas, Texas

James M. Cross, MD, FACS
Professor of Surgery
Director, Burn Center
University of Texas Health Science Center at Houston
Houston, Texas

Stephen W. Davies, MD
Department of Surgery
University of Virginia
Charlottesville, Virginia

Priya H. Dedhia, MD, PhD
Endocrine Surgery Fellow
Department of Surgery
University of Wisconsin School of Medicine and Public Health
University of Wisconsin Hospital and Clinics
Madison, Wisconsin

Ronald P. DeMatteo, MD
Vice Chair
Department of Surgery
Memorial Sloan-Kettering Cancer Center
New York, New York

Danielle K. DePeralta, MD
Surgical Oncology Fellow
Moffitt Cancer Center
Tampa, Florida

Emilia J. Diego, MD, FACS
Assistant Professor
Department of Surgery
University of Pittsburgh School of Medicine
Section Chief
Breast Surgery
Magee Women's Hospital–University of Pittsburgh
    Medical Center
Pittsburgh, Pennsylvania

Charles S. Dietrich III, MD
Associate Professor
Department of Obstetrics and Gynecology
Uniformed Services University of the Health Sciences
Bethesda, Maryland
Chief
Gynecologic Oncology Service
Tripler Army Medical Center
Honolulu, Hawaii

Anastasia Dimick, MD
Laing & Dimick Dermatology
Ann Arbor, Michigan

Justin B. Dimick, MD, MPH
George D. Zuidema Professor of Surgery
Chief, Division of Minimally Invasive Surgery
Department of Surgery
University of Michigan
Ann Arbor, Michigan

Sharmila Dissanaike, MD, FACS, FCCM
Peter C. Canizaro Chair & Professor
Department of Surgery
Texas Tech University Health Sciences Center
Chief, University Medical Center
Lubbock, Texas

Gerard M. Doherty, MD
Moseley Professor of Surgery, Harvard Medical School
Surgeon-in-Chief, Brigham and Women's Health Care
Boston, Massachusetts

Michael J. Englesbe, MD
Darling Professor of Surgery
Associate Professor of Surgery – Transplantation
University of Michigan Medical School
Ann Arbor, Michigan

Cecilia G. Ethun, MD, MSCR
Post-Doctoral Research Fellow
Division of Surgical Oncology, Department of Surgery
Winship Cancer Institute, Emory University
Resident in General Surgery
Emory University
Atlanta, Georgia

David A. Etzioni, MD, MSHS
Associate Professor
Surgery, Mayo Clinic College of Medicine
Consultant, Mayo Clinic Arizona
Phoenix, Arizona

Heather Leigh Evans, MD, MS
Professor
Department of Surgery
Medical University of South Carolina
Vice Chair of Clinical Research and Applied Informatics
Charleston, South Carolina

Carole Fakhry, MD, MPH
Associate Professor
Department of Otolaryngology-Head and Neck Surgery
Johns Hopkins University
Baltimore, Maryland

Gavin A. Falk, MD
Pediatric Surgery
Kalispell Regional Medical Center
Kalispell, Montana

Anna Z. Fashandi, MD
Department of Surgery
University of Virginia
Charlottesville, Virginia

Joseph Fernandez-Moure, MD, PhD
Division of Trauma, Critical Care and Emergency Surgery
Department of Surgery
Perelman School of Medicine, University of Pennsylvania
Philadelphia, Pennsylvania

Cristina R. Ferrone, MD
Associate Professor and Director of Liver Program
Department of Surgery
Massachusetts General Hospital
Boston, Massachusetts

Jonathan F. Finks, MD
Associate Professor of Surgery
University of Michigan
Ann Arbor, Michigan

Emily Finlayson, MD, MS
Professor in Residence
Department of Surgery, Medicine, and Health Policy
University of California
Professor of Surgery
Division of General Surgery
UCSF Medical Center
San Francisco, California

Samuel R.G. Finlayson, MD, MPH, FACS
Chair and Professor
Department of Surgery
University of Utah School of Medicine
University of Utah Health
Salt Lake City, Utah

Emily M. Fontenot, MD
Department of Surgery
University of North Carolina at Chapel Hill
Chapel Hill, North Carolina

Danielle M. Fritze, MD
Assistant Professor of Surgery
Transplant Surgery
University of Texas Health Science Center
San Antonio, Texas

Sara Amelia Gaines, MD
General Surgery Resident
Department of Surgery
University of Chicago Medical Center
Chicago, Illinois

Wolfgang B. Gaertner, MD, MSc, FACS, FASCRS
Assistant Professor
Division of Colon & Rectal Surgery
Department of Surgery
University of Minnesota
Minneapolis, Minnesota

Paul G. Gauger, MD
Professor of Surgery, Professor of Learning Health Sciences
Dept of Surgery, Michigan Medicine
Attending Surgeon, University of Michigan Hospital
Ann Arbor, Michigan

Mitchell J. George, MD
General Surgery Resident
Department of Surgery
McGovern Medical School
Memorial Herman Hospital
Houston, Texas

Tonya George, PA-C, PhD
Instructor of Surgery
McGovern Medical School
University of Texas Health Science Center at Houston
Houston, Texas

Amir A. Ghaferi, MD, MS
Associate Professor
Department of Surgery
University of Michigan Medical School
University of Michigan
Ann Arbor, Michigan

Ian C. Glenn, MD
Department of Surgery
Akron Children's Hospital
Akron, Ohio

Philip P. Goodney, MD
Associate Professor of Vascular Surgery
Dartmouth-Hitchcock Medical Center
Lebanon, New Hampshire

Zhen Gooi, MBBS
Assistant Professor
Section of Otolaryngology-Head and Neck Surgery
Department of Surgery
University of Chicago
Chicago, Illinois

Jessica S. Koller Gorham, MD
Instructor of Surgery
Geisel School of Medicine
Hanover, New Hampshire
Fellow, Minimally Invasive Surgery
Dartmouth-Hitchcock Medical Center
Lebanon, New Hampshire

Jon Gould, MD
Chief and Alonzo P. Walker Chair of General Surgery
Vice Chair for Quality, Department of Surgery
Professor of Surgery, Medical College of Wisconsin
Senior Medical Director for Clinical Affairs
Froedtert Hospital
Milwaukee, Wisconsin

Jacob A. Greenberg, MD, EdM
Associate Professor of Surgery
Department of Surgery
University of Wisconsin
Madison, Mississippi

Sarah E. Greer, MD
Director
Institute for Trauma Research and Injury Prevention
Princeton, New Jersey

Chasen J. Greig, MD
Research Fellow, Pediatric Surgery
Yale School of Medicine
New Haven, Connecticut

Tyler R. Grenda, MD
Fellow, Cardiothoracic Surgery
Section of Thoracic Surgery
Department of Surgery
University of Michigan
Ann Arbor, Michigan

Rebecca L. Gunter, MD, MS
General Surgery Resident
Department of Surgery
University of Wisconsin
Madison, Wisconsin

Oliver L. Gunter Jr., MD
Assistant Professor of Surgery
Director, Emergency General Surgery
Vanderbilt University Medical Center
Nashville, Tennessee

Adil H. Haider, MD, MPH, FACS
Kessler Director and Associate Chair for Research
The Center for Surgery and Public Health
Brigham and Women's Hospital
Harvard Medical School, and the Harvard T.H. Chan School of
    Public Health
Boston, Massachusetts

Ihab Halaweish, MD
House Officer VII, General Surgery
University of Michigan
Ann Arbor, Michigan

Amy L. Halverson, MD
Professor of Surgery
Chief, Section of Colon and Rectal Surgery
Northwestern University, Feinberg School of Medicine
Northwestern Memorial Hospital
Chicago, Illinois

Allen Hamdan, MD
Associate Professor of Surgery
Department of Surgery
Harvard Medical School
Attending Surgeon
Division of Vascular and Endovascular Surgery
Beth Israel Deaconess Medical Center
Boston, Massachusetts

Audrey F. Hand, MD
General Surgery Resident
Texas tech University Health Sciences Center
university Medical Center
Lubbock, Texas

Natasha Hansraj, MD
Department of Surgery, Baltimore VA Medical Center and
University of Maryland School of Medicine
Baltimore, Maryland

John A. Harvin, MD, FACS
Assistant Professor
Division of Acute Care Surgery, Department of Surgery
McGovern Medical School at UT Health
University of Texas Health Science Center at Houston
Houston, Texas

Elliott R. Haut, MD, PhD, FACS
Vice Chair of Quality, Safety & Service, Department of Surgery
Associate Professor of Surgery, Anesthesiology/Critical Care
    Medicine (ACCM) and Emergency Medicine
Division of Acute Care Surgery, Department of Surgery
The Johns Hopkins University School of Medicine
Associate Professor of Health Policy & Management
The Johns Hopkins University Bloomberg School of Public Health
Core Faculty, The Armstrong Institute for Patient Safety and
    Quality, JHM
Baltimore, Maryland

Harold Heah, MBBS, M Med, MRCSEd
Adjunct Instructor, Head & Neck Centre
Duke-NUS Medical School
Consultant, Department of Otolaryngology
Singapore General Hospital
Singapore

David W. Healy, MD, MRCP, FRCA
Assistant Professor
Anesthesiology
University of Michigan
Director, Head & Neck Anesthesia
Department of Anesthesiology Health Systems
University of Michigan Hospital and Health Systems
Ann Arbor, Michigan

Mark R. Hemmila, MD, FACS
Professor of Surgery
Trauma Medical Director
University of Michigan Medical School
Michigan Medicine
Ann Arbor, Michigan

Samantha Hendren, MD, MPH
Associate Professor of Surgery
University of Michigan
Attending Surgeon
University Hospital
Ann Arbor, Michigan

Richard J. Hendrickson, MD, FACS, FAAP
Department of Surgery, Children's Mercy Hospital
Kansas City, Missouri

Peter K. Henke, MD
Leland Ira Doan Professor of Surgery
Section of Vascular Surgery
Department of Surgery
University of Michigan
Ann Arbor, Michigan

H. Andrew Hopper, MD
Instructor in Clinical Surgery
Vanderbilt University Medical Center
Nashville, Tennessee

Michael G. House, MD
Associate Professor of Surgery
Department of Surgery
Indiana University School of Medicine
Indianapolis, Indiana

Thomas S. Huber, MD, PhD
Professor and Chief
Department of Surgery
Division of Vascular Surgery
University of Florida
Gainesville, Florida

David T. Hughes, MD
Assistant Professor of Surgery
Division of Endocrine Surgery
Department of Surgery
University of Michigan Hospitals and Health Centers
Ann Arbor, Michigan

JoAnna L. Hunter-Squires, MD
Assistant Professor of Surgery
Indiana University School of Medicine
Indianapolis, Indiana
Indiana University Health
Avon, Indiana

Justin B. Hurie, MD, MBA
Associate Professor
Dept of Vascular and Endovascular Surgery
Wake Forest university
Attending Surgeon
Wake Forest University Hospital
Winston-Salem, North Carolina

Todd F. Huzar, MD, FACS
Assistant Professor of Surgery
University of Texas Health Science Center at Houston
Houston, Texas

Neil Hyman, MD
Professor
Department of Surgery
University of Chicago School of Medicine
Chief, Colorectal Surgery
Codirector, Digestive Disease Center
Chicago, Illinois

Kenji Inaba, MD, FRCSC, FACS
Professor
University of Southern California
Vice Chair & Program Director of Surgery
LAC and USC Medical Center
Department of Surgery
Los Angeles, California

Angela M. Ingraham, MD, MS
Assistant Professor of Surgery
Trauma and Acute Care Surgery
University of Wisconsin
Madison, Wisconsin

Alexis D. Jacob, MD
Assistant Professor
Department of Surgery/Vascular
University of Texas Southwestern Medical Center and Hospital
Dallas, Texas

Kevin N. Johnson, MD
Clinical Lecturer
Department of Surgery
University of Michigan
Staff, Mott Children's Hospital
Ann Arbor, Michigan

Lily E. Johnston, MD, MPH
Department of Surgery
University of Virginia
Charlottesville, Virginia

Douglas Jones, MD
Boston Medical Center
Boston, Massachusetts

Jussuf T. Kaifi, MD, PhD
Assistant Professor of Surgery
Chief, Thoracic Surgery
Department of Surgery
University of Missouri

Jeffrey Kalish, MD
Laszlo N. Tauber Assistant Professor
Department of Surgery
Boston University School of Medicine
Director of Endovascular Surgery
Department of Surgery
Boston Medical Center
Boston, Massachusetts

Bartholomew J. Kane, MD, PhD, FACS
Assistant Professor
Department of Surgery
Kansas University Medical Center
Kansas City, Kansas

Arielle E. Kanters, MD, MS
General Surgery Resident
Department of Surgery
University of Michigan - Michigan Medicine
Ann Arbor, Michigan

Lillian S. Kao, MD, MS
Professor
Department of Surgery
McGovern Medical School at the University of Texas Health
    Science Center at Houston
Houston, Texas

Muneera R. Kapadia, MD
Clinical Associate Professor
Department of Surgery
University of Iowa Carver College of Medicine
University of Iowa Hospital & Clinics
University of Iowa
Iowa City, Iowa

Lewis J. Kaplan, MD, FACS, FCCM, FCCP
Associate Professor of Surgery
Division of Trauma, Critical Care and Emergency Surgery
Department of Surgery
Perelman School of Medicine, University of Pennsylvania
Philadelphia, Pennsylvania
Section Chief, Surgical Critical Care
Corporal Michael J Crescenz VA Medical Center
Philadelphia, Pennsylvania

Alex C. Kim, MD, PhD
Chief Resident
Division of General Surgery
Department of Surgery
University of Michigan Medical School
Ann Arbor, Michigan

Eric T. Kimchi, MD, MBA
Associate Professor of Surgery
Chief, Division of Oncologic and General Surgery
Medical Director, Ellis Fischel Cancer Center
Department of Surgery
University of Missouri
Columbia, Missouri

Martyn Knowles, MD
Adjunct Assistant Professor
Department of Surgery
University of North Carolina
Holly Springs, North Carolina
Attending Vascular Surgeon
University of North Carolina Rex Hospital
Raleigh, North Carolina

Bona Ko, MD
Resident
Department of Surgery
Northwestern University
Northwestern University Hospital
Chicago, Illinois

Lisa M. Kodadek, MD
Fellow, Department of Surgery
Johns Hopkins University School of Medicine
Baltimore, Maryland

Carla Kohoyda-Inglis, MPA
Program Director, International Center for Automotive
    Medicine
Department of General Surgery
University of Michigan Health System
Ann Arbor, Michigan

Geoffrey W. Krampitz, MD, PhD
Fellow, Complex General Surgical Oncology
Department of Surgical Oncology
University of Texas, MD Anderson Cancer Center
Houston, Texas

David M. Krpata, MD
Assistant Professor
Department of Surgery
Cleveland Clinic Lerner College of Medicine
Cleveland, Ohio

Henry Kuerer, MD, PhD, FACS
Robinson Distinguished Endowed Professor
Executive Director, Breast Programs
Department of Surgical Oncology Program
MD Anderson Cancer Center
Houston, Texas

Michael E. Kupferman, MD, MBA
Senior Vice President, Clinical and Academic Network
    Development, Cancer Network
Professor, Head & Neck Surgery
The University of Texan MD Anderson Cancer Center
Houston, Texas

Kate Lak, MD
Attending Physician
Department of Surgery
Froedtert Memorial Lutheran Hospital
Milwaukee, Wisconsin

Christine L. Lau, MD
Associate Professor of Surgery
Division of Thoracic and Cardiovascular Surgery
University of Virginia
Charlottesville, Virginia

Anne Laux, MD
Texas Vascular Associates
Dallas, Texas

Yeranui Ledesma, MD
General Surgery Resident
Department of Surgery
University of California
UCSF Bakar Cancer Hospital
San Francisco, California

Marie Catherine Lee, MD
Associate Professor
Departments of Interdisciplinary Oncology and Surgery
University of South Florida Morsani School of Medicine
Associate Member
Comprehensive Breast Program
Moffitt Cancer Center
Tampa, Florida

Suzie S. Lee, MD
Transplant Fellow
Washington University School of Medicine
St. Louis, Missouri

Anthony J. Lewis, MD, MSc
Chief Resident
Department of Surgery
University of Pittsburgh Medical Center
Pittsburgh, Pennsylvania

Patric Liang, MD
Beth Israel Deaconess Medical Center
Boston, Massachusetts

Jules Lin, MD, FACS
Associate Professor, Mark B. Orringer Professor
Surgical Director, Lung Transplant
Section of Thoracic Surgery
University of Michigan
University of Michigan Hospital
Ann Arbor, Michigan

Pamela A. Lipsett, MD, MHPE, MCCM
Warfield M. Firor Endowed Professorship in Surgery
Professor of Surgery, Anesthesiology, and Critical Care Medicine
Program Director, General Surgery and Surgical Critical Care
Co-Director, Surgical Intensive Care Units
Johns Hopkins University School of Medicine
Baltimore, Maryland

Roy Lirov, MD
General and Endocrine Surgeon
Department of Surgery
Seton Medical Center
Austin, Texas

Ann C. Lowry, MD
Clinical Professor of Surgery
Division of Colon and Rectal Surgery
University of Minnesota
St. Paul, Minnesota

Hubert Yiu-Wei Luu, MD, MS
Resident Physician
Department of Surgery
University of California
San Francisco, California

Paul M. Maggio, MD, MBA, FACS
Associate Professor of Surgery
Vice Chair of Surgery for Clinical Affairs
Associate Chief Medical Officer
Stanford University Medical Center
Stanford, California

Shishir K. Maithel, MD, FACS
Associate Professor of Surgery
Scientific Director, Emory Liver and Pancreas Center
Winship Cancer Institute, Division of Surgical Oncology
Department of Surgery, Emory University
Atlanta, Georgia

Julie A. Margenthaler, MD
Professor of Surgery
Department of Surgery
Washington University School of Medicine
Attending Physician
Barnes-Jewish Hospital
St. Louis, Missouri

Linda W. Martin, MD, MPH
Associate Professor
Division of Thoracic Surgery, Department
    of Surgery
University of Virginia School of Medicine
Charlottesville, Virginia

Kazuhide Matsushima, MD
Assistant Professor of Clinical Surgery
Division of Acute Care Surgery
University of Southern California

Jeffrey B. Matthews, MD, FACS
Surgeon-in-Chief and Chairman
Dallas B. Phemister Professor of Surgery
The University of Chicago Medicine
Chicago, Illinois

Anne E. Mattingly, MD
Breast Surgical Oncologist
Hendricks Regional Health Breast Center
Danville, Indiana

Haggi Mazeh, MD
Associate Professor with tenure
Department of Surgery
Hadassah-Hebrew University Medical Center
Jerusalem, Israel

Greg J. McKenna, MD, FRCS(C), FACS
Associate Professor of Surgery
Texas A&M College of Medicine
Multiorgan Abdominal Transplant Surgeon
Simmons Transplant Institute
Baylor University Medical Center
Dallas, Texas

Sean E. McLean, MD
Associate Professor
Division of Pediatric Surgery
Department of Surgery
University of North Carolina at Chapel Hill
University of North Carolina Children's Hospital
Chapel Hill, North Carolina

Ashley D. Meagher, MD, MPH
Assistant Professor
University of Indiana School of Medicine
Indianapolis, Indiana

Benjamin D. Medina, MD
Research Fellow
Department of Surgery
Memorial Sloan-Kettering Cancer Center
New York, New York

Patrick D. Melmer, MD
General Surgery Resident, PDY-2
Department of Surgery
University of South Carolina
Columbia, South Carolina
Grand Strand Medical Center
Myrtle Beach, South Carolina

Genevieve B. Melton-Meaux, MD, PhD
Professor of Surgery and Health Informatics Core
    Faculty
University of Minnesota
Chief Data and Health Informatics Officer
Fairview Health Services
Minneapolis, Minnesota

Joseph Melvin, MD
Chief Surgical Resident
Department of Surgery
University of Missouri
Columbia, Missouri

David E. Meyer, MD, MS, FACS
Assistant Professor of Surgery
McGovern Medical School at UT Health
Memorial Hermann Hospital - Texas Medical Center
Houston, Texas

Stacey A. Milan, MD, FACS
Assistant Professor of Surgery
Texas Tech University Health Sciences Center, El Paso
El Paso, Texas

Barbra S. Miller, MD, FACS
Assistant Professor
Department of Surgery
University of Michigan
Michigan Medicine
Ann Arbor, Michigan

Katrina B. Mitchell, MD
Clinical Assistant Professor
Department of Surgery
University of New Mexico
Breast Surgical Oncologist
Surgical Oncology
Presbyterian Healthcare Services-MD Anderson Cancer
    Network
Albuquerque, New Mexico

Omeed Moaven, MD
Clinical Fellow
Division of Surgical Oncology
Department of Surgery
Wake Forest University
Winston-Salem, North Carolina

Adeyiza O. Momoh, MD, FACS
Associate Professor of Surgery
Section of Plastic Surgery
Department of Surgery
University of Michigan
Ann Arbor, Michigan

Derek Moore, MD, MPH
Associate Professor
University of Tennessee Health Science Center
Program Director
St. Thomas West
Nashville, Tennessee

Arden M. Morris, MD, MPH
Professor and Vice Chair for Clinical Research
Section of Colorectal Surgery
Department of Surgery
Stanford University School of Medicine
Stanford Hospital
Stanford, California

Monica Morrow, MD
Professor of Surgery
Weill Medical College of Cornell University
New York, New York
Chief, Breast Service
Department of Surgery
Anne Burnett Windfohr Chair of Clinical Oncology
Memorial Sloan-Kettering Cancer Center
New York, New York

Rori E. Morrow, MD
Vascular Fellow
Division of Vascular and Endovascular Surgery
University of Virginia
Charlottesville, Virginia

Michael W. Mulholland, MD, PhD
Professor of Surgery
Chair, Department of Surgery
University of Michigan
Ann Arbor, Michigan

Shilpa S. Murthy, MD, MPH
Oncology Fellow
Fox Chase Cancer Center
Philadelphia, Pennsylvania

Alykhan S. Nagji, MD
General Thoracic Surgeon
Assistant Professor
Department of Cardiovascular and Thoracic Surgery
Associate Program Director – Cardiothoracic Surgery
   Fellowship
The University of Kansas Health System
Kansas City, Kansas

Avery B. Nathens, MD, MPH, PhD
Professor
Department of Surgery
University of Toronto
Chief of Surgery
Sunnybrook Health Sciences Centre
Toronto, Ontario, Canada

Nicole Nevarez, MD
Surgical Resident
University of Texas – Southwestern
Dallas, Texas

Lisa A. Newman, MD, MPH, FACS, FASCO
Director, Henry Ford Health System Breast Oncology Program
Medical Director, International Center for the Study
   of Breast Cancer Subtypes
Adjunct Professor of Surgery, MD Anderson Cancer Center
Adjunct Professor, Health Management and Policy, University of
   Michigan School of Public Health
Detroit, Michigan

Erika A. Newman, MD
Assistant Professor, Pediatric Surgery
University of Michigan
C.S. Mott Children's Hospital
Ann Arbor, Michigan

Stephanie Nitzschke, MD
Instructor of Surgery
Harvard Medical School
Associate Surgeon
Brigham and Women's Hospital
Boston, Massachusetts

Jeffrey A. Norton, MD
Professor of Surgery
Stanford University, School of Medicine
Stanford, California

Yuri W. Novitsky, MD, FACS
Professor of Surgery
Director, Columbia Comprehensive Hernia Center
Columbia University Medical Center
New York, New York

Nabeel R. Obeid, MD
Assistant Professor of Surgery
Minimally-Invasive and Bariatric Surgeon
University of Michigan Medical School
Michigan Medicine
Ann Arbor, Michigan

Robert W. O'Rourke, MD
Professor
Department of Surgery
University of Michigan Medical School
Chief, Division of General Surgery
Ann Arbor Veteran's Administration Hospital
Ann Arbor, Michigan

Carlos H. Palacio, MD
Fellow Surgical Critical Care
Division of Acute Care Surgery
Michael E. DeBakey Department of Surgery
Baylor College of Medicine
Houston, Texas

Lucian Panait, MD
Minimally Invasive Surgeon
Department of Surgery
AtlantiCare Regional Medical Center
Atlantic City, New Jersey

Timothy M. Pawlik, MD, MPH, PhD
Professor and Chair
The Ohio State University School of Medicine
Chair of Surgery
Department of Surgery
Wexner Medical Center
Columbus, Ohio

Christian Perez, MD
Medical Director of Metabolic and Bariatric Surgery
Department of Surgery, Carle Foundation Hospital
Urbana, Illinois

Lindsay Petersen, MD
Surgeon, Henry Ford Health System Breast Oncology Program
Clinical Assistant Professor, Wayne State University School of Medicine
Detroit, Michigan

Benjamin K. Poulose, MD, MPH
Robert M. Zollinger Lecrone-Baxter Professor of Surgery
Chief, Division of General and Gastrointestinal Surgery
The Ohio State University College of Medicine, Wexner Medical Center
Columbus, Ohio

Michael J. Pucci, MD, FACS
Assistant Professor of Surgery
Department of Surgery
Sidney Kimmel Medical College
Thomas Jefferson University
Philadelphia, Pennsylvania

Jennifer Racz, MD
Assistant Professor of Surgery
Department of Surgery
Mayo Clinic
Mayo Clinic Hospital, Methodist Campus
Rochester, Minnesota

Krishnan Raghavendran, MD
Professor of Surgery; Division Chief, Acute Care Surgery
Director, Michigan Center for Global Surgery
Department of Surgery, Michigan Medicine
University of Michigan
Ann Arbor, Michigan

Matthew W. Ralls, MD
Assistant Professor, Pediatric Surgery
Department of Surgery
University of Michigan
Ann Arbor, Michigan

Sara K. Rasmussen, MD, PhD, FACS
Assistant Professor of Surgery
Department of Surgery
University of Virginia Health System
Charlottesville, Virginia

Scott E. Regenbogen, MD, MPH
Department of Colon and Rectal Surgery
Lahey Clinic
Burlington, Massachusetts

William P. Robinson III, MD
Associate Professor
Division of Vascular and Endovascular Surgery
University of Virginia School of Medicine
University of Virginia Health System
Charlottesville, Virginia

Michael J. Rosen, MD, FACS
Professor of Surgery
Department of General Surgery
Cleveland Clinic Foundation
Cleveland, Ohio

Kelly Joyce Rosso, MD
Breast Surgical Oncologist
Department of Surgical Oncology
Banner MD Anderson Cancer Center
Gilbert, Arizona

Campbell S. Roxburgh, PhD, FRCS
Clinical Senior Lecturer
Institute of Cancer Sciences
University of Glasgow
Consultant Colorectal Surgeon
Department of Colorectal Surgery
Glasgow Royal Infirmary
Glasgow, United Kingdom

Michael S. Sabel, MD
William W. Coon Collegiate Professor of Surgery
Chief of Surgical Oncology
Division of Surgical Oncology, Department of Surgery
University of Michigan Health Systems
Ann Arbor, Michigan

Ian C. Sando, MD
Plastic and Reconstructive Surgery
St. Vincent Medical Group
Carmel, Indiana

George A. Sarosi Jr., MD
Robert H. Hux Professor of Surgery
Vice Chairman for Education
University of Florida College of Medicine
Gainesville, Florida

Brian D. Saunders, MD, FACS
Associate Professor of Surgery and Medicine
Penn State College of Medicine
Penn State Milton S. Hershey Medical Center
Hershey, Pennsylvania

Sara Scarlet, MD
Department of Surgery
University of North Carolina at Chapel Hill
Chapel Hill, North Carolina

Samuel A. Schechtman, MD
Clinical Assistant Professor
Director of Head and Neck Anesthesiology & Airway Management
Faculty Anesthesiologist
Michigan Medicine—University of Michigan
Department of Anesthesiology
Ann Arbor, Michigan

Randall P. Scheri, MD
Associate Professor of Surgery
Department of Surgery
Duke University Medical Center
Duke University
Durham, North Carolina

Andrew B. Schneider, MD
General Surgery Resident
Department of Surgery
The University of Chicago Medicine
Chicago, Illinois

Stephanie Sea, MD
Critical Care Fellow
University of Southern California
Los Angeles, California

Shinil K. Shah, DO, FACS
Assistant Professor of Surgery
Department of Surgery
University of Texas Health McGovern Medical School
Houston, Texas

Mihir M. Shah, MD
Department of Surgery
Emory University Hospital
Atlanta, Georgia

Miraj G. Shah-Khan, MD, FACS
Assistant Professor of Surgery
Division of Surgical Oncology
Medical College of Wisconsin
Milwaukee, Wisconsin

Scott S. Short, MD
Assistant Professor of Pediatric Surgery
Primary Children's Hospital
University of Utah School of Medicine
Salt Lake City, Utah

Sarah P. Shubeck, MD, MS
House Officer, General Surgery
Department of Surgery
University of Michigan
Ann Arbor, Michigan

Matthew J. Sideman, MD
Associate Professor
Department of Surgery
University of Texas Health Science Center at San Antonio
San Antonio, Texas

Rebecca S. Sippel, MD
Associate Professor of Surgery
University of Wisconsin School of Medicine and Public Health
Chief of Division of Endocrine Surgery
Department of Surgery
University of Wisconsin Hospitals and Clinics
Madison, Wisconsin

Jeffrey J. Skubic, DO
Instructor of Surgery
Harvard Medical School
Fellow in Trauma and Acute Care Surgery
Brigham and Women's Hospital
Boston, Massachusetts

Oliver S. Soldes, MD, FACS, FAAP
Associate Professor of Surgery
Division of Pediatric Surgery
Dayton Children's Hospital
Dayton, Ohio

Carmen C. Solórzano, MD
Professor of Surgery
Chief, Division of Surgical Oncology & Endocrine Surgery
Vanderbilt University Medical Center
Nashville, Tennessee

Vernon K. Sondak, MD
Department of Cutaneous Oncology
H. Lee Moffitt Cancer Center
Tampa, Florida

Christopher J. Sonnenday, MD, MHS
Associate Professor of Surgery, Health Management & Policy
Department of Surgery
University of Michigan
Ann Arbor, Michigan

Julie Ann Sosa, MD, MA, FACS
Leon Goldman MD Distinguished Professor of Surgery
and Chair
Department of Surgery
University of California, San Francisco
San Francisco, California

Jason L. Sperry, MD, MPH
Professor of Surgery and Critical Care
Director of Acute Care Surgery Fellowship
University of Pittsburgh Medical Center
Pittsburgh, Pennsylvania

Kevin F. Staveley-O'Carroll, MD, PhD
Professor of Surgery, Medicine, Microbiology and Immunology
Department of Surgery
Penn State College of Medicine
Penn State Hershey Medical Center
Hershey, Pennsylvania

Scott R. Steele, MD
Professor of Surgery
Chairman, Department of Colorectal Surgery
Cleveland Clinic Lerner College of Medicine at Case Western Reserve University
Cleveland, Ohio

Melissa K. Stewart, MD
Instructor
Acute and Critical Care Surgery
Washington University
Barnes Jewish Hospital
St. Louis, Missouri

Kimberly S. Stone, MD
Clinical Assistant Professor
Department of Surgery
Stanford University Medical Center
Stanford, California
Medical Director
Stanford Cancer Center South Bay
San Jose, California

Erin A. Strong, MD, MBA, MPH
Resident in Surgery, Department of Surgery
Medical College of Wisconsin Affiliated Hospitals
Milwaukee, Wisconsin

Ryan M. Svoboda, MD
Resident, Vascular Surgery
Dartmouth-Hitchcock Medical Center
Lebanon, New Hampshire

John F. Sweeney, MD
W. Dean Warren Distinguished Professor of Surgery
Department of Surgery
Emory University School of Medicine
Atlanta, Georgia

Dana A. Telem, MD, MPH
Associate Professor of Surgery
Division of Minimally-Invasive Surgery
Michigan Medicine
Ann Arbor, Michigan

Pierre R. Theodore, MD
Vice President, Thoracic Surgical Oncology
Johnson & Johnson Medical Devices Companies
UCSF Health Sciences Associate Professor of Surgery
UCSF Van Auken Endowed Chair, Thoacic Surgery
San Francisco, California

Jonathan R. Thompson, MD
Assistant Professor of Surgery
Associate Program Director, Vascular Surgery Fellowship
University of Nebraska Medical Center
Omaha, Nebraska

Nirav C. Thosani, MD, MHA
Artilla Ertan MD Chair in Gastroenterology, Hepatology & Nutrition
Assistant Professor, Gastroenterology, Hepatology & Nutrition
McGovern Medical School, University of Texas Health Science Center at Houston
Houston, Texas

Carlos H. Timaran, MD
Professor
Department of Surgery
UT Southwestern Medical Center
Dallas, Texas
Adjunct Assistant Professor
Department of Surgery
University of North Carolina Rex Hospital
Raleigh, North Carolina

Thadeus Trus, MD
Associate Professor of Surgery
Department of Surgery
Dartmouth Medical School
Lebanon, New Hampshire

Susan Tsai, MD, MHS
Associate Professor
Division of Surgical Oncology
Department of Surgery
Medical College of Wisconsin
Froedtert Memorial Lutheran Hospital
Milwaukee, Wisconsin

Douglas J. Turner, MD, FACS
Division of General Surgery
Baltimore VA Medical Center
Baltimore, Maryland

Anna Tyson, MD, MPH
Chief Surgical Resident
Carolinas Medical Center
Charlotte, North Carolina

Gilbert R. Upchurch Jr., MD
Woodward Professor & Chair
Department of Surgery
University of Florida
Professor of Surgery
Vascular Surgery Division
UF Health Shands Hospital
Gainesville, Florida

Eva Maria Urrechaga, MD
Resident in General Surgery
Department of Surgery
University of Miami
Miami, Florida

Kyle J. Van Arendonk, MD, PhD
Assistant Professor
Department of Surgery
Medical College of Wisconsin
Pediatric Surgeon, Children's Hospital of Wisconsin
Milwaukee, Wisconsin

Oliver A. Varban, MD
Assistant Professor of Surgery
Michigan Medicine, University Hospital
University of Michigan
Ann Arbor, Michigan

Seth A. Waits, MD
Clinical Lecturer of Surgery – Transplantation
University of Michigan
Ann Arbor, Michigan

Peter A. Walker, MD
Assistant Professor, Surgery
McGovern Medical School, University of Texas Health Science Center at Houston
Houston, Texas

Stewart C. Wang, MD, PhD
Endowed Professor of Burn Surgery & Professor of Surgery
Department of General Surgery
University of Michigan Health Systems
Ann Arbor, Michigan

Jeremy L. Ward, MD
Assistant Professor of Surgery
Michael E. DeBakey Department of Surgery
Baylor College of Medicine
Attending Surgeon, General Surgery, Ben Taub Hospital
Houston, Texas

Martin R. Weiser, MD
Professor
Department of Surgery
Weill Cornell Medical College
Vice Chairman
Department of Surgery
Memorial Sloan Kettering Cancer Center
New York, New York

Bradford P. Whitcomb, MD
Associate Professor of Obstetrics and Gynecology
UConn School of Medicine
Division Chief, Gynecologic Oncology, Obstetrics and
  Gynecology
Carole and Ray Neag Comprehensive Cancer Center UConn
  Health
Farmington, Connecticut

Joseph M. White, MD, FACS
MAJ(P), United States Army
Associate Program Director, Vascular Surgery Fellowship
Assistant Professor of Surgery
Department of Surgery at Uniformed Services University of the
  Health Sciences
Walter Reed National Military Medical Center
Bethesda, Maryland

David R. Whittaker, MD, FACS
Chief of Vascular and Endovascular Surgery
Uniformed Services University of the Health Sciences and
Walter Reed National Military Medical Center
Bethesda, Maryland

Carlin Williams, MD
University of Virginia
Charlottesville, Virginia

Emily R. Winslow, MD, FACS
Associate Professor of Surgery
Department of Surgery
University of Wisconsin Health
University of Wisconsin
Madison, Wisconsin

Kevin B. Wise, MD
Assistant Professor of Surgery
Department of Surgery
Mayo Clinic
Rochester, Minnesota

Sandra L. Wong, MD, MS
Professor of Surgery
Chair, Department of Surgery
Geisel School of Medicine
Dartmouth-Hitchcock Medical Center
Lebanon, New Hampshire

Derek T. Woodrum, MD
Associate Professor, Attending Anesthesiologist
Department of Anesthesiology
University of Michigan Medical School, Michigan Medicine
Ann Arbor, Michigan

Charles J. Yeo, MD, FACS
Samuel D. Gross Professor
Department of Surgery
Thomas Jefferson University
Chair, Department of Surgery
Thomas Jefferson University Hospital
Philadelphia, Pennsylvania

Jason B. Young, MD, PharmD
Assistant Professor of Surgery (Clinical Track)
Division of General Surgery, Department of Surgery
University of Utah School of Medicine
Surgeon, University of Utah Health
Salt Lake City, Utah

Jennifer Yu, MD
Resident, General Surgery
Washington University School of Medicine
Housestaff, General Surgery
Barnes-Jewish Hospital
Department of Surgery
St. Louis, Missouri

Brian S. Zuckerbraun, MD, FACS
Henry T. Bahnson Professor of Surgery
Chief, Division of General and Trauma Surgery
University of Pittsburgh
University of Pittsburgh Medical Center and
VA Pittsburgh Healthcare System
Pittsburgh, Pennsylvania

● CONTRIBUTORS TO THE PREVIOUS EDITION

Edouard Aboian, MD

Daniel Albo, MD, PhD

Amy K. Alderman, MD, MPH

Steven R. Allen, MD

John B. Ammori, MD

Christopher D. Anderson, MD

Stanley W. Ashley, MD

Samir S. Awad, MD

Douglas C. Barnhart, MD, MSPH

William C. Beck, MD

Natasha S. Becker, MD, MPH

Filip Bednar, MD

Jessica M. Bensenhaver, MD

Noelle L. Bertelson, MD, FACS, FASCRS

Avi Bhavaraju, MD

James H. Black III, MD, FACS

Brendan J. Boland, MD

Melissa Boltz, DO, MBA

Tara M. Breslin, MD

Adam S. Brinkman, MD

Malcolm V. Brock, MD

James T. Broome, MD

Steven W. Bruch, MD, MSc

Terry Lynn Buchmiller, MD

Richard E. Burney, MD

Marisa Cevasco, MD, MPH

Alfred E. Chang, MD

Anthony G. Charles, MD, MPH

Herbert Chen, MD, FACS

Steven Chen, MD, MBA

Hueylan Chern, MD

Albert Chi, MD

Sara E. Clark, MD

Robert A. Cowles, MD

Eric J. Culbertson, MD

Lillian G. Dawes, MD

Sebastian G. De la fuente, MD

Ronald P. DeMatteo, MD

Charles S. Dietrich III, MD

Anastasia Dimick, MD

Justin B. Dimick, MD, MPH

Paul D. Dimusto, MD

Gerard M. Doherty, MD

Bernard J. Dubray, MD

Gregory Ara Dumanian, MD

Guillermo A. Escobar, MD

David A. Etzioni, MD, MSHS

Heather L. Evans, MD, MS

Gavin A. Falk, MD

Jonathan F. Finks, MD

Emily Finlayson, MD, MS

Samuel R.G. Finlayson, MD, MPH, FACS

Emily M. Fontenot, MD

Heidi L. Frankel, MD

Timothy L. Frankel, MD

Michael G. Franz, MD

Danielle Fritze, MD

Samir K. Gadepalli, MD

Wolfgang B. Gaertner, MS, MD

Paul G. Gauger, MD

James D. Geiger, MD

Philip P. Goodney, MD, MS

Sarah E. Greer, MD, MPH

Tyler Grenda, MD, MS

Erica R. Gross, MD

Travis E. Grotz, MD

Oliver L. Gunter, MD, MPH

Jeffrey S. Guy, MD, MSc, MMHC

Adil H. Haider, MD, MPH

Ihab Halaweish, MD

A.L. Halverson, MD

Allen Hamdan, MD

James Harris Jr., MD

Elliott R. Haut, MD

A.V. Hayman, MD

David W. Healy, MD, MRCP, FRCA

Mark R. Hemmila, MD, FACS

Samantha Hendren, MD, MPH

Peter K. Henke, MD

Richard Herman, MD

Michael G. House, MD

Gina M.S. Howell, MD

Thomas S. Huber, MD, PhD

David T. Hughes, MD

Alicia Hulbert, MD

Justin Hurie, MD

Neil Hyman, MD

Angela M. Ingraham, MD, MS, FACS

Kamal M.F. Itani, MD

Alexis D. Jacob, MD

Lisa K. Jacobs, MD

James W. Jakub, MD

Jennifer E. Joh, MD

Jussuf T. Kaifi, MD, PhD

Jeffrey Kalish, MD

Lillian S. Kao, MD, MS

Muneera R. Kapadia, MD, MME

Srinivas Kavuturu, MD, FRCS

Sajid A. Khan, MD

Hyaehwan Kim, MD

Andrew S. Klein, MD, MBA

Carla Kohoyda-Inglis, MPA

Geoffrey W. Krampitz, MD

Andrew Kroeker, MD

Hari R. Kumar, MD

Adriana Laser, MD

Christine L. Lau, MD, MBA

Constance W. Lee, MD

Marie Catherine Lee, MD

Jules Lin, MD

Peter H. Lin, MD

Pamela A. Lipsett, MD, MHPE

Ann C. Lowry, MD

Dennis P. Lund, MD

Paul M. Maggio, MD, MBA

Ali F. Mallat, MD, MS

Sean T. Martin, MD

Jeffrey B. Matthews, MD, FACS

Haggi Mazeh, MD

Timothy W. McCardle, MD

Erin McKean, MD

Sean E. McLean, MD

Michelle K. McNutt, MD

Genevieve Melton-Meaux, MD, MA

April E. Mendoza, MD

Evangelos Messaris, MD, PhD

Stacey A. Milan, MD

Barbra S. Miller, MD

Judiann Miskulin, MD

Derek Moore, MD, MPH

Arden M. Morris, MD

Monica Morrow, MD

John Morton, MD, MPH

Michael Mulholland, MD, PhD

Alykhan S. Nagji, MD

Lena M. Napolitano, MD

Avery B. Nathens, MD, MPH, PhD

Erika Newman, MD

Lisa A. Newman, MD, MPH

Jeffrey A. Norton, MD

Babak J. Orandi, MD, MSc

Mark B. Orringer, MD

Paul Park, MD, MA

Pauline K. Park, MD

Timothy M. Pawlik, MD, MPH

Shawn J. Pelletier, MD

Peter D. Peng, MD, MS

Catherine E. Pesce, MD

Rebecca Plevin, MD

Benjamin K. Poulose, MD, MPH

Sandhya Pruthi, MD

Krishnan Raghavendran, MD

Julie Ann Sosa, MD, MA

Matthew W. Ralls, MD

John Rectenwald, MD

Scott E. Regenbogen, MD, MPH

Amy L. Rezak, MD

William P. Robinson III, MD

Michael J. Rosen, MD

Michael S. Sabel, MD

Vivian M. Sanchez, MD

George A. Sarosi Jr., MD

Brian D. Saunders, MD

C. Max Schmidt, MD, PhD, MBA

Maureen K. Sheehan, MD

Terry Shih, MD

Andrew Shuman, MD

Sabina Siddiqui, MD

Matthew J. Sideman, MD

Rebecca S. Sippel, MD

Alexis D. Smith, MD

Vance L. Smith, MD, MBA

Oliver S. Soldes, MD

Vernon K. Sondak, MD

Christopher J. Sonnenday, MD, MHS

Matthew Spector, MD

Jason L. Sperry, MD, MPH

Kevin F. Staveley-O'Carroll, MD, PhD

John F. Sweeney, MD

Kevin E. Taubman, MD

Daniel H. Teitelbaum, MD

Pierre Theodore, MD

Thadeus Trus, MD

Douglas J. Turner, MD

Gilbert R. Upchurch Jr., MD

Kyle J. Van Arendonk, MD

Chandu Vemuri, MD

Jon D. Vogel, MD

Wendy L. Wahl, MD

Thomas W. Wakefield, MD

Jennifer F. Waljee, MD, MS

Stewart C. Wang, MD, PhD

Joshua A. Waters, MD

Sarah M. Weakley, MD

Walter P. Weber, MD

Martin R. Weiser, MD

Bradford P. Whitcomb, MD

Elizabeth C. Wick, MD

Sandra L. Wong, MD, MS

Derek T. Woodrum, MD

Leslie S. Wu, MD

Charles J. Yeo, MD

Barbara Zarebczan, MD

FOREWORD

In preparing a generation of surgical residents to enter practice, there are some thoughts on reading that I may offer. There are also some rules that I have found useful while writing and editing chapters for surgical textbooks. Most of us are not born surgeons; we become surgeons through dedicated effort. If you are the exception—accomplished, articulate, and confident; if surgical principles come effortlessly, you may stop reading now. Still, you might want to take a look. Here are three thoughts:

1. Start reading right away

For most surgeons, the most difficult reading assignment is the first assignment. The problem lies not in realizing the high stakes of a board exam; the trouble comes with the commitment that board preparation requires. The form of most contemporary texts is part of the problem. A glance shows the chapters to be long, devoid of illustrations, a daunting proposition. *Clinical Scenarios in Surgery* is so inviting with its crisp writing, generous illustrations, and telegenic presentation that it begs to be read. Get started.

2. Look to the future

Modern surgery is forward looking, seeking to improve the care of current patients and to prevent disease in potential future patients. Given the pace of modern biomedical research, no individual can be expected to find, read, synthesize, and apply all new knowledge relevant to any clinical problem. All surgeons need an occasional guide through the surgical literature. In the midst of this information overload, the experienced, energetic editors of *Clinical Scenarios in Surgery* strike just the right balance. Keep going.

3. Keep reading, even just a little bit, every day

Reading is a skill, sharpened with practice, perfected by *continuous* practice. Operative surgery reinforces this notion. The physical skills, sense of prioritized organization, personal confidence, and intuition of the accomplished surgeon result from attention to the craft. That is the reason it is called the practice of surgery. A book becomes much friendlier with frequent use. Enjoy the journey.

Michael W. Mulholland, MD, PhD

PREFACE

Despite remarkable technical advances and rapid scientific progress, it has never been more challenging to become a safe and proficient surgeon.

Young surgeons are challenged both by the pace of change and the subspecialization of surgery. Traditional surgical textbooks, which have grown to keep pace with these changes, are becoming encyclopedic reference books, which we turn to only when we need a comprehensive overview. With the vast amount of information available, it is often difficult to sort out the basic principles of safe surgery for a given clinical scenario. The mismatch between existing education materials and the need for a solid understanding of general surgical principles becomes most apparent when young surgeons sit down to prepare to take their written and oral board exams.

Young surgeons also learn differently than those in the past. Modern surgical trainees do not sit down and read for hours at a time. They are multitaskers who demand efficiency and immediate relevance in their learning materials. Most medical schools have responded to these changes by transitioning to curricula based on case-based learning.

Clinical narratives are extremely effective learning tools because they use patient stories to teach essential surgical principles. Most existing surgical textbooks have not kept pace with these broader changes in medical education.

We wrote this book to fill these gaps. We have created a case-based text that communicates core principles of general surgery and its specialties. We believe the patient stories in these clinical scenarios will provide context to facilitate learning the principles of safe surgical care. Students, residents, and other young surgeons should find the chapters short enough to read between cases or after a long day in the hospital. We hope this book will be particularly useful for senior surgical residents and recent graduates as they prepare for the American Board of Surgery oral examination.

Justin B. Dimick
Gilbert R. Upchurch Jr.
Christopher J. Sonnenday
Lillian S. Kao

CONTENTS

SECTION 14: TRANSPLANT

SECTION 15: HEAD AND NECK

Abdominal Wall

Symptomatic Primary Inguinal Hernia

REBECCA L. GUNTER AND JACOB A. GREENBERG

Based on the previous edition chapter "Symptomatic Primary Inguinal Hernia" by Evangelos Messaris

1

Presentation

A 47-year-old man with a history of hypertension and no previous abdominal surgeries presents to clinic with a bulge in his left groin. The bulge has been present for 6 months and gives him occasional discomfort but does not interfere with his daily activities. He denies fevers, chills, nausea, vomiting, and changes in bowel or bladder habits. On physical exam, the bulge is easily reducible without tenderness to palpation but easily recurs after reduction.

● DIFFERENTIAL DIAGNOSIS

It is important to differentiate hernias from other pathologies that may lead to pain in the affected groin. While groin discomfort is a common complaint among patients with inguinal hernias, not all hernias are symptomatic. Inguinal lymphadenopathy, which may represent metastatic disease, primary lymphoma, or an inflammatory reaction, can present with a palpable mass and groin discomfort. Testicular and scrotal pathologies, such as varicocele, spermatocele, hydrocele, testicular torsion, testicular tumors, epididymitis, and epididymal cysts should be ruled out, as these can cause scrotal swelling and may even extend into the inguinal canal. Groin discomfort in the absence of a palpable mass or bulge may be related to musculoskeletal pathology, including sports hernia (athletic pubalgia), ligamentous injury, ilioinguinal strain, and hip abnormalities, such as bursitis, labral tears, femoroacetabular impingement, or avascular necrosis.

● WORKUP

Upon more extensive physical examination, our patient is found to have a reducible inguinal mass at the level of the external ring of the inguinal canal on the left side. This bulge extends into his scrotum but reduces easily with manual palpation. There are no overlying skin changes. Examination of the inguinal region on his right side is unremarkable.

The diagnosis of inguinal hernia is based primarily on a good physical examination, which has a reported sensitivity and specificity of 75% and 95%, respectively. In a male patient, the examiner invaginates the scrotum and places a finger through the external ring or directly palpates the inguinal canal. Upon Valsalva, the examiner will feel the hernia sac and any contents at the tip or on the pad of the finger. Classically, an indirect hernia is felt at the tip of the finger, and a direct hernia is felt with the pad of the finger, though the reliability of this finding is questionable. In a female patient, the inguinal area just lateral to the pubic tubercle is palpated for a bulge suggestive of a hernia. The examiner should take care to note the location of the bulge in relation to the inguinal ligament, as hernias below the inguinal ligament are by definition femoral hernias. Both sides should be examined carefully to rule out bilateral hernias. Laboratory studies are not indicated in the diagnosis of inguinal hernias.

When the diagnosis is uncertain, imaging studies may be helpful to confirm the presence of a hernia and to determine its contents. Routine imaging is not necessary and is most helpful in patients in whom physical examination is particularly challenging, as in the obese patient. Ultrasound is helpful in diagnosing testicular or scrotal pathology as well as inguinal lymphadenopathy. A skillful ultrasonographer may also be able to detect a hernia sac and identify its contents (Figure 1-1). Computed tomography (CT) is useful in cases of very large inguinal hernias when the contents cannot be identified and the anatomy may be significantly distorted (Figure 1-2). Finally, magnetic resonance imaging (MRI) may be used for those patients with groin discomfort in the absence of a bulge or palpable mass to assess for musculoskeletal pathology.

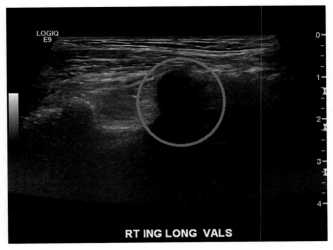

FIGURE 1-1. An ultrasound of the groin with a hernia noted within the *red circle*.

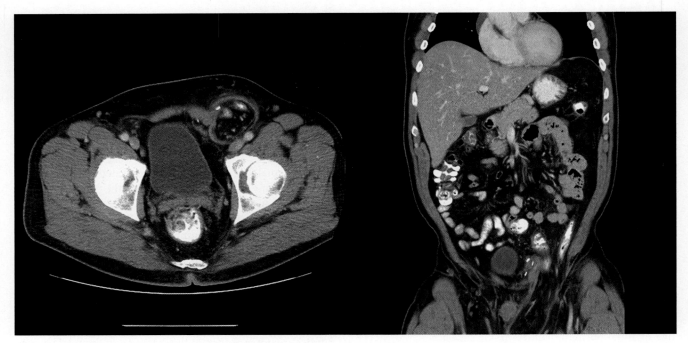

FIGURE 1-2. Axial and coronal computed tomographic views of a large recurrent left inguinal hernia.

● DIAGNOSIS AND TREATMENT

Once an inguinal hernia has been diagnosed, the decision to repair it is based primarily on the presence of symptoms and patient preference. In asymptomatic and minimally symptomatic patients, a strategy of watchful waiting is acceptable. Long-term results of randomized clinical trials have demonstrated the safety of this approach; however, patients should be counseled that they are likely to develop symptoms if the hernia is not repaired, particularly if they have an active lifestyle at baseline. Thus, it is reasonable to offer repair to patients who are asymptomatic at the time of initial surgical consultation.

For patients whose hernia causes discomfort that limits their activity, or those that have evidence of incarceration or strangulation, surgical repair is the appropriate treatment. Patients with incarceration or strangulation may have more severe pain or pain that acutely worsens. In advanced cases, there may be overlying skin changes indicating strangulation of hernia contents (e.g., small bowel, colon, or omentum). The timing of surgical repair depends on the danger posed to the patient. Symptomatic, but reducible, hernias may be repaired electively on an outpatient basis. Incarcerated hernias should be repaired more urgently, and strangulated hernias should be repaired emergently to prevent tissue loss and limit ischemia to the hernia contents.

● SURGICAL APPROACH

Inguinal hernias may be repaired using an open technique, or may be repaired laparoscopically. Open repairs are suture based (McVay, Bassini, and Shouldice repairs) or use mesh to bolster the repair (e.g., Lichtenstein repair). Laparoscopic repair is performed using one of the following techniques: total extraperitoneal (TEP) or transabdominal preperitoneal (TAPP). A TEP repair does not enter the peritoneal cavity, whereas a TAPP repair does. Additionally, TAPP may be performed robotically. Mesh is used in all laparoscopic and robotic approaches.

The choice of approach is determined by patient and surgeon factors. Meta-analyses of published clinical trials indicate equivalence between laparoscopic and open techniques in terms of hernia recurrence rates. Laparoscopic repairs result in slightly lower rates of postoperative groin pain and numbness, and a quicker return to normal activities. However, there may be slightly higher rates of perioperative complications following laparoscopic repair. Surgeon experience and comfort should guide the choice of approach; this author prefers the TAPP laparoscopic repair. In patients who have bilateral hernias, laparoscopic repair is often preferred as both sides may be fixed through one set of incisions. Prior prostatic or other pelvic surgery (e.g., prostatectomy) or radiation can complicate a laparoscopic approach, making open repair the optimal approach in these patients.

Ultimately, the goal is a tension-free repair to prevent recurrence and minimize postoperative pain or discomfort. To that end, mesh should be used in most cases, as it reduces recurrence rates following repair of primary inguinal hernias. However, mesh should be avoided in contaminated cases in favor of a suture repair (Bassini, McVay, or Shouldice repair). Some authors have advocated the use of biologic mesh in contaminated cases, but this author recommends a suture-based technique for the initial repair followed by a laparoscopic repair if the hernia recurs.

● PREOPERATIVE CARE

Prior to arriving in the operating room, all patients should empty their bladder. Spontaneous voiding in the preoperative area immediately prior to surgery is clearly preferable to bladder decompression with a Foley catheter, though this may be necessary to ensure adequate visualization and prevent intraoperative bladder injury. This is particularly essential when a laparoscopic approach is used.

Regardless of approach, the patient is placed supine on the operating table. Knee-high pneumatic sequential compression devices (SCDs) should be placed. We do not routinely administer preoperative heparin. Controversy exists surrounding the utility of preoperative antibiotics to prevent surgical site infection in elective inguinal hernia repair. It is our practice to administer a first-generation cephalosporin preoperatively to cover skin flora. In cases of urgent or emergent inguinal hernia repair for incarcerated or strangulated viscera, antibiotics should be given within 1 hour of incision.

A variety of anesthetic approaches may be used. For elective inguinal hernia repair, local anesthesia either by nerve block or by direct infiltration into the skin may be adequate. Alternatively, spinal or general anesthesia may be administered. For urgent and emergent cases, general anesthesia will be required.

● REPAIR TYPES

Open Inguinal Hernia Repair

The "gold standard" for inguinal hernia repair has historically been the open, tension-free Lichtenstein repair using mesh (Table 1-1). Using the pubic tubercle and the anterior superior iliac spine (ASIS) as anatomic landmarks to approximate the course of the inguinal ligament, an oblique incision is made two fingerbreadths superior to the inguinal ligament, angling the incision slightly cephalad as it progresses laterally. The incision is carried down through the subcutaneous tissue until the external oblique aponeurosis is reached. The aponeurosis is incised sharply with a knife and then cut in line with the direction of the muscle fibers using scissors, taking care to elevate the fascia as it is cut to protect the ilioinguinal nerve, which runs just deep to the external oblique aponeurosis along the spermatic cord. The superior and inferior external oblique flaps are dissected free and held in place with a self-retaining retractor. Once the flaps have been raised, the iliohypogastric nerve should be identified running along the interior oblique aponeurosis, superior to the spermatic cord. The spermatic cord is dissected free from the surrounding tissues, taking care to preserve the vessels and vas deferens. The genital branch of the genitofemoral nerve runs posterior to the cord and should be identified and preserved. In female patients, the round ligament may be transected and the internal ring closed. Once the hernia sac has been identified, it may be either reduced through the internal ring or ligated at the level of the internal ring.

Table 1-1	Open Lichtenstein Tension-free Herniorrhaphy

Key Technical Steps

1. An oblique skin incision is made two fingerbreadths superior to the inguinal ligament and carried through the subcutaneous tissues.
2. The external oblique is cut in the direction of its muscle fibers.
3. The cord structures are dissected free from the hernia sac.
4. The hernia sac and its contents are returned to the abdomen.
5. Polypropylene mesh is secured to the pubic tubercle medially, the inguinal ligament inferiorly, and the rectus sheath and internal oblique muscle superiorly.
6. The external oblique is reapproximated and the skin closed.

Potential Pitfalls

- The pubic tubercle must be completely covered by the mesh and the mesh well secured to avoid recurrence.
- All three nerves (ilioinguinal, iliohypogastric, and genital branch of the genitofemoral nerve) must be identified and protected throughout the operation.
- Mesh fixation must be tension free.
- Avoid injury to the cord structures, and return them to their proper position at the end of the operation.

Once the spermatic cord has been skeletonized and the hernia has been reduced, attention is then turned to placement of the mesh. A piece of polypropylene mesh is cut large enough to reach from the inguinal ligament to an overlap of the rectus by 1 to 2 cm. In male patients, a slit is cut on the lateral edge of the mesh to accommodate the spermatic cord. In female patients, no slit is required if the round ligament has been ligated and the internal ring closed. The mesh is placed under the spermatic cord and the medial edge secured to the pubic tubercle using 2-0 polydiaxanone. The inferior edge of the mesh is then secured to the inguinal ligament with a running or interrupted 2-0 polydiaxanone suture. The superior edge is secured to the rectus sheath and internal oblique muscle. The internal ring is then reconstructed by securing the two ends of the cut slit of the lateral edge of the mesh. The lateral tails of the mesh are tucked under the external oblique. The external oblique is reapproximated using 2-0 absorbable suture in a running fashion, again taking care to avoid injuring the ilioinguinal and iliohypogastric nerves.

Total Extraperitoneal Laparoscopic Hernia Repair

The TEP repair aims not to violate the peritoneal cavity (Table 1-2). An incision is made just inferior to the umbilicus. The subcutaneous tissues are dissected down to the level of the rectus sheath. The rectus sheath is sharply incised, and the rectus

Table 1-2	Laparoscopic Totally Extraperitoneal Repair of Inguinal Hernia

Key Technical Steps

1. An infraumbilical incision is made down to the anterior rectus sheath through which a balloon dissector is introduced into the retromuscular space.
2. The balloon dissector is slowly inflated to bluntly dissect the preperitoneal space.
3. Two 5-mm trocars are placed in the lower midline.
4. Careful and complete dissection is performed to adequately identify the relevant anatomy (the inferior epigastric vessels superiorly, Cooper's ligament medially, and the iliopubic tract laterally).
5. The hernia sac is dissected from the cord structures and returned to the peritoneal cavity.
6. Mesh is introduced and positioned to cover the entire myopectineal orifice.
7. Fixation may be used but is not necessary.

Potential Pitfalls

- A complete understanding of the anatomy and its orientation from this perspective is critical.
- Inadequate dissection or dissection in the wrong plane can lead to poor visualization of key anatomy.
- Injury to major vascular structures (epigastric and iliac vessels) should be carefully avoided.

Table 1-3	Laparoscopic Transabdominal Preperitoneal Repair of Inguinal Hernia

Key Technical Steps

1. The first port is placed at the umbilicus. Two additional ports are placed on either side lateral to the rectus sheath.
2. The peritoneum is incised from the ipsilateral medial umbilical fold to the level of the ASIS.
3. The preperitoneal space is bluntly dissected from the anterior iliac spine laterally, to the medial umbilical fold medially, and below Cooper's ligament inferiorly.
4. The hernia sac is dissected from the cord structures and returned to the peritoneal cavity.
5. Mesh is introduced and positioned to cover the entire myopectineal orifice.
6. The peritoneal defect is closed using tacks or sutures.

Potential Pitfalls

- As in TEP repair, a complete understanding of the relevant anatomy from the laparoscopic perspective is critical for safe completion of the operation.
- The mesh should not be allowed to curl or shift during closure of the peritoneal defect.
- Avoid injuring the epigastric vessels during closure of the peritoneal defect, especially if using tacks.

muscle is bluntly dissected laterally to expose the retrorectus space. An endoscopic balloon dissector is introduced into the retrorectus space and advanced to the pubic symphysis. A 10-mm 0° laparoscope is introduced and the balloon dissector is slowly inflated under direct visualization. The balloon is removed and replaced with a standard blunt port. The preperitoneal space is then insufflated to 12 mm Hg. Two additional 5-mm trocars are placed in the lower midline, one 2 cm cranial to the pubic symphysis and the other at least 4 cm cranial to the lower trocar. Complete dissection is performed to clearly identify the inferior epigastric vessels superiorly, Cooper's ligament medially, and the iliopubic tract laterally. The hernia sac is dissected off the spermatic cord structures and reduced into the peritoneal cavity, taking care not to injure the vas deferens or gonadal vessels. Mesh is then introduced and positioned from medial to lateral under the cord structures paying particular attention to cover the entire myopectineal orifice. The mesh may be fixated using tacks, staples, or fibrin glue, or it may be left in place without fixation. If tacks or staples are used for fixation, they should not be placed below Cooper's ligament medially or below the iliopubic tract laterally.

Transabdominal Preperitoneal Laparoscopic Hernia Repair

The TAPP laparoscopic hernia repair is the author's preferred approach (Table 1-3). It may be performed laparoscopically

or robotically. The first trocar is placed at the level of the umbilicus via a Hasson technique. Two additional 5-mm ports are placed lateral to the rectus sheath, 1 to 2 cm cranial to the umbilicus. A 5-mm 30° laparoscope is placed in the port ipsilateral to the hernia. The peritoneum is grasped at the medial umbilical fold and incised out laterally with laparoscopic scissors (Figure 1-3). Two blunt graspers are then introduced into the created preperitoneal space and spread to bluntly dissect the space. Care should be taken to avoid inadvertent entry into the retrorectus space. The preperitoneal space is dissected laterally to the level of the ASIS, medially to the ipsilateral medial umbilical fold, and inferiorly to the level of the iliopubic tract. Cooper's ligament is identified and cleared for about 2 cm in anticipation of mesh fixation

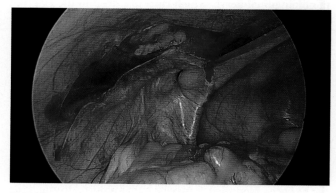

FIGURE 1-3. The peritoneal incision during a laparoscopic TAPP repair.

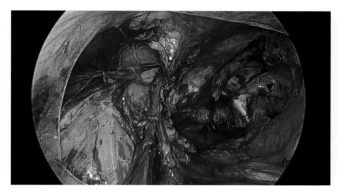

FIGURE 1-4. The exposed myopectineal orifice after hernia completed dissection during a TAPP repair.

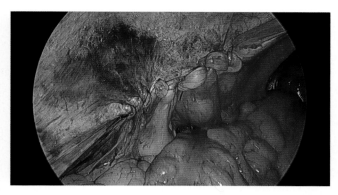

FIGURE 1-6. Sutured peritoneal closure at the end of a TAPP repair.

at its superior aspect. The hernia sac is dissected free of the spermatic cord contents and reduced into the peritoneal space, taking care not to injure the vas deferens or gonadal vessels. Once the hernia sac has been reduced, the peritoneum is further dissected free from the iliac vessels, vas deferens, and gonadal vessels, providing generous exposure of the myopectineal orifice in preparation for mesh placement (Figure 1-4). Mesh is then introduced and positioned similarly to a TEP repair (Figure 1-5). Once the mesh has been placed to satisfaction, the peritoneal defect is closed using tacks or self-retaining sutures (Figure 1-6).

● SPECIAL INTRAOPERATIVE CONSIDERATIONS

A complete understanding of the complex anatomy of the inguinal canal and its surrounding structures is essential to the successful repair of inguinal hernias. This is particularly true for laparoscopic approaches as the anatomy of this approach is far different from that of the traditional anterior approach that most surgeons are comfortable performing. Complete dissection and identification of relevant anatomy is crucial in laparoscopic repairs and open repairs.

Careful attention must be paid to identify all three nerves (ilioinguinal, iliohypogastric, genital branch of the

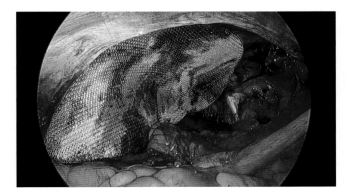

FIGURE 1-5. Mesh placement to cover the entire myopectineal orifice.

genitofemoral) during open repairs. Nerve injury or entrapment can cause significant postoperative groin neuralgia. If nerve injury is detected intraoperatively, the nerve should be ligated and excised proximally to allow retraction into the muscle or preperitoneal space.

Peritoneal violation during laparoscopic repair, whether inadvertent during TEP repair or intentional during TAPP repair, should be closed, when possible, using absorbable suture. Regardless of approach, intraoperative complications, including vascular injury (e.g., femoral vessels or inferior epigastric vessels), bladder or testicular injuries, vas deferens injury, and nerve injury should be carefully avoided.

● POSTOPERATIVE MANAGEMENT

Elective, uncomplicated inguinal hernia repair may be done on an outpatient basis, with patients leaving the surgery center within a few hours following the procedure. Prior to discharge, patients should have adequate pain control, and should be ambulating and voiding without difficulty. Urinary retention following inguinal surgery is the most common complication, and higher risk is associated with narcotic administration, older age, prolonged anesthesia time, bilateral hernia repair, and obesity. Patients who had incarcerated or strangulated visceral contents in the hernia sac should be admitted for observation and may be discharged upon return of normal bowel function.

Following discharge, patients may resume their normal activities as their pain level allows. We do not place weight restrictions on postoperative patients, but rather counsel them to be mindful of their own comfort level. Common postoperative complications include seromas and inguinal neuralgia. Seromas generally resolve spontaneously without further intervention. Especially in the presence of mesh, they should not be aspirated or otherwise violated unless there is a high index of suspicion for an infection. Chronic groin pain has been reported in as many as 10% to 14% of cases, and may be caused by nerve injury, by injury to the structures within the inguinal canal, or by anchoring sutures placed too deeply into the pubic tubercle periosteum. Nerve injury is characterized by hypo- or hyperesthesia, allodynia, and paresthesia, most often in the distribution of the affected nerve(s). Risk factors for postoperative groin pain include young age, operation for recurrent hernia, preoperative groin pain, use of heavyweight mesh, and female sex. Treatment ranges from medical management, including pharmacologic therapies and peripheral nerve blocks, to operative management, including neurectomy of one to all three nerves.

Case Conclusion

Our patient underwent a TAPP laparoscopic hernia repair at an outpatient surgery center 1 month after his initial consultation. He had an uneventful recovery and was seen in clinic 3 weeks later. His incisions had healed well, and he had no postoperative pain. He was back at work and had resumed his normal activities. On exam, there was no evidence of recurrence, seroma, or hematoma.

TAKE HOME POINTS

- Inguinal hernias are common, and their repair is one of the most common surgical procedures performed worldwide.
- Asymptomatic and minimally symptomatic inguinal hernias may be safely managed nonoperatively, but are likely to become symptomatic. Symptomatic inguinal hernias should be repaired to relieve symptoms and prevent future incarceration or strangulation.

- Inguinal hernias may be repaired open, laparoscopically, or robotically, depending on patient factors and surgeon comfort. Regardless of approach, the goal is a tension-free repair, almost always involving mesh.
- Seromas, groin neuralgia, and hernia recurrence are the most common postoperative complications.

SUGGESTED READINGS

Bjurstrom MF, Nicol AL, Amid PK, Chen DC. Pain control following inguinal herniorrhaphy: current perspectives. *J Pain Res.* 2014;29(7):277-290.
Fitzgibbons RJ, Giobbie-Hurder A, Gibbs JO, et al. Watchful waiting vs repair of inguinal hernia in minimally symptomatic men: a randomized clinical trial. *JAMA.* 2006;295(3):285-292.
Fitzgibbons RJ, Ramanan B, Arya S, et al. Long-term results of a randomized controlled trial of a nonoperative strategy (watchful waiting) for men with minimally symptomatic inguinal hernias. *Ann Surg.* 2013;258(3):508-515.
McCormack K, Scott NW, Go PM, et al. Laparoscopic techniques versus open techniques for inguinal hernia repair. *Cochrane Database Syst Rev.* 2003;(1):CD001785.
Neumayer L, Giobbie-Hurder A, Jonasson O, et al. Open mesh versus laparoscopic mesh repair of inguinal hernia. *N Engl J Med.* 2004;350(18):1819-1827.
Nguyen DK, Amid PK, Chen DC. Groin pain after inguinal hernia repair. *Adv Surg.* 2016;50(1):203-220.
O'Reilly EA, Burke JP, O'Connell PR. A meta-analysis of surgical morbidity and recurrence after laparoscopic and open repair of primary unilateral inguinal hernia. *Ann Surg.* 2012;255(5):846-853.

Recurrent Inguinal Hernia (Transabdominal Preperitoneal Repair)

JONATHAN F. FINKS

2

Based on the previous edition chapter "Recurrent Inguinal Hernia" by Jonathan F. Finks

Presentation

A 60-year-old man presents with a 6-month history of a right groin bulge. Although reducible, the patient has noted increasing discomfort associated with the bulge over the last few weeks. He denies any obstructive symptoms and has had no symptoms on the left side. He has a history of two previous open right inguinal hernia repair procedures with mesh, most recently 5 years ago. He also has a history of a robotic-assisted prostatectomy 2 years ago for prostate cancer and remains cancer-free. The patient has a body mass index of 35. Physical exam demonstrates some fullness in the right groin, but the exam is limited by the patient's body habitus.

● DIFFERENTIAL DIAGNOSIS

The leading diagnosis based on these symptoms is a recurrent right inguinal hernia. Other considerations would include hydrocele; lymphadenopathy; soft tissue mass, such as a lipoma or sarcoma; and hematoma related to trauma.

● WORKUP

The most appropriate study to evaluate for a recurrent hernia is a computed tomography (CT) of the abdomen and pelvis with an hernia protocol that includes both standard and Valsalva images. This approach allows for better identification of hernia contents within the inguinal canal. Groin ultrasound is an alternative imaging option. However, these studies can be difficult to interpret, especially in the setting of obesity, and may be user-dependent.

● DIAGNOSIS AND TREATMENT

In this case, cross-sectional imaging demonstrated a recurrent right inguinal hernia containing a nonobstructed loop of small bowel. The left inguinal canal was normal in appearance. Given the symptomatic nature of this hernia, repair is warranted.

There are several options for surgical management. An open or anterior approach would be very difficult and unlikely to produce durable results, given the patient's body habitus and significant scarring from the previous open repairs. A preperitoneal approach is preferred in this case because it would allow for the repair to be done in an unviolated tissue plane. The preperitoneal approach also allows access to the entire myopectineal orifice, ensuring identification of occult femoral hernia that may not be appreciated with open repairs. Preperitoneal repairs can be done with an open technique using a Pfannenstiel incision. In this case, however, the open approach would be difficult given the patient's obesity. A laparoscopic total extraperitoneal (TEP) repair would be contraindicated because of the previous prostatectomy, which would greatly increase the risk for a bladder injury during development of the preperitoneal space.

In this case, the optimal repair would entail a laparoscopic transabdominal preperitoneal (TAPP) approach. This method would facilitate safe dissection of the preperitoneal space, starting lateral to the bladder to promote better visualization of this structure and lower risk for injury. The transabdominal route also allows the surgeon to avoid the lower abdominal wall pannus that can be present in patients with obesity. A TAPP approach can also be useful in cases of large scrotal hernias, as these can be more easily reduced from the peritoneal cavity than from the preperitoneal space. Moreover, the transabdominal approach also allows for assessment of bowel viability in cases of acutely incarcerated hernias. Finally, conversion to TAPP repair is a good fallback option if technical difficulties arise during a TEP procedure.

● SURGICAL TECHNIQUE

The TAPP procedure for inguinal hernia repair involves entry into the preperitoneal space via a transverse incision of the lower abdominal wall peritoneum. Once in the preperitoneal space, assessment of the entire myopectineal orifice is made. This includes the direct, indirect, femoral, and obturator spaces. Hernia contents are reduced, and the peritoneum is dissected well off of the cord structures or round ligament to make room for the mesh. The mesh is then placed such that it adequately covers all of the potential hernia defects. The peritoneum is then secured up to the abdominal wall to cover the mesh.

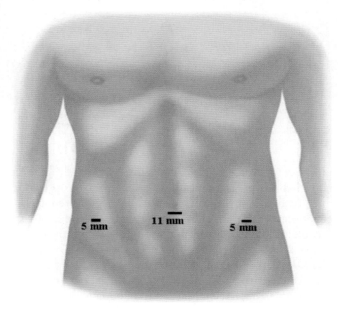

FIGURE 2-1. Port placement for transabdominal preperitoneal (TAPP) hernia repair. (Reprinted under Creative Commons License from Carter J, Duh QY. Laparoscopic repair of inguinal hernias. *World J Surg.* 2011;35(7):1519-1525.)

The procedure is performed under general anesthesia with the patient supine, both arms tucked to the side, and in slight Trendelenburg position. It is important to ensure that the patient's thumbs are up in order to prevent ulnar nerve injury and that the elbows and wrist are adequately padded.

The patient should void in the preoperative area to empty the bladder, as a Foley catheter is usually not required. There should be at least one monitor at the head of the table for visualization during access to the abdomen and one at the foot of the table to be used during the repair.

Access to the peritoneal cavity is obtained using a Veress needle below the left costal margin (Palmer's point) and pneumoperitoneum is established. The surgeon stands on the side opposite the hernia, with the assistant on the ipsilateral side. An 11-mm trocar is placed above the umbilicus in the midline for placement of the laparoscope and later insertion of the mesh into the peritoneal cavity. Some surgeons prefer to work through 5-mm ports on both sides of the midline so as to effect proper triangulation (Figure 2-1). However, in the obese individual, the surgeons' working ports (both 5 mm in diameter) should both be on the side contralateral to the hernia, usually on either side of the midclavicular line and below the level of the umbilicus. In some cases, an additional 5-mm assistant's port may be placed on the ipsilateral side, at the midclavicular line above the level of the umbilicus. In the case of bilateral inguinal hernia repair, the working trocars are generally placed at or above the level of the umbilicus. A 10-mm 30° laparoscope is placed in the midline supraumbilical port.

The procedure begins with an inspection of the lower abdominal wall bilaterally. The median umbilical ligaments and epigastric vessels should be identified on either side of the bladder. A direct or indirect hernia may be seen from within the peritoneal cavity (Figure 2-2), although smaller defects may not be apparent until the peritoneum

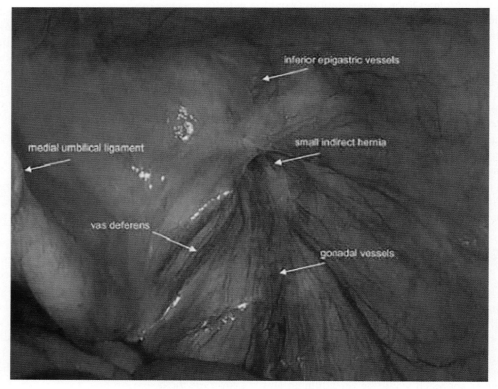

FIGURE 2-2. Transabdominal view of the right inguinal region with a small indirect inguinal hernia. (Reprinted under Creative Commons License from Carter J, Duh QY. Laparoscopic repair of inguinal hernias. *World J Surg.* 2011;35(7):1519-1525.)

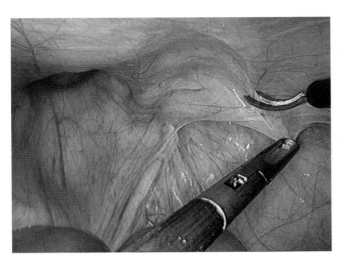

FIGURE 2-3. Incision of the peritoneum in the right inguinal region in a patient with a direct inguinal hernia. (Reprinted from Kapiris S. Laparoscopic transabdominal preperitoneal hernia repair (TAPP): stapling the mesh is not mandatory. *J Laparoendosc Adv Surg Tech A.* 2009;19(3):419-422, with permission.)

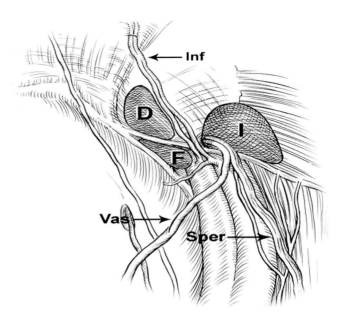

FIGURE 2-4. Preperitoneal anatomy of the right inguinal region. D, direct hernia; I, indirect hernia; F, femoral hernia; Inf, inferior epigastric vessels; Sper, spermatic (testicular) vessels. (Reprinted from Takata MC, Duh QY. Laparoscopic inguinal hernia repair. *Surg Clin North Am.* 2008;88(1):157-178, with permission.)

is taken down. The preperitoneal space is then developed beginning with an incision in the peritoneum using electrocautery (Figure 2-3). The incision begins laterally at the level of the anterior superior iliac spine and is carried transversely above the level of the hernia defects to the median umbilical ligament. The incision is then carried cephalad along the ipsilateral median umbilical ligament. In cases of a bilateral inguinal hernia, a mirror incision is made on the opposite side. Bilateral hernia are repaired through separate dissections and using separate pieces of mesh. Blunt and sharp dissection is then used to develop the preperitoneal space, staying close to the peritoneum. This dissection begins lateral to the cord structures, in Bogros' space, and extends medially toward the retropubic space. Medially, the bladder is carefully dissected off of the anterior abdominal wall, exposing the symphysis pubis and Cooper's ligament. Care must be taken not to injure *corona mortis*, which refers to the venous connection between the inferior epigastric and obturator veins. This structure courses inferiorly along the lateral aspect of Cooper's ligament and can be difficult to control if lacerated or avulsed.

At this point, the myopectineal orifice is evaluated to identify any hernia defects (Figure 2-4). Indirect hernias are located superior to the inguinal ligament and lateral to the epigastric vessels. Direct hernias occur through Hesselbach's triangle, bordered laterally by the inferior epigastric vessels, medially by lateral edge of the rectus muscle, and inferiorly by the inguinal ligament. Femoral hernias occur through the femoral space, bordered laterally by the femoral vein, posteriorly by Cooper's ligament, and anteriorly by the inguinal ligament. Obturator hernias occur posterior to Cooper's ligament through the obturator foramen.

An assessment for femoral and direct hernia defects occurs during the medial dissection. Careful attention

is paid to identify the critical structures: inferior epigastric vessels, Cooper's ligament, and the femoral vein. Direct and femoral hernias may contain a peritoneal sac, although more commonly the hernia contents include only preperitoneal fat. It is not uncommon for direct hernias to contain the urinary bladder. The hernia contents are reduced with gentle blunt dissection. With a direct hernia, there is usually a clear transition between transversalis fascia and the hernia contents. These structures can often be separated by applying cephalad and posterior retraction of the hernia contents and anterior and caudad retraction of the transversalis fascia.

In the setting of a large direct defect, large seromas may develop. To help minimize the risk for seroma formation, the transversalis fascia may be reduced from within Hesselbach's triangle and tacked to Cooper's ligament. When reducing femoral hernia, care must be taken to carefully delineate between hernia contents and the adipose/lymphatic tissue intimately associated with the femoral vein. Injudicious dissection can lead to injury to the femoral vein. The medial dissection may also reveal an obturator hernia, which can be reduced by blunt dissection and may require an additional medially placed mesh to cover the defect.

An indirect hernia is identified during the lateral dissection. The hernia sac is bluntly dissected away from the underlying spermatic cord structures, namely, the vas deferens and the testicular vessels, in a man or the round ligament in a woman. The sac must be dissected free from the cord structures prior to reduction of the sac from within the deep inguinal ring to avoid inadvertent laceration or transection of the vas deferens or testicular vessels. It is critical to avoid dissection posterior to the spermatic cord or round ligament in the "triangle of doom," as this can risk injury to the femoral vessels. The hernia sac is then reduced by application of cephalad and posterior retraction on the hernia sac, with anterior and caudad retraction of the transversalis fascia. One should minimize use of cautery during this dissection, especially in the space lateral to the cord structures, the "triangle of pain," as this can risk injury to the genital branch of the genitofemoral nerve, which courses anterior to the psoas muscle in the pelvis and passes through the inguinal canal along with the cord in the lateral bundle of the cremasteric fascia.

Care must be taken to ensure that the hernia sac remains free from the cord structures along its entire length during the reduction process, particularly in the setting of a large scrotal sac. If the peritoneal sac is very large and cannot be easily reduced, it may be transected, with the distal aspect allowed to retract into the scrotum. The proximal aspect of the sac must then be closed during reperitonealization following the mesh repair to prevent bowel adhesions to the mesh. Transection of the sac is safe but may lead to development of a hydrocele in some cases. Preperitoneal fat within the deep inguinal ring (cord lipomas) should be completely reduced from that space in order to prevent the patient's sensation of a persistent bulge following hernia repair.

Once the hernia sac has been reduced, the peritoneum is dissected further off of the cord structures in a cephalad direction. Adequate parietalization of the cord is essential, as it prevents the peritoneum from slipping underneath the bottom edge of the mesh, which can lead to indirect hernia recurrence. Similarly, herniated preperitoneal fat must also be dissected well off of the cord so that it cannot slip beneath the mesh. This dissection continues cephalad to the level of the anterior superior iliac spine and laterally to the iliac wing, allowing for exposure of the psoas muscle. Medially, this continues to the transition to the urinary bladder, which is then itself dissected off of Cooper's ligament and the pubis in order to clear a space for placement of the mesh. Gentle medial retraction on the bladder allows for better delineation between prevesicular fat and fat associated with the femoral vein and helps reduce the risk of inadvertent injury to the vein.

Once hemostasis has been assured, the next step involves placement of a large piece of nonabsorbable mesh (Figure 2-5). We employ a contoured woven polypropylene mesh that is 4 inches in height by 6 inches in width. The mesh must be large enough to cover the direct, indirect, and femoral spaces (myopectineal orifice) and the posterior aspect of Cooper's ligament. The mesh is rolled and inserted into the abdomen through the 11-mm port. It is inserted into the preperitoneal space and unrolled such that the posterior aspect is draped over the cord structures and psoas muscle laterally and Cooper's ligament and pubic

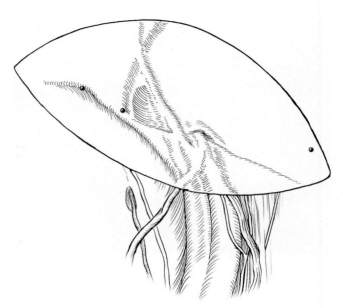

FIGURE 2-5. Repair of the right inguinal hernia with a contoured polypropylene mesh. (Reprinted from Takata MC, Duh QY. Laparoscopic inguinal hernia repair. *Surg Clin North Am.* 2008;88(1):157-178, with permission.)

symphysis medially. The anterior aspect of the mesh then covers the anterior abdominal wall above the level of the iliopubic tract, including the inferior epigastric vessels and the rectus muscle medially. We tack the mesh medially to Cooper's ligament with a single 5-mm spiral tack to prevent the mesh from sliding and will tack to the rectus muscle in cases of a large direct hernia to prevent the mesh from herniating through the defect. One should avoid tack placement laterally to prevent injury to the ilioinguinal and iliohypogastric nerves.

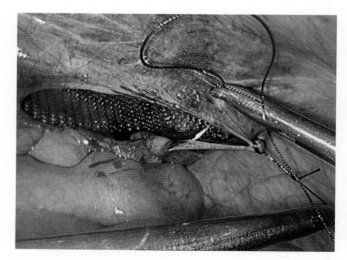

FIGURE 2-6. Suture closure of the peritoneal defect following TAPP inguinal hernia repair. (Reprinted from Kapiris S. Laparoscopic transabdominal preperitoneal hernia repair (TAPP): stapling the mesh is not mandatory. *J Laparoendosc Adv Surg Tech A.* 2009;19(3):419-422, with permission.)

Table 2-1	Recurrent Inguinal Hernia (Transabdominal Preperitoneal Repair)

Key Technical Steps

1. Incision of the peritoneum and development of the preperitoneal space
2. Reduction of direct, femoral or obturator hernias medially
3. Dissection of an indirect hernia sac off of the cord structures/round ligament and subsequent reduction of the sac and cord lipoma from within the deep inguinal ring
4. Extensive peritoneal dissection with parietalization of the cord
5. Placement of nonabsorbable mesh to cover the entire myopectineal orifice
6. Closure of the peritoneum

Potential Pitfalls

- Injury to femoral vessels from dissection in the "triangle of doom" deep to the cord structures
- Injury to genital branch of the genitofemoral nerve from injudicious use of cautery in the "triangle of pain" lateral to the cord structures
- Injury to the cord structures during reduction of an indirect hernia if the sac is not adequately dissection off of the cord prior to reduction of the sac
- Early recurrence if the peritoneum is not adequately dissected prior to mesh placement

Once the mesh has been placed, the peritoneum is closed. This is facilitated by reducing the pneumoperitoneum pressure as low as possible while still permitting adequate visualization. The entire peritoneum must be secured and the mesh covered to prevent bowel adhesions to the mesh or incarceration of a bowel loop within the preperitoneal space. This can be accomplished using absorbable tacks, absorbable suture, or a combination of these. The 11-mm port should be removed and a transfascial absorbable suture placed using a suture passing device, with a 5-mm laparoscope in one of the lateral ports (Figure 2-6). The suture should not be tied down, as the port will be reinserted. The laparoscope is then placed in the 11-mm port so that the 5-mm ports can be removed under direct visualization. This added step is done to ensure that there is no bleeding from inadvertent port injury to the epigastric vessels or branches thereof (Table 2-1).

SUGGESTED READINGS

Carter J, Duh QY. Laparoscopic repair of inguinal hernias. *World J Surg.* 2011;35(7):1519-1525.

Castorina S. An evidence-based approach for laparoscopic inguinal hernia repair: lessons learned from over 1,000 repairs. *Clin Anat* 2012;25(6):687-96.

Hussain A. Technical tips following more than 2000 transabdominal preperitoneal (TAPP) repair of the groin hernia. *Surg Laparosc Endosc Percutan Tech.* 2010;20(6):384-388.

Kapiris S., et al. Laparoscopic transabdominal preperitoneal hernia repair (TAPP): stapling the mesh is not mandatory. *J Laparoendosc Adv Surg Tech A.* 2009;19(3):419-422.

Incarcerated/Strangulated Inguinal Hernia

3

SARAH P. SHUBECK, MATTHEW W. RALLS, AND JUSTIN B. DIMICK

Based on the previous edition chapter "Incarcerated/Strangulated Inguinal Hernia" by Matthew W. Ralls

Presentation

A 61-year-old man presents to the emergency department with obstipation and left groin mass for 3 days. His past medical history was notable for chronic obstructive pulmonary disease, type 2 diabetes, obesity, hyperlipidemia, and schizophrenia. His surgical history was significant for two prior inguinal hernia repairs on the left side. Due to his schizophrenia, he resides in an assisted living facility and comes in with a caregiver today. He describes an increase in abdominal pain and distention over the 3-day period. His oral intake has decreased, and he reports minimal urine output over the past 2 days. Physical exam is notable for a well-healed scar in the right lower quadrant at McBurney's point and a large, 12 × 12-cm bulge in the left inguinal region. The mass is tender to palpation, erythematous, and nonreducible. Although the bulge has intermittently been present, both the patient and caregiver state that the size and tenderness are new in the past 2 days. Laboratory values were notable for a WBC of 8.7 and hematocrit of 42.4.

● DIFFERENTIAL DIAGNOSIS

In a patient with an intermittent groin bulge that is now fixed, tender, and erythematous, complications of a groin hernia should be the first consideration in the differential diagnosis. However, there are several other possible etiologies to consider. Subcutaneous pathology can also present as a groin mass, including lipoma, groin abscess, or inguinal adenopathy. Testicular pathology including torsion and epididymitis should also be considered, especially when the mass involves the scrotum. Vascular etiologies, such as aneurysmal or pseudoaneurysmal disease, should be considered in patients with a history of vascular disease and/or previous interventions at or near the femoral vessels.

Once the surgeon suspects groin hernia, it is important to discern inguinal from femoral hernia. To some degree, this can be ascertained on physical exam. For patients presenting with a femoral hernia, the bulge is below the inguinal ligament. In contrast, in an inguinal hernia, the bulge would be above the inguinal ligament (Figure 3-1). However, this distinction can be difficult to assess if the bulge is large, tender, and inflamed, or if the patient is obese and/or has a large overhanging pannus.

Early identification of groin hernia complications, such as incarceration or strangulation, is essential. Patients presenting with these complications require immediate intervention. Incarcerated hernias by definition cannot be reduced and therefore may progress to strangulation, if not already present on presentation. Strangulated hernias occur when the blood supply of the viscus is compromised. In contrast, for an easily reducible groin hernia, surgical intervention can be delayed and scheduled electively and therefore performed under more controlled circumstances. Suspected incarceration and/or strangulation are surgical emergencies.

● WORKUP

History and physical examination in patients with suspected incarcerated and/or inguinal hernia are often diagnostic. The decision to operate is often made without further evaluation (Figure 3-2). Laboratory values such as complete blood count, comprehensive metabolic panel, and lactate level can provide information about the patient's hydration status and whether there is systemic inflammatory response, which are important in assessing the likelihood of strangulation. However, these tests have a high sensitivity and low specificity, that is, many patients with incarceration and strangulation (especially if presenting early) will have normal or near-normal laboratory values. To avoid a high false-negative rate (i.e., missing the diagnosis when

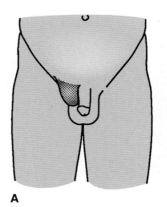 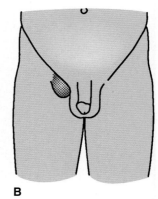

A   B

FIGURE 3-1. Landmarks in discerning inguinal **(A)** versus femoral **(B)** hernia. (Reprinted from Mulholland MW, et al. *Greenfield's Surgery: Scientific Principles & Practice.* 4th ed. Philadelphia, PA: Lippincott Williams & Wilkins; 2011, with permission.)

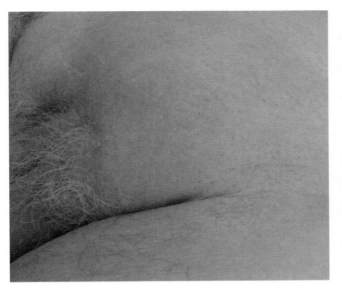

FIGURE 3-2. Erythema and swelling over left groin concerning for incarcerated hernia. This exam finding, coupled with appropriate presentation, is sufficient cause for exploration.

it is present), surgeons should err on the side of exploring patients when incarceration/strangulation are suspected.

If there is substantial uncertainty regarding the diagnosis, imaging studies can be obtained. If the patient is obstructed at the site of incarceration, plain films of the abdomen will show signs of distended loops of bowel and air–fluid levels if the patient is obstructed (Figure 3-3). Computed tomography (CT) imaging is the standard in emergency evaluation (Figure 3-4) if the clinical diagnosis is in question

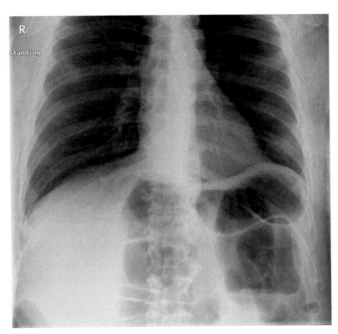

FIGURE 3-3. Plain film of patient described in this clinical scenario. Distended loops of large bowel are concerning for a distal large bowel obstruction.

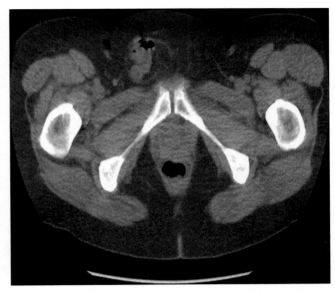

FIGURE 3-4. CT showing left inguinal hernia.

after history, physical, and plain abdominal radiographs. It is important to note that it should be the rare patient who obtains a CT scan to diagnose an incarcerated hernia. Most cases will be diagnosed by history and physical examination, and obtaining a CT scan may often be viewed as an unnecessary delay.

● DISCUSSION

Inguinal hernia repair is one of the most commonly performed surgical procedures worldwide. Over 800,000 inguinal hernia repairs are performed in the United States each year. Despite being a very common operation, the relevant anatomy is complex and often difficult for students and surgical trainees to fully understand. An intimate knowledge of this anatomy is important, especially for addressing incarcerated or recurrent inguinal hernias. In these settings, the distortion of the tissues makes operative repair extremely challenging. In 1804, Astley Cooper stated, "no disease of the human body, belonging to the province of the surgeon, requires in its treatment a greater combination of accurate anatomic knowledge, with surgical skill, than hernia in all its varieties."

Over the past two centuries, there have been many advances in groin hernia repair. The most frequently used technique in contemporary surgical practice is the tension-free mesh repair or Lichtenstein's repair. Laparoscopic techniques including totally extraperitoneal (TEP) and transabdominal preperitoneal (TAPP) are minimally invasive approaches that allow for quicker recovery, less pain, and similar or lower recurrence rates in experienced hands. Primary tissue repairs, such as the Bassini and McVay, are rarely used. However, in certain settings, such as contaminated fields with infection or bowel resection, a working knowledge of primary tissue repairs is essential.

Symptomatic inguinal hernias that are reducible should be repaired on an elective basis. As discussed above, incarcerated or strangulated hernias should be addressed more expeditiously as surgery within 6 hours may prevent loss of bowel. Emergent repair differs little from elective repair. Either open or laparoscopic techniques are acceptable, although it is the preference of the author to utilize the transabdominal preperitoneal laparoscopic approach if at all possible. The rationale for using this approach is that a laparoscopic exploration can be used to assess the viability of the bowel before and after reduction. A peritoneal flap can then be created to repair the hernia in the preperitoneal space. After completion of the repair, the viability of the bowel can be reassessed. Moreover, with adequate closure of the peritoneum, a laparoscopic bowel resection can be performed without contaminating the mesh.

● DIAGNOSIS AND TREATMENT

The patient in our case presents with a scenario worrisome for incarcerated or strangulated inguinal hernia. He has a fixed bulge that is tender to palpation, which is typical of incarceration. He also presents with erythema in the overlying skin, which suggests possible strangulation. The patient also presents with radiographic evidence of large bowel obstruction (Figure 3-3) with resultant obstipation, abdominal pain, and associated nausea and vomiting. This hernia can be approached by either open or laparoscopic procedures depending on surgeon preference and expertise.

● SURGICAL APPROACH FOR OPEN MESH REPAIR OF INCARCERATED INGUINAL HERNIA REPAIR (TABLE 3-1)

Open repair can often be done under general, spinal, or local anesthetic with sedation. Regardless of the anesthesia, the patient is placed in the supine position. Reverse Trendelenburg's position is advocated by some to aid in reduction of the hernia. The patient is prepped and draped in the standard sterile fashion. Local anesthetic is injected in the subcutaneous space above and parallel to the inguinal ligament. The patient can be further anesthetized with varying forms of nerve block if necessary. A 6- to 8-cm incision is made above and parallel to the inguinal ligament. The incision is deepened through the soft tissue with a combination of blunt dissection and Bovie electrocautery to the level of the external oblique aponeurosis. The muscle is then cut along the line of the external oblique fibers from the level of the internal ring and through the external ring.

At this point, groin exploration is warranted in the case of suspected incarceration/strangulation. If the viability of the bowel is in question, a resection can be performed via the inguinal incision. If that is not feasible, it may be necessary to perform laparotomy (see Special Intraoperative

Table 3-1	Open Inguinal Hernia Repair with Mesh

Key Technical Steps

1. Verify laterality.
2. Prophylaxis with antibiotics.
3. Groin incision.
4. Expose and incise the external oblique in the direction of the fibers to the external ring.
5. Identify and protect the ilioinguinal nerve.
6. Mobilize flaps of external oblique.
7. Attempt reduction of hernia contents to better establish anatomical landmarks.
8. Encircle the spermatic cord (round ligament if female) at the external ring with a Penrose drain.
9. Identify the hernia sac on the anteromedial surface of the cord and dissect it free from the surrounding structures.
10. In the case of an indirect hernia, open the sac, reduce the contents, and highly ligate with suture ligature.
11. If direct hernia, free sac from surrounding attachments and reduce into the abdomen.
12. Assess the floor of the canal and prepare the mesh.
13. Begin medially at the pubic tubercle and secure the mesh in place to the shelving edge inferiorly and the conjoined tendon superiorly.
14. Avoid narrowing the internal ring or incorporating nervous tissue into the repair.
15. Ensure hemostasis.
16. Close the external oblique aponeurosis and Scarpa's fascia in layers.
17. Approximate the skin edges and apply a dressing.

Considerations). Great care is taken to not injure the ilioinguinal nerve that is underlying this layer. Tissue flaps are mobilized. Through blunt finger dissection, the cord (and hernia sac) are freed circumferentially and encircled in a Penrose drain. If there is no bowel compromise, the procedure moves forward as with an uncomplicated hernia repair.

The dissection is now turned to identification and separation of the hernia sac from the cord structures with division of the cremasteric fibers. Classically, the sac of an indirect hernia will be anterior and medial with respect to the cord. The internal ring is inspected for evidence of indirect hernia. If found, the sac is dissected free and ligated under direct vision. Care is taken to avoid injury to the contents of the hernia prior to reducing the contents back into the peritoneal cavity. If a direct hernia is encountered, the hernia is reduced. The inguinal floor should be inspected for weakness.

Attention is then turned to repairing the ring and floor with mesh. A polypropylene mesh (precut or 6 inch²) is typically used. The medial point is secured to the lateral aspect of the pubic tubercle, suturing to the periosteum and not the bone itself. The prosthesis is positioned over the inguinal

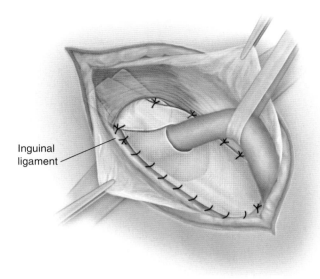

FIGURE 3-5. Mesh placement during standard open (Lichtenstein) hernia repair. (From Mulholland MW, et al. *Operative Techniques in Surgery*. Wolters Kluwer Health. Philadelphia, PA; 2015.)

floor and secured to the lateral edge of the rectus sheath (i.e., the conjoint tendon or area). The cord structures are placed through a slit in the lateral portion of the mesh, and the two tails are secured to each other to create a new internal ring. The inferior leaflet of the mesh is secured to the shelving edge of the inguinal ligament (Figure 3-5). The external oblique aponeurosis and Scarpa's fascia are closed in layers. The skin is approximated.

● SURGICAL APPROACH TO LAPAROSCOPIC REPAIR OF INCARCERATED INGUINAL HERNIA (TABLE 3-2)

Depending on a surgeon's experience and preference, it is reasonable to approach incarcerated or strangulated hernias laparoscopically. If the hernia is recurrent, or multiply recurrent, laparoscopic hernia repair is more likely to produce better long-term results including lower rates of recurrence, as a laparoscopic repair allows for repair of the hernia through tissue planes that are undisturbed by prior surgery.

As discussed above, the author's preference is to approach incarcerated/strangulated hernias via a TAPP approach. The patient is placed in the supine position and then prepped and draped in standard sterile fashion. General anesthesia is induced. The first trocar is placed at the umbilicus to establish pneumoperitoneum, and two 5-mm ports are placed on either side of the umbilicus just lateral to the rectus sheath (Figure 3-6). The surgeon then performs an initial exploration with assessment of the viability of the potentially incarcerated bowel and hernia contents. Once this step is complete, and we are convinced

Table 3-2	TAPP Inguinal Hernia Repair with Mesh

Key Technical Steps

1. Verify laterality.
2. Prophylaxis with antibiotics.
3. Infraumbilical incision for the 10- to 12-mm trocar followed by insufflation.
4. Placement of two 5-mm trocars at the level of the umbilicus, lateral to the rectus sheath.
5. Creation of peritoneal flap starting lateral to inferior epigastric vessels.
6. Dissection of contents of inguinal canal and identification of a hernia sac.
7. Skeletonize the cord structures.
8. If direct: reduce the sac and preperitoneal from the internal ring by gentle traction.
9. If indirect: mobilize the sac from the cord structures, and reduce into the peritoneum.
10. Place precut lateralized mesh in proper orientation to completely cover direct, indirect, and femoral spaces.
11. Place tacking suture on the medial aspect of the mesh in Cooper's ligament securing mesh in place.
12. Tack peritoneal flap back to the abdominal wall to fully cover newly introduced mesh.
13. Desufflation and trocar removal under direct visualization.

the bowel is viable, a peritoneal flap is created to enter the preperitoneal space (Figure 3-7). The peritoneum is then incised starting lateral to the inferior epigastric vessels to establish a preperitoneal plane that extends laterally to the anterior superior iliac spine.

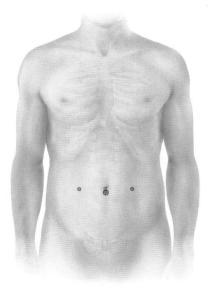

FIGURE 3-6. Port placement for TAPP inguinal hernia repair. (From Mulholland MW, et al. *Operative Techniques in Surgery*. Philadelphia, PA: Wolters Kluwer Health; 2015.)

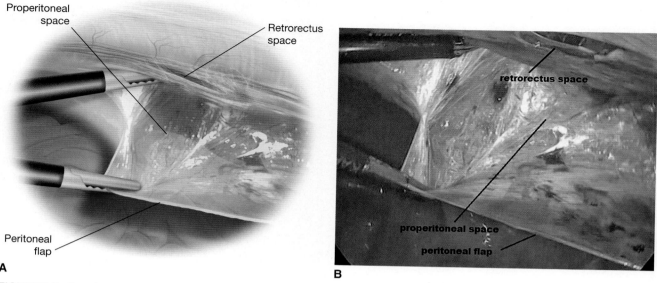

FIGURE 3-7. Creation of peritoneal flap during TAPP. **A:** Illustration. **B:** Intraoperative Laparoscopic Image. (From Mulholland MW, et al. *Operative Techniques in Surgery.* Philadelphia, PA: Wolters Kluwer Health; 2015.)

Dissection then proceeds identify a possible indirect hernia sac. Once identified, the sac and contents can be reduced to facilitate identification of the remaining cord structures. After dissecting cord structures free from the hernia sac and determining bowel contents of the hernia sac are viable, mesh is introduced via the umbilical port. The mesh will again be placed covering direct, indirect, and femoral spaces. The mesh is tacked in place with minimal points of fixation (Figure 3-8). The peritoneal flap is then closed with tack fixation followed by desufflation, previously incarcerated bowel reexamined for viability, and trocar removal under direct visualization. The procedure is finished with closure of the port sites and skin approximation.

The complex anatomy must be well understood by the surgeon (Figure 3-9). Blunt graspers are used to free the cord and hernia sac from the surrounding areolar tissue.

Two pitfalls of this portion of the operation are to dissect in the triangle of doom and the triangle of pain. The triangle of doom is bordered by the vas deferens medially, spermatic vessels laterally, and external iliac vessels inferiorly. The contents of this space comprise the external iliac artery and vein and the deep circumflex iliac vein. Damage to these vessels

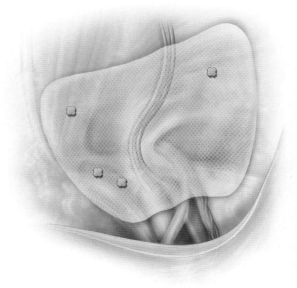

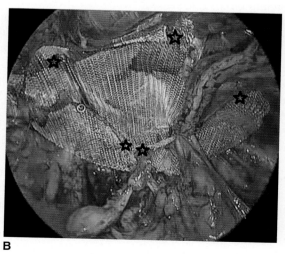

FIGURE 3-8. Mesh fixation. **A:** Illustration. **B:** Intraoperative Laparoscopic Image. (From Mulholland MW, et al. *Operative Techniques in Surgery*. Philadelphia, PA: Wolters Kluwer Health; 2015.)

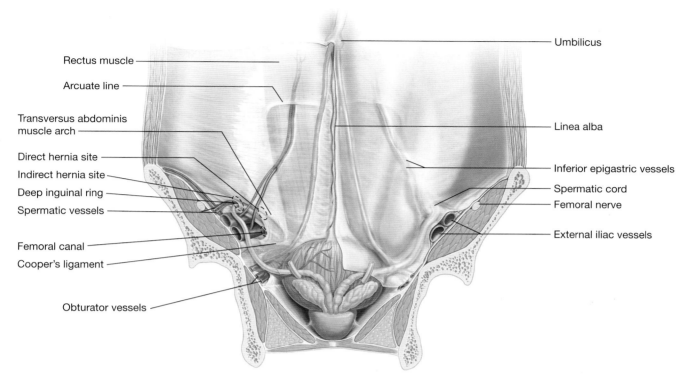

Rectus muscle

Arcuate line

Transversus abdominis muscle arch

Direct hernia site

Indirect hernia site

Deep inguinal ring

Spermatic vessels

Femoral canal

Cooper's ligament

Obturator vessels

Umbilicus

Linea alba

Inferior epigastric vessels

Spermatic cord

Femoral nerve

External iliac vessels

FIGURE 3-9. Anatomy of inguinal canal. (From Mulholland MW, et al. *Operative Techniques in Surgery*. Wolters Kluwer Health. Philadelphia, PA; 2015.)

can cause major bleeding and should be avoided. The triangle of pain is defined as spermatic vessel medially, the iliopubic tract laterally, and inferiorly the inferior edge of skin incision. This triangle contains the lateral femoral cutaneous nerve and anterior femoral cutaneous nerve of the thigh. Manipulation, dissection, and tacking should be avoided as nerve damage or entrapment can cause neuralgia.

● SPECIAL INTRAOPERATIVE CONSIDERATIONS

As with many urgent or emergent general surgery situations, intraoperative decision-making is essential to optimize outcomes. Incarceration or strangulation increases the odds of gross spillage of bowel contents. In the case of bowel resection or other contamination, the surgeon will need to utilize biologic mesh or primary tissue repair. For a straightforward primary inguinal hernia with contamination, a Bassini repair would be a good choice. For this procedure, the lateral edge of the rectus sheath (i.e., conjoined tendon) is approximated to the inguinal ligament. A relaxing incision is made if there is any tension. For a femoral hernia with contamination, a Bassini repair will not be adequate because the femoral canal has not been addressed. In this case, a McVay (Cooper's ligament) repair is appropriate. With a McVay repair, the lateral edge of the rectus sheath (i.e., conjoined tendon) is approximated to Cooper's ligament. To perform these primary tissue repairs, the surgeon must be able to correctly identify these

anatomical structures. In recurrent hernias or where acute inflammation obscures the anatomy, an alternative is to perform a Lichtenstein repair with biologic mesh. However, using biologic mesh will likely result in recurrent hernia as it is incorporated and weakens.

In certain circumstances, a laparotomy may be necessary. If there is any question of bowel compromise during inguinal exploration that cannot be managed with evaluation or resection via the inguinal incision, a laparotomy should be performed to further inspect the bowel and perform resection. In some cases, intra-abdominal adhesions may be too dense to adequately reduce the hernia through an inguinal incision. When forced to make a laparotomy, a lower midline laparotomy below the umbilicus is usually adequate. With this approach, the operator can choose to enter the peritoneal cavity or stay preperitoneal. Once a laparotomy is performed, it is also possible to perform an open preperitoneal repair, which is useful in recurrent hernias with anterior scarring and distortion of the relevant anatomy.

● POSTOPERATIVE MANAGEMENT

Postoperative care for patients undergoing surgery for incarcerated inguinal hernias is mostly supportive, including correcting lab aberrations, providing intravenous hydration, optimizing pain control, and awaiting the return of bowel function. The period of observation should be dictated by the severity of presenting illness as well as postoperative clinical progression. It is important to avoid the reduction of necrotic bowel into the peritoneal cavity. If this is the case, the patient will likely have continued or worsening bowel obstruction with overall deterioration of the clinical picture. If left untreated, abdominal sepsis will ensue.

Case Conclusion

The patient was taken emergently to the operating room (OR) for laparoscopic evaluation and repair. Upon initial diagnostic laparoscopy, portions of the small bowel as well as the sigmoid colon were found to be in a large direct hernia sac. Once fully reduced, it was apparent that all bowel was viable. Given the distorted anterior anatomy from previous hernia repair, a transabdominal preperitoneal approach with placement of prosthetic mesh was performed. A laparoscopic transabdominal preperitoneal approach is an excellent option for multiply recurrent hernias. Following the procedure, the patient was monitored, resuscitated, and had an uneventful postoperative course.

TAKE HOME POINTS

- Suspected incarceration or strangulation mandates immediate surgical intervention.
- The gold standard approach to suspected incarceration or strangulation is groin exploration to assess bowel viability and repair hernia.
- If the hernia cannot be managed through a groin incision, due to questionable bowel viability, intra-abdominal adhesions, or an inability to safely reduce the hernia contents, a lower midline laparotomy should be made.
- When bowel resection is necessary due to strangulation, prosthetic mesh should not be used. Instead, a primary tissue repair (e.g., Bassini or McVay) can be performed.
- Laparoscopic or open preperitoneal approaches can be used for multiply recurrent hernias, but it is essential to ensure viability of hernia contents before proceeding with these techniques.

SUGGESTED READINGS

Bittner J. Incarcerated/strangulated hernia: open or laparoscopic? *Adv Surg.* 2016;50:67-78.

Eklund AS, Montgomery AK, Rasmussen IC, et al. Low recurrence rate after laparoscopic (TEP) and open (Lichtenstein) inguinal hernia repair: a randomized, multicenter trial with 5-year follow-up. *Ann Surg.* 2009;249:33-38.

Ferzli G, Shapiro K, Chaudry G, et al. Laparoscopic extraperitoneal approach to acutely incarcerated inguinal hernia. *Surg Endosc.* 2004;18:228-231.

Kouhia ST, Huttunen R, Silvasti SO, et al. Lichtenstein hernioplasty versus totally extraperitoneal laparoscopic hernioplasty in treatment of recurrent inguinal hernia—a prospective randomized trial. *Ann Surg.* 2009;249:384-387.

Pisanu A, Podda M, Saba A, Porceddu G, Uccheddu A. Meta-analysis and review of prospective randomized trials comparing laparoscopic and Lichtenstein techniques in recurrent inguinal hernia repair. *Hernia.* 2015;19:355-366.

Sevonius D, Gunnarsson U, Nordin P, et al. Repeated groin hernia recurrences. *Ann Surg.* 2009;249:516-518.

Ventral Incisional Hernia

4

MELISSA K. STEWART AND BENJAMIN K. POULOSE

Based on the previous edition chapter "Ventral Incisional Hernias" by
Vivian M. Sanchez and Kamal M.F. Itani

Presentation

A 73-year-old woman with a medical history notable for rheumatoid arthritis requiring immunologic therapy presents to outpatient surgery clinic with complaints of an abdominal bulge with associated discomfort. The symptoms have been present for more than 2 years with escalating severity. The pain occurs daily and is described as a constant, nonradiating, ache centered about the bulge that is worsened with standing and straining. No associated gastrointestinal obstructive symptoms are elicited. The patient is very active and works extensively in her community and exercises routinely. The bulge affects her ability to perform these activities. Her past surgical history is notable for total abdominal hysterectomy complicated by vaginal vault prolapse resulting in three subsequent operative interventions: anterior/posterior colporrhaphy, perineorrhaphy and retropubic urethropexy; cystocele repair; and abdominal sacral colpopexy with abdominal fascial harvest. All operations were done through a Pfannenstiel incision. On examination, her vital signs were within normal limits and her body mass index (BMI) is 28. She has a well-healed low transverse incision with an underlying ventral incisional hernia. The hernia is nontender and reducible with a palpable abdominal wall defect of approximately 5 cm. No overlying skin changes were noted.

● DIFFERENTIAL DIAGNOSIS

The diagnosis of a ventral incisional hernia is usually straightforward, simply requiring the presence of an abdominal bulge with associated fascial defect in a patient with a prior history of an abdominopelvic operative intervention. The ascertainment of a fascial defect can be difficult in obese patients or with hernias that are chronically incarcerated. Incarceration generally describes the inability to completely reduce the hernia contents through the hernia defect.

Hernias can be chronically or acutely incarcerated. Chronically incarcerated hernias may remain asymptomatic for years, whereas an acute incarceration episode is often an emergent event. Reducibility generally describes the ability to spontaneously or manually place the hernia contents through the hernia orifice. A reducible and/or chronically incarcerated hernia usually does not merit an urgent operation, whereas acute incarceration of a hernia often warrants urgent evaluation and intervention to prevent progression of dire sequelae including strangulation or bowel obstruction. Strangulation refers to the condition in which the blood supply of the herniated viscus is so constricted by swelling and congestion as to compromise its circulation. Combining patient history and physical exam can most often lead to the accurate distinction between incarceration/reducibility and associated chronicity. Patients exhibiting signs and symptoms of acute incarceration/strangulation will often complain of acutely worsened pain over the site of the hernia and possibly obstructive gastrointestinal symptoms (nausea, emesis, obstipation, constipation). Concomitant physical exam will reveal an acutely tender bulge that is not reducible. Overlying skin inflammatory changes may also be present. Patients with chronic incarceration usually will not exhibit signs and symptoms of acute inflammation yet the hernia contents itself will not reduce.

Additionally, when evaluating a patient for a ventral incisional hernia, it is important to distinguish a ventral hernia from rectus diastasis. As opposed to a hernia, rectus diastasis refers to separation of the rectus abdominis muscles from the midline without a concomitant fascial defect. Diastasis recti will clinically present as a symmetric protrusion of the midline, extending from xiphoid to the umbilicus. This entity should be distinguished from incision-associated diastasis where no fascial defect may be discernable, but a previous operation has occurred in the area of a bulge. These entities are poorly understood in terms of best management. Treatment should be individualized and should generally include compression garments and physical therapy if impacting a patient's quality of life. The benefit of surgical intervention is unclear in diastasis recti, and most surgeon do not offer repair.

● DIAGNOSIS AND TREATMENT

Though the diagnosis of ventral incisional hernia may appear obvious based on history and physical exam, it is prudent to entertain a differential diagnosis for the presenting symptoms, primarily abdominal pain. Among others, such diagnoses include small bowel obstruction, biliary processes (symptomatic cholelithiasis, chronic cholecystitis, and choledocholithiasis), pancreatitis, and urogynecologic pathologies. Abdominal and abdominal wall tumors should also be considered.

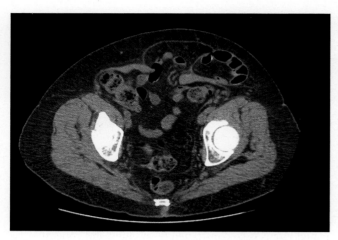

FIGURE 4-1. CT scan revealing a 4 cm fascial defect of the lower midline with a 15 cm hernia sac containing multiple loops of nonobstructed small bowel with a septation propagating through the midportion of the sac.

Adjunct imaging for ventral incisional hernia management is usually employed in two situations: to establish the diagnosis of ventral incisional hernia and for operative planning. Surgeon-performed ultrasound has been shown to be an effective way to diagnose and characterize ventral incisional hernia with comparable results to computed tomography (CT) evaluation. This offers the benefit of reduced radiation exposure and quick assessment of the abdominal wall. Surgeon physical exam often has a higher false-negative rate in obese patients. In this patient, hernia repair by open approach with myofascial release via retromuscular repair is planned. The risks and benefits were thoroughly outlined and accepted. Medical optimization strategies prior to surgery, including weight loss and perioperative cessation of immunologically active rheumatologic medications, were initiated. Based on known medical history and current physiologic status, no further preoperative studies to assess cardiac and/or pulmonary status were felt necessary for the patient.

The patient in our case study underwent biochemical evaluation that revealed normal white blood cell count, liver function, and pancreatic enzymes. Subsequently, she underwent CT to confirm the diagnosis of ventral incisional hernia, to rule out concomitant pathologic processes, and to assist with operative planning. The CT revealed a 4 cm fascial defect of the lower midline with a 15 cm hernia sac containing multiple loops of nonobstructed small bowel with a septation propagating through the midportion of the sac (Figure 4-1). Notably, there was no radiographic evidence of bowel, gynecologic, urinary, biliary, or pancreatic pathology. The diagnosis of a symptomatic ventral incisional hernia was confirmed.

● DISCUSSION

Ventral incisional hernias are an important entity to all surgeons who operate in the abdomen and pelvis, because they occur up to 30% of the time following laparotomy.

As such, ventral incisional hernia repair is the most common reason for reoperation following laparotomy. The cost of hernia repair in the United States is approximately $4,000 to $16,000 for outpatient and inpatient repairs, respectively. Both the cumulative incidence and estimated costs are rising over time.

Ventral incisional hernias occur as a result of a combination of patient, perioperative, and technical factors. Patient factors increasing the risk of hernia formation include obesity, tobacco abuse, diabetes mellitus, malnourishment, connective tissue disorders, chronic obstructive pulmonary disease, use of immunosuppressant medications, and repeat abdominal operations. Perioperative and technical factors include surgical wound classification, surgical site infection, and technique for abdominal closure. Regarding technique, one of the most effective preventive measures is a "small bites" technique, which has been shown to reduce subsequent hernia formation.

Indications for acute operative repair of a ventral incisional hernia include strangulation and/or acute incarceration. Indications for elective repair of a ventral incisional hernia include bothersome symptoms (pain, discomfort, respiratory dysfunction, cosmetic concerns) and/or functional concerns (impact on quality of life, impairment of abdominal wall function). The majority of hernia operations are performed electively.

Though the approach to ventral incisional hernia repair will be discussed at length in the subsequent section, most agree that utilization of mesh in ventral incisional hernia repair is necessary to minimize the risk of recurrence. In a prospective study of ventral incisional hernia <6 cm, the recurrence rate was 24% and 43% (at 3 years) and 32% and 63% (at 10 years) for primary repair and repair with mesh, respectively. Beyond health benefit to the patient, recurrence minimization is important, for data reveal that a global 1% reduction in hernia recurrence would result in a $32 million yearly savings in procedural costs alone. Though use of mesh is widely utilized and endorsed, it should be noted that as outcomes are longitudinally tracked and assessed, mesh-related complications occur approximately 5% of the time.

● SURGICAL REPAIR OF VENTRAL INCISIONAL HERNIAS

Approach

When planning an operative repair of a ventral incisional hernia, the surgeon must decide between a minimally invasive versus open repair and type of mesh. If an open technique is chosen, the location of mesh placement must also be considered.

The minimally invasive approach, typically performed laparoscopically, currently accounts for close to 30% of ventral incisional hernia repairs. When performing a laparoscopic approach, the mesh is typically placed in an intraperitoneal, sublay, position. Technically, the operative approach requires safe peritoneal entry, careful lysis of adhesions with minimal use of thermal energy, placement of mesh with appropriate mesh/fascial overlap (>4 cm), and mesh fixation. The type of mesh utilized is dictated by sublay position. Typically, a permanent mesh that has an antiadhesive barrier is used for intraperitoneal placement. The repair is based on the principle of transmission of fluid pressure. Application of this principle dictates that as intra-abdominal pressure increases, the applied force is displaced equally across the mesh. Advantages to the laparoscopic approach include shorter operative time, decreased length of hospital stay, quicker patient recovery, and decreased wound complications. Disadvantages of a laparoscopic approach mainly concern the low but increased risk of unrecognized hollow viscus injury, which can lead to potentially catastrophic sequelae. Contraindications to laparoscopic repair include inability to tolerate general anesthesia or abdominal insufflation, strangulated hernia, hostile/frozen abdomen, and/or infected/contaminated field. Controversies yet to be resolved include the need for fascial closure, type of mesh fixation required, and the utility of robotically assisted minimally invasive approaches.

Beyond decreased recurrence rates, proponents of open repair often cite better functional outcome with restoration of normal abdominal wall anatomy and the reduced risk of unrecognized hollow viscus injury. Open ventral incisional hernia mesh placement techniques include inlay (bridging the defect with mesh), onlay (covering the defect with mesh and fascia overlap), and sublay repair (placing the mesh in a retromuscular, preperitoneal, or intraperitoneal position). Although mesh inlay and onlay techniques have benefit in specific settings, the sublay repair with retromuscular mesh placement has been deemed as the Americas Hernia Society preferred method of repair. Such preference is secondary to decreased recurrence rates and mesh-related complications. Technically, the repair requires peritoneal entry, adhesiolysis, retromuscular dissection, reconstruction of the posterior sheath, mesh placement, and reconstruction of the anterior layer. If further mobilization is required, transversus abdominis or external oblique releases may be required. The type of mesh utilized in this reconstruction is dependent largely on risk of wound complications. In low-risk wounds (typically clean), midweight or heavyweight permanent meshes are usually employed. In higher-risk wounds (clean contaminated or contaminated), an array of mesh types can be considered including biologics, bioabsorbables, or lightweight/midweight macroporous polypropylene products. In heavily contaminated settings, permanent prosthetics and slowly resorbable meshes should be avoided.

Postoperative Management

The postoperative management following ventral incisional hernia repair starts with preoperative planning. Patients often benefit from preoperative placement of an epidural or regional nerve block for adjunctive pain management. These patients not only benefit from improved pain control, but narcotic minimization also has multiorgan system benefits. Diet advancement is often based on the extent of lysis of adhesions and need for concomitant procedures (e.g., bowel resection). In general, most patients can tolerate a clear liquid diet when awake with advancement of diet upon return of bowel function. To distribute tension across the abdominal wall, all patients should wear an abdominal binder for the first four weeks after operation. Following Surgical Care Improvement Project (SCIP) guidelines, preoperative antibiotics are given prior to incision and are generally carried out for the remainder of the 24 hour perioperative setting. Additionally, patients are provided both mechanical and pharmacologic venous thromboembolism prophylaxes. Most often, operative drains are left superficial to inserted mesh and deep to created lipocutaneous flaps, if present. Retromuscular drains are usually left until output is <50 mL per day and/or the patient is discharged from the hospital (usually 3 to 5 days). Subcutaneous drains are usually left in place until output is <30 mL per day.

Postoperative Complications

Wound complications are the most common issues after ventral incisional hernia repair. Surgical site infections and surgical site occurrences have been well defined for this clinical entity. Infections should be treated with antibiotics and drainage, as indicated. Depending on clinical response and degree of infection, mesh excision may be required, but mesh salvage can usually be achieved depending on prosthetic type and patient factors. Noninfectious wound complications (hematoma, seroma, flap necrosis, etc.) should be managed expectantly. Pulmonary complications following ventral incisional hernia repair are not uncommon. Postintubation status, poor respiratory effort and clearance secondary to inadequate pain control, and decreased compliance given increased intra-abdominal pressure often lead to plugging, pneumonia, hypoxia, and hypercarbia. Hernia repair patients are also at risk for aspiration given likelihood of ileus secondary to concomitant bowel manipulation during adhesiolysis. Another feared complication is the creation of intra-abdominal hypertension (IAH). The acute increase in intra-abdominal pressure may adversely affect venous return/cardiac output, pulmonary compliance, and renal blood flow and function. The management of IAH first requires appropriate recognition and diagnosis. Most surgeons advocate following intraoperative change in plateau airway pressures as a marker of dynamic changes in intra-abdominal pressures. The postoperative management of IAH is supportive: continued mechanical ventilation with paralysis for elevated airway pressures with consequent hypercarbia and judicious fluid management to augment the decrease in preload and subsequent decrease in cardiac output. Decompressive laparotomy is rarely needed to treat IAH induced by abdominal wall reconstruction.

Case Conclusion

The patient underwent an open ventral incisional hernia repair with posterior rectus sheath mobilization and mesh insertion. First, a lower midline incision was created and the abdomen was entered sharply through the hernia sac. Adhesions from the omentum and transverse colon to the anterior abdominal wall were lysed. A 9 × 5 cm hernia defect was noted. The fascia was noted to be of good quality bilaterally. The space of Retzius was entered inferiorly and the preperitoneal space was developed to the pubis. Similarly, the preperitoneal space in the midline was mobilized toward the upper abdomen. Next, bilateral retromuscular mobilizations were performed by separating the posterior rectus sheath from the rectus muscle (Figure 4-2). This facilitated advancement of the linea alba to midline. The posterior rectus sheath was reapproximated using running absorbable suture. Next, a 25 × 15 cm midweight, macroporous, polypropylene mesh was inserted into the retromuscular and preperitoneal spaces and sutured to the abdominal wall.

Two closed suction drains were then placed over the mesh. The linea alba was closed with running absorbable suture. The subcutaneous tissue and skin were then closed in successive layers with running absorbable suture.

The patient underwent epidural insertion preoperatively. Postoperatively, given the minimal amount of adhesiolysis required, she was given a clear liquid diet. As her bowel function returned, her diet was advanced to a regular diet. Her pain control was weaned from an epidural to a multimodal oral pain regimen. She was able to void spontaneously after catheter removal. Following her clinical progression, she was discharged to home on postoperative day 4. Her drains were removed prior to discharge, as is usually the case in patients undergoing open retromuscular ventral incisional hernia repair. Routine follow-up after this type of repair includes postoperative visits at 4 weeks with continued evaluation for 1 to 3 years after operation depending on practice preference.

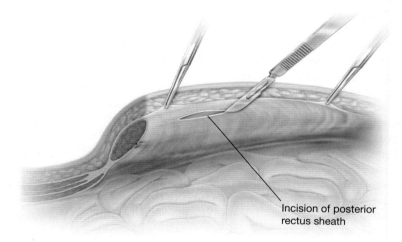

Incision of posterior rectus sheath

A

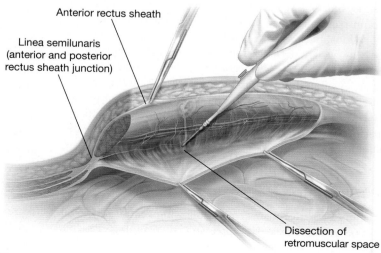

Anterior rectus sheath

Linea semilunaris (anterior and posterior rectus sheath junction)

Dissection of retromuscular space

FIGURE 4-2. **A:** The posterior rectus sheath is incised 1 cm lateral to the linea alba to gain access to the retrorectus space. **B:** The posterior rectus sheath is separated off the rectus muscle until the lateral edge of the rectus is identified by the presence of the perforating neurovascular bundles. (Reprinted from Hawn M. *Operative Techniques in Foregut Surgery*. Philadelphia, PA: Wolters Kluwer; 2015, with permission.)

B

TAKE HOME POINTS

- Incisional hernia is a common consequence of laparotomy.
- Laparoscopic and open incisional hernia repair are both reasonable options. Laparoscopic repair is associated with decreased wound complications and shorter hospitalizations/recovery. Open repair via retromuscular sublay technique offers decreased recurrence rates and improved abdominal wall function.
- Use of mesh is recommended in the repair of an incisional hernia. The type of mesh utilized is dictated by anatomic location of insertion and wound risk.

SUGGESTED READINGS

Alexander AM, Scott DJ. Laparoscopic ventral hernia repair. *Surg Clin North Am.* 2013;93:1091-1110.

Baucom RB, et al. Comparative evaluation of dynamic abdominal sonography for hernia and computed tomography for characterization of incisional hernia. *JAMA Surg.* 2014;149:591-596.

Baucom RB, et al. Prospective evaluation of surgeon physical examination for detection of incisional hernias. *J Am Coll Surg.* 2014;218:363-366.

Beck WC, et al. Comparative effectiveness of dynamic abdominal sonography for hernia versus computed tomography in the diagnosis of incisional hernia. *J Am Coll Surg.* 2013;216:447-453.

Carlson MA, Frantzides CT, Laguna LE, et al. Minimally invasive ventral herniorrhaphy: an analysis of 6,266 published cases. *Hernia.* 2008;12:9-22.

Eker HH, et al. Laparoscopic versus open incisional hernia repair: a randomized clinical trial. *JAMA Surg.* 2013;148:259-263.

Flum DR, Horvath K, Koepsell T. Have outcomes of incisional hernia repair improved with time? A population-based analysis. *Ann Surg.* 2003;237(1):129-135.

Itani KMF, Hawn MT, eds. Advances in abdominal wall hernia repair. *Surg Clin North Am.* 2008;88:17-19.

Itani KMF, Hur K, Neumayer L, et al. Comparison of laparoscopic and open repair with mesh for the treatment of ventral incisional hernia: a randomized trial. *Arch Surg.* 2010;145:322-328.

Kokotovic D, Bisgaard T, Helgstrand F. Long-term recurrence and complications associated with elective incisional hernia repair. *JAMA.* 2016;316:1575.

Luijendijk RW, Hop WCJ, van den Tol MP, et al. A comparison of suture repair with mesh repair for incisional hernia. *N Engl J Med.* 2000;343(6):392-398.

Pauli EM, Rosen MJ. Open ventral hernia repair with component separation. *Surg Clin North Am.* 2013;93:1111-1133.

Poulose BK, et al. Epidemiology and cost of ventral hernia repair: making the case for hernia research. *Hernia.* 2011;16:179-183.

Complex Abdominal Wall Reconstruction

DAVID M. KRPATA AND MICHAEL J. ROSEN

5

Based on the previous edition chapter "Complex Abdominal Wall Reconstruction" by Michael J. Rosen

Presentation

The patient is a 56-year-old obese (BMI 41 kg/m²) male with a past medical history of hypertension and non–insulin-dependent diabetes. Three years prior to this presentation, he underwent an elective sigmoid colectomy for multiply recurrent sigmoid diverticulitis. He developed a postoperative wound infection and his wound healed by secondary intention. Within 1 year, he noted a bulge along his incision that was becoming increasing uncomfortable. He was noted to have an incisional hernia and underwent elective repair. He was repaired in an open fashion with a 10 × 15-inch piece of Composix mesh (polypropylene and PTFE). He initially did well and was discharged on postoperative day 3. However, on his 2-week postoperative visit, he was noted to have erythema of the wound and purulent drainage. He was explored in the operating room, the wound was opened, the fascia appeared intact, and cultures revealed MRSA. He was placed on a negative pressure wound therapy for approximately 6 months and presents to you with a chronic draining sinus. An abdominal computerized tomography scan reveals fluid around the mesh. The patient reports generalized malaise, denies fevers, and has no erythema on exam. His laboratory evaluation is unremarkable.

● DIFFERENTIAL DIAGNOSIS

This case presentation considers the workup of a patient with a chronic draining sinus after an open ventral hernia repair with prosthetic mesh. The differential diagnosis of a draining sinus after an open ventral hernia repair depends on the time of presentation. In the early postoperative period, multiple factors can lead to wound issues. Superficial surgical site infections are common and often are a result of skin flora contamination. Deep space infections involving the mesh in the early postoperative period are more concerning. While these are most often associated with prosthetic contamination with skin flora, potential bowel injury and missed enterotomy must be considered. Culture results revealing gram-negative or anaerobic bacteria should raise concern for the surgeon. Patients presenting

with chronic draining sinuses many months after open ventral hernia repair often represent some form of an infected foreign body. Occasionally, these can be the result of a suture sinus abscess, and removal of the suture can be curative. Unfortunately, most often this involves contamination of the graft, signaling lack of incorporation, and will not resolve without surgical intervention. If patients present with a draining sinus long after their initial surgery, the possibility of mesh erosion into the viscera should be entertained. Careful evaluation for a fistula is imperative to guide preoperative planning.

● DISCUSSION

Abdominal wall reconstruction represents a broad spectrum of disease. Patients can range from those with a small umbilical hernia (<2 cm) up to some of the most challenging reconstructive problems such as patients with massive hernias and an enterocutaneous fistula. The reconstructive surgeon dealing with the full spectrum of these problems must have multiple reconstructive techniques at hand. It is impossible for one procedure or one form of prosthetic to address all of the unique problems these patients can display. This chapter focuses on the complex spectrum of these scenarios. It is important to mention that there is no single definition of a "complex" ventral hernia. In fact, multiple factors can make a ventral hernia complex, and often recognizing these issues preoperatively can avoid potential postoperative morbidity. In general, ventral hernias become complex based on certain patient, defect, and surgical technique characteristics. Patient comorbidities linked to postoperative complications include obesity, smoking, COPD, immunosuppression, malnutrition, and diabetes. Optimization of each of these parameters preoperatively is important for ultimate success of the repair. Complex defect characteristics include the presence of contamination or infection (i.e., infected prosthetic material, enterocutaneous fistulas, or concomitant elective bowel surgery), large defects with substantial tissue loss, massive hernias with loss of abdominal domain (more viscera outside the abdominal cavity than within it), and multiply recurrent hernias with fixed noncompliant abdominal walls. Finally, at times, the reconstructive techniques chosen by the surgeon can complicate the repair. For instance, a commonly performed procedure, component separation, typically involves elevation of large subcutaneous flaps that can be associated with wound morbidity of up to 40% in some series. In this chapter, I will address a common clinical scenario of a complex abdominal wall problem: infected prosthetic mesh.

● WORKUP

The initial workup of any patient presenting with problem after surgery is to obtain all operative reports and determine exactly what was done before. It is important to identify what mesh was placed and in what compartment in the abdominal wall. The management of an onlay mesh can be significantly different than an intraperitoneally placed mesh. Likewise, the composition of the mesh material can have implications in management. For example, macroporous mesh (polypropylene and polyester mesh) can often be salvaged with partial mesh excision. However, microporous mesh (ePTFE, GORE-TEX) can almost never be salvaged and requires complete mesh excision. I obtain an abdominal computerized tomography scan for all patients with complex abdominal wall problems. This imaging test gives important information with regard to whether there is uncontrolled infection (i.e., undrained fluid collections), the size of the mesh, the layer of the abdominal wall where the mesh was placed, whether bowel is involved, and the extent of remaining uninvolved abdominal wall that can be used for eventual reconstruction.

It is never an emergency to remove an infected piece of prosthetic material from the abdominal wall. If there is extensive soft tissue inflammation/erythema, a course of antibiotics is warranted. If there are undrained fluid collections causing systemic inflammatory response, these should be drained surgically or by interventional radiology. Although it is not likely that this will cure the infection, these measures will reduce soft tissue inflammation and preserve these important structures for eventual abdominal wall reconstruction. Appropriate treatment of any skin breakdown is also important. Optimization of nutrition prior to formal abdominal wall reconstruction is paramount. In patients with a chronic nidus of infection, it is often impossible to normalize their metabolic profile, but maximizing nutrition is important for a successful result. If a fistula is present, I rarely keep patients NPO unless they are high output and cannot control the effluent with an ostomy appliance.

● DIAGNOSIS AND TREATMENT

In this patient, the timing of the early wound infection followed by a chronic draining sinus and the presence of MRSA suggests a deep surgical site infection involving the prosthetic. Given the fact that it is a PTFE-based mesh,

complete surgical excision of the graft is warranted. In these situations, it is important to have clear goals between the surgeon and the patient as to what must be accomplished and what would be the ideal situation if possible. After 6 months of conservative therapy, it is not necessary to continue with any other nonoperative measures, and the patient should be optimized for resection of the mesh as previously mentioned. The most important principle in managing infection of a prosthetic device regardless of its location is complete resection of all foreign material whenever possible. Fortunately, in cases of infected microporous mesh, the graft is often not well incorporated and can be easily removed.

When planning the operation, the surgeon will be faced with several potential scenarios. Occasionally, the peritoneal cavity is not violated during resection of the mesh. In this case, I often will leave the wound open, allow it to heal by secondary intention, and perform my formal reconstruction 6 months to 1 year later in a clean field. Alternatively, if the peritoneal cavity is violated, the surgeon must stabilize the abdominal wall. Rapidly absorbable synthetic mesh (Vicryl or Dexon) are reasonable alternatives; however, they often result in very large defects to repair in the future. Single-staged reconstruction with biologic mesh is another alternative. There are multiple products available, and it is beyond the scope of this chapter to evaluate these differences, but certain reconstructive principles remain constant. These materials do not function as an interposition graft to prevent hernias. They should be used with advanced reconstructive techniques such as a Rives-Stoppa or component separation to function as a reinforcement of a primary facial repair. When used accordingly, they have reported successful reconstructions in up to 80% of contaminated single-staged repairs.

● VENTRAL HERNIA STAGING

Recent developments in classification and staging of ventral hernias have played a key role in allowing for an informed discussion with patients about expectations regarding wound morbidity and hernia recurrence. Ventral hernia staging is based on surgical wound contamination (clean vs. contaminated) and hernia width. A stage I ventral hernia is defined as a hernia that is <10 cm and clean. Stage I hernias are at low risk of wound morbidity and hernia recurrence with quoted rates of 10% for both surgical site occurrence and hernia recurrence. Stage II ventral hernias are contaminated cases that are <10 cm in hernia width or clean cases that have a hernia width of 10 to 20 cm. Surgical site occurrence and hernia recurrence rates are 20% and 15%, respectively. Stage III ventral hernias are high risk and include hernias that are >10 cm in width and contaminated or any hernia with a width >20 cm. Wound morbidity significantly increases in these high-risk patients with a surgical site occurrence rate of 42% and hernia recurrence rate of 26%.

With this staging system, surgeons can define expectations better for patients undergoing complex abdominal wall reconstruction.

● SURGICAL APPROACH

As described above, the principles of the operation are to perform complete excision of all prosthetic material. This often requires a full midline laparotomy to expose the entire abdominal wall to ensure complete mesh removal and definitive abdominal wall reconstruction if necessary. Key technical points of the reconstruction are described in Table 5-1.

Table 5-1	Component Separation

Key Technical Steps

1. Remove all prosthetic material, and address any bowel issues as necessary.
2. Perform complete adhesiolysis of the entire anterior abdominal wall to the paracolic gutters to allow muscular components to slide to the midline during reconstruction.
3. Elevate lipocutaneous flaps 2 cm lateral to the linea semilunaris, edge of the rectus muscle.
4. Incise the external oblique fascia and separate the external and internal oblique muscles in their avascular plane.
5. Continue the dissection 3–4 cm above the costal margin and inferiorly to the inguinal ligament.
6. Release the posterior rectus sheath by making an incision 1 cm lateral to the linea alba.
7. Develop the retromuscular plane out to the linea semilunaris while preserving the neurovascular bundles to the rectus muscle.
8. Place an appropriately sized biologic graft as an underlay, redistributing tension across the graft to help medialize the rectus complex.
9. Drains placed over the mesh.
10. Midline fascia reapproximated with interrupted figure-of-8 sutures.
11. Remove excess devascularized skin, and close over multiple drains.

Potential Pitfalls

- Not dissecting the adhesions free from the undersurface of the abdominal wall, which prevents the muscular blocks from medializing after release.
- Inadvertent injury to the linea semilunaris, which results in full-thickness defect in the lateral abdominal wall and a troublesome hernia to repair.
- Skin flap necrosis from excessive undermining and division of the medial row (periumbilical) perforators.

● COMPONENT SEPARATION

Begin by performing a complete laparotomy and removing all prosthetic material, and address any bowel issues as necessary. Perform a complete adhesiolysis of the entire anterior abdominal wall to the paracolic gutters. This will allow muscular components to mobilize toward the midline during reconstruction. Elevate lipocutaneous flaps 2 cm lateral to the linea semilunaris to the lateral edge of the rectus muscle. Take care to avoid the periumbilical perforators during this mobilization by leaving an "island" of subcutaneous tissue in the middle of the flap. This maneuver will prevent problems with abdominal wall ischemia (Table 5-1).

Incise the external oblique fascia just lateral to the rectus sheath and separate the external and internal oblique muscles in their avascular plane (Figure 5-1A). Continue the dissection 3 to 4 cm above the costal margin and inferiorly to the inguinal ligament. Release the posterior rectus sheath by making an incision 1 cm lateral to the linea alba along the posterior abdominal wall. Develop the retromuscular plane out to the linea semilunaris while preserving the neurovascular bundles to the rectus muscle. Releasing the external oblique and posterior rectus sheath can add up 10 cm of myofascial advancement in the midabdomen (Figure 5-1B). Place an appropriately sized biologic graft as an underlay, redistributing tension across the graft to help medialize the rectus complex. Place closed suction drains over the mesh. Reapproximate the midline fascia with interrupted figure-of-8 sutures. Remove excess devascularized skin, and close in several layers.

● SPECIAL INTRAOPERATIVE CONSIDERATIONS

In certain cases of infected and contaminated abdominal wall reconstruction, the field will be grossly contaminated. It is imperative that appropriate bioburden reduction techniques are employed, including debridement of all devitalized tissue and copious pulse lavage irrigation of the wound. If the wound cannot be grossly decontaminated, then reconstructive efforts should be postponed. The patients can be placed on dressings for several days and formal reconstruction performed after the wound has been decontaminated.

● POSTOPERATIVE MANAGEMENT

These reconstructive procedures performed in the setting of infection and contaminations are fraught with postoperative wound complications. Recognizing and managing these appropriately is important to eventual success of the operation. In cases of MRSA prosthetic infections, I feel there is often a biofilm present in the wound that cannot be eradicated. Therefore, I place these patients on suppressive

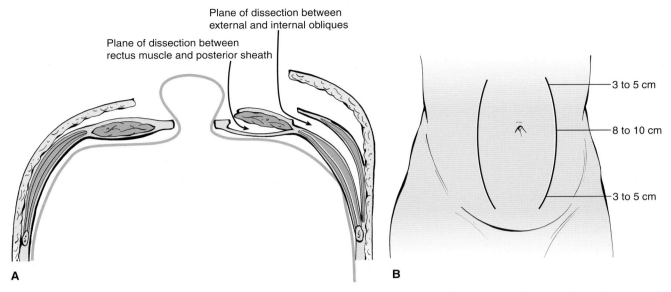

Plane of dissection between external and internal obliques

Plane of dissection between rectus muscle and posterior sheath

3 to 5 cm

8 to 10 cm

3 to 5 cm

A   B

FIGURE 5-1. **A:** For maximal advancement during an anterior component separation, the external oblique and posterior rectus sheath should be released and separated from adjacent tissue. **B:** A myofascial advancement of up to 10 cm can obtained on each side of the abdominal wall after complete release of the external oblique and posterior rectus sheath. The upper and lower thirds of the abdomen have less advancement than the middle abdominal wall. (Adapted from Nguyen VT, Shestak KC. "Separation of anatomic components" method of abdominal wall reconstruction. *Oper Tech Gen Surg.* 2006;8(4):183-191. Copyright © 2006 Elsevier, with permission.)

antibiotic therapy for at least 6 months after removal of the graft (Bactrim SS QD). I also feel it is important to keep the drains in place in cases of biologic mesh utilization. Despite the term "mesh," these are actually grafts that are often not perforated and therefore are prone to fluid buildup around the graft. This fluid will prevent incorporation and often contains collagenases that will degrade the graft. Therefore, I leave the drains in place for at least 2 weeks in most cases. These reconstructive procedures are also major surgical endeavors, and epidurals can help pain management, and most patients should be observed in an intensive care unit setting for the immediate postoperative period.

TAKE HOME POINTS

- Set realistic expectations for the patients and the surgeons about what can actually be accomplished in one setting in these difficult problems.
- Remove all infected prosthetic material whenever possible.
- Single-staged reconstruction of infected and contaminated fields is reasonable in most patients, although it

does not always have to be performed. Know when you are in a difficult situation and know when to bail out.
- Optimize patients preoperatively with adequate nutrition, infection control, and preservation of soft tissues.
- Do not wait forever to remove infected synthetic mesh. If the wound is not healed by 3 to 6 months, the prosthetic is almost always infected.

SUGGESTED READINGS

Kanters AE, et al. Modified hernia grading scale to stratify surgical site occurrence after open ventral hernia repairs. *J Am Coll Surg.* 2012;215(6):787-793.

Krpata DM, et al. Posterior and open anterior components separations: a comparative analysis. *Am J Surg.* 2012;203(3):318-322.

Petro CC, et al. Designing a ventral hernia staging system. *Hernia.* 2016;20(1):111-117.

Ramirez OM, Ruas E, Dellon AL. Components separation method for closure of abdominal wall defects: an anatomical and clinical study. *Plast Reconstr Surg.* 1990;86(3):519-526.

Rosen M, et al. A 5-year clinical experience with single-staged repairs of infected and contaminated abdominal wall defects utilizing biologic mesh. *Ann Surg.* 2013;257(6):991-996.

Enterocutaneous Fistula

LUCIAN PANAIT AND YURI W. NOVITSKY

6

Based on the previous edition chapter "Enterocutaneous Fistula" by Eric J. Culbertson and Michael G. Franz

Presentation

65-year-old female with history of morbid obesity and Hartmann's procedure for diverticulitis was admitted to the surgical service for small bowel obstruction. She failed conservative management and underwent laparoscopy converted to open lysis of adhesions and small bowel resection with primary anastomosis. Several inadvertent serosal injuries were repaired with Lembert sutures. She developed a postoperative wound infection, and a few staples were removed at the inferior pole of the wound for wet-to-dry packing. Due to persistent foul-smelling wound drainage, the wound was completely opened on postoperative day 7. A loop of small intestine with two openings was noticed in the middle aspect of the wound.

● DIFFERENTIAL DIAGNOSIS

Differential diagnosis of copious fluid drainage through an abdominal wound includes superficial or deep surgical site infection, fascial dehiscence, and enterocutaneous fistulas. The later diagnosis is confirmed by visualization of succus entericus and/or intestinal mucosa through the wound. Even if no bowel mucosa is visualized, but drainage of intestinal succus is suspected, the presence of a fistula can be confirmed with measurement of amylase level from the fluid and additional imaging studies.

Most enterocutaneous fistulas are devastating complications of abdominal surgery. They generally happen through three main mechanisms: missed enterotomy or partial-thickness small bowel injury progressing to full thickness often as a result of enterolysis; leak from a gastrointestinal anastomosis; and bowel injury during prolonged open abdomen. The latter leads to development of enteroatmospheric fistulas, a subset that represents fistulization of a segment of the intestine through a fascial dehiscence, without soft tissue coverage. Less often, enterocutaneous fistulas may appear spontaneously, as a consequence of intrinsic bowel disease (foreign body, radiation, local infection, neoplasm, distal obstruction, appendicitis, diverticulitis, etc.).

● WORKUP

A thorough history and review of prior operative reports are necessary when evaluating a patient with enterocutaneous fistula. On physical examination, one can assess the degree of fistula maturation by the resolution of the redness of the skin surrounding the fistula or the ability to pinch the migrated epithelial tissue or a skin graft, if present, off the underlying intestines. Measurement of markers of inflammation and assessment of nutrition status are essential in assessing the patient's general condition.

The workup generally continues with a CT scan of the abdomen and pelvis. This will give information regarding location of the fistula in the GI tract, the presence of foreign bodies (i.e., mesh), distal obstruction, other intrinsic bowel disease, presence of intra-abdominal collection, and extent of associated fascial defect (Figure 6-1). Adjunct imaging studies are represented by fistulogram with or without small bowel follow-through, which can give more precise information regarding location of the fistula and length of distal small bowel.

● DIAGNOSIS AND TREATMENT

Treatment priorities in management of enterocutaneous fistulas include wound care with preservation of the skin, nutritional support, and delayed surgical intervention.

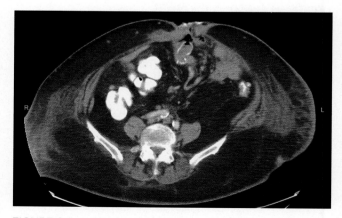

FIGURE 6-1. A CT scan reveals separation of the midline fascia and loops of small bowel underlying the disrupted wound, suggesting an enterocutaneous fistula.

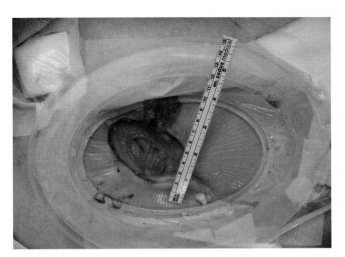

FIGURE 6-2. Wound manager used to collect fistula effluent and protect the skin around the wound.

Wound care and skin protection: Wound managers are useful in collecting the fistula effluent and protecting surrounding skin. These devices can be custom fit to accommodate the edges of normal skin and allow contact between the fistula effluent and the granulation tissue in the bed of the wound, thus stimulating wound contraction (Figure 6-2). Negative-pressure wound therapy is also beneficial in achieving wound contraction and reepithelialization around the fistula, if an interface can be achieved between the sponge and tissues surrounding the fistulized end of the bowel. Although skin grafts may also be used to decrease the wound surface around the fistula, wound contraction is less pronounced than in the other strategies mentioned above. The role of intraluminal stents to bridge the fistula opening is still evolving, but in selected cases, they may allow healing of the surrounding wound and independence from TPN. Other reported technologies used to decrease the burden of enterocutaneous fistulas include biologic fistula plugs, endoscopic suturing or clipping devices, and endoscopic vacuum-assisted therapy.

Nutrition: Almost all high-output fistulas (>500 mL per day) will require TPN for maintenance of a positive nitrogen balance and correction of fluid and electrolyte losses. Patients with low-output fistulas (<500 mL per day) may receive oral diet and supplements either alone or in combination with parenteral nutrition, if the fistula output does not increase once oral diet is initiated. When feasible, tube feedings into the distal end of the fistula (fistuloclysis) with or without reinfusion of the chyme from the afferent end are beneficial in maintaining the villous integrity of the distal small bowel, preventing intestinal atrophy and preserving immune function (Figure 6-3). Lastly, proton-pump inhibitors and somatostatin analogues may help decrease the output of fistulas, although their use has not been shown to expedite spontaneous closure of fistulas.

Surgical treatment: There are three phases in the evolution of an enterocutaneous fistula, and operative principles differ with each of them:

1. Development phase (the first 7 to 10 days after the index operation): In the rare event a fistula becomes apparent

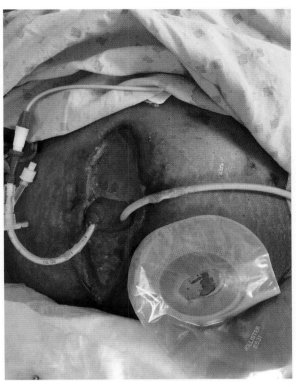

FIGURE 6-3. Attempt at controlling the fistula output (left catheter in afferent limb) and nutrition by fistuloclysis (right catheter in efferent limb).

during this phase, an early reintervention may be possible if the original operation did not involve significant enterolysis. However, if extensive enterolysis has been performed, then it is likely that the small intestine loops will be significantly adhered again, which may increase the risk for inadvertent enterotomy and development of new fistulas; therefore, a more cautious, conservative approach is recommended.

2. Early phase: An operation is contraindicated. The focus of this period is to achieve patient optimization in preparation for the definitive therapy, which will happen months down the road, after the fistula maturation. A multidisciplinary approach is necessary for achieving best results. Under surgeon's leadership, other health care providers should play important roles, including an experienced dietician, wound care nurse/stoma therapist, physical therapist, and sometimes a psychologist to assist with depression related to the presence of the fistula or prolonged hospitalization. Efforts in this phase should focus on correction of intravascular volume deficits, aggressive nutrition intervention, drainage of abscesses and control of sepsis, control of fistula effluent, and protection of the skin. With adequate support, some fistulas may spontaneously close.

3. Late phase (3 to 12 months): Fistula maturation. Once the acute and subacute inflammation has resolved, the surgeon can focus on planning the definitive operation. Nutrition efforts should be maximized in order to achieve an albumin level of at least 3 g/dL and a prealbumin level of

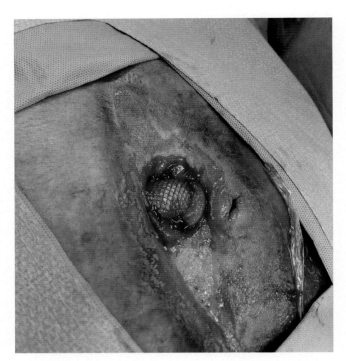

FIGURE 6-4. Endoscopic stent placed percutaneously to bridge the two openings of the fistula.

20 mg/dL. CRP/prealbumin ratio is another useful marker of nutrition assessment, especially in patients with ongoing inflammation. Delineation of the anatomy is mandatory in order to assist in preoperative planning. This involves review of all prior operative records, imaging of the GI tract (if not already done) with CT scan and sometimes fistulogram with small bowel follow-through, and assessment of the abdominal wall and any associated fascial defects.

In the case scenario presented, once the diagnosis of enterocutaneous fistula was made, we initiated TPN and attempted tube feeding through the distal end of the fistula (fistuloclysis)—as shown in Figure 6-3. Negative-pressure therapy was used around the two fistulous orifices. However, the abdominal wound was difficult to manage, due to the high fistula output and constant wound soiling. An endoscopic stent was subsequently placed percutaneously in order to bridge the two opening of the fistulas; this proved successful in decreasing the fistula output, allowing wound contraction and resolution of skin infection, and weaning the patient off TPN to a regular diet (Figure 6-4).

● SURGICAL APPROACH

Certain fistulas will require definitive operative intervention. These include (1) fistulas that *have not* closed in 30 to 45 days in spite of maximal supportive measures, (2) fistulas that *are not likely* to close due to eversion of the mucosa or their large size (greater than one-third of the bowel circumference), and (3) fistulas that *cannot* close because of associated conditions precluding closure, such as distal obstruction, presence of

foreign body, neoplasm, inflammatory bowel disease, radiation enteritis, or local infection.

The surgeon needs to make two important decisions regarding the definitive treatment: when to operate and if a reconstructive (single-stage) hernia operation should be undertaken at the time of fistula takedown. In spite of pressure from the patient or other health care providers, it is very important to wait until the patient is optimized for surgery and fistula is mature, which sometimes may take up to 1 year. The main goal of the surgical intervention is fistula closure with re-establishment of gastrointestinal continuity. Creation of a stable abdominal wall closure is only a secondary goal. Therefore, a staged repair is a completely acceptable outcome. This involves bridging the fascial defect with a biologic or bioabsorbable mesh, or closing the defect primarily at the initial operation, thus accepting a potential subsequent recurrence of the hernia, which can be addressed at a later time.

The operation starts with entry into the abdomen at a midline location remote from the fistula, ideally in an area where the fascia is intact. A thorough abdominal exploration is necessary to assess the state of the intestines and decide the operative strategy. Complete adhesiolysis is recommended in order to isolate the fistulous segment of the intestine and relieve any potential distal obstruction. The dissection should be very meticulous in order to avoid accidental bowel injury, which could compromise the success of the operation. Any undrained abscesses should be addressed at this time. The affected segment of bowel is dissected off the healthy organs and viscera with the goal to preserve as much normal intestine as possible. En bloc resection of the fistula and any involved abdominal wall is subsequently performed. This should also include any foreign material present (i.e., old mesh, permanent sutures, etc.), which otherwise could serve as nidus for chronic infection, bowel adherence, and potential refistulization. Intestinal continuity is restored with a side-to-side anastomosis if enough normal intestine is present. In cases involving resection of a large segment of small bowel, an end-to-end anastomosis may be beneficial in order to maximize the absorptive capacity of the remaining GI tract. Proximal protective jejunostomy/ileostomy may be necessary when there are concerns with the integrity of the anastomosis, particularly when the distal segment of intestine has not been used for feeding and is atrophic. If the fascial defect is small, primary closure should be attempted without use of mesh (Table 6-1).

In patients with associated large fascial defects, a reconstructive operation at the time of fistula takedown may be undertaken only if the surgeon is an expert in advanced hernia repair. This may involve separation of abdominal components with use of sublay mesh in a potentially contaminated field (ideally, mesh should not be placed intraperitoneally). If significant soft tissue deficit is present in addition to the fascial defect, an advanced plastic surgical flap (i.e., thigh flaps) may need to be utilized. Preoperative consultation with a plastic surgeon is highly recommended in order to assist with difficult abdominal wall closure in the presence of soft tissue deficits. However, for most patients, we advocate a staged approach with resection of the fistula initially with

Table 6-1	Enterocutaneous Fistula

Key Technical Steps

1. Elliptical incision to encompass the enterocutaneous fistula and any inflamed tissue
2. Careful entry into the abdomen in an area with intact fascia, either superior or inferior to the fistula
3. Thorough abdominal exploration with complete lysis of adhesions and circumferential dissection of the fistulized segment of the intestine
4. Resection of the enterocutaneous fistula and any involved abdominal wall, including all foreign body material while preserving as much normal intestine as possible
5. Drainage of any intra-abdominal abscess
6. Restoration of GI continuity by side-to-side or end-to-end anastomosis
7. Abdominal wall closure

Potential Pitfalls

- Inadvertent enterotomies or serosal tears during enterolysis
- Uncertainty about the integrity of the small bowel anastomosis due to significant peritoneal contamination either secondary to unaddressed abscesses or spillage at the time of fistula takedown, necessitating protective loop enterostomy
- Inability to primarily close the fascia at the end of the operation

primary or bridged fascial closure, followed by abdominal wall reconstruction at a subsequent operation. In this staged approach, strategies for managing a large abdominal wall defect at the time of fistula takedown should be individualized to patient's anatomy and include use of retention sutures or dynamic fascial closure devices, partial fascial bridging with nonpermanent mesh, local cutaneous flaps, etc.

● SPECIAL INTRAOPERATIVE CONSIDERATIONS

In the presence of significant inflammatory bowel disease, neoplastic process involving multiple bowel loops, or intraperitoneal infection is present, the surgeon may be faced with the need to resect a significant portion of the intestine, which would put the patient at risk for short-gut syndrome. Therefore, meticulous enterolysis is necessary in order to preserve at least 100 cm of the small bowel in a patient with competent ileocecal valve and functional colon, or 180 cm otherwise.

● POSTOPERATIVE MANAGEMENT

Nutrition support efforts should continue in the postoperative period. If TPN was used preoperatively, it should continue

after the operation until the patient tolerates a regular diet. Sometimes, a prolonged postoperative ileus is present; therefore, diet should be advanced slowly, particularly in patients who have not received enteral nutrition for a long period of time.

Postoperative wound infection should be addressed promptly with local wound care. Negative-pressure therapy should be used judiciously, especially in cases in which complete fascial closure has not been achieved. Refistulization may occur, therefore a high index of suspicion should be present. If faced with this postoperative complication, the surgeon should maximize supportive efforts and not attempt immediate reoperation.

Upon discharge from the hospital, the patient should be followed in the office until the wounds are completely healed. If a protective loop enterostomy was created, this could be reversed in 3 to 6 months from the operation for fistula resection.

Case Conclusion

After 6 months of supportive treatment with negative-pressure therapy around the fistula site, and regular diet with occasional TPN supplementation, the fistula matured (Figure 6-5). The patient underwent resection of the enterocutaneous fistula, including the endoscopic stent, with side-to-side anastomosis, and primary repair of the fascial defect (Figure 6-6). Her postoperative course was uneventful and was discharged from the hospital on postoperative day 7, tolerating regular diet. Her staples were removed in the office 2 weeks after the operation, and the wound was adequately healed.

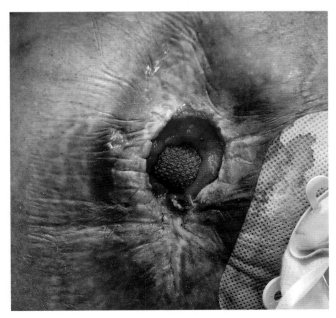

FIGURE 6-5. Appearance of the wound after 6 months of endoscopic stent bridging and negative-pressure therapy.

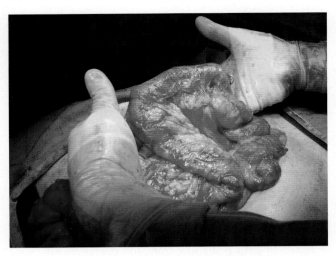

FIGURE 6-6. Laparotomy with en bloc excision of the entero-cutaneous fistula and endoscopic stent. (Photograph courtesy of Eric Pauli, MD.)

TAKE HOME POINTS

- A multidisciplinary approach should be used in treating patients with enterocutaneous fistulas.
- Correction of nutritional deficits and fluid and electrolyte losses, control of sepsis, protection of the skin, wound management, and psychological support are paramount in achieving optimal outcomes.
- One-third of the fistulas will close with adequate supportive measures. For the ones that do not close, a careful surgical strategy should be employed. Understanding fistula anatomy plays a very important role in the preoperative planning.

- Fistula maturation may take up to 6 to 12 months. It is imperative not to rush to operate.
- New technologies like intraluminal stents, biologic plugs, endoscopic suturing, or clipping devices show promise in decreasing the burden of enterocutaneous fistulas. Their role is still not fully established.
- The main goal of the operation is resection of the fistula with restoration of the intestinal continuity. Definitive repair of the associated fascial defect is a secondary goal. A planned hernia or recurrence of a hernia is not a failure of the operation. If mesh is used for fascial reinforcement, intraperitoneal mesh placement should be avoided.
- Postoperative supportive efforts should continue until the wounds are completely healed.

SUGGESTED READINGS

Chapman R, Foran R, Dunphy JE. Management of intestinal fistulas. *Am J Surg.* 1964;108:157-164.

Cheesborough JE, Park E, Souza JM, Dumanian GA. Staged management of the open abdomen and enteroatmospheric fistulae using split-thickness skin grafts. *Am J Surg.* 2014;207(4):504-511.

Dudrick SJ, Panait L. Metabolic consequences of patients with gastrointestinal fistulas. *Eur J Trauma Emerg Surg.* 2011;37(3):215-125.

Krpata DM, Stein SL, Eston M, Ermlich B, Blatnik JA, Novitsky YW, et al. Outcomes of simultaneous large complex abdominal wall reconstruction and enterocutaneous fistula takedown. *Am J Surg.* 2013;205(3):354-358.

Saar MG. Abdominal wall surgery in the setting of an enterocutaneous fistula: combined versus staged definitive repair. In: Novitsky YV, ed. *Hernia Surgery: Current Principles.* Springer International Publishing, Switzerland 2016:379-385.

Slade DA, Carlson GL. Takedown of enterocutaneous fistula and complex abdominal wall reconstruction. *Surg Clin North Am.* 2013;93(5):1163-1183.

Infected Ventral Hernia Mesh

7

JEFFREY A. BLATNIK

Based on the previous edition chapter "Infected Ventral Hernia Mesh" by Gregory Ara Dumanian

Presentation

A 58-year-old female with a BMI of 27 kg/m² and past history of hypertension, Roux-en-Y gastric bypass, laparoscopic cholecystectomy, and open appendectomy is referred for a multiply recurrent hernia. Her hernia repair history includes four previous open repairs; the first three were repaired using a hybrid PTFE/polypropylene permanent synthetic mesh. Her most recent repair 1 year prior to presentation involved open component separation with biologic mesh reinforcement. She initially developed some purulent drainage from the wound requiring local exploration and removal of a suture sinus. However, since that time, she has had ongoing drainage from her wound despite attempts at local wound care and antibiotic therapy. At the time of evaluation, she had a 2 × 1-cm opening in the midportion of her abdomen with chronic granulation tissue and mild drainage (Figure 7-1).

● DIFFERENTIAL DIAGNOSIS

The differential diagnosis for this patient includes a prosthetic mesh infection, a persistent seroma or an enterocutaneous fistula (ECF) to the mesh. The most likely of those diagnosis is a prosthetic mesh infection given her multiple previous operations, the chronicity of the drainage, and

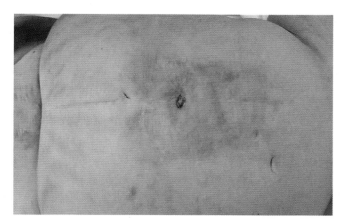

FIGURE 7-1. Shows area of chronic wound and drainage following previous hernia repair. This area had never healed following her last operation and was plagued by continuous drainage.

the low volume of drainage. Prosthetic mesh infection can be further differentiated into acute and chronic. Acute mesh infections are defined as occurring immediately after the procedure and have a potential for mesh salvage. Chronic infections can occur at any time after surgery but typically develop in the first few weeks after surgery and fail to resolve. In this scenario, it is a chronic problem as it has been going on for nearly 1 year. Mesh infections are frequently seen in patients who had an initial postoperative course that was complicated by a surgical site infection. They often give a history of the wound intermittently draining then stopping for several weeks only to start draining again. In this scenario, the patient did have a postoperative surgical site infection that required a surgical wound debridement. If this was an ECF, you would expect to see a higher volume of output with potentially a more feculent characteristic. A persistent seroma in this scenario would be more of a diagnosis of exclusion as a mesh infection or ECF is much more likely to be the problem.

● WORKUP

Workup for a patient like this should include a CT scan to help further delineate the underlying anatomy. Often times, you may see a tract of inflammation from the skin opening leading back to the underlying mesh. In addition, you want to look for any evidence of undrained fluid collection that may require interval drainage or evidence of an ECF. If your concern for ECF is high, you can consider obtaining a CT scan with oral contrast to look for any extravasation from the bowel. A culture of the wound can also be of some assistance as the presence of enteric bacteria may point more toward an ECF. However, a negative culture does not rule out an underlying infectious problem as often time a chronic mesh infection may be related to low-grade colonization and biofilm of the mesh. Finally, if a patient has been on chronic suppressive antibiotics, this may also limit the value of a fluid culture.

In this scenario, the patient had undergone multiple previous hernia repairs with at least three pieces of synthetic mesh and one piece of biologic mesh. The amount of fluid draining from her wound was low (~10 to 15 mL per day). Her CT scan (Figure 7-2) demonstrated the known prosthetic mesh as well significant inflammation and a small fluid collection consistent with her suspected mesh infection.

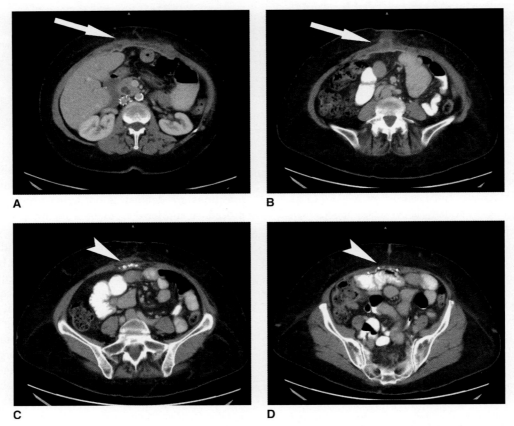

FIGURE 7-2. Demonstrates the patient's CT scan. **A:** Inflammation and fluid (*arrow*) surrounding her previous biologic mesh. **B:** Fluid collection (*arrow*) and location of chronic drainage sinus. **C:** Metallic tacks (*arrow head*) from previous laparoscopic repair. **D:** Additional tacks (*arrow head*) showing the extent of previous mesh within this patient.

There was no clear evidence of intraperitoneal involvement decreasing the likelihood of this being related to an ECF. Her laboratory evaluation was negative for any significant abnormality (i.e., normal white blood cell count), which is usually the case in low-grade chronic infections. Culture from her wound was positive for methicillin-sensitive *Staphylococcus aureus*.

● DIAGNOSIS AND TREATMENT

The most likely diagnosis for the patient in the scenario is a chronic mesh infection given her history and the findings on her CT scan. This patient had undergone initial attempts at conservative treatment including antibiotics; however, her symptoms have persisted. In addition, although an ECF is felt to be less likely, this should still be discussed with the patient as a possible intraoperative finding, which may require bowel resection.

Depending on the location of the previous mesh, the chronicity of the infection and potentially the type of mesh, initial attempts at conservative management are appropriate. This may include antibiotic therapy, minimal local debridement, or negative pressure wound therapy. If this is an early mesh infection and the mesh has physical properties such as monofilament material and a microporous design, this can occasionally be managed without need for surgical mesh excision. However, if the infection has been present for a prolonged period of time and has failed previous attempts at conservative management, surgical removal is necessary.

Once it is decided that surgical intervention is necessary, the surgeon should approach the operation with an appropriate plan in place. The ultimate goal is for removal of the infected mesh and if necessary treatment of any possible gastrointestinal issue. The surgeon should also keep in mind the long-term goals for the patient and the status of the abdominal wall musculature. After mesh removal, the patient is at high risk for recurrent hernia, and one should try to preserve as much of the muscle as possible, while ensuring you remove all of the previous mesh. Finally, it is important to minimize the risk for significant abdominal wall issues during the period between mesh resection and definitive hernia repair. This may require temporary reinforcement of the abdominal wall with a biologically derived or biosynthetic mesh. Single-staged removal of infected mesh and definitive abdominal wall hernia repair have been described, although great care should be taken when implanting a new permanent synthetic mesh at the same time of removal of infected mesh.

● SURGICAL APPROACH

The goal at the time of operation is for removal of all mesh if possible. If that is not feasible, the removal of all grossly infected mesh is a minimum. I also discuss with the patient the potential for gastrointestinal tract issues (bowel resection and possible ostomy) if the concern for an ECF is high. Broad-spectrum antibiotic prophylaxis is appropriate as is routine deep vein thrombosis prophylaxis. In general, I utilize an open surgical exploration, although minimally invasive approaches have been performed successfully. I plan my incision around the location of the mesh to be removed. For example, if the infected mesh was from a midline hernia repair, I will approach through a midline incision. If the mesh of concern was initially implanted through a flank incision, I will approach it through the flank. I feel this is important to provide the greatest access to the mesh and the best chance for complete removal.

In the operating room, after opening the incision down to and exposing the affected mesh, I extend the incision above and below out to noninvolved tissue if possible (Figure 7-3). A bacterial culture of the mesh is obtained at this point if not available preoperatively. I will divide the mesh in the midportion to facilitate adhesiolysis of any underlying abdominal contents if necessary (Figure 7-4). After freeing up all the adhesions to the bowel, I will place a towel in the abdomen to protect the viscera during mesh excision. Clamps are placed on the mesh and surrounding native tissue to provide generous tension and counter tension, which facilitates mesh removal. Using electrocautery, great care is taken to remove all the mesh while preserving as much of the native abdominal wall as possible. Landmarks, including transfascial sutures and surgical tacks, are used to help identify the borders of the mesh and ensure complete excision. Depending on the location of the mesh, extreme caution must be taken around critical structures (i.e., iliac vessels in the groin and the ureter if removing mesh from the flank). It can be difficult depending on the mesh type and severity of inflammation to differentiate scar from prosthetic mesh. Following complete removal of all mesh

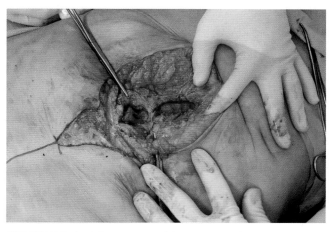

FIGURE 7-3. Initial exposure of the grossly infected mesh.

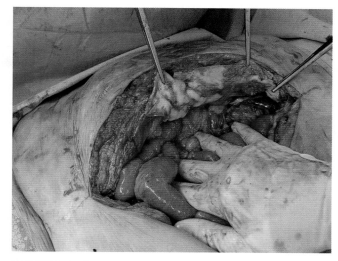

FIGURE 7-4. Completion of adhesiolysis demonstrating no evidence of underlying fistulous connection to the bowel. This figure also demonstrates clamps placed on the mesh to facilitate adequate traction necessary for mesh removal.

(Figure 7-5), subsequent repair of the abdominal wall must be considered. It is my practice in general to delay definitive repair of the abdominal wall. For this reason, if possible, I will close the fascia at this operation with figure-of-8 slowly absorbable sutures. If too much tension is present, then I

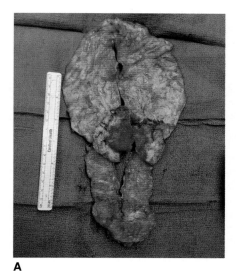

A

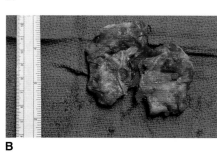

B

FIGURE 7-5. Completely removed surgical mesh. **A:** All meshes placed in original anatomic orientation. **B:** Close-up of grossly infected mesh after removal.

will bridge the abdominal wall with a resorbable mesh. Any affected subcutaneous tissue and skin are excised and then closed loosely.

Potential pitfalls include the discovery of a fistula to the underlying bowel, which should be addressed in the standard manner of small bowel resection and anastomosis. If the entire mesh cannot be excised due to concern for significant damage to the surrounding muscle, then at minimum removal of all grossly infected mesh must be performed back to well-incorporated mesh. Although the potential for recurrent infection of the remaining mesh is a possibility, preservation of the abdominal wall is critical. Finally, insufficient soft tissue and skin coverage should ideally be considered preoperatively, and the potential for soft tissue or muscle flap repair should be undertaken (Table 7-1).

In this scenario, the patient had several pieces of infected mesh as a result of her multiple previous hernia repairs. After obtaining abdominal access and complete adhesiolysis, there was no evidence of gastrointestinal involvement. All of the mesh was able to be completely removed (Figure 7-5), and the resulting hernia defect was repaired with slowly resorbable suture.

● SPECIAL INTRAOPERATIVE CONSIDERATIONS

In general, most patients have undergone extensive imaging prior to presenting to the operating room for mesh excision. The concern for an ECF should be high and considered as a potential pitfall that may be encountered. Rarely, at the time of the operation, you may find something that was not reported in prior operative report such as additional pieces of mesh or other foreign material. This should be addressed in a similar manner, and all efforts should be made to remove the mesh.

● POSTOPERATIVE MANAGEMENT

Initial postoperative management revolves around general management following a laparotomy. Care should be taken to minimize the risk for early postoperative complication, include dehiscence or evisceration. Following initial recovery from surgery, ongoing close follow-up is critical. In addition, patient education on the signs of symptoms of recurrent hernia should be given. In the event of recurrent hernia, definitive repair should be delayed for at least 6 months to minimize the risk for encountering a significantly adhesed abdomen.

Case Conclusion

This patient developed a recurrent hernia 9 months after surgery (Figure 7-6). This was ultimately repaired with an open transversus abdominis release and abdominal wall reconstruction with permanent synthetic mesh. Her postoperative course was unremarkable following the second operation, and she was discharged home on postoperative day 3.

Table 7-1	Infected Ventral Hernia Mesh

Key Technical Steps

1. Laparotomy in the area of infected mesh
2. Complete adhesiolysis and evaluation of bowel and surrounding structures
3. Repair any gastrointestinal issues as appropriate
4. Excision of all prosthetic mesh taking care to preserve abdominal wall muscles
5. Utilize landmarks such as transfascial sutures or tacks to identify periphery of the mesh
6. Repair the resulting hernia defect with primary closure versus resorbable mesh

Potential Pitfalls

- Underlying gastrointestinal fistula to the mesh
- Unable to remove all prosthetic material due to concern for significant damage to the abdominal wall
- Insufficient soft tissue or skin coverage

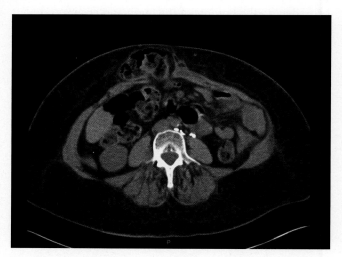

FIGURE 7-6. Follow-up CT at 9 months after complete mesh removal demonstrating a recurrent hernia. Subsequent repair in a clean setting was performed successfully.

TAKE HOME POINTS

- Persistent drainage following hernia repair with mesh in the postoperative period should raise the concern for a mesh infection.
- Initial attempts at conservative management including antibiotics are warranted.
- Keep the possibility of enterocutaneous fistula within your differential diagnosis, especially if cultures are consistent with enteric contents.
- Failure of conservative management will require excision of infected mesh.
- At the time of mesh excision, avoid excess damage to the abdominal wall muscles to facilitate incisional hernia repair at a later date.
- Ongoing follow-up is needed as there is a very high rate of recurrent hernia formation following mesh excision and primary hernia repair.

SUGGESTED READINGS

Baharestani MM, Gabriel A. Use of negative pressure wound therapy in the management of infected abdominal wounds containing mesh: an analysis of outcomes. *Int Wound J.* 2011;8(2):118-125.

Blatnik JA, Krpata DM, Jacobs MR, Gao Y, Novitsky YW, Rosen MJ. In vivo analysis of the morphologic characteristics of synthetic mesh to resist MRSA adherence. *J Gastrointest Surg.* 2012;16(11):2139-2144.

Chung L, Tse GH, O'Dwyer PJ. Outcome of patients with chronic mesh infection following abdominal wall hernia repair. *Hernia.* 2014;18(5):701-704.

Meagher H, Clarke Moloney M, Grace PA. Conservative management of mesh-site infection in hernia repair surgery: a case series. *Hernia.* 2015;19(2):231-237.

Rosen MJ, Krpata DM, Ermlich B, Blatnik JA. A 5-year clinical experience with single-staged repairs of infected and contaminated abdominal wall defects utilizing biologic mesh. *Ann Surg.* 2013;257(6):991-996.

Slater NJ, Knaapen L, Bökkerink WJ, et al. Large Contaminated Ventral Hernia Repair Using Component Separation Technique with Synthetic Mesh. *Plast Reconstr Surg.* 2015;136(6):796e-805e.

Postoperative Dehiscence

ANGELA M. INGRAHAM AND AVERY B. NATHENS

8

Based on the previous edition chapter "Postoperative Dehiscence" by Angela M. Ingraham and Avery B. Nathens

Presentation

A 59-year-old male with a history of type 2 diabetes mellitus, hypertension, and a 30-pack-year smoking history underwent a left colectomy for an obstructing colon cancer. He tolerated the procedure well except for some hypotension in the operating room due to bleeding. On postoperative day 5, he was febrile to 38.7°C, was found to have a leukocytosis of 12.3, and was noted to have some erythema of the inferior aspect of the wound for which he was started on cefazolin. On postoperative day 6, he was getting out of bed when he noticed the abrupt onset of copious serosanguineous drainage from the wound.

● DIFFERENTIAL DIAGNOSIS

Postoperative fascial dehiscence is easily diagnosed if evisceration is present. On the other end of the spectrum, when evisceration is not the presenting sign, there may be a delay in the recognition of a fascial dehiscence, as the superficial layers of the wound remain intact while there remains a defect in the abdominal wall. Other issues regarding the wound, such as seroma or infection, may make the identification of a postoperative fascial dehiscence more challenging.

Fascial dehiscence is the postoperative separation of the reapposed musculoaponeurotic layers of the abdomen. Failure of acute surgical wounds occurs when the load being placed across the wound exceeds the resistive capacity of the suture line and temporary matrix. Surgical wound strength increases rapidly from the first week until the 4th to 6th week postoperatively. At that time, the wound strength is between 50% and 80% of unwounded tissue. Wound strength following this initial postoperative period increases at a slower rate and never achieves the strength of unwounded tissue.

The incidence of postoperative fascial dehiscence varies depending on the study but has been reported to be between 1% and 5%. Despite the advances in antimicrobial prophylaxis, anesthesia, and suture materials, the incidence of this complication has not significantly decreased over time.

Fascial dehiscence is typically recognized within several days of the index procedure. Postoperative fascial dehiscence has been reported between postoperative days 1 and 21 with

the average occurrence being on postoperative day 7. Patients often report that "something has given way" or experiencing a "ripping sensation." In 23% to 84% of cases, serosanguineous fluid drains from the wound prior to a dehiscence. Rarely, and most commonly in late fascial dehiscence (>7 to 10 days), the fascia separates while the superficial wound layers remain intact.

● WORKUP

A thorough examination of the wound, including opening a draining wound, is performed. The role of advanced imaging in the diagnosis of fascial dehiscence is limited. However, a CT scan may be useful if the dehiscence is identified late in the postoperative course, a subfascial fluid collection is suspected, or operative management is not planned. In the latter scenario, it is noteworthy that the rate of intra-abdominal infection among patients with a fascial dehiscence is as high as 44% and thus might justify the use of diagnostic imaging in this context.

When evaluating a patient for postoperative fascial dehiscence, the risk factors predisposing to the complication should also be considered. Risk factors for fascial dehiscence fall into two broad categories, those related to the patient's comorbidities and those indicative of surgeon technique and decision-making. Patient characteristics identified as predictors of postoperative fascial dehiscence include age >65, wound infection, pulmonary disease, hemodynamic instability, presence of an ostomy within the incision, hypoproteinemia, sepsis, obesity, uremia, use of hyperalimentation, malignancy, ascites, steroid use, and hypertension. In a case–control study, patients with five risk factors were reported to have an incidence of 30%, while those with eight or more comorbidities all had postoperative dehiscence.

Characteristics of the incision have also been proposed as risk factors for fascial dehiscence, although this remains controversial. Retrospective data have suggested that upper abdominal incisions are at higher risk for dehiscence than those in the lower abdomen. Retrospective data have also found a higher incidence of fascial dehiscence in midline as compared to transverse incisions due to abdominal wall contractions approximating the edges of transverse incisions while separating those of midline incisions.

Although patient factors are important in dehiscence, there are important technical factors to also consider. The most common cause of postoperative fascial dehiscence is the suture tearing through fascia. "Bites" of tissue should reapproximate the fascia without impeding perfusion of the healing tissue. Excessive suture tension impedes blood flow causing muscle/fascial necrosis. Failure of the suture to hold occurs in the area just adjacent to the wound edge. In this area, the native tissue integrity is reduced due to proteases, which have been activated during the tissue repair process. Other causes of postoperative fascial dehiscence include a broken suture, a slipped knot, a loose stitch, and excessive travel between stitches. Lastly, whether continuous versus interrupted, closure techniques to decrease the risk of postoperative fascial dehiscence continue to be debated in the literature. A meta-analysis of 23 randomized, controlled studies found that interrupted closure is associated with a significantly decreased risk of dehiscence (odds ratio: 0.58, $P = 0.014$). However, a second meta-analysis of 15 randomized studies with at least 1 year of follow-up found no difference in the risk of fascial dehiscence using continuous versus interrupted suture. Furthermore, a multicenter randomized trial comparing three parallel groups (interrupted sutures with an absorbable braided material [Vicryl USP 2], continuous suture with a slowly absorbable monofilament material with longitudinal elasticity [MonoPlus USP 1], and continuous suture with a slowly absorbable monofilament material without longitudinal elasticity [PDS II USP 1]) found no significant difference in the incidence of fascial dehiscence.

In addition to the manner of closure, the utilization of external retention sutures has been debated in the literature. A randomized controlled trial of prophylactic retention sutures was undertaken in 300 high-risk patients with at least two risk factors for dehiscence who underwent midline laparotomy. Fascia was continuously repaired using a running looped no. 1 nylon suture with or without retention sutures that included the skin, subcutaneous tissue, rectus muscle, and abdominal fascia. Wound dehiscence occurred in 6 patients (4%) in the intervention group and 20 patients in the control group (13.3%) ($P = 0.007$). Retention sutures have been criticized previously due to the potential for skin and subcutaneous tissue trauma under the retention suture itself.

● DIAGNOSIS AND TREATMENT

As fascial dehiscence can be complicated to treat, attention should be directed toward preventing fascial dehiscences and making a prompt diagnosis when appropriate. Surgical techniques that can minimize the incidence of fascial dehiscence include appropriate antibiotic coverage, improved operative technique (minimizing dead space, appropriate use of electrocautery currents in making incisions), controlling intraoperative risk factors (minimizing operative time, avoiding hypothermia), and proper closure technique (appropriate choice of suture material, utilization of drains). Proper suture placement improves bursting strength of abdominal incisions.

Decreased tissue strength along the border of the acute wound has prompted investigations into the identification of an ideal suture length to wound length (SL-to-WL) ratio for primary closure of midline celiotomies. An SL-to-WL ratio of 4:1 has been reported to reduce the occurrence of fascial dehiscence and incisional hernia formation. This is the basis for the surgical dogma of 1-cm "bites" with progress between bites of 1 cm. The dogma of 1 cm back and 1 cm apart has come under investigation. Using a standardized procedure of closing emergency midline laparotomies by using a "small steps" technique of continuous suture with a slowly absorbable (polydioxanone) suture material in a wound–suture ratio of minimum 1:4, the rate of dehiscence in one study that prospectively enrolled patients and compared outcomes to a retrospective cohort was reduced from 6.6% to 3.8% ($P = 0.03$). The ideal SL-to-WL ratio allows the wound to be approximated with an appropriate amount of tension along the suture line. Increased tension causes the wound to fail at the suture–native tissue interface.

While not specifically addressing wound dehiscence, two randomized controlled trials have focused on the effect of type of fascial closure on incisional hernia formation. A prospective, multicenter, double-blind, randomized controlled trial of adult patients undergoing elective abdominal surgery at 10 hospitals in the Netherlands randomized patients to receive small tissue bites of 5 mm every 5 mm or large bites of 1 cm every 1 cm. At 1-year follow-up, 35 (13%) of 268 patients in the small bites group and 57 (21%) of 277 patients in the large bites group had incisional hernias ($P = 0.0220$). The PRImary Mesh Closure of Abdominal Midline Wound (PRIMA) trial was a double-blinded, international, multicenter, randomized controlled trial comparing running slowly absorbable suture closure with the same closure augmented with a sublay or onlay mesh in elective midline laparotomy for patients with abdominal aortic aneurysm and/or patients with a BMI of more than 27. Of the 480 patients included in the primary analysis, 92 patients were identified with an incisional hernia, 33 (30%) had been assigned to the primary suture-only group, 25 (13%) had been assigned to onlay mesh reinforcement, and 34 (18%) had been assigned to sublay mesh reinforcement (onlay mesh reinforcement vs primary suture, OR 0.37, 95% CI 0.20–0.69; $P = 0.0016$; sublay mesh reinforcement vs. primary suture, 0.55, 0.30–1.00; $P = 0.05$).

Studies have found no difference in acute fascial wound dehiscence with mass abdominal wall closures versus layered closures. Randomized trials comparing one-layer (peritoneum not reapproximated) and two-layer closures (peritoneum reapproximated) have found no difference in the rate of fascial dehiscence of paramedian and midline incisions.

● SURGICAL APPROACH

Management of dehiscence follows several surgical principles with customization of the treatment based upon the patient's condition and the available resources. The management of fascial dehiscence must take into account the most probable cause of the complication. Primary closure is acceptable if the cause of the dehiscence was technical in nature and occurred in an otherwise healthy patient. In more complicated patients where tension precludes primary closure, options include component release, temporary packing with an overlying plastic silo or packs, use of mesh or bioprosthesis, and skin closure only.

In less complicated cases of fascial dehiscence (i.e., without evisceration), the operative management of fascial dehiscence is dependent upon when the dehiscence occurs in the postoperative course. Dehiscence in the early postoperative period when adhesions are at a minimum potentially warrants immediate operative repair. However, if a dehiscence has occurred later in the postoperative course when new adhesions are more likely to be encountered, the risks of inadvertent enterotomies and fistulas may outweigh the development of a hernia that can be repaired at a later date.

When early repair of the dehiscence is pursued, intestinal decompression via a nasogastric tube is often utilized to facilitate closure. The patient is placed under general anesthesia with adequate use of muscle relaxants to minimize abdominal wall tension. The abdomen should be explored to identify any intra-abdominal infection or any injury secondary to the dehiscence. Wide debridement of compromised fascia and subcutaneous tissues is carried out. Fascial edges should be debrided back to healthy/bleeding tissue. Debridement should not be compromised due to a concern of having inadequate tissue for closure. If adequate healthy tissue is present and primary closure can be accomplished without tension, the fascia can be primarily repaired. Closure technique (use of internal and external retention sutures and running versus interrupted stitches) is primarily surgeon dependent.

When there is inadequate tissue for primary repair, the placement of an absorbable mesh (e.g., polyglycolic acid—Vicryl or Dexon) or a bioprosthesis (e.g., Surgisis or AlloDerm) can be considered. Since most wounds are contaminated, an absorbable or biologic mesh is usually used after acute wound failure. This is especially true for patients with perforation, gross spillage, or intra-abdominal abscess. Although the use of an absorbable or biologic mesh may result in hernia formation, using prosthetic mesh could result in chronic mesh infection, a dreaded complication. Similar to the use of mesh in elective general surgical cases, when using mesh to treat a fascial dehiscence, an attempt should be made to place omentum between the bowel and the mesh to minimize the development of fistula.

SPECIAL INTRAOPERATIVE CONSIDERATIONS

The intraoperative management of fascial dehiscence is heavily directed by individual patient factors. Due to excessive tension on the wound, primary closure may not be feasible in patients with significant intra-abdominal visceral edema.

Table 8-1	Postoperative Dehiscence

Key Technical Steps

1. Debride nonviable fascia.
2. Reinforce wound with an absorbable or biologic mesh if necessary to achieve tension-free closure.
3. Consider temporary abdominal closure for patients at risk for abdominal compartment syndrome.

Potential Pitfalls

- Inadequate wound debridement due to a concern of not being able to primarily close the wound.
- Excessive tension on the wound as this promotes fascial necrosis.

Closing an abdominal wall under excess tension predisposes the patient to a repeated dehiscence, respiratory compromise, and even compartment syndrome. Therefore, in patients with anasarca or visceral edema, a temporary wound closure, such as the ABThera™ Open Abdomen Negative Pressure Wound Therapy System, should be considered.

POSTOPERATIVE MANAGEMENT

Patients whose index surgery was complicated by fascial dehiscence will often require intensive care and will often have prolonged hospital stays. It is important to note that the same comorbidities that placed the patient at risk for fascial dehiscence predispose them to developing other postsurgical complications.

After closure of a fascial dehiscence, particular attention should be paid to modifying risk factors to prevent repeat dehiscence. Patients should be educated regarding their postoperative surgical and wound care. They should be instructed to avoid straining and heavy lifting for a minimum of 6 weeks. An abdominal binder is often prescribed to reduce tension of the wound. Finally, the patient's nutritional status should be optimized to promote healing (Table 8-1).

Case Conclusion

The patient's wound was opened at the bedside. Examination of the wound revealed an approximately 10-cm area where the fascia had dehisced and the suture had torn through the fascia. The patient was taken back to the operating room emergently. No visceral injuries from the fascial dehiscence were identified. After debridement of some of the fascial edges, the musculoaponeurotic layer was reapproximated without tension using interrupted, figure-of-8 stitches with 0-Prolene suture, paying special attention to suture placement. The superficial wound was packed with moist gauze.

TAKE HOME POINTS

- The incidence of postoperative fascial dehiscence has not decreased significantly despite advances in surgical care.
- Both patient- and surgeon-dependent factors contribute to postoperative fascial dehiscence.
- Emphasis on appropriate surgical technique will decrease the modifiable risk of fascial dehiscence.

SUGGESTED READINGS

Carlson MA. Acute wound failure. *Surg Clin North Am.* 1997;77(3):607-636.

Cliby WA. Abdominal incision wound breakdown. *Clin Obstet Gynecol.* 2002;45(2):507-517.

Deerenberg EB, et al. Small bites versus large bites for closure of abdominal midline incisions (STITCH): a double-blind, multicentre, randomised controlled trial. *Lancet.* 2015;386:1254-1260.

Diener MK, Voss S, Jensen K, et al. Elective midline laparotomy closure: the INLINE systematic review and meta-analysis. *Ann Surg.* 2010;251(5):843-856.

Dubay DA, Franz MG. Acute wound healing: the biology of acute wound failure. *Surg Clin North Am.* 2003;83(3):463-481.

Graham DJ, Stevenson JT, McHenry CR. The association of intra-abdominal infection and abdominal wound dehiscence. *Am Surg.* 1998;64(7):660-665.

Gupta H, Srivastava A, Menon GR, et al. Comparison of interrupted versus continuous closure in abdominal wound repair: a meta-analysis of 23 trials. *Asian J Surg.* 2008;31(3):104-114.

Jairam AP, Timmermans L, Eker HH, et al.; PRIMA Trialist Group. Prevention of incisional hernia with prophylactic onlay and sublay mesh reinforcement versus primary suture only in midline laparotomies (PRIMA): 2-year follow-up of a multicentre, double-blind, randomised controlled trial. *Lancet.* 2017;390(10094):567-576. doi: 10.1016/S0140-6736(17)31332-6. Epub 2017 Jun 20. Erratum in: Lancet. 2017 Aug 5;390(10094):554.

Khorgami Z, et al. Prophylactic retention sutures in midline laparotomy in high-risk patients for wound dehiscence: a randomized controlled trial. *J Surg Res.* 2013;180(2):238-243.

Nieuwenhuizen J, et al. A double blind randomized controlled trial comparing primary suture closure with mesh augmented closure to reduce incisional hernia incidence. *BMC Surg.* 2013;13:48.

Seiler CM, Bruckner T, Diener MK, et al. Interrupted or continuous slowly absorbable sutures for closure of primary elective midline abdominal incisions: a multicenter randomized trial. *Ann Surg.* 2009;249(4):576-582.

Timmermans L, et al. Short-term results of a randomized controlled trial comparing primary suture with primary glued mesh augmentation to prevent incisional hernia. *Ann Surg.* 2015;261(2):276-281.

Tolstrup MB, Watt SK, Gögenur I. Reduced rate of dehiscence after implementation of a standardized fascial closure technique in patients undergoing emergency laparotomy. *Ann Surg.* 2017;265:821-826.

van't Riet M, Steyerberg EW, Nellensteyn J, et al. Meta-analysis of techniques for closure of midline abdominal incisions. *Br J Surg.* 2002;89(11):1350-1356.

Webster C, Neumayer L, Smout R, et al. Prognostic models of abdominal wound dehiscence after laparotomy. *J Surg Res.* 2003;109(2):130-137.

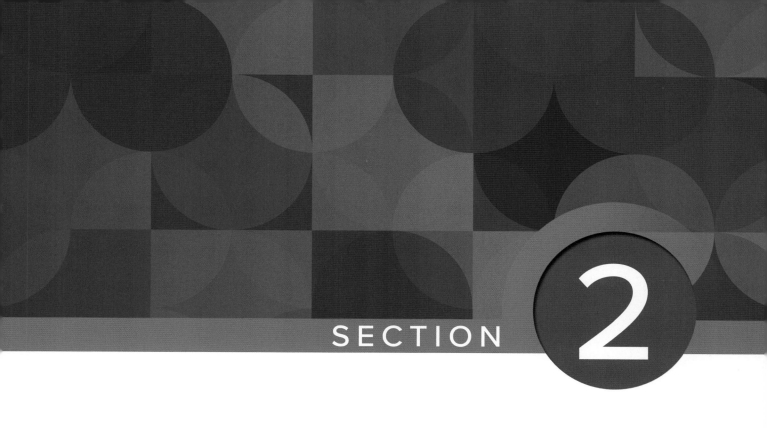

Upper Gastrointestinal

Paraesophageal Hernia

9

THADEUS TRUS AND JESSICA S. KOLLER GORHAM

Based on the previous edition chapter "Paraesophageal Hernia" by ThadeusTrus

Presentation

A 65-year-old woman presents to clinic for evaluation of a large hiatal hernia. She has a significant history of gastroesophageal reflux disease (GERD) controlled by a proton pump inhibitor, which she takes daily. She was noted on her annual lab work to be slightly anemic with a hemoglobin of 9.8. She endorses mild but progressive shortness of breath with activity. She also notes early satiety and occasional dysphagia. More recently, she has experienced mild postprandial epigastric discomfort and has lost 10 lb. On exam, she appears well and in no distress. Heart sounds are normal and lung fields are clear to auscultation. Her abdomen is soft and nontender without palpable masses or lymphadenopathy. Stool guaiac is positive. Her symptoms prompted a chest x-ray (CXR), which reveals a retrocardiac air–fluid level due to her large intrathoracic stomach. Recent colonoscopy was negative.

● DIFFERENTIAL DIAGNOSIS

The patient's nonspecific symptoms can be associated with a variety of conditions such as GERD, esophagitis, esophageal dysmotility, peptic ulcer disease, delayed gastric emptying, cardiopulmonary disease, biliary disease such as cholelithiasis or colic, and malignancy. Her heartburn may be due to her hiatal hernia. Her overall clinical picture is most consistent with a paraesophageal hernia (PEH).

● WORKUP

All patients, particularly older and comorbid patients, who present with atypical chest pain or dyspnea with exertion, should undergo evaluation for coronary artery disease as the cause of their symptoms. Further workup for GERD, dysphagia, and anemia should include upper gastrointestinal (UGI) barium swallow and upper and lower endoscopy (esophagogastroduodenoscopy [EGD] and colonoscopy). The barium swallow provides a "snap shot" of the esophagogastric anatomy and allows for evaluation of reflux, characterization of a hiatal hernia, and can identify areas of benign or malignant structuring and diverticulum. In the case of PEH, it can define the type of hernia (I to IV) and rotation (organoaxial vs. mesoaxial) if present. It is less sensitive for esophageal motility and mucosal pathology. EGD assesses for esophagitis, intestinal metaplasia (Barrett's esophagus), stricture, Cameron's ulcers, and malignancy. The PEH is visualized adjacent to the gastroesophageal junction (GEJ) on retroflexion as an additional gastric pouch above the level of the diaphragm (Figure 9-1). This can be dynamic and difficult to accurately quantify. Cameron's ulcers may also be identified; however, these are transient in nature. One-third of patients with PEH have anemia, and the absence of Cameron's ulcers on endoscopy does not rule out their presence. Peptic strictures, if found, should be biopsied and dilated as needed preoperatively. Esophageal manometry can be considered as an adjunct during workup; however, it is often difficult to pass the probe effectively, and the results may not be accurate given the distorted gastric anatomy.

The patient in this scenario undergoes further workup of her hiatal hernia. Barium swallow demonstrates a giant type III PEH with a foreshortened esophagus and the entire stomach herniating into the chest (Figure 9-2A). Compare this to the adjacent image of a type II PEH, where the GEJ is in its normal anatomic location at the level of the diaphragm, with gastric antrum herniating into the chest (Figure 9-2B). EGD confirms a large hiatal hernia with a paraesophageal component. A Cameron's ulcer is found along the level of the diaphragm (Figure 9-3). The surveyed mucosa is otherwise normal.

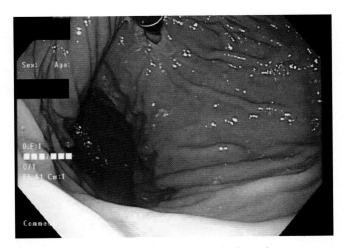

FIGURE 9-1. Upper endoscopy demonstrating a large paraesophageal hernia and otherwise normal mucosa.

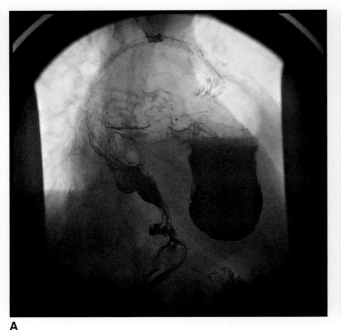
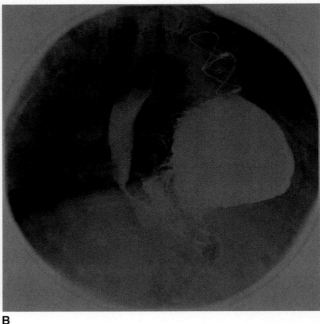

A   **B**

FIGURE 9-2. **A:** Barium contrast study showing a large type III paraesophageal hernia. **B:** Barium contrast study showing a type II paraesophageal hernia.

● DISCUSSION

The patient in this scenario has a type III hiatal hernia. There are four types of hiatal hernias. Type I or the sliding hiatal hernia is the most common, accounting for 90% to 95% of hiatal hernias. It is characterized by migration of the GEJ through the hiatus while maintaining the normal anatomic relationship of the esophagus, GEJ, and stomach. Type II hernias are true PEHs. The GEJ remains in its normal anatomic position below the diaphragm, while a portion of the stomach herniates above the GEJ through the hiatus. Type III PEHs are characterized by herniation of both the GEJ and gastric fundus above the diaphragm with a portion of the

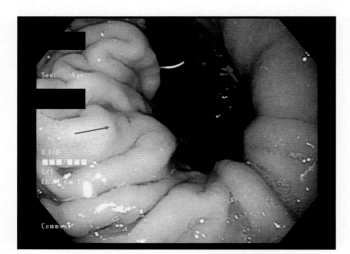

FIGURE 9-3. Upper endoscopy demonstrating a paraesophageal hernia with Cameron's ulcer (*arrow*).

stomach located cephalad to the GEJ. Type IV hernias are characterized by another intra-abdominal organ such as the colon migrating into the thorax alongside a PEH.

Paraesophageal hernias tend to occur in patients greater than 60 years old. It is unclear as to why certain individuals develop PEHs, but it is likely related to the progression of a hiatal hernia in the setting of increased intra-abdominal pressure, such as obesity.

● DIAGNOSIS AND TREATMENT

Evaluation for PEH should be considered in patients with GERD and dysphagia, atypical chest pain or shortness of breath with negative cardiac workup, and chronic anemia in patients with otherwise unknown etiology. Patients with PEH may also present with regurgitation, cough, or pneumonia. Symptomatic patients with PEHs warrant surgical repair. Rarely, patients present with acute obstruction secondary to gastric volvulus (Figure 9-4). These patients present with severe epigastric or substernal chest pain and should be decompressed with a nasogastric tube or, if necessary, endoscopy. This often provides relief of the patient's symptoms and allows for preoperative resuscitation. The patients should be definitively repaired within a few days of presentation. If an unstable patient requires emergent surgical intervention, reduction with crural closure and gastropexy is a mediating alternative until definitive repair can be safely performed.

Controversial data exists regarding the management of asymptomatic PEHs. Historically, studies suggested that up to 30% of asymptomatic patients with PEHs will develop

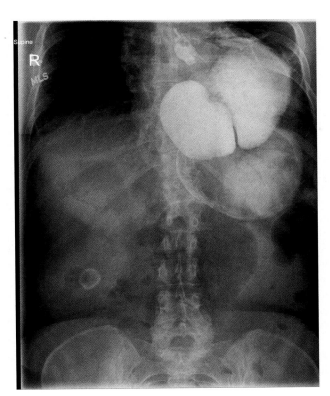

FIGURE 9-4. Barium contrast study revealing an incarcerated paraesophageal hernia due to gastric volvulus.

potentially life-threatening complications such as strangulation or perforation; however, recent data suggests this incidence is far lower. The mortality associated with emergency surgical repair remains as high as 22%. Given that most patients are found to have at least mild symptoms and the morbidity of emergent repair is so high, we advocate for early elective repair in patients who are appropriate surgical candidates.

● SURGICAL APPROACH

Various approaches to PEH repair have been described, including open transabdominal, thoracotomy, laparoscopic, video-assisted thoracoscopic surgery (VATS), and robotic. The laparoscopic transabdominal approach is currently the preferred method of repair. Over three-fourths of PEH repairs in the United States are performed minimally invasively, which carries significantly less morbidity, mortality, and length of hospital stay than the open approach. There still remain a few debates when discussing surgical PEH repair. Some advocate for an open transabdominal or transthoracic approach in the setting of foreshortened esophagus or herniation of >75% of the stomach. Some surgeons use esophageal lengthening techniques such as Collis gastroplasty. The use of expensive biologic mesh has also been shown to decrease recurrence rates in the short term; however, it is equivalent in longer-term follow-up. It is also notable that not all recurrences have clinical significance, as many are asymptomatic, significantly

smaller than at the time of original presentation, and do not require reoperative intervention. Because of the less invasive approach, we advocate laparoscopic repair without routine use of biomesh and find that gastroplasty is not required to achieve adequate length for durable repair.

Regardless of surgical approach, there are four fundamental steps to PEH repair:

1. Complete reduction of the stomach, GEJ, and distal esophagus into the abdominal cavity without tension
2. Complete reduction and excision of the hernia sac
3. Crural closure
4. Fixation of the stomach in the abdomen with fundoplication or gastropexy

Laparoscopic PEH repair is performed with the patient supine, split-legged or in lithotomy, in steep reverse Trendelenburg, with the surgeon standing between the patient's legs or on the patient's left. Access to the abdominal cavity can be obtained with an open or closed technique. The camera port should be placed approximately 15 mm inferior to the xiphoid process and to the left of midline, through the rectus muscle. After achieving insufflation, 5 mm ports are placed under direct vision. The surgeon's working ports are placed along the right and left costal margin approximately 10 cm away from the xiphoid process. A right lateral port is used for a liver retractor to elevate the left lobe and expose the hiatus. One or two left upper quadrant 5 mm ports are placed laterally for the assistant. The hernia is first reduced with gentle traction. Excessive traction can lead to injury to the stomach and should be avoided. Dissection of the hernia sac begins along the inner border of the crura—we prefer starting this dissection along the left crus, continuing over the crural arch to the right crus. The gastrohepatic ligament is incised to improve access to the right crus. The plane between the hernia sac and crura is developed bluntly and dissection proceeds into the mediastinum. Care must be taken to identify the pleural edges and reflect them laterally. The anterior and posterior vagal nerves should be identified and preserved. A posterior esophageal fat pad often exists and requires complete reduction. Caution should be used during posterior dissection of the crural base as a branch of the inferior phrenic vein often courses in this location. Once complete, a Penrose drain is placed around the esophagus and vagus nerves to improve retraction. This allows for improved mediastinal dissection to achieve adequate esophageal length.

Once reduced intra-abdominally, any excess sac should be removed from its gastric attachments. Caution that injury to the anterior vagus nerve, which is often lifted off the esophagus, can occur during excision of the sac if not recognized. The short gastric vessels are then divided. This can be done prior to completion of the crural dissection to allow for improved exposure to the posterior sac and crural base if preferred. The crural defect is then closed posterior to the esophagus using multiple, nonabsorbable pledgeted sutures, incorporating peritoneum over the crural edges. Caution must be exercised as the vena cava can be pulled quite close to the right crus. A partial or full fundoplication over a 60-French bougie is then fashioned. Any large defect or muscular attenuation should be reinforced with a U-shaped biologic mesh sutured to the apices of the crura. Synthetic mesh should not be used given the risk of erosion.

Potential pitfalls of the operation include pneumothorax or injury to the vagus nerves, an accessory or replaced left hepatic artery, the gastric serosa, and the esophagus (Table 9-1). If a pneumothorax is recognized, often by billowing of the affected hemidiaphragm, one can usually continue the operation with the patient on positive-pressure ventilation without difficulty. These more often occur on the left, where it can be difficult to identify pleural edge from hernia sac. At the completion of the case, the pneumothorax can be evacuated with a red-rubber catheter placed through the hiatal closure and put to water seal. These rarely require thoracostomy for evacuation. An accessory or replaced left hepatic artery can be injured during division of the gastrohepatic ligament if unrecognized. Excessive traction on the stomach during reduction can result in serosal tears. These should be primarily repaired at the time of injury. Finally, although esophageal perforations are rare, inadvertent myotomy during dissection are not infrequent.

Table 9-1	**Laparoscopic Paraesophageal Hernia Repair**

Key Technical Steps

1. Gentle reduction of herniated intra-abdominal contents as able.
2. Dissection of the hernia sac along the inner border of the crura.
3. Identification of the anterior and posterior vagus nerves.
4. Circumferential control of the distal esophagus and vagus nerves with a Penrose drain.
5. Careful mediastinal dissection for complete hernia reduction including 3 cm of intra-abdominal esophagus.
6. Division of the short gastric vessels if performing fundoplication.
7. Closure of the crural defect with nonabsorbable pledgeted sutures.
8. Fundoplication or gastropexy.

Potential Pitfalls

- Pneumothorax during mediastinal dissection if the pleural edges are not recognized and reflected laterally.
- Injury to the anterior or posterior vagus nerves; these should be contained within the Penrose drain and particular caution used during dissection and division of the anterior and posterior hernia sac.
- Undue traction on the stomach can result in serosal tears.
- Esophageal injury can occur during mechanical dissection or from heat injury secondary to inappropriate use of energy.

SPECIAL INTRAOPERATIVE CONSIDERATIONS

A shortened esophagus can pose a challenge to obtaining the desired 3 to 4 cm of tension-free, intra-abdominal esophagus. We find that a high mediastinal dissection can achieve this goal. Rarely, a Collis gastroplasty can be considered.

Gastric perforation can occur in the patient with acute gastric volvulus. This can often be avoided with early decompression and surgical intervention. These perforations usually occur on the anterior surface of the fundus and can be repaired primarily laparoscopically.

Management of the critically ill patient can be difficult. If the patient cannot tolerate extensive surgery, the surgeon should attempt separation of the sac from the esophagus and stomach, crural closure, and gastropexy (G-tube or suture pexy).

POSTOPERATIVE MANAGEMENT

If a Foley catheter was placed during the case, it can typically be removed at its completion. Routine nasogastric decompression is not warranted. Postoperative CXR is not routinely performed unless clinically indicated. Small pneumothoraces are common and generally do not require intervention. Patients are started on a limited clear liquid diet without carbonation on the evening after surgery or postoperative day 1. They can be advanced to a mechanical soft diet as tolerated over the next 24 to 48 hours. Medications that come as tablets or capsules should be crushed, opened, or converted to a liquid form if available. These changes should be maintained for 2 to 4 weeks. Dietitian consultation is recommended for education and compliance. Patients are typically discharged home on postoperative day 1 or 2, depending on PO intake and mobility.

Unexplained tachycardia or shortness of breath mandates immediate UGI study with gastrograffin followed by barium to evaluate for an esophageal perforation. If a leak is found, immediate exploration with primary repair and drainage is warranted. Exploratory laparoscopy can also be liberally used to rule out postoperative bleeding or leak.

TAKE HOME POINTS

- Paraesophageal hernias commonly occur in the elderly.
- Symptoms may be vague and nonspecific.
- Consider PEH in the setting of chronic anemia when no other source is found.
- Most PEHs should be repaired electively.
- Paraesophageal hernias can be safely repaired through a laparoscopic approach with good outcomes.
- Principles of repair include complete reduction of the hernia sac, crural closure, and fundoplication or gastropexy.

SUGGESTED READINGS

Carrott PW, Hong J, Kuppusamy MK, Low DE, et al. Repair of giant paraesophageal hernias routinely produces improvement in respiratory function. *J Thorac Cardiovasc Surg.* 2012;143:398-404.

Edye MB, Canin-Endres J, Gattorno F, et al. Durability of laparoscopic repair of paraesophageal hernia. *Ann Surg.* 1998;228(4):528-535.

Lal DR, Pellegrini CA, Oelschlager BK. Laparoscopic repair of paraesophageal hernia. *Surg Clin North Am.* 2005;85:105-118.

McLaren PJ, Hart KD, Hunter JG, et al. Paraesophageal hernia repair outcomes using minimally invasive approaches. *JAMA Surg.* 2017;152:1176. doi: 10.1001/jamasurg.2017.2868.

Oelschlager BK, Pellegrini CA. Paraesophageal hernias: open, laparoscopic or thoracic repair?. *Chest Surg Slin North Am.* 2001;11(3):589-603.

Skinner DB, Belsey RH. Surgical management of esophageal reflux and hiatus hernia. Long term results with 1030 patients. *J Thorac Cardiovasc Surg.* 1967;53(1)33-54.

Gastroesophageal Reflux Disease

JONATHAN F. FINKS

10

Based on the previous edition chapter "Gastroesophageal Reflux Disease" by Jonathan F. Finks

Presentation

A 55-year-old otherwise healthy, mildly obese (body mass index 33) woman is referred for evaluation of refractory heartburn and regurgitation. Her symptoms have been present for approximately 10 years. She initially attempted lifestyle changes, including cessation of smoking and caffeine use, as well as weight loss, but did not have significant relief. Her symptoms have improved with use of twice daily proton pump inhibitors (PPIs), but she continues to have breakthrough symptoms, especially after eating and when lying down.

● DIFFERENTIAL DIAGNOSIS

The leading diagnosis based on these symptoms is gastroesophageal reflux disease (GERD). An important consideration is whether or not there is an accompanying hiatal hernia, as this can influence the choice of treatment. The differential diagnosis also includes achalasia. Patients with achalasia often present with dysphagia, but may predominantly complain of regurgitation and retrosternal burning. Whereas heartburn usually occurs within 30 minutes of eating in patients with GERD, with achalasia, the burning usually does not begin until several hours after eating and is the result of fermentation of undigested food within the esophagus. Alarm symptoms, such as dysphagia, odynophagia, weight loss, anemia, and gastrointestinal bleeding, should prompt a search for esophagogastric malignancy.

● WORKUP

For patients with classic symptoms (heartburn and regurgitation), a good response to a trial of proton pump inhibitor therapy is diagnostic of GERD. Further workup is indicated, however, in patients over 50, those with frequent breakthrough symptoms or whose symptoms have persisted for over 5 years, and those with alarm symptoms as mentioned above.

For patients with dysphagia, a *barium swallow* is a good first study, as it allows for assessment of esophageal strictures (benign and malignant) and diverticula. Furthermore, a barium swallow provides a detailed view of the anatomic relationships of the stomach, esophagus, and diaphragm, allowing for identification of hiatal hernia (Figure 10-1). A barium swallow also provides useful information with regard to esophageal motility and serves as a good confirmatory study for patients with manometric evidence of achalasia.

Upper endoscopy offers direct visualization of esophageal mucosa, allowing for identification of esophagitis, Barrett's esophagus, and esophagogastric malignancies. It is especially useful for patients with atypical, or extraesophageal, symptoms, such as cough, wheezing, and hoarseness and is indicated in any patient for whom antireflux surgery is considered. The presence of esophagitis on upper endoscopy, in association with typical reflux symptoms (heartburn and regurgitation), is generally considered adequate evidence of reflux disease to justify antireflux surgery without any further testing.

Ambulatory esophageal pH testing is indicated for patients with atypical symptoms and those with nonerosive disease

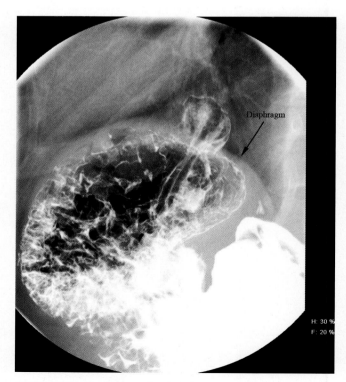

FIGURE 10-1. Barium swallowing demonstrating a sliding hiatal hernia.

for whom antireflux surgery is being considered. It involves placement of a catheter, or endoscopically placed sensor, in the esophagus, 5 cm from the lower esophageal sphincter. Esophageal pH is measured at several points in the esophagus over a 24- or 48-hour period, and information is provided on the extent of acid exposure during the test as well as correlation of symptoms with acid events. Generally, this study should be performed with the patient off of any antacid medicine, especially PPIs, for the duration of the study and 1 week prior.

Esophageal pH monitoring may be combined with *esophageal impedance testing*. These catheters measure changes in electrical impedance at multiple points along the esophagus, which allows for detection of a liquid bolus passage, with a determination of the direction of flow. When combined with pH monitoring, impedance can detect both acid and non-acid reflux. This study is particularly useful for patients with persistent symptoms despite the use of maximum medical therapy, as well as those with extraesophageal symptoms, both of whom may suffer from significant volume reflux.

Esophageal manometry offers a functional assessment of the upper and lower esophageal sphincters (LES) as well as the motility of the body. Manometry can detect motility disorders, such as achalasia, and is indicated for patients with dysphagia, where malignancy, stricture and hiatal hernia have been ruled out by other studies. Most surgeons also consider esophageal manometry essential before antireflux surgery in order to rule out a significant motility disorder, where dysphagia could be exacerbated by fundoplication. As with pH testing, manometry can be combined with impedance testing, which provides more information about the functional ability of esophageal contractions to move a bolus forward through the esophagus.

● TREATMENT

The patient from our clinical scenario had classic symptoms of reflux and demonstrated improvement with the use of PPIs. However, because of her age and the duration of symptoms, she underwent an upper endoscopy, that demonstrated a small hiatal hernia but no evidence of esophagitis. Ambulatory pH testing demonstrated that the fraction of time with a pH < 4 was 8% (upper limit of normal is <4%), and manometry demonstrated normal esophageal motility and LES function. All of these findings are consistent with GERD.

● MEDICAL THERAPY

Lifestyle modification can often lead to significant improvement and even resolution of GERD symptoms. Important steps include weight loss, smoking cessation, limiting alcohol and caffeine, and changes in eating habits. For example, patients should be encouraged to avoid eating within 3 hours

of bedtime. For patients who have persistent symptoms despite behavioral changes, proton pump inhibitors are the mainstay of treatment for patients with GERD. For most patients, they are highly effective at controlling symptoms and resolving esophagitis. PPIs are also generally safe medications, although long-term use has been associated with increased susceptibility to *Clostridium difficile* colitis, bone loss, and dementia.

● ANTIREFLUX PROCEDURES

Despite the effectiveness and popularity of PPIs, there are patients who do not tolerate these medications or are concerned about long-term side effects. Moreover, a number of patients will have breakthrough symptoms while on PPIs, often at night, or when lying down. These symptoms may indicate the presence of a hiatal hernia, in which case PPIs may neutralize the fluid entering the esophagus and reduce heartburn symptoms, but do not necessarily lower the volume of fluid and the associated regurgitation-related symptoms. These patients will often benefit from an antireflux procedure, which can favorably alter the foregut anatomy to better control reflux symptoms.

Over the past two decades, there have been a number of endoluminal and minimally invasive surgical devices developed to treat GERD. The EsophyX is used to place full-thickness plication sutures in the gastroesophageal junction in order to restore the angle of His and recreate a competent antireflux valve. The Stretta device uses radiofrequency energy to thicken the smooth muscle of the LES, thereby improving its barrier capability. Short-term studies with these devices demonstrate a reduction in reflux symptoms and PPI use, but there is little long-term evidence to support their effectiveness and no trials comparing them to laparoscopic fundoplication.

More recently, however, the LINX procedure has grown in popularity. This operation involves laparoscopic placement of magnetic beads in a ring around the lower esophageal sphincter to help augment contraction in this area. This procedure has been shown to control GERD symptoms and reduce esophageal acid exposure in short- and medium-term studies. It also compares favorably to fundoplication at 1 year. However, long-term effectiveness of the procedure is still uncertain and it may not be appropriate for patients with more than a small hiatal hernia.

● LAPAROSCOPIC FUNDOPLICATION

For now, laparoscopic esophagogastric fundoplication remains the gold standard in the surgical treatment of GERD. Fundoplication procedures have proven safe and effective in reducing GERD symptoms, resolving esophagitis, and reducing the need for antacid medication. However, long-term studies do show at least some symptom recurrence in up to

20% of patients. What underlies the success of antireflux surgery is that it restores the normal anatomic position of the stomach and gastroesophageal junction. Reduction of hiatal hernia ensures that the LES is aligned with the diaphragm, which serves to augment its contractility and enhance its barrier effect. Furthermore, the fundoplication recreates the flap valve mechanism of the angle of His, which acts to limit the reflux that occurs with postprandial distension of the cardia.

Patient selection is crucial to success with antireflux surgery. Patients with typical GERD symptoms and those who respond to PPIs tend to have better results after fundoplication than do those with predominantly extraesophageal symptoms and poor response to antacid medication. Before proceeding to the OR, surgeons should ensure that patients have objective evidence of GERD, which includes either esophagitis at endoscopy, an abnormal esophageal pH study, or evidence of a large hiatal hernia on barium swallow. Finally, preoperative manometry is helpful to rule out the presence of significant dysmotility.

● SURGICAL APPROACH

There is some controversy over the choice of Nissen (360°) fundoplication versus a partial fundoplication, such as a Toupet (270°) procedure. There have been a number of comparison studies over the past two decades, including a number of randomized clinical trials. Most of the studies demonstrate equipoise between the two operations, although the Toupet procedure may reduce early dysphagia rates and the Nissen fundoplication may have an edge with long-term reflux control. For patients with any preoperative dysphagia and/or evidence of esophageal dysmotility, a Toupet fundoplication may be the better approach.

There are several technical elements that are key to successful antireflux surgery. First, any hiatal hernia must be completely reduced. This process involves extensive mediastinal dissection to ensure full esophageal mobilization and adequate closure of the diaphragmatic crura. These steps will help reduce the risk for recurrent hiatal hernia, by far the most common cause for failure of these operations. Furthermore, the fundus should be completely mobilized by division of the short gastric vessels in order to prevent twisting of the wrap. Finally, a 2-cm long "floppy" posterior fundoplication (Nissen) is performed around the distal esophagus over a large dilator, in order to minimize postoperative dysphagia.

The procedure is performed under general anesthesia with the patient in the split-leg position. This allows the surgeon to operate from between the legs, which may enhance operative ergonomics. Alternatively, the patient can remain supine, with the primary surgeon operating from the patient's right side. An orogastric tube is inserted, but a Foley catheter is not usually necessary.

Access to the peritoneum is obtained using a closed (Veress) or open (Hasson) technique and pneumoperitoneum is established. We employ a 5-port approach with a camera port placed 15 cm below the junction of the right and left costal margins. The surgeon's working ports are placed in the upper abdomen. The assistant stands to the patient left, using a port in the left upper quadrant and operating the laparoscope. The bed is then put into the steep reverse Trendelenburg position, and a Nathanson retractor is placed through a 5-mm port site in the subxiphoid position to elevate the left lateral segment of the liver and expose the diaphragmatic hiatus.

First, the stomach is manually reduced into the abdomen in the event of a hiatal hernia. The gastrohepatic ligament is then incised using bipolar electrocautery (or ultrasonic dissector). Division of the ligament begins in the avascular portion and extends toward the diaphragm in order to expose the right crus. We recommend preserving the hepatic branch of the vagus nerve where possible, both to reduce risk for subsequent gallstone formation and also to avoid injury to the accessory left hepatic artery, which can be present in up to 12% of patients (Figure 10-2).

Next, the phrenoesophageal ligament anterior to the esophagus is opened, with care taken to avoid injury to the underlying esophagus and anterior vagus nerve. Blunt dissection is then used to develop a plane between the right crus and the esophagus. This dissection is continued posteriorly until the decussation of the left and right crura is visualized. Some retroesophageal dissection may be done from the right side during this portion of the procedure. Care should be taken to prevent injury to the posterior vagus nerve and keep the nerve up with the esophagus during the dissection.

Attention then turns to mobilization of the fundus (Figure 10-3). The short gastric vessels are divided, beginning at the level of the inferior pole of the spleen and extending toward the left crus. The posterior attachments of the stomach should also be divided to ensure full mobilization of the fundus. At this point, the retroesophageal dissection is completed from the left side and a Penrose drain is placed around the esophagus, with the ends anchored anteriorly

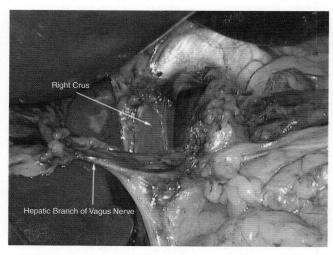

Right Crus

Hepatic Branch of Vagus Nerve

FIGURE 10-2. Exposure of the right crus of the diaphragm.

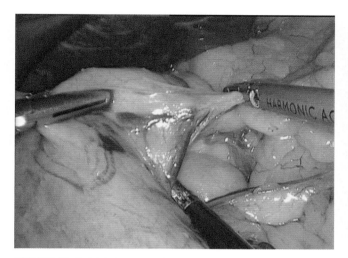

FIGURE 10-3. Mobilization of the fundus.

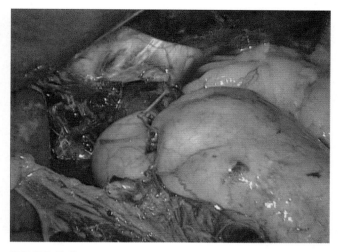

FIGURE 10-5. Fundoplication.

using an endoscopic ligating loop. The Penrose drain facilitates retraction of the esophagus.

What follows is an extensive mediastinal mobilization, using both blunt and sharp dissection with bipolar electrocautery or ultrasonic dissection to free the esophagus from its mediastinal attachments (Figure 10-4). This dissection continues until at least 2.5 to 3 cm of distal esophagus remains within the abdomen without having to apply traction to the stomach. The diaphragmatic crura are then approximated using nonabsorbable suture. The closure should be snug, as radial dilation around the esophagus will occur with time and can lead to recurrent hiatal hernia. At the same time, calibration with a 56 to 60 French dilator may be helpful during the closure to prevent dysphagia.

The fundus of the stomach is brought behind the esophagus and a 360° (Nissen) fundoplication is then performed over a large dilator (56 to 60 French) (Figure 10-5). The fundoplication is secured at the right anterolateral aspect of the esophagus with 3 nonabsorbable sutures. The sutures are placed 1 cm apart, with the superior-most suture placed

2 cm above the gastroesophageal junction. Each suture incorporates a full-thickness bite of stomach on either side of the esophagus, as well as a partial thickness bite of esophagus, in order to prevent slippage of the fundus behind the wrap. Should the surgeon opt to perform a Toupet procedure, both the right and left aspects of the fundoplication are anchored separately to the esophagus with three nonabsorbable sutures (Table 10-1).

Table 10-1 Gastroesophageal Reflux Disease

Key Technical Steps

1. Incision of the gastrohepatic ligament through the avascular space to expose the right crus.
2. Blunt dissection to develop a plane between the esophagus and the crus until the crural decussation is visualized.
3. Complete mobilization of the fundus.
4. Extensive mediastinal dissection to deliver at least 2.5–3 cm of distal esophagus into the abdomen.
5. Snug closure of the crural defect with nonabsorbable sutures.
6. Creation of a 2-cm long posterior fundoplication (Nissen or Toupet) over a dilator, using nonabsorbable suture.

Potential Pitfalls

- Injury to accessory or replaced left hepatic artery running with the hepatic branch of the vagus nerve in the gastrohepatic ligament.
- Injury to anterior and posterior vagus nerves. The posterior nerve often falls away from the esophagus and is most susceptible to injury.
- Injury to the proximal short gastric vessels. These are fragile and difficult to control if avulsed off the spleen.
- Esophageal injury from inadvertent contact with energy source during mediastinal dissection.

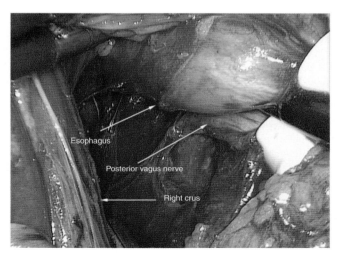

FIGURE 10-4. Mediastinal dissection.

● SPECIAL INTRAOPERATIVE CONSIDERATIONS

During the mediastinal dissection, especially in the setting of a large hiatal hernia, the pleura can be adherent to the hernia sac and is then susceptible to injury. A pleural tear can result in capnothorax with resultant hypercarbia, hypoxia, and possibly hemodynamic compromise from tension capnothorax. Should the patient develop any compromise, there are several steps that will help remedy the situation. First, the tear is enlarged and a 14 French red rubber catheter is inserted into the abdomen after cutting small holes near the narrow end of the catheter. The narrow end is then inserted into the pleural space and the larger end is left in the abdomen. This will help equalize the pressure between the two cavities. At the end of the procedure, the abdominal end of the catheter is pulled out through the left subcostal port while the pneumoperitoneum is released. This end of the catheter is placed into a water seal while deep Valsalva breaths are administered by the anesthesiologist. This will allow for evacuation of any remaining gas from the affected pleural space. The red rubber catheter may then be removed. In some cases, the pneumoperitoneum may need to be periodically released to allow for resolution of hypercapnia.

● POSTOPERATIVE MANAGEMENT

Patients initially receive scheduled IV acetaminophen, ketorolac (selectively) and ondansetron for pain and nausea control with IV morphine for breakthrough pain. Opiates are minimized to help reduce nausea and retching, which may lead to early recurrent hiatal hernia or disruption of the fundoplication. On the first postoperative night or the following day, patients are started on a clear liquid diet and then advanced to a full liquid diet. They are typically discharged on the 1st or 2nd postoperative day and may advance to a mechanical soft diet within the first week after surgery.

● SIDE EFFECTS

Side effects of antireflux procedures include dysphagia and gas-bloat symptoms. Mild dysphagia is not uncommon in the first few weeks after surgery. For this reason, patients are advised to avoid tough or dry meat, raw vegetables, and bread for at least 4 to 6 weeks following the operation. In the case of severe or persistent dysphagia (>4 weeks), patients should undergo a barium swallow to rule out a recurrent hiatal hernia and assess for narrowing at the diaphragm or within the fundoplication. In the absence of a recurrent hiatal hernia, symptoms will often improve with empiric endoscopic dilation.

The cause of gas-bloat symptoms after antireflux surgery is not clear, but may relate to vagal stretch during the dissection. Many patients complain of an inability to belch after fundoplication, and this can also contribute to these symptoms. Gas-bloat symptoms usually resolve spontaneously after several weeks. However, patients can also minimize these symptoms by avoiding carbonated beverages and eating small meals five to six times per day.

KEY POINTS

- Careful patient selection is essential. Those scheduled for surgery should have objective evidence for reflux and symptoms that are attributable to GERD.
- Preoperative workup for all surgical patients should include upper endoscopy and esophageal manometry. Ambulatory 24-hour pH/ impedance testing should be reserved for patients with nonerosive disease and those with atypical symptoms. A barium swallow may better define anatomy and is a must for patients with dysphagia.
- Dysphagia is a common complaint following antireflux surgery. The risk for this complaint can be reduced by full mobilization of the fundus and creation of a "floppy" fundoplication over a 56 to 60 French dilator or by selection of a Toupet fundoplication.
- Recurrent hiatal hernia is the most common cause for failure of antireflux surgery. Adequate crural closure and a thorough mediastinal mobilization of the esophagus, allowing for a minimum of 2.5 to 3 cm of intra-abdominal esophageal length, will help reduce the risk for this complication.

SUGGESTED READINGS

Campos GM, Peters JH, DeMeester TR, et al. Multivariate analysis of factors predicting outcome after laparoscopic nissen fundoplication. *J Gastrointest Surg.* 1999;3(3):292-300.

Hunter JG, Trus TL, Branum GD, et al. A physiologic approach to laparoscopic fundoplication for gastroesophageal reflux disease. *Ann Surg.* 1996;223(6):673-685.

Jobe BA, Kahrilas PJ, Vernon AH, et al. Endoscopic appraisal of the gastroesophageal valve after antireflux surgery. *Am J Gastroenterol.* 2004;99(2):233-243.

Malhi-Chowla N, Gorecki P, Bammer T, et al. Dilation after fundoplication: timing, frequency, indications and outcome. *Gastrointest Endosc.* 2002;55(2):219-223.

Gastric Cancer

JOSEPH MELVIN, JUSSUF T. KAIFI, ERIC T. KIMCHI, AND KEVIN F. STAVELEY-O'CARROLL

11

Based on the previous edition chapter "Gastric Cancer" by Srinivas Kavuturu, Jussuf T. Kaifi, and Kevin F. Staveley-O'Carroll

Presentation

A 52-year-old male presents with a history of epigastric discomfort and dysphagia for 6 months. He describes two previous episodes of black tarry stools and a 30-lb weight loss over the past 3 months. His past medical history is significant for hypertension, hypercholesterolemia, and benign prostatic hypertrophy. His past surgical history is only significant for an open appendectomy as a child. He drinks about eight beers a day and has a 30-pack-year history of smoking cigarettes. He has a family history of heart disease and hypertension. His medications include tamsulosin, metoprolol, omeprazole, and Lipitor. He is not allergic to any known medications.

● DIFFERENTIAL DIAGNOSIS

Based on the patient's age and clinical presentation (e.g., dysphagia, weight loss, and melena) in conjunction with a social history significant for a 30-pack-year smoking history, esophageal/gastric cancer should be considered as the leading differential diagnosis but the following alternative diagnoses could also be taken into account. Benign diseases to consider include esophagitis, gastritis, peptic ulcer disease, or esophageal varices given the substantial ETOH history. Malignant diseases to consider include gastric or esophageal carcinoma, MALT (mucosa lymphoid tissue) lymphoma of the stomach, primary gastric lymphoma (non-MALT type), and gastrointestinal stromal tumor (GIST).

● WORKUP

Workup includes a thorough history and physical examination, laboratory testing, diagnostic imaging, and invasive tests (e.g., endoscopy). In cases concerning for malignancy, the diagnostic workup should have two goals: (1) determine the extent of disease (clinical staging) and (2) risk stratification for any proposed surgery.

Environmental factors, previous surgical history, and family history all play a significant role in assessing a patient's risk of gastric cancer. Personal history of smoking, ETOH abuse, *Helicobacter pylori* (*H. Pylori*), previous gastric surgery, and a family history of upper GI cancers (e.g., hereditary diffuse gastric cancer [HDGC], Lynch syndrome II, BRCA2 mutation, and familial polyposis coli) are associated with malignancy.

Most patients with malignancy have normal physical exams. Positive findings on physical examination are most often associated with locally advanced or metastatic disease. These findings may include a palpable abdominal mass from a large primary tumor, liver or ovarian metastases (Krukenberg's tumor), palpable left supraclavicular node (Virchow's node), periumbilical nodule (Sister Mary Joseph node), pelvic deposits (rectal Blummer's shelf), jaundice, or ascites. Paraneoplastic syndromes associated with gastric cancer include acanthosis nigricans, thrombophlebitis, circinate erythema, dermatomyositis, pemphigoid, and seborrheic keratosis.

When malignancy is suspected, flexible endoscopy is the diagnostic modality of choice. The diagnostic accuracy of upper GI endoscopy for gastric cancer approaches 98%. In a study of 100 randomly selected patients, endoscopy was more sensitive (92% vs. 54%) and specific (100% vs. 91%) than double-contrast barium studies. Barium studies also cannot distinguish benign from malignant ulcers. Once a malignancy is identified, it is categorized by its location using the Siewert classification. Siewert 1 lesions are above the gastroesophageal (GE) junction, Siewert 2 lesions are at the true GE junction, and Siewert 3 lesions are in the gastric cardia.

Preoperative staging evaluates local extent of the tumor, resectability, lymph node involvement, and presence of metastasis. Imaging modalities include computerized tomography (CT) scan, upper endoscopy, endoscopic ultrasound (EUS), positron emission tomography (PET), magnetic resonance imaging (MRI), and laparoscopic exploration. CT and MRI scans of the abdomen are valuable in determining hepatic metastasis, bulky lymphadenopathy, visceral metastasis, ascites, and extragastric extension to surgically unresectable structures. These scans can also help in planning the extent of surgery (e.g., if en bloc resection of nearby organs is necessary). However, the value of imaging is limited in detecting peritoneal disease and smaller hepatic metastasis (<1 cm in size). CT scan of the chest should be included for tumors at the GE junction to evaluate the extent of disease in the mediastinum. EUS can assess the depth of the tumor (T stage) and local nodal status (N stage) with overall accuracy ranging from 57% to 88%. EUS-guided fine needle aspiration (FNA) biopsy of the regional lymph nodes, aspiration of small volume ascites,

57

and accessible distant metastatic sites (e.g., mediastinal lymph nodes, liver) improve the accuracy of lymph nodal staging and could prove distant metastasis avoiding noncurative laparotomy. However, EUS can be technically challenging and is user dependent. PET-CT improves preoperative staging of gastric adenocarcinoma and can alter treatment options in up to 20% of patients. PET combined with CT is more accurate for preoperative staging than either modality alone (combined PET/CT 68%, PET alone 47%, or CT alone 53%). Furthermore, PET/CT can facilitate the selection of patients for a curative resection by confirming a nodal status identified by CT and is also the most sensitive noninvasive imaging modality for the diagnosis of hepatic metastases from gastric cancer.

Performing diagnostic laparoscopy prior to definitive surgery has several advantages. Laparoscopy detects small metastases (<0.5 cm) of the peritoneum and liver in up to 40% patients who are eligible for potentially curative resection based on CT scan alone. Laparoscopy also allows for staging by cytopathologic analysis of peritoneal fluid, placement of a feeding jejunostomy tube in patients with an obstructing GE junction mass, and avoids unnecessary laparotomies in patients with metastatic gastric cancer. Currently, staging laparoscopy is recommended in select patients with high probability of having distant metastatic disease in the abdomen, based on suspicious radiographic findings and patient presentation. The role of intraoperative laparoscopic ultrasonography to stage the gastric cancer is still to be defined by systematic studies.

Preoperative risk stratification for surgery includes nutritional, cardiovascular, pulmonary, central nervous system, and functional assessment should be assessed both clinically and with appropriate testing to optimize patient selection and outcomes.

The patient described in the scenario above had an unremarkable clinical examination and no relevant family history regarding malignancies. Evaluation with an upper endoscopy revealed an irregular Siewert type III GE junction tumor (i.e., tumor lying within 2 to 5 cm distal to the GE junction). Biopsies from the mass were consistent with moderately differentiated adenocarcinoma. A multiphase CT scan of his chest, abdomen, and pelvis with contrast revealed thickening of stomach wall at the GE junction and a few perigastric lymph nodes <1 cm in size. There was no evidence of invasion/encasement of any major vascular structures, distant metastasis, or peritoneal seeding. PET-CT showed an FDG (fluorodeoxyglucose) avid lesion in the proximal stomach corresponding to the lesion seen on the CT scan. The subcentimeter lymph nodes seen on the CT scan were also FDG avid on the PET-CT, indicating metastatic spread to these regional lymph nodes. EUS demonstrated that the lesion invaded muscularis propria (T2), and EUS-guided FNA of the perigastric lymph nodes were positive for adenocarcinoma (N1). Lastly, diagnostic laparoscopy was performed with no gross evidence of distant metastasis and peritoneal cytology negative for malignancy.

● DIAGNOSIS AND TREATMENT

The diagnosis of gastric cancer is established by histopathologic assessment of biopsies or cytology from gastric washes/brushing. The two most commonly used pathologic classifications of gastric cancer based on microscopic configuration are that of Lauren and World Health Organization (WHO) systems. The Lauren classification divides gastric cancer into two major histologic types: intestinal and diffuse. The intestinal form is often seen arising in a setting of chronic atrophic gastritis (e.g., *Helicobacter pylori* and autoimmune gastritis), whereas the diffuse form is less related to environmental influences and may arise as single cell mutations within normal gastric glands. The WHO classification has five subtypes: adenocarcinoma (intestinal and diffuse), papillary, tubular, mucinous, and signet-ring cell. Staging of gastric cancer is currently based on the *American Joint Committee on Cancer Recommendation of the TNM Staging* (7th edition, 2010) with the addition of the term "R status" denoting the status of resection margins after surgery (R0, negative margins; R1, microscopic residual disease; R2, gross residual disease).

Surgical resection is the mainstay of treatment of gastric cancer. However, a multidisciplinary team approach with combined modality therapy (surgery, chemotherapy, and radiation) is most effective especially in patients who have locoregional disease. Clinically, gastric cancer can be classified into early, locoregionally advanced (but resectable), nonresectable, and metastatic.

For patients with early gastric cancer (Tis, T1 tumors limited to mucosa), gastrectomy with D1/D2 lymphadenectomy remains the treatment of choice. Endoscopic mucosal resection (EMR) is being performed on select patients, particularly those deemed nonsurgical candidates, but is not yet the standard of care. Per NCCN Guidelines, EMR may be considered when the lesion is ≤2 cm in diameter, well or moderately differentiated, does not penetrate beyond the superficial submucosa, has no evidence of lymphovascular invasion, and has clear lateral and deep margins.

For patients with locoregionally advanced resectable gastric cancer, recent evidence supports neoadjuvant therapy prior to surgery. The MAGIC trial was the first to demonstrate improved progression-free survival and overall survival among those patients undergoing perioperative chemotherapy. A more recent study from Ychou et al. demonstrated that perioperative chemotherapy with fluorouracil and cisplatin significantly increased the curative resection rate, disease-free survival, and overall survival in patients with resectable cancer (FNCLCC/FFCD Trial). Furthermore, the ACTS GC trial and the CLASSIC trial have since supported the use of adjuvant chemotherapy after curative D2 gastrectomy and should be considered as a treatment option for patients with operable gastric cancer.

For patients with locally advanced but initially nonresectable disease, neoadjuvant chemotherapy or chemoradiotherapy

Table 11-1	Siewert Classification	
Siewert	**Description**	**Surgical Approach**
I	Tumor center located between 1 and 5 cm above the anatomic EGJ	Managed as esophageal or EGJ cancer
II	Tumor center located between 1 cm proximal and 2 cm distal to the EGJ	Managed as esophageal or EGJ cancer
III	Tumor center located between 2 and 5 cm below the EGJ	Managed as gastric cancer

has also been tried with an intention to downstage tumors into potentially resectable disease with a curative intent, but the approach has not yet been standardized. Patients with metastatic disease are only candidates for palliative therapy, depending on their symptoms and functional status.

Postoperatively, for patients undergoing gastric resection who have not received preoperative chemotherapy or chemoradiation, current NCCN Clinical Practice Guidelines In Oncology (NCCN Guidelines®) recommend adjuvant chemotherapy with a fluoropyrimidine (5-FU or capecitabine) before and after fluoropyrimidine-based chemoradiation following R0 resection of T3, T4, and node-positive pT1-T2 tumors in patients who had less than a D2 lymph node dissection. For patients who have undergone a D2 lymph node dissection, postoperative chemotherapy with combined capecitabine and oxaliplatin is recommended.

● SURGICAL APPROACH

The extent of gastric resection is a crucial part of surgical plan. Since gastric carcinoma has the propensity to spread via submucosal and subserosal lymphatics, a resection margin of at least 5 cm is advocated. Curative resection with microscopically negative margins (R0 resection) involves resection of the tumor with lymphatics and lymph nodes and any adjacent organ involved by direct extension of the tumor (e.g., tail of pancreas, spleen). Hence, selection of appropriate surgical procedure is determined by location of the tumor, lymph node status, and extragastric extension into the adjacent organs.

A total gastrectomy with esophagojejunostomy is appropriate for proximal (upper third) gastric tumors. GE junction tumors predominantly involving cardia (Siewert type III) should be treated by an extended total gastrectomy with a segment of esophagus to provide an adequate margin. On the other hand, GE junction tumors with predominant involvement of the esophagus (Siewert type I) should be treated by transhiatal/transthoracic esophagectomy with proximal gastrectomy and

gastric pull-up with cervical/thoracic esophagogastrostomy. The necessary extent of resection for Siewert type II has been controversial, and intraoperative assessment of the tumor by an experienced surgeon and frozen section of the resected margins help decide the course—either a total gastrectomy or a esophagectomy (Table 11-1). For tumors in the distal stomach (lower two-thirds), a subtotal gastrectomy with Bilroth II or Roux-en-Y reconstruction is appropriate (Tables 11-2 and 11-3).

Previously, western studies were unable to replicate the survival benefit of a D2 lymph node dissection (lymph nodes along the named arteries of the stomach) over D1 (immediate perigastric lymph nodes) demonstrated by randomized controlled trials out of Japan. Multiple western studies have since provided additional evidence to support the claim of a long-term survival benefit for those patients undergoing a D2 lymph node dissection. Additionally, there is growing evidence against resection of the pancreas or spleen in conjunction with a D2 dissection. Thus, for patients with localized resectable gastric cancer, current NCCN Guidelines®

Table 11-2	Total Gastrectomy

Key Technical Steps

1. Midline laparotomy and full exploration.
2. Mobilize GE junction and esophagus, taking a margin of diaphragmatic crura.
3. Separate the omentum and lesser sac lining en bloc from the transverse colon.
4. Divide the short gastric vessels, and skeletonize the celiac, splenic, and common hepatic arteries, taking their lymph nodes.
5. Ligate left and right gastric and gastroepiploic arteries at their bases.
6. Divide esophagus, stomach, and jejunum.
7. Reconstruction with esophagojejunostomy and jejunojejunostomy.

Table 11-3	Total Gastrectomy

Potential Pitfalls

1. Accessory/replaced left hepatic artery arising from the left gastric artery (15%–20%)
2. Injury to the spleen
3. Positive tumor margins of the esophagus and stomach
4. Ischemic-looking duodenal stump

recommend gastrectomy with D1 or a modified D2 lymph node dissection, with the aim of evaluating a minimum of 15 lymph nodes reserving splenectomy for only those instances when the spleen or hilum is directly involved.

It is our preference and practice to perform gastrectomy with D2 lymphadenectomy after neoadjuvant chemotherapy. Depending on the extent of tumor, a splenectomy and/or a distal pancreatectomy is performed selectively when it is felt necessary to achieve negative margins (R0 resection). This strategy maximizes the chances of R0 resection and provides an adequate number of lymph nodes for accurate staging of the disease.

The patient in our case scenario has a moderately differentiated adenocarcinoma of the stomach (Siewert type III) with T3, N1, M0—stage IIB, that is locally advanced but resectable. Hence, as a part of multimodality treatment, he underwent neoadjuvant chemotherapy with etoposide, cisplatin, and 5-FU. He then underwent a total gastrectomy with Roux-en-Y esophagojejunostomy.

● OPERATIVE PROCEDURE

The patient is placed in a supine position. The skin from the chin to the pubic symphysis is prepared and draped. Prepping the patient in this manner allows for an esophagectomy to be performed with a cervical anastomosis if the need arises. We prefer a midline incision extending from the xiphoid process to just below the umbilicus for most patients undergoing a total gastrectomy. An extra large wound protector/retractor followed by placement of a fixed retractor (e.g., Thomson) are used for adequate exposure of the GE junction. Careful methodical exploration of the abdomen is performed to exclude metastasis, assess resectability, and local extension to other viscera. The gastrohepatic omentum is divided close to the liver. Evaluation for the presence of an accessory left hepatic artery is performed, and when one is present, it should be preserved in most cases. Dissection in the region of the esophagus and the fundus of the stomach starts by taking a ring of diaphragmatic crura, dividing the phrenic vein en route and taking the pericardial lymph node packet en bloc with the specimen (Figure 11-1). An omental bursectomy is performed. This includes resection of the omentum and the lesser sac with the lining are separated en bloc from the transverse colon. The short gastric vessels along

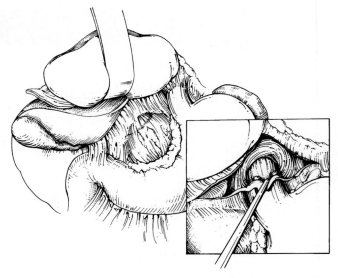

FIGURE 11-1. Mobilization of esophageal hiatus is completed by detaching the peritoneal reflection from the diaphragm. (From Fischer JE, et al. *Mastery of Surgery*. 5th ed. Philadelphia, PA: Lippincott Williams & Wilkins; 2007, with permission.)

the greater curvature of the stomach are divided close to the spleen (Figure 11-2). This dissection is facilitated by a vessel-sealing device. The celiac, splenic, and common hepatic arteries are skeletonized, and the nodal tissue swept up the left gastric artery (D2 dissection). The left and right gastric arteries and the gastroepiploic vessels are ligated at their bases, and the lymph nodes are taken with the specimen. The duodenum is then divided with a GIA stapler 2 to 3 cm distal to the pyloric vein (Figure 11-3). The GE junction is mobilized, and esophagus is divided with a transverse anastomosis (TA) stapler. The specimen is sent to pathology and a frozen section obtained from the proximal and distal margins of the specimen to check for adequacy of resection. Reconstruction after a standard

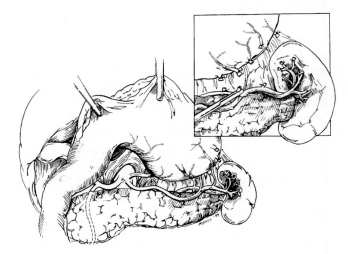

FIGURE 11-2. Omental bursectomy and division of the short gastric vessels adjacent to the spleen. (From Fischer JE, et al. *Mastery of Surgery*. 5th ed. Philadelphia, PA: Lippincott Williams & Wilkins; 2007, with permission.)

D2 total gastrectomy is performed utilizing a Roux- en-Y esophagojejunostomy (Figure 11-4). We prefer to perform this with an end-to-end anastomosis (EEA) stapling device. Alternately, a hand-sewn anastomosis or anastomosis to a jejunal pouch could also be performed. A jejunostomy feeding tube is placed routinely. We use closed suction drains to drain the duodenal stump and the esophagojejunal anastomosis.

There are several potential pitfalls during a routine gastrectomy. The gastrohepatic ligament might contain an accessory left hepatic artery (15% to 20%) and sometimes it represents the only arterial flow to the left lobe of the liver. Proximal ligation of left gastric artery in such case may result in hepatic ischemia. Injury to the spleen or its vessels may sometimes necessitate splenectomy to control hemorrhage. Positive esophageal resection margin may require reresection of the distal esophageal margin. The stapled duodenal stump often does not require further reinforcement with additional sutures; however, if there is concern for ischemia, we recommend oversewing it with Lembert sutures to prevent duodenal stump leak, which is a difficult postoperative complication.

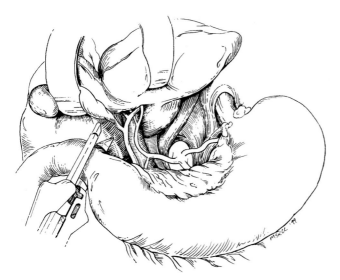

FIGURE 11-3. The duodenum being divided with the GIA stapler. (From Fischer JE, et al. *Mastery of Surgery*. 5th ed. Philadelphia, PA: Lippincott Williams & Wilkins; 2007, with permission.)

● SPECIAL INTRAOPERATIVE CONSIDERATIONS

In situations when a gastric tumor extends for a substantial distance up the esophagus and down the stomach, a total gastrectomy or esophagectomy alone may not provide a proper oncologic resection. In these cases, a total esophagogastrectomy with colon/jejunum interposition should be performed. The left colonic segment based on the ascending branch of the left colic vessels is used, or alternatively, this segment may be based on the middle colic vessels. When the colon is absent or has extensive diverticulosis, a jejunal conduit can be used.

● POSTOPERATIVE MANAGEMENT

We place a nasogastric tube (threaded beyond the gastrojejunal anastomosis intraoperatively), which is maintained on low intermittent suction. Postoperative pain control and early ambulation are critical to an expedited recovery. Jejunostomy feeding is started on postoperative day 2. Drains are removed on the 4 postoperative day if the bilirubin and amylase in the drain fluid is less than three times the serum values. Patients are typically discharged home on postoperative day 5 to 7 on jejunal tube feeds. Patients return to clinic 2 weeks after discharge and have a contrast swallow study to evaluate for a potential leak at the esophagojejunostomy. Provided that there is no leak seen at this time, oral feedings are initiated, and the tube feeds are weaned off over the course of a week. A dietitian can help the patient adapt to the change in eating habits to frequent small meals. Multivitamin, B_{12}, and iron supplementation will be needed for life in cases of total gastrectomy.

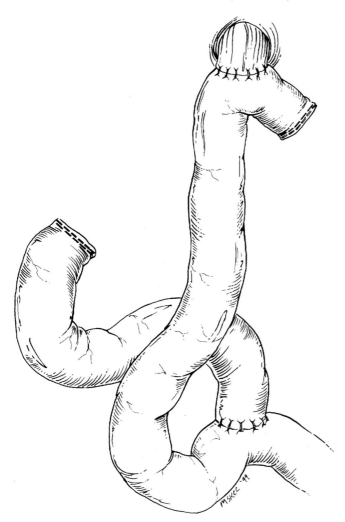

FIGURE 11-4. Completed Roux-en-Y reconstruction. (From Fischer JE, et al. *Mastery of Surgery*. 5th ed. Philadelphia, PA: Lippincott Williams & Wilkins; 2007, with permission.)

● POSTOPERATIVE SURVEILLANCE

Although there are no strict guidelines for postoperative follow-up, it is important to develop a systematic approach within your practice. This should include a history and physical exam every 3 to 6 months for the first 2 years and every 6 to 12 months for years 3 to 5 followed by annual evaluation per NCCN Guidelines. Laboratory, imaging, and endoscopic evaluation should be performed when clinically indicated.

Case Conclusion

The patient in our case scenario had a Siewert type III adenocarcinoma, T3, N1, M0—stage IIB, that was locally advanced but resectable. He underwent neoadjuvant chemotherapy with etoposide, cisplatin, and 5-FU (ECF) followed by a total gastrectomy with Roux-en-Y esophagojejunostomy with D2 lymphadenectomy. Pathology revealed the tumor was a 3-cm moderately differentiated gastric adenocarcinoma which had invaded the muscularis propria (resected with negative margins) with 2 out of 32 lymph nodes positive for malignancy and no evidence of metastasis (T2N1M0, stage IIA). He progressed well postoperatively with J-tube feeding initiated on postoperative day 2, drains removed on postoperative day 4, and discharge to home on postoperative day 6. At his 2-week follow-up appointment, his contrast upper GI was negative for a leak and he was transitioned to oral feedings. He subsequently underwent adjuvant chemotherapy with ECF, and he remains disease free to this day (5 years at the time of this publication).

TAKE HOME POINTS

- Upper GI endoscopy is diagnostic, and EUS provides the tumor and lymph node stage.
- PET-CT is emerging as a vital diagnostic tool in diagnosing regional as well as distant metastasis.
- Most Siewert type II GE junction tumors are staged and treated like an esophageal cancer. Neoadjuvant chemotherapy has shown to improve survival rate in locally advanced tumors and is being recommended by many surgeons and oncologists.
- Total gastrectomy with Roux-en-y esophagojejunostomy remains the operation of choice for locally advanced resectable proximal (upper one-third) gastric carcinoma.
- Current NCCN Guidelines recommend that at least 15 lymph nodes should be retrieved for adequate staging

(Tables 11-3 and 11-4), predominantly achieved through a D2 lymph nodal dissection.
- Postoperative chemotherapy and radiation are advised for locally advanced cancers (Table 11-5).

Table 11-4 — American Joint Committee on Cancer (AJCC) TNM Staging Classification for Staging of the Stomach (8th ed., 2018)

Primary Tumor (T)	
TX	Primary tumor cannot be assessed
T0	No evidence of primary tumor
Tis	Carcinoma in situ: intraepithelial tumor without invasion of the lamina propria
T1a	Tumor invades lamina propria or muscularis mucosae
T1b	Tumor invades submucosa
T2	Tumor invades muscularis propria
T3	Tumor penetrates subserosal connective tissue without invasion of visceral peritoneum or adjacent structures
T4a	Tumor invades serosa (visceral peritoneum)
T4b	Tumor invades adjacent structures
Regional Lymph Nodes (N)	
NX	Regional lymph node(s) cannot be assessed
N0	No regional lymph node metastasis
N1	Metastasis in 1–2 regional lymph nodes
N2	Metastasis in 3–6 regional lymph nodes
N3	Metastasis in 7 or more regional lymph nodes
N3a	Metastasis in 7–15 regional lymph nodes
N3b	Metastasis in 16 or more regional lymph nodes
Distant Metastasis (M)	
M0	No distant metastasis
M1	Distant metastasis
Histologic Grade (G)	
GX	Grade cannot be assessed
G1	Well differentiated
G2	Moderately differentiated
G3	Poorly differentiated
G4	Undifferentiated

From Edge SB, Byrd DR, Compton CC, et al. eds. *AJCC cancer staging manual.* 7th ed. New York, NY:Springer;2010. Copyright © 2010 American Joint Committee on Cancer. Reproduced with permission of Springer in the format Book via Copyright Clearance Center.

Table 11-5 — American Joint Committee on Cancer (AJCC) TNM Staging Classification for Staging of the Stomach (8th ed., 2018, Table 2)

Stage	T	N	G
Stage 0	Tis	N0	M0
Stage IA	T1	N0	M0
Stage IB	T1	N1	M0
	T2	N0	M0
Stage IIA	T1	N2	M0
	T2	N1	M0
	T3	N0	M0
Stage IIB	T1	N3a	M0
	T2	N2	M0
	T3	N1	M0
	T4a	N0	M0
Stage IIIA	T2	N3a	M0
	T3	N2	M0
	T4a	N1	M0
	T4a	N2	M0
	T4b	N0	M0
Stage IIIB	T1	N3b	M0
	T2	N3b	M0
	T3	N3a	M0
	T4a	N3a	M0
	T4b	N1	M0
	T4b	N2	M0
Stage IIIC	T3	N3b	M0
	T4a	N3b	M0
	T4b	N3a	M0
	T4b	N3b	M0
Stage IV	Any T	Any N	M1

From Edge SB, Byrd DR, Compton CC, et al. eds. *AJCC cancer staging manual.* 7th ed. New York, NY:Springer;2010. Copyright © 2010 American Joint Committee on Cancer. Reproduced with permission of Springer in the format Book via Copyright Clearance Center.

SUGGESTED READINGS

Ajani JA, Komaki R, Putnam JB, et al. A three-step strategy of induction chemotherapy then chemoradiation followed by surgery in patients with potentially resectable carcinoma of the esophagus or gastroesophageal junction. *Cancer.* 2001;92(2):279-286.

Avella D, Garcia L, Staveley-O'Carroll K, et al. Esophageal extension encountered during transhiatal resection of gastric or gastroesophageal tumors: attaining a negative margin. *J Gastrointest Surg.* 2009;13(2):368-373.

Bang YJ, et al. Adjuvant capecitabine and oxaliplatin for gastric cancer after D2 gastrectomy (CLASSIC): a phase 3 open-label, randomised controlled trial. *Lancet.* 2012;379(9813):315-321.

Bonenkamp JJ, Hermans J, Sasako M, et al. Extended lymph-node dissection for gastric cancer. *N Engl J Med.* 1999;340(12):908-914.

Bozzetti F, Bonfanti G, Bufalino R, et al. Adequacy of margins of resection in gastrectomy for cancer. *Ann Surg.* 1982;196(6):685-690.

Cardoso R, Coburn N, Seevaratnam R, et al. A systemic review and meta-analysis of the utility of EUS for preoperative staging for gastric cancer. *Gastric Cancer.* 2012;15(suppl 1):S19-S26.

Cascinu S, Scartozzi M, Labianca R, et al. High curative resection rate with weekly cisplatin, 5-fluorouracil, epidoxorubicin, 6S-leucovorin, glutathione, and filgrastrim in patients with locally advanced, unresectable gastric cancer: a report from the Italian Group for the Study of Digestive Tract Cancer (GISCAD). *Br J Cancer.* 2004;90(8):1521-1525.

Chen J, Cheong JH, Yun MJ, et al. Improvement in preoperative staging of gastric adenocarcinoma with positron emission tomography. *Cancer.* 2005;103(11):2383-2390.

Chua YJ, Cunningham D. The UK NCRI MAGIC trial of perioperative chemotherapy in resectable gastric cancer: implications for clinical practice. *Ann Surg Oncol.* 2007;14(10):2687-2690.

Cunningham D, Allum WH, Stenning SP, et al. Perioperative chemotherapy versus surgery alone for resectable gastroesophageal cancer. *N Engl J Med.* 2006;355(1):11-20.

Cuschieri A, Fayers P, Fielding J, et al. Postoperative morbidity and mortality after D1 and D2 resections for gastric cancer: preliminary results of the MRC randomized controlled surgical trial. The Surgical Cooperative Group. *Lancet.* 1996;347(9007):995-999.

Dooley CP, Larson AW, Stace NH, et al. Double-contrast barium meal and upper gastrointestinal endoscopy. A comparative study. *Ann Intern Med.* 1984;101(4):538-545.

Ganpathi IS, So JB, Ho KY. Endoscopic ultrasonography for gastric cancer: does it influence treatment? *Surg Endosc.* 2006; 20(4):559-562.

Gotoda T, Iwasaki M, Kusano C, et al. Endoscopic resection of early gastric cancer treated by guideline and expanded National Cancer Centre criteria. *Br J Surg.* 2010;97(6):868-871.

Karpeh MS, Leon L, Klimstra D, Brennan MF. Lymph node staging in gastric cancer: is location more important than Number? An analysis of 1,038 patients. *Ann Surg.* 2000;232:362-571.

Kinkel K, Lu Y, Both M, et al. Detection of hepatic metastases from cancers of the gastrointestinal tract by using noninvasive imaging methods (US, CT, MR imaging, PET): a meta-analysis. *Radiology.* 2002;224(3):748-756.

Lee YT, Ng EK, Hung LC, et al. Accuracy of endoscopic ultrasonography in diagnosing ascites and predicting peritoneal metastases in gastric cancer patients. *Gut.* 2005;54(11):1541-1545.

NCCN Clinical Practice Guidelines in Oncology (NCCN Guidelines®) for Gastric Cancer V.2.2018. © 2016 National Comprehensive Cancer Network, Inc. 2018. All rights reserved. Accessed (August 14, 2018). To view the most recent and complete version of the guideline, go online to NCCN.org.

Power DG, Schattner MA, Gerdes H, et al. Endoscopic ultrasound can improve the selection for laparoscopy in patients with localized gastric cancer. *J Am Coll Surg.* 2009;208(2):173-178.

Rosenbaum SJ, Sterg H, Antoch G, et al. Staging and follow-up of gastrointestinal tumors with PET/CT. *Abdom Imaging.* 2006;31:25-35.

Saikawa Y, Kubota T, Kumagai K, et al. Phase II study of chemoradiotherapy with S-1 and low-dose cisplatin for inoperable advanced gastric cancer. *Int J Radiat Oncol Biol Phys.* 2008;71(1):173-179.

Sakuramoto S, Sasako M, Yamaguchi T, et al. Adjuvant chemotherapy for gastric cancer with S-1, an oral fluoropyrimidine. *N Engl J Med.* 2007;357:1810-1820.

Sarela AI, Lefkowitz R, Brennan MF, et al. Selection of patients with gastric adenocarcinoma for laparoscopic staging. *Am J Surg.* 2006;191(1):134-138.

Schwarz RE, Smith DD. Clinical impact of lymphadenectomy extent in resectable gastric cancer of advanced stage. *Ann Surg Oncol.* 2007;14:317-328.

Siewert JR, Feith M, Werner M, Stein HJ. Adenocarcinoma of the esophagogastric junction. Results of surgical therapy based on anatomical/topographic classification in 1,002 consecutive patients. *Ann Surg.* 2000;232:353-361.

Siewert JR, Stein HJ. Adenocarcinoma of the gastroesophageal junction: classification, pathology and extent of resection. *Dis Esophagus.* 1996;9:173-182.

Siewert JR, Stein HJ, Feith M. Adenocarcinoma of the esophagogastric junction. *Scand J Surg.* 2006;95:260-269.

Smith JW, Moreira J, Abood G, et al. The influence of (18) flourodeoxyglucose positron emission tomography on the management of gastroesophageal junction carcinoma. *Am J Surg.* 2009;197(3):308-312.

Songun I, Putter H, Kranenbarg EM, et al. Surgical treatment of gastric cancer: 15-year follow-up results of the randomized nationwide Dutch D1D2 trial. *Lancet Oncol.* 2010;11:439-449.

Yang SH, Zhang YC, Yang KH, et al. An evidence-based medicine review of lymphadenectomy extent for gastric cancer. *Am J Surg.* 2009;197(2):246-251.

Ychou M, Boige V, Pignon J-P, et al. Perioperative chemotherapy compared with surgery alone for resectable gastroesophageal adenocarcinoma: an FNCLCC and FFCD multicenter phase III trial. *J Clin Oncol* 2011;29:1715-1721.

Gastrointestinal Stromal Tumor

12

BENJAMIN D. MEDINA AND RONALD P. DeMATTEO

Based on the previous edition chapter "Gastrointestinal Stromal Tumor" by
John B. Ammori and Ronald P. DeMatteo

Case Presentation

A 70-year-old male has 4 months of early satiety. His past medical and surgical history are unremarkable. Review of systems is negative for any other symptoms. On physical examination, he has a palpable left, upper abdominal mass. There is no adenopathy. Contrast-enhanced CT scan of the abdomen and pelvis demonstrates a large, heterogenous mass associated with the gastric fundus without evidence of liver or peritoneal metastasis or adenopathy (Figure 12-1).

● DIFFERENTIAL DIAGNOSIS

The differential diagnosis of a gastric mass includes gastric adenocarcinoma, gastrointestinal stromal tumor (GIST), leiomyosarcoma, leiomyoma, gastric lymphoma, and neuroendocrine tumor. Given the exophytic growth pattern of the mass, gastric adenocarcinoma and neuroendocrine tumor are unlikely. Gastric lymphoma is unlikely since there was no lymphadenopathy on clinical or radiologic

examination. Leiomyomas are typically homogenous, and leiomyosarcomas are rare, making the most likely diagnoses a GIST.

● WORKUP

Endoscopy demonstrates a submucosal mass in the gastric body without any ulceration. Biopsy of the mucosa overlying the mass revealed no pathologic abnormality. Endoscopic ultrasound (EUS) showed a large heterogeneous mass contiguous with the gastric wall without perigastric lymphadenopathy. Fine needle aspiration (FNA) biopsy showed spindle cells, and immunohistochemistry was not performed.

As in this case, endoscopic biopsies are often unable to render a diagnosis since the mass is submucosal. If the tumor has eroded into the gastric mucosa, biopsy is more likely to yield a diagnosis. EUS is not mandatory in the workup of the extent of these tumors. In a patient with a resectable tumor who is fit for surgery, preoperative biopsy is not always necessary if the degree of suspicion of GIST is high. FNA or core needle biopsy is useful for tumors that are metastatic or clearly unresectable, if neoadjuvant therapy is considered, or if the

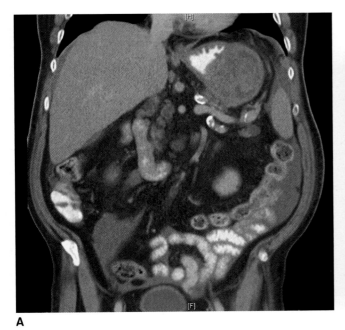

A

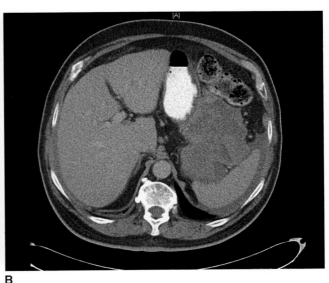

B

FIGURE 12-1. CT scan demonstrating a **(A)** large, heterogenous, partially necrotic left upper quadrant mass inseparable from the gastric fundus and **(B)** spleen and (not shown) the distal pancreas. There is a small amount of fluid behind the spleen.

diagnosis of lymphoma is strongly suspected. High-quality cross-sectional imaging of the abdomen and pelvis is crucial to evaluate the local and distant extent of disease. CT is preferred over MRI. PET scan is rarely required. The typical imaging finding is a large, hypervascular, exophytic, heterogeneous mass, often with central necrosis.

● DIAGNOSIS AND MEDICAL TREATMENT

The estimated annual number of GIST cases in the United States is 3 to 5,000. The stomach is the most common (60%) primary site of GIST, followed by the small intestine (30%), rectum, and extraintestinal. GIST rarely occurs in the colon.

The clinical presentation of GIST depends on both its size and location. Nearly 30% of GISTs are asymptomatic and discovered incidentally. Symptoms generally result from mass effect and are usually nonspecific, such as nausea, emesis, early satiety, abdominal distension, or pain. The median size of GIST in symptomatic patients is approximately 9 cm compared with nearly 3 cm in asymptomatic patients. Patients may also present with microcytic anemia due to subclinical gastrointestinal bleeding from erosion into the gastrointestinal tract. Overt hemorrhage can also occur from gastrointestinal erosion or intraperitoneal tumor rupture.

GISTs have three principal histologic patterns—spindle (70%), epithelioid (20%), and mixed. The definitive diagnosis of GIST is made by immunohistochemical expression of KIT (CD117 antigen) and consistent morphology. Approximately 95% of GISTs stain positive for KIT, with the remainder often having a *PDGFRA* mutation. The most frequent site of *KIT* mutation is exon 11 (70%), followed by exon 9 (10%), and exons 13 and 17 (rare). GISTs with an exon 9 mutation have a poorer clinical course compared to those with an exon 11 mutation.

Imatinib is a tyrosine kinase inhibitor that inhibits the KIT and PDGFRA oncoproteins and is the first-line therapy for metastatic GIST. Approximately 60% of patients have a partial response and 25% have disease stability. Tumors with *KIT* exon 11 mutations are more sensitive to imatinib therapy than tumors with *KIT* exon 9 mutations, with approximately 75% achieving a partial response compared to 45%, respectively. Adjuvant (i.e., postoperative) imatinib following complete resection of primary GIST increases recurrence-free survival (RFS) but does not appear to increase the chance of cure compared with surgery alone, which is about 70%. The optimal duration of adjuvant imatinib is unknown, but there is a suggestion that chronic therapy may be advisable for patients at high risk of recurrence. Neoadjuvant imatinib should be considered in clinical situations in which tumor downsizing would facilitate achieving negative resection margins, such as with large tumors that may require adjacent organ resection, gastroesophageal tumors, duodenal GISTs, and rectal GISTs. The tumor is reassessed with cross-sectional imaging, and surgery is often performed after 6 months of treatment, after which continued tumor shrinkage is often minimal.

Response to imatinib is readily assessed with CT. Initially, tumors may not decrease substantially in size, but the tumor appearance changes from heterogeneous and hypervascular to homogeneous, hypoattenuating, and cystic (Figure 12-2). Primary resistance to imatinib therapy is seen in 15% of tumors. Secondary resistance to imatinib occurs after approximately 18 months of therapy, often due to additional mutations in the *KIT* gene. Resistance may manifest as a new solid enhancing focus within a responding mass (Figure 12-2). Patients who develop resistance to imatinib may respond to second-line sunitinib therapy or third-line therapy regorafenib.

The most common sites of metastatic disease are the liver and peritoneum. The three major factors predicting metastases following resection of the primary are tumor site of origin, size, and mitotic rate (Table 12-1). These variables have

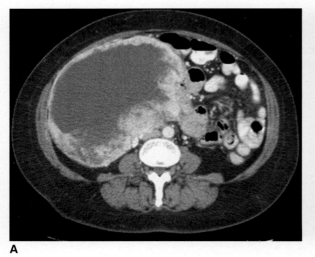

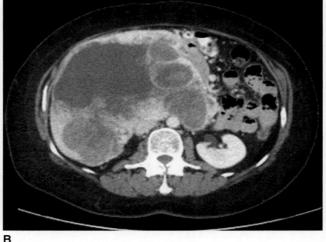

A   **B**

FIGURE 12-2. CT imaging of imatinib response and secondary resistance. **A:** Characteristic response of a GIST to imatinib, showing a homogenous, cystic center of the tumor. **B:** After several months of imatinib, new peripheral, enhancing foci within a responding mass indicates the development of secondary resistance.

Table 12-1	Miettinen Risk of Recurrence Following the Resection of Primary GIST				
Tumor Parameters		**Risk for Progressive Disease (%), Based on Site of Origin**			
Mitotic Rate	**Size**	**Stomach**	**Jejunum/Ileum**	**Duodenum**	**Rectum**
≤5 per 50 HPFs	≤2 cm	0%	0%	0%	0%
	>2, ≤5 cm	1.9%	4.3%	8.3%	8.5%
	>5, ≤10 cm	3.6%	24%	Insufficient data	Insufficient data
	>10 cm	10%	52%	34%	57%
>5 per 50 HPFs	≤2 cm	0%	50%	Insufficient data	54%
	>2, ≤5 cm	16%	73%	50%	52%
	>5, ≤10 cm	55%	85%	Insufficient data	Insufficient data
	>10 cm	86%	90%	86%	71%

HPFs, high-power fields.

Reprinted from Miettinen M, Lasota J. Gastrointestinal stromal tumors: pathology and prognosis at different sites. *Semin Diagnostic Pathol.* 2006; 23(2): 70-83. Copyright © 2006 Elsevier, with permission.

been incorporated into a nomogram to predict RFS after resection of localized, primary GIST (Figure 12-3). There is also a risk scoring system (Table 12-1) that serves as the basis for the AJCC staging system for GIST. While the standard treatment for metastatic disease is imatinib, there are three main indications for cytoreductive surgery in metastatic or recurrent GIST. These are: (1) emergencies such as hemorrhage, bowel perforation, or rarely obstruction; (2) resectable disease that is stable or responsive to imatinib; and (3) focal progression defined as the development of secondary drug resistance to imatinib in one or a few sites while other sites of metastatic disease remain stable. In the latter case, one may consider resecting only the drug resistant tumors if complete resection of all disease is not possible.

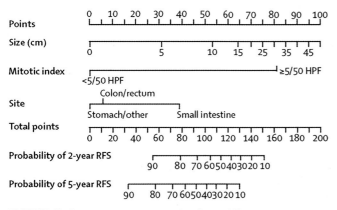

FIGURE 12-3. Nomogram to predict 2- and 5-year recurrence-free survival. The nomogram is available at https://www.mskcc.org/nomograms/gastrointestinal. (Used from Gold JS, Gönen M, Gutiérrez A, et al. Development and validation of a prognostic nomogram for recurrence-free survival after complete surgical resection of localised primary gastrointestinal stromal tumour: a retrospective analysis. *Lancet Oncol.* 2009;10:1045-1052, with permission.)

Cytoreductive surgery does not confer a survival advantage for unresectable, progressive disease or diffuse progression during tyrosine kinase therapy.

● SURGICAL APPROACH

Surgery is the principal treatment for resectable primary GIST. Complete surgical resection with negative microscopic margins is the treatment of choice for resectable tumors without evidence of metastasis. Segmental resection of the stomach or small intestine is appropriate. Formal gastrectomy, for example, for wider clearance of uninvolved tissue is unnecessary. Since lymph node metastases are rare, lymphadenectomy is unnecessary unless there is clinical suspicion of lymph node involvement. GISTs are often exophytic from the stomach or small bowel and can typically be lifted away from adjacent organs. Some tumors can become densely adherent to surrounding organs requiring en bloc resection in order to achieve complete resection. In general, one may approach surgical resection of GIST by either a laparoscopic (up to about 8-cm tumors) or open approach depending on technical concerns, as well as surgeon preference and experience.

The key technical steps for resection of a gastric GIST are as follows (Table 12-2). The abdomen is explored to exclude the presence of peritoneal or liver metastases. The lesser sac is entered through the gastrocolic ligament. The tumor is identified. A partial gastrectomy is performed with 1-cm gross margins. This can often be done with GIA stapling devices. Care should be taken to avoid narrowing the gastric lumen. If the tumor is located near the pylorus, gastrointestinal reconstruction with a gastroduodenal or gastrojejunal anastomosis may be necessary. Total gastrectomy is rarely needed, especially if neoadjuvant imatinib is used for a gastroesophageal GIST.

Table 12-2	Gastrointestinal Stromal Tumor

Key Technical Steps

1. Midline incision or laparoscopy
2. Abdominal exploration for metastatic disease
3. Partial gastrectomy for complete tumor clearance
4. Remove portions of organs that adhere to the tumor if necessary
5. Gastrointestinal reconstruction is usually unnecessary as wedge resections can often be performed

Potential Pitfalls

- Tumor bleeding
- Tumor rupture

The patient presented in this chapter underwent laparotomy due to the large tumor size and anticipated need for a complex resection. At laparotomy, there was no evidence of peritoneal or liver metastases. A large tumor arising from the greater curvature of the stomach was identified. It was densely adherent to the pancreatic tail and splenic hilum. A complete resection was achieved with an en bloc resection including wedge partial gastrectomy, splenectomy, and distal pancreatectomy.

● SPECIAL INTRAOPERATIVE CONSIDERATIONS

Meticulous and careful intraoperative handling of GISTs is critical. GISTs are usually fragile with extensive necrosis or hemorrhage. If the pseudocapsule is torn, bleeding and tumor rupture may occur, increasing the risk of peritoneal recurrence. GISTs also tend to parasitize blood supply from surrounding structures, so numerous vessels supplying the tumor may be encountered.

Metastatic disease may be discovered at exploration. If there are limited and resectable metastases, resection of all diseases should be performed, and postoperative imatinib should be used. If there is extensive metastatic disease, it is a clinical judgment as to whether the primary GIST should be resected or not, depending on the difficulty of doing so and the presence of symptoms.

● POSTOPERATIVE MANAGEMENT

Routine postoperative care for abdominal surgery is recommended. Postoperative bleeding is a rare complication and may occur early in the postoperative period if feeding vessels were not adequately controlled. Gastrointestinal leakage is rare and usually presents approximately 1 week postoperatively. It can often be controlled with percutaneous drainage and antibiotics, but reoperation is necessary for free intraperitoneal leaks. Long-term follow-up after full postoperative recovery includes history and physical as well as CT scan every 3 to 6 months for 3 to 5 years and annually thereafter, depending on the risk of tumor recurrence.

Case Conclusion

The patient in the case presented in this chapter recovered well without surgical complication. He is taking adjuvant imatinib and is without recurrence several years following surgery.

TAKE HOME POINTS

- GIST is the most common sarcoma.
- GIST nearly always expresses the KIT protein by immunohistochemistry.
- *KIT* mutation occurs in 75% of tumors while *PDGFRA* mutation occurs in about 12%.
- Patients may present with nonspecific symptoms, abdominal fullness, or gastrointestinal hemorrhage.
- Tumors tend to grow in an exophytic fashion, and lymph nodes are rarely involved.
- Endoscopy may show a submucosal mass, occasionally with an overlying ulcer.
- Surgery with negative margins is the goal for localized, primary GIST and results in cure about 70% of the time.
- Patients at high risk for recurrence should receive adjuvant imatinib for at least 1 year.
- Imatinib is the first-line agent for metastatic GIST, although resistance commonly develops.
- Surgery plays a role in selected patients with resectable, metastatic disease that is stable or responsive to imatinib and in selected patients with focal progression.

SUGGESTED READINGS

Agulnik M, Asare EA, Baldini EH, et al. Soft tissue sarcoma. *American Joint Commission on Cancer (AJCC) Staging Manual*, 7th ed. Springer, 2016.

Corless CL, Ballman KV, Antonescu CR, et al. Pathologic and molecular features correlate with long-term outcome after adjuvant therapy of resected primary GI stromal tumor: the ACOSOG Z9001 trial. *J Clin Oncol.* 2014;32(15):1563-1570.

Demetri GD, von Mehren M, Antonescu CR, et al. NCCN Task Force report: update on the management of patients with gastrointestinal stromal tumors. *J Natl Compr Canc Netw.* 2010;8(suppl 2):S1-S41.

Joensuu H, DeMatteo RP. The management of gastrointestinal stromal tumors: a model for targeted and multidisciplinary therapy of malignancy. *Annu Rev Med.* 2012;63:247-258.

Splenectomy for Hematologic Disease

13

MIHIR M. SHAH AND JOHN F. SWEENEY

Based on the previous edition chapter "Splenectomy for Hematologic Disease" by John F. Sweeney

Presentation

Case 1: A 44-year-old female presented to her primary care doctor several months ago complaining of a recent onset of easy bruising and gum bleeding. A complete blood count (CBC) demonstrated a platelet count <10 × 10⁹/L. She was diagnosed with immune thrombocytopenic purpura (ITP) and admitted to the hospital for treatment. She was started on high-dose intravenous immunoglobulin and high-dose corticosteroids with an excellent response in her platelet count. She was discharged home on a gradual prednisone taper. As her prednisone doses were weaned below 20 mg per day, the patient experienced a recurrence in her thrombocytopenia with associated recurrence of easy bruising.

Case 2: A 71-year-old gentleman with idiopathic myelofibrosis (IMF) for several years started complaining of intermittent episodes of intense left upper quadrant pain and decrease in appetite within the last 2 months. He also complained of worsening fatigue, and laboratory analysis revealed mild anemia (hemoglobin 11.3 g/dL). A computed tomography of the abdomen revealed a 26-cm (anteroposterior) × 13 cm (transverse) × 30 cm (craniocaudal) spleen consistent with massive splenomegaly.

● DIFFERENTIAL DIAGNOSIS

Case 1: Excluding trauma, benign hematologic diseases are the most common indication for splenectomy (Table 13-1). ITP is the most common indication for splenectomy and constitutes >70% of patients undergoing splenectomy for benign disease. ITP is a disorder characterized by antiplatelet antibodies to platelet membrane glycoprotein. This results in opsonization of platelets and their premature removal from the circulation by the spleen. Adult patients typically present with petechiae, purpura, and bruising tendency. Mucosal bleeding, including epistaxis and hematuria, tend to be more frequent when the platelet count decreases to <20 × 10⁹/L. The incidence of severe bleeding (e.g., intracranial hemorrhage) increases with platelet counts below 10 × 10⁹/L.

Case 2: Hematologic and nonhematologic conditions associated with myelofibrosis include polycythemia vera, essential thrombocythemia, chronic myelogenous leukemia, Hodgkin's/non-Hodgkin's lymphoma, other hematologic malignancies, toxins, infections, and carcinoma.

Additional benign hematologic conditions that are indications for splenectomy include patients with congenital hemolytic anemia, metabolism abnormalities, hemoglobinopathies, and erythrocyte structure abnormalities (e.g., hereditary spherocytosis and elliptocytosis). Splenectomy may be indicated as a diagnostic tool or for palliation in patients with malignant hematologic disease. Surgical staging is utilized most often in Hodgkin's disease, resulting in a change in diagnosis and subsequent impact on therapy and prognosis in up to 30% to 40% of patients. Splenectomy can also provide relief to patients with symptomatic splenomegaly, which may or may not be accompanied by hypersplenism and cytopenias. Patients with malignant hematologic diseases are more likely to have massively enlarged spleens (>1,000 g), resulting in significant discomfort and pain as well as early satiety. When splenomegaly is accompanied by cytopenias (hypersplenism), the cytopenia is often improved or sometimes cured by removal of the spleen.

● WORKUP

Case 1: Although the presumptive diagnosis is ITP, the patient undergoes a bone marrow aspirate that demonstrates normal marrow cellularity with specific mention of adequate megakaryocytes. Review of the peripheral blood smear does not demonstrate platelet clumping.

Case 2: Physical exam would usually reveal splenomegaly. Bone marrow aspirate is the gold standard for diagnosis. This patient previously had a bone marrow aspirate at the time of diagnosis. However, a bone marrow aspirate was repeated to check for progression and stage his disease, and was deemed stable based on unchanged quantity of CD-34–positive blasts (<5% of total nucleated cell population).

● DISCUSSION

Case 1: First-line therapy for ITP includes oral corticosteroids and IV immunoglobulin. The majority of patients will initially respond to medical management of ITP, but recurrent thrombocytopenia is common. The indication and timing of splenectomy is often individualized according to response to treatment and patient and physician preferences. Splenectomy is indicated for ITP in patients with episodes of severe bleeding related to thrombocytopenia, patients who

Table 13-1	Hematologic Indications for Splenectomy

Diagnosis	Incidence
Benign	
Immune thrombocytopenic purpura (ITP)	21%–68%
Thrombocytopenic thrombotic purpura (TTP)	2%–6%
Hereditary spherocytosis	4%–13%
Autoimmune hemolytic anemia	3%–10%
Evan's syndrome	1%
Hemoglobinopathies	1%
Sickle cell anemia	
Beta thalassemia	
Hemoglobin S/C disease	
Malignant	
Lymphoma	10%–55%
Hodgkin's disease	
Non-Hodgkin's lymphoma	
Leukemia	7%–10%
Chronic lymphocytic leukemia	
Chronic myelogenous leukemia	
Hairy cell leukemia	3%–6%
Other	
Myeloproliferative disorders (myelofibrosis)	
Idiopathic hypersplenism	
Sarcoidosis	
Splenomegaly with portal hypertension	
Splenic tumor/cyst	

fail to respond to 4 to 6 weeks of medical therapy, patients who require toxic doses of immunosuppressive medication to achieve remission, or patients who relapse following an initial response to steroids. Patients with ITP are ideal candidates for a minimally invasive approach because they are frequently young, otherwise healthy patients with normal-sized spleens.

Case 2: Degree of anemia is the most important prognostic factor for chronic IMF (CIMF). Hemoglobin <10 g/dL is associated with poor prognosis. Primary treatment is medical with excellent advances in target-specific directed therapy and immunotherapy. Splenectomy does not cure myeloproliferative diseases. It is associated with increased perioperative morbidity and mortality when performed for malignant diseases compared to benign disease, mainly due to patient risk factors and technical challenges in these patients. Hence, it should be performed very selectively. Indications include symptomatic portal hypertension, severely symptomatic splenomegaly, transfusion-dependent anemia, severe thrombocytopenia, and uncontrollable hemolysis. Due to significant symptoms and massive splenomegaly, this patient was offered splenectomy.

Table 13-2	Laparoscopic Splenectomy

Key Technical Steps

1. Patient positioned in modified right lateral decubitus position.
2. Abdominal access via open Hasson technique with 12-mm trocar ~3–4 cm below the left costal margin in the midclavicular line.
3. Two 5-mm trocars are placed along the costal margin between xiphoid process and Hasson trocar.
4. Divide the splenocolic ligament and mobilize the splenic flexure caudad.
5. Additional 12-mm trocar is placed in the left anterior axillary line below the costal margin.
6. The short gastric vessels are divided in their entirety up to the level of the superior pole of the spleen.
7. Mobilize inferior pole of the spleen by dividing splenorenal ligament.
8. Mobilize the superior pole of the spleen to isolate the splenic hilum.
9. The splenic hilar vessels are divided with an endoscopic stapler.
10. Spleen is placed in endobag, which is exteriorized through the Hasson trocar site so the spleen can be morcellated.
11. Upon completion, the abdomen is then reinspected laparoscopically to ensure hemostasis.
12. All ports are withdrawn under direct vision. The lateral 12-mm port is closed with absorbable suture using an endoclose device, and the Hasson Trocar site is close in layers with absorbable sutures.

Potential Pitfalls

- Injury to the splenic artery or vein results in significant and rapid blood loss, mandating conversion to HALS or open splenectomy.
- Injury to the short gastric vessels results in significant and rapid blood loss; if not controlled quickly, mandates conversion to HALS or open splenectomy.
- Injury to the tail of the pancreas leads to pancreatic leak, with resulting pancreatitis, pancreatic abscess, or pancreatic fistula.

● TECHNIQUE FOR MINIMALLY INVASIVE SPLENECTOMY

Removal of the spleen in a minimally invasive fashion is facilitated by the fact that the anatomic landmarks are relatively consistent, the operation is extirpative, and in most cases, the spleen does not need to be preserved for pathology so it can be morcellated in the abdominal cavity prior to removal (Table 13-2). Laparoscopic splenectomy (LS) has been shown in several retrospective studies to have equivalent or superior short- and long-term outcomes when compared to open splenectomy.

● PREOPERATIVE PREPARATION

The patient's preoperative preparation includes administration of pneumococcal vaccine (PCV13), Haemophilus influenzae type b vaccination (Hib), and meningococcal vaccines (MenACWY and MenB) at least 2 weeks before surgery. The evening before surgery, patients commence a clear liquid diet and take a mild laxative several hours before bedtime to decompress the colon and facilitate laparoscopic visualization of the left upper quadrant and spleen. Several units of packed red blood cells are crossmatched, and in patients with idiopathic thrombocytopenic purpura, platelets are crossmatched for administration after the splenic artery has been ligated intraoperatively if there is failure of clot formation.

Immediately preoperatively, pneumatic compression boots are applied, and a preoperative antibiotic (2 g cefazolin; 3 g if weight is >120 kg) is given. Patients who have been receiving corticosteroids within 6 months of surgery are given stress doses of intravenous corticosteroids. Before transport to the operating room, a beanbag-stabilizing device is placed on the operating table to enable subsequent patient positioning and stabilization. After endotracheal induction of general anesthesia, a Foley catheter and an orogastric tube are placed.

The patient is positioned in the incomplete right lateral decubitus position at an angle of 45°. This allows the patient's position to be changed from nearly supine to nearly lateral by tilting the operating table. In this way, a combined supine and lateral approach can be realized. It is important to position the patient with the iliac crest immediately over the table's kidney rest and mid-breakpoint. The kidney rest is elevated and the table flexed, allowing more distance between the iliac crest and the left lower costal margin in the midaxillary line. The beanbag-stabilizing device is activated, and the patient's hip is secured to the table with loosely applied tape. Legs are padded with pillows, and an axillary roll is placed. The left arm is hung over the chest on a sling. The arm must be far enough cephalad to clear the operative field and allow obstruction-free use of the laparoscopic instruments. All pressure points are adequately padded.

The skin is prepared and draped so that either laparoscopy or open surgery can be performed. The table is tilted 30° to the left to place the patient in the near-supine position. Before incisions are made, the area is anesthetized with long-lasting local anesthetic.

● LAPAROSCOPIC SPLENECTOMY

We prefer to obtain intra-abdominal access via an open technique with placement of a 12-mm Hasson trocar approximately 3 to 4 cm below the costal margin in the left midclavicular line (Figure 13-1). The abdomen is then insufflated to a pressure of 15 mm Hg with carbon dioxide and

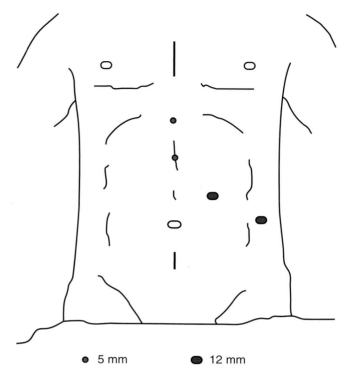

● 5 mm   ⬤ 12 mm

FIGURE 13-1. Laparoscopic splenectomy port placement.

a 10-mm, 30° laparoscope is introduced into the abdomen. Two 5-mm trocars are then placed in the upper midline or to the left of the midline along the costal margin. The first 5-mm trocar is placed 3 to 4 cm below the xiphoid process, and the second 5-mm trocar is placed in between the subxiphoid 5-mm trocar and the Hasson trocar. The abdomen is inspected with special attention paid to the splenic hilum, greater omentum, and splenocolic regions that are common locations for accessory splenic tissue. Accessory spleens are found in 10% to 15% of patients with hematologic disease and have been associated with disease recurrence in patients with ITP when they are not removed.

Following division of the splenocolic ligament and mobilization of the splenic flexure, an additional 12-mm trocar is placed in the left anterior axillary line, below the costal margin. The patient is then placed in steep reverse Trendelenburg position and the table rolled to the patient's right giving a true left lateral decubitus position. Ultrasonic shears are used to divide the gastrosplenic ligament and short gastric blood vessels, allowing the stomach to fall to the patient's right and providing excellent exposure to the splenic hilum. The splenic artery can then be easily identified and ligated with hemoclips if desired at this point of the case. Attention is then turned toward mobilization of the lower pole of the spleen. The splenophrenic and the splenorenal ligaments are divided using ultrasonic shears. If a lower pole vessel is encountered at this point, it is divided using an endoscopic stapling device with a vascular cartridge. This approach allows for visualization of the splenic hilum and the tail of the pancreas by retracting the spleen toward the abdominal wall. The superior splenophrenic attachments to the upper pole of the spleen are left intact to prevent torsion of the spleen during division of the hilum. The endoscopic stapling device with a vascular cartridge is then used to divide the well-exposed splenic hilum. Several fires of the stapler may be necessary. Following division of the remaining upper pole attachments, the spleen is placed into a specimen retrieval bag. The mouth of the bag is brought through the 12-mm Hasson trocar site, and the spleen is then morcellated with sponge forceps and removed in pieces. Special care must be taken to avoid ripping the endoscopic bag during this process in order to prevent spillage of splenic tissue in the abdomen. The left upper quadrant is irrigated and inspected for hemostasis. A second search for accessory splenic tissue is undertaken before the 12-mm fascial openings are securely closed with absorbable suture and the skin incisions are closed. The orogastric tube is removed in the operating room, and the patient is taken to the recovery room.

● HAND-ASSISTED LAPAROSCOPIC SPLENECTOMY

The LS can be converted to hand-assisted laparoscopic splenectomy (HALS) if difficult anatomy, dense adhesions due to a previous upper abdominal surgery or excessive splenomegaly, is encountered. Preoperatively, the decision to proceed with HALS is made for patients with very large spleens or if the spleen must be removed intact for pathologic examination. When HALS is indicated preoperatively, we still place all trocars as described for a LS and proceed with division of the gastrosplenic ligament and short gastric blood vessels (Table 13-3). This provides excellent exposure to the splenic hilum and allows for early ligation of the splenic artery, which we feel is an essential step in patients with significant splenomegaly. We then create an incision connecting the two 5-mm trocars about 7 cm in size in the left paramedian position (Figure 13-2). The left hand is then placed into the abdomen, which is then reinsufflated. There are several commercially available hand-port devices that can be used for HALS. The spleen is then mobilized as described for a total LS with the left hand providing gentle traction while at the same time preventing injury to the splenic capsule by the ultrasonic shears or a laparoscopic grasper. After the splenic hilum is divided and the spleen completely mobilized, it is placed in a specimen retrieval bag. A sterile radiograph cassette bag can be placed in the abdomen through the hand incision to retrieve those spleens that do not fit in the large specimen retrieval bags. The fascia is closed with appropriate strength suture and the abdomen then reinsufflated and inspected for hemostasis as described above.

● INTRAOPERATIVE CONSIDERATION

It should be considered standard of care to perform this operation with <1% mortality and <4% incidence of pancreatic injury. It is also prudent to place a closed suction drain, when

| Table 13-3 | Hand-Assisted Laparoscopic Splenectomy |

Key Technical Steps

1. Patient is positioned in modified right lateral decubitus position.
2. Abdominal access via open Hasson technique with 12-mm trocar ~3–4 cm below the left costal margin in the midclavicular line.
3. Two 5-mm trocars are placed in the paramedian position ~7–8 cm apart with the first being just below xiphoid process.
4. Divide the splenocolic ligament and mobilize of the splenic flexure caudad.
5. Additional 12-mm trocar is placed in the left anterior axillary line below the costal margin.
6. The short gastric vessels are divided in their entirety up to the level of the superior pole of the spleen.
7. Connect the 5-mm skin incisions and open the subcutaneous tissue and fascia.
8. Place hand port. Utilize left hand to protect and retract the spleen and the right hand to use dissecting instruments.
9. Mobilize inferior pole of the spleen by dividing splenorenal ligament.
10. Mobilize the superior pole of the spleen to isolate the splenic hilum.
11. The splenic hilar vessels are divided with an endoscopic stapler.
12. Spleen placed in large endobag or sterile x-ray cassette cover and exteriorized through the hand-port site, so the spleen can be morcellated or removed in its entirety.
13. Close hand-port site with heavy monofilament suture. Upon completion, the abdomen is then reinspected laparoscopically to ensure hemostasis. All ports are withdrawn under direct vision. The lateral 12-mm port is closed with absorbable suture using an endoclose device, and the Hasson Trocar site is close in layers with absorbable sutures.

Potential Pitfalls

- Injury to the splenic artery or vein results in significant and rapid blood loss, mandating conversion to open splenectomy.
- Injury to the short gastric vessels results in significant and rapid blood loss; if not controlled quickly, mandates conversion to open splenectomy.
- Injury to the tail of the pancreas leads to pancreatic leak, with resulting pancreatitis, pancreatic abscess, or pancreatic fistula.
- Hand-port site at increased risk for development of incisional hernia over time.

there is a specific concern about the pancreatic tail integrity. During reexploration for splenic tissue retention, intraoperative gamma probe scanning may be useful in locating small foci of splenic tissue.

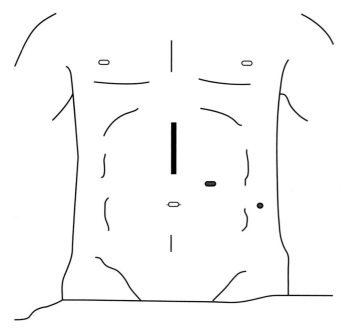

FIGURE 13-2. Hand-assisted laparoscopic splenectomy (HALS) port placement.

● POSTOPERATIVE CARE

Postoperatively, the patient is allowed clear liquids orally and ambulates the day of surgery. The Foley catheter is removed the following morning. Pain is controlled with intermittent parenteral narcotics until the patient is able to take oral pain medication. Diet is advanced on postoperative day 1, and the patient is discharged when oral intake is tolerated and pain is controlled with oral analgesics, usually on postoperative day 2.

Postsplenectomy, up to 50% of the patients may experience thrombocytosis. Hemorrhage and thromboembolic phenomena may occur from thrombocytosis. It is reasonable to consider aspirin 81 mg for platelet counts in excess of 750,000 mm³.

Postsplenectomy, the patient should receive pneumococcal (PPSV23) vaccination at least 8 weeks after PCV13, followed by PPSV23 revaccination 5 years later, and again after the age of 65 (5 years from the last dose, if the other doses were given prior to 65 years of age). There is currently no recommendation for PCV13 revaccination. If the patient has already received PPSV23 but not PCV13, PCV13 should be given at least 1 year after the PPSV23 dose.

In addition, the patient should receive a total of two initial doses of meningococcal (MenACWY) vaccination. If a dose has been given preoperatively, the next dose of MenACWY should be a minimum of 8 weeks after the first dose and then revaccinate with one dose every 5 years. Also, the series of meningococcal B (MenB) vaccination should be completed. There is no recommendation on MenB revaccination at this time.

Case Conclusion

Case 1: The patient does very well after LS. Her platelet count returns to the normal range before discharge from the hospital. At 6- and 12-month follow-up, the patient has no clinical evidence of thrombocytopenia and has normal platelet counts.

LS has become the "gold standard" for removal of the spleen in the setting of ITP. Although the increase in platelet number that defines a complete response to splenectomy varies between studies, numerous retrospective reviews and prospective nonrandomized trials have determined that the response rates (80% to 89%) and long-term remission rates (50% to 70%) to LS are comparable to those following open splenectomy, despite initial concern about the accuracy of accessory spleen identification using laparoscopy. LS also provides patients with improved short-term morbidity. Reductions in postoperative morbidity characteristic of minimally invasive procedures such as reduced length of hospital stay and reduced postoperative ileus have been consistently demonstrated in patients with ITP who undergo LS.

Case 2: Postoperative visit confirmed resolution of the left upper quadrant pain after HALS. The spleen weighed 3,670 g. The patient continued to follow-up with his hematologist close to his residence.

TAKE HOME POINTS

- Immune thrombocytopenic purpura (ITP) is the most common indication for splenectomy excluding trauma.
- Splenectomy is indicated for treatment of ITP in patients with episodes of severe bleeding related to thrombocytopenia, patients who fail to respond to 4 to 6 weeks of medical therapy, patients who require toxic doses of immunosuppressive medications to achieve remission, or patients who relapse following an initial response to steroids.
- Laparoscopic splenectomy (LS) is the optimal approach for removal of the spleen in the setting of ITP. It is associated with a shorter hospital stay, decreased postoperative pain, and earlier return to regular activities.
- Accessory spleens are found in 10% to 15% of patients and if not removed at the time of splenectomy will lead to recurrence of ITP.
- LS for ITP is associated with short-term response rates of 80% to 89% and complete long-term remission rates of 50% to 70% that are compatible with outcomes for open splenectomy.
- Splenectomy is not curative for myeloproliferative diseases and should be performed selectively after thorough discussion with the patient and the patient's hematologist.
- Severe thrombocytosis after splenectomy may have implications, and it may be reasonable to treat it prophylactically for platelet counts >750,000 mm³.

SUGGESTED READINGS

Ahmed A, Chang CC. Chronic idiopathic myelofibrosis: clinico-pathologic features, pathogenesis, and prognosis. *Arch Pathol Lab Med.* 2006;130(8):1133-1143.

Bagrodia N, Button AM, Spanheimer PM, et al. Morbidity and mortality following elective splenectomy for benign and malignant hematologic conditions: analysis of the American College of Surgeons National Surgical Quality Improvement Program Data. *JAMA Surg.* 2014;149(10):1022-1029.

Bresler L, Guerci A, Brunaud L, et al. Laparoscopic splenectomy for idiopathic thrombocytopenic purpura: outcome and long-term results. *World J Surg.* 2002;26:111-114.

Brunt LM, Langer JC, Quasebarth MA, et al. Comparative analysis of laparoscopic versus open splenectomy. *Am J Surg.* 1996;172:596-599; discussion 599-601.

Centers for Disease Control and Prevention. (2016). Recommended adult immunization schedule. Retrieved from http://www.cdc.gov/vaccines/schedules/downloads/adult/adult-schedule.pdf

Friedman RL, Fallas MJ, Carroll BJ, et al. Laparoscopic splenectomy for ITP. The gold standard. *Surg Endosc.* 1996;10:991-995.

Mikhael J, Northridge K, Lindquist K, et al. Short-term and long-term failure of laparoscopic splenectomy in adult immune thrombocytopenic purpura patients: a systematic review. *Am J Hematol.* 2009;84(11):743-748.

Rescorla FJ, Engum SA, West KW, et al. Laparoscopic splenectomy has become the gold standard in children. *Am Surg.* 2002;68:297-301; discussion 301-302.

Targarona EM, Espert JJ, Cerdan G, et al. Effect of spleen size on splenectomy outcome. A comparison of open and laparoscopic surgery. *Surg Endosc.* 1999;13:559-562.

Morbid Obesity

NABEEL R. OBEID AND DANA A. TELEM

14

Based on the previous edition chapter "Morbid Obesity" by John Morton

Presentation

A 42-year-old female with hypertension managed with two antihypertensive agents, dyslipidemia on a statin, obstructive sleep apnea, and depression presents for consultation due to concerns about her weight. She states that she has struggled with her weight for most of her life, beginning in early adolescence, and has been unsuccessful with multiple attempts at weight loss including formal dieting programs. She describes a cyclical pattern of losing 10 to 20 pounds with a strict diet, followed by weight regain despite her best efforts. She is now at her heaviest weight, and her body mass index (BMI) is 47.5 kg/m². Her primary care provider is concerned that her obesity is significantly and negatively affecting her overall health, including her numerous comorbid conditions. She is referred to your office for evaluation.

● DIFFERENTIAL DIAGNOSIS

Overweight, obesity, and morbid obesity are chronic disease conditions that are diagnosed and classified based on BMI, which is calculated using measurements of weight in kilograms divided by height in meters squared. The healthy range for BMI is 18 to 25 kg/m², and Table 14-1 lists the World Health Organization (WHO) designations for overweight and obesity based on BMI. A BMI > 35 kg/m² is commonly referred to as morbid obesity, and a BMI above 50 kg/m² is termed super obesity.

The etiology of obesity is multifactorial, including both genetic and environmental influences. Some common conditions associated with weight gain include hypothyroidism,

Table 14-1	WHO Classification for Overweight and Obesity Based on BMI
BMI (kg/m²)	**Classification**
18.5–24.9	Healthy
25–29.9	Overweight
30–34.9	Obesity Class 1
35–39.9	Obesity Class 2
≥40	Obesity Class 3

Cushing syndrome, polycystic ovarian syndrome, and the use of certain medications. A minority of obese patients may have other, more specific and relatively uncommon conditions that may also affect their weight, such as Prader-Willi syndrome.

● WORKUP

The primary workup begins with a comprehensive history. It is important to gain an understanding of the chronicity and severity of the disease, as well as documentation of prior weight loss attempts. Many times, this will include formal diet programs, and one should inquire about the weight loss results related to these attempts. Functional status, level of independence, and current physical activity level are also important. Obesity-related comorbidities are common and should detail the extent of the disease (e.g., poorly-controlled diabetes requiring insulin or daily gastroesophageal reflux symptoms requiring maximal medical therapy). Past medical and surgical histories may identify risk factors like chronic kidney disease and venous thromboembolic events (VTE) or relative contraindications to certain bariatric procedures such as inflammatory bowel disease, recent or current neoplastic process, or previous gastrointestinal tract surgery. Medications should be reviewed, with specific attention to any aspirin, nonsteroidal anti-inflammatory drugs (NSAIDs), steroids, anticoagulant, or weight loss medication usage. Family history should be reviewed for diseases such as neoplasia or VTE. A comprehensive social history is essential, which includes psychosocial factors, family and social support system, and detailed substance use or abuse history (including all nicotine products). It is also wise to inquire about the patient's specific motivations for pursuing bariatric surgery.

A thorough physical examination should then be performed, including vital sign, height, and weight measurements. This will allow for calculation of the patient's BMI. The main focus will be the abdominal exam, which includes inspection for any scars or deformities in addition to palpation for masses, organomegaly, hernias, and to assess for tenderness. Patients are usually enrolled in a multidisciplinary bariatric program, which includes adjuncts such as a psychological assessment and nutrition evaluation. Laboratory analysis is performed and often includes a complete blood count, hepatic panel, thyroid function tests, and vitamin and micronutrient levels. Controversy exists regarding the need for routine preoperative evaluation of the foregut via esophagogastroduodenoscopy (EGD) or upper gastrointestinal series (UGIS). Patients also attend support group meetings to gain a better understanding of the lifelong commitment and to set realistic expectations.

Presentation Continued

The patient states she has tried formal diet programs with only modest, transient results. She is fully independent and walks for 30 minutes three to four times per week. She denies any history of diabetes or reflux symptoms, and does not take any NSAIDs or anticoagulation. Her past surgical history is significant for two Cesarean sections. She is married with two children, and her husband and extended family are very supportive of her decision, which she state is motivated by her desire to live a more active lifestyle with her children. She has never smoked and states she drinks alcoholic beverages in social settings, approximately one to two times per month. Her BMI is 47.5 kg/m², and there is a well-healed Pfannenstiel scar. There were no reservations from her psychological evaluation, and she demonstrated comprehension of her dietary instructions. Blood work revealed a vitamin D deficiency, for which she was started on supplementation.

● DIAGNOSIS AND TREATMENT

The surgeon will be able to diagnose a patient with morbid obesity on the basis of BMI as well as exclusion of atypical causes of weight gain. In addition, one will determine whether or not a patient is an appropriate surgical candidate based on the information gathered from the workup described previously. Coverage for bariatric surgery is many times limited to those patients with BMI ≥ 40 kg/m² or BMI ≥ 35 kg/m² with comorbidities.

The most durable and effective treatment for morbid obesity is bariatric surgery, which not only results in substantial weight loss but also aids in improvement or resolution of obesity-related comorbidities. Bariatric surgery has been demonstrated to extend life expectancy and improve overall quality of life as well. New procedural options are on the horizon, mostly endoluminal in nature, but lack of robust clinical experience and long-term data have limited the role of such therapies at present time, and further description is beyond the scope of this text.

● SURGICAL APPROACH

The two most commonly performed operations for the treatment of morbid obesity are laparoscopic sleeve gastrectomy (LSG) and laparoscopic Roux-en-Y gastric bypass (LRYGB). There are relative indications and contraindications for each procedure that should guide the surgeon

when recommending surgery. Active nicotine use is a relative contraindication to bariatric surgery. The need for regular administration of aspirin or NSAIDs is a contraindication for LRYGB because of the increased risk of marginal ulceration. Inflammatory bowel disease is another contraindication given the need to perform anastomoses involving the small intestine. Patients with poorly-controlled diabetes may have an added metabolic benefit from LRYGB as compared to LSG, although both procedures improve glycemic control. The relationship between acid reflux and sleeve gastrectomy is variable, with resolution in some patients and severe exacerbation of disease in others. Thus, intractable reflux or severe disease including Barrett's esophagus (BE) are considered relative contraindications for sleeve gastrectomy. In particular, patients with BE are generally counseled toward LRYGB because of the procedure's antireflux properties.

Presentation Continued

The patient was deemed to be an appropriate candidate for surgery, and after an extensive discussion regarding surgical options, she and her surgeon agreed to proceed with LSG.

The LSG begins with mobilization of the greater curvature of the stomach, extending from the angle of His to several centimeters proximal to the pylorus (Figure 14-1). This usually begins at the midbody of the stomach where vessels are less dense, resulting in easier entry to the lesser sac. Proximal gastric mobilization must be complete with visualization of the entire left crus. If a hiatal hernia is identified, it is repaired at this time. Any retrogastric attachments to the pancreas or retroperitoneum are divided (Figure 14-2). A bougie or endoscope (34 French minimum) is passed and positioned along the lesser curvature (Figure 14-3), which serves as a guide during the longitudinal gastrectomy. Transection of the stomach using a linear cutting stapler

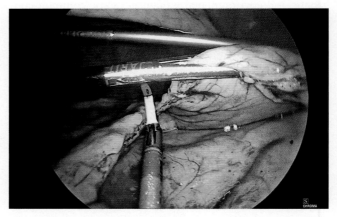

FIGURE 14-1. Mobilization of the greater curvature of the stomach. (Photo courtesy of Nabeel R. Obeid, MD.)

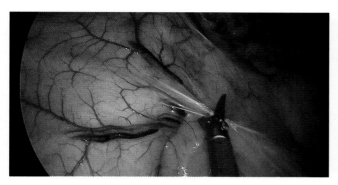

FIGURE 14-2. Division of retrogastric adhesions. (Photo courtesy of Nabeel R. Obeid, MD.)

(Figure 14-4) begins 5 to 7 cm proximal to the pylorus along the greater curvature, continues proximally, and is completed at the angle of His (Figure 14-5). This can be performed with or without reinforced staple loads. The specimen is removed and, depending on surgeon preference, an intraoperative leak test may be performed. The staple line and divided edge of the omentum are inspected for hemostasis.

There are several potential pitfalls during a sleeve gastrectomy. Lack of exposure or improper use of the energy device during ligation of the short gastric vessels may result in vessel retraction and hemorrhage that is difficult to control. If the proximal gastric mobilization is inadequate, a hiatal hernia—usually Type 1 (sliding)—may be missed with resultant postoperative exacerbation or new onset of GERD. Without careful attention during lysis of retrogastric adhesions, the lesser curvature vessels may be inadvertently ligated, while incomplete lysis may result in difficulty with staple firing, injury to the pancreas, or redundant fundus. During gastric transection, the surgeon may excessively narrow the gastric sleeve which could result in stricture causing dysphagia or chronic nausea with PO intolerance. This is most susceptible at the level of the incisura angularis. During proximal transection, inadequate lateral retraction may result in retained fundus on the sleeve, which is

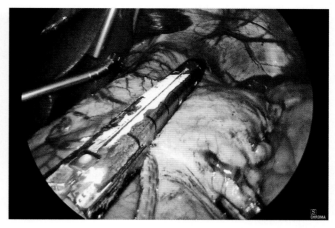

FIGURE 14-4. Longitudinal transection using a linear cutting stapler. (Photo courtesy of Nabeel R. Obeid, MD.)

occasionally associated with inadequate weight loss due to lack of restriction and orexigenic hormonal influences. Finally, if the gastroesophageal junction is not clearly delineated, the proximal-most staple fires may encroach the distal esophagus (Table 14-2).

Presentation Continued
The patient underwent a LSG and hiatal hernia repair with an uneventful intraoperative course.

● SPECIAL INTRAOPERATIVE CONSIDERATIONS

In rare instances, there may be an excess of visceral adiposity, extremely large and boggy liver despite preoperative liquid diet, or other factors that make exposure and dissection exceedingly difficult. In these circumstances, it is wise to abort the procedure and plan for additional weight loss before re-attempting surgery. During longitudinal stapling, if the sleeve is narrowed or twisted significantly at any point along its length, this should be investigated with

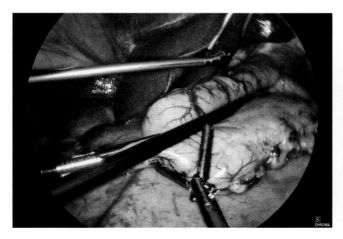

FIGURE 14-3. Passage of the bougie along the lesser curvature of the stomach. (Photo courtesy of Nabeel R. Obeid, MD.)

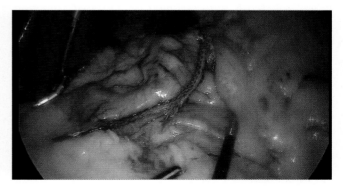

FIGURE 14-5. Completed sleeve gastrectomy. (Photo courtesy of Nabeel R. Obeid, MD.)

Table 14-2	Laparoscopic Sleeve Gastrectomy

Key Technical Steps

1. Mobilization of the greater curvature of the stomach
2. Proximal and complete mobilization of the fundus with exposure of the left crus
3. Evaluation of the hiatus and hiatal hernia repair, as indicated
4. Assessment and lysis of retrogastric adhesions
5. Passage of the bougie with placement along the lesser curvature of the stomach
6. Longitudinal gastrectomy using a linear cutting stapler
7. Removal of the specimen

Potential Pitfalls

- Bleeding from the short gastric vessels or splenic hilum
- Narrowing of the sleeve at the level of the incisura angularis
- Retained fundus on the sleeve

nutrient deficiencies. Counseling regarding appropriate dietary choices and highlighting the importance of regular, moderate physical activity are of utmost importance to help maintain durable results.

Case Conclusion

Following surgery, the patient had significant nausea and was given ondansetron and metoclopramide on a scheduled basis with improvement. She was eventually able to tolerate her diet, was ambulating, voiding, and pain controlled, and was discharged to home on POD 1. She was seen as an outpatient and has recovered well. The patient was last seen at her 2-year post-surgery visit and is at her lowest weight with a BMI 33 kg/m^2 and is compliant with her bariatric multivitamin administration. She no longer requires anti-hypertensive medications, her sleep apnea has resolved, and only remains on a statin. She states her quality of life is wonderful and is able to enjoy more activities with her family.

intraoperative endoscopy, and may require prophylactic stenting or conversion to LRYGB. If the intraoperative leak test is positive, the area in question should be repaired with sutures to imbricate this portion of the staple line, and the leak test should then be repeated with consideration for drain placement.

● POSTOPERATIVE MANAGEMENT

Patients are started on a bariatric clear liquid diet with protein supplements on the day of surgery, with advancement to full liquids as tolerated. Routine UGIS are no longer performed. Acetaminophen and opioid analgesics are administered as needed, as well as anti-emetics on a scheduled basis. Early ambulation is expected within 6 hours of surgery, most importantly for the preventions of venous thromboembolism. Most patients may be discharged by postoperative day (POD) 1. The most common postoperative complications include intractable nausea usually managed with several anti-emetics, but an UGIS should be performed if there is intolerance of diet or dysphagia. Early, sustained tachycardia is an ominous sign, usually suggestive of hemorrhage, leak, or VTE. Fevers, hypoxia, or acute anemia may help identify the etiology. For evaluation of leak, some prefer UGIS to assess the gastrojejunostomy for extravasation, while others utilize computed tomography (CT) due to the ability to identify hematomas, fluid collections, or vascular filling defects.

Long term, patients are followed on an annual basis with weight monitoring, comorbidity assessment, symptom evaluation, and laboratory analysis especially for vitamin/

TAKE HOME POINTS

- Morbid obesity is a chronic disease that requires attention and treatment
- Surgery is the most efficacious and durable treatment for morbid obesity
- Laparoscopic sleeve gastrectomy and Laparoscopic Roux-en-Y gastric bypass are currently the most common bariatric procedures performed
- Important steps during sleeve gastrectomy include full mobilization of the fundus, evaluation for a hiatal hernia, retrogastric adhesiolysis, proper placement of the bougie, and meticulous staple firing
- Pitfalls include short gastric vessel or splenic hilar bleeding, narrowing or twisting at the incisura angularis, and inadvertently retaining fundus
- Dietary counseling and laboratory assessment are essential components of lifelong follow-up

SUGGESTED READINGS

Birkmeyer NJ, Dimick JB, Share D, et al. Hospital complication rates with bariatric surgery in Michigan. *JAMA.* 2010;304(4):435-442.

Colquitt JL, Pickett K, Loveman E, et al. Surgery for weight loss in adults. *Cochrane Database Syst Rev.* 2014;(8):CD003641.

Gagner M, Deitel M, Erickson AL, et al. Survey on laparoscopic sleeve gastrectomy (LSG) at the Fourth International Consensus Summit on Sleeve Gastrectomy. *Obes Surg.* 2013; 23(12):2013-2017.

Hutter MM, Schirmer BD, Jones DB, et al. First report from the American College of Surgeons Bariatric Surgery Center Network: laparoscopic sleeve gastrectomy has morbidity and effectiveness positioned between the band and the bypass. *Ann Surg.* 2011;254(3):410-420.

Ibrahim AM, Ghaferi AA, Thumma JR, et al. Variation in outcomes at bariatric surgery centers of excellence. *JAMA Surg.* 2017;152(7):629-636.

Parikh M, Issa R, McCrillis A, et al. Surgical strategies that may decrease leak after laparoscopic sleeve gastrectomy: a systematic review and meta-analysis of 9991 cases. *Ann Surg.* 2013; 257(2):231-237.

Rosenthal RJ. International Sleeve Gastrectomy Expert Panel, Diaz AA, et al. International Sleeve Gastrectomy Expert Panel Consensus Statement: best practice guidelines based on experience of >12,000 cases. *Surg Obes Relat Dis.* 2012;8(1):8-19.

Schauer PR, Bhatt DL, Kirwan JP, et al. Bariatric surgery versus intensive medical therapy for diabetes—5-year outcomes. *N Engl J Med.* 2017;376(7):641-651.

Telem DA, Gould J, Pesta C, et al. American Society for Metabolic and Bariatric Surgery: Care Pathway Development for Laparoscopic Sleeve Gastrectomy. ASMBS Professional Resource Center. https://asmbs.org/resources/care-pathway-laparoscopic-sleeve-gastrectomy. Accessed on February 15, 2018.

Varban OA, Sheetz KH, Cassidy RB, et al. Evaluating the effect of operative technique on leaks after laparoscopic sleeve gastrectomy: a case-control study. *Surg Obes Relat Dis.* 2017;13(4):560-567.

Surgical Treatment of Gastroesophageal Reflux Disease in the Obese Patient

AMIR A. GHAFERI AND ROBERT W. O'ROURKE

15

Presentation

A 42-year-old woman presents with a 20-year history of progressive obesity and a body mass index (BMI) that has increased over the past decade from 37 to 45 kg/m². She remains morbidly obese despite multiple attempts at diet-induced weight loss. She reports an 8-year history of diabetes, a 12-year history of hypertension, and a 5-year history of obstructive sleep apnea. She also reports a 10-year history of episodic "burning" epigastric pain that has increased in frequency and severity in the last 3 years. She now reports daily pain not only that is often post-prandial but also wakes her at night. Her nighttime pain is often associated with "fluid in her mouth." The pain is partially relieved with antacid therapy, and nighttime frequency is reduced by sleeping on a wedge. Medications include insulin, metformin, lisinopril, and omeprazole. She is compliant with CPAP therapy. Her omeprazole dosing was increased from once daily to twice daily last year. Her past surgical history includes appendectomy 20 years ago and bilateral tubal ligation 6 years ago.

● DIFFERENTIAL DIAGNOSIS

The differential diagnosis for obesity is relatively straight-forward. The vast majority of cases are polygenic in origin, the result of multiple poorly defined genetic polymorphisms, so-called common human obesity. Rare cases of monogenic obesity exist, including patients with mutations in the genes that encode for leptin, leptin receptor, melanocortin 4 receptor, POMC, and PCSK1 among others. A family history combined with thorough history and physical exam to identify corollary signs associated with rare monogenic disorders usually confirms diagnosis of these rare cases. Finally, contributing factors to common polygenic human obesity, while rarely the sole cause of excess body mass, must be sought and treated, including hypothyroidism, Cushing's syndrome, and hypothalamic disorders.

The differential diagnosis for epigastric pain is broad, including but not limited to gastroesophageal reflux disease (GERD), peptic ulcer disease, gastritis, gallbladder disease, pancreatitis, adhesive bowel obstruction, and myocardial ischemia. Symptom relief with antacid therapy supports a diagnosis of GERD but may also be observed with PUD and gastritis. Nighttime symptoms relieved by positioning also support a diagnosis of GERD, as do associated symptoms of globus, water brash, and dysphagia.

A preponderance of data support obesity as a risk factor for GERD, the prevalence of which in bariatric surgery patients ranges from 40% to 60% depending on diagnostic definitions and methods used. The mechanisms underlying this association are not well-understood. Elevated BMI is also a risk factor for hiatal hernia, a dominant contributor to GERD. Increased intra-abdominal pressure may predispose to hiatal hernia and thus contribute to lower esophageal sphincter (LES) failure and GERD. Data regarding the association between obesity and LES failure independent of hiatal hernia are conflicting, with some studies demonstrating decreased LES pressures in obese compared to lean subjects, while others demonstrate the opposite, that is increased LES pressures in the obese. These latter observations have been rationalized as a compensatory response to increased abdominal pressures which in turn induces increased LES pressure and suggest that antireflux surgery (ARS), which is directed toward repairing a defective LES, may be less effective in the context of obesity.

● WORKUP

The diagnostic evaluation for the obese patient with abdominal pain should proceed sequentially. EGD is an appropriate initial test and will diagnose peptic ulcer disease or gastritis, as well as provide information about GERD-related pathology including esophagitis, Barrett's esophagus, and hiatal hernia. Any pathologic lesions identified on EGD should be biopsied. Testing for *Helicobacter pylori* is an appropriate next step, especially in the presence of gastritis or ulcer disease. UGI provides information regarding anatomic defects including hiatal hernia. Ultrasound and CT scan may be used to diagnose gallbladder disease and other intra-abdominal pathology based on history and symptoms. In the absence of other pathology, a history of classic symptoms, including heartburn, globus, dysphagia, and water brash, especially if relieved by antacid therapy, supports a diagnosis of GERD. While some argue that a history of typical GERD symptoms precludes the need for further testing, consensus opinion is that definitive diagnosis of GERD is made with 24-hour pH study. Finally, esophageal manometry and gastric emptying studies should be obtained if dysphagia or emesis symptoms suggestive of esophageal or gastric dysmotility are present.

● DIAGNOSIS AND TREATMENT

A trial of antacid therapy, usually a proton pump inhibitor, is an appropriate first step in all patients with an initial diagnosis of GERD. Dosing may be daily or twice daily, and addition of a QHS H2-antagonist further reduces acid secretion. Treatment for concomitant *H. pylori* infection if present is recommended. Patients in whom medical therapy fails and who experience significant breakthrough symptoms despite antacid therapy should be considered for surgery. Preoperative optimization of obesity-related comorbidities is an important safety measure, including appropriate treatment of diabetes with glycemic control as evidenced by hemoglobin A1c ≤7%, hypertension controlled on antihypertensive medications, and sleep apnea adequately treated with CPAP. Screening for cardiopulmonary, hepatic, and psychiatric disease is also recommended when indicated.

The choice of operation for the obese patient with GERD is controversial. Options include primary ARS or bariatric surgery; primary bariatric operations include Roux-en-Y gastric bypass (GBP), sleeve gastrectomy, and adjustable gastric banding. Finally, bariatric operations may be combined with an antireflux procedure.

Primary ARS (e.g., fundoplication) is generally reserved for the treatment of GERD in nonobese patients, due to a preponderance of data demonstrating high rates of failure in the obese. Despite these data, however, debate persists, as a minority of studies demonstrate good outcomes for primary fundoplication in the obese, although many of these studies include small number of patients with relatively low BMI. In addition, combining bariatric surgery operations with fundoplication procedures has been reported, most commonly cardiopexy, less commonly modified fundoplication, but rigorous outcome data for such operative strategies are lacking. Overall, consensus opinion supports bariatric surgery rather than primary ARS as a treatment for GERD in the morbidly obese. Bariatric surgery not only is effective therapy for GERD but also provides treatment or prevention for other prevalent metabolic diseases such as diabetes, hypertension, hyperlipidemia, and sleep apnea.

Gastric banding has decreased dramatically over the past decade due to evolving data demonstrating a high rate of late morbidity and failure, with late band explant rates as high as 20% to 30%. While data are conflicting, gastric banding is generally considered to exacerbate GERD and induce esophageal motility dysfunction. That said, it is important to note that some studies demonstrate improvement in GERD with gastric banding. It is possible that GERD in the context of gastric banding may be associated with complications such as slippage and pouch dilation, in the absence of

which gastric banding may improve GERD. Hiatal hernia, either preexisting or induced by gastric banding, may also contribute to GERD, and repair of hiatal hernia concomitant with gastric banding may reduce postoperative GERD risk. These considerations aside, however, gastric banding in patients with significant GERD is controversial, and combined with its high late morbidity, is generally not considered appropriate for the obese patient with GERD.

Application of sleeve gastrectomy as a primary treatment for morbid obesity has increased dramatically over the past decade, due to its efficacy and low long-term morbidity. However, data regarding sleeve gastrectomy and GERD are conflicting and evolving. A subset of patients experience improvement in GERD after sleeve gastrectomy, with remission ranging from 10% to over 65%. There is another subpopulation that appears to be at risk for de novo or worsening GERD symptoms, ranging in incidence from 3% to over 60%. Similar to gastric banding, aggressive repair of hiatal hernia may reduce postoperative GERD risk in patients undergoing sleeve gastrectomy. Mechanisms that may contribute to worsening GERD after sleeve gastrectomy include disruption of the angle of His and/or creation of a high pressure conduit that predisposes to retrograde reflux. In contrast, increased gastric emptying after sleeve gastrectomy, along with reduction in parietal cell mass as a result of the gastric resection, may contribute to improvement in GERD. Distinguishing between procedure-independent beneficial effects of weight loss on GERD and the beneficial and adverse procedure-specific effects of sleeve gastrectomy on GERD is challenging as reliable predictors of outcome remain elusive. The advantages of sleeve gastrectomy, including a lower lifetime risk of reoperations for complications compared to gastric bypass or gastric banding, must be weighed against what are currently poorly understood risks of persistent or worsening reflux symptoms. Sleeve gastrectomy nonetheless remains an important option in patients with relative contraindications to GBP, including a prior history of lower abdominal surgery, significant intestinal adhesions, and oxalate nephrolithiasis. Further research will define the role of sleeve gastrectomy in the treatment of the obese patient with GERD.

GBP is generally considered the optimal operation for the obese patient with severe GERD. In patients with Barrett's esophagus, GBP is preferred as the remnant stomach is preserved for use as a conduit in the unlikely event that the patient requires esophagectomy in the future. The mechanisms by which GBP improves GERD are likely multiple and include reduction in acid reflux due to divorce of the parietal cell mass from the gastric pouch, and a long Roux limb that prevents retrograde biliary reflux. Weight loss also contributes to GERD remission via less well-defined mechanisms that may include reduced intra-abdominal pressures with improved function of the anatomic antireflux mechanism. GERD remission rates in response to GBP range from 85% to over 95% in most studies, depending on the diagnostic methods used that far exceeds response rates from gastric banding and sleeve gastrectomy. For these reasons, GBP remains the dominant surgical treatment for obese patients with severe GERD.

● SURGICAL APPROACH

Key Technical Steps

1. *Patient positioning*: Obese surgical patients are at higher risk of positioning injuries, including brachial plexus and peroneal nerve injuries. A split-leg or closed leg positioning may be used. The surgeon may stand on the patient's right if a closed leg position is used, or between the legs if a split-leg position is used. The assistant stands on the patient's left.

2. *Laparoscopic access* is obtained. A camera is placed through a right middle quadrant port. The jejunojejunostomy is created using two working ports in the right upper and lower quadrants. The gastrojejunostomy is created using the right upper quadrant port and a left upper quadrant port. An assistant port is placed in the left lateral midabdomen (Figure 15-1). Variations on trocar arrangement exist.

3. *Exploration*: Upon gaining laparoscopic access, limited exploration of the abdomen is performed. Liver size and pathology (steatosis, cirrhosis) should be assessed to ensure that adequate liver retraction is possible to permit safe creation of a gastric pouch and a gastrojejunostomy. The hiatus should be explored to determine if a hiatal hernia is present. The small intestine should be examined, ensuring normal anatomy (e.g., no malrotation, significant adhesions, or mesenteric shortening).

4. *Jejunojejunostomy*: The operation begins with creation of a Roux-en-Y jejunojejunostomy. The jejunum is traced 50 to 75 cm distal from the ligament of Treitz and divided with a stapler. The jejunal mesentery is divided with sequential staple firings to its root, taking care to divide the mesentery centrally such that neither intestinal limb is devascularized. This mesenteric division provides length to bring the Roux limb to the pouch, reducing tension on the gastrojejunostomy. A 100 to 150 cm Roux/alimentary limb is then traced, starting at the distal staple line of the transected jejunum and proceeding distally. Stay sutures are then placed 5 cm apart between the biliary limb and the Roux limb. Cautery is used to create enterotomies in each limb just distal to the proximal stay suture, and a linear stapler is passed and used to create the side-to-side jejunojejunostomy. The resultant enteral defect created by the stapler is then closed with running suture (Figure 15-2).

5. *Closure of the mesenteric defect*: The mesenteric defect is closed, suturing the stapled edge of the mesentery of the biliary limb to the adjacent sheet of Roux limb mesentery (Figure 15-3).

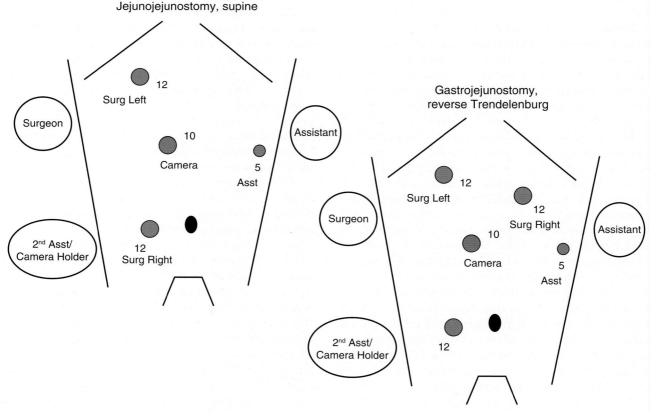

FIGURE 15-1. Gastric bypass trocar arrangement.

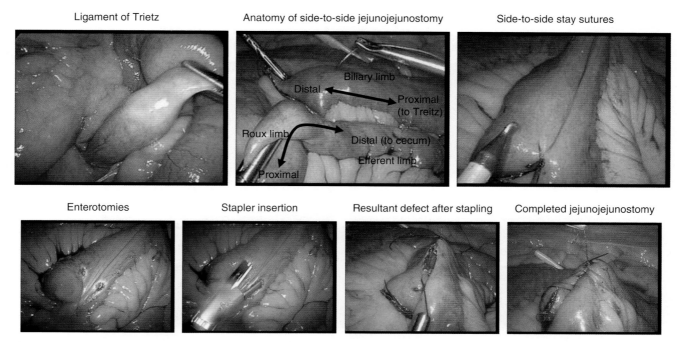

FIGURE 15-2. Jejunojeunostomy.

6. *Divide the omentum*: The omentum is divided with a harmonic scalpel from its distal end to its junction with the transverse colon, to provide a path through which the antecolic Roux limb travels, reducing tension on the gastrojejunostomy.

7. *Pouch gastroplasty*: A liver retractor is placed to expose the upper stomach and hiatus. A 25-mL lesser curve-based pouch gastroplasty is created using serial stapler firings, starting with horizontal stapler firing 5 cm below the gastroesophageal junction, then carrying stapler firings vertically, dividing the pouch from the remnant stomach at the left crus. A sizing balloon may be used to size the pouch (Figure 15-4).

8. *Gastrojejunostomy*: The Roux limb is brought up to the pouch in an antecolic configuration (Figure 15-5)

between the divided leaves of the omentum, ensuring that the limb is not twisted (Figure 15-6). A back row of interrupted sutures is used to secure the Roux limb to the distal pouch staple line over a length of 5 cm. A gastrotomy and a jejunotomy are created with cautery, dilated gently with a grasper, then the blades of a 45-mm linear stapler are passed through the enterotomies and the stapler is fired, creating the gastrojejunostomy. A 32 French tube is then passed per os through the anastomosis, and the enteral defect created by the stapler is sutured closed over the tube with running suture. A leak test is then performed with methylene blue through the oral tube, or a bubble test via endoscopy. The gastrojejunostomy may also be created using circular stapler or fully hand-sewn techniques. No clear difference in

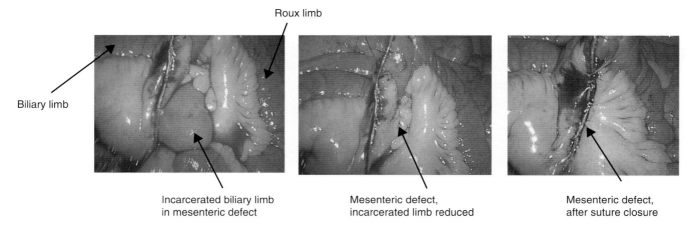

FIGURE 15-3. Mesenteric defect closure. (Adapted by permission from Springer: O'Rourke RW. Management Strategies for Internal Hernia after Gastric Bypass. *J Gastrointest Surg.* 2011; 15(6):1049-1054. Copyright © 2010 The Society for Surgery of the Alimentary Tract.)

Hiatal exposure

Starting pouch dissection on lesser curve,
5 cm distal to gastroesophageal junction;
note sizing balloon in place

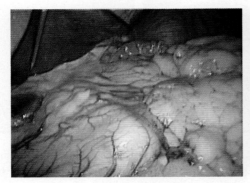
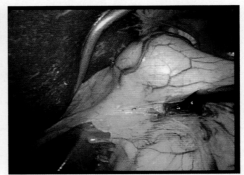

After first staple firing

Just prior to final staple firing

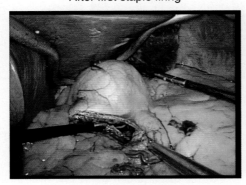
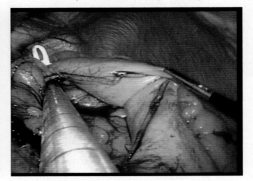

FIGURE 15-4. Pouch gastroplasty.

outcomes has been demonstrated between these anastomotic techniques, with the exception that some data suggest higher rates of anastomotic stricture with circular
stapler anastomosis. Absorbable suture should be used,
as nonabsorbable suture acts as a nidus for ulcer formation (Figure 15-7).

9. *Closure of Petersen's defect*: After completion of the gastrojejunostomy, the Petersen's mesenteric defect is closed
with a running stitch by reflecting the Roux limb to the
patient's left and sewing the staple line of the Roux limb
to the underlying mesentery of the transverse colon
(Figure 15-8).

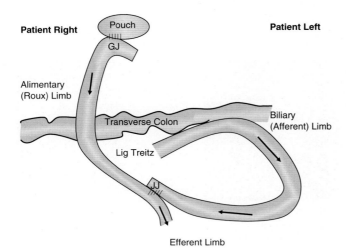

FIGURE 15-5. Gastric bypass configuration.

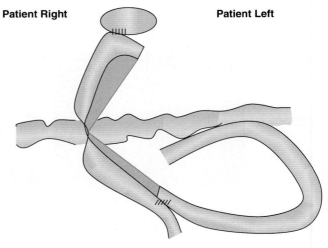

FIGURE 15-6. Pitfall: Twisted Roux Limb and mesentery.

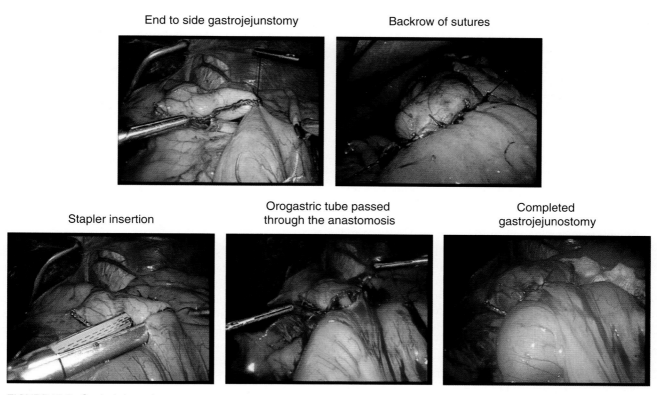

FIGURE 15-7. Gastrojejunostomy.

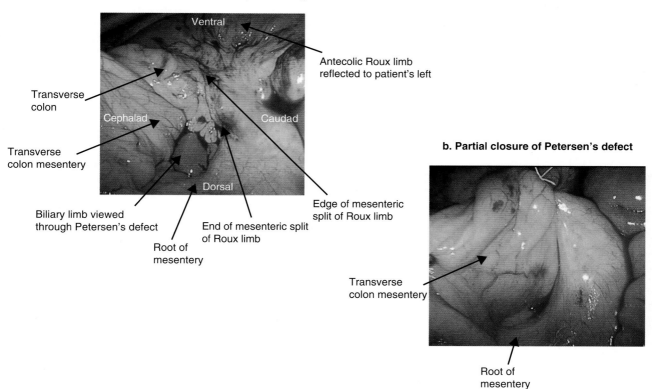

FIGURE 15-8. Petersen's defect. (Adapted by permission from Springer: O'Rourke RW. Management Strategies for Internal Hernia after Gastric Bypass. *J Gastrointest Surg.* 2011; 15(6):1049-1054. Copyright © 2010 The Society for Surgery of the Alimentary Tract.)

Pitfalls

1. *Pitfalls during creation of the Roux-en-Y jejunojejunostomy*: When tracing the biliary and Roux limbs, it is critical to clearly identify the ligament of Treitz and to maintain instrument control of the intestine at all times to prevent creation of aberrant intestinal anatomy (e.g., "Roux-en-O" or antiperistaltic limbs) (Figure 15-9). Once created, diagnosis may be challenging unless index of suspicion is high, and restoration to functional anatomy is fraught with difficulty. Another dysfunctional anatomy is the so-called "candy cane syndrome", in which the distal stump of the Roux limb in the end-to-side gastrojejunostomy is excessively long, resulting delayed emptying. Patients may provide a history of positional bloating and relief with emptying of the limb, a phenomenon that may be observed during dynamic upper gastrointestinal series. EGD may also aid in diagnosis, as cannulation of the long excluded limb is generally possible. Treatment is straightforward and involves resection of the redundant Roux limb stump. Excessively long Roux and afferent intestinal limbs may be associated with higher rates of internal hernia and malabsorptive complications. Standard limb lengths are 50 to 70 cm for the afferent/biliary limb and 100 cm for the Roux limb.

2. *Closure of mesenteric defects*: Data are conflicting regarding whether routine closure of mesenteric defects reduces the risk of internal hernia. Closure of such defects is tenuous, and reduction of mesenteric adipose tissue with weight loss may lead to opening of previously closed defects. Nonetheless, despite some studies demonstrating no reduction in internal hernia rates with routine closure, recent meta-analyses support that closure reduces late internal herniation rates. The risks involved in mesenteric defect closure are low; as such, routine closure of mesenteric defects is recommended.

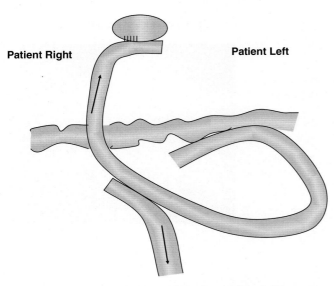

Patient Right   **Patient Left**

FIGURE 15-9. Pitfall: "Roux en O": Reversed Biliary, Roux limbs.

3. *Clinical implications of pouch morphology*: The gastric pouch is created by serial stapler firings beginning with a single lateral staple firing 5 cm below the gastroesophageal junction, then proceeding with cephalad stapler firings ending at angle of His and the left crus, creating a lesser curve-based gastric pouch. This pouch morphology avoids inclusion of lateral fundus, which can lead to a distensible pouch prone to dilation and stasis. Larger pouches that extend beyond 5 cm below the gastroesophageal junction may also be associated with an increased risk of anastomotic ulcers and GERD symptoms, possibly due to inclusion in the pouch of parietal cells along the distal lesser curvature. Estimation of pouch size may be accomplished by measuring 5 cm distal from the gastroesophageal junction as a starting point for the first staple firing. Sizing balloon catheters may be used as well. Complete division of the pouch from the remnant stomach is critical to avoid gastrogastric fistula.

4. *Hemorrhage during creation of the gastric pouch*: Three potential sources of hemorrhage may be encountered during creation of the gastric pouch: ultrasonic dissection is used to divide tissues along the lesser curve of the upper stomach to create space for initial horizontal staple firing, and *branches of the left gastric artery* may be encountered at this point. As the dissection is carried laterally and cephalad with serial firings of the stapler, the *splenic vessels* may be encountered deep to the posterior stomach. Finally, as the dissection is carried toward the angle of His and the left crus, *high short gastric vessels* may be encountered. Keeping the dissection close to the stomach at all times will reduce the likelihood of hemorrhage. In addition, initial blunt dissection is used to take down the peritoneal attachments of the upper stomach/fundus to the left crus. This provides a window for the final stapler firing that completely divides the pouch from the remnant stomach and identifies a landmark that aids in keeping the dissection medial to the high short gastric vessels (Figure 15-10).

5. *Pitfalls during creation of the gastrojejunostomy*: Excessive tension on the gastrojejunostomy increases the risk of anastomotic dehiscence. Carrying the jejunal mesenteric division to the root of the mesentery provides length on the Roux limb, allowing it to reach the hiatus with minimal tension (Figure 15-11). Complete mobilization of the gastric pouch from its peritoneal attachments to left crus and diaphragm will provide length on the gastric pouch, also reducing anastomotic tension.

   Suture closure of the gastrojejunostomy over a 32 to 36 French tube or stent minimizes the risk of narrowing the anastomosis. This technique is not necessary or possible with a circular sitapler technique but is important for linear stapler or hand-sewn techniques.

   Routine intraoperative testing of the gastrojejunal anastomosis with EGD–air insufflation or methylene blue may be associated with reduced anastomotic dehiscence rates and is advisable.

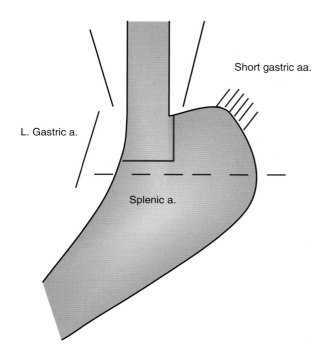

FIGURE 15-10. Pitfall: Sources of hemorrhage during pouch gastroplasty.

Drain placement at the gastrojejunal anastomosis is practiced selectively. No clear data demonstrate that routine drain placement neither increases early detection or reduces morbidity of anastomotic dehiscence nor does compelling data exist suggesting that drains increase the risk of such events. Some data suggest that drains may allow for nonoperative management of anastomotic dehiscence.

6. *The gallbladder*: Significant weight loss increases the risk of cholelithiasis. Reported incidences of postoperative cholelithiasis ranges from 15% to 70%, and approximately 7% of patients will require postoperative

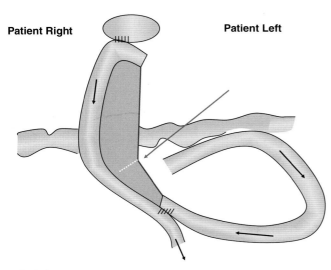

FIGURE 15-11. Pitfall: Inadequate mesenteric division leading to unnecessary tension.

cholecystectomy. Nonetheless, risk–benefit analyses do not support prophylactic cholecystectomy at the time of laparoscopic bariatric surgery unless symptomatic cholelithiasis is present. Prophylactic treatment with ursodeoxycholic acid during the first 6 postoperative months reduces the risk of postoperative cholelithiasis, from 28% to 9% in one recent meta-analysis (Uy et al.). Such therapy entails little morbidity and is common practice, but no clear data demonstrate that this practice reduces cholecystectomy rates or is cost-effective.

SPECIAL INTRAOPERATIVE CONSIDERATIONS

1. The prevalence of *hiatal hernia* in bariatric surgery patients ranges from 35% to 60%. This wide range reflects variable definitions and methods of diagnosis, with preoperative diagnosis reflecting the lower range of prevalence, while intraoperative diagnosis suggests higher rates. Debate exists regarding the threshold for repair, with some arguing that dissection and crural approximation should be performed in all patients, while others argue for repair only if a clearly visible hiatal hernia is present. Most surgeons agree that hiatal hernia repair should be pursued on a selective basis, but that the threshold for repair of small hernias should be low.

2. The prevalence of *cirrhosis* secondary to steatohepatitis in the bariatric surgery population ranges from 1% to 5%. When encountered, the surgeon must decide whether to abort or proceed with GBP. If intra-abdominal varices or significant splenomegaly are present, risks of proceeding are likely elevated, although small series demonstrate reasonable safety of bariatric surgery in such patients. Alternatively, the operation may be aborted, and portal pressure measurements may be obtained to guide further decision-making, although the threshold for elevated portal pressures that define an acceptable margin safety for surgery is not well-defined.

3. A minority of patients may have a *foreshortened small intestine mesentery* that places tension on the Roux limb during creation of the gastrojejunostomy. Carrying the mesenteric division to the root of the mesentery, as stated above, will reduce anastomotic tension. Bringing up the Roux limb in retrocolic, retrogastric position may also reduce tension in such situations. Finally, while potentially increasing the risk of anastomotic ulcer, creation of a longer gastric pouch may reduce tension as well.

POSTOP MANAGEMENT

Postoperative management after GBP includes dietary management to prevent impaction and to maintain hydration as anastomotic edema resolves in the few weeks after surgery. Patients start a clear liquid diet on the first postoperative day, with progression to full liquids within the first week after surgery. Hospital stays range from 1 to 4 days after a laparoscopic operation. Solid foods are progressively incorporated into the diet starting 3 weeks after surgery.

Early postoperative complications include anastomotic dehiscence, most often within 2 weeks of operation with published incidences of 0.1% to 2%. Anastomotic dehiscence requires prompt operative intervention with washout and drainage; select cases may be amenable to percutaneous drainage and nonoperative management, but the threshold for operative intervention should be low. Postoperative hemorrhage, usually from staple lines, occurs with an incidence of 1% to 4% and may be intraperitoneal or intraluminal. Intraluminal bleeding presents with melena and is often self-limited, requiring only transfusion and observation. Infrequently, endoscopic or operative intervention may be necessary to treat hemorrhage. Early postoperative bowel obstruction (due to trocar herniation, internal herniation, or adhesions) occurs with published incidences of 0.5% to 3%. Obesity is a risk factor for DVT. Aggressive DVT prophylaxis should be employed. Optimal prophylaxis regimens are not defined, but unfractionated or low molecular weight heparin prior to surgery and continued throughout the hospitalization is typical. Subtherapeutic dosing of these agents is common in obese patients; the American College of Chest Physicians recommends weight-based dosing.

TAKE HOME POINTS

- Obesity increases the risk of GERD.
- Diagnosis and management of the obese patient with GERD is complex.
- Predictors of outcome after bariatric surgery with respect to postoperative GERD remission and exacerbation remain elusive.
- Gastric bypass is the mainstay of surgical care, but evolving data suggest that sleeve gastrectomy may play a role in a subset of patients.

SUGGESTED READINGS

Anvari M, Bamehriz F. Outcome of laparoscopic Nissen fundoplication in patients with body mass index >or=35. *Surg Endosc.* 2006;20:230-234.

Ayazi S, Hagen JA, Chan LS, et al. Obesity and gastroesophageal reflux: quantifying the association between body mass index, esophageal acid exposure, and lower esophageal sphincter status in a large series of patients with reflux symptoms. *J Gastrointest Surg.* 2009;13:1440-1447.

Bello B, Zoccali M, Gullo R, Allaix ME, Herbella FA, Gasparaitis A, Patti MG. Gastroesophageal reflux disease and antireflux surgery-what is the proper preoperative work-up? *J Gastrointest Surg.* 2013;17(1):14-20.

Crawford C, Gibbens K, Lomelin D, Krause C, Simorov A, Oleynikov D. Sleeve gastrectomy and anti-reflux procedures. *Surg Endosc.* 2017;31:1012-1021.

Frantzides CT, Carlson MA, Madan AK, Stewart ET, Smith C. Selective use of esophageal manometry and 24-hour pH monitoring before laparoscopic fundoplication. *J Am Coll Surg.* 2003;197(3):358-363.

Frezza EE, Ikramuddin S, Gourash W, Rakitt T, Kingston A, Luketich J, Schauer P. Symptomatic improvement in gastroesophageal reflux disease (GERD) following laparoscopic Roux-en-Y gastric bypass. *Surg Endosc.* 2002;16(7):1027-1031.

Hendricks L, Alvarenga E, Dhanabalsamy N, Lo Menzo E, Szomstein S, Rosenthal R. Impact of sleeve gastrectomy on gastroesophageal reflux disease in a morbidly obese population undergoing bariatric surgery. *Surg Obes Relat Dis.* 2016; 12(3):511-517.

Hirsh J, Bauer KA, Donati MB, Gould M, Samama MM, Weitz JI; American College of Chest Physicians. Parenteral anticoagulants: American College of Chest Physicians Evidence-Based Clinical Practice Guidelines (8th Edition). *Chest.* 2008;133(6 suppl): 141S-159S.

Jobe BA, Richter JE, Hoppo T, et al. Preoperative diagnostic workup before antireflux surgery: an evidence and experience-based consensus of the Esophageal Diagnostic Advisory Panel. *J Am Coll Surg.* 2013; 217(4):586-597.

Madalosso CA, Gurski RR, Callegari-Jacques SM, Navarini D, Mazzini G, Pereira Mda S. The impact of gastric bypass on gastroesophageal reflux disease in morbidly obese patients. *Ann Surg.* 2016; 263(1):110-116.

Gastroesophageal Reflux Disease After Sleeve Gastrectomy

KATE LAK AND JON GOULD

16

Presentation

A 45-year-old obese female presents to your office 13 months after she underwent a laparoscopic sleeve gastrectomy for morbid obesity. Her BMI prior to surgery was 50 kg/m². Preoperative comorbidities included obstructive sleep apnea managed on continuous positive airway pressure (CPAP), hypertension, and gastroesophageal reflux disease. She had been on a daily dose of a proton pump inhibitor for years with excellent control of GERD symptoms. Her BMI has dropped to 35 kg/m², and her weight has been stable for a few months. She no longer requires CPAP, and her hypertension is under better control. Her GERD symptoms appeared once again shortly after surgery despite the fact she never stopped taking her proton pump inhibitor (PPI). Her GERD symptoms have been so severe for her this past year that she is now on a BID PPI and well as an H2 blocker at night. She takes TUMS often throughout the day and has severe persistent heartburn and regurgitation. These symptoms often wake her up at night. She has minor dysphagia.

● DIFFERENTIAL DIAGNOSIS

The differential diagnosis in this patient includes GERD and stenosis/stricture of the sleeve. A stenosis or stricture typically presents earlier as epigastric pain, dysphagia, and inability to tolerate oral intake. Many of these patients have a difficult time drinking enough fluid and may require supplemental IV fluid administration in the first few weeks following surgery. The presence of significant heartburn partially responsive to a PPI and the protracted and evolving course makes this condition likely to be worsening GERD following sleeve gastrectomy.

Obesity and increasing BMI has been shown to be risk factors for GERD. Several studies have demonstrated that as many as 50% or more of patients to undergo bariatric surgery suffer from some degree of GERD, and many are taking acid reduction medications at the time of surgery. Studies comparing bariatric surgical procedures have documented that resolution of GERD following bariatric surgery occurs at a much higher rate following Roux-en-y gastric bypass (RYGB) when compared to sleeve gastrectomy. In fact, some patients to undergo sleeve gastrectomy have reported the onset of de novo GERD following surgery. The link between obesity and GERD is multifactorial and likely related to factors more common in the obese including increased abdominal pressure, decreased lower esophageal sphincter pressures, esophageal motility disorders, and an increase in anatomical abnormalities such as hiatal hernia. While many studies have reported that there is a high incidence of new-onset GERD and worsening GERD following sleeve gastrectomy, others have reported that with subsequent weight loss, GERD resolves at a high rate following sleeve gastrectomy. A systematic review and meta-analysis examining the relationship between sleeve gastrectomy and GERD included 33 studies. The authors of this study concluded "because of high heterogeneity among available studies and paradoxical outcomes of objective esophageal function tests, the exact effect of laparoscopic sleeve gastrectomy on the prevalence of GERD remains unanswered." In a study evaluating hospitals across the state of Michigan, it was found that acid reduction medication use after sleeve gastrectomy was widely variable and not associated with other traditional short- or long-term quality indicators. The authors suggest that this may imply that details in the surgical technique rather than the procedure itself may be responsible for new or worsening reflux after sleeve gastrectomy.

It has been suggested that a preexisting or undiagnosed hiatal hernia not addressed at the time of sleeve gastrectomy may be responsible for postoperative GERD. Several investigators have suggested that hiatal hernias can be difficult to recognize at the time of sleeve gastrectomy unless specifically sought with a crural dissection and repair. In fact, the incidence of hiatal hernia at the time of sleeve gastrectomy may be as high as 40% according to some studies. Several studies suggest that routine hiatal hernia repair and crural repair can decrease the incidence of GERD in sleeve gastrectomy patients. How the sleeve is created at the original operation may also contribute to the risk of postoperative GERD. When the staple line for the sleeve at the proximal margin includes the angle of His and esophageal mucosa, the incidence of postoperative GERD may be higher. When too much fundus is left behind, GERD has also been demonstrated to be more prevalent. The most likely diagnosis in our patient is therefore GERD. The etiology may relate to a variety of factors described above including a new or unrecognized hiatal hernia and an excessively large fundus/neofundus.

● WORKUP

Patients who underwent sleeve gastrectomy and present in a similar fashion to the patient in our vignette are typically treated with acid reduction medications empirically. H2 blocker, PPIs, and antacids (TUMS for example) can all be employed alone or in combination. Lifestyle modifications (avoid foods that exacerbate symptoms, sleep with the head of the bed elevated, avoid eating late at night, avoid laying supine immediately after eating) should also be employed. Weight loss may also help with symptoms in some patients, and for this reason, most surgical procedures for GERD after sleeve gastrectomy take place well after the original operation. If medication and lifestyle changes fail to adequately address GERD symptoms, further evaluation and management is appropriate.

The first diagnostic step in most patients will be an upper gastrointestinal (UGI) esophagram. This test is useful to sort through the differential diagnosis (can rule out a sleeve stricture or stenosis) and may point to anatomic factors leading to GERD. A hiatal hernia or an excessively large proximal sleeve (retained fundus or neofundus) are two common findings on UGI in patients with GERD after sleeve that ultimately may require surgical management to correct. Figure 16-1 is an image from an UGI that demonstrates a hiatal hernia and an enlarged proximal sleeve. Not apparent on this single still image is the fact that contrast freely refluxes to the thoracic inlet.

Upper endoscopy is an essential step in any patient being considered for antireflux in surgery. A hiatal hernia may be identified, and the gastroesophageal junction (GEJ) can be evaluated. The mucosa should be inspected for evidence of esophagitis. The gastric mucosa should be inspected for evidence of ulceration or stenosis and even twisting of the sleeve. Most patients who have been on a PPI for some period of time will have nonerosive reflux and normal-appearing esophageal mucosa.

A 24-hour pH testing is the gold standard for diagnosing GERD in patients with normal foregut anatomy. This test can also be of value in a patient with a prior sleeve gastrectomy when diagnostic uncertainty exists. In patients with severe dysphagia—especially without a clear stricture or obstruction to explain this symptom, esophageal manometry can be useful to evaluate for an underlying motility disorder.

● DIAGNOSIS AND TREATMENT

Our patient underwent an UGI that demonstrated a 3-cm hiatal hernia, a patulous GEJ, an enlarged proximal sleeve, free reflux of contrast back up to the thoracic inlet, and no evidence of a sleeve stricture. The motility pattern of the UGI appeared normal. A barium soaked marshmallow passed through the GE junction after a mild delay. Upper endoscopy revealed Los Angeles Grade A esophagitis and a Grade III GEJ valve. The gastric mucosa was of normal appearance, and the pylorus was easily visualized and intubated.

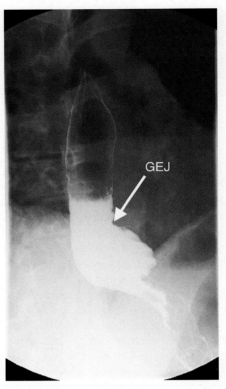

FIGURE 16-1. UGI demonstrating a hiatal hernia and an enlarged proximal sleeve. The *arrow* indicates the gastroesophageal junction (GEJ).

A biopsy of the GE junction revealed evidence of chronic inflammation consistent with GERD. Prepyloric biopsy was negative for *Helicobacter pylori*. Esophageal manometry and pH studies were not attained as the diagnosis of GERD following sleeve was felt to be secure.

Initial management of GERD following a sleeve gastrectomy is with acid reduction medications. In medically refractory cases, surgery should be considered. Considering the anatomic findings on endoscopy and UGI, there are three primary options for surgical treatment of medically refractory GERD to consider. The most commonly performed procedure in this circumstance would be a conversion of the sleeve to a Roux-en-Y gastric bypass and hiatal hernia repair. Another option would be a hiatal hernia repair alone. A final option would be implantation of a magnetic sphincter augmentation device. All of these procedures could be performed laparoscopically depending on the skills and experience of the surgeon.

Laparoscopic implantation of a magnetic sphincter augmentation device (LINX, Torax Medical, Shoreview, MN) has been reported as a treatment for GERD following sleeve gastrectomy in a very small case series (*n* = 7) at the time of this writing with limited follow-up. In this small case series, there was minimal morbidity and good short-term clinical results. Use of LINX following sleeve is currently considered off label and will therefore not be discussed in additional detail.

While laparoscopic hiatal hernia repair alone could be considered as an option in this patient, there are limited data to support the efficacy of this approach. Rather than subject the patient to a potential third operation, it is this author's opinion that a concurrent hiatal hernia repair and conversion of a sleeve gastrectomy to a gastric bypass is the best option for this patient.

Another potential treatment option in this patient would be radiofrequency ablation (Stretta, Mederi Therapeutics, Norwalk, CT). There are anecdotal reports of using this treatment in postsleeve GERD patients. A multicenter registry to study the benefits of Stretta following sleeve was recently established, and objective data to support this as an option are forthcoming. If this patient had a retained fundus or a neofundus and GERD, another potential option is fundectomy or a "resleeve." This has been described in small case series. While the reported short-term results in terms of GERD control are encouraging, the postoperative morbidity (10% leak rate in a series of 19 patients) is a concern. Fundoplasty or anterior fundoplication with the residual fundus has also been described in very small case series with good very short-term results in terms of GERD control.

● SURGICAL APPROACH

We had a long and informed discussion with our patient about many of the options described above. We ultimately recommended laparoscopic conversion of her sleeve gastrectomy to a Roux-en-Y gastric bypass with concurrent hiatal hernia repair. In addition to addressing her medically refractory GERD, our secondary goal was additional weight loss given the fact that she was still obese. From among the different options, we felt that this was the most definitive option with the highest likelihood of success in achieving our treatment goals. Informed discussion regarding the proposed procedure included the fact that her rate of perioperative complications such as leak, reoperation, stenosis, deep venous thrombosis/pulmonary embolism (DVT/PE) was higher than would be expected in a primary gastric bypass.

At the time of surgery, we chose to use a Veress needle inserted in the left costal margin at the midclavicular line—Palmer's point. We insufflated the abdomen to 15 mm Hg and gained entry to the abdomen under direct vision using a 5-mm optical trocar and a 0° laparoscope. Upon confirming safe entry, we exchanged our scope for a 5-mm, 30° laparoscope. A 5-mm trocar was placed to the left and slightly above the umbilicus for the camera. The initial access point in the left upper quadrant was upsized to 12 mm to accommodate an endoscopic linear cutting stapler. A right subcostal 12-mm port was placed for a stapler as well. Additional ports included a left-sided 5-mm and a right-sided 5-mm accessory port. A 5-mm subxiphoid incision was made, and a Nathanson liver retractor was placed to retract the left lobe of the liver anteriorly and expose the GEJ.

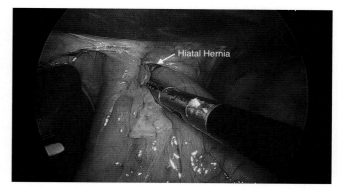

FIGURE 16-2. Intraoperative image indicating a hiatal hernia after prior sleeve gastrectomy.

To begin, the greater omentum is elevated, and the ligament of Treitz was identified at the base of the transverse mesocolon. The jejunum is divided 50 cm distal to the ligament of Treitz, and the mesentery between each segment is divided with a vascular load of the stapler. A Roux limb 100 cm in length is then measured, and the jejunojejunostomy is created with a 60-mm laparoscopic stapler after aligning the Roux limb to the biliopancreatic limb with a stay suture. We chose to perform a double-stapled jejunojejunostomy. The mesenteric defect at the jejunojejunostomy is closed with a running, locking, permanent suture. The omentum is split with an ultrasonic shears in the midtransverse colon, and the Roux limb is placed in the proximal abdomen.

Attention is then turned to the hiatus. Any adhesions are carefully lysed. The base of the right crus is identified, and the phrenoesophageal membrane is opened. A circumferential hiatal dissection is conducted until the entire hiatal hernia (Figure 16-2) is reduced and at least 2 cm of intra-abdominal esophageal length without tension is attained. Closure of the hiatus is deferred until later in the case.

The left gastric artery is identified. A window into the lesser sac is made medial to the lesser curve neurovascular bundle and distal to the insertion of the left gastric artery. Transecting the sleeve in this location with an endoscopic stapler creates a 20 to 30 mL gastric pouch (Figure 16-3).

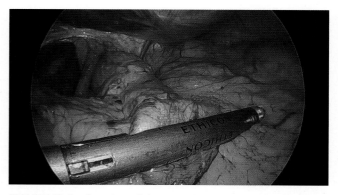

FIGURE 16-3. Creation of the gastric pouch with an endoscopic stapler. The stapler is inserted into the lesser sac distal to the left gastric artery.

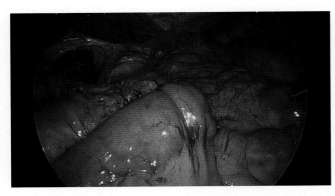

FIGURE 16-4. Completion of a linear stapled gastrojejunostomy. The anterior staple line is oversewn with interrupted 2-0 Vicryl sutures prior to removing the bougie.

In patients with a retained fundus or neofundus, this should be trimmed at the time of pouch creation. Once a well-perfused pouch has been created, we perform a linear stapled gastrojejunostomy. To do this, we make an enterotomy approximately 2-cm proximal to the tip of the Roux limb on the antimesenteric side. We then make a gastrotomy in the lateral corner of the gastric pouch staple line. The endoscopic linear cutting stapler is brought in from the right-sided 12-mm port side, and about 25 to 30 mm of the stapler is passed into the Roux limb and gastric pouch through the gastrotomy. Once the stapler is fired, 3 stay sutures are placed across the opening. A 32-French bougie is then passed across the anastomosis, and an additional load of the endoscopic stapler is fired to complete the anastomosis. We choose to leave the bougie in place as we oversew the staple line with interrupted 2-0 Vicryl sutures (Figure 16-4). Upon completion of this anastomosis, an endoscopy is performed. The gastric pouch is evaluated as well as patency through the anastomosis. A leak test is performed after placing a bowel clamp on the jejunum distal to the anastomosis. The gastric pouch is then insufflated, while the anastomosis is submerged in saline laparoscopically. At this time, a posterior cruroplasty can be performed. The endoscope can be used to calibrate the closure. We place interrupted, permanent sutures in the hiatus to complete the hiatal hernia repair (Figure 16-5).

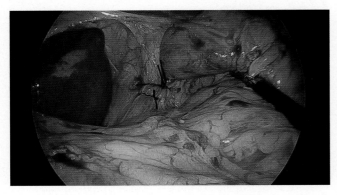

FIGURE 16-5. Posterior cruroplasty with interrupted permanent sutures.

We typically perform an omentoplasty of the gastrojejunostomy in reoperative cases as well. For this, we select a mobile piece of healthy omentum and loosely wrap this around the gastrojejunostomy. This is secured with interrupted, absorbable sutures. Placement of a drain is at the surgeon's discretion—but we tend not to place a drain in most cases.

There are several potential pitfalls that may be encountered in a case like this. The gastric tissue near the potential staple line may be thicker than in a primary gastric bypass. Consideration should be given to using a stapler load appropriate for thicker tissue if needed. Adhesions are always encountered, but considering the fact that the original procedure was laparoscopic, these adhesions are typically not extensive. It is important to ensure that the pouch has an adequate blood supply, especially considering the mobilization of the proximal pouch and esophagus that needs to take place to repair the hiatal hernia. For this reason, we always identify the left gastric artery and visualize as well as preserve the arterial vessels going to the lesser curve of the proposed pouch before transecting the sleeve. A poorly vascularized pouch is more likely to result in leak, stenosis, or marginal ulcer (Table 16-1).

Table 16-1	Conversion of a Sleeve Gastrectomy to Roux-en-Y Gastric

Key Technical Steps

1. Pneumoperitoneum, trocar placement, and exploration
2. Create the biliopancreatic limb. Elevate the greater omentum, identify the ligament of Treitz, and transect the jejunum at 50 cm
3. Create a 100- to 150-cm Roux limb. Perform a jejunojejunostomy between the biliopancreatic and the more distal jejunum at the measured location
4. Close the mesenteric defect at the jejunojejunostomy
5. Place a liver retractor to expose the hiatus
6. Perform lysis of adhesions and crural dissection. Reduce hiatal hernia and mobilize esophagus
7. Transect the stomach to create an ~20–30 mL gastric pouch
8. Perform gastrojejunostomy
9. Perform endoscopy to evaluate the proximal anastomosis and perform a leak test
10. Perform a primary posterior cruroplasty with permanent sutures

Potential Pitfalls

- Injury to the left gastric artery or its branches causing devascularization of the pouch
- Failed staple lines on the pouch or during creation of the gastrojejunostomy due to thickened gastric tissue related to previous surgery

SPECIAL INTRAOPERATIVE CONSIDERATIONS

A large abdominal wall hernia may be identified in some patients at the time of exploration, especially if the patient has had a previous laparotomy. While this hernia may have been identified and not repaired at the time of sleeve gastrectomy, the risk of leaving some hernias behind following Roux-en-Y gastric bypass is potentially greater. This is especially true in the case of an antecolic Roux limb. In these patients, the omentum is split and laid to the side along each pericolic gutter. The Roux limb is therefore in the central abdomen and immediately under the fascia. In a patient with a periumbilical or upper midline hernia defect, the Roux limb may become incarcerated in the perioperative period—especially for small- to moderate-sized defects. This is especially dangerous considering the fresh anastomosis directly upstream of the Roux limb. An incarcerated hernia with Roux limb may lead to an anastomotic leak, a very serious complication. Considering the clean-contaminated nature of the procedure described, permanent synthetic mesh should not be placed in the abdomen for hernia repair. We typically perform a primary sutured repair of these defects, often in an open manner for small hernias for this reason. The hernia repair is likely to fail in the long run, but definitive repair can be conducted in a setting where the GI tract is not violated, and hopefully in a less obese person with a subsequently decreased risk of hernia recurrence.

POSTOPERATIVE MANAGEMENT

Postoperative management is similar to following primary gastric bypass. While upper GI studies are not routinely indicated following primary Roux-en-Y gastric bypass (not sensitive for leak), UGI following these revision procedures may be helpful to document the resolution of a preexisting hiatal hernia and to document gastric pouch size. Given a negative intraoperative leak test in a patient without tachycardia and a good urine output, there is minimal value in an early post-op upper GI to rule out leak. We recommend routine DVT prophylaxis and progression in accord with standard pathways.

The most common complications postoperatively include wound infection, bleeding, GI leak, and DVT/PE. In a primary gastric bypass, leak rates are well under 1%. The true rate of anastomotic leak in cases of conversion of sleeve to gastric bypass is difficult to determine but is likely higher than 1%. Leak can present in the early postoperative period (first 48 to 72 hours) or in a delayed manner (in the first 10 days and after discharge). Leak presents with pain, tachycardia, and low urine output that does not respond to appropriate fluid resuscitation. These are all nonspecific signs and symptoms in a fresh postoperative patient, and so a high index of suspicion for leak in these patients is needed. If a leak is strongly suspected, the best management is often to proceed to the operating room for a diagnostic laparoscopy and concurrent endoscopy. If a leak is identified, over-sew, omental patch, and wide drainage is the treatment of choice. Consideration should be given to whether some form of enteral access may be needed in the first few weeks postoperatively. If there is enough of the distal sleeve left in situ, a gastrostomy can be placed into the remnant. In most patients, a jejunostomy tube in the proximal common channel distal to the Roux limb is the best choice.

Case Conclusion

Our patient underwent laparoscopic conversion to Roux-en-Y gastric bypass as described. An upper GI was not attained. We were able to advance her along a standard gastric bypass care pathway, and she was discharged on a pureed postgastric bypass diet on postoperative day 2. She was discharged home on a single dose of a PPI for 6 months. Postoperative prophylaxis with a PPI may decrease the rate of marginal ulcers following gastric bypass. She was able to stop her PPI at 6 months post-op and reported that her GERD symptoms were completely resolved. She lost additional weight, and at 6 months postop, her BMI had decreased to 28 kg/m^2.

TAKE HOME POINTS

- Morbidly obese patients have a high incidence of gastroesophageal reflux.
- Morbidly obese patients who undergo sleeve gastrectomy are at risk for de no GERD or exacerbation of GERD symptoms after sleeve gastrectomy.
- At the time of primary sleeve gastrectomy, surgeons should carefully evaluate for the presence of a hiatal hernia and should perform a concurrent hiatal hernia repair at the time of sleeve gastrectomy when a hernia is identified.
- In patients with GERD following sleeve gastrectomy, primary and first-line therapy is acid suppression with medications.
- In sleeve gastrectomy patients with medically refractory GERD, an evaluation including a minimum of an upper endoscopy and upper GI esophagram should be conducted to determine if surgery is indicated.
- Although a variety of alternative treatments have been identified in sleeve patients with refractory GERD, conversion to Roux-en-Y gastric bypass is the procedure of choice. Further investigation is needed to determine if magnetic sphincter augmentation (LINX), radiofrequency ablation (Stretta), or plication procedures are safe and effective in these patients.
- When compared to primary gastric bypass, conversion of a sleeve to a gastric bypass is technically more complex and associated with increased rates of patient morbidity.

SUGGESTED READINGS

Crawford C, Gibbens K, Lomelin D, Krause C, Simorov A, Oleynikov D. Sleeve gastrectomy and anti-reflux procedures. *Surg Endosc.* 2017;31:1012.

Daes J, Jimenez ME, Said N, Daza JC, Dennis R. Laparoscopic sleeve gastrectomy: symptoms of gastroesophageal reflux can be reduced by changes in surgical technique. *Obes Surg.* 2012;22 (12):1874-1879.

DuPree CE, Blair K, Steele SR, Martin MJ. Laparoscopic sleeve gastrectomy in patients with preexisting gastroesophageal reflux disease: a national analysis. *JAMA Surg.* 2014;149(4):328-334.

Oor JE, Roks DJ, Ünlü Ç, Hazebroek EJ. Laparoscopic sleeve gastrectomy and gastroesophageal reflux disease: a systematic review and meta-analysis. *Am J Surg.* 2016;211(1):250-267.

Quezada N, Hernández J, Pérez G, Gabrielli M, Raddatz A, Crovari F. Laparoscopic sleeve gastrectomy conversion to Roux-en-Y gastric bypass: experience in 50 patients after 1 to 3 years of follow-up. *Surg Obes Relat Dis.* 2016;12:1611.

Varaban OA, Hawasli AA, Carlin Am, et al. Variation in utilization of acid reducing medication at 1 year following bariatric surgery: results from the Michigan Bariatric Surgery Collaborative. *Surg Obes Relat Dis.* 2015;11(1):222-228.

Leak After Bariatric Surgery

17

OLIVER A. VARBAN

Presentation

A 45-year-old male presents to the emergency room with left chest and back pain, nausea, shortness of breath, and subjective fever. He underwent an uncomplicated laparoscopic bariatric procedure 10 days earlier, and his current body mass index (BMI) is 58 m/kg².

On exam, the patient is diaphoretic, and vital signs are notable for a temperature of 38.5°C, pulse of 114 beats per minute, blood pressure of 114/75, respiratory rate of 20 breaths per minute, and an oxygen saturation of 94%. His abdomen is nontender and incision sites are dry and intact without signs of erythema or drainage.

● DIFFERENTIAL DIAGNOSIS

The differential diagnosis for a patient with tachycardia and tachypnea after bariatric surgery includes gastrointestinal (GI) leak, postoperative bleeding, missed bowel or pancreatic injury, pulmonary embolism, and myocardial infarction. Although the incidence of gastrointestinal leak after primary bariatric surgery is an increasingly uncommon event, it remains a disastrous complication resulting in significant patient morbidity and mortality. Given their body habitus, it is important to recognize that patients undergoing bariatric surgery may not develop clinically apparent peritonitis in the face of a leak. It is also important to recognize that bariatric surgery patients often suffer from numerous weight-related comorbidities such as heart disease, hypertension, diabetes, and obstructive sleep apnea, resulting in a higher rate of overall complications as well as prolonged complex hospitalizations when leaks occur. As such, early detection of leaks is pivotal for successful management.

Gastrointestinal leaks can occur after either type of stapled primary bariatric procedures such as sleeve gastrectomy (SG) or gastric bypass (GB). Male gender, older age (>65 years old), and a BMI of 50 kg/m² or greater are risk factors. Leaks may occur due to technical complications of surgery, due to staple misfire, or as a result of ischemia compounded by distal obstruction. After sleeve gastrectomy, leaks most commonly occur along the staple line at the gastroesophageal (GE) junction. After gastric bypass, leaks may occur along the gastric pouch or remnant stomach staple line or at either the gastrojejunostomy or jejunojejunostomy.

In the modern era, the majority of bariatric procedures are performed laparoscopically, and surgeons typically perform an intraoperative leak test with insufflation, methylene blue, and/or endoscopy. Some surgeons may also perform an upper gastrointestinal contrast study on postoperative day 1. Although widely used, perioperative testing has not been found to reduce the incidence of leaks. Thus, one must continue to have a high suspicion for leaks even if all of the initial perioperative studies are negative.

● WORKUP

The workup of this patient needs to be performed in a thorough yet expeditious manner so as to establish the correct diagnosis and initiate treatment. Patients with severe obesity often lack the cardiopulmonary reserve to withstand hemodynamic instability from shock due to their numerous underlying comorbidities. Moreover, they are more prone to dehydration during the initial postoperative period as their diet consists primarily of liquids/protein shakes. Patients should be asked about their oral intake, symptoms of nausea or emesis, urine output, and orthostatic hypotension in order to gain insight into their level of hydration after bariatric surgery.

After obtaining vital signs, a thorough physical exam may reveal signs of a cardiac arrhythmia or pleural effusion in addition to their presenting signs of tachycardia and tachypnea. An abdominal exam may be unrevealing given the patient's large habitus, and peritoneal signs are not always present. Nevertheless, after a leak, patients can experience pain particularly in the left upper quadrant or left subscapular region as a fluid collection or abscess may collect in the left subdiaphragmatic space. A lower extremity exam should be performed in order to evaluate for unilateral edema, which would increase one's suspicion for a deep venous thrombosis or pulmonary embolism, which may present in a similar manner as a GI leak.

Initial laboratory studies should include a complete blood count, metabolic panel, liver profile, amylase, lipase, urinalysis, and cardiac enzymes. These studies can help delineate whether the patient's symptoms represent hypovolemic, cardiogenic, or septic shock.

In a clinically stable patient with a suspected leak, computed tomography (CT) scan of the abdomen and pelvis with water-soluble oral and intravenous (IV) contrast is the

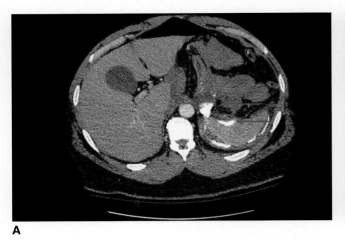
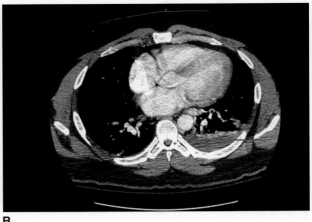

A   **B**

FIGURE 17-1. **A:** CT scan (sagittal) of the abdomen demonstrating extraluminal oral contrast and air (*arrows*), consistent with a leak after sleeve gastrectomy. **B:** CT scan (sagittal) of the chest and abdomen demonstrating a left pleural effusion and atelectasis (*arrows*) secondary to leak after sleeve gastrectomy.

preferred imaging modality (Figure 17-1). It is more sensitive and specific in identifying a leak when compared to upper gastrointestinal contrast studies and has the added benefit of identifying associated intra-abdominal abscesses, hematomas, and/or obstruction. Evidence of extraluminal air and/or contrast extravasation is diagnostic, and if the type of procedure is unknown (i.e., gastric bypass vs. sleeve gastrectomy), postsurgical anatomy can be delineated. A CT angiogram of the chest can also be included to rule out a pulmonary embolism and/or identify a pulmonary effusion, which can be associated with a subdiaphragmatic abscess secondary to a leak.

In our case, the patient underwent a sleeve gastrectomy, and laboratory studies demonstrate a leukocytosis, elevated creatinine, and normal cardiac enzymes. The CT scan demonstrates oral contrast extravasation and extraluminal air along with a complex fluid collection located in the left subdiaphragmatic space (Figure 17-2).

● DIAGNOSIS AND TREATMENT

The most likely diagnosis for the patient in this scenario is a gastric staple line leak after sleeve gastrectomy. This patient is presenting with early signs of septic shock and has evidence of extraluminal air and contrast. Initial management consists of obtaining two large-bore IVs and providing resuscitation. If a patient with a suspected leak presents with hemodynamic instability, operative management should be considered over an imaging study because surgical exploration remains the diagnostic test with the highest sensitivity and specificity and also yields the most expeditious source control.

Principles of treatment for a patient with a leak after bariatric surgery include (1) drainage of fluid collection/abscess, (2) antibiotics, and (3) nutritional support. As discussed in more detail below, primary suture repair of the defect can be attempted but is usually not feasible, and an omental patch

with wide drainage is preferred. While the leak is healing, an alternative means of nutrition should be provided, usually by inserting a feeding jejunostomy well beyond the site of the leak.

Over time, leaks will seal without any further management or develop into a chronic fistula. Average closure time for leaks may be 4 to 6 weeks for either gastric bypass or sleeve gastrectomy. However, closure times of 3 to 6 months are not uncommon after sleeve gastrectomy given the higher pressures within the lumen of the stomach. Definitive management of a chronic fistula is technically challenging and should be attempted only after enough time has lapsed and nonoperative treatment has failed. Several surgical procedures have been described including conversion of sleeve gastrectomy to gastric bypass, total gastrectomy with esophagojejunostomy, and T-tube placement. Such procedures can be performed laparoscopically or open depending on the level of experience and technical skill. Complication rates and recurrent leaks remain high (>50%), and given the paucity of data, there is no preferred approach that can be advocated at this time.

Nonoperative management is appropriate and even optimal in the clinically stable patient. The same principles of drainage, antibiotics and nutritional support are pursued. However, management requires a multidisciplinary approach that involves interventional radiology as well as advanced endoscopy. In the nonoperative setting, abscesses can usually be drained adequately with CT-guided drain placement. However, it should be noted that a transpleural approach may be necessary to place a drain in the subdiaphragmatic space. Endoluminal stents have been used with a healing success rate of 55% to 100% with the added benefit of maintaining oral nutrition. However, management involves numerous endoscopies, and complications include migration, kinking, erosion, and patient intolerance due to pain, nausea, and emesis. Many patients do not tolerate stents due to reflux or intolerance. Other endoscopic

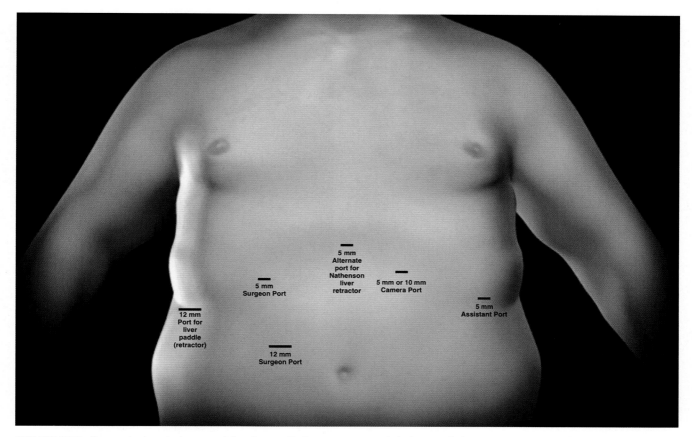

FIGURE 17-2. Suggested port placement for diagnostic laparoscopy and drainage of abscess cavity secondary to leak after sleeve gastrectomy.

modalities such as placement of clips, fibrin sealant, and endoscopic suturing are additional maneuvers that may be used; however, they are rarely used as a stand-alone treatment. Finally, endoscopy offers the opportunity to dilate distal strictures that may contribute to the presence of the fistula.

The patient in this scenario was experiencing early signs of septic shock and underwent operative management via laparoscopic exploration, thorough irrigation, and drain placement. After the patient stabilized, endoscopic stent placement was performed several weeks later; however, due to stent migration, pain, and excessive vomiting, the stent was subsequently removed.

● SURGICAL APPROACH

This patient has evidence of a leak on imaging studies and is clinically unstable, which requires immediate operative drainage. A laparoscopic approach is preferred as it spares the patient the morbidity of a laparotomy, which is significant in patients who are obese. Moreover, exposure and visualization of the hiatus and subdiaphragmatic space can be challenging during open surgery in patients with a BMI > 50 kg/m^2.

Access to the abdominal cavity is achieved using a Veress needle at Palmer's point in the usual fashion. After adequate abdominal insufflation, a port is placed in the left upper quadrant, and an angled laparoscope (5 or 10 mm) is entered in the abdominal cavity. After initial inspection for needle or trocar injury, the patient is placed in the steep reverse Trendelenburg position, and additional ports are placed. Port placement should allow for optimal access for the surgeon to operate with two instruments, an assistant to assist with at least one instrument, and a fixed liver retractor (Figure 17-3). Careful exploration of the left upper quadrant should be performed with blunt atraumatic graspers. The main goal is to identify and drain any abscess cavity, irrigate copiously with warm saline, and then place one or more drains into the cavity spaces. In most cases, abscesses form in the left upper quadrant of the abdomen in the most dependent space of the abdominal cavity. In the case of a gastric bypass leak, the lesser sac should be examined as well. Identification of the exact location of the leak is not necessary as primary repair is often not feasible, and narrowing by overzealous attempts at repair of a sleeve or gastric bypass pouch leak can result in a stricture. An omental patch may be placed over the site of the leak if identified by placing seromuscular sutures through healthy gastric tissue and omentum. Typically, three sutures are adequate

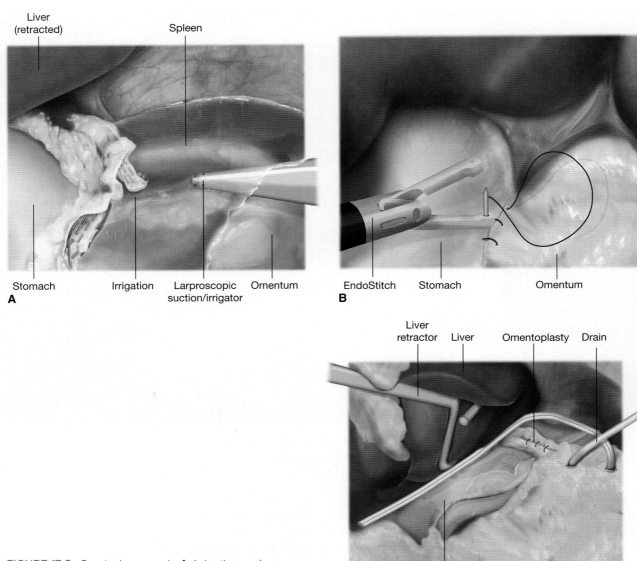

FIGURE 17-3. Surgical approach. **A:** Irrigation and debridement of abscess cavity. **B:** Omentoplasty. **C:** Drain placement.

to approximate the omentum to the location of the leak. Finally, large (>10 Fr) round channel drains are placed in the dependent spaces of all abscess cavities.

After adequate irrigation, debridement, and drain placement, the next goal is to establish access for long-term enteral feeding as leak closure can take as long as 3 to 6 months. In the case of a leak after sleeve gastrectomy, enteral feeding can be established via nasojejunal feeding tube or operatively, via a feeding jejunostomy tube. For patients who sustain a leak after gastric bypass surgery, a feeding gastrostomy tube can be placed in the remnant stomach, assuming the source of leak is not along the remnant stomach staple line. Alternatively, a feeding jejunostomy may be placed in the common channel, distal to the jejunojejunostomy. Placing a feeding jejunostomy involves placing four sutures (2-0 braided absorbable sutures are used typically) in a diamond formation along the antimesenteric portion of the small bowel. Next, an

enterotomy is created in the middle of the four sutures, and a 12- to 14-Fr silastic feeding tube is advanced into the bowel directing it distally along the jejunum. The four sutures are anchored to the abdominal wall using a Carter-Thomason suture passer to grasp each tail of the sutures through the fascia. The tails are tied extracorporeally with the knots lying in the subcutaneous space of the incision where the drain exits the skin. The drain is then sutured to the skin with a 3-0 nylon suture.

When exploring the left upper quadrant and debriding associated abscess cavities, it is imperative to avoid injuring the spleen, tail of the pancreas, or colon. Intraoperative hemorrhage from a splenic injury is potentially life threatening, and splenectomy may be required to obtain hemostasis. A pancreatic injury may present postoperatively when persistent drainage from one of the drains is recorded to have an abnormally high level of amylase and lipase. The splenic flexure of the colon may form adhesions along the leak site, and aggressive adhesiolysis may result in deserosalization, a full-thickness injury, or an ischemic injury to the colon. If the site of colonic injury is small, it may be repaired primarily. Gastrocolic fistulas have been reported as a long-term complication after a sleeve leak. Judicious use of drains is important as poor drain placement or drain migration can lead to inadequate drainage and ongoing abdominal sepsis (Table 17-1).

● POSTOPERATIVE MANAGEMENT

After surgery, the patient is admitted to the hospital for management of abdominal sepsis. Initially, the patient may need intensive care for advanced monitoring, continued ventilatory support, and vasopressors if necessary. The typical hospital stay is 6 to 7 days, and the patient may be discharged when hemodynamically stable, tolerating tube feeds, and ambulating and has adequate pain management. Antibiotics are continued and can be discontinued when abscesses have resolved and the patient no longer has a leukocytosis. In most tertiary institutions, an infectious disease consult is place to manage antibiotics after surgery.

Clinic follow-up can be made at 2- to 4-week intervals in order to assess the volume and consistency of the drain output. A repeat CT scan is performed when the drain output has decreased <30 cc/d in order to assess for a residual leak or abscess. An upper GI study or drain injection study can also be performed to confirm resolution of the leak or identify a fistula.

The patient recovers well after undergoing laparoscopic drainage and inpatient hospitalization for sepsis. After 3 months, an upper gastrointestinal contrast study is performed, and there is no evidence of a residual leak. As such, the patient is advanced to a clear diet initially followed by a regular diet.

TAKE HOME POINTS

- Leaks after bariatric surgery can occur along a staple line or anastomosis.
- Patients presenting with a leak may not exhibit peritonitis. Common signs of a leak include fever, tachycardia, and/or tachypnea.
- Diagnosis can be confirmed by CT scan with IV and PO water-soluble contrast.
- CT angiogram of the chest should be performed as well to rule out pulmonary embolism as patients may present with similar symptoms.
- Management consists of resuscitation, antibiotics, effective drainage of the leak, and nutritional support.
- Placement of drains can be performed surgically (laparoscopic or open) or by interventional radiology.
- Feeding jejunostomy is ideal for long-term nutritional support.
- Most leaks will seal without further management; however, closure times may vary from 4 weeks to 6 months.
- Endoscopic stents, clips, or sealant materials have been attempted with various success rates.
- Definitive management of a chronic fistula is challenging. Surgical options include revisional surgery or conversion of sleeve gastrectomy to gastric bypass. Complication rates for these procedures remain high and should only be attempted after nonoperative therapy has failed.

Table 17-1 Leak After Bariatric Surgery

Key Technical Steps

1. Veress needle entry in the left upper quadrant followed by abdominal insufflation.
2. Placement of laparoscopic ports and a liver retractor. For optimal visualization of the left upper quadrant of the abdominal cavity, the patient is also positioned in steep reverse Trendelenburg.
3. Careful exploration of left upper quadrant and subdiaphragmatic space with copious irrigation and debridement of all abscess cavities.
4. If the location of the leak is identified, an omental patch may be performed.
5. Large, round channel drains (>10 Fr) are placed in the dependent portions of the abscess cavity.
6. Surgical feeding jejunostomy is placed for long-term enteral access.

Potential Pitfalls

- Splenic injury
- Pancreatic injury
- Colonic injury
- Inadequate drainage or drain placement

SUGGESTED READINGS

AbouRached A, Basile M, El Masri H. Gastric leaks post sleeve gastrectomy: review of its prevention and management. *World J Gastroenterol.* 2014;20:13904-13910.

Aurora AR, Khaitan L, Saber AA. Sleeve gastrectomy and the risk of leak: a systematic analysis of 4,888 patients. *Surg Endosc.* 2012;26:1509-1515.

Kim J, Azagury D, Eisenberg D, DeMaria E, Campos GM; American SFMABSCIC. ASMBS position statement on prevention, detection, and treatment of gastrointestinal leak after gastric bypass and sleeve gastrectomy, including the roles of imaging, surgical exploration, and nonoperative management. *Surg Obes Relat Dis.* 2015;11:739-748.

Spyropoulos C, Argentou MI, Petsas T, Thomopoulos K, Kehagias I, Kalfarentzos F. Management of gastrointestinal leaks after surgery for clinically severe obesity. *Surg Obes Relat Dis.* 2012 Sep-Oct;8(5):609-615. doi: 10.1016/j.soard.2011.04.222. Epub 2011 Apr 27.

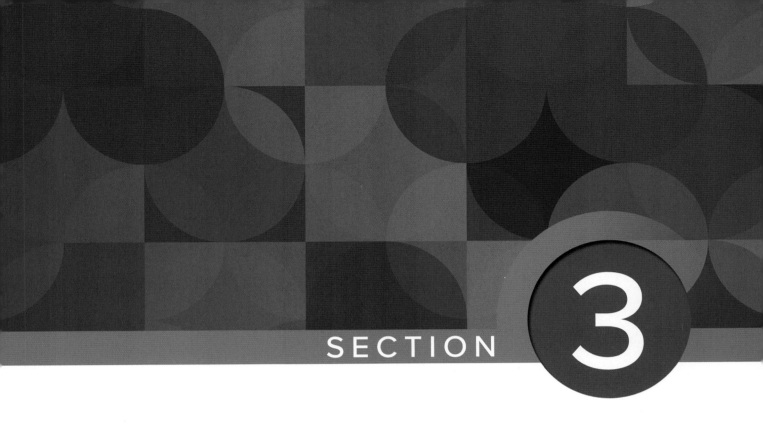

SECTION 3

Emergency General Surgery

Acute Appendicitis

JASON B. YOUNG, SARAH E. GREER, AND SAMUEL R.G. FINLAYSON

18

Based on the previous edition chapter "Acute Appendicitis" by Sarah E. Greer and Samuel R.G. Finlayson

Presentation

A 24-year-old woman presents to the emergency department with abdominal pain, nausea, vomiting, and anorexia that began the previous evening. She describes her abdominal pain as initially periumbilical, but now localized to the right lower quadrant (RLQ). Her temperature is 37.9. Her vital signs are otherwise normal. On abdominal exam, her abdomen is soft and nondistended, but tender to palpation over McBurney's point. She has no signs of peritonitis.

● DIFFERENTIAL DIAGNOSIS

In the United States, acute appendicitis is the most common time-sensitive surgical problem. The signs and symptoms of acute appendicitis are believed to develop as a result of obstruction of the appendiceal lumen. This obstruction leads to bacterial proliferation, which can result in appendiceal necrosis and perforation.

While the classic symptoms of abdominal pain migrating to the RLQ, nausea, and anorexia occur in a majority of patients with acute appendicitis, symptoms may be less specific, requiring clinicians to consider a broad differential diagnosis, including gastrointestinal, urologic, and gynecologic pathology. Alternative gastrointestinal diagnoses that must be considered include gastroenteritis, colitis, ileitis, diverticulitis, and inflammatory bowel disease. Infectious causes, such as mesenteric adenitis, urinary tract infection, and pyelonephritis, should also be considered. In women, it is important to include mittelschmerz, salpingitis, tubo-ovarian abscess, ovarian torsion, and ruptured ovarian cyst in the differential diagnosis.

● WORKUP

A full history and physical exam must be performed to help establish the diagnosis. In addition to eliciting a history of symptoms and their temporal evolution, the surgeon should ask the patient about any family history of inflammatory bowel disease and a complete menstrual and pregnancy history in women.

On physical exam, pain over McBurney's point (one-third the distance from the anterior superior iliac spine to the umbilicus) is a classic presenting sign of acute appendicitis. Additional physical exam findings may suggest appendicitis as a diagnosis. *Rovsing's sign* is pain in the RLQ when pressure is applied in the left lower quadrant (LLQ); an obturator sign is pain with passive rotation of the flexed right hip; and a psoas sign describes pain on extension of the right hip, the latter commonly present in patients with a retrocecal appendix that lies in contact with the iliopsoas muscle. A pelvic exam in women of childbearing age must not be omitted, as it may reveal gynecologic conditions to which the patient's symptoms can be attributed.

Laboratory tests that should be obtained include a complete blood count, which will typically reveal a low-grade leukocytosis. Other laboratory tests that should be ordered include a coagulation profile, type and screen (if an operation is anticipated), and a urinalysis to exclude urinary pathology. A pregnancy test should also be performed in women of childbearing age.

In the patient above, pelvic exam reveals no adnexal mass or cervical motion tenderness. Laboratory evaluation reveals a leukocytosis of 16,000. The patient is otherwise healthy, with no history of previous abdominal surgery and no pertinent family history.

In 1986, Alvarado published a practical scoring system for the early diagnosis of acute appendicitis. The scoring system helps clinicians predict which patients can be safely observed and which should undergo operative intervention based on symptoms (migration of pain, anorexia or urine acetone, and nausea–vomiting), signs (tenderness in the RLQ, rebound pain, and elevation of temperature), and laboratory findings (leukocytosis, and shift to the left).

● DIAGNOSTIC IMAGING

In young males with symptoms and signs consistent with acute appendicitis, imaging studies to confirm the diagnosis are generally unnecessary prior to proceeding to surgery. In many cases, however, when the diagnosis is not clear after thorough history taking and physical examination, imaging may be helpful in making the decision whether or not to proceed with surgery. Many clinicians are more liberal in the use of imaging in young female patients, both because of the presence of gynecologic conditions in the differential diagnosis and because of the risk of infertility associated with ruptured appendicitis that might result from a delay in diagnosis.

The two most common imaging modalities used in the diagnosis of appendicitis are ultrasound and computed tomography (CT). CT has demonstrated significantly higher sensitivity for the diagnosis of appendicitis, 94% versus 83% to 88%. However, because CT scans expose patients to ionizing radiation, this modality should be used judiciously, especially in children.

Although CT scans are an expensive technology, a focused contrast CT scan limited to the appendix may actually be cost saving. A study by Rao et al. found that routine appendix-focused CT in patients with suspected appendicitis prevented unnecessary appendectomies as well as unnecessary hospitalization for observation, with a net reduction in use of hospital resources and cost per patient.

In the patient in this case, a CT scan was performed that demonstrates a dilated, thickened appendix with surrounding inflammatory changes, consistent with acute appendicitis (Figure 18-1).

● DIAGNOSIS AND TREATMENT

Although a few studies in the surgical literature support nonoperative management of nonperforated acute appendicitis, surgical appendectomy represents the standard of care in the United States. A systematic review by Wilms et al. evaluating appendectomy versus antibiotic treatment for acute appendicitis concluded that results from available studies must be interpreted with caution, and definite conclusions about the acceptability of nonoperative treatment cannot be made.

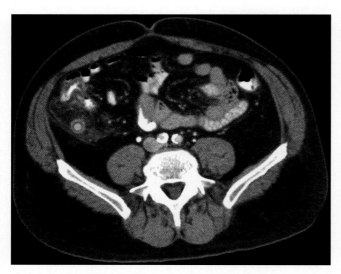

FIGURE 18-1. CT radiograph showing appendiceal dilation, wall thickening, and periappendiceal fat stranding consistent with acute appendicitis.

Management of the 15% to 30% of patients who present with perforated appendicitis is controversial. Perforated appendicitis with abscess can be treated initially with antibiotics and image-guided percutaneous drainage, with interval appendectomy 6 to 12 weeks later to prevent recurrence. This approach has been advocated to decrease complication and reoperation rates associated with immediate appendectomy for perforated appendicitis. However, others have argued that an immediate operative approach to perforated appendicitis may improve long-term outcomes and consume fewer health care resources. A randomized controlled trial by Mentula et al. in adult patients undergoing laparoscopic surgery versus conservative treatment for appendiceal abscess found no difference in hospital length of stay, and patients in the laparoscopic surgery group had significantly fewer readmissions and additional interventions than did the conservative treatment group.

A study by Skarda et al. found that implementation of a uniform doctor's preference card and technical standardization for laparoscopic appendectomy in pediatric patients with appendicitis was associated with a significant reduction in cost without dramatically increasing operative times, hospital length of stay, or postoperative complications. An additional study by the same group found that implementing a criteria-based postoperative protocol designed to eliminate postoperative antibiotics and facilitate timely discharge in pediatric patients undergoing appendectomy (laparoscopic or open) for nonruptured appendicitis was associated with a decrease in hospital length of stay, cost of care, and antibiotic use without significantly affecting adverse events.

● SURGICAL APPROACH

The technique for open appendectomy was described by McBurney in 1894 and has been used with little modification throughout the 20th century. In 1983, Semm introduced the option of laparoscopic appendectomy. Since then, there has been much debate regarding the superiority of one approach versus the other. Advantages of laparoscopic appendectomy include the ability to perform diagnostic laparoscopy if the appendix is found to be normal. Laparoscopic appendectomy is also associated with less postoperative pain, faster recovery, and lower wound infection rates. In contrast, open appendectomy has been found to be less costly and less time-consuming.

● OPEN APPENDECTOMY

Following administration of preoperative antibiotics and induction of general anesthesia, with the patient in a supine position, an incision is made in an oblique or transverse direction overlying McBurney's point. The subcutaneous fat and Scarpa's fascia are divided to expose the external oblique aponeurosis. The aponeurosis is sharply opened along the direction of its fibers. The fibers of the internal oblique muscle and transversus abdominis are then bluntly separated. The

Table 18-1	Open Appendectomy

Key Technical Steps

1. Incise the skin and subcutaneous tissues in a transverse (Rocky-Davis) or oblique (McBurney) orientation over McBurney's point.
2. Divide the external oblique aponeurosis, internal oblique muscle, and transversus abdominis muscle in the direction of their fibers.
3. Elevate and sharply divide the peritoneum.
4. Digitally explore the abdomen and deliver the appendix into the wound.
5. Divide the mesoappendix.
6. Ligate and divide the appendix at its base.
7. Close the abdominal wall layers.

Table 18-2	Laparoscopic Appendectomy

Key Technical Steps

1. Incise the skin adjacent to the umbilicus and create pneumoperitoneum using Hassan or Veress needle technique.
2. Place an 11-mm trocar at the umbilical incision.
3. Inspect the abdominal cavity laparoscopically to confirm the diagnosis.
4. Place two additional trocars (5 mm) in positions that facilitate access to the RLQ.
5. Dissect open a "window" in the mesoappendix adjacent to the base of the appendix.
6. Divide the base of the appendix.
7. Divide the mesoappendix.
8. Remove the appendix through the 11-mm trocar incision.
9. Close the trocar incisions.

underlying peritoneum is then elevated into the wound and sharply opened along the length of the incision (Table 18-1).

Upon entering the abdominal cavity, presence of purulent fluid or foul smell should be noted. If the appendix is not immediately visualized, exploration with the index finger may reveal an inflammatory mass. Alternately, the teniae coli of the right colon can be followed proximally to the base of the appendix, which is then delivered into the wound with gentle traction, taking care not to avulse the appendix.

The mesoappendix including the appendiceal artery is divided between clamps and ligated. The base of the appendix once free of the mesentery is doubly ligated close to the cecum and sharply divided. The stump mucosa is often cauterized to prevent the development of a mucocele. Although invagination of the stump into the cecum with a purse-string suture or Z-stitch can be performed, there are no high-quality data demonstrating that invagination improves outcomes as compared to simple ligation.

After copious irrigation and ensuring hemostasis, the wound is closed in layers with absorbable suture. The skin may be closed primarily with a subcuticular suture or may be left open for a delayed primary closure in the setting of significant contamination.

● LAPAROSCOPIC APPENDECTOMY

Similar to an open approach, the patient receives preoperative antibiotics and general anesthesia and is positioned supine on the operating table. Gastric decompression should be accomplished with an orogastric tube, and a urinary catheter should be placed to decompress the bladder. In cases of uncomplicated appendicitis, a urinary catheter may not be necessary if the patient has voided preoperatively. Once the abdomen has been sterilely prepped and draped, a three-port-site approach is used: one at the umbilicus and the other two according to surgeon preference.

The abdomen is systematically explored to confirm the diagnosis and rule out other pathology (Table 18-2).

The appendix is then mobilized to expose its base. A window in the mesoappendix is created near the base of the appendix using blunt dissection, and then an endoscopic stapler may be used to divide the appendix. If the tissue at the base of the appendix is not deemed viable, a small portion of the cecum may be removed with the appendix to ensure that the staple line traverses tissue that will heal well. The mesoappendix and appendiceal artery are then divided with cautery and clips, or with a stapler using a vascular load. Alternatively, a combination of an electrothermal device and a ligature can be used to divide the mesoappendix and appendix and to secure the appendiceal stump respectively. A specimen bag is typically used to remove the appendix through the largest port site.

The RLQ may be irrigated with saline, although prospective randomized trials in both pediatric and adult patients undergoing laparoscopic appendectomy for perforated appendicitis have shown no advantage to irrigation of the peritoneal cavity over suction alone to prevent postoperative intra-abdominal abscess. Once hemostasis at the surgical site is assured, and provided no other pathology is noted, the ports are removed under direct vision to ensure the absence of abdominal wall bleeding. The fascia is reapproximated with absorbable suture at port sites larger than 5 mm. The skin is then closed with a subcuticular suture.

● SPECIAL INTRAOPERATIVE CONSIDERATIONS

When the appendix is found to be normal, the abdominal cavity must be searched diligently for an alternative explanation for the patient's symptoms. In female patients, the ovaries and uterus should be inspected carefully for pathologic findings, such as tubo-ovarian abscess, ovarian torsion, tumor, or cyst. The small bowel should be systematically inspected for sources of inflammation, such as Crohn's disease or Meckel's diverticulitis. The gallbladder should also be inspected for signs of cholecystitis.

Traditionally, a normal appendix is removed when it is discovered during open appendectomy, mainly to prevent future surgeons from assuming that the appendix is absent on the basis of an RLQ scar. This traditional approach has been called into question since the advent of laparoscopic appendectomy.

Appropriate management of the normal appendix requires judgment when Crohn's disease is found as the cause of the patient's illness. If the base of the appendix and cecum appear to be uninvolved in the inflammatory process, appendectomy is likely safe. The major benefit of appendectomy in the setting of Crohn's disease is that subsequent episodes of RLQ pain will not be confused with appendicitis.

Appendiceal tumors are rare, but given the prevalence of appendectomy, most surgeons will occasionally encounter them. Carcinoid tumors constitute the majority of appendiceal tumors. If a carcinoid tumor is suspected at the time of surgery, the appendix should be sent to the pathology laboratory for a frozen section histologic diagnosis. For carcinoids <2 cm, simple appendectomy is sufficient. For larger carcinoids, right hemicolectomy with ileocolic lymphadenectomy is recommended. If the histology shows adenocarcinoma of the appendix, a right hemicolectomy is also warranted.

● POSTOPERATIVE MANAGEMENT

For patients with acute appendicitis in the absence of perforation, abscess, or gangrene, a single dose of prophylactic antibiotics is sufficient. Prolonged postoperative antibiotics in this patient population do not alter the incidence of superficial, deep, or organ space surgical site infections, and do correlate with higher rates of *Clostridium difficile* infection, urinary tract infection, postoperative diarrhea, and prolonged hospital stay. Empirically, antimicrobial therapy for appendicitis with perforation, abscess, or gangrene is often continued until after the resolution of all clinical signs of infection, including resolution of leukocytosis and fever. However, recent evidence from the open-label multicenter randomized STOP-IT trial found that treatment of complicated intra-abdominal infections, including

perforated appendicitis, with a fixed duration of antibiotic therapy (median of 4 days) after adequate source control has similar surgical site infection, recurrent intra-abdominal infection, and mortality outcomes when compared to an antibiotic course that extends until after resolution of physiologic abnormalities (median of 8 days).

SUGGESTED READINGS

Addiss DG, Shaffer N, Fowler BS, et al. The epidemiology of appendicitis and appendectomy in the United States. *Am J Epidemiol.* 1990;132:910-925.

Alvarado A. A practical score for the early diagnosis of acute appendicitis. *Ann Emerg Med.* 1986;15:557-564.

Chung RS, Rowland DY, Li P, et al. A meta-analysis of randomized controlled trials of laparoscopic versus conventional appendectomy. *Am J Surg.* 1999;177:250-256.

Coakley BA, Sussman ES, Wolfson TS, et al. Postoperative antibiotics correlate with worse outcomes after appendectomy for nonperforated appendicitis. *J Am Coll Surg.* 2011;213:778-783.

Mentula P, Sammalkorpi H, Leppaniemi A. Laparoscopic surgery or conservative treatment for appendiceal abscess in adults? A randomized controlled trial. *Ann Surg.* 2015;262:237-242.

Rao PM, Rhea JT, Novelline RA, et al. Effect of computed tomography of the appendix on treatment of patients and use of hospital resources. *N Engl J Med.* 1998;338:141-146.

Sawyer RG, Claridge JA, Nathens AB, et al. Trial of short-course antimicrobial therapy for intraabdominal infection. *N Engl J Med.* 2015;372:1996-2005.

Silen W, ed. *Cope's Early Diagnosis of the Acute Abdomen.* 19th ed. New York, NY: Oxford University Press; 1996.

Simillis C, Symeonides P, Shorthouse AJ, et al. A meta-analysis comparing conservative treatment versus acute appendectomy for complicated appendicitis. *Surgery.* 2010;147:818-829.

Skarda DE, Rollins M, Andrews S, et al. One hospital, one appendectomy: the cost effectiveness of a standardized doctor's preference card. *J Pediatr Surg.* 2015;50:919-922.

Skarda DE, Schall K, Rollins M, et al. A dynamic postoperative protocol provides efficient care for pediatric patients with non-ruptured appendicitis. *J Pediatr Surg.* 2015;50:149-152.

Snow HA, Choi JM, Cheng MW, et al. Irrigation versus suction alone during laparoscopic appendectomy; a randomized controlled equivalence trial. *Int J Surg.* 2016;28:91-96.

St Peter SD, Adibe OO, Iqbal CW, et al. Irrigation versus suction alone during laparoscopic appendectomy for perforated appendicitis: a prospective randomized trial. *Ann Surg.* 2012;256:581-585.

Wilms IM, de Hoog DE, de Visser DC, et al. Appendectomy versus antibiotic treatment for acute appendicitis. *Cochrane Database Syst Rev.* 2011;11:CD008359.

Perforated Appendicitis

19

BENJAMIN DAVID CARR AND MARK R. HEMMILA

Based on the previous edition chapter "Perforated Appendicitis" by
Terry Shih, Mark R. Hemmila, and Justin B. Dimick

Presentation

A 25-year-old man with no previous medical or surgical history presents to the emergency room with 5 days of abdominal pain. His pain was initially periumbilical, but has since migrated to his right lower quadrant (RLQ), and finally became diffuse. For the past 3 days, he has had nausea, vomiting, and fevers. He presents now as he could no longer tolerate oral intake. His vital signs include a fever of 39.2°C, tachycardia with a heart rate in the 110s, and a normal blood pressure. On physical examination, his abdomen is nondistended and he has tenderness to palpation in the RLQ with focal rebound tenderness and voluntary guarding.

● DIFFERENTIAL DIAGNOSIS

RLQ pain with fevers, nausea, and vomiting with localized tenderness is the classic presentation of acute appendicitis. In a young, otherwise healthy male, there is a limited list of other potential diagnoses, such as gastroenteritis or the initial presentation of Crohn's disease. In a female patient, gynecologic pathologies must be considered, including ovarian torsion, ectopic pregnancy, ruptured ovarian cyst, or pelvic inflammatory disease.

This patient has a delayed presentation (5 days) with a high fever, which raises suspicion for perforated appendicitis, as perforation typically occurs 24 to 36 hours following onset of symptoms. Patients with perforation often also present with a more extensive systemic inflammatory response, including higher fevers and tachycardia. Patients may have more substantial abdominal pain and tenderness as the underlying inflammatory process may be more significant (e.g., phlegmon or abscess). Because of the delayed presentation, the differential diagnosis is different than for early acute appendicitis and should include right-sided diverticulitis, perforated right-sided colon cancer, cecal perforation due to a distal obstruction (cancer or diverticular stricture), and typhlitis in immunosuppressed patients.

● WORKUP

Patients with suspected appendicitis, either early or late in their course, should undergo laboratory tests, including a complete blood count (CBC) and basic metabolic panel (i.e., electrolytes, BUN, and creatinine). In our patient, the CBC and basic metabolic panel reveal a leukocytosis with a white blood cell count of 18,000 and an elevated creatinine to 1.8 mg/dL. All other laboratory tests are within normal limits.

In young healthy males who present with signs and symptoms of classic early appendicitis, further imaging with computed tomography (CT) scan may not be necessary before proceeding to surgery. However, female patients should be evaluated with additional imaging such as a CT scan or transabdominal and transvaginal ultrasound, as pathology of RLQ structures may mimic the presentation of appendicitis.

This case demonstrates several key differences from early appendicitis. The patient has had pain for 5 days with high fevers and tachycardia, increasing the chance of perforation, abscess, or phlegmon. Contrary to early appendicitis, where CT scan is used selectively, cross-sectional imaging is always warranted when perforation is suspected. In our patient, a CT scan of the abdomen and pelvis reveals a dilated appendix to 1.2 cm with extraluminal air and fat stranding surrounding the appendix. There is a periappendiceal fluid collection that measures 4 × 5 cm with rim enhancement (Figure 19-1).

● DISCUSSION

Once the diagnosis of perforated appendicitis is established, treatment depends on the extent of the inflammatory process. Patients with evidence of perforated appendicitis without a large abscess may benefit from appendectomy at the time of presentation. However, if the patient has evidence of a large amount of inflammation (i.e., periappendiceal phlegmon or abscess), immediate surgical intervention may do more harm than good. In this setting, appendectomy is associated with a significantly higher rate of complications and concomitant bowel resection (e.g., ileocecectomy or right colectomy) than an operation performed for nonperforated appendicitis.

Patients with phlegmon but no definitive abscess (Figure 19-2) will often improve with intravenous antibiotics alone. Patients with evidence of abscess (e.g., contained collections of air and fluid on CT scan) (Figures 19-1 and 19-3A–C) may benefit from radiology-guided percutaneous drainage, in addition to intravenous antibiotics. Figure 19-1A–D demonstrate CT-guided percutaneous

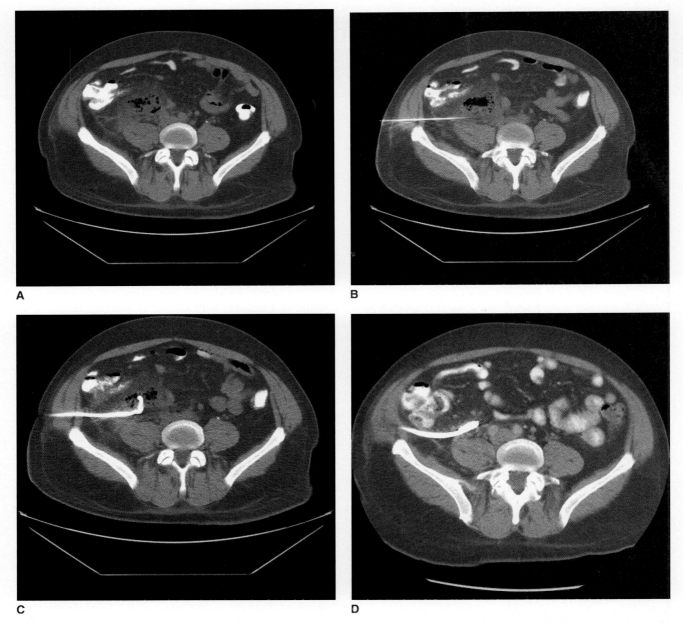

FIGURE 19-1. **A:** Right lower quadrant abscess. **B:** Drain placement for abscess 1. **C:** Drain placement 2. **D:** Drain placement with resolution of abscess.

aspiration with placement of a drain. Resolution of symptoms and leukocytosis will determine the duration of IV antibiotics. Typically, antibiotics may be transitioned to an oral regimen for the patient to complete a 1- or 2-week course as an outpatient.

After allowing inflammation to subside (6 to 8 weeks), an interval appendectomy may be performed as an outpatient procedure. Pain is usually controlled with oral narcotics or NSAIDs. The patient should be educated to monitor for signs of postoperative infection: fevers, chills, fatigue, nausea, vomiting, or diarrhea from possible pelvic abscess.

Recent studies suggest that interval appendectomy is likely not warranted in an asymptomatic patient, but select patients may benefit from surgery to eliminate the risk of recurrent appendicitis or malignancy. Patients with the following risk factors are appropriate candidates for interval appendectomy: recurrent appendicitis, persistent RLQ pain, fecalith, age over 40 years, and symptoms concerning for malignancy (change in bowel habits, rectal bleeding, anemia, suspicious imaging findings). Patients who are of appropriate age (>50 years) or have suspicious findings on imaging should undergo colonoscopy to rule out malignancy.

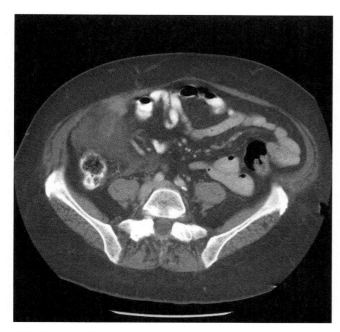

FIGURE 19-2. Phlegmon without definite abscess.

● SURGICAL APPROACH

The decision to operate in a patient with perforated appendicitis should be made after a careful assessment of the degree of inflammation. Most patients will be managed nonoperatively with intravenous antibiotics with (abscess) or without (phlegmon) percutaneous drainage. Operation in patients with advanced degrees of inflammation could result in a

much larger operation (e.g., ileocecectomy) because the base of the appendix may be involved in the process, making it unsafe to remove the appendix in isolation.

There are two specific clinical scenarios where surgery should be considered in perforated appendicitis. First, prompt exploratory laparotomy should be pursued in patients who present with diffuse peritonitis due to free perforation of appendicitis. Often the precise diagnosis will be unknown at the time of exploration. However, if a patient with perforated appendicitis becomes clinically worse (e.g., develops diffuse peritonitis and/or worsening systemic inflammatory response) despite medical management, emergent laparotomy should be undertaken. Exploratory laparotomy, ileocecectomy, and irrigation are usually necessary in this scenario. Second, appendectomy can be pursued in patients with early perforation (e.g., insignificant inflammation but small amounts of extra-appendiceal fluid and air on CT scan). This latter scenario is somewhat controversial, and clinical practice varies across surgeons. In our practice, we believe that a laparoscopic appendectomy in early perforated appendicitis will be less bothersome to the patient than a long hospital stay for intravenous antibiotics and bowel rest.

As with early acute appendicitis, appendectomy can be performed via an open or laparoscopic approach. Studies comparing these approaches have shown a decrease in the incidence of wound infection but an increase in the incidence of intra-abdominal abscess with the laparoscopic approach. Patients who undergo laparoscopic appendectomy also experience less postoperative pain, have shortened hospital stays, and return to normal activity earlier. However, the advantages in this regard are small.

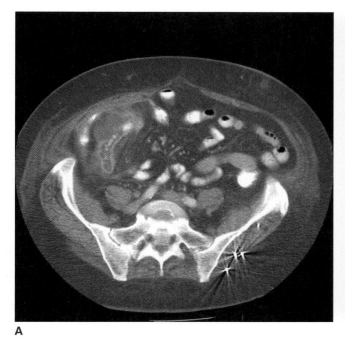

A

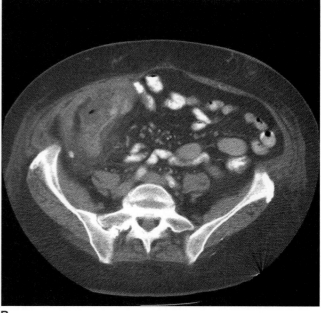

B

FIGURE 19-3. **A:** Small perforation on lateral wall of appendix. **B:** Perforation with small pocket of air.

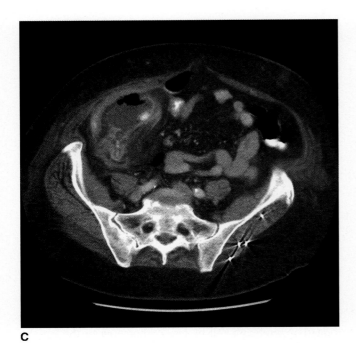

C

FIGURE 19-3. (*Continued*) **C:** Periappendiceal abscess.

There are several clinical scenarios where laparoscopy may be favored over an open approach. Laparoscopy may be favored in women or in men with an unclear diagnosis because it allows more thorough abdominal exploration relative to the size of the incision made. In patients with obesity, an open approach may be difficult due to the depth of the incision, potentially requiring a large incision to navigate successfully into the peritoneal cavity. Laparoscopy allows for easier access to the peritoneal cavity in such cases.

● LAPAROSCOPIC APPENDECTOMY

The procedure is performed under general anesthesia, in the supine position with the left arm tucked. An orogastric tube and Foley catheter are placed. The entire abdomen is prepped and draped. A 12-mm infraumbilical incision can be made either curvilinearly or vertically in the midline. Access to the abdomen is made with either Veress needle or open Hasson technique. The abdomen is insufflated with CO_2 to 15 mm Hg. A 5-mm 30° laparoscope is then inserted and diagnostic laparoscopy is performed.

Thorough exploration is crucial in patients with perforation. The degree of inflammation should be assessed carefully. In case of abscess or phlegmon or if it looks like a "bomb went off" in the RLQ, the procedure can be aborted and the patient treated medically with antibiotics and percutaneous drainage, if indicated.

If the decision is made to proceed, two additional 5-mm ports are placed, one in the midline above the pubic symphysis and another in the left lower quadrant. Transillumination of

the abdominal wall is recommended to avoid abdominal wall blood vessels during the additional port placement process.

Port placement may vary with position of the appendix and the patient's body habitus. For example, in young, thin patients, ports should be placed further away from the appendix to ensure adequate working room. Placement of the patient in Trendelenburg's position with right side up will improve exposure of the cecum and appendix. Attention is turned to the RLQ, and the appendix may be identified by following the teniae of the cecum toward its base. The terminal ileum and all loops of small bowel are swept away from the pelvis and periappendiceal region. Adhesions may be encountered, especially in the case of previous perforated appendicitis (i.e., interval appendectomy). These adhesions can often be divided using blunt dissection, but may require sharp dissection or cautery. Once free of adhesions, the appendix is retracted anteriorly and a window in the mesentery at the base of the appendix is created using a Maryland dissector. Prior to dividing the appendix, carefully assess the degree of inflammation at its base. If the base is inflamed, a cuff of uninvolved cecum should be included. If this is not possible, ileocecectomy should be considered. The mesoappendix is divided with an Endo GIA with a 2.5-mm (vascular) staple load, and the appendix is then divided at its base with 3.5-mm staples (bowel load). The appendix is retrieved with an Endo Catch bag and removed through the infraumbilical incision. The appendiceal and mesoappendiceal staple lines are thoroughly inspected to assure hemostasis. If the appendix is perforated, the RLQ should be evacuated of pus. Extensive use of irrigation is controversial and has questionable benefit. The 5-mm ports are removed under camera visualization followed by desufflation of the abdomen. The infraumbilical port is then removed, and the fascia is closed with absorbable sutures. Skin is closed with either monofilament suture or Indermil glue (Table 19-1).

● OPEN APPENDECTOMY

The patient is placed in supine position under general anesthesia. The entire abdomen is prepped and draped. A transverse skin incision is made at McBurney's point, two-thirds the distance from the umbilicus to the anterior superior iliac spine. The incision is carried down to the external oblique aponeurosis using Bovie electrocautery. The aponeurosis is opened sharply parallel to the direction of its fibers to expose the internal oblique muscle. The muscle fibers are bluntly separated at right angles. The peritoneum is identified, elevated, and incised sharply, avoiding abdominal viscera.

The appendix is then identified and delivered into the incision. The appendix can often be found by locating the cecum and grasping the teniae with Babcock forceps, and following the teniae down to their convergence at the base of the cecum. The mesoappendix is then divided between clamps and ligated with silk sutures. A silk purse-string suture is placed at the base of the appendix.

Table 19-1	Laparoscopic Appendectomy

Key Technical Steps

1. Infraumbilical 12-mm incision and abdominal access via Veress needle or open Hasson technique.
2. Insert two 5-mm ports in low midline above pubic symphysis and left lower quadrant.
3. Divide adhesions in RLQ to expose appendix.
4. Create mesenteric window at base of appendix with Maryland dissector.
5. Divide mesoappendix and appendix with endoscopic GIA stapler.
6. Retrieve appendix with Endo Catch device.
7. Remove ports, close fascia at infraumbilical incision, and close skin.

Potential Pitfalls

- Injury to inferior epigastric vessels or abdominal viscera during port placement
- Dense adhesions requiring conversion to open appendectomy
- Injury to cecum, small bowel, or iliac vessels during dissection
- Division of the appendix with inflammation at the base, resulting in staple line leak

Table 19-2	Open Appendectomy

Key Technical Steps

1. Skin incision at McBurney's point or point of maximal tenderness.
2. Open external oblique aponeurosis and bluntly separate internal oblique and transverse abdominis muscles.
3. Incise peritoneum.
4. Identify appendix and deliver into operative field.
5. Divide mesoappendix.
6. Place purse-string suture around base of appendix.
7. Clamp crush base of appendix and ligate and divide appendix at its base.
8. Invaginate appendiceal stump into base of cecum.
9. Close peritoneum, fascia, and skin in individual layers.

Potential Pitfalls

- Damage to cecum
- Difficult exposure due to retrocecal appendix
- Inability to inspect other abdominal structures with limited incision

A straight clamp is used to crush the appendix at its base and then moved distally and applied again. The appendix is then ligated with absorbable suture and divided sharply proximal to the clamp. Electrocautery is used to obliterate the mucosa of the appendiceal stump. The appendiceal stump is then invaginated into the cecum with the purse-string silk suture.

The surgical field is then irrigated and the peritoneum, fascia, and skin are closed in layers. In cases with gross contamination, leaving the wound open or a loose closure may be a better option (Table 19-2).

● SPECIAL INTRAOPERATIVE CONSIDERATIONS

If extensive inflammation is encountered involving the base of the appendix or cecum, it may be necessary to perform a larger resection such as an ileocecectomy or right colectomy. The resection should extend to healthy noninflamed bowel both proximally and distally. This may be performed laparoscopically, depending on the surgeon's experience. The anastomosis may be either stapled or hand-sewn based on surgeon preference.

Leaving surgical drains after appendectomy for perforation has not been shown to prevent abscess, and prolongs length of stay.

● POSTOPERATIVE MANAGEMENT

In the setting of acute perforation, the patient often has an ileus. Broad-spectrum intravenous antibiotics are administered, and the patient is kept NPO. The patient's diet may be advanced as tolerated once symptoms improve. There is no advantage to prolonged courses of antibiotics, as outcomes are equivalent between short-course therapy (3 days) and longer-course (5 days or more).

Case Conclusion

The patient undergoes ultrasound-guided percutaneous drain placement upon admission. He is made NPO, given fluid hydration, and treated with IV piperacillin/tazobactam for broad-spectrum coverage of enteric flora. This is transitioned to oral amoxicillin/clavulanic acid when his leukocytosis resolves after 3 days and he is able to tolerate an oral diet. He is discharged home to complete a 2-week course of antibiotics and seen in clinic in 2 weeks. His drain is discontinued in clinic as its output is <30 mL per day. He is seen 8 weeks after initial presentation, at which time a CT scan reveals no residual abscess. He elects to undergo an interval laparoscopic appendectomy and is discharged home on the same day of his procedure. He is seen in clinic 2 weeks after surgery and is noted to be doing well.

TAKE HOME POINTS

- Patients with RLQ pain with delayed presentation, high fevers, or marked leukocytosis should undergo CT scan as they may have perforated rather than early appendicitis.
- Perforated appendicitis with intra-abdominal abscess should initially be managed medically with percutaneous drain placement and intravenous antibiotics.
- There is no significant difference in patient outcomes between laparoscopic and open appendectomy in perforated appendicitis.
- Interval appendectomy may no longer be routinely indicated for carefully selected patients.

SUGGESTED READINGS

Andersson RE, Petzold MG. Non-surgical treatment of appendiceal abscess or phlegmon. A systematic review and meta-analysis. *Ann Surg.* 2007;246:741-748.

Brown CV, Abrishami M, Muller M, et al. Appendiceal abscess: immediate operation or percutaneous drainage? *Am Surg.* 2003;69:829.

Cheng Y, Zhou S, Zhou R, et al. Abdominal drainage to prevent intra-peritoneal abscess after open appendectomy for complicated appendicitis. *Cochrane Database Syst Rev.* 2015;2: CD010168.

Forsyth J, Lasithiotakis K, Peter M. The evolving management of the appendix mass in the era of laparoscopy and interventional radiology. *Surgeon.* 2017;15:109-115. http://dx.doi.org/10.1016/j.surge.2016.08.002

Hemmila MR, Birkmeyer NJ, Arbabi S, et al. Introduction to propensity scores: a case study on the comparative effectiveness of laparoscopic vs open appendectomy. *Arch Surg.* 2010;145:939-945.

Kaminski A, Liu IL, Applebaum H, et al. Routine interval appendectomy is not justified after initial nonoperative treatment of acute appendicitis. *Arch Surg.* 2005;140:897-901.

Oliak D, Yamini D, Udani VM, et al. Initial nonoperative management for periappendiceal abscess. *Dis Colon Rectum.* 2001;44:936-941.

Sauerland S, Lefering R, Neugebauer EA. Laparoscopic versus open surgery for suspected appendicitis. *Cochrane Database Syst Rev.* 2004;4:CD001546.

Sawyer RG, Claridge JA, Nathens AB, et al. Trial of short-course antimicrobial therapy for intraabdominal infection. *N Engl J Med.* 2015;372:1996-2005.

Simillis C, Symeonides P, Shorthouse AJ, et al. A meta-analysis comparing conservative treatment versus acute appendectomy for complicated appendicitis (abscess or phlegmon). *Surgery.* 2010;147:818-829.

St. Peter SD, Adibe OO, Igbal CW, et al. Irrigation versus suction alone during laparoscopic appendectomy for perforated appendicitis: a prospective randomized trial. *Ann Surg.* 2012;256:581-585.

Van Rossem CC, Schreinemacher MH, Treakes K, et al. Duration of antibiotic treatment after appendicectomy for acute complicated appendicitis. *Br J Surg.* 2014;101:715-719.

Perforated Duodenal Ulcer

20

GEORGE A. SAROSI JR.

Presentation

A 70-year-old man presents to the emergency department (ED) with a 1-hour history of generalized abdominal pain that began abruptly and now radiates to both shoulders. The patient has a prior history of peptic ulcer disease but is not currently on acid suppression therapy, and he is on low-dose aspirin for peripheral vascular disease. He has never had an abdominal surgery. He has no known drug allergies. He does not smoke tobacco or drink alcohol.

On examination by the ED physician, his temperature is 36.5°C, heart rate is 100 bpm, blood pressure is 125/70 mm Hg, and his abdomen is diffusely tender to palpation.

● DIFFERENTIAL DIAGNOSIS

The differential diagnosis includes perforated hollow viscus secondary to PUD, carcinoma, gastrinoma, mesenteric ischemia, small bowel obstruction, Crohn's disease, Boerhaave syndrome, pancreatitis, appendicitis, diverticulitis, ruptured abdominal aortic aneurysm, ruptured ectopic pregnancy, pneumonia, pulmonary infarction, and renal or biliary colic.

Peptic ulcers in the stomach and duodenum are defects that extend through the muscularis mucosa. They are most often associated with *Helicobacter pylori* infection or the use of nonsteroidal anti-inflammatory drugs (NSAIDs), including aspirin. Risk factors for the development of NSAID-related ulcers include advanced age, history of prior ulcer, serious systemic illness, concomitant use of anticoagulants or corticosteroids, and high NSAID doses. Less common causes of PUD include gastrinoma, systemic mastocytosis, carcinoma, sarcoidosis, Crohn's disease, and carcinoid syndrome.

Ulcer complications include perforation, obstruction, bleeding, and rarely, enteroenteric fistulas. The most common location of perforation is the duodenal bulb, followed by the pyloric region of the antrum and then the gastric body. Ulcer perforation is associated with prior history of ulcer disease and use of NSAIDs. In the setting of NSAID therapy, the risk factors associated with ulcer perforation include a history of prior ulcer, age > 60 years, and the concomitant use of steroids, anticoagulants, selective serotonin reuptake inhibitors, or alendronate.

The classic clinical presentation of a perforated peptic ulcer has been described as a 3-stage process:

1. Early (onset to 2 hours): the abdominal pain begins abruptly, with the patient often being able to remember the exact time the pain started. The pain may first localize to the epigastrium but quickly becomes generalized. The pain may radiate to the shoulders if the diaphragm is irritated. On examination, the patient may be tachycardic, have a low body temperature, and have a tender abdomen to palpation.
2. Intermediate (2 to 12 hours): the patient may report an improvement in pain. However, on physical exam, the patient often displays increased pain with movement, and the abdominal wall is rigid. In addition, there may be significant pain with palpation of the hypogastrium and right lower quadrant secondary to drainage of succus from the perforation. Immunosuppressed patients or those on steroids may not present with the clinical findings of peritonitis.
3. Late (after 12 hours): the patient may complain of increased pain and display temperature elevation, signs of hypovolemia, and abdominal distension. In addition, though the patient may vomit during any stage, typically vomiting is most severe at this stage.

Presentation Continued

The patient's presenting signs and symptoms, combined with his risk factors for ulcer perforation, place the diagnosis of a perforated peptic ulcer high on the list of differential diagnoses.

● WORKUP

It is important to quickly diagnose a perforated peptic ulcer because the prognosis is good if treatment is provided within the first 6 hours, whereas delay in treatment beyond 12 hours after perforation is associated with increased morbidity and mortality.

Imaging Studies

An upright chest x-ray or an abdominal x-ray may reveal the presence of intraperitoneal free air; however, free intraperitoneal air is seen on chest x-ray with roughly 75% of perforated ulcers. Computed tomography (CT) scanning may also be used to identify intraperitoneal free air or free fluid and is the most sensitive test for the diagnosis of perforated ulcer. Approximately 10% to 20% of patients with a perforated duodenal ulcer will not have direct findings of perforation. If free air is present, no other test is required to confirm the diagnosis. An upper GI study or an abdominal CT scan with water soluble contrast may demonstrate the leak if free air is not present and a confirmatory test is required for diagnosis.

Laboratory Studies

Laboratory studies are not necessary for the diagnosis of a perforated duodenal ulcer. However, they contribute to the complete evaluation and appropriate management of the patient. A basic metabolic panel will assist in fluid and electrolyte resuscitation. A complete blood count may demonstrate leukocytosis with a left shift in a patient with a perforated ulcer. A serum gastrin level may assist in the diagnosis of gastrinoma, though the result of the test will likely not return in time to influence the operative strategy. Given that *Helicobacter pylori* infection is present in 70% to 90% of duodenal ulcers and 30% to 60% of gastric ulcers, patients with PUD ought to be tested for *H. pylori* infection. Noninvasive testing for *H. pylori* infection includes urea breath testing, stool antigen testing, and serology. Ideally, *H. pylori* infection is identified preoperatively, as it can influence operative strategy. A monoclonal stool antigen test is available that has 94% sensitivity, 97% specificity, and may be performed in about an hour. There is also a rapid stool antigen test for the diagnosis of *H. pylori* which can be done in 5 minutes. However, its sensitivity and specificity have been shown to be 76% and 98%, respectively.

Presentation Continued

An upright chest x-ray demonstrates free intraperitoneal air. A stool antigen test is positive for *H. pylori* infection.

● DIAGNOSIS AND TREATMENT

Presentation Continued

A diagnosis of a perforated peptic ulcer is made based on the patient's presenting symptoms, the past history of PUD, multiple risk factors for ulcer complications, and presence of intraperitoneal free air on upright chest x-ray. The ED physician consults general surgery, starts fluid resuscitation, initiates nasogastric decompression, places a urinary catheter, and administers omeprazole, ampicillin, metronidazole, ceftriaxone, and fluconazole.

The medical/nonoperative management of a perforated peptic ulcer includes fluid resuscitation, nasogastric decompression, acid suppression, and empiric antibiotic therapy for coverage of enteric gram-negative rods, oral flora, anaerobes, and fungus. In the setting of a perforated duodenal ulcer without peritonitis, the application of a nonoperative management strategy has been proposed, especially for patients at high risk for operative complications. However, delaying the surgical repair of a perforated peptic ulcer over 12 hours after presentation has been associated with increased morbidity and mortality. Therefore, operative management is the preferred treatment strategy in most patients who are able to tolerate surgery, with nonoperative management reserved for patients whose clinical presentation suggests a perforated ulcer that has sealed spontaneously.

● SURGICAL APPROACH

Presentation Continued

You evaluate the patient 2 hours after the start of the symptoms, at which time the patient notes an improvement in generalized pain. However, on examination, the heart rate is 110 bpm, the blood pressure is 90/50 mm Hg, and the abdomen is rigid, with the patient more sensitive to changes in position. You decide to proceed to the operating room for management of this problem.

Elective operations for PUD have become uncommon with the successful medical management of acid and *H. pylori* infection. However, surgical management is almost always indicated for a perforated ulcer, but especially when the patient is hemodynamically unstable, has signs of peritonitis, or has evidence of free contrast extravasation on imaging. Although operative treatment is the appropriate plan, the patient should receive fluid resuscitation and antibiotic treatment prior to going to the operating room. Emergency surgery for peptic ulcer perforation has a 6% to 30% risk of mortality, and the presence of comorbid disease has been shown to increase the risk of death. In patients requiring emergency surgery, variables identified as being independently associated with 20-day mortality include age, ASA (American Society of Anesthesiologists) class, shock on admission, hypoalbuminemia on admission, preoperative metabolic acidosis, liver disease, and an elevated serum creatinine.

Presentation Continued

On exploration, you identify a 1 cm anterior duodenal perforation.

Surgical Procedure(s) for the Management of Perforated Duodenal Ulcers

1. *Omental patch repair*: The safest technique for the management of a perforated duodenal ulcer, especially in the setting of delayed repair (>24 hours after presentation), hemodynamic instability or significant intra-abdominal contamination is a patch repair with an omental pedicle. This technique combined with the appropriate medical therapy is likely sufficient in the case of a patient with a history of *H. pylori* infection or NSAID use.

Table 20-1	Omental Patch
Key Technical Steps	
1. Laparoscopic or open approach	
2. Fix omental pedicle in place	
3. No need to suture the perforation closed	
4. Irrigate peritoneal cavity	

Omental patch repair procedure (Table 20-1): The repair may be performed laparoscopically or open, with laparoscopic repair having a slightly shorter hospital stay and less postoperative pain. The perforation is repaired by taking a seromuscular bite from one side of the perforation, taking a bite of omentum, followed by another seromuscular bite from the other side of the perforation, and then tying to fix the omental pedicle in place. Typically, three to four sutures are required to secure the patch. Following repair, the peritoneal cavity is irrigated with large volumes of warm saline.

Pitfalls:

- The optimal repair of duodenal ulcer perforations >2 cm can be challenging, and the omental patch repair may be associated with increased risk of failure. Performing a definitive ulcer operation has been suggested, as have less standard repairs, including tube duodenostomy.
- On exploration, the omentum, liver, or gallbladder may have already "patched" the perforation. If this is the case, the surgeon must decide whether to remove the natural patch and surgically repair the defect, or to simply irrigate the peritoneal cavity.
- If the ulcer perforation is located at the distal end of the pyloric channel, the duodenum may need to be mobilized to provide adequate exposure of the defect.

2. A definitive ulcer procedure may be performed if the patient is hemodynamically stable, has minimal intra-abdominal contamination, and either (1) has a history of PUD with unknown *H. pylori* status or (2) is unable to stop NSAID therapy.

   a. *Truncal vagotomy and pyloroplasty (drainage) (V&D)* (Table 20-2): A truncal vagotomy reduces basal acid secretion by 80% and stimulated acid secretion by 50%. It reduces acid secretion by preventing direct cholinergic stimulation for acid secretion and by decreasing the response of parietal cells to histamine and gastrin. Unfortunately, a truncal vagotomy also damages the stomach's receptive relaxation and antral grinding, in addition to the pyloric sphincter's coordination required for gastric emptying. To compensate for these changes, a pyloroplasty is performed to facilitate gastric drainage. The benefit of V&D is that it is safe and may be done relatively quickly. The drawbacks of the procedure are that 10% of patients later report diarrhea or dumping syndrome, and 10% have a recurrent ulcer.

Table 20-2	Truncal Vagotomy and Pyloroplasty
Key Technical Steps	
1. Isolate the distal esophagus	
2. Identify, dissect, and transect the vagal trunks—send nerve biopsy to pathology	
3. Dissect the distal 6-cm of the esophagus to ensure complete division of vagal fibers	
4. Mobilize the duodenum	
5. Make a longitudinal incision from the antrum onto the proximal duodenum	
6. Place stay sutures at either end of the incision to facilitate transverse closure	

Procedure: Access the esophageal hiatus by dividing the left triangular ligament and retracting the left lateral lobe of the liver. Open the peritoneum overlying the esophagus by dividing the lesser omentum and the esophagophrenic ligament. Use blunt dissection between the esophagus and the adjacent crux to allow two fingers behind the esophagus. Careful dissection is critical to avoid iatrogenic esophageal perforation. Downward traction on the gastroesophageal junction facilitates identification of the vagus nerve. Identify the anterior and posterior vagal trunks, dissect them from the esophagus, and then transect them (Figure 20-2). Mark the transected vagal margins with hemoclips and send biopsies of both nerves to pathology to confirm that the transected structures were nerves. Note that the criminal nerve of Grassi, coming off the posterior vagus trunk, can be missed if the vagotomy is performed lower on the esophagus. To avoid this, complete circumferential dissection of the distal 6 cm of the esophagus ensures division of these nerve fibers.

A Heineke-Mikulicz pyloroplasty is begun by mobilizing the second part of the duodenum using a Kocher maneuver. Then a 5-cm incision is made from the antrum, over the pyloric sphincter, and onto the proximal duodenum. Place seromuscular tacking sutures to the cephalad and caudad ends of the incision to facilitate the transverse closure of the wound (Figure 20-1).

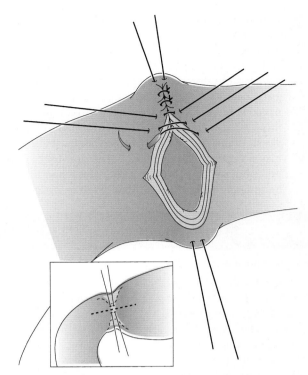

FIGURE 20-1. Pyloroplasty. (Reprinted from Mulholland MW. Gastroduodenal ulceration. In: Mulholland MW, Lillemoe KD, Doherty GM, et al., eds. *Greenfield's Surgery: Scientific Principles and Practice*. 5th ed. Baltimore, MD: Lippincott Williams & Wilkins; 2011:704-705, with permission).

Table 20-3	Antrectomy

Key Technical Steps

1. Free the greater curvature of the stomach
2. Dissect the first part of the duodenum from the pancreas
3. Divide the stomach
4. Ligate the right gastric artery at the level of the pylorus
5. Divide the duodenum just distal to the pylorus—send duodenal stump margin for pathology
6. Complete with either a Billroth I or Billroth II anastomosis

The incision is closed in one or two layers. If closed in two, start with an inner layer of full-thickness interrupted absorbable sutures, followed by a seromuscular layer of Lembert sutures. Alternatively, a stapled closure may be performed using a thoracoabdominal (TA) stapler containing 4.8 mm staples. Note that if the duodenum is severely scarred or inflamed, then a gastrojejunostomy may be used in place of a pyloroplasty.

Pitfalls:
- Deliberate care ought to be taken during the dissection of the esophagus to avoid esophageal injury.
- Biopsies of the vagal nerves should be sent to pathology for confirmation of the appropriate resection of nerve tissue.
- Splenic injury may occur with traction of the stomach to the patient's right side.
- Avoid a postoperative hiatal hernia by repairing any defects at the esophageal hiatus at the time of vagotomy.

b. *Vagotomy and antrectomy* (Table 20-3): The combination of the vagotomy and antrectomy eliminates basal acid secretion and decreases stimulated acid secretion by 80%. The benefits of a vagotomy with antrectomy are that the procedure may be applied to a variety of situations, including larger ulcers, and that the ulcer recurrence rate is very low. The disadvantages are that the operative mortality is higher than with V&D or parietal cell vagotomy (also known as highly selective vagotomy) and that there may be complications associated with the subsequent Billroth I or Billroth II reconstructions.

Procedure: The vagotomy proceeds as described above. The antrectomy is begun by separating the distal half of the greater curvature by dissecting the greater omentum from the proximal half of the transverse colon, carefully isolating and ligating the branches from the gastroepiploic arcade. Then the posterior wall of the first part of the duodenum is dissected from the pancreas. The gastrohepatic ligament is divided proximally along the lesser curvature, and the left gastric vessels along the lesser curvature are ligated and divided. The stomach is divided with the goal to remove all the antral mucosa. The upper margin of the antrum may be approximated by identifying the halfway point along the lesser curvature between the gastroesophageal junction and the pylorus. The stomach is divided with a gastrointestinal anastomosis (GIA)ar stapler using 4.8 mm staples. Next, the right gastric artery is identified above the pylorus, ligated and divided. To facilitate manipulation of the duodenum, approximately 1.5 cm of the posterior duodenum is dissected off of the pancreas. The duodenum is divided just distal to the pylorus with a GIA-style linear stapler. A frozen section biopsy of the margin of duodenal stump should be sent to confirm the presence of duodenal Brunner's glands to avoid retained antrum. Following the antrectomy, either a Billroth I gastroduodenal anastomosis or a Billroth II gastrojejunostomy is constructed. A Billroth I requires at least 1 cm of healthy duodenum, and in the case of significant scarring, it is difficult to perform. A Billroth II is the default reconstruction and can almost always be performed. For a Billroth I reconstruction, the staple line of the transected duodenum is excised and an end-to-end gastroduodenal anastomosis is performed in two layers. The inner layer consists of full-thickness continuous sutures. The outer layer consists of interrupted seromuscular Lembert sutures. A crown stitch is placed at the "angle of sorrow" of the gastroduodenal anastomosis.

Table 20-4	Parietal Cell Vagotomy

Key Technical Steps

1. Divide the lesser omentum from the lesser curvature
2. Encircle the trunks with Penrose drain and apply tension to facilitate exposure of branches
3. Dissect and ligate neurovascular branches of the vagal trunks proximal to the crow's foot of the nerve of Latarjet
4. Skeletonize the distal 6 cm of the esophagus to ensure complete division of criminal nerve of Grassi

If a Billroth II is to be constructed, then the duodenal stump is closed in two layers. The Billroth II gastrojejunostomy is begun by choosing a loop of proximal jejunum and bringing it antecolic or retrocolic to the stomach. If a retrocolic approach is chosen, care must be taken to close the mesenteric defect to reduce the risk of a future internal hernia. The jejunum is aligned along the gastric pouch, and a two-layered gastrojejunostomy is performed. A crown stitch is placed at the "angle of sorrow" at the medial margin of the gastrojejunal anastomosis. Any exposed staples from the antrectomy should be oversewn.

Pitfalls:

- Incomplete removal of the antrum increases the risk of developing a marginal ulcer.
- For the Billroth II reconstruction, it is important to properly close the duodenal stump to prevent future leaks that could be complicated by fistula formation or pancreatitis.
- Splenic injury may occur secondary to downward traction on the greater curvature of the stomach.

c. *Parietal cell vagotomy* (Table 20-4) (Figure 20-2): The goal of the parietal cell vagotomy is to eliminate vagal stimulation of the acid-secreting portion of the stomach, while retaining motor innervation to the antrum and pylorus. The receptive relaxation of the stomach is still affected by this procedure, and liquid emptying from the stomach is accelerated, but solid emptying is normal. This procedure reduces the basal acid secretion by 75% and the stimulated acid secretion by 50%. The highly selective vagotomy has low mortality (risk <0.5%) and morbidity but has a high ulcer recurrence rate especially with inexperienced surgeons.

Procedure: The initial exploration is as described for truncal vagotomy. The anterior nerve of Latarjet, which is the termination of the left vagus nerve, is identified and encircled. The lesser sac is examined for adhesions to the pancreas and then entered by dividing the gastrocolic ligament, while preserving the gastroepiploic arcade. Next, the lesser omentum is divided from the lesser curvature between the incisura angularis and the cardia, by dividing all of the blood vessels and nerves that enter the lesser curvature. The dissection begins just proximal to the crow's foot of the nerve of Latarjet and proceeds proximally along the lesser curvature to the left side of the gastroesophageal junction. The neurovascular branches should be ligated with 3 to 0 or 4 to 0 silk sutures and divided. The stomach is reflected upward, and the posterior denervation is conducted in a similar manner. Lastly, the nerve fibers and blood vessels on the lower 5 to 7 cm of the esophagus must be dissected and ligated.

Pitfalls:

- Recurrent ulcers may be the consequence of an inadequate proximal vagotomy.

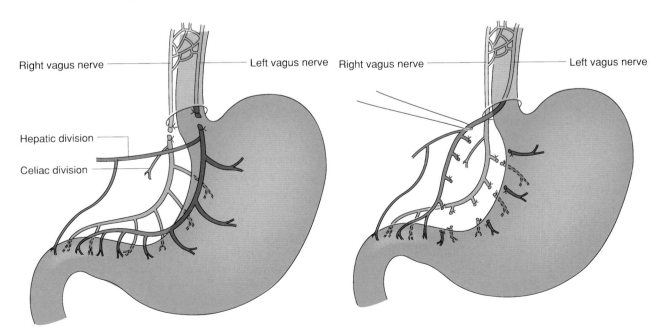

FIGURE 20-2. Truncal and parietal cell vagotomy. (Reprinted with permission from Mulholland MW, Lillemoe KD, Doherty GM, et al. *Greenfield's Surgery: Scientific Principles and Practice*. 4th ed. Baltimore, MD: Lippincott Williams & Wilkins; 2006:722-735.)

- Careful dissection around the lesser curvature of the stomach is important to decrease the risk of injury to the lesser curve.

> **Presentation Continued**
> You performed an omental patch repair.

● SPECIAL INTRAOPERATIVE CONSIDERATIONS

Giant perforated ulcers: There is no standard management for giant perforated ulcers (>2 to 3 cm). Recommendations for repair have included omental patch, controlled tube duodenostomy, jejunal pedicled graft, jejunal serosal patch, free omental plug, partial gastrectomy, and gastric disconnection. The choice of repair will be influenced by the patient's status, the size of the perforation, the degree of intraperitoneal contamination, and the surgeon's experience.

Posterior perforation: Spontaneous posterior perforation of a duodenal ulcer is rare. A definitive ulcer operation is typically undertaken, though there is no standard treatment.

Perforated gastric cancer: Though perforation is a rare complication (<1%) of gastric cancer, a biopsy and frozen section should be taken during surgery for all gastric perforations. Options for the surgical repair of a perforated gastric cancer include omental patch, emergency gastrectomy, and a two-stage radical gastrectomy.

Perforation at the gastroesophageal junction: The operative approach to perforation of an ulcer located next to the esophagogastric junction may include a subtotal gastrectomy to include the ulcer with a Roux-en-Y esophagogastrojejunostomy or a vagotomy with antrectomy.

● POSTOPERATIVE MANAGEMENT

Helicobacter pylori infection should be treated with triple therapy for 10 to 14 days; a common treatment regimen is clarithromycin, amoxicillin, and omeprazole. Following treatment conclusion, *H. pylori* eradication should be confirmed. Patients should receive counseling regarding NSAID use.

Postoperative complications include the following:

1. An early ulcer recurrence with leak is often treated with reexploration and may require gastric resection to adequately repair.
2. An uncontained leak after omental patch may require reexploration and gastric resection with a Billroth II.
3. Subphrenic and subhepatic abscesses are associated with a treatment delay >12 hours.
4. A patient should be evaluated for duodenal obstruction if gastric emptying is not normal by the 8th postoperative day.
5. Wound infection.
6. Pneumonia.
7. Pancreatitis.

In patients following a definitive ulcer surgery, there are also risks of the following:

1. Diarrhea following truncal vagotomy occurs in 5% to 10% of patients. It typically occurs 1 to 2 hours following a meal. This problem usually resolves without intervention. Persistent symptoms may be improved by cholestyramine and/or loperamide. If medical therapy does not improve symptoms, a surgical option includes placement of a reversed jejunal interposition placed 100 cm distal to the ligament of Treitz.
2. Dumping syndrome occurs in 5% to 10% of patients following distal gastrectomy, pyloroplasty, or pyloromyotomy. It is classified as either early dumping, occurring within 30 to 60 minutes of eating; or late dumping, occurring 2 to 3 hours following a meal. Symptoms of early dumping include fatigue, facial flushing, lightheadedness, diaphoresis, palpitations, cramping abdominal pain, nausea, vomiting, and diarrhea. Symptoms of late dumping are typically limited to vasomotor symptoms. Treatment of these symptoms with dietary manipulation is often successful. Octreotide may be useful in severe cases. Octreotide, administered prior to meals, has been shown to improve both gastrointestinal and vasomotor symptoms. Remedial surgery is an option for patients with dumping symptoms resistant to medical management; however, this approach is typically not used because most patient do eventually respond to conservative therapy.
3. Following elimination of the pyloric sphincter, bile can reflux into the stomach. Alkaline reflux gastritis develops in 2% of patients. It is characterized by epigastric pain and nausea that is provoked by meals. Medical therapy with cholestyramine may improve symptoms. Cases resistant to medical management may be treated surgically with a Billroth II gastrojejunostomy with Braun enteroenterostomy, Roux-en-Y gastrojejunostomy, or an isoperistaltic jejunal interposition procedure (Henley loop).
4. Early satiety with epigastric fullness and emesis with meals may develop secondary to gastric stasis, having a small gastric remnant, or from postsurgical atony. Atony may be confirmed with a solid food emptying test and then treated with a prokinetic agent, or if that fails, gastric pacing or completion gastrectomy. Symptoms of a small gastric remnant typically improve with small frequent meals.
5. Following Billroth II construction, the limb may become obstructed and cause afferent and efferent loop syndromes. Afferent loop syndrome is characterized by postprandial epigastric pain and nonbilious vomiting that is relieved following bilious vomiting. Efferent loop syndrome is characterized by epigastric pain, distention, and bilious vomiting. Both syndromes are treated with a surgical approach.

TAKE HOME POINTS

- Early diagnosis and operation is associated with improved outcome.
- It is important to identify prior NSAID use.
- It is important to identify *H. pylori* infection.
- Surgical goals are to control the perforation and lavage the abdominal cavity.
- Although rarely required, definitive ulcer operation may be required in select patients.
- Gastric perforation should prompt consideration of underlying gastric cancer.

ACKNOWLEDGMENTS

The author would like to acknowledge Constance W. Lee, MD for her contribution to a previous version of this chapter.

SUGGESTED READINGS

Crofts TJ, Park KG, Steele RJ, Chung SS, Li AK. A randomized trial of nonoperative treatment for perforated peptic ulcer. *N Engl J Med.* 1989;320(15):970-973.

Huang JQ, Sridhar S, Hunt RH. Role of Helicobacter pylori infection and non-steroidal anti-inflammatory drugs in peptic-ulcer disease: a meta-analysis. *Lancet.* 2002;359(9300):14-22.

Ng EK, Lam YH, Sung JJ, et al. Eradication of Helicobacter pylori prevents recurrence of ulcer after simple closure of duodenal ulcer perforation: randomized controlled trial. *Ann Surg.* 2000;231(2):153-158.

Sanabria A, Villegas MI, Morales Uribe CH. Laparoscopic repair for perforated peptic ulcer disease. *Cochrane Database Syst Rev.* 2013;2:CD004778

Silen W. *Cope's Early Diagnosis of the Acute Abdomen.* 19th ed. New York: Oxford University Press; 1996. xiv, 315 p., 24 p. of plates.

Siu WT, Leong HT, Law BKB, et al. Laparoscopic repair for perforated peptic ulcer: a randomized controlled trial. *Ann Surg.* 2002;235(3):313-319.

Søreide K, Thorsen K, Harrison EM, et al. Perforated peptic ulcer. *Lancet.* 2015;386(10000):1288-1298.

Wang YR, Richter JE, Dempsey DT. Trends and outcomes of hospitalizations for peptic ulcer disease in the United States, 1993 to 2006. *Ann Surg.* 2010;251(1):51-58.

Gynecologic Causes of Lower Abdominal Pain

21

CHARLES S. DIETRICH III, BRADFORD P. WHITCOMB, AND
CHRISTOPHER J. CRELLIN

Based on the previous edition chapter "Gynecologic Causes of Lower Abdominal Pain"
by Charles S. Dietrich III and Bradford P. Whitcomb

Presentation

A 35-year-old female with no significant prior history presents to the emergency department with acute-onset severe right lower-quadrant pain that started earlier that day and has been progressively worsening. Her vital signs are significant for a low-grade temperature, mild tachycardia, and a normal blood pressure. On abdominal examination, tenderness to deep palpation is noted in the right pelvic region, and rebound tenderness is elicited. Her pelvic examination is remarkable for exquisite right adnexal tenderness that further precludes adequate examination.

DIFFERENTIAL DIAGNOSIS

Acute pelvic pain can be caused by a number of possible diagnoses that include not only gynecologic causes but also gastrointestinal, urologic, and musculoskeletal etiologies. The most common gynecologic causes for lower abdominal pain include complications of pregnancy (ectopic pregnancy or spontaneous abortion), hemorrhagic or ruptured ovarian cysts, pelvic inflammatory disease (PID), ovarian torsion, dysmenorrhea, degenerating uterine leiomyomas, endometriosis, and pelvic adhesive disease. Nongynecologic causes that should be considered include appendicitis, diverticulitis, acute cystitis, and urinary calculi (Table 21-1).

WORKUP

The patient undergoes ultrasound evaluation of the pelvis revealing an 8 cm solid/cystic right ovarian mass resting anterior to the uterus (Figure 21-1). Doppler studies reveal no internal ovarian flow. A small amount of pelvic fluid surrounds the ovary and fills the pelvic cul-de-sac. The endometrial lining is approximately 8 mm in maximal diameter. The uterus and left adnexa are normal in shape and size. Serum laboratory assessment is notable for a white blood count of $12.2 \times 10^3/\mu L$, hemoglobin of 12 g/dL, and a normal platelet count. Quantitative β-hCG is <2 mIU/mL. Serum chemistries, liver function tests, and urinalysis are unremarkable. Tumor markers including a CA125, AFP, LDH, and inhibin levels are collected but are pending. Computed tomography (CT) imaging is ordered for further evaluation confirming the right complex ovarian mass (Figure 21-2). Further findings include a normal caliber appendix, no suspicious pelvic or para-aortic lymphadenopathy, and no evidence of metastatic disease.

DISCUSSION

Female patients presenting with acute pelvic pain should be initially evaluated with a thorough history and physical exam. An accurate menstrual history should be collected including age of menarche, start date of the last menstrual period, duration of menstrual flow, quantification of flow, and time interval between menses. Any intermenstrual bleeding should also be documented. Other important aspects of the history include a sexual history, contraceptive techniques, and a history of prior pregnancies, sexually transmitted diseases, abnormal cervical cytology, or other gynecologic problems. Trauma resulting from sexual abuse

Table 21-1	Common Causes for Acute Pelvic Pain	
Gynecologic	**Urologic/ Gastrointestinal**	
Spontaneous abortion	Urinary tract infections	
Ectopic pregnancy	Nephroureterolithiasis	
Pelvic inflammatory disease	Interstitial cystitis	
Endometritis	Gastrointestinal	
Salpingitis	Appendicitis	
Tubo-ovarian abscess	Diverticulitis	
Degenerating uterine leiomyomas	Inflammatory bowel disease	
Endometriosis	Irritable bowel syndrome	
Dysmenorrhea	Gastroenteritis	
Mittelschmerz		
Ruptured ovarian cysts		
Hemorrhagic ovarian cysts		
Ovarian torsion		
Pelvic adhesive disease		

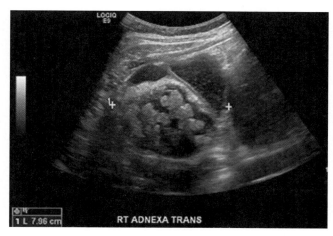

FIGURE 21-1. Ultrasound image showing an 8 cm complex solid/cystic right ovarian mass.

or assault may not be evident based on a patient interview alone, and should be specifically questioned if clinical suspicion is high. Abdominal examination should be performed to assess for signs of a surgical abdomen. Pelvic examination should include direct visualization of the cervix, assessment for cervical motion tenderness, and bimanual examination to determine uterine size and the presence of pelvic masses as well as regions of tenderness. Rectovaginal examination is also useful to help localize any masses that may be found.

All women of reproductive age presenting with acute pain should have pregnancy testing. If qualitative testing is positive, further clarification with a quantitative β-hCG is warranted. Other important laboratory assessments include a complete blood count, basic chemistries, liver function tests, and urinalysis.

The best initial imaging modality for assessing pelvic pain is ultrasound because it can accurately identify ovarian pathology. Morphology indexing to stratify the risk for malignancy can be performed if an ovarian mass is noted. Ultrasound is invaluable in assessing early pregnancy

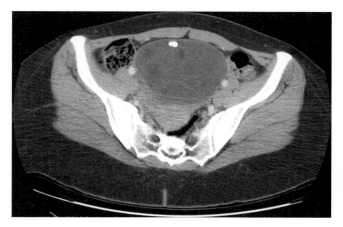

FIGURE 21-2. CT image of the complex right ovarian mass. The calcific density within the mass is suggestive of a teratoma.

complications as well. Doppler studies are often used to establish the presence of ovarian blood flow and to further assess the risk for a malignant process. CT imaging may also be useful to exclude other diagnoses such as appendicitis.

● DIAGNOSIS AND TREATMENT

The findings in this case are most consistent with acute ovarian torsion. Following ectopic pregnancy, hemorrhagic ovarian cyst, PID, and appendicitis, ovarian torsion is the fifth most common emergency room presentation for acute pain in females. While it can occur in all age groups, the majority of females affected are under 50 years. In most cases involving adnexal torsion, an ovarian or tubal tumor is present. The risk for torsion increases linearly with ovarian size. In one series, 83% of affected patients had an ovarian tumor ≥5 cm. Conversely, very large tumors become less likely to undergo torsion because of decreasing mobility. Normal-sized ovaries can also undergo torsion, but this presentation is more prevalent in children and early adolescents. Histologically, any ovarian tumor can twist; however, dermoid tumors are more commonly seen secondary to their prevalence and greater tissue density when compared to other diagnoses. Fortunately, malignancy is rarely encountered in cases of ovarian torsion, occurring in <2% of adult patients.

When an ovarian torsion occurs, the ovary's vascular pedicle becomes compromised. Initially, venous flow is more affected than arterial flow, causing ovarian engorgement. As the torsion becomes more complete, ischemia results, which eventually leads to necrosis and peritonitis. Pain is the most common presenting complaint and is often associated with nausea. If an intermittent torsion is present, the pain can come in waves, especially with activity. Fevers occasionally are noted and are usually low grade. Mild leukocytosis is often the only laboratory abnormality, although mild anemia can also occur from secondary hemorrhage. Unfortunately, the clinical presentation is often nonspecific, making diagnosis challenging in many cases. Ultrasound is highly sensitive for identifying ovarian masses, and the presence of an adnexal mass should raise the suspicion for torsion if acute pain is present. Doppler studies are usually reported when a tumor is identified; however, diminished or absent flow can be found in normal adnexa. Conversely, the presence of flow does not exclude an intermittent torsion. Maintaining a high index of suspicion with early operative intervention confirms the diagnosis and maximizes the chance for ovarian conservation.

● FURTHER DISCUSSION

Other diagnoses to consider for acute gynecologic pain that can mimic ovarian torsion include ectopic pregnancy, PID, and hemorrhagic ovarian cysts. Pain associated with an ectopic pregnancy can be similar to a torsion presentation.

The key difference, however, is an elevated human chorionic gonadotropin (hCG) level. Ultrasound, again, is critical to the diagnosis. Although a gestational sac can often be identified once the hCG level exceeds 1,500 mIU/mL, when no intrauterine gestational sac is noted with an hCG level over 3,000 mIU/mL, then an ectopic pregnancy should be strongly considered. If the hCG level rests below this discriminatory zone, then serial hCG levels can be helpful as long as the patient is stable. Ninety-nine percent of symptomatic patients with a viable intrauterine pregnancy will demonstrate at least a 53% increase in hCG levels over 48 hours. While an adnexal mass can be found with an ectopic pregnancy, it is usually smaller than those associated with torsion and often is paraovarian in location. Historically, surgical removal was the standard approach to treatment. With accurate hCG assays and improving ultrasound technology, earlier diagnosis has made medical management with methotrexate more prevalent.

Acute PID can also have a similar presentation to torsion, although the onset of pain tends to be more insidious. Severe cases of PID are often associated with a tubo-ovarian abscess, which on ultrasound can be quite sizable and associated with diminished Doppler flow. Fevers and leukocytosis tend to be more prominent in PID. A mucopurulent cervical discharge and cervical motion tenderness are also typically seen. Most acute cases are associated with gonorrhea or chlamydia, although many presentations are polymicrobial. Antibiotics, in most cases, quickly lead to resolution. Occasionally, surgical or percutaneous drainage of a tubo-ovarian abscess is required.

Hemorrhagic or ruptured ovarian cysts also present similarly to ovarian torsion. Pain often has an acute onset, and an adnexal mass is obviously noted on ultrasound. Fevers and leukocytosis are typically absent, while anemia may be more pronounced if active bleeding is ongoing. On ultrasound, pelvic fluid may also be more prominent. Management is usually conservative with ultrasound abnormalities often resolving within 6 weeks, although cases involving hemodynamic instability require urgent surgical intervention.

● SURGICAL APPROACH

Surgical management of ovarian pathology in the acute setting can be accomplished by several routes including laparoscopy, minilaparotomy, and laparotomy. The decision on the approach should be based on operator experience, available resources, ovarian size and mobility, the risk for a malignant process, and patient comorbidities. Relatively large ovarian masses can be removed laparoscopically if they are predominantly cystic and can be decompressed once placed inside a specimen retrieval system. If there is concern for a malignant process, care should be taken not to rupture the tumor, as this upstages the malignancy and usually necessitates postoperative chemotherapy. Predominantly solid tumors cannot be adequately decompressed and are more amenable to removal

via open laparotomy. When performing a laparotomy, most benign pelvic pathology can be addressed via a Pfannenstiel incision. If further lateral exposure is needed, conversion to a Cherney incision can be accomplished by detaching the rectus muscles from their tendinous insertions on the pubic symphysis. If malignancy is suspected, or if distorted fixed anatomy is anticipated, then a midline vertical approach is preferred. Maximal pelvic exposure is achieved by developing the space of Retzius, and ensuring the fascial incision extends completely to the pubic symphysis.

When faced with twisted adnexa, the primary intraoperative decision to make revolves around ovarian salvage. Historically, salpingo-oophorectomy was the procedure of choice as it was thought that reduction of the torsion would release clots or inflammatory cells into the ovarian vein. Recent reports, however, have confirmed the efficacy of conservative, ovarian-sparing approaches. Conservation is significantly more common in children, adolescents, and women early in their reproductive years. Timing is critical, as the risk for ovarian necrosis significantly increases after 24 hours of torsion. Following conservation, the ovary will often remain dark or dusky, but subsequent ovarian function is usually noted. Adjuncts to assess ovarian perfusion intraoperatively include intravenous fluorescein injection and ovarian bivalving. The primary risk associated with ovarian conservation is necrosis in cases where irreversible ischemic injury has occurred, leading to peritonitis and systemic infection. Fortunately, this risk is low but necessitates close surveillance immediately following surgery. Oophoropexy is sometimes performed following ovarian conservation, especially in cases of recurrent torsion, and in children or adolescents.

Ovarian cystectomy is a relatively simple surgical procedure allowing for ovarian conservation in reproductive-aged individuals. It should be reserved for benign pathology or for an interval procedure where the diagnosis is uncertain. Initially, either a linear or elliptical incision over the antimesenteric portion of the ovarian mass is created in the serosa with either a scalpel or electrocautery. Blunt and sharp dissection with Metzenbaum scissors or Endo Shears is then used to identify the underlying tumor and to separate it from the surrounding stroma. The ease of dissection is highly variable, depending on tumor histology and other cofactors such as infection or prior surgeries. Bleeding is usually minimal until the base of the tumor is reached where the ovarian vessels enter the ovarian hilum. Care should be taken to avoid tumor rupture; however, this is not an uncommon event, especially with thin-walled tumors. Once the tumor is removed, bleeding is controlled with suture ligation and cautery. The ovarian serosa can either be left open or reapproximated with fine suture (Table 21-2).

Salpingo-oophorectomy is also a relatively straightforward procedure. It is indicated for malignant pathology, nonviable ovarian tissue following torsion, definitive management of recurrent benign pathology, and electively in postmenopausal patients undergoing gynecologic procedures. The first step is to develop the pararectal space to

Table 21-2	Ovarian Cystectomy

Key Technical Steps

1. Expose and stabilize the ovarian mass.
2. Create a superficial incision in the ovarian serosa over the anterior surface of the mass.
3. Use blunt and sharp dissection to identify the mass and to separate it from its serosal and stromal attachments.
4. Hemostasis within the remaining ovarian cavity is achieved with either ligation using fine absorbable suture or with cautery.
5. The ovarian serosa can either be left open or reapproximated with absorbable suture.

Potential Pitfalls

- Avoid tumor rupture if possible.
- If rupture occurs, ensure that all portions of the cyst wall are removed.
- Most significant bleeding occurs at the base of the tumor where ovarian vessels enter the ovarian hilum. If hemostasis cannot be achieved with conservative approaches, oophorectomy may be indicated.

allow for identification of important retroperitoneal structures (Figure 21-3). The infundibulopelvic ligament is located on the pelvic sidewall, and the peritoneum 1 cm lateral to this structure is incised in a parallel fashion from the round ligament toward the line of Toldt. The external iliac artery and vein can then be identified. Careful blunt dissection of the loose areolar tissue medial to these vessels will open up the pararectal space, which can be further developed inferiorly until the sacrum is reached. The ureter should then be directly visualized as it courses along the medial peritoneal reflection. By following the iliac vessels cephalad and gently lifting anteriorly on the infundibulopelvic ligament, it is usually easy to locate the ureter as it crosses over the external

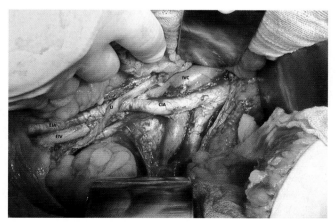

FIGURE 21-3. Retroperitoneal pelvic anatomy. IVC, inferior vena cava; CIA, common iliac artery; U, Ureter; EIA, external iliac artery; EIV, external iliac vein.

iliac artery and vein near the bifurcation of the common iliac vessels. Once the ureter has been positively identified, a window is then made between the ureter and ovarian vessels. The ovarian vessels can then be safely transected with suture ligation or laparoscopic vessel sealant devices. Once the ovarian vessels are ligated and divided, the ovary and fallopian tube should be placed on anterior traction and the remainder of the sidewall peritoneum skeletonized toward the utero-ovarian ligament. Finally, the fallopian tube and utero-ovarian ligament are transected close to the uterus, freeing the remaining ovarian attachments in the process (Table 21-3).

● SPECIAL INTRAOPERATIVE CONSIDERATIONS

While ovarian cystectomy and salpingo-oophorectomy are relatively straightforward procedures, several dilemmas may arise intraoperatively regarding management of adnexal masses. The first issue that is commonly encountered is management of an incidental adnexal mass found during surgical evaluation for a separate indication. Key issues surrounding this problem include consent parameters, the impact intervention might have on reproductive potential, the risk for malignant

Table 21-3	Salpingo-Oophorectomy

Key Technical Steps

1. Expose the pelvic sidewall and identify the infundibulopelvic and round ligaments.
2. Incise the peritoneum approximately 1 cm lateral to the infundibulopelvic ligament and develop the pararectal space.
3. Identify important retroperitoneal structures including the ureter, external and internal iliac arteries, and the external iliac vein.
4. Create a window through the peritoneum isolating the ovarian vessels from the ureter.
5. Ligate and divide the ovarian vessels.
6. Place the ovary and fallopian tube on anterior traction while transecting the inferior peritoneal attachments toward the utero-ovarian ligament.
7. Ligate the fallopian tube and utero-ovarian ligaments close to the uterine cornua.

Potential Pitfalls

- Failure to properly develop the pararectal space and identify the ureter can lead to ureteral injury.
- Adherent pathology may necessitate radical dissection with ureterolysis to the bladder insertion.
- Avoid tumor rupture if possible.
- If tumor size or adhesions prohibit adequate visualization, controlled tumor decompression may be needed.

pathology, and the potential morbidity associated with non-intervention (future tumor rupture, hemorrhage, or torsion). While there is no definitive answer, several guiding principles can be used to help make decisions. Simple ovarian cysts in reproductive-aged females <5 cm in diameter are usually functional in nature and will resolve on their own. Solid tumors, masses ≥10 cm, or those associated with excrescences are more likely to be malignant, and removal should be considered. Finally, any mass found intraoperatively in a postmenopausal patient should be considered for removal. Intraoperative consultation with a gynecologist is recommended if possible. If the indications are unclear or resources unavailable for management, it is always appropriate to refer the patient postoperatively for treatment counseling. While this approach may result in a second operation, it allows for better planning and gives the patient time to deal with potential impacts on fertility, hormonal status, or a malignant diagnosis.

Another potential challenge that may arise when dealing with pelvic pathology is distorted or fixed masses. In this case, rushing into the surgery without a well-thought-out approach can lead to unintended injuries and hemorrhage. In this event, the operative team should be alerted of the situation, and blood products should be readily available. Experienced assistance should be called. The first step should be to optimize exposure. If a large tumor is present that limits pelvic sidewall exposure, controlled tumor decompression or partial debulking may be necessary to improve visualization. Development of avascular pelvic spaces will improve visualization of important retroperitoneal structures. Vascular control should be obtained as early in the surgical process as is feasible. Ureteral stenting can help with identification of the ureters; however, the risk for injury is not decreased, and ureterolysis is often required to ensure ureteral integrity. During this process, care should be taken as the tunnel of Wertheim is entered since the uterine artery crosses over the ureter near this point. Bowel adhesions usually can be freed from the pelvis; however, on occasion, en bloc resection may be necessary if there are dense intestinal adhesions.

● POSTOPERATIVE MANAGEMENT

Postoperative care for a patient who has recently undergone laparoscopic or open ovarian cystectomy or oophorectomy is relatively straightforward and is similar to any patient having abdominal surgery. Postoperative complications such as bleeding, venous thromboembolism, or infection occur at rates comparable to other similarly classed procedures. Pelvic rest is often recommended during the convalescent period. In general, most patients recover quickly and are able to resume normal activities in 4 to 6 weeks after open procedures or sooner after laparoscopic procedures.

Questions that often arise in the postoperative setting in patients who have had a unilateral salpingo-oophorectomy include the impact on future fertility in reproductive-aged women as well as the possibility for earlier menopause. In most

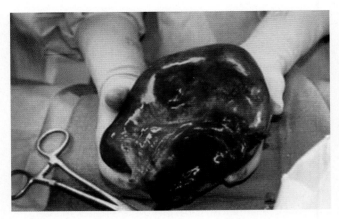

FIGURE 21-4. A necrotic right ovarian mass following salpingo-oophorectomy. Final pathology was consistent with a mature teratoma.

cases, fertility is minimally impacted as long as the contralateral ovary and fallopian tube are normal. However, fertility rates are challenging to generalize as the disease process requiring surgery in the first place can impact reproductive potential. There are a number of studies that suggest patients who have had unilateral oophorectomy reach menopause slightly earlier than those who did not; however, in many of these studies, the patients also had concurrent hysterectomy.

Case Conclusion

The patient was taken to the operating room for a diagnostic laparoscopy, where a right ovarian torsion was noted to be associated with an 8 cm mass. Following reduction, no vascular flow was identified and necrotic tissue was evident. Conversion to an open laparotomy was necessary as the tumor was predominantly solid. A right salpingo-oophorectomy was performed without complications (Figure 21-4). The patient's final pathology was consistent with a mature cystic teratoma with significant regions of necrosis. Her postoperative course was uneventful and she was released from the hospital 2 days later.

TAKE HOME POINTS

- Leading diagnoses for acute pelvic pain in females include ectopic pregnancy, hemorrhagic ovarian cyst, PID, appendicitis, and adnexal torsion.
- All women of reproductive potential with pelvic pain should have hCG testing as part of their initial evaluation.
- Ultrasound is the best initial modality for imaging pelvic pathology.
- Adnexal torsion can be difficult to diagnose. Therefore, any patient presenting with acute pain in the presence of an ovarian mass should raise suspicion. Early surgical intervention confirms the diagnosis and increases the chance for ovarian conservation.

- Reducing adnexal torsion does not increase the risk for clot embolization and will help determine if ovarian salvage is possible.
- Optimal pelvic exposure and development of the avascular pelvic spaces minimize the risk for adjacent structural injury during salpingo-oophorectomy.

● DISCLAIMER

The views expressed in this manuscript are those of the authors and do not reflect the official policy or position of the Department of the Army, Department of Defense, or the United States Government.

SUGGESTED READINGS

American College of Obstetricians and Gynecologists' Committee on Practice Bulletins-Gynecology. Practice Bulletin No. 174: evaluation and management of adnexal masses. *Obstet Gynecol.* 2016;128:e210-e226.

Baggish MS, Karram MM, eds. *Atlas of Pelvic Anatomy and Gynecologic Surgery.* 4th ed. Philadelphia, PA: Saunders Elsevier; 2016.

Brunham RC, Gottlieb SL, Paavonen J. Pelvic inflammatory disease. *N Engl J Med.* 2015;372:2039-2048.

Crochet JR, Bastian LA, Chireau MV. Does this woman have an ectopic pregnancy? The rational clinical examination systematic review. *JAMA.* 2013;309:1722-1729.

Dietrich CS, Martin RF. Obstetrics and gynecology for the general surgeon. *Surg Clin North Am.* 2008;88(2):223-440.

Sasaki KJ, Miller CE. Adnexal torsion: review of the literature. *J Minim Invasive Gynecol.* 2014;21(2):196-202.

Small Bowel Obstruction

DAVID E. MEYER

22

Based on the previous edition chapter "Small Bowel Obstruction" by Sara E. Clark and Lillian G. Dawes

Presentation

A 78-year-old man with a history of hypertension, diabetes, and coronary artery disease presents with a two-day history of diffuse abdominal pain, nausea, and several episodes of emesis. He has not been able to tolerate any oral intake. His bowel movements had been normal until yesterday when he had a liquid bowel movement. He has not had any flatus for at least 2 days. On physical exam, his abdomen is distended and tympanitic, and he has mild diffuse abdominal tenderness without guarding. He has a well-healed midline laparotomy scar and a right subcostal scar. He has had multiple abdominal surgeries, including an open aortic aneurysm repair, a cholecystectomy, and a right hemicolectomy for colon cancer.

● DIFFERENTIAL DIAGNOSIS

The constellation of abdominal pain, nausea, vomiting, and decreased flatus/bowel movements is nonspecific but may represent a small bowel obstruction. The presence of obstipation and abdominal distension should increase suspicion. Bowel obstructions may occur for a variety of reasons including but not limited to adhesions, hernias, and malignancy. Determining the likely cause of obstruction can inform the treatment plan, as some causes of obstruction are more likely to respond to a particular strategy than others. Additionally, aperistaltic causes of bowel dilatation (such as a paralytic ileus) can cause distention due to a lack of bowel motility and mimic obstruction. In this patient with a history of multiple abdominal surgeries, a mechanical bowel obstruction is a concern.

Adhesions from prior surgery are the most common cause of a mechanical small bowel obstruction, accounting for up to two-thirds of all bowel obstructions. Incarcerated hernias are the next most common cause, followed by neoplastic/malignant processes. Inflammatory bowel disease (e.g., Crohn's disease) can cause a mechanical obstruction in diseased segments of bowel. Less common causes of a small bowel obstruction include volvulus, bezoar, gallstone ileus, and intussusception (Table 22-1).

Small bowel neoplasms can progressively occlude the bowel lumen or serve as a lead point for intussusception.

Symptoms may be insidious, as the onset is slow, and patients may have chronic anemia. Extrinsic neoplasms may entrap loops or cause external compression. If the obstruction is due to a solitary mass that is amenable to resection, surgical intervention should be performed without delay. Obstruction caused by diffuse or metastatic cancer is often multifocal, and surgical intervention is fraught with complications. A comprehensive physical exam that includes evaluation for hernia is imperative in any patient presenting with signs of obstruction. Patients with incarcerated hernias can present with small bowel obstruction that may progress to ischemia. Internal hernias, which may not be apparent on physical examination, can occur from acquired adhesive defects or lateral to surgical defects (e.g., parastomal hernias). Volvulus results from rotation of bowel loops about a fixed point due to congenital anomalies or acquired adhesions. Patients with volvulus will usually have acute onset of symptoms, and strangulation may occur rapidly. Malrotation of the intestine is a cause of midgut volvulus in children but is very rare in adults.

Other rare causes of obstruction include foreign bodies (bezoar, ingested), gallstone ileus (passage of large stone through cholecystoenteric fistula), and inflammatory bowel disease (secondary to inflammation and fibrosis of small bowel wall).

Table 22-1	Causes of Small Bowel Obstruction
Causes	**Incidence (%)**
Adhesions	60%–74%
External hernia	8%–15%

Neoplasms
  Intrinsic (*i.e.*, primary small bowel - 20%)
  Extrinsic (*i.e.*, metastatic - 80%)
	8%–10%

Inflammatory bowel disease	5%
Miscellaneous (*e.g.*, intussusception, volvulus, gallstone ileus, infection/abscess, foreign body, bezoar)	10%

● WORKUP

The patient undergoes further evaluation with laboratory workup, which is significant for a mild leukocytosis, hypokalemia, and hypochloremia. He has no evidence of acidosis, and his creatinine is normal. Upright, supine, and lateral decubitus films of the abdomen demonstrate air–fluid levels and dilated loops of small bowel with no evidence of free intraperitoneal air. He undergoes computed tomography (CT) scan of the abdomen and pelvis, which demonstrates a large, fluid-filled stomach, dilated loops of proximal small bowel, and a possible transition point in the pelvis. The distal ileum and colon are decompressed (Figure 22-1).

When presented with this clinical scenario, several questions should be considered.

- Are these findings the result of an obstruction or a motility disorder (such as paralytic ileus)?
- If due to obstruction, is the blockage partial or complete? (Do you see bowel gas distal to the point of proposed obstruction?)
- Is the obstruction simple or complicated (i.e., is there suspicion of bowel ischemia or perforation)?

A complete workup for obstruction should include a combination of radiographic and laboratory investigations. If the diagnosis of obstruction is in question, an acute abdominal series (i.e., upright, supine, and left lateral decubitus abdominal x-rays +/− upright chest) may be performed to evaluate for free air, dilated small bowel or stomach, air–fluid levels, and the presence or absence of gas in the colon. Air–fluid levels are never a normal finding in the small or large bowel.

Unfortunately, the diagnostic scope of plain films is limited, and additional imaging will likely be necessary. If the diagnosis is certain or if there are multiple, competing diagnoses, computed tomography (CT) can provide enhanced diagnostic capability. Whenever possible, CT should be obtained with intravenous and enteric contrast, as this will provide the most information regarding the integrity of small bowel, the presence or absence of signs of bowel ischemia (e.g., pneumatosis intestinalis), the location (if any) of a transition point, and the presence or absence of volvulus, intussusception, hernias, and neoplasms. If adhesive small bowel obstruction is suspected, a small bowel follow-through with water-soluble contrast such as Gastrografin may be an alternative imaging option. Data from randomized trials suggest that water-soluble contrast studies may predict clinical resolution and accelerate recovery in adhesive, partial small bowel obstructions.

Laboratory evaluation may reveal a mild leukocytosis, anemia if there is a bleeding mass, or elevated hematocrit if the patient is volume contracted. The presence of a significant leukocytosis or bandemia should raise concerns for the possibility of strangulated/ischemic bowel. Likewise, an abnormal lactate may also indicate compromised bowel. However, both of these values can be normal even in the presence of frankly necrotic bowel, so normal values do not preclude the diagnosis. Electrolyte abnormalities may be present because of gastric losses or fluid shifts, and the creatinine may be elevated if the patient is dehydrated.

An ileus may mimic a small bowel obstruction. Conditions that may cause an ileus are listed in Table 22-2. Ileus tends to affect the entire gastrointestinal tract, so there should not be a transition point on CT scan. With an ileus, the large bowel is often dilated as well as the small bowel.

● DIAGNOSIS AND TREATMENT

In the patient from our scenario, a nasogastric tube (NGT) is placed, and 1 L of bilious fluid is immediately drained. He has partial resolution of his abdominal pain following

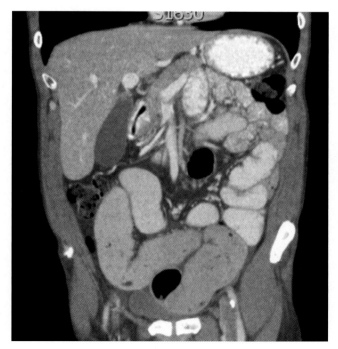

FIGURE 22-1. Dilated small bowel is evident as is a collapsed colon. A transition point was found to be in the pelvis.

Table 22-2	Causes of Ileus
Causes	
Postoperative
Metabolic and/or electrolyte imbalance
Hypokalemia
Hyponatremia
Hypomagnesemia
Uremia
Drugs (especially opioids and antimotility agents like loperamide and atropine/diphenoxylate) Inflammation (e.g., acute pancreatitis)
Sepsis

placement. Nonoperative management with nasogastric decompression and bowel rest is elected, and he is placed on intravenous fluids and kept nil per os.

Mechanical small bowel obstructions caused by adhesions respond especially well to nonoperative management, so this treatment modality is usually pursued initially. This includes NGT decompression, bowel rest, intravenous fluid resuscitation, and correction of electrolyte abnormalities. If the patient fails to improve clinically over 48 hours, it is likely that he will require an operation.

The challenge in treating a small bowel obstruction is deciding when to operate; 65% to 85% of partial small bowel obstructions will resolve without an operation. For this reason, a strategy of early surgical intervention may result in unnecessary procedures. In fact, the surgical truism of "never let the sun rise or set on a bowel obstruction" has largely been supplanted by the new paradigm of nonoperative management. However, early surgical intervention is imperative in cases of complete small bowel obstruction or large bowel obstruction or when there is concern for strangulation or ischemia. Here, delays in surgical therapy can lead to irreversible bowel ischemia and necrosis.

Indications for immediate operation include peritonitis, sepsis, hemodynamic instability, acidosis, radiographic evidence of bowel compromise (such as pneumatosis), perforation, internal hernia, and volvulus. Physical exam findings suggesting the need for early operation are fever, tachycardia, hypotension, and pain out of proportion to physical findings. Cross-sectional imaging may provide additional useful information. Although the presence of a transition point on CT scan has failed to reliably predict the need for operation, there are some findings that should alert the surgeon that earlier surgery is warranted. Bowel compromise is associated with intraperitoneal fluid and decreased enhancement of the bowel wall. Pneumatosis and portal venous air can also be seen with bowel ischemia. The presence of a "whirl sign" is concerning for a volvulus or internal hernia (Figure 22-2).

One special case worth mentioning is concern for obstruction following bariatric surgery. Because of the mesenteric defects that result from the creation of the gastrojejunostomy (often antecolic) and the jejunojejunostomy, as well as the rapid postoperative weight loss, bariatric surgery patients are at increased risk for internal hernias. Due to body habitus and the nature of the hernia, physical exam findings may be subtle leading to a delay in diagnosis. Such delays may result in bowel necrosis and, in extreme cases, catastrophic midgut volvulus. In these patients, the surgeon should look carefully for evidence of internal hernia or volvulus (e.g., mesenteric "swirl" sign on CT scan) and have a high index of suspicion to explore patients with any suggestion of an obstruction.

Small bowel obstruction due to intussusception in adults is often due to a tumor of the small bowel that serves as a lead point. The hallmark of intussusception on CT scan is the presence of a "target sign." A target sign on CT scan may at times be seen with normal peristalsis. However, when evidence of intussusception on CT scan is associated with

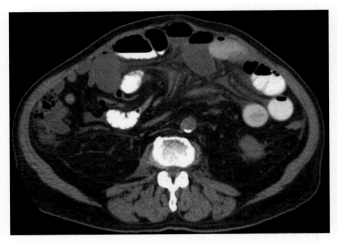

FIGURE 22-2. In the center of this CT scan image, there are mesenteric vessels that move in a circular pattern to the left. This is known as a "swirl sign" and is concerning for a potential volvulus. At operation, a loop of bowel twisted around an internal hernia was found. Untwisting of the mesentery restored blood flow and relieved the obstruction.

a bowel obstruction, hematochezia or melena, or a mass (Figure 22-3), operative intervention and small bowel resection with removal of the abnormal segment are indicated.

● SURGICAL APPROACH

The usual operative approach to patients with bowel obstruction is through a midline laparotomy incision (Table 22-3). Entering the abdomen away from a prior incision may be beneficial if possible (e.g., entering the midline just above or below a prior laparotomy site). The abdomen is entered carefully with sharp dissection in order to avoid bowel injury. The bowel is freed from the anterior abdominal wall and carefully inspected. All adhesions should be divided and the small bowel

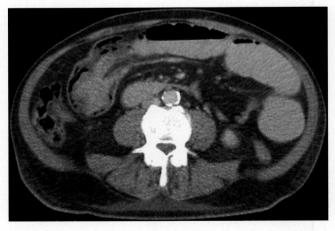

FIGURE 22-3. Small bowel intussusception is demonstrated here with a mass as the lead point. A spindle cell tumor was found at operation causing the intussusception and bowel obstruction.

Table 22-3	Small Bowel Obstruction

Key Technical Steps

1. Run the entire small bowel; multiple points of obstruction can be present.
2. Assess the bowel blood supply. If there is uncertainty, consider a "second look" operation.
3. Carefully inspect for potential enterotomy. Missed enterotomy is a devastating postoperative complication.
4. Preserve as much bowel as possible. With an intact duodenum and colon, 200 cm or more of residual small bowel is usually sufficient to prevent symptoms of short gut syndrome. If extensive small bowel must be resected, the remaining length should be measured to aid in identification of patients at risk for short gut.

Potential Pitfalls

- Missed enterotomy.
- Missed intraluminal lesion.
- Lack of recognition of compromised bowel.
- Recurrent bowel obstruction in the future.

inspected in its entirety. It is important to try and identify the point of obstruction or "transition point" where the bowel goes from dilated to decompressed. However, oftentimes, the transition point will not be obvious. For very dense adhesions, dissection with a scalpel is often useful. Enterotomies can be repaired primarily if the bowel is viable and the edges are clean and amenable to such a repair. If the bowel is ischemic or the damage is extensive, a small bowel resection should be performed. In order to determine viability, the vascular supply of the small bowel should be evaluated. This can be done by standard clinical judgment (i.e., color and appearance), Doppler ultrasound of mesentery, or, if the adequacy of perfusion remains unclear, fluorescein dye evaluation.

The less common causes of small bowel obstruction are usually apparent upon operative inspection of the bowel. Volvulus may require manual reduction and lysis of adhesions. If recurrent volvulus seems likely, the affected segment of bowel should be resected. Intussusception can be reduced with gentle traction and by milking the intussusceptum from the intussuscipiens. Any masses or lead points should be resected. In all circumstances, bowel viability must be assessed. Hernias can be approached through an incision over the hernia (e.g., umbilical, inguinal) with low threshold for conversion to laparotomy if the herniated bowel cannot be reduced or if there is concern ischemia of the unseen intra-abdominal bowel. For hernias where strangulation is suspected, manual reduction of the hernia should not be attempted prior to operative intervention, as it may preclude inspection of the involved loop of bowel.

During the operation, it is essential to be aware of any enterotomies or spillage from the bowel. Contamination of the peritoneal cavity by enteric contents can lead to postoperative intra-abdominal abscess, sepsis, and other complications.

SPECIAL INTRAOPERATIVE CONSIDERATIONS

During exploration for small bowel obstruction, it is important to be aware of findings of Crohn's disease. Laparotomy findings consistent with Crohn's disease include creeping fat, thickening of the bowel wall (especially in the terminal ileum), free perforation from full-thickness ulceration, and fibrotic strictures. Opening resected bowel on the back table may reveal extensive mucosal ulceration interspersed with areas of normal-appearing mucosa (so-called "skip" lesions). Strictures from Crohn's disease can cause obstruction and abdominal pain and often are managed with strictureplasty rather than resection to avoid excessive loss of small bowel and the development of short gut syndrome.

If an obstructing stone is found in the ileum just proximal to the ileocecal valve, a "gallstone ileus" is likely the cause. Inspection of the gallbladder is warranted to investigate the possibility of a cholecystoenteric fistula. Often this is diagnosed preoperatively due to the presence of air in the bile ducts without any history of endoscopic or surgical intervention. Inspection of the entire small bowel for multiple stones should be performed as there are frequently additional stones present. The obstruction is relieved by performing a proximal enterotomy and milking the stone retrograde for retrieval. Repair of the cholecystoenteric fistula is usually not necessary and should be deferred.

POSTOPERATIVE MANAGEMENT

Postoperatively, nasogastric decompression should be continued until there is return of bowel function with flatus. Care should be taken to maintain the patient's volume status, and all electrolyte abnormalities should be aggressively corrected. If the patient has been without nutrition for a prolonged period, consideration should be given to starting parenteral nutrition. Patients with chronic obstructive problems may have a prolonged ileus following lysis of adhesions. Optimizing the nutritional status is important to prevent complications, including wound infection and dehiscence.

Case Conclusion

Two days after admission, the patient continues to have 1,200 mL of bilious drainage per day from his NGT, and he has not passed any flatus. He is taken to surgery where he is found to have dense adhesions of the proximal ileum with an obvious transition point in the pelvis. The adhesions are divided, the bowel is inspected and found to be normal, and the abdomen is closed. Bowel function returns on postoperative day 3, and his diet is slowly advanced. The remainder of his postoperative course is uneventful and he is discharged to home on postoperative day 6.

TAKE HOME POINTS

- Early surgical intervention should be considered when the obstruction is complete or when bowel ischemia is a concern.
- Partial small bowel obstructions can be managed initially with NGT decompression, intravenous fluids, and close observation. Surgical intervention should be reconsidered in cases that do not begin to demonstrate resolution by 48 hours.
- Computed tomography can be helpful in distinguishing between ileus and obstruction (i.e., by determining the presence of a "transition point") and can identify complications that require immediate operative intervention (e.g., internal hernia, volvulus, ischemic bowel).
- Inspect the bowel carefully for injuries/enterotomies at the conclusion of adhesiolysis. Missed enterotomies can become a source of significant morbidity and mortality.
- Evaluation of the bowel's blood supply is important. Resect if ischemic, or if in doubt, consider a "second look" operation.
- Preserve as much small bowel as possible, especially when operating in the setting of inflammatory bowel disease. Operative techniques such as stricturoplasty and internal bypass can be used to preserve length if necessary.

SUGGESTED READINGS

Colon MJ, Telem DA, Wong D, et al. The relevance of transition zones on computed tomography in the management of small bowel obstruction. *Surgery.* 2010;147(3):373-377.

Diaz JJ Jr, Bokhari F, Mowery NT, et al. Guidelines for management of small bowel obstruction. *J Trauma.* 2008;64(6):1651-1664.

Kendrick ML. Partial small bowel obstruction: clinical issues and recent technical advances. *Abdom Imaging.* 2009;34:329-334.

O'Day BJ, Ridgway PF, Keenan N, et al. Detected peritoneal fluid in small bowel obstruction is associated with the need for surgical intervention. *Can J Surg.* 2009;52(3):201-206.

Olasky J, Moazzez A, Barrera K, et al. In the era of routine use of CT scan for acute abdominal pain, should all adults with small bowel intussusceptions undergo surgery?. *Am Surg.* 2009;75(10):958-961.

Zielinski MD, Eiken PW, Bannon MP, et al. Small bowel obstruction-who needs an operation? A multivariate prediction model. *World J Surg.* 2010;34(5):910-929.

Acute Cholecystitis

MEREDITH BARRETT AND DANIELLE M. FRITZE

Based on the previous edition chapter "Acute Cholecystitis" by Danielle Fritze and Justin B. Dimick

23

Presentation

A 50-year-old woman presents to the emergency room with right upper quadrant pain. The pain awakened her from sleep approximately 8 hours ago and is accompanied by nausea. She has had prior episodes of postprandial abdominal pain that she describes as similar but less severe. Notable history includes a laparoscopic Roux-en-Y gastric bypass, with more than 100 lb weight loss. On exam, she appears uncomfortable but not toxic. She is febrile to 38.6°C; all other vital signs are within normal range. Her abdomen is soft, with marked tenderness to palpation in the right subcostal region and a positive Murphy's sign.

● DIFFERENTIAL DIAGNOSIS

This patient's history of acute postprandial right upper quadrant (RUQ) pain with fever is a classic presentation of acute cholecystitis. Still, other pathology can yield similar symptoms and must be considered. The differential diagnosis for acute abdominal pain is broad and includes not only etiologies within the abdomen but also the chest. Notably, acute coronary syndromes can manifest as upper abdominal pain and may be deadly if overlooked. Gastroenteritis, gastroesophageal reflux disease, ulcer disease, and bowel obstruction are among the intra-abdominal processes to consider. This patient's history of a Roux-en-Y procedure also confers a risk of internal hernia.

Most commonly, acute cholecystitis must be distinguished from other biliary disease. A thorough understanding of biliary pathology is essential for an accurate and expedient diagnosis. Biliary colic results from temporary impaction of a gallstone in the gallbladder neck. This leads to postprandial abdominal pain, nausea, and vomiting that characteristically resolves over several hours. Signs of systemic inflammation, such as fever and leukocytosis, are absent. With sustained obstruction, systemic inflammation develops and acute cholecystitis ensues. Downstream passage of stones with obstruction of the common bile duct (CBD) can cause the more serious complication of ascending cholangitis; pancreatic duct obstruction leads to biliary pancreatitis.

Acalculous biliary disease is also a diagnostic consideration. Sphincter of Oddi dysfunction or biliary dyskinesia with low gallbladder ejection fraction often mimics the symptoms of biliary colic. Acute acalculous cholecystitis is usually limited to critically ill patients. It is thought to be the end result of relative gallbladder ischemia in the setting of global organ hypoperfusion.

● WORKUP

This patient's history and physical exam findings are classic for acute cholecystitis. Constant RUQ abdominal pain is the most common presenting symptom and often occurs following ingestion of a high fat meal. Many patients have known gallstones; nearly half report prior episodes of biliary colic. Additionally, this patient's bariatric surgery with rapid weight loss is a risk factor for stone formation. Physical exam commonly reveals fever in a stable patient. While hemodynamic derangements are possible, significant instability should raise concern for acute cholangitis, pancreatitis, or severe acute cholecystitis. There is often marked tenderness in the RUQ and epigastrium. Occasionally, an inflamed and dilated gallbladder may be palpable just inferior to the ribcage. Inspiratory arrest with deep palpation in the right subcostal region, known as Murphy's sign, is a classic finding in acute cholecystitis.

Despite the strong likelihood of acute cholecystitis based upon this patient's history and physical exam, further evaluation is needed to confirm the diagnosis. Notable laboratory values included a white blood count of 14,000/mm^3, transaminases just above the normal range, bilirubin of 1 mg/dL, and normal pancreatic enzymes. Leukocytosis with a predominance of neutrophils is common in acute cholecystitis. Marked leukocytosis >18,000/mm^3 distinguishes moderate from mild acute cholecystitis by the 2013 Tokyo Guidelines (Table 23-1). Pancreatic and liver enzymes are most commonly normal; elevated levels should prompt consideration of choledocholithiasis, cholangitis, or pancreatitis.

There are numerous imaging options available in the evaluation of possible cholecystitis. Ultrasound is the first-line imaging modality. It is a low cost, noninvasive imaging tool readily available in most settings; in trained hands, its sensitivity for acute cholecystitis is >80%. This patient's ultrasound revealed classic findings of acute cholecystitis including gallstones with gallbladder wall thickening, pericholecystic fluid, and a normal caliber CBD (Figure 23-1). Occasionally, the culprit stone can be visualized, impacted in

Table 23-1	TG13 Severity Grading for Acute Cholecystitis

Grade I Mild
- Does not meet below criteria for moderate or severe

Grade II Moderate
Meets any of the following criteria
- Gangrenous or emphysematous cholecystitis
- Pericholecystic or hepatic abscess
- Biliary peritonitis
- Palpable, tender RUQ mass
- WBC >18,000/mm^3
- Symptom duration >72 h

Grade III Severe
- Hemodynamic instability or other organ dysfunction

the gallbladder neck. The sonographer also reported a sonographic Murphy's sign—pain with the ultrasound probe situated directly over the inflamed gallbladder. While ultrasound is useful in demonstrating gallstones and the presence of gallbladder inflammation, choledocholithiasis is much less readily detected. Indirect signs of CBD stones such as CBD dilation may be present but are neither sensitive nor specific.

While characteristic ultrasound findings are sufficient to diagnose acute cholecystitis in this patient with concordant history and exam findings, other imaging modalities may be useful in cases of diagnostic uncertainty. Hepatobiliary iminodiacetic acid (HIDA) scan is considered the gold standard for diagnosis of acute cholecystitis, with sensitivity and specificity >95%. It is particularly useful in distinguishing cholecystitis from biliary colic and nonbiliary pain but may have false-positive results in the setting of chronic cholecystitis. Nonvisualization of the gallbladder at 60 minutes is diagnostic (Figure 23-2). Gallbladder contraction may be stimulated by morphine or cholecystokinin to further improve accuracy.

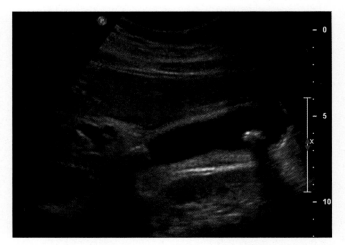

FIGURE 23-1. US with classic findings of cholecystitis: cholelithiasis, thickened gallbladder wall, and pericholecystic fluid.

HIDA can also be used to identify biliary dyskinesia, defined by a gallbladder ejection fraction of <35% to 40%.

The role of computed tomography (CT) in the evaluation of suspected acute cholecystitis is limited by inferior sensitivity and specificity. While CT may be used to diagnose complications of acute cholecystitis such as gallbladder gangrene or perforation, its primary utility is in the exclusion of nonbiliary etiologies of abdominal pain. Findings suggestive of acute cholecystitis include cholelithiasis, an enhancing and thickened gallbladder wall, pericholecystic fluid, and surrounding fat stranding (Figure 23-3).

In patients for whom choledocholithiasis is suspected, further evaluation of the biliary tree is warranted, either pre- or intra-operatively. Magnetic resonance cholangiopancreatography (MRCP) provides a noninvasive means of visualizing the biliary tree and is useful in diagnosing choledocholithiasis (Figure 23-4). Therapeutic sphincterotomy and stone extraction may be accomplished by endoscopic retrograde cholangiopancreatography (ERCP) in those patients with signs or symptoms of persistent biliary obstruction.

● DIAGNOSIS AND TREATMENT

The initial management of acute cholecystitis includes *nil per os* NPO status with systemic antibiotics and resuscitation as dictated by the patient's clinical condition. The 2013 Tokyo Guidelines (TG13) are useful in stratifying patients with acute cholecystitis by severity. Moderate disease is distinguished from mild acute cholecystitis by evidence of significant inflammation (Table 23-1). Hemodynamic instability and end-organ dysfunction characterize severe acute cholecystitis.

Those patients with mild disease and most patients with moderate disease should undergo cholecystectomy during the index admission, preferably within the first 24 hours. Although traditionally patients with symptoms lasting >72 hours have been treated with delayed cholecystectomy, randomized trials now suggest that such delay is not warranted. Associated morbidity, hospital length of stay, and overall costs are lower for those who undergo prompt operative intervention.

If there is significant concern for choledocholithiasis, the CBD should be evaluated. The decision between preoperative ERCP and intraoperative cholangiography (IOC) (with CBD exploration or postoperative ERCP if warranted) should be tailored to patient presentation and surgeon expertise. Preoperative ERCP should be followed by cholecystectomy prior to hospital discharge.

Patients with severe acute cholecystitis and those with prohibitive operative risk related to comorbidities require gallbladder drainage to achieve source control. Decompensated cardiac failure, unstable angina, and severe or poorly controlled chronic lung disease are among the conditions that may render surgical risk prohibitively high. Traditionally, gallbladder drainage is accomplished via a percutaneous cholecystostomy tube. This may be used as

CHAPTER 23 • Acute Cholecystitis

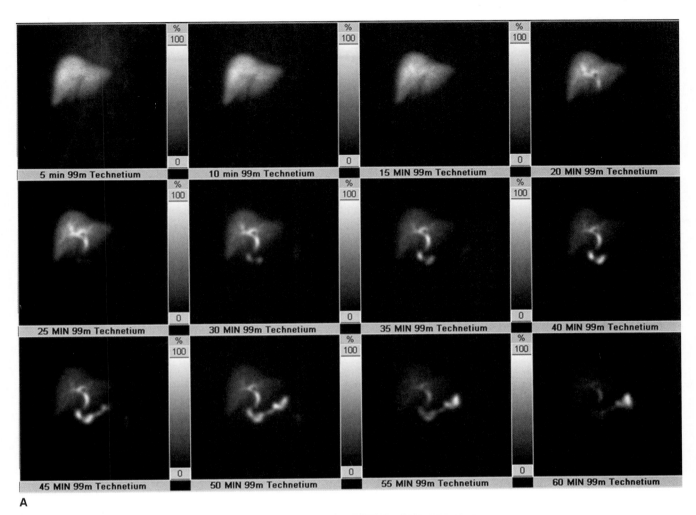

A

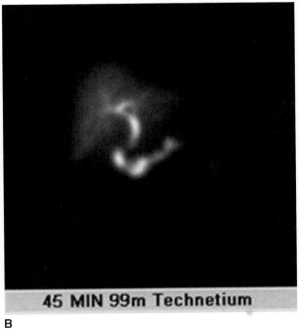

B

FIGURE 23-2. **A:** HIDA scan consistent with acute cholecystitis. **B:** At 45 minutes after injection of contrast, there is opacification of the intra- and extrahepatic biliary tree and duodenum. The gallbladder is not visualized.

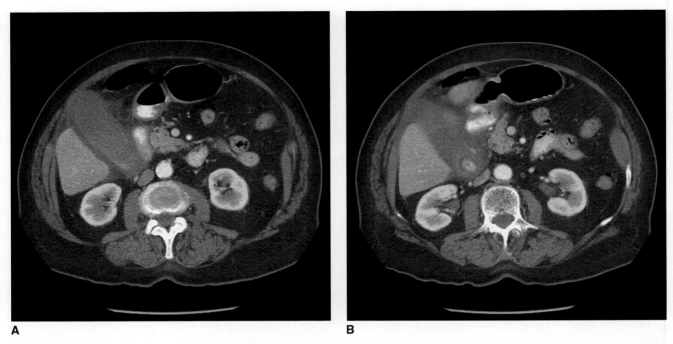

A   **B**

FIGURE 23-3. A: CT scan consistent with acute cholecystitis demonstrating a dilated, thick-walled gallbladder with surrounding inflammatory stranding. **B:** A large gallstone is lodged in the gallbladder neck.

a bridge to cholecystectomy when the patient's condition improves, or it may remain in place indefinitely. Any trial of tube removal must be preceded by contrast injection to confirm a patent cystic duct. Up to 50% of patients will still develop recurrent cholecystitis; the risk is lower in patients with acalculous disease.

In recent years, various endoscopic gallbladder drainage procedures have emerged as alternatives to percutaneous cholecystostomy. Where available, these options offer the advantage of source control without requiring an external drain. In patients with end-stage liver disease and ascites, in whom operation carries a high mortality rate and

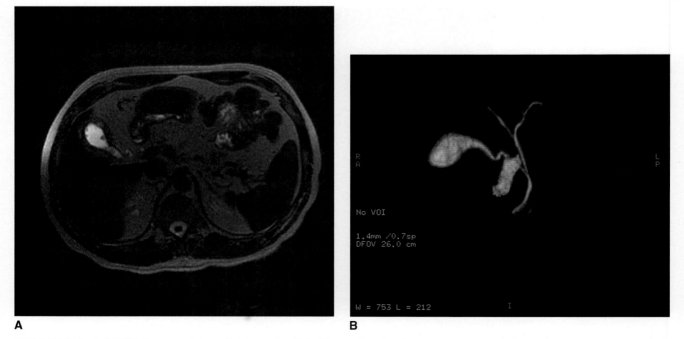

A   **B**

FIGURE 23-4. A: MRCP demonstrating a thickened gallbladder wall and gallstones within the cystic duct, but no biliary dilation or choledocholithiasis. **B:** The filling defects within the gallbladder likely represent small polyps. Reformatted images delineate the patient's biliary anatomy.

percutaneous tubes are particularly problematic, cystic duct stenting offers a significant therapeutic advantage. Long-term data will be useful in guiding future practice.

Fortunately, this patient's cholecystitis is mild, and she has few comorbidities. She was made NPO, provided intravenous fluids and pain control, and started on broad spectrum antibiotics. Plans were made for urgent laparoscopic cholecystectomy. Given her elevated liver enzymes and the relative inaccessibility of her biliary tree via ERCP (due to her roux anatomy), informed consent was also obtained for intraoperative cholangiogram and CBD exploration as needed.

● SURGICAL APPROACH

Cholecystectomy may be accomplished via either a laparoscopic or an open approach. Laparoscopic cholecystectomy is associated with decreased length of hospital stay, less patient discomfort, and shorter recovery time. Relative contraindications include a hostile abdomen, known aberrant anatomy, or severe inflammation. For these patients, one must have a low threshold for open conversion or IOC to confirm anatomy.

Laparoscopic cholecystectomy is performed under general anesthesia with the patient in supine position (Table 23-2). Access to the abdomen is generally obtained at the umbilicus via open Hassan or closed Veress needle technique. Pneumoperitoneum is established and a 30° laparoscope inserted. Two additional operating ports are inserted in the RUQ and one in the epigastrium. Adjusting the operating table to a left side down and reverse Trendelenburg position facilitates displacement of the bowel and omentum out of the operative field. The fundus of the gallbladder is grasped and retracted cephalad over the edge of the liver via the lateral subcostal port. The remainder of the operation is conducted through the subxiphoid and medial right subcostal ports. Any adhesions to the gallbladder are taken down to reveal the triangle of Calot. The infundibulum is retracted laterally to open the triangle, separating the cystic duct from the common hepatic duct. The overlying peritoneum is incised, and the triangle of Calot is cleared of soft tissue. Dissection continues until the cystic duct and cystic artery are the only remaining structures in the triangle and can be seen directly entering the gallbladder, and the distal 1/3 of the gallbladder has been elevated off of the liver. This constitutes the "critical view of safety" (Figure 23-5). Opening the peritoneal reflections over the gallbladder and retracting the infundibulum medially to expose the posterior aspect of the triangle may facilitate this portion of the operation. Only after the critical view of safety has been definitively achieved, the cystic duct and artery are doubly clipped and divided. The gallbladder is dissected off of the liver with electrocautery, placed into a specimen bag, and removed from the abdomen. After hemostasis is assured, pneumoperitoneum is released, all port sites are closed, and the patient is allowed to emerge from anesthesia.

Table 23-2	Laparoscopic Cholecystectomy

Key Technical Steps

1. Access the peritoneum.
2. Place ports: umbilical, subxiphoid, medial, and lateral right subcostal.
3. Retract the gallbladder fundus cranially and the infundibulum laterally to open the triangle of Calot.
4. Incise and divide the peritoneum overlying the gallbladder and the triangle of Calot.
5. Establish the critical view of safety: completely dissect the triangle of Calot until the cystic duct and the cystic artery are the only structures remaining. Elevate the lower third of the gallbladder off of the liver.
6. Clip and divide the cystic duct and artery only after the critical view of safety has been definitively achieved.
7. Elevate the gallbladder off of the liver bed with electrocautery.
8. Place the gallbladder in a specimen bag and then remove from the abdomen.
9. Assure hemostasis, release the pneumoperitoneum, and close all port sites.

Potential Pitfalls

- Complicated abdominal entry with damage to abdominal viscera or great vessels.
- Aberrant biliary or vascular anatomy.
- Inability to define the relevant anatomy.
- Injury to portal structures, liver, or duodenum.
- Choledocholithiasis.
- Perforation of the gallbladder.

The most problematic pitfall in any cholecystectomy is failure to accurately identify relevant structures. One of the most common causes of biliary injury is mistaking the CBD for the cystic duct. The CBD is then ligated and divided before the injury is appreciated. Concomitant vascular injuries are common. This is more likely to occur in the setting of severe inflammation, a short broad cystic duct, or Mirizzi syndrome where a stone in the cystic neck or duct extrinsically compresses the common hepatic duct or CBD. Strict delineation of biliary and vascular anatomy, coupled with a low threshold for open conversion, is mandatory for safe conduct of the operation.

● SPECIAL INTRA-OPERATIVE CONSIDERATIONS

Approximately 5% to 10% of attempts at laparoscopic cholecystectomy for acute cholecystitis result in conversion to an open operation. The primary indication for conversion is

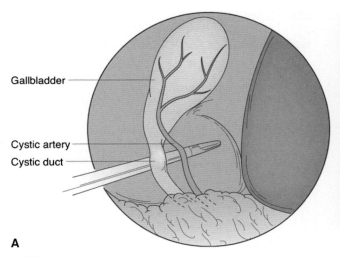
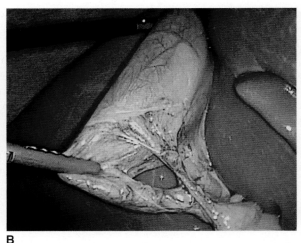

A   **B**

FIGURE 23-5. **A:** The critical view of safety. The triangle of Calot has been neatly cleared of all tissue except the cystic artery and cystic duct. **B:** These two remaining structures are seen directly entering the gallbladder and may be safely divided. (Intraoperative photo courtesy of Dr. Filip Bednar.)

an inability to clearly define the anatomy of the biliary tract. Failure to establish the critical view of safety mandates conversion. Other indications include significant inflammation, failure to make satisfactory progress, any suspicion of injury to ductal or vascular structures, and concern for gallbladder cancer (Table 23-3).

Intraoperative cholangiography (IOC) may be used routinely in cholecystectomy or reserved for select circumstances (Table 23-4). Direct imaging of the biliary tree may demonstrate choledocholithiasis in patients suspected of having common duct stones due to elevated liver enzymes, biliary dilatation, or pancreatitis (Figure 23-6). Stones may be removed via CBD exploration or ERCP, either during the operation or postoperatively. Additionally, IOC may aid in delineating biliary anatomy or identifying a biliary injury.

Patients with severe inflammation pose a particular challenge. A thick-walled, tightly distended, or hydropic gallbladder may be extremely difficult to grasp. Needle aspiration of gallbladder contents facilitates grasping the gallbladder for more effective retraction. Occasionally, delineation of relevant anatomy may be easier with a top down approach. The gallbladder fundus is elevated off of the liver and dissection carried along the gallbladder wall down toward the triangle of Calot. Again, no structures are divided until the critical

view of safety is achieved. If it is not possible to definitively attain the critical view of safety, conversion to open is the safest option. Subtotal cholecystectomy is an additional consideration but requires confirmation that the gallbladder remnant and cystic duct are clear of stones. The proximal gallbladder is resected, and the gallbladder neck can be stapled or oversewn (reconstituting) or left open (fenestrating). If severe inflammation or anatomical distortion renders any form of cholecystectomy dangerous, a cholecystostomy tube may be placed intraoperatively to accomplish gallbladder drainage.

● POSTOPERATIVE MANAGEMENT

Most patients with acute cholecystitis are able to return home the day after laparoscopic cholecystectomy. Regular diet may be resumed immediately after surgery. Oral pain medications usually provide ample analgesia, with the patient quickly transitioning from opioid therapy to over the counter pain medications. Antibiotics are not indicated beyond the immediate perioperative period. Some patients experience diarrhea associated with altered bile salt storage after cholecystectomy, but this is typically mild and temporary.

Table 23-3	Indications for Conversion to Open

1. Inability to define relevant biliary and vascular anatomy
2. Suspected injury to the biliary tree, vasculature, or bowel
3. Uncontrolled hemorrhage
4. Suspicion of gallbladder cancer
5. Failure to make satisfactory progress
6. Patient intolerance of pneumoperitoneum

Table 23-4	Indications for Intraoperative Cholangiogram

1. Inability to define relevant biliary anatomy
2. Suspicion of biliary injury
3. Suspicion of choledocholithiasis:
   - Dilated CBD
   - Elevated liver or pancreatic enzymes
   - CBD stones identified on preoperative imaging
4. Routine use

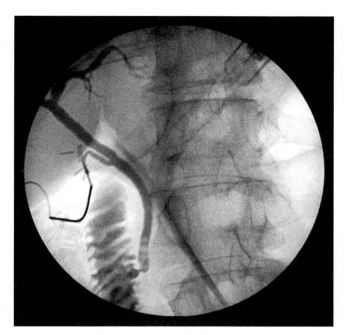

FIGURE 23-6. IOC with choledocholithiasis. This intraoperative cholangiogram revealed stones stacked within the CBD.

Persistent abdominal pain, fever, or hyperbilirubinemia should prompt evaluation for retained CBD stone, biliary leak, or biliary injury. US should be the initial imaging study as it noninvasively demonstrates biliary dilation and fluid collections. Similar information may be derived from abdominal CT. Biliary dilation should be further evaluated with ERCP to identify a retained CBD stone or biliary injury causing obstruction. During the same procedure, interventions such as stent placement, stone extraction, or sphincterotomy may be accomplished. Postoperative fluid collections may represent hematoma, biloma, or abscess. Percutaneous image-guided drain placement allows for adequate drainage of the collection as well as identification of its source. Return of bilious fluid should prompt ERCP to pinpoint the leak. During ERCP, an endobiliary stent may then be placed to encourage bile flow through the biliary tree into the duodenum rather than into the peritoneum (Figure 23-7). For patients such as ours with Roux-en-Y anatomy, initial MRCP or drain injection should be considered for localization of leak or injury. If the biliary tree cannot be reached by transoral endoscopy due to Roux anatomy, laparoscopy can provide direct access to the gastric remnant or small intestine, allowing for intraoperative ERCP. Alternatively, open surgery remains an option.

Case Conclusion

This patient underwent laparoscopic cholecystectomy, IOC, and CBD exploration with stone extraction. Her diet was resumed immediately postoperatively, and her pain was well controlled on oral agents. She was discharged the following day. At her postoperative follow-up visit, she was recovering well without evidence of complication or recurrent pain.

TAKE HOME POINTS

- Acute cholecystitis presents with RUQ pain, fever, and leukocytosis.
- RUQ ultrasound is the first-line diagnostic test.
- Acute cholecystitis must be distinguished from other biliary pathology such as biliary colic, choledocholithiasis, cholangitis, or biliary pancreatitis.
- Acute cholecystitis may be stratified by severity according to the 2013 Tokyo Guidelines.
- Urgent laparoscopic cholecystectomy is the treatment of choice for most patients with mild and moderate cholecystitis, even those presenting after 72 hours.
- Patients with severe acute cholecystitis, characterized by instability and organ dysfunction, merit resuscitation and percutaneous or endoscopic gallbladder drainage.
- During laparoscopic cholecystectomy, no structures may be divided until the critical view of safety is definitely established.
- Inability to achieve the critical view of safety mandates conversion to open operation.
- Intraoperative cholangiogram may be useful in defining the patient's biliary anatomy and identifying choledocholithiasis or biliary injury.
- Persistent postoperative pain, fever, or hyperbilirubinemia are concerning for retained CBD stone or biliary leak.

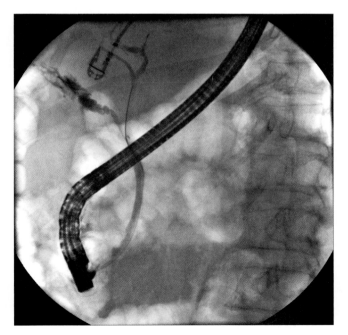

FIGURE 23-7. ERCP with bile leak. Postoperative ERCP demonstrating a cystic duct stump leak. A wire is seen within the common hepatic duct, which traverses the CBD and terminates in the duodenum. A stent is placed across this wire to encourage bile flow into the duodenum rather than through the leak.

SUGGESTED READINGS

Baron TH, Grimm IS, Swanstrom LL. Interventional approaches to gallbladder disease. *N Engl J Med.* 2015;373(4):357-365.

de Mestral C, Rotstein OD, Laupacis A, Hoch JS, Zagorski B, Nathens AB. A population-based analysis of the clinical course of 10,304 patients with acute cholecystitis, discharged without cholecystectomy. *J Trauma Acute Care Surg.* 2013;74(1):26-30; discussion 30-21.

Demehri FR, Alam HB. Evidence-based management of common gallstone-related emergencies. *J Intensive Care Med.* 2016; 31(1):3-13.

Gutt CN, Encke J, Köninger J, et al. Acute cholecystitis: early versus delayed cholecystectomy, a multicenter randomized trial (ACDC study, NCT00447304). *Ann Surg.* 2013;258(3):385-393.

Kiriyama S, Takada T, Strasberg SM, et al. TG13 guidelines for diagnosis and severity grading of acute cholangitis (with videos). *J Hepatobiliary Pancreat Sci.* 2013;20(1):24-34.

Peitzman AB, Watson GA, Marsh JW. Acute cholecystitis: when to operate and how to do it safely. *J Trauma Acute Care Surg.* 2015;78(1):1-12.

Roulin D, Saadi A, Di Mare L, Demartines N, Halkic N. Early versus delayed cholecystectomy for acute cholecystitis, are the 72 hours still the rule?: a randomized trial. *Ann Surg.* 2016;264:717.

Strasberg SM. Error traps and vasculo-biliary injury in laparoscopic and open cholecystectomy. *J Hepatobiliary Pancreat Surg.* 2008;15(3):284-292.

Törnqvist B, Waage A, Zheng Z, Ye W, Nilsson M. Severity of acute cholecystitis and risk of iatrogenic bile duct injury during cholecystectomy, a population-based case–control study. *World J Surg.* 2016;40(5):1060-1067.

Yamashita Y, Takada T, Strasberg SM, et al. TG13 surgical management of acute cholecystitis. *J Hepatobiliary Pancreat Sci.* 2013; 20(1):89-96.

Cholangitis

MICHAEL W. CRIPPS

24

Based on the previous edition chapter "Cholangitis" by William C. Beck and
Benjamin K. Poulose

Presentation

A 68-year-old man with a history of adult-onset diabetes, obesity, and tobacco use presents to the emergency department. He is febrile on arrival with a temperature of 102.7, a blood pressure of 95/50, and a heart rate of 106. His primary complaint is of right upper quadrant pain of 24-hour duration. He notes that he has had similar pain on occasion before but always had complete resolution of pain within a couple of hours. He reports his urine has been very dark for the last 12 hours. On exam, he has tenderness of his right upper quadrant with voluntary guarding. His sclerae are mildly icteric. No jaundice is present.

● DIFFERENTIAL DIAGNOSIS

Ascending cholangitis is the most likely diagnosis for a patient with these constellation of symptoms. Ascending cholangitis, the result of ascending bacterial infection from the bowel into the biliary tree, should not be confused with other inflammation-associated biliary diseases that utilize the term "cholangitis" such as primary sclerosing cholangitis. The typical presentation of ascending cholangitis involves the combination of right upper quadrant pain, fever, and jaundice, commonly known as Charcot's triad. However, while Charcot's triad has a high specificity, the sensitivity is low, with only 50% to 70% of patient presenting with all three elements. The addition of mental status changes and hypotension comprise Reynolds' pentad, which is indicative of systemic sepsis. A complaint of right upper quadrant pain necessitates the consideration of biliary colic, but patients with cholangitis usually manifest with fever and jaundice. In a patient presenting with a history of gallstones or right upper quadrant pain, the presence of jaundice, hypotension, or altered mental status should alert the provider to the diagnosis of cholangitis. Acute cholecystitis should also be a strong consideration within the differential diagnosis, with care taken to delineate it from cholangitis as the immediate treatment would differ considerably. Factors that predispose a patient to ascending cholangitis that should be elucidated in the patient's history include biliary interventions such as endoscopically or radiologically placed biliary stents or history of chronic biliary conditions (i.e., primary sclerosing cholangitis). Malignancy can also be a cause of biliary

obstruction, but pain is usually less of a component of the presentation and the onset is more insidious. Peritonitis is uncommon in cholangitis and, if present, should prompt the examiner to look for other causes of abdominal pain such as diverticulitis, perforated ulcer, or pancreatitis.

Presentation Continued

This patient undergoes further evaluation of his abdominal pain, fevers, and jaundice with a complete blood count (CBC), comprehensive metabolic panel (CMP), amylase, lipase, coagulation profile, and two sets of blood cultures. He has a leukocytosis of 13,300/μL with a left shift, a bilirubin of 4.4 mg/dL, and alkaline phosphatase of 500 IU/L. Both the AST and the ALT are elevated at 210 and 334 IU/L, respectively.

● WORKUP

There is no imaging modality that can directly reveal infection of the biliary tree. Instead, indirect evidence of blockage of intra- and extrahepatic ducts lends data toward a diagnosis of ascending cholangitis. An abdominal ultrasound (US) is often the preferred *initial* imaging study, as it is quick, painless, and radiation-free and can detect signs of cholecystitis. US utility can be limited by bowel gas patterns, inability to evaluate the distal common bile duct, and operator skill set. Computed tomography (CT) scans can identify biliary dilation and detect inflammation but requires patient transport and increased time for image acquisition. In the above patient, imaging reveals cholelithiasis with mild intra- and extrahepatic biliary duct dilation. CT scan and magnetic resonance cholangiopancreatography (MRCP) may also prove helpful to identify the underlying etiology of the biliary obstruction that predisposed the patient to cholangitis, such as benign or malignant biliary strictures, or periampullary mass. MRCP is particularly helpful in identifying noncalcified biliary stones. In general, a single, good-quality, noninvasive study (US, CT, or MRCP) can suffice to establish biliary ductal dilation and provide clues to the etiology of biliary obstruction. A high suspicion for common bile duct stones is present with ascending cholangitis without other obvious etiology or total bilirubin >4 mg/dL. Other strong predictors of common bile duct stones include a dilated common bile duct (>6 mm) on US with gallbladder *in situ* and bilirubin between 1.8 and 4 mg/dL.

Blood test results can vary in patients with acute cholangitis and must be taken in the context of the history and physical exam of the individual patient. The white blood cell count is elevated above 10,000/μL in 60% to 80% of patients with acute cholangitis and is the most often noted abnormal result. Total bilirubin is only elevated in 60% to 70% of patients with cholangitis, so it is important to remember that the diagnosis can still be made in the absence of jaundice. While liver enzymes (AST, ALT, GGT) are usually elevated, there is no specific pattern that has been demonstrated. Alkaline phosphatase is also usually elevated and is typically more elevated in biliary obstruction due to malignant etiologies as compared to choledocholithiasis.

● DIAGNOSIS AND TREATMENT

Although Charcot's triad remains the classic definition of ascending cholangitis, many patients do not present with the triad. In 2006, an international consensus meeting was held in Tokyo, Japan, with the goal of developing guidelines useful in establishing the diagnosis of acute cholangitis. These guidelines have been twice updated, with the most recent in 2018. The consensus was reached that while Charcot's triad has a low sensitivity, the high specificity is sufficient to diagnose acute cholangitis. Additionally, the Tokyo guidelines suggest that the diagnosis of cholangitis can be made if two of the three elements of Charcot's triad are present along

with (1) laboratory evidence of inflammatory response, (2) abnormal liver function tests, and (3) abnormal imaging studies demonstrating biliary dilatation, inflammatory findings, or the presence of an etiology such as a biliary stricture, calculus, stent, or mass (Figure 24-1).

The 2013/2018 Tokyo Guidelines recommend that the severity of cholangitis should be categorized into three grades to help in its management: mild (grade 1), moderate (grade 2), and severe (grade 3). The grades are based on the response to therapy and by the onset of organ failure. Mild or grade 1 acute cholangitis is characterized as acute cholangitis that responds to initial medical treatment and does not meet the criteria for grade 2 or 3 cholangitis. Moderate or grade 2 acute cholangitis is defined as acute cholangitis that has any two of the following: abnormal WBC count (>12,000/mm³ or <4,000/mm³), high fever (≥39°C), old age (≥75 years old), hyperbilirubinemia (total bilirubin ≥5 mg/dL), or hypoalbuminemia. Grade 2 can also include any patient with cholangitis who does not respond to initial therapy, but does not have organ failure. Severe or grade 3 acute cholangitis is regarded as acute cholangitis that does not respond to initial medical treatment and is accompanied by the onset of organ failure. The 2018 guidelines indicated that those patients who are in grade 2 have a significant mortality benefit from urgent or early (within 48 hours) drainage.

In this patient presenting with two elements of Charcot's triad (fever, abdominal pain, and jaundice), biliary disease should be at the top of the differential diagnosis. In the setting of altered mental status and relative hypotension in a normally hypertensive man, the provider should strongly

Charcot's triad: (1) Fever
(2) Jaundice
(3) Right upper quadrant pain

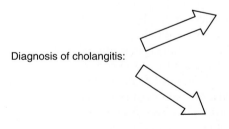

Diagnosis of cholangitis:

Tokyo Criteria

(1) Presence of 2/3 elements of Charcot's triad +
(2) Laboratory evidence of inflammation: +

i. Elevated WBC
ii. Elevated CRP
iii. Increased ESR

(3) Abnormal LFT's +
(4) Abnormal imaging studies

i. Biliary dilatation
ii. Inflammation
iii. Etiology

1. Stones
2. Stents
3. Mass

FIGURE 24-1. Diagnosis of cholangitis may be made using either the traditional Charcot's triad or Tokyo criteria.

suspect cholangitis as the diagnosis. Many patients have a history of prior calculous biliary disease or biliary operation. In Western countries, choledocholithiasis is the most common etiology of cholangitis, followed by benign and malignant biliary strictures. Other etiologies include autoimmune cholangitis, parasitic infections, prior biliary operations, indwelling stents, and chronic pancreatitis.

When cholangitis is suspected, fluid resuscitation and empiric antibiotic therapy should be initiated immediately, regardless of the ability to make the initial diagnosis. The patient should be admitted to the hospital for intravenous fluid resuscitation, initiation of appropriate antibiotics, hemodynamic monitoring, and prompt biliary decompression if indicated. Blood cultures should be sent prior to the initiation of antibiotics to allow for the tailoring of antibiotic therapy after the causative organism is identified. Timely initiation of empiric intravenous antibiotic therapy is crucial to successful treatment. Those with grade 3 cholangitis or who show signs of septic shock should have antibiotic therapy started within 1 hour, while those who are less ill should begin antibiotics within 6 hours. Therapy should target gram-negative bacteria and anaerobes, and local antibiograms should be evaluated prior to selecting antibiotic agents. Additionally, history of antimicrobial usage, renal and hepatic function, and a history of allergies and other adverse events should be considered. A cephalosporin plus metronidazole or extended-spectrum beta-lactam (piperacillin–tazobactam) can provide adequate empiric coverage, but *Escherichia coli* resistance patterns must be considered. For those with beta-lactam allergies, a fluoroquinolone with added metronidazole can be used, being cautious of increasing fluoroquinolone resistance patterns. Occasionally, coagulopathy is present, which needs to be corrected prior to undergoing any intervention. If the patient responds well to antibiotic therapy, and there is no hemodynamic instability, further imaging (CT or MRCP) may be performed to better elucidate the underlying cause of the cholangitis. However, if the patient appears septic, urgent biliary decompression is required either by endoscopic, percutaneous, or surgical means.

Source control of infection remains the mainstay of therapy for patients with acute cholangitis, but antimicrobial therapy may temporize the patient and allow for elective, rather than urgent, decompression. Those who respond well to initial resuscitation and antibiotic therapy without biliary drainage are deemed as having mild (grade 1) cholangitis. With continued clinical improvement, the urgency of biliary decompression may be delayed as the etiology for biliary obstruction is sought. Patients who do not respond to resuscitation and antibiotics alone will need urgent biliary decompression.

● SURGICAL APPROACH

Urgent endoscopic decompression of the biliary tree has been established as the treatment of choice for the management of acute cholangitis. Endoscopic retrograde cholangiopancreatography (ERCP) is successful in over 90% of patients in decompressing the biliary tree. The timing of endoscopic biliary decompression should be individualized and often occurs within 24 to 48 hours of initial admission. The urgency of intervention should be dictated by the patient's clinical response to resuscitation and antibiotic therapy. An initial good response followed by clinical deterioration prompts urgent biliary decompression. The 2013 and 2018 Tokyo guidelines report significant improvement in mortality for those with grade 2 ascending cholangitis as a result of more timely decompression. More urgent or emergent decompression is required in patients who remain hypotensive despite aggressive resuscitation and antibiotic therapy. When ERCP expertise is not readily available and urgent biliary decompression is needed, percutaneous or surgical biliary decompression should be employed.

ERCP can be performed under moderate or deep sedation and is associated with decreased rates of postoperative mechanical ventilation and death as opposed to traditional open bile duct exploration. ERCP is typically performed with the patient in the prone or semiprone position. The duodenoscope is advanced through the oropharynx, esophagus, and stomach to the second portion of the duodenum. The ampulla is visualized and engaged with a cannula or sphincterotome. Wire access to the biliary tree is achieved and the cannula advanced into the bile duct. Before a large volume of contrast in instilled into the biliary tree, bile is aspirated to assist with decompression and to obtain biliary cultures. The act of biliary cannulation alone will often result in rapid biliary decompression in patients with acute suppurative cholangitis (Figure 24-2), and cultures should be obtained. Radiopaque contrast is then injected into the bile duct and cholangiography performed to ascertain the etiology of biliary obstruction. Should a common bile duct calculus be discovered, a judgment is made regarding appropriateness of biliary sphincterotomy prior to stent placement. If the

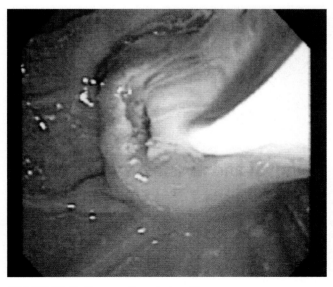

FIGURE 24-2. Suppurative cholangitis.

calculus is relatively small and there is little associated ampullary edema, biliary sphincterotomy can usually be safely performed to help facilitate ductal clearance either with a biliary extraction balloon or a Dormia basket. However, for grade 3 cholangitis or those with coagulopathy, sphincterotomy should be avoided at the initial endoscopy. A temporary transampullary biliary stent is then placed to ensure continued biliary drainage (Figure 24-3). If during cholangiography, a large, challenging stone or complex stricture is encountered, the main priority should be biliary decompression with stenting to quickly improve the patient's clinical condition. This is done at the expense of repeated diagnostic and therapeutic procedures to help define the precise etiology of biliary obstruction and definitively treat the patient, although cultures taken at this time may help guide antibiotic therapy. However, these additional procedures can often be performed on an elective basis. In experienced hands, ERCP can be performed with minimal risk. Post-ERCP pancreatitis is the most frequently encountered complication, followed by hemorrhage, cholangitis, and perforation. In patients with severe sepsis and hypotension who do not have suppurative cholangitis at the time of ERCP, serious consideration should be given to an alternate diagnosis.

If ERCP is not available, other options for biliary decompression include percutaneous transhepatic drainage and surgical decompression. If the intrahepatic ducts are dilated, thus providing a transhepatic target for biliary access, a percutaneous route to biliary drainage is favored as it is less invasive than surgical decompression and provides adequate drainage. In addition, a percutaneously placed biliary drain drainage can usually be converted to an internal endoscopically placed stent once acute issues have resolved via a rendezvous technique.

Surgical decompression of the biliary tree is largely of historical interest given the high success of ERCP and percutaneous techniques, avoiding the additional physiologic insult of a major operation. There are a few atypical scenarios that arise in patients with altered upper gastrointestinal anatomy (e.g., post Roux-en-Y gastric bypass) that limit endoscopy and traditionally indicate the need for surgical decompression. However, recent reports have demonstrated that balloon-assisted enteroscopy has been successful in patients with altered upper gastrointestinal anatomy. If this or any endoscopic techniques are not available, decompression may need to be performed surgically, with more than one option available. If a patent cystic duct can be demonstrated with an *in situ* gallbladder, an open or laparoscopic cholecystostomy tube may be an efficient, lifesaving intervention until further expertise can be obtained. If common bile duct access is necessary, an open approach is usually employed for common bile duct exploration and T-tube placement (Table 24-1). Surgeons with advanced laparoscopic skills and experience may consider a laparoscopic approach. If a laparotomy is performed, an upper midline or right subcostal incision is utilized to approach the biliary tree. A self-retaining retractor is used to retract the liver cephalad and colon caudally. If a gallbladder is present, it is mobilized in a dome-down fashion until the cystic duct is identified. Calot's triangle is defined and the cystic artery is ligated and divided. The anterior surface of the cystic duct is dissected toward the common bile

Table 24-1	Open Biliary Decompression

Key Technical Steps

1. An upper midline or right subcostal laparotomy is performed.
2. A self-retaining retractor is used to lift liver cephalad and retract colon caudally.
3. If present, gallbladder is dissected using "dome-down" technique until Calot's triangle is identified. The cystic artery is ligated and divided.
4. Cystic duct is followed antegrade to the common bile duct, which is dissected anteriorly.
5. The cholecystectomy is completed.
6. A longitudinal choledochotomy is made 1–2 cm distal to the confluence of the cystic duct and the common bile duct.
7. The common bile duct is cleared with irrigation or a Fogarty catheter.
8. The choledochotomy is closed using absorbable suture over a T tube and a closed-suction drain is left in the area of the choledochotomy.

Potential Pitfalls

- Dissection on the common bile duct laterally, thereby compromising the blood supply.
- Rigid instrumentation of the CBD, causing injury.
- Failure to correctly identify the CBD prior to making choledochotomy.

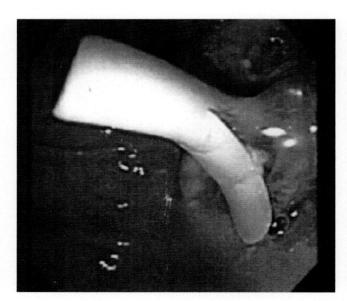

FIGURE 24-3. Transampullary stent placement.

duct, which usually is readily identified. Care is then taken to dissect the anterior surface of the bile duct only to avoid the flanking blood supply coursing at the 3 and the 9 o'clock positions. The caliber of the bile duct and associated inflammation are assessed to help further guide surgical intervention. The cholecystectomy is completed. The intended area of choledochotomy should be 1 to 2 cm distal to the insertion of the cystic duct toward the ampulla. Two separate mural sutures, using a fine 4-0 or 5-0 suture, are placed on either side of the anterior portion of the bile duct and a longitudinal choledochotomy made with a no. 15 blade scalpel. At this point, a decision is made to proceed with common bile duct exploration or to insert a T-tube for decompression in the unstable patient. If common bile duct stones are suspected, simple irrigation of the ductal lumen with a small bore red rubber catheter is usually adequate to mobilize most calculi out through the choledochotomy. The red rubber catheter can be advanced both proximally and distally to clear the bile duct. A balloon-tipped catheter ("biliary Fogarty") may also be used. Rigid instrumentation and extraction forceps should be avoided, especially with inflamed tissues increasing the chance of ductal injury. Choledochoscopy is a very useful adjunct to ensure ductal clearance. A 3- or 5-mm choledochoscope can be used with continuous saline irrigation to adequately and efficiently visualize the ductal lumen. Difficult stones can be retrieved with wire baskets placed through the scope. It is essential that the surgeon be familiar with the equipment intended for choledochoscopy prior to the procedure. In addition, biliary endoscopy can be challenging even for experienced surgical endoscopists; familiarity with endoscopic techniques in general greatly facilitates this procedure, especially when through-the-scope therapeutics are employed. Once the duct is cleared, a T-tube is usually placed in the setting of acute cholangitis. For adequate drainage, a 14 F or 16 F guttered T tube should be placed within the bile duct. The choledochotomy is closed using absorbable sutures over the T tube, which is brought through the abdominal wall. Some redundancy of the tubing should be left within the abdomen to avoid tension, but a long and tortuous course should be avoided to help facilitate possible future percutaneous techniques. If time and resources permit, a completion T-tube cholangiogram can be performed to confirm bile duct clearance and integrity of the ductal closure. A closed-suction drain is placed in the area of the choledochotomy and the abdomen closed in the standard fashion.

● SPECIAL INTRAOPERATIVE CONSIDERATIONS

The surgical approach to the common bile duct should be avoided in patients with smaller ducts (<5 mm) where identification and manipulation would be technically difficult, especially in an inflamed field. In these situations, cholecystostomy tube placement may be an ideal method of biliary decompression, should endoscopy not be feasible. Should the surgeon encounter severely inflamed tissues around the main portal triad, every effort to minimize dissection and safely enter the common bile duct need to be employed. Keen judgment should be used to avoid injury to the portal vein, hepatic artery, or duodenum in the inflamed field. Identification of the common bile duct can be facilitated by using a small needle (22 to 25 g) to aspirate bile from the duct before an incision is made within it. This technique is especially helpful in patients who have had prior cholecystectomy. Laparoscopy has limited use in the acute decompression of the common bile duct except among surgeons and surgical teams who have considerable expertise with these techniques.

● POSTOPERATIVE MANAGEMENT

Following biliary decompression, patients are observed in the hospital for resolution of their symptoms. Antibiotics may be tailored following the results of cultures and continued for 4 to 7 days. If bacteremia with gram-positive cocci such as *Enterococcus* spp., *Streptococcus* spp. is present, duration of minimum 2 weeks is recommended. If, after the initial management strategy, there remains obstruction of the biliary tree (i.e., residual stones or mass), antibiotic treatment should be continued until these anatomic problems are resolved. A CBC and CMP may be sent to follow improving white blood cell counts and liver profile. Definitive therapy is dictated by the underlying cause of biliary obstruction. In most patients who undergo ERCP for choledocholithiasis, elective cholecystectomy can be performed at a later date with ductal clearance usually achieved via ERCP.

For those patients in whom a T tube was placed, the tube is initially left to gravity drainage in the acute setting. After discharge, a contrast study is obtained via the tube to confirm clearance of the bile duct and patency of the biliary tree. With this study, usually performed 2 to 3 weeks after insertion, the decision can then be made to "internalize" biliary drainage (i.e., cap the T tube). Another study is repeated at 4 to 6 weeks, and the tube is removed should this study demonstrate normal patency and drainage of the biliary system.

Case Conclusion

In the patient presented, a high suspicion of common bile duct stones existed based on documented cholelithiasis, extrahepatic biliary ductal dilation, clinical ascending cholangitis, and a total bilirubin level greater than 4 mg/dL. The patient underwent successful ERCP with biliary sphincterotomy and extraction of common bile duct stones. Once discharged, an elective laparoscopic cholecystectomy was performed.

TAKE HOME POINTS

- Prompt diagnosis, antibiotic administration, and fluid resuscitation are of utmost importance in the patient with acute cholangitis.
- The most common cause of acute cholangitis in Western countries is choledocholithiasis, followed by malignancy.
- Urgent biliary decompression is the essential treatment in acute cholangitis not responsive to resuscitation and antibiotics.
- Endoscopic biliary decompression is associated with lower morbidity and mortality than with conventional surgical bile duct exploration.
- Percutaneous or surgical decompression should be employed when endoscopic intervention is not feasible.

SUGGESTED READINGS

ASGE Standards of Practice Committee, Maple JT, Ben-Manachem T, et al. The role of endoscopy in the evaluation of suspected choledocholithiasis. *Gastrointest Endosc.* 2010;71:1-9.

Gomi H, et al. Tokyo Guidelines 2018: antimicrobial therapy for acute cholangitis and cholecystitis. *J Hepatobiliary Pancreat Sci.* 2018 Jan;25(1):3-16. doi: 10.1002/jhbp.518. Epub 2018 Jan 9.

Kiriyama S, et al. Diagnostic and severity grading criteria for acute cholangitis in the Tokyo Guidelines 2018. *J Hepatobiliary Pancreat Sci.* 2018 Jan;25(1):31-40. doi: 10.1002/jhbp.50

Lai EC, Mok FP, Tan ES, et al. Endoscopic biliary drainage for severe acute cholangitis. *N Engl J Med.* 1992;326:1582-1586.

Miura F, et al. Tokyo Guidelines 2018: initial management of acute biliary infection and flowchart for acute cholangitis. *J Hepatobiliary Pancreat Sci.* 2018 Jan;25(1):17-30.

Tsuchiya T, et al. Endoscopic management of acute cholangitis according to the TG13. *Dig Endosc.* 2017;29(suppl 2):94-99

Symptomatic Cholelithiasis in Pregnancy

25

KIMBERLY S. STONE AND PAUL M. MAGGIO

Based on the previous edition chapter "Symptomatic Cholelithiasis in Pregnancy"
by Vance L. Smith and Paul M. Maggio

Presentation

A 32-year-old woman, 28 weeks pregnant with her second child, with no significant past medical history presents to the emergency department with a 2-day history of right upper quadrant (RUQ) abdominal pain and nausea. Her obstetrician–gynecologist, who had evaluated her earlier in the day, thought it was unlikely that her symptoms were related to her pregnancy. In the emergency department, she is afebrile and her vital signs are remarkable for mild tachycardia of 102. Her pain is episodic, lasting approximately 90 minutes after eating. On abdominal examination, the fundal height measures 29 weeks and is consistent with her pregnancy. She has focal tenderness in the RUQ and reports that the pain radiates through to her back on the same side. She is anorexic but has been able to keep liquids down.

● DIFFERENTIAL DIAGNOSIS

Symptomatic cholelithiasis is a common cause of RUQ abdominal pain and is second only to appendicitis as a cause of abdominal emergencies during pregnancy. Although gallstones and sludge have been reported in up to 10% to 30% of patients during pregnancy, symptomatic cholelithiasis is only seen in 0.5% to 2%. Gallstone-related complications occur in <1% of pregnancies and include cholecystitis, choledocholithiasis, cholangitis, and pancreatitis. When complications related to gallstones occur, there is an increased risk of morbidity and mortality for both the mother and fetus. The risk of gallstone formation increases with increased number of pregnancies and body mass index (BMI). Contributing factors include hormonal changes that occur during pregnancy and are associated with increased bile stone formation and altered gallbladder contractility.

Diagnosing symptomatic cholelithiasis during pregnancy can be a challenge for any physician, particularly when compounded by efforts to limit radiologic exposure. The presenting signs and symptoms of symptomatic cholelithiasis may be nonspecific and difficult to distinguish from those associated with pregnancy itself, and the changing position of intra-abdominal contents during pregnancy may complicate the examination of the gravid abdomen. For example, the appendix is typically located at McBurney's point early in pregnancy but is later displaced laterally and upward into the RUQ by the enlarging uterus (Figure 25-1). As a consequence, appendicitis may present as RUQ pain in the pregnant patient, especially in patients late in their pregnancy. Less common causes of RUQ pain during pregnancy include peptic ulcer disease, pancreatitis, pyelonephritis, HELLP syndrome (syndrome of hemolysis, elevated liver enzymes, and low platelets), acute fatty liver, and hepatitis.

● WORKUP

Laboratory evaluation including a complete blood count and liver function tests was obtained. The white blood cell count was mildly elevated at $13 \times 10^3/\mu L$. Liver and pancreatic

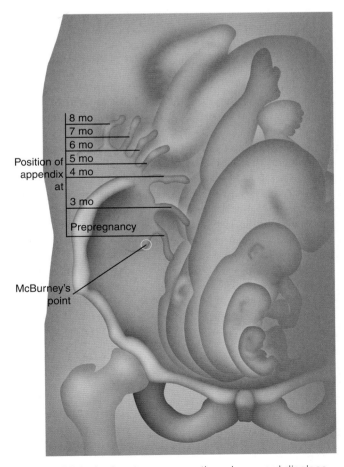

FIGURE 25-1. As the uterus grows, there is upward displacement of the appendix in counterclockwise fashion.

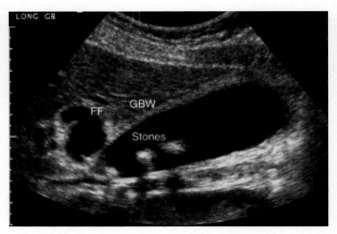

FIGURE 25-2. RUQ abdominal ultrasound revealing cholelithiasis.

enzymes were normal (total bilirubin 1.0 mg/dL, indirect bilirubin 0.5 mg/dL, alkaline phosphatase 90 U/L, lipase 35 U/L). An RUQ abdominal ultrasound was performed (Figure 25-2) and demonstrated a normal gallbladder wall with multiple hyperechoic shadows consistent with gallstones. The common bile duct measured 0.7 cm.

● DIAGNOSIS AND TREATMENT

The imaging modality of choice in diagnosing symptomatic cholelithiasis is ultrasonography. Transabdominal ultrasound is sensitive (>95% for gallstones), inexpensive, and safe without exposing the patient to radiation. For the diagnosis of acute cholecystitis, it yields a sensitivity of 88% and a specificity of 80%.

When choledocholithiasis is suspected (e.g., bilirubin or alkaline phosphatase is elevated), an MRCP can be used as a diagnostic modality. Once choledocholithiasis is confirmed, an ERCP or operative bile duct exploration are therapeutic considerations, but the benefits must be weighed against the risks of radiation exposure to the developing fetus. Some centers offer radiation-free evaluation of the CBD using endoscopic ultrasound and/or cholangioscopy.

Surgical intervention for symptomatic cholelithiasis in the pregnant patient is safe, decreases the likelihood of gallstone related complications, and prevents future hospitalizations. Historical recommendations were to delay surgical intervention until the second trimester. In the intervening time, these patients were managed with intravenous fluids, bowel rest, narcotics, broad-spectrum antibiotics, and a fat-restricted diet. More recent evidence suggests that an operation can be performed safely during any trimester of pregnancy. In fact, some surgeons have argued that delaying surgery may have devastating consequences for the fetus. When managed nonoperatively, symptomatic cholelithiasis has a high recurrence rate, and its associated complications, such as gallstone pancreatitis, can lead to spontaneous abortion and preterm labor. Recurrence rates for symptomatic patients have been

reported to be as high as 92% in the first trimester, 64% in the second trimester, and 44% in the third trimester.

Once the decision has been made to perform an operation, laparoscopic cholecystectomy is the preferred approach. It carries the same benefits of laparoscopy performed in the nonpregnant patient, including decreased requirement for narcotics, a lower rate of wound complications, shorter hospital stays, and a decreased risk of venous thromboembolism secondary to early ambulation. An obstetric consultation should be obtained for all cases involving a viable fetus (>24 weeks of gestation) and will typically include preoperative and postoperative monitoring of fetal heart rate and uterine activity.

● SURGICAL APPROACH FOR LAPAROSCOPIC CHOLECYSTECTOMY

The patient is placed supine on the operating table. For the gravid patient, she can lie in the left lateral recumbent position to decrease compression of the vena cava. Access to the abdomen is obtained via an open Hasson, Veress needle, or optical trocar, depending on surgeon preference and level of experience. While there is no evidence that any of the above options is superior to others, many surgeons would opt to enter via an open Hasson technique. This allows direct visualization of the abdominal wall and intra-abdominal viscera prior to trocar insertion. Port location should be adjusted for fundal height, which should be measured before and after induction of general anesthesia. More recent advances such as single-port laparoscopy should be reserved for high-volume centers with surgeons experienced in this technique, and only in pregnant patients whose fundal height permits entry at the umbilicus.

Pneumoperitoneum can usually be achieved by CO_2 insufflation of 10 to 15 mm Hg, although it is important to remember that some pregnant patients may demonstrate restrictive lung physiology due to elevation of their diaphragm. These patients are prone to arterial desaturation and may be better managed with insufflation pressures <12 mm Hg. In all cases, adequate visualization of the gallbladder and biliary anatomy must be maintained.

Once all ports are placed, the fundus of the gallbladder is retracted toward the abdominal wall and superiorly over the liver, and the peritoneum is dissected from the gallbladder neck. Dissection should be carried out from the gallbladder neck to the common bile duct in order to gain the critical view of safety (Figure 25-3). The critical view is achieved by clearing all fat and fibrous tissue in Calot's triangle, after which the cystic structures can be clearly identified, occluded, and divided. This helps to avoid bile duct injuries, and failure to successfully create this view is an indication for conversion to an open cholecystectomy.

The cystic duct and artery are then clipped and divided, and the gallbladder is removed from its fossa using electrocautery or the Harmonic scalpel. If there is spillage of bile from the gallbladder, the abdomen should be irrigated and the fluid aspirated. The ports are withdrawn under direct visualization and the abdomen desufflated. Each incision is closed (Table 25-1).

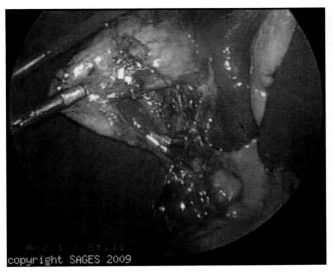

FIGURE 25-3. Critical view during laparoscopic cholecystectomy. Note the clear delineation of the junction of the cystic duct with the gallbladder as well as the clear space between the gallbladder and liver, devoid of any other structure other than the cystic artery.

Table 25-2	Open Cholecystectomy in the Pregnant Patient

Key Technical Steps

1. Make a right subcostal incision.
2. Pack viscera and uterus from the operative field.
3. Grasp gallbladder and dissect via a top-down approach.
4. Use electrocautery to dissect the gallbladder from the liver fossa.
5. Identify the cystic duct and artery just beyond gallbladder neck.
6. Ligate and divide the cystic duct and cystic artery.
7. Close the abdomen in two layers.

cystic duct and artery are identified, ligated, and divided. Once adequate hemostasis is obtained, the viscera are returned to their normal anatomic position and the incision is closed in two layers (Table 25-2).

● SURGICAL APPROACH FOR OPEN CHOLECYSTECTOMY

For patients in whom laparoscopic cholecystectomy cannot be performed safely, an open cholecystectomy is indicated. This is accomplished through a right subcostal incision. After retractors are placed and the bowel and gravid uterus packed away from the surgical field, the gallbladder is grasped and dissection is performed via a top-down approach. The

● POSTOPERATIVE MANAGEMENT

After undergoing laparoscopic cholecystectomy, patients are usually admitted overnight for observation. Fetal monitoring is required in cases that involve a viable fetus to evaluate fetal heart rate and uterine activity. An oral diet can be started on the day of surgery and oral pain medications shortly thereafter. Patients undergoing an open cholecystectomy typically require a 3- to 5-day hospital stay to achieve adequate pain control and sufficient oral intake.

Table 25-1	Laparoscopic Cholecystectomy in the Pregnant Patient

Key Technical Steps

1. Position the patient in the supine position, and a left lateral recumbent position for third-trimester patients.
2. Appropriate port placement based on fundal height of uterus preferably through an open Hasson technique.
3. Insufflate abdomen to 10–15 mm Hg, 12 mm Hg in patients with restrictive lung physiology.
4. Adequately retract gallbladder toward abdominal wall.
5. Dissect peritoneum from the gallbladder neck to the common bile duct in order to gain the critical view of safety.
6. Identify the cystic artery as it courses from the right hepatic artery to the gallbladder.
7. Divide and ligate both the cystic duct and the cystic artery.
8. Use electrocautery or Harmonic scalpel to dissect the gallbladder from the liver fossa.
9. Remove ports under direct visualization and close port sites.

Potential Pitfalls

- Improper port placement
- Failure to achieve the critical view
- Failure to recognize replaced right hepatic artery

Case Conclusion

Once diagnosed with symptomatic cholelithiasis, the patient is admitted to the Obstetrics Antepartum unit for preoperative pain control and fetal monitoring. That afternoon, she undergoes a laparoscopic cholecystectomy and is admitted postoperatively for 24 hours of fetal monitoring. After an uneventful stay, she is discharged on postoperative day 1. Her follow-up visit reveals no further pain, and her pregnancy progressed uneventfully to term.

TAKE HOME POINTS

- The presenting signs and symptoms of symptomatic cholelithiasis may be nonspecific and difficult to distinguish from those associated with pregnancy.
- The changing position of intra-abdominal contents during pregnancy complicates the examination of the gravid abdomen.
- Asymptomatic cholelithiasis, even found during pregnancy, is not an indication for cholecystectomy.
- For symptomatic cholelithiasis, a cholecystectomy can be safely performed in all trimesters of pregnancy.
- Nonoperative management of symptomatic cholelithiasis exposes the patient to a high rate of recurrence and associated complications.
- Laparoscopic cholecystectomy is preferred to an open procedure and carries the same benefits as in the nonpregnant patient with lower rate of maternal and fetal complications.

- An obstetric consultation should be obtained for all cases involving a viable fetus (>24 weeks of gestation) and will typically include preoperative and postoperative fetal monitoring.

SUGGESTED READINGS

Basso L, McCollum PT, Darling MR, et al. A study of cholelithiasis during pregnancy and its relationship with age, parity, menarche, breast-feeding, dysmenorrhea, oral contraception and a maternal history of cholelithiasis. *Surg Gynecol Obstet.* 1992;175:41-46.

Chan CHY, Enns RA. ERCP in the management of choledocholithiasis in pregnancy. *Curr Gastroenterol Rep.* 2012;14:504-551.

Date RS, Kaushal M, Ramesh A. A review of the management of gallstone disease and its complications in pregnancy. *Am J Surg.* 2008;196:599-608.

Ellington SR, Flowers L, Legardy-Williams JK, Jamieson DJ, Kourtis AP. Recent trends in hepatic diseases during pregnancy in the United States. *Am J Obstet Gynecol.* 2015;212:524.e1-524.e7.

Jorge AM, Keswani RN, Veerappan A, Soper NJ, Gawron AJ. Nonoperative management of symptomatic cholelithiasis in pregnancy is associated with frequent hospitalizations. *J Gastrointest Surg.* 2015;19:598-603.

Ko CW. Risk factors for gallstone-related hospitalization during pregnancy and the postpartum. *Am J Gastroenterol.* 2006;101:2263-2268.

Oto A, Ernst RD, Ghulmiyyah LM, et al. MR imaging in the triage of pregnant patients with acute abdominal and pelvic pain. *Abdom Imaging.* 2009;34:243-250.

Sedaghat N, Amy Cao BM, Guy Eslick BD, Michael Cox BR, Eslick BD. Laparoscopic versus open cholecystectomy in pregnancy: a systematic review and meta-analysis. *Surg Endosc.* 2017;31:673-679.

Shea JA, Berlin JA, Escarce JJ, et al. Revised estimates of diagnostic test sensitivity and specificity in suspected biliary tract disease. *Arch Intern Med.* 1994;154:2573-2581.

Surgery and *Clostridium Difficile* Colitis

26

EVA MARIA URRECHAGA AND BRIAN S. ZUCKERBRAUN

Based on the previous edition chapter "Fulminant *Clostridium difficile* Colitis" by Natasha S. Becker and Samir S. Awad

Case Presentation

The patient is 72-year-old woman with a history of diabetes and hypertension. One week ago, she completed a course of moxifloxacin for community-acquired pneumonia. Her pulmonary symptoms have resolved, and she was otherwise well, until she noted having significant diarrhea that started 3 days prior to presentation. She now reports crampy abdominal pain as well as watery diarrhea up to 15 times per day. She denies any associated nausea, vomiting, melena, or hematochezia. She denies any recent travel, sick contacts, or changes in diet. She denies having fevers at home over the past day. On exam, she is afebrile with a heart rate of 102 and a blood pressure of 132/86. Her lips appear cracked and oral mucosa appears dry. Her abdomen is soft, mildly distended, diffusely tender to deep palpation, but without peritoneal signs.

● DIFFERENTIAL DIAGNOSIS

The diagnosis of a patient with acute diarrhea includes infectious versus noninfectious etiologies. By far, infection is the more common cause of acute diarrhea and can be due to viruses, bacteria, or parasites. Common bacterial pathogens include *Campylobacter, Salmonella, Shigella*, and multiple strains of *Escherichia coli*. However, if presenting after completion of a course of antibiotics (usually within the last 2 weeks but up to within the last 3 months) as in this case, the differential should always include *Clostridium difficile* infection (CDI). The most common viral pathogens include rotavirus (particularly in infants), norovirus, and astrovirus. Parasitic infections, like many bacterial infections, are commonly associated with travel or ingestion of contaminated water and include *Giardia lamblia, Cryptosporidium*, and *Entamoeba histolytica*. Noninfectious etiologies should also be considered, especially if the clinical history does not point to an infectious cause or the symptoms persist longer than 2 weeks. Noninfectious causes of diarrhea include causes of malabsorption, drug effects, inflammatory bowel disease, endocrine tumors, or hyperthyroidism.

● WORKUP AND TREATMENT

The patient above was admitted for further workup to the medicine service. She was started on intravenous fluids for volume resuscitation. Labs were significant for creatinine of 1.5 mg/dL, white blood cell count of 14,000/µL, albumin of 3.0 g/dL, and a lactate of 2.2 mmol/L. Given the history of recent antibiotic use, the patient was started on empiric oral metronidazole 500 mg three times a day for possible CDI, and testing for CDI by polymerase chain reaction (PCR) was sent. PCR was positive for CDI the next morning, and the patient was continued on metronidazole. There was no significant change over the first 3 days. By hospital day 4, the patient reported resolution of the diarrhea but endorses increased distension, worsening abdominal pain, and fevers to 38.4°C. Her white blood cell was increased to 27,500/µL and creatinine to 2.7 mg/dL, and her heart rate was 115 with a blood pressure of 85/55. The patient was transferred to the intensive care unit. A computed tomography (CT) scan of the abdomen and pelvis was obtained (without intravenous contrast secondary to the acute kidney injury) and demonstrated pancolitis and ascites (Figure 26-1). The patient was made NPO and started on intravenous metronidazole 500 mg three times per day and oral vancomycin 500 mg four times per day. Surgical consultation was obtained.

Patients initially presenting as in this scenario are often found to be hypovolemic due to fluid loss from diarrhea and require volume resuscitation. Laboratory workup should include evaluation of electrolytes, creatinine, lactate, basic coagulation studies, and complete blood count. Additionally, we advocate checking serum albumin, although it is nonspecific; serum albumin levels can decrease secondary to protein losses from severe and/or chronic diarrhea. Diagnostic workup of profuse, watery diarrhea should include tests for the abovementioned pathogens as appropriate given the clinical history; these tests should include stool cultures and ova and parasite exam. If there is suspicion for CDI, as in the above case, initial evaluation should focus on this specific diagnosis and testing for other pathogens can be delayed. Empiric treatment for CDI should begin prior to receiving results for CDI infection if this is the leading clinical diagnosis. However, the rapidity of PCR as a diagnostic tool to confirm the diagnosis should allow practitioners to confirm the diagnosis in a timely fashion.

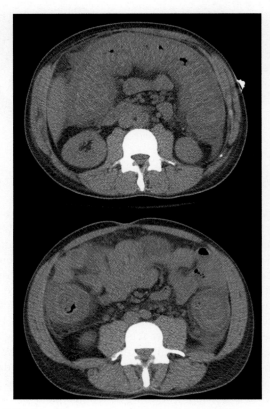

FIGURE 26-1. CT scan of the abdomen and pelvis demonstrating pancolitis with thickened loops of edematous colon and pericolonic ascites.

Clostridium difficile is an anaerobic, gram-positive, spore-forming bacteria that can be cultured as part of the normal human colonic flora in <10% of the adult population. Increased environmental exposure to *C. difficile* and dysregulation of other normal gut flora, most commonly by broad-spectrum antibiotics, is believed to result in colonization by *C. difficile*. Not all those who become colonized go on to develop infection, and the risk of development of infection increases with age, pharmacologic immunosuppression, and increased comorbidities. The infection and clinical syndrome is secondary to toxin production. Toxins A (enterotoxin) and B (cytotoxin) are the best known toxins produced by *C. difficile*. These toxins are believed to cause secretory diarrhea by compromising intercellular bond integrity and via inactivation of Rho proteins that are responsible for cytoskeleton construction. This causes fluid secretion into the digestive tract. Furthermore, there can be pronounced neutrophil chemotaxis. Together this can cause a large local and systemic inflammatory response. The prevalence of CDI, particularly severe infections, has been on the rise over the last decades, rapidly becoming the most common cause of nosocomial infection in the United States and affecting up to 10% of all hospital admissions. Concurrently, there has been identification of more virulent strains of the pathogen such as BI/NAP1/ribotype 027, which has been linked to as much as a 23-fold higher toxin production, longer hospital stays, increased mortality, and antibiotic resistance.

Diagnosis of CDI is often based on the history and symptoms. Major risk factors include exposure to pathogen and antibiotic use, while extended hospital stay, gastric acid suppression, and major comorbidities are other well-known contributors. While enzyme immunoassay (EIA) for toxins A and B in stool has classically been the mainstay for testing of *C. difficile*, many facilities have begun using DNA-based testing like nucleic acid amplification tests (NAATs) such as PCR. NAATs can provide higher sensitivity and specificity than EIA, and results take hours as opposed to days. Other tests include stool culture or glutamate dehydrogenase (GDH) screening. However, these tests alone are not sufficient for diagnosis since not all strains of *C. difficile* make toxins, although they could aid in screening or confirming diagnosis.

Once diagnosis is confirmed or if clinical suspicion is high, therapy should begin immediately. This includes cessation of any current antibiotics when possible in order to promote proliferation of the normal colonic flora. If antibiotics cannot be discontinued for the treatment of a concurrent infection, the antibiotic regimen should be changed to not include the inciting antibiotic. Cephalosporins, fluoroquinolones, and clindamycin should be avoided. Exposure of pathogens to other at-risk hospitalized patients can be limited by proper infection control among staff. Alcohol-based sanitizers often used in hospitals are ineffective against *C. difficile* spores, and contact precautions plus handwashing with soap and water is essential to minimize spread to other patients.

CDI causes a spectrum of disease ranging from a simple diarrheal illness to progression in 3% to 8% of patients to full-blown, life-threatening ileus with sepsis (sometimes referred to by the catch-all phrase "megacolon"). The American College of Gastroenterology has a simple severity scoring system that classifies CDI into mild, moderate, severe, severe–complicated, and recurrent (Table 26-1). Severe–complicated disease is characterized by ileus, mental status changes, hypotension, or organ failure. In these cases such as our patient, immediate surgical consultation is crucial. Severe–complicated CDI carries a mortality rate as high as 80% in some reports.

Metronidazole remains the appropriate first-line therapy for mild to moderate disease, although treatment depends on the severity of infection. For mild to moderate cases, oral metronidazole 500 mg three times a day is the treatment of choice. Intravenous metronidazole is effective against CDI as well secondary to enterohepatic secretion but is dependent upon decreased intestinal transit time in the setting of diarrhea to make it to the colon at an effective concentration. Oral vancomycin 125 mg four times a day is usually reserved for cases that fail to respond to metronidazole or severe cases of the disease. Severe–complicated disease is often treated with both intravenous metronidazole 500 mg three times per day plus oral vancomycin 500 mg four times a day. Furthermore, if a patient is classified as severe–complicated secondary to the development of ileus or significant distention, vancomycin enemas should be added to guarantee delivery into

Table 26-1	CDI Severity Scoring System and Summary of Recommended Treatments	

Severity	Criteria	Treatment
Mild	Diarrhea	Metronidazole 500 mg PO tid
Moderate	Diarrhea plus any additional signs or symptoms not meeting severe or complicated criteria	Metronidazole 500 mg PO tid
Severe	Any two of the following: • WBC ≥ 15,000 cells/mm³, • Serum albumin < 3 g/dL • Abdominal tenderness	Vancomycin 125 mg PO qid
Complicated	Any one of the following: • Admission to intensive care unit for CDI • Hypotension with or without required use of vasopressors • Fever ≥38.5° • Ileus or significant abdominal distention • Mental status changes • WBC ≥ 35,000 cells/mm³ • Serum lactate levels > 2.2 mmol/L • End-organ failure (mechanical ventilation, renal failure, etc)	Metronidazole 500 mg IV tid + vancomycin 125 mg PO qid + vancomycin 500 mg in 500 mL saline as enema qid (if ileus or distended) + surgical consultation

Adapted from Guidelines of the American College of Gastroenterology (Surawicz CM, Brandt LJ, Binion DG, et al. Guidelines for diagnosis, treatment, and prevention of *Clostridium difficile* infections. *Am J Gastroenterol.* 2013;108:478-498).

the colon.[1] Of note, the dose for vancomycin enemas is usually 500 mg in at least 500 mL of diluent (we prefer lactated Ringer's to decrease the risk of hyperchloremia secondary to colonic absorption). The volume must be substantial enough to reflux into the proximal colon. Data would suggest that any patient with severe–complicated disease warrants immediate surgical consultation to decrease associated mortality.[2]

Indications for emergent surgery include generalized peritonitis, worsening abdominal tenderness or distention on CDI-targeted therapy, hypotension despite adequate volume resuscitation, significant mental status changes, acute kidney failure, need for endotracheal intubation and ventilation not secondary to another known cause, serum lactate ≥5 mmol/L, signs of abdominal compartment syndrome, or findings of intraperitoneal free air. Surgical therapy should be considered in patients with severe–complicated disease that do not meet these above criteria but do not improve after 5 to 6 days or have an escalating white blood cell count above 50,000/µL despite adequate therapy. The need for earlier surgical intervention is recognized, and several scoring systems have been developed to predict which patients will progress require surgery.[3,4] These scoring systems utilize factors associated with poor prognosis such as advanced age, recent surgery, severely increased WBC (>50,000/µL), elevated lactate, immunosuppression, pressor requirement, and multiple comorbidities.

As CDI is usually a pancolonic disease, total abdominal colectomy with end ileostomy emerged as the standard of care in the 1990s; however, mortality rates even after surgery have been reported to range from 30% to 80%. Additionally, the colon is usually not necrotic or perforated and has the ability to recover. Based upon this, a colon preservation surgery was developed by our group using diverting loop ileostomy with on table colonic lavage with a high volume of polyethylene glycol–based solution and postoperative antegrade colonic vancomycin treatment through the ileostomy.[5,6] This can most often be achieved by laparoscopy. This treatment strategy was associated with improved mortality and a higher restoration of gastrointestinal continuity and ostomy reversal. There does not appear to be any contraindication to this procedure, and our current intraoperative treatment strategy is highlighted in Figure 26-2. Ongoing studies to validate this technique are currently in progress.

SURGICAL APPROACH

The patient in the above scenario became hypotensive and was transferred to the ICU requiring pressor support. Surgical consultation was obtained, and the decision for surgical treatment was offered secondary to her ongoing hypotension, worsening exam, and acute kidney injury.

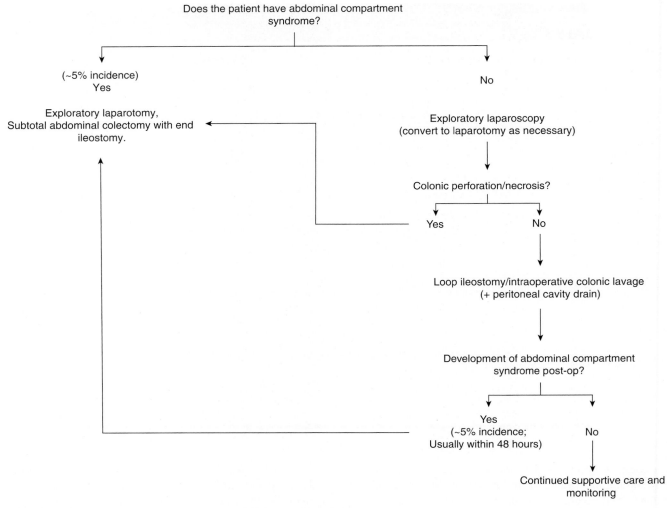

FIGURE 26-2. Operative management strategy for complicated CDI.

Consent was obtained for exploratory laparoscopy, possible laparotomy, possible ileostomy, and possible total colectomy. She was taken for immediate surgery and underwent a loop ileostomy and colonic lavage.

Surgery for fulminant *C. difficile* colitis carries with it high morbidity and mortality, which is in part related to the comorbidities often found in patients who progress to this severe disease. These patients are also usually unstable and profoundly ill with multisystem failure driven by toxin-mediated inflammatory response. Total abdominal colectomy is effective because it achieves rapid elimination of the disease-causing bacteria and toxins by removing most of the colon, without a challenging pelvic dissection in an extremely sick patient. While the rectal stump can also harbor toxin-producing bacteria, the risks of extensive pelvic dissection often outweigh the benefits, particularly since the rectum often clears the infection postoperatively. Rectal vancomycin can additionally be used to support rectal clearance.[7] End ileostomy is necessary as the patient's inflammatory state leads to high risk of leak in reanastomosis. We favor leaving a well-vascularized, long stump if possible with postoperative vancomycin flushes through the anus (50 mg in 50 to 100 mL

instilled gently). This can also result in an improved functional outcome after future potential ileostomy reversal.

Again, we believe most patients are candidates for loop ileostomy without resection (Table 26-2). Contraindications include findings of full-thickness ischemia or perforation, but these are not common. Additionally, if a patient has abdominal compartment syndrome, we advocate colectomy, as loop ileostomy and lavage would not address the compartment syndrome and would require leaving an open abdomen. Most individuals treated with loop ileostomy will show immediate improvement, but some will continue to demonstrate high white blood cell counts, abdominal tenderness, and hypotension for up to 5 days. From our experience, this operative approach treats the bacterial infection by decreasing bacterial load and toxin production, but this critical illness may persist for several days as the neutrophil-laden colon is still present and can drive an ongoing inflammatory response.

Prior to operative treatment, the patient is identified and marked, and an ileostomy site is identified. The patient is placed under general anesthesia. When planning a loop ileostomy, we place a 28-French rectal Malecot and drainage

Table 26-2	Loop Ileostomy

Key Technical Steps

1. Cut down technique for laparoscopy
2. Abdominal exploration
3. Steep table positioning to identify terminal ileum
4. Assurance of correct proximal and distal orientation of the ileostomy
5. Irrigation by gravity drainage into the colon
6. Closed-suction drain for ascites collection
7. Maturation of ileostomy

Potential Pitfalls

- Perforation of enlarged colon at incision
- Failure to keep the orientation of ileostomy
- Kinking of distal ileum at point of possible retroperitoneal fixation in creation of ileostomy to prevent forward irrigation.
- Failure to recognize impending abdominal compartment syndrome

system to collect the effluent from the lavage. Modified lithotomy position can be chosen if there is uncertainty of the diagnosis, and intraoperative colonoscopy may be considered as an adjunct in the evaluation. When performing a planned loop ileostomy, usually we perform an open cut down technique to gain access to the peritoneum. The abdomen is insufflated, and 1 to 2 additional 5-mm ports are placed. The peritoneal cavity is inspected for signs of perforation or necrosis. Use of steep Trendelenburg position can aid in easy identification of the terminal ileum and a loop of ileum that can easily be brought up as a loop ileostomy is identified. An incision is made at the ileostomy site and the loop of ileum is brought through this, assuring the correct proximal and distal orientation. Pneumoperitoneum is relieved, and ports are left in place. A purse string suture and enterotomy is performed on the loop of bowel, and a large-bore (26-French) Foley catheter is placed into the efferent loop toward the colon. The balloon portion is placed below the fascia and blown up with 10 cc of water. The colonic lavage is then performed with 8 L of warmed (at least body temperature to prevent hypothermia) polyethylene glycol solution. Usually rectal effluent will begin to drain after instillation of the first 1 to 1.5 L of irrigant. Once the irrigation is complete, a quick laparoscopic inspection is performed. We usually place an intraperitoneal closed-suction drain to remove ascites and prevent compartment syndrome. Gloves are then changed, and the ports are removed. These incisions are closed and dressed. The Foley is then removed and the ileostomy matured. We favor leaving a 22-French Malecot catheter in the efferent loop of the ileostomy below the level of the fascia. This does not have to be in the colon. We do not like to leave the ballooned catheter, as this is more prone to pressure necrosis and can be more confusing for the care team given the two proximal ports for instillation.

Vancomycin is instilled at a dose of 500 mg in 500 mL of lactated Ringer's every 8 hours for 7 to 10 days.

In the case of colectomy, a midline incision in made for exploratory laparotomy (Table 26-3). Laparoscopic colectomy is rarely possible given the distention and edema of the colon and is not advocated. The abdomen should be inspected for further pathology or evidence of contamination, and attention should quickly be turned to the colon. Intraoperative findings may be nonspecific as this is a mucosal disease; however, this should not dissuade the surgeon from carrying out a total colectomy since this could misleadingly hide pancolonic involvement. When possible, attempts should be made for early devascularization of the colon to potentially minimize further systemic inflammatory response. The major vascular stalks, including the ileocolic, right colic, middle colic, left colic, and sigmoid vessels, are identified, clamped, and transected. The colon is mobilized by freeing the retroperitoneal attachments beginning at the ileocecal junction. Care should be taken to avoid damage to the ureter, as in all colon surgery. The colon is then transected with a linear stapler at the terminal ileum and the rectosigmoid junction. Inspection to ensure that the remaining distal stump is healthy enough to hold a staple line and remains well vascularized should be performed. The ileum is then brought up for end ileostomy creation. Risk of leak from the staple line at the rectal stump is a concern if inflammation extends into the rectum, so the staple line may be oversewn. We advocate leaving a small-bore

Table 26-3	Total Abdominal Colectomy

Key Technical Steps

1. Colonoscopy
2. Midline incision
3. Abdominal exploration
4. Ligation of the colonic vessels
5. Mobilization of the colon
6. Transection at the ileum and rectosigmoid junction
7. Removal of the colon
8. Bringing up the ileum and optional oversewing of rectal stump
9. Irrigation if contamination or perforation
10. Closure of incision
11. Maturation of ileostomy

Potential Pitfalls

- Perforation of enlarged colon at midline incision
- Damage to the ureter during mobilization of the colon
- Failure to resect entire colon due to normal intra-abdominal appearance, likely leaving diseased mucosa
- Failure to resect entire sigmoid colon if sigmoid vessels have been ligated
- Failure to oversewn rectal stump or create mucous fistula if high risk of leak

rectal tube for low-volume vancomycin enemas for 72 hours postoperatively. If there is a concern about the integrity of the rectal stump (which may be more common in the setting of severe–complicated CDI in a patient with inflammatory bowel disease), then the Hartmann's pouch may be brought up as a mucous fistula that is matured through a separate incision or brought out through the lower portion of the incision and left intact below the surface of the skin closure. Otherwise, the fascia is closed and the ileostomy is then matured, with possible anastomosis at a later date.

● POSTOPERATIVE MANAGEMENT

As previously discussed, mortality even after operative therapy is high. Patients require close monitoring in the ICU and continued supportive care. Bowel function may be delayed postoperatively, so patients need to be kept NPO until there are signs of ileostomy function. Care should be taken to observe for progression of rectal infection or recurrent infection, and close monitoring for sepsis should continue. In the case of loop ileostomy and lavage, attention to the possible development of compartment syndrome in the postoperative period should be performed, particularly in patients with ongoing substantial intravenous volume requirements and acute kidney failure. However, this is not common and has occurred in <5% of our patients. Restorative procedure and reanastomosis could be considered several months later once the patient has recovered and is a candidate for an elective operative procedure.

Case Conclusion

The patient tolerated her operative procedure. She was taken to the ICU postoperatively and extubated on postoperative day (POD) 1. Her ileostomy began to function on POD 1. She required intermittent vasopressors for 48 hours. A diet was initiated on POD 2. Her closed-suction drain was draining 50 to 200 cc of clear ascites per day and was removed on POD 5. She was discharged to home on POD 10.

TAKE HOME POINTS

- Patients presenting with diarrhea and abdominal pain with a history of recent antibiotic use should cause suspicion for *C. difficile* infection (CDI).
- Metronidazole is the treatment of choice for mild to moderate infection, with oral vancomycin reserved for severe disease.
- Surgical consultation should be obtained for every patient with severe–complicated CDI.
- Indications for surgery include generalized peritonitis, worsening abdominal tenderness or distention on CDI-targeted therapy, hypotension despite adequate volume resuscitation, significant mental status changes, acute kidney failure, need for endotracheal intubation and ventilation not secondary to another known cause, serum lactate ≥5 mmol/L, signs of abdominal compartment syndrome, or findings of intraperitoneal free air.
- The decision for surgical management should be made early to improve survival.
- Loop ileostomy and colonic lavage can be considered in patients without perforation or necrosis.
- When performing colonic resection, total colectomy is preferred even when the serosal surface of the colon appears relatively bland.

REFERENCES

1. Kim PK, Huh HC, Cohen HW, et al. Intracolonic vancomycin for severe *Clostridium difficile* colitis. *Surg Infect (Larchmt).* 2013; 14(6):532-539.
2. Sailhamer EA, Carson K, Chang Y, et al. Fulminant *Clostridium difficile* colitis patterns of care and predictors of mortality. *Arch Surg.* 2009;144(5):433-439.
3. Julien M, Wild JL, Blansfield J, et al. Severe complicated *Clostridium difficile* infection: can the UPMC proposed scoring system predict the need for surgery?. *J Trauma Acute Care Surg.* 2016;81(2): 221-228.
4. Van der Wilden GM, Chang Y, Cropano C, et al. Fulminant *Clostridium difficile* colitis: prospective development of a risk scoring system. *J Trauma Acute Care Surg.* 2014;76(2):424-430.
5. Neal MD, Alverdy JC, Hall DE, Simmons RL, Zuckerbraun BS. Diverting loop ileostomy and colonic lavage. *Ann Surg.* 2011; 254:423-429.
6. Kautza, B, Zuckerbraun, BS. The surgical management of complicated *Clostridium difficile* infection: alternative to colectomy. *Surg Infect.* 2016;17(3):337-342.
7. Van der Wilden GM, Subramanian MP, Chang Y, et al. Antibiotic regimen after a total abdominal colectomy with ileostomy for fulminant *Clostridium difficile* colitis: a multi-institutional study. *Surg Infect (Larchmt).* 2015;16(4):455-460.

SUGGESTED READINGS

Butala P, Divino CM. Surgical aspects of fulminant *Clostridium difficile* colitis. *Am J Surg.* 2010;200:131.

Campion EW, Dupont HL. Acute infectious diarrhea in immunocompetent adults. *N Engl J Med.* 2014;16370(17):1532-1540.

Jaber MR, Olafsson S, Fung WL, Reeves ME. Clinical review of the management of fulminant *clostridium difficile* infection. *Am J Gastroenterol.* 2008;103:3195.

Julien M, Wild JL, Blansfield J, et al. Severe complicated *Clostridium difficile* infection: can the UPMC proposed scoring system predict the need for surgery?. *J Trauma Acute Care Surg.* 2016;81(2):221-228.

Kaiser AM, Hogen R, Bordeianou L, et al. *Clostridium difficile* infection from a surgical perspective. *J Gastrointest Surg.* 2015;19:1363-1377.

Kazanowski M, Smolarek S, Kinnarney F, Grzebieniak Z. Clostridium difficile: epidemiology, diagnostic and therapeutic possibilities— a systematic review. *Tech Coloproctol.* 2014;18:223-232.

Kautza, B, Zuckerbraun, BS. The surgical management of complicated *Clostridium difficile* infection: alternative to colectomy. *Surg Infect (Larchmt).* 2016;17(3):337-242.

Kim PK, Huh HC, Cohen HW, et al. Intracolonic vancomycin for severe *Clostridium difficile* colitis. *Surg Infect (Larchmt).* 2013;14(6):532-539.

Leffler DA, Lamond JT. *Clostridium difficile* infection. *N Engl J Med.* 2015;372:1539-1548.

Lim SK, Stuart RL, MacKin KE, et al. Emergence of a ribotype 244 strain of *clostridium difficile* associated with severe disease and related to the epidemic ribotype 027 strain. *Clin Infect Dis.* 2014;58:1723.

Neal MD, Alverdy JC, Hall DE, Simmons RL, Zuckerbraun BS. Diverting loop ileostomy and colonic lavage. *Ann Surg.* 2011;254: 423-429.

Ofosu A. *Clostridium difficile* infection: a review of current and emerging therapies. *Ann Gastroenterol.* 2016;29:147-154.

Portela F, Lago P. Fulminant colitis. *Best Pract Res Clin Gastroenterol.* 2013;27:771.

Sailhamer EA, Carson K, Chang Y, et al. Fulminant *Clostridium difficile* colitis patterns of care and predictors of mortality. *Arch Surg.* 2009;144(5):433-439.

Seltman A. Surgical management of *Clostridium difficile* colitis. *Clin Colon Rectal Surg.* 2012;25:204.

Surawicz CM, Brandt LJ, Binion DG, et al. Guidelines for diagnosis, treatment, and prevention of *Clostridium difficile* infections. *Am J Gastroenterol.* 2013;108:478-498.

Van der Wilden GM, Subramanian MP, Chang Y, et al. Antibiotic regimen after a total abdominal colectomy with ileostomy for fulminant *Clostridium difficile* colitis: a multi-institutional study. *Surg Infect (Larchmt).* 2015;16(4):455-460.

Van der Wilden GM, Chang Y, Cropano C, et al. Fulminant *Clostridium difficile* colitis: prospective development of a risk scoring system. *J Trauma Acute Care Surg.* 2014;76(2): 424-430.

Complicated Diverticulitis

BONA KO AND SCOTT R. STEELE

Based on the previous edition chapter "Complicated Diverticulitis" by Sean T. Martin and Jon D. Vogel

Presentation

The patient is a 62-year-old obese man who presents with a history of recurrent urinary tract infections and pneumaturia in the setting of a live donor kidney transplant performed two decades ago for IgA nephropathy. His medical history is also notable for ureteral strictures that were treated with stent placement, gout, hypertension, and cholecystectomy. His current immunosuppressive regimen includes azathioprine, cyclosporine, and prednisone. He is also taking metoprolol and terazosin. On examination, the patient was afebrile, his heart rate was 95 bpm, and he was hypertensive to 160/100 mm Hg. His examination was otherwise normal. He denied any abdominal pain, back pain, fevers, chills, nausea, vomiting, and diarrhea. A colonoscopy from 6 years ago showed diverticulosis in the sigmoid colon (Figure 27-1).

● DIFFERENTIAL DIAGNOSIS

Given the patient's age, cluster of symptoms (i.e., pneumaturia) and previous colonoscopy findings (diverticular disease), the most likely diagnosis is diverticulitis with an associated

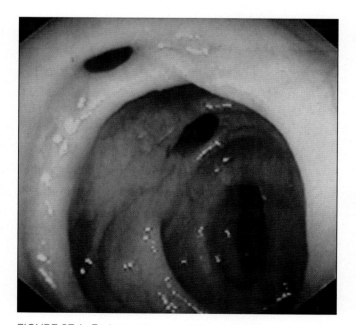

FIGURE 27-1. Endoscopic view of diverticulosis.

complication: a colovesicular fistula. Although this particular patient presented only with genitourinary signs and symptoms, other cases of complicated diverticulitis (i.e., stricture, abscess, perforation) are usually associated with left lower quadrant abdominal pain and potentially sepsis. When considering older age and left lower quadrant pain, patient evaluation should always rule out colorectal cancer, as well as (though lower on the differential) irritable bowel syndrome, colonic volvulus, intestinal ischemia, infectious colitis, and inflammatory bowel disease. Outside of the GI track, primary genitourinary problems such as nephrolithiasis and pyelonephritis should be included in the differential as well. Additionally, in the female patient, gynecologic causes of pain should be taken into consideration. In older women, ovarian mass and torsion, fibroids, and less commonly pelvic inflammatory disease should be noted as causes for lower abdominal pain. Most of these (outside of fistulous Crohn's disease or malignancy) typically do not present with concomitant pneumaturia.

Within the diagnosis of a complicated diverticulitis, the differential diagnosis can be further expanded to consider the etiology of complication. A colovesicular fistula is merely one of a myriad of ways a case of complicated diverticulitis can present. Approximately 15% to 25% of patients with acute diverticulitis have associated acute and chronic complications such as abscess, stricture, perforation, or less commonly, bleeding. Diverticular abscesses occur in about 10% to 20% of hospitalized patients with acute diverticulitis. Other patients experience colonic obstruction due to luminal narrowing from pericolonic inflammation or from an abscess. Perforations can occur as well from a ruptured abscess or from the free rupture of an inflamed diverticulum. And finally, fistulas can form between the colon and any adjacent viscera: bladder, urethra, vagina, uterus, skin, or other regions of the gastrointestinal tract.

● WORKUP

Diverticulitis can often be readily diagnosed with a thorough history and physical examination. Approximately half of all patients who present with a colovesicular fistula have a history of diverticulitis. The other half are diagnosed with underlying diverticulosis when the fistula becomes clinically evident and a workup is commenced. Because the physical examination is often unremarkable, a detailed history is necessary if the patient is suspected to have a fistula. Common symptoms include pneumaturia, dysuria, irritative genitourinary symptoms, recurrent urinary tract infections, and fecaluria. Other symptoms, though uncommon, include crampy abdominal pain, diarrhea, hematuria, and the passage of urine through the rectum. In contrast, patients with diverticular abscesses, strictures, or frank bowel perforation are often febrile, tachycardic, hypotensive, and complain of generalized or focal abdominal pain on examination. They may also complain of recurrent attacks of diverticulitis.

Laboratory tests provide additional support for the diagnosis and its associated complications. For febrile patients, pan cultures should be obtained prior to starting the patient on empiric antibiotic therapy. Blood chemistries are necessary to assess renal function and electrolyte abnormalities that can come secondary to vomiting or diarrhea. A white blood cell count should be noted for the presence of leukocytosis with a left shift, which indicates infection. However, the absence of leukocytosis should not rule out diverticulitis, especially if the patient is elderly, is immunocompromised, or has less severe disease. Hemoglobin and hematocrit levels should be assessed to address possible blood loss, though is not typically from diverticulitis or those with a colovesicular fistula. In patients with possible bowel perforation and/or diffuse peritonitis, serum aminotransferases, alkaline phosphatase, bilirubin, amylase, and lipase levels can also be obtained to rule out other causes of acute abdominal pain. Finally, stool studies should be performed in patients with diarrhea to rule out infectious etiologies. As in the present case, those with a suspected colovesicular fistula should also get a urinalysis and urine culture.

Imaging studies can also establish the diagnosis of acute diverticulitis and rule out other causes of abdominal pain. A plain radiograph series of the abdomen with supine and upright films are helpful in the setting of an acute abdomen where perforation (free air), bowel obstruction (air–fluid levels with distal decompression), or ileus (pan dilation) is suspected. While an x-ray may easily confirm an emergent complication from an acute diverticulitis, it does not typically help in confirming the source. Fluoroscopic images may confirm the presence of a fistula to the bladder with the instillation of Gastrografin through the rectum and identify filling of the bladder (Figure 27-2). More commonly, an abdominal and pelvic CT scan with intravenous contrast has become the best imaging modality to confirm a diagnosis of diverticulitis (Figure 27-3). Patients who likely have a fistula can receive a CT with oral or rectal contrast without intravenous contrast. A CT can confirm the diagnosis, but one should proceed with caution in patients with renal compromise. Imaging findings characteristic of a diverticulitis include the presence of colonic diverticula, presence of localized bowel wall thickening, increase in soft tissue density with pericolonic fat secondary to inflammation or fat stranding, abscesses, air–fluid levels, tissue with low attenuation (suggestive of necrotic debris), and extracolonic air

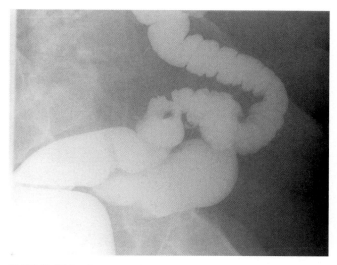

FIGURE 27-2. Gastrografin view of a colovesical fistula.

(suggestive of a fistula). On a CT, local colonic thickening adjacent to the area of thickened bladder or other visceral tissue and bubbles or contrast within organs other than the bowel are also indicative of a fistula. Finally, cystoscopy can be performed that can identify a fistula, sometimes visualized as a "cherry-red spot" or other feculent debris within the bladder (Figure 27-4).

The present patient presented with a normal-range WBC of $7.3 \times 10^3/mm^3$ without a left shift, a BUN of 25, and creatinine of 1.73 (around his baseline). His urinalysis was positive for blood, bacteria, and leukocyte esterase, and the urine culture grew vancomycin-resistant enterococcus. The abdominal x-ray demonstrated air within the bladder with efflux of air into the ureter of the transplanted kidney, and

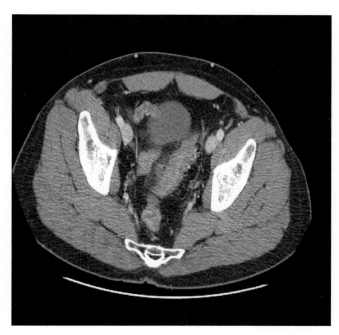

FIGURE 27-3. CT demonstrating acute diverticulitis with stranding adjacent to bladder and possible fistula.

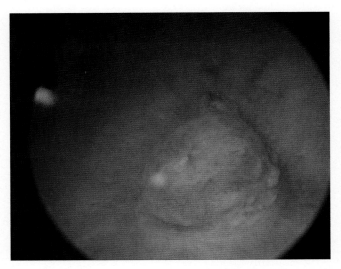

FIGURE 27-4. Cystoscopic view of colovesical fistula.

the abdominopelvic CT revealed sigmoid colon diverticulosis with evidence of fistulous communication between the sigmoid colon and the posterior bladder wall.

● DIAGNOSIS AND TREATMENT

Treating this patient, or any other case of complicated diverticulitis, ultimately depends on the patient's overall clinical status. Complicated diverticulitis has a broad spectrum of disease presentation, with anywhere from a small pericolic abscess or fistula formation to feculent peritonitis. In order to help stratify, the Hinchey's classification is a helpful guide to grade disease severity and eventually help to determine treatment (Table 27-1).

Initial management follows standardized guidelines of resuscitation, regardless of the underlying diagnosis. Septic patients with peritonitis mandate a surgical exploration. For stable patients, medical management with appropriate fluid resuscitation and antibiotic therapy with or without percutaneous drain placement often suffices for those whose disease can be classified under Hinchey I and II and an amenable abscess. This will do nothing for the colovesical fistula but often will allow the inflammation to subside and make the

Table 27-1	Hinchey's Classification

Classification	Description
I	Localized pericolic abscess or phlegmon
II	Pelvic abscess in the retroperitoneum or distant to the inflamed phlegmon
III	Purulent peritonitis
IV	Feculent peritonitis

corresponding surgery easier and perhaps more amenable to a minimally invasive approach. Many patients with routine or uncomplicated diverticulitis can be managed as an outpatient with oral antibiotics alone. Hospitalization should be considered if they are unable to tolerate oral hydration, fail outpatient antibiotic therapy, are immunocompromised, or have comorbidities that also require hospitalization. In the latter group of patients, it is appropriate to begin with conservative nonoperative therapy if they are hemodynamically stable. Treatment begins with bowel rest, intravenous fluid hydration, venous thromboembolic chemoprophylaxis, and intravenous gram-negative and anaerobic coverage. Patients should also receive adequate analgesia for their pain, though not too much that could mask a worsening of the clinical diagnosis. It is often helpful to enlist the support of an enterostomal therapist, who can educate and mark a patient appropriately prior to surgery should a temporary or permanent stoma be required. While immunocompromised patients are often at higher risk for surgical complications and invoke an inherent response to always pursue a nonoperative course, it is important to realize that many of these have higher risk of recurrence, often with worse outcomes, and surgery is many times the optimal long-term solution. In the immediate setting, they should have adequate *Enterococcus* and *Pseudomonas* coverage. Proceeding further with surgical treatment after nonoperative management will depend on the patient's clinical condition, underlying presentation, and risk stratification. Patients who will be proceeding with operative therapy should undergo preoperative evaluation by anesthesia or medicine, when appropriate, along with the aforementioned stoma marking, to help reduce complication rates.

● SURGICAL APPROACH

The definition of complicated diverticulitis is changing and encompasses a broad disease spectrum, which adds additional complexity to the decision-making. Recent clinical practice guidelines define complicated disease as free perforation, abscess, fistula, obstruction, or stricture. However, most practitioners agree that not all abscesses constitute complicated disease. With the ability to percutaneously drain most clinically significant abscesses, and with abscesses <3 to 4 cm often responding to antibiotics alone, it is increasingly unclear where the line is that separates the two. Nevertheless, sigmoid colectomy is recommended after the resolution of most abscesses (especially larger ones) due to high rates of recurrence.

The indications for surgery are clear in that the patient who presents in extremis with free perforation and peritonitis requires an emergent surgery. These patients need to undergo abdominal exploration and likely a Hartmann's procedure (i.e., sigmoid resection and end colostomy). A stoma, whether end or diverting, should be performed when there are contraindications for an anastomosis, such as severe sepsis, frank peritonitis, and lack of viable healthy bowel, or technical problems arise during the course of surgery. In a hemodynamically stable patient with a complicated episode, including free perforation, one can proceed with nonoperative management followed by a delayed elective or semielective resection and primary anastomosis +/− proximal diversion. Resection is also recommended if there is fistula formation or stricturing disease. Eventually, elective colon resection is advised due to the high incidence of medical treatment failure, recurrence, and late complications. Those who do not respond to nonoperative management within 72 hours will typically require an exploration and sigmoid colectomy during the same admission.

An exception to delay is made in those who are significantly immunocompromised. Despite their increased risk for operative morbidity, these patients should again typically be offered a colectomy on the initial admission since they are more likely to fail a nonoperative approach in the long term. The recommendation for colectomy in this population is independent of the presence of uncomplicated or complicated disease or initial response to antibiotics.

The patient in our present case has a colovesicular fistula, which is a late complication of acute diverticulitis. Operative management is guided by the etiology, location, and condition of the patient. Diverticular fistulas do not generally close spontaneously; however, their presence is rarely an indication for urgent surgery. A single-stage bowel resection with primary anastomosis, with takedown of the fistula, but without diversion is suitable for treating most patients. Multistaged procedures are reserved for those who are at high risk of developing an anastomotic leak or cannot undergo a prolonged operation. Risk factors include gross fecal contamination, large abscesses, malnutrition, corticosteroid use, history of pelvic radiation therapy, and hemodynamic instability—to name a few. Management of the bladder depends on the size of the defect. A small defect can be "pinched off" during the bowel resection (Figures 27-5 and 27-6). Larger defects

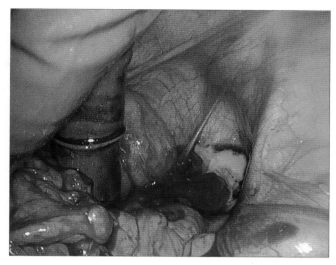

FIGURE 27-6. Blunt takedown of the fistula and adjacent pus in the pelvis.

require a simple closure, often in several layers. The bladder can be filled with several hundred cubic centimeters of sterile saline at the time of the operation to ensure watertight closure. In addition, it is the authors' preference to leave a JP drain in the pelvis for additional drainage, as well as leave the Foley catheter in for 7 days. A CT cystogram prior to Foley removal may also be considered at the discretion of the attending surgeon or urologist. In our 62-year-old patient with two decades of immunosuppressive therapy and other concomitant factors, he underwent a two-stage operation—laparoscopic sigmoid colectomy with a diverting loop ileostomy followed by closure of the ostomy 6 weeks later following a Gastrografin enema that demonstrated no sign of leak, stricture or re-formation of the fistula (Table 27-2).

For a laparoscopic sigmoid colectomy, the patient should be positioned in low lithotomy and secured to the table to allow for extremes of positioning changes, which are necessary with laparoscopic surgery. The Hasson technique or the Veress technique may be used for abdominal entry and to establish pneumoperitoneum. Port placement can vary depending on patient's body habitus, the individualized anatomy of the sigmoid colon, and any adhesions present from prior procedures. The senior author's preference is shown in Figure 27-7. A 12-mm right lower quadrant port should be positioned such that the angle of the stapler will be appropriate for the distal transection point past the point where the teniae splay (i.e., upper rectum). A 5-mm right upper quadrant port should be positioned to facilitate appropriate triangulation. Many times a left lower quadrant port is used to aid left colon and splenic flexure mobilization and left-sided pelvic dissection. As such, the port must be positioned to allow the instruments to easily reach the splenic flexure.

Once pneumoperitoneum is achieved and ports are placed, for a lateral approach the rectosigmoid is retracted medially and the peritoneum is incised at the white line of Toldt. This lateral peritoneal incision is then taken to the

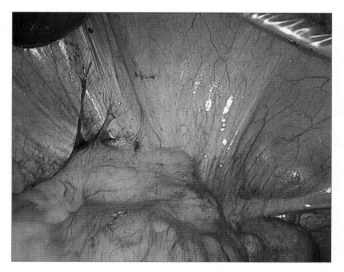

FIGURE 27-5. Laparoscopic view of the sigmoid colon attached to the bladder in a patient with a colovesical fistula.

Table 27-2	Laparoscopic Sigmoid Colectomy

Key Technical Steps

1. Position the patient in lithotomy.
2. Place the patient in slight Trendelenburg's position.
3. Maintain pneumoperitoneum and insert ports.
4. Inspect the four quadrants of the abdomen and pelvis.
5. Retract rectosigmoid and dissect along the plane behind the mesosigmoid to the level of the IMA.
6. Identify the left ureter and then define the vascular pedicle.
7. Continue medial-to-lateral dissection from the posterolateral edge of the descending colon down into the rectosigmoid.
8. Determine the proximal transection point. Splenic flexure may need to be mobilized. Clamp the colon and divide it at this point.
9. Distal transection is divided at the proximal rectum.
10. The mesentery of the specimen is then divided.
11. Remove the specimen.
12. Create an anastomosis and follow with an air-leak test.
13. Conclude with a final inspection of the abdomen. Then close the extraction site and port site.

Potential Pitfalls

- The margin of resection is the most important contributor to the likelihood of recurrent diverticulitis. While there is no need to resect past inflamed tissue in the proximal bowel, distal resection should extend below the rectosigmoid junction.
- Severe inflammation of the sigmoid colon can cause damage to surrounding structures (left ureter, bladder, iliac vessels). A colostomy and drainage should be considered.

level of the splenic flexure. Full splenic flexure mobilization includes takedown of the lateral, omental, and retroperitoneal attachments. This typically includes visualization of the inferior border of the pancreas to ensure full mobilization. Distally, the lateral-to-medial dissection should be continued until the ureter is identified, most commonly at the point of crossing the bifurcation of the common iliac, and the upper rectum is dissected.

If the procedure is to be completed intracorporeally, the sigmoid colon is then retracted anteriorly and the peritoneum is incised on the right side of the colon from the sacral promontory towards the ligament of Treitz. A window is created, through which the ureter can again be identified. The inferior mesenteric vascular pedicle is identified and is divided with either a vascular staple load or a vessel sealing device.

A medial-to-lateral approach may also be employed from the onset. For this, the sigmoid colon's lateral attachments are initially preserved and the rectosigmoid is retracted anterolaterally. The dissection plane is identified and the peritoneum is scored along that plane from the sacral promontory to the inferior mesenteric vascular pedicle. Blunt dissection is then used to develop the avascular plane behind the mesosigmoid and mesentery to the descending colon, along the sacral promontory anterior to the iliac vessels and sympathetic trunks, and extending to the level of the IMA. The left ureter must be identified at this point to ensure it is not injured when ligating the vasculature. Once the ureter is clearly identified and traced, the vascular pedicle is dissected out and divided between clips, with a stapler, or with an energy device. The medial-to-lateral dissection is then continued to the posterolateral edge of the descending colon and the sigmoid colon and extending down into the pelvis. The partially mobilized colon is then brought medially. The rectosigmoid is retracted medially and the lateral peritoneal

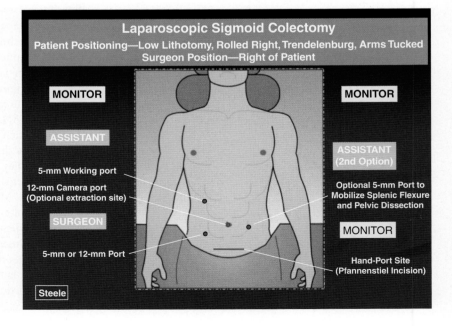

FIGURE 27-7. Port placement for a laparoscopic sigmoid colectomy.

attachments are released using electrocautery or a vessel sealing device. The lateral dissection extends from the true pelvis to the splenic flexure.

The proximal transection point can be identified at this point. Based on the length and mobility of the remainder of the descending colon, a decision should be made regarding the necessity of splenic flexure mobilization, though it is the senior author's preference to routinely perform this step. If additional length is required to facilitate a tension-free anastomosis, the splenic flexure should be taken down. Omental attachments to the anterior transverse colon are also divided at least to the level of the mid-transverse colon. The planned proximal transection point is grasped and brought into the pelvis to confirm adequate length. If additional length is needed, it may be necessary to perform a higher division of the inferior mesenteric vein at the level of the pancreas.

The authors often prefer an alternative method to a medial approach—the sub-IMV approach. In this method, we start with a patient in the reverse Trendelenburg's position with the left side elevated. The avascular plane medial to the IMV and just lateral to the ligament of Treitz is accessed using sharp dissection (Figure 27-8). Medial-to-lateral dissection continues in a superior-to-inferior fashion. Care should be taken to avoid dissecting underneath the pancreas. Dividing the attachments right above the pancreatic tail will allow access to the lesser sac. Dissection inferiorly will lead to the superior aspect of the IMA. The patient is then placed in a head down position, and the sacral promontory is identified. The peritoneum is then scored similar to above, with dissection and ligation of the IMA.

With either approach, the colon is then divided at the proximal transection point either using a linear stapling device or by sharp division after clamping the colon with a laparoscopic bulldog Glassman clamp. The distal transection is similarly carried out at the level of the proximal rectum at the sacral promontory using a linear laparoscopic stapler (Figure 27-9). The mesentery of the specimen is then divided.

The specimen may then be removed typically in one of a few ways. Transanal removal may be carried out by placing the specimen in an endoscopic retrieval bag and bringing

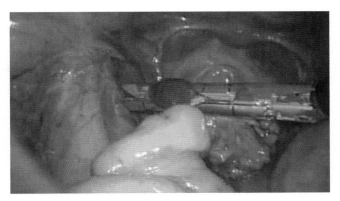

FIGURE 27-9. Distal transection of the sigmoid colon on the upper rectum.

the bag out through the opened rectal stump (sharp distal transection is preferred over stapled if this is the intended method of extraction). This approach is not preferred, especially with the distal division carried out with a laparoscopic stapler. Alternatively, the specimen may be removed via a small Pfannenstiel incision, or through an extended lower abdominal port-site incision, or through the umbilical port, generally with the use of a wound protector.

Similar to an open procedure, the proximal bowel may be extracorporealized and the anvil secured into position using a purse-string suture. The proximal colon is then placed back into the abdomen and the port is closed either temporarily with sutures on Rumel tourniquets or by closing off the wound protector with the aid of a clamp. The anvil is then grasped with an anvil grasper placed through a 12-mm port and the anvil with its attached proximal colon is brought into the pelvis (Figure 27-10). This is done carefully in order to ensure no twisting of the colon, which inherently compromises the blood supply. The mesentery should be oriented posteriorly. Meanwhile, the assistant serially dilates the anus before inserting the head of the circular stapler. While maintaining constant communication with the surgeon, the assistant brings the point of the stapler head out of the rectal stump adjacent to

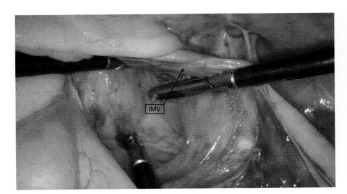

FIGURE 27-8. Sub-IMV approach underneath the inferior mesenteric vein (IMV) towards the pancreas and splenic flexure.

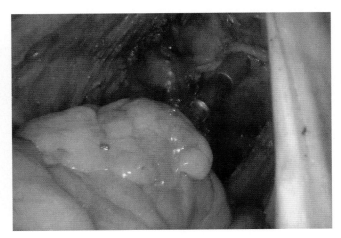

FIGURE 27-10. Intracorporeal stapled end-to-end anastomosis.

the staple line. The anvil and head are then brought together, and the stapler is fired. We then proceed with a proctoscopic examination and air-leak test. If a leak is identified, the anastomosis is redone if possible, or the leak is oversewn with a simple suture. If any question remains regarding the fidelity of the anastomosis, a diverting loop ileostomy should be performed.

Approaching a Perforated Diverticulitis

In patients with perforated diverticulitis and abdominal sepsis where an anastomosis may be unsafe, the Hartmann's procedure has become the gold standard operation for the treatment of perforated diverticulitis. The technique involves resection of the affected sigmoid colon with an end colostomy proximally and an oversewn rectal stump distally.

In many cases, the procedure is similar to above. To begin, the patient is placed in the modified lithotomy position. For an open approach, a midline laparotomy incision is made. The abdomen is inspected, and any free fluid is evacuated. The sigmoid colon is retracted medially and the peritoneum is incised at the white line of Toldt. The peritoneal incision is carried from the rectosigmoid junction to the splenic flexure. The sigmoid colon is then medialized and the left ureter is identified. The sigmoid colon is then run proximally until healthy, noninflamed tissue is identified. A window is created in the mesentery immediately adjacent to the colon wall and the colon is transected with a GIA stapler. The rectosigmoid is then mobilized and divided with a GIA stapler at the sacral promontory. The diseased sigmoid colon is then resected by dividing the remaining mesenteric attachments from the colon wall. Before determining whether to leave the distal rectal segment as a Hartmann's pouch, it is essential that the rectum be evaluated for obstructing masses. If no distal obstruction is present, the rectal stump should achieve adequate drainage via the anus. If an obstructing lesion is identified, a mucus fistula should be created.

Provided the rectum is not distally obstructed, the rectal pouch staple line should be oversewn. Marking sutures should also be placed into the rectal stump to facilitate retraction and identification at subsequent colostomy reversal. The abdomen and pelvis should then be copiously irrigated. Attention is again turned to the descending colon and proximal staple line. Enough colon should be mobilized such that the stapled end can easily pass through the abdominal wall in the previously marked stoma site. The skin of the left lower quadrant is then grasped with a Kocher clamp just inferior to the umbilicus and lateral to the rectus sheath. The skin is lifted and a circular skin incision about the size of a fifty-cent piece is created. The skin is left attached to the underlying subcutaneous tissue and is retracted anteriorly. The subcutaneous fat is divided down to the level of the external oblique fascia where the skin and attached fat are amputated. A cruciate incision is then made in the anterior fascia. The underlying muscle is split, and the posterior fascia and peritoneum are likewise divided. The opening in the abdominal wall should be large enough to easily accommodate two fingers.

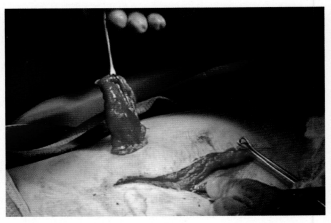

FIGURE 27-11. Hartmann's procedure with end descending colostomy.

The descending colon staple line is then brought out through the abdominal wall defect (Figure 27-11). At least 2 cm of colon are needed above the skin to create an adequate stoma. Then the colon wall is secured to the adjacent abdominal wall fascia using several sutures of 3-0 Vicryl to help prevent prolapse or parastomal hernia. The abdomen is then closed in standard fashion prior to maturation of the stoma. The staple line of the exteriorized descending colon is then resected with electrocautery and the stoma is matured with Brooke sutures of 4-0 Vicryl placed in the cardinal directions. Gaps between the colon and skin are closed with full-thickness simple sutures of 4-0 Vicryl. In certain situations, such as morbid obesity or a foreshortened mesentery due to inflammation, it is difficult to have the stoma adequately reach the anterior abdominal wall. Ensuring proper mobilization, "defatting" the subcutaneous tissue, ligation of additional vessels (without creating further ischemia), or resiting the stoma may be required to avoid a "sunken stoma."

● SPECIAL INTRAOPERATIVE CONSIDERATIONS

Intraoperative management of the patient may deviate from the routine under numerous circumstances. For example, difficulties can arise when constructing a stoma for the obese patient. Obese patients have a thick abdominal wall and a shortened, thick mesentery that makes it difficult to construct a tension-free and well-vascularized stoma. Constructing a well-functioning stoma begins with a preoperative evaluation and stoma marking. Intraoperatively, the segment of colon used for the colostomy should be free of any inflamed or damaged tissue. The colon should be completely mobilized medially and laterally so that it is free of peritoneal attachments at the base of the colonic mesentery under the inferior mesenteric artery. The splenic flexure should be mobilized and the mesenteric artery ligated at its base to ensure collateral flow is preserved. Subsequently, a large abdominal trephine should be made to allow the thick colonic mesentery to pass through and prevent venous congestion and subsequent stomal ischemia. The upper abdomen, above the umbilicus, can also be used for the stoma site since it tends to be thinner in obese patients. Abdominal wall contouring through subcutaneous lipectomy or by removing an elliptical segment of skin and subcutaneous tissue can aid in the formation of a tension-free stoma as well. If a healthy stoma is still not possible, an ileostomy can be created.

Additional consideration should also be taken to monitor the immunocompromised transplant patient, such as the gentleman in our case, during a nontransplant procedure such as the laparoscopic colectomy or Hartmann's procedure. A comprehensive preoperative evaluation should occur prior to the surgery. During the surgery, several clinical factors should be taken into consideration. Most importantly, these patients require proper management of their immunosuppressant regimen. Glucocorticoids can theoretically blunt the response of the hypothalamic–pituitary–adrenal axis under surgical stress. However, clinically relevant hypotension secondary to adrenal insufficiency is uncommon and is responsive to rescue treatment if it does occur. Additional steroids are unnecessary, and continuation of preoperative doses is recommended. Supplemental doses should be considered in patients who have recently withdrawn from therapy or if they are steroid dependent. Azathioprine decreases and cyclosporine increases the duration of muscle relaxants. Perioperative drugs such as diltiazem, phenobarbital, and phenytoin can alter cyclosporine and tacrolimus levels. Immunosuppressants should be adjusted accordingly depending on the patient's regimen and clinical condition (Table 27-3).

● POSTOPERATIVE MANAGEMENT

The postoperative stage of management should focus on expediting patient discharges and decreasing complication rates. Enhanced recovery (i.e., fast track) programs are an integrated multimodal approach that begins in the preoperative setting. It reduces the physiologic stress of surgery by minimizing pain, lowers ileus rates and duration, and decreases hospital length of stay. In the postoperative stage, the patient should continue the antibiotic regimen, which should be tailored to culture results and sensitivities. To promote early gastrointestinal recovery, early mobilization, early urinary catheter removal, early feeding, limiting intravenous fluid administration, controlling nausea, and chewing gum should be encouraged. An exception to this would be patients who underwent repair for fistula. As stated, these patients typically require an indwelling bladder catheter for 7 days and a suction drain placement in the bladder after fistula closure.

In addition to early gastrointestinal recovery, patients should have multimodal analgesics available with minimal narcotics. The enhanced recovery should also include avoidance of nasogastric tubes and pelvic drains, as well as early removal of urinary catheters. Enhanced recovery protocols

Table 27-3	Hartmann's Procedure

Key Technical Steps

1. Place the patient in the modified lithotomy position.
2. Make a midline laparotomy incision.
3. Explore the abdomen and evacuate any free fluid.
4. Mobilize the colon. Incise the white line of Toldt. Carry the peritoneal incision from the rectosigmoid junction to the splenic flexure.
5. Blunt dissection should be used to dissect the sigmoid colon if there is severe inflammation.
6. Identify and protect the ureters.
7. After the colon is mobilized, determine the proximal and distal points of bowel transection.
8. Resect the diseased colon by dividing the mesenteric attachments from the colon wall. Ligate the mesenteric vessels.
9. Remove the specimen.
10. Create an end colostomy and close the rectal stump.
11. Irrigate the abdomen and pelvis. Close the abdomen.
12. Allow colostomy to mature.

Potential Pitfalls

- Excessive mobilization of the colon should be avoided. This may result in a redundant stoma, and increase the risk of prolapse and parastomal hernias.
- Severe inflammation of the sigmoid colon can cause damage to surrounding structures (left ureter, bladder, iliac vessels). A colostomy and drainage should be considered.
- The margin of resection is the most important contributor to the likelihood of recurrent diverticulitis. While there is no need to resect past inflamed tissue in the proximal bowel, distal resection should extend below the rectosigmoid junction.

overall have shown a tendency to reduce postoperative ileus as well as length of stay. In addition, patients should be evaluated for postoperative complications such as wound infections, intraabdominal sepsis, or abscesses. Education regarding ostomy teaching should also be involved prior to patient discharge.

Case Conclusion

The patient successfully underwent a laparoscopic takedown of colovesical fistula, sigmoid and upper rectal resection with primary anastomosis, and a diverting loop ileostomy. His ostomy began to function on day 7. Throughout his stay, he continued on IV antibiotics for urosepsis and maintained his immunosuppressive regimen. He was discharged without complications. He returned approximately 1 month later for reversal of his loop ileostomy.

TAKE HOME POINTS

- About 50% who present with a colovesicular fistula have a history of diverticulitis. The other half are diagnosed with diverticulosis when the fistula becomes clinically evident.
- Complicated diverticulitis has a broad spectrum of disease presentation: free perforation, abscess, fistula, obstruction, or stricture. The Hinchey's classification can aid in grading disease severity and determining treatment.
- Patients with complicated disease who present with an abscess (Hinchey I and II) are recommended to undergo antibiotic treatment with an abscess <3 cm, or percutaneous drainage for a clinically significant abscess. Sigmoid colectomy is recommended after the resolution of an abscess ≥5 cm due to high rates of recurrence.
- Emergent abdominal exploration and sigmoid resection with end colostomy is necessary for patients who present with free perforation and peritonitis.
- Most patients with complicated diverticulitis who require hospitalization are treated with nonoperative therapy followed by elective colon resection.
- Immunocompromised patients should be immediately offered surgical intervention instead of nonoperative management, even if the patient is clinically stable.
- Stoma construction is difficult in obese patients. Adequate splenic mobilization, abdominal modeling, and stoma placement in the upper abdomen can aid in the formation of a tension-free stoma.

SUGGESTED READINGS

Angenete E, Thornell A, Burcharth J, et al. Laparoscopic lavage is feasible and safe for the treatment of perforated diverticulitis with purulent peritonitis. The first results from the randomized controlled trial DILALA. *Ann Surg.* 2014;00(00):1-6.

Chapman J, Dozois E, Wolff B, et al. Diverticulitis: a progressive disease? Do multiple recurrences predict less favorable outcomes? *Ann Surg.* 2006;243:876-883.

Feingold D, Steele S, Lee S, Kaiser A, Boushey R, Buie D, et al. Practice parameters for the treatment of sigmoid diverticulitis. *Dis Colon Rectum.* 2014;57:284-294.

Hall J, Roberts P, Ricciardi R, et al. Long-term follow-up after an initial episode of diverticulitis: what are the predictors of recurrence? *Dis Colon Rectum.* 2011;54(3):283-288.

Hannaman MJ, Erti MJ. Patients with immunodeficiency. *Med Clin North Am.* 2013;97(6):1139-1159.

Colonic Volvulus

ARDEN M. MORRIS

Based on the previous edition chapter "Colonic Volvulus" by Arden M. Morris

Presentation

A 28-year-old, nonobese, woman presents to the emergency department with complaints of recurrent, severe upper abdominal pain for the third time in 1 month. Prior to her recurrent symptoms of crampy abdominal pain, nausea, and vomiting, the patient had a normal 8-month intrauterine pregnancy and was otherwise healthy except for long-standing constipation.

● PRESENTATION

Colonic volvulus is a rare cause of bowel obstruction in the developed world, with an estimated annual incidence of about 3/10,000 in the United States. Although volvulus is unusual, it is the most common cause of bowel obstruction in pregnant women and the third leading cause of colonic obstruction after cancer and diverticulitis. Patients present with symptoms of excruciating abdominal pain out of proportion to the clinical examination, absence of flatus, and an empty rectal vault. Often, the minimal distension present during early volvulus increases dramatically over time.

The mechanical etiology of volvulus is axial rotation of the colon, functionally resulting in a closed loop obstruction. Axial rotation usually arises by one of two alternative mechanisms. First, in the case of a congenitally unfixed or partially unfixed colon, any portion of the colon—particularly the cecum—is at risk. During peristalsis, an unfixed ileocecal area on a narrow mesentery can twist, resulting in right lower quadrant pain and symptoms of small bowel obstruction with minimal distension. Second, and more commonly, the sigmoid colon may elongate due to chronic constipation and then twist on a relatively narrow mesentery. Major risk factors for sigmoid volvulus include advanced age, neurologic and psychiatric disease, lifelong high-fiber diet, and other causes of chronic constipation or elevated intraluminal pressure. Patients with compromised communication, such as those with dementia, previous stroke, or psychiatric disorders, are particularly susceptible to a delayed diagnosis.

If colonic volvulus does not self-reduce or otherwise resolve, the increased luminal pressure, thinning colon wall, and compromised venous outflow will lead over time to ischemic compromise of the bowel wall with necrosis and perforation.

● DIFFERENTIAL DIAGNOSIS

Colonic obstruction in an adult should be considered cancer until proven otherwise. Other items in the differential diagnosis are pseudo-obstruction, constipation, obstipation, diverticulitis, intussusception, external compression by adhesions, and external compression by an extraluminal mass. Rarely, patients may present with late symptoms of volvulus including colonic ischemia, necrosis, and perforation. Therefore, the differential diagnosis of late volvulus includes the conditions listed above as well as mesenteric ischemia.

● WORKUP

The diagnosis of volvulus is usually based on the clinical history and physical examination and confirmed radiologically. Volvulus pain can be intermittent, with initial self-reducing episodes of partial torsion. The pain tends to be diffuse and crampy in nature, which may differ from the constant pain of obstructing rectal cancer. Most patients present with symptoms several times before they receive a diagnosis. Important history and physical exam findings include elderly, frail, or chronically institutionalized patients; the presence of long-standing constipation; vague recurrent discomfort; signs of obstruction; and no stool in the rectal vault on digital examination. The exception to this general picture is the young, otherwise healthy pregnant woman with intermittent bouts of increasing abdominal pain and obstructive symptoms during progression into the third trimester.

Laboratory tests are not diagnostic but may indicate secondary sequelae of obstruction such as electrolyte abnormalities, nonanion gap acidosis, and an elevated white blood count. High lactic acid levels are rare and indicate a more advanced disease process.

Radiologic imaging is the key to the diagnosis, starting with a flat and upright abdominal x-ray. The classic appearance of sigmoid volvulus on x-ray is a "bent inner tube sign," with an inverted, distended sigmoid loop; absence of the normal haustral folds; and pointing toward the right upper quadrant (Figure 28-1). If the patient is stable and there is any doubt about the diagnosis based on regular abdominal x-ray, a water-soluble radio-opaque enema may be performed. Barium is contraindicated in this setting due to risk

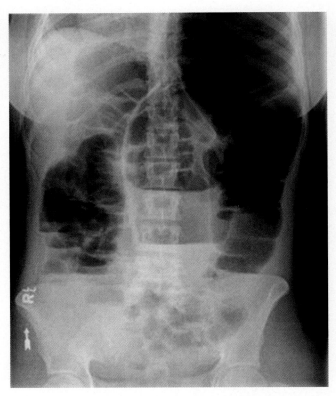

FIGURE 28-1. Abdominal x-ray displaying a distended sigmoid in an inverted U, directed superiorly, with loss of haustral folds and proximal distended bowel. (Image supplied courtesy of Charles O. Finne.)

of perforation. The classic finding on contrast enema of a "bird's beak" appearance to the bowel lumen (Figure 28-2A and B) should result in resuscitation, colonic decompression, and elective operation. If a contrast enema is nondiagnostic or not feasible, a computed tomography (CT) scan with intravenous contrast should be performed. Skipping the contrast enema and going immediately to a CT scan is a reasonable practice. The CT scan can help to identify alternative diagnoses and can demonstrate the sine qua non "swirl sign" indicating a torsed mesentery. Rigid or flexible lower endoscopy can play either a diagnostic or more often a (usually temporary) therapeutic role for the patient with volvulus.

DIAGNOSIS AND TREATMENT

If free intraperitoneal air is present on abdominal radiographs, no further studies are needed. The patient and family should be warned that this is an ominous sign, and, after obtaining informed consent, the patient should be resuscitated with normal saline or lactated ringers and electrolyte repletion before urgently performing an open exploratory celiotomy with Hartmann procedure and peritoneal irrigation.

Presentation Continued

In the scenario described above, the patient was clinically stable and her diagnosis remained in doubt despite a suggestive abdominal x-ray (Figure 28-3). The abdominal x-rays showed a severely distended colon and an empty rectum but no characteristic signs. Therefore, lower endoscopy was performed, revealing a combination of spiral narrowing of the sigmoid colon with associated mucosal erythema, edema, and ulcerations (Figure 28-4). The endoscopist was able to advance the scope beyond this segment without significant effort, revealing proximal colonic dilation.

If no free intraperitoneal air is present and the patient is clinically stable, she can be resuscitated and the colon decompressed preferably with a flexible or rigid sigmoidoscope. Particularly in frail or elderly patients, rigid sigmoidoscopy is preferable due to lower risk of colonic perforation and the ability to pass a rectal tube through the scope lumen to continue proximal decompression for several days. After supportive care and resolution of symptoms, an elective operation should be undertaken within 3 months as up to 70% of cases will recur without an operation.

In the case of an unsuccessful attempt at decompression, the patient should be taken urgently to the operating room for an exploratory celiotomy and sigmoid resection. The decision to perform an anastomosis versus colostomy will depend upon the presence of ischemia, stool spillage, and the general health of the patient.

Although sigmoid volvulus is the most common cause of colon obstruction during pregnancy, fewer than 100 cases have been reported in the literature. Based upon these cases, the consensus is that, in the absence of peritonitis, nonoperative decompression is preferred in the first trimester, sigmoid colectomy is preferred in the second trimester, and nonoperative treatment is again preferred in the third trimester until delivery. After delivery, a sigmoid colectomy is recommended.

SURGICAL APPROACH

As noted above, if the patient is unstable or has free intraperitoneal air, she should be resuscitated and taken to the operating room urgently for an open exploration (Table 28-1). Laparoscopic exploration is not judicious during an urgent operation for volvulus given the extensive dilated bowel and negligible working space. A laparoscopic or an open approach could be used for a patient who has undergone successful endoscopic decompression.

For sigmoid volvulus, the appropriate operation is a sigmoid colectomy. For cecal volvulus, the definitive operation is a right colectomy with primary anastomosis. In both cases, intraoperative judgment should inform the decision for an

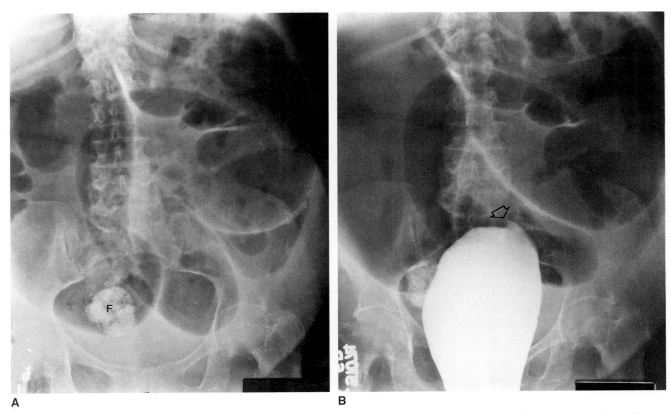

FIGURE 28-2. Radio-opaque enema displaying the classic "bird's beak" of narrowed lumen at the distal site of torsion, without contrast **(A)** and with contrast **(B)**.

ostomy versus primary anastomosis. Cecopexy to the right lower quadrant also has been described as a way to speed the operation and limit anastomotic complications. However, this advantage may be lost due to increased risk when placing suture in a distended, thinned cecal wall. Additionally, cecopexy for volvulus has historically been associated with a high recurrence rate. Placement of a cecostomy tube is also described for extremely frail patients. Advantages are the avoidance of an abdominal wound and tethering of the cecum that theoretically prevents recurrent torsion.

For the most part, the key technical steps in operating urgently for sigmoid volvulus also apply to a resection for cecal volvulus. Fist, a midline laparotomy and full abdominal exploration are performed with the goal of identification of potential areas of bowel ischemia or other causes of obstruction. Warm saline-soaked sponges are applied to any dusky bowel. Areas of torsed bowel are identified, as well as areas of ischemia extending beyond the obvious torsion. Before detorsing, identify appropriate proximal and distal sites for current or future anastomosis. Divide the mesentery prior to detorsing in order to avoid exposing the circulation to accumulated cytokines or bacteria in the ischemic segment. The bowel is then divided proximally and distally and the specimen is removed from the field.

Intraoperative judgment regarding whether to anastomose the bowel or to create an end ostomy and mucus fistula depends upon the patient's cardiovascular function, nutritional status, and absence of bowel necrosis or gross contamination. As well, the remaining bowel must be healthy-appearing and the ends must abut without tension. If an anastomosis is performed, it should be scrutinized for adequate perfusion and patency and if possible undergo a leak test prior to closing the abdomen. Adequate perfusion can be established based on presence of a pulse in the mesentery abutting the anastomosis, evaluation of intraoperative indocyanine green fluorescence angiography, or by carefully inspecting the color of the intestine and ensuring that it is pink and not dusky or injected-appearing. A leak test can be performed for a sigmoid resection but is problematic for a right colectomy. A straightforward approach to the leak test is to fill the pelvis with sterile saline, gently compress the bowel proximal to the anastomosis, and insufflate the rectum with air using a rigid sigmoidoscope. The presence of bubbles indicates a leak. Other options for leak test include instillation of Betadine or indigo carmine in the rectum and a search for discoloration of surrounding lap sponges applied to the anastomosis.

● SPECIAL INTRAOPERATIVE CONSIDERATIONS

Occasionally, a severely demented or otherwise noncommunicating patient with severe colonic distension and radiographic free air will undergo celiotomy and no evidence of perforation can be identified. If the bowel appears pink and viable and no evidence of a perforation site, succus,

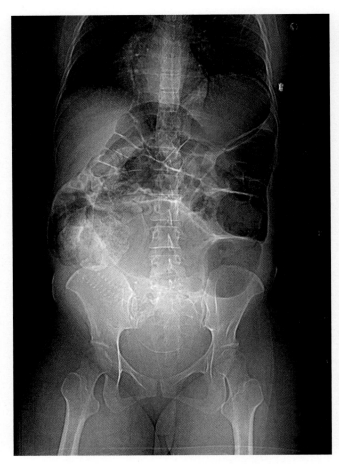

FIGURE 28-3. Abdominal radiograph of patient displaying distended sigmoid colon with loss of haustral markings and proximal distension, as well as a third-trimester fetus.

purulence, or other spilled bowel contents can be identified, resection is not warranted. If the colon can be decompressed endoscopically, this may be advantageous but will likely be temporary.

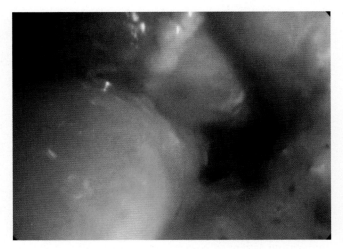

FIGURE 28-4. Endoscopic appearance of the sigmoid mucosa with a swirl pattern confirming volvulus and ulcerations and erythema consistent with ischemia.

Table 28-1	Operating for Sigmoid Volvulus

Key Technical Steps

1. Midline laparotomy and full exploration, examining for viability of bowel.
2. Place warm saline-soaked laparotomy sponges on any dusky-appearing bowel and recheck periodically for improving perfusion.
3. Identify areas of torsed mesentery and redundant bowel and prepare to resect, including areas of nonresolving ischemia.
4. Identify an appropriate proximal and distal anastomotic site and divide the sigmoid vessels and the intervening mesentery without detorsing.
5. Divide the bowel proximally and distally, passing off the specimen.
6. Perform anastomosis if clinical parameters are suitable (cardiovascular function, nutritional status, absence of bowel necrosis, or gross contamination) and remaining bowel appears healthy and without tension.
7. If the clinical parameters for an anastomosis are not suitable, perform an end ostomy and mucus fistula.
8. If an anastomosis was performed, examine it closely for evidence of adequate perfusion, anastomotic patency, and absence of leaks if possible.

Potential Pitfalls

- Inflammatory cytokines or bacteria released to the circulation during detorsion of twisted mesentery.
- Nonresolving venous congestion.
- Placement of suture in distended, thinned colonic wall during a pexy procedure.

● POSTOPERATIVE MANAGEMENT

Patients who have undergone a bowel resection for colonic volvulus should be managed expectantly with intravenous hydration, electrolyte repletion, and bowel rest until the

Case Conclusion

After decompression of the colon, the patient was initially taken to the operating room for a transverse loop colostomy by the emergency surgery service. Six weeks later, she had a normal spontaneous vaginal delivery of a healthy baby. At 6 weeks postpartum, she underwent an uneventful closure of the transverse colostomy closure and resection of approximately 18 inches of sigmoid colon with a primary anastomosis through a small Pfannenstiel incision by the colorectal surgery service.

return of peristalsis. Intravenous nutrition should be considered if the patient is initially malnourished or if more than a week passes without oral intake. Routine postcolectomy care is appropriate in the absence of clinical instability. For patients with an end ileostomy, waiting at least 6 to 12 weeks before performing an ostomy closure is prudent.

TAKE HOME POINTS

- Colonic volvulus, an axial rotation of the colon resulting in a closed loop obstruction, can occur at any nonfixed portion of the colon, most commonly in the sigmoid colon and cecum.
- Conditions such as chronic constipation or treatment for neurologic or psychiatric conditions are associated with chronically increased intraluminal pressure and ultimately elongation of the sigmoid colon, resulting in greater risk of volvulus.
- Colonic volvulus is typically diagnosed based on radiographic studies, including upright abdominal radiograph ("bent inner tube sign" or "coffee bean sign"), radio-opaque enema ("bird's beak"), or computed tomography ("swirl sign").
- The first line of treatment for volvulus in a stable patient is endoscopic decompression and placement of a decompressing rectal tube, followed by supportive hydration and electrolyte correction.
- Patients who cannot be treated successfully with endoscopic decompression or who exhibit worsening clinical signs should be taken to the operating room for an open procedure.
- Prior to intraoperative detorsion of the volvulus, the mesentery should be divided to prevent circulation of inflammatory cytokines or septicemia.
- Even among stable, successfully decompressed patients, an elective laparoscopic or open sigmoidectomy is recommended due to recurrence rates ranging from 30% to 70%.

SUGGESTED READINGS

Alshawi JS. Recurrent sigmoid volvulus in pregnancy: report of a case and review of the literature. *Dis Colon Rectum.* 2005;48(9): 1811-1813.

Ballantyne GH, Brandner MD, Beart RW Jr, et al. Volvulus of the colon. Incidence and mortality. *Ann Surg.* 1985;202(1):83-92.

Renzulli P, Maurer CA, Netzer P, et al. Preoperative colonoscopic derotation is beneficial in acute colonic volvulus. *Dig Surg.* 2002; 19(3):223-229.

Necrotizing Soft Tissue Infections (NSTIs)

29

AUDREY F. HAND AND SHARMILA DISSANAIKE

Based on the previous edition chapter "Necrotizing Soft Tissue Infections" by Michelle K. McNutt and Lillian S. Kao

Presentation

A 43-year-old man with no significant past medical or surgical history presents to the emergency room with a toothache and subjective fevers for 1 week. His vital signs are as follows: systolic blood pressure of 118 mm Hg, heart rate of 122 beats per minute, and temperature of 99.3°F. On physical exam, he has erythema, induration, and tenderness extending from the angle of the mandible and palpable crepitus. His laboratory values include a white blood cell (WBC) count of 19 with 7% bands, serum sodium concentration of 133 mmol/L, creatinine of 2.0, glucose of 136 mg/dL, and lactic acid of 2.6.

● DIFFERENTIAL DIAGNOSIS

The differential diagnosis of necrotizing soft tissue infections (NSTIs) includes nonnecrotizing cellulitis, drug rash, impetigo, furuncles, carbuncles, folliculitis, skin changes of chronic venous/arterial insufficiency, insect and spider bites, or malignancy.

● DISCUSSION

NSTIs are a broad spectrum of necrotizing infections, which include clostridial myonecrosis, gas gangrene, Meleney's ulcer, and flesh-eating infections. These terms refer to an aggressive soft tissue infection that involves necrosis of skin, subcutaneous fat, superficial/deep fascia, and/or muscle. Prompt recognition and aggressive early treatment including surgery are essential for good outcomes; if there is a delay in diagnosis, sepsis, multiple organ failure (MOF), and death may ensue. Despite improvement in medical and surgical care, the average mortality ranges from 10% to 23.5%. Poorer outcomes are reported for patients with diabetes mellitus, advanced age, immunosuppression, and shock on presentation.

NSTIs are divided into three clinical subtypes. Type I infections are the most common form of disease and are polymicrobial in nature. The causative microbes are a combination of Gram-positive/negative aerobes, and fungi (Table 29-1). These organisms work synergistically and may produce virulent toxins that increase tissue destruction. Type II NSTIs are monobacterial and are caused by either β-hemolytic streptococci, *Clostridium perfringens*, or *Staphylococcus aureus*. Type III NSTIs are acquired with a saltwater-associated skin wound infected with *Vibrio vulnificus*.

● WORKUP

The evaluation for possible NSTIs starts with a high index of suspicion. The physician must start with a thorough history and physical exam. An evaluation of disease time course and patient history is important. Risk factors for NSTIs include chronic renal insufficiency, diabetes, coronary artery disease, peripheral vascular disease, intravenous drug use, advanced age, traumatic injury, or steroid/nonsteroidal anti-inflammatory drug (NSAID) use. However, NSTIs may develop without significant risk factors. If a patient develops systemic toxicity with progression of infection despite antibiotic therapy, the physician should be on high alert for NSTI. Physical exam findings for NSTIs include erythema, tense edema, ulcers/vesicles or bullae, necrosis, grayish or "dishwater" wound drainage, crepitus, paresthesia, and pain out of proportion to physical exam findings. In early NSTIs, the cutaneous manifestations (bullae, vesicles, crepitus or skin necrosis) may be absent or subtle, which may result in a dangerous delay of diagnosis. Laboratory evaluation may aid in the diagnosis of NSTI. The physician should obtain an electrolyte panel, complete blood cell count with differential, C-reactive protein (CRP), and blood gas analysis. It is advised not to obtain superficial wound cultures for they are not helpful in directing antibiotic therapy. The laboratory risk indicator for necrotizing fasciitis (LRINEC) score was developed to assist in recognition of NSTIs (see table).

Radiographic evaluation should never delay prompt surgical debridement and is not required in diagnosing NSTIs, although it may be helpful on occasion. Soft tissue gas may be seen on plain radiographs and CT scan; however, while highly specific, this is not a sensitive sign and its absence does not exclude the diagnosis. Magnetic resonance imaging (MRI) findings of thickened fascia, fluid collection, and fascial rim enhancement can help differentiate NSTI from cellulitis, but should be combined with clinical findings for diagnostic accuracy.

Table 29-1	**Causative Microbes in Type I (Polymicrobial) NSTIs**		
Gram-Positive Aerobes	**Gram-Negative Aerobes**	**Anaerobes**	**Fungi**
Staphylococcus	Pseudomonas	Bacteroides	Candida
Streptococcus	Escherichia coli	Clostridium	Mucormycoses
Enterococcus	Enterobacter		
	Klebsiella		

DIAGNOSIS AND TREATMENT

Prompt diagnosis and differentiation of nonnecrotizing from necrotizing soft tissue infection is essential to decide the treatment course. Adjunctive tests to history and physical exam findings are not necessary for the diagnosis of NSTI and may contribute to delaying definitive surgical treatment. Surgical exploration may be both diagnostic and therapeutic, and if there is doubt as to the diagnosis, a small incision down to fascia performed at bedside under local anesthetic may be the most appropriate diagnostic test. Emergent surgical exploration and institution of broad-spectrum antibiotics remains the gold standard for treatment.

Intraoperative findings suggestive of an NSTI include thrombosis of small blood vessels (obliterative endarteritis), swollen gray fascia (liquefactive necrosis), and the ability to easily dissect fascia away from normally adherent tissue (loss of tissue planes). If the diagnosis is still uncertain, deep tissue fascial biopsy with frozen section analysis may be confirmatory. Histologic changes consistent with NSTIs include tissue necrosis, fibrinous vascular thrombosis, polymorphonuclear infiltration, and microorganisms within destroyed tissue.

The LRINEC score measures nonspecific biochemical and inflammatory markers and can aid in the early recognition of necrotizing infections (Table 29-2). A numerical score is assigned based on six laboratory parameters: CRP, total WBC count, hemoglobin concentration, sodium level, creatinine, and glucose. A score of ≥6 should raise the suspicion of necrotizing fasciitis (positive predictive value, 92% and negative predictive value, 96%), and a score of ≥8 is strongly predictive of the disease. The LRINEC score was derived from a single-center retrospective study and requires further validation with prospective studies. Despite this limitation, the LRINEC score remains a useful tool for the early detection of NSTI, and an elevated score should alert the physician to a patient at increased risk of having an NSTI.

Patients with NSTI often present with systemic toxicity and vital sign abnormalities that require optimization in concert with surgical debridement. Electrolyte abnormalities should be corrected, hyperglycemia treated with insulin, intravascular volume status optimized with fluid

resuscitation, and broad-spectrum antibiotics initiated. Operative exploration should not be delayed in the unstable patient.

NSTI patients should be treated initially with broad-spectrum antibiotics that can then be narrowed, based on cultures. Historical front-line agents included penicillins or cephalosporins with an aminoglycoside or a fluoroquinolone, plus an antianaerobic agent, such as clindamycin or metronidazole. More recently, these combination regimens have been replaced by a single broad-spectrum agent, such as a carbapenem or piperacillin–tazobactam. As the incidence of methicillin-resistant *S. aureus* NSTIs is increasing,

Table 29-2	**Laboratory Risk Indicator for Necrotizing Fasciitis Score**
Variables, Units	**Score**
C-reactive protein, mg/L	
<150	0
≥150	4
Total white cell count, per mm³	
<15	0
15–25	1
>25	2
Hemoglobin, g/dL	
>13.5	0
11–13.5	1
<11	2
Sodium, mmol/L	
≥135	0
<135	2
Creatinine, µmol/L	
≤141	0
>141	2
Glucose, mmol/L	
≤10	0
>10	2

vancomycin or linezolid should be used empirically until culture results are available. Clindamycin has theoretical additional benefits against endotoxemia and streptococcal toxins in particular, in additional to its antimicrobial properties, and is often added to the regimen for that indication. Patients with cirrhosis or saltwater and seafood exposure are at increased risk for developing *Vibrio* infections. *Vibrio* is a Gram-negative bacillus and is susceptible to doxycycline, as well as other antibiotics, with Gram-negative activity. Once culture results are available, antibiotics should be de-escalated and tailored as appropriate.

SURGICAL APPROACH

Definitive therapy for NSTIs requires urgent surgical debridement with excision of all infected tissue to a margin of grossly normal healthy tissue. The initial incision should be extensive and the patient draped so as to allow the surgeon to extend the incision if needed. The underlying soft tissue destruction is often more severe than the findings on physical exam would suggest. The initial incision should be taken down to and through the fascia to ensure that a deep myonecrosis or true necrotizing fasciitis is not overlooked. The margins of excision are carried to noninflamed, nonpurulent tissue with normal bleeding. The "push test" where a finger pushing on the margins of the wound does not cause the tissue to yield easily, should be performed. If the tissue gives way easily, then debridement should be extended until firm subcutaneous tissue or fascia is encountered, with no further "give" to manual pressure. A large segment of tissue as well as a sample of fluid should be sent for culture and Gram stain. This will aid to confirm the presumptive NSTI diagnosis and de-escalate the antibiotic regimen postoperatively. If there is doubt regarding the diagnosis, a specimen may be sent for histologic confirmation as well. The wound should be copiously irrigated and surgical hemostasis obtained.

There are several approaches to postsurgical wound care, without clear evidence of benefit of one over the other. The senior author's preference is to leave the wound completely open for 48 hours, which allows for assessment at bedside rather than requiring reoperation. A water-based ointment may be applied to hydrate the exposed muscle, or a spritz of antimicrobial solution may be used. Surprisingly, this approach also reduces pain since there is no need for frequent dressing changes and no adherent gauze is used. More commonly, the wound is packed with Kerlix or gauze soaked in saline or an antimicrobial solution such as sodium hypochlorite.

Following adequate control of the infection, a negative pressure wound therapy system may be utilized to expedite healing either by contracture or to prepare an optimal bed for subsequent skin grafting. Wound closure may require a combination of rotational flaps and skin grafting depending on the size of the soft tissue defect (Table 29-3).

Table 29-3	Surgical Debridement for NSTI

Key Technical Steps

1. Extensive incision.
2. Aggressive excision of all necrotic tissue.
3. Excision margin to grossly normal tissue.
4. Consideration of guillotine amputation or disarticulation in presence of systemic toxicity and hemodynamic instability.
5. Frequent assessment of wound for progression of infection despite initial debridement.
6. Repeat surgical debridement until infection controlled.
7. Reconstruction with skin graft or flap.

Potential Pitfalls

- Delay in diagnosis.
- Inadequate debridement either at the margins or depth of wound.
- Delayed recognition of disease progression despite debridement

SPECIAL INTRAOPERATIVE CONSIDERATIONS

With aggressive infections involving the extremities, a damage-control guillotine amputation or disarticulation may be indicated in the setting of systemic toxicity and hemodynamic instability. Heart disease, shock (systolic blood pressure <90), and clostridial infections have been identified as three independent predictors of limb loss with NSTIs. It is advised to discuss the possibility of amputation with the patient and their family preoperatively.

POSTOPERATIVE MANAGEMENT

Patients with an NSTI are best monitored in the intensive care unit. Aggressive fluid resuscitation and broad-spectrum antibiotic therapy should continue in the postoperative period. Continuous invasive hemodynamic monitoring with the use of arterial and central lines may be necessary, and standard sepsis treatment guidelines should be followed. Hemoglobin, renal function, glucose control, and acid–base status should also be carefully monitored. Rapid clinical resolution frequently occurs following appropriate surgical debridement of the necrotic tissue, especially if the infection is diagnosed early. Clinical deterioration or lack of clinical improvement should raise the suspicion of progressive spread of infection and prompt repeat surgical exploration. Once a microbiologic diagnosis is made, the broad-spectrum antibiotics should be de-escalated. Antibiotics may be discontinued after clinical resolution of symptoms.

Case Conclusion

The patient was treated with broad-spectrum antibiotics, intravenous fluid resuscitation and was taken to the operating room within 4 hours of initial evaluation by the surgery team. Patient underwent radical soft tissue incision and debridement of his neck, anterior torso, and abdomen by the General Surgery team (Figure 29-1). All necrotic, friable, tissue was excised and the wound was copiously irrigated. Tissue samples were sent to pathology along with grossly apparent dishwater fluid expressed from the wound. An oral surgeon assisted in the initial operation and extracted five teeth, performed an alveoloplasty, and incised and drained an intraoral abscess. The patient required vasopressors and ventilator support. Furthermore, two additional operations were performed as the surgical margins rapidly showed stigma of infection and clinically there was nonresolution of his sepsis. After gross healthy surgical margins were finally obtained and improvement of his sepsis, pressure support was weaned and patient was extubated. Negative pressure wound therapy was used for coverage of his wound, and his antibiotics were tailored to culture sensitivities. He was discharged on hospital day 31. He was readmitted for definitive coverage of his soft tissue deficit with split-thickness skin grafting. He had 99% skin graft take (Figure 29-2) and is doing well.

TAKE HOME POINTS

- The surgeon must maintain a high index of suspicion for prompt diagnosis.

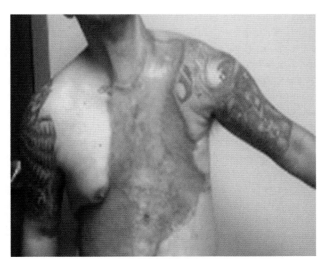

FIGURE 29-2. Healed split-thickness skin graft with good take; there is evidence of contracture at the edges that will likely require scar revision at a later date.

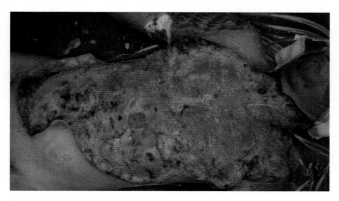

FIGURE 29-1. Radical debridement of all infected tissue until healthy margins are achieved.

- Delay in diagnosis and treatment increases morbidity and mortality.
- The most important therapy is immediate source control through surgical debridement.
- Supportive therapy includes aggressive fluid resuscitation and broad-spectrum antibiotics to cover Gram-negative, Gram-positive, and anaerobic bacteria.
- Repeat surgical debridements as needed until infection is controlled.
- Mortality remains relatively high, ranging from 10% to 23.5% despite aggressive therapy.
- Definitive treatment for soft tissue deficit can be done with negative pressure therapy, contraction, skin grafts, or rotational flaps.

SUGGESTED READINGS

Cocanour CS, Chang P, Huston JM, et al. Management and novel adjuncts of necrotizing soft tissue infections. *Surg Infect (Larchmt).* 2017;18(3):250-272. doi:10.1089/sur.2016.200.

Faraklas I, Yang D, Eggerstedt M, et al. A multi-center review of care patterns and outcomes in necrotizing soft tissue infections. *Surg Infect (Larchmt).* 2016;17(6):773-778.

Fernando SM, Tran A, Cheng W, et al. Necrotizing soft tissue infection: diagnostic accuracy of physical examination, imaging, and LRINEC score: a systematic review and meta-analysis. *Ann Surg.* 2018, doi: 10.1097/SLA.0000000000002774.

Gelbard RB, Ferrada P, Yeh DD, et al. Optimal timing of initial debridement for necrotizing soft tissue infection: a practice management guideline from the Eastern association for the surgery of trauma. *J Trauma Acute Care Surg.* 2018;85(1):208-214. doi: 10.1097/TA.0000000000001857.

Kobayashi L, Konstantinidis A, Shackelford S, et al. Necrotizing soft tissue infections: delayed surgical treatment is associated with increased number of surgical debridements and morbidity. *J Trauma.* 2011;71(5):1400-1405.

Moore SA, Levy BH, Prematilake C, Dissanaike S. The Prediction predicament: rethinking necrotizing soft tissue infections mortality. *Surg Infect (Larchmt).* 2015;16(6):813-821. doi:10.1089/sur.2015.002.

Bleeding Gastric Ulcer

30

ALEX C. KIM AND MICHAEL W. MULHOLLAND

Based on the previous edition chapter "Bleeding Gastric Ulcer" by Danielle Fritze and Michael Mulholland

Presentation

A 58-year-old man presents to the emergency room following several episodes of coffee ground emesis. While awaiting evaluation, he suddenly vomits a large volume of bright red blood. As he is urgently transported to a resuscitation bay, his wife explains that he is generally healthy except for a stomach ulcer he had the previous year. He completed a course of two antibiotics for the ulcer. He has never had an operation and takes no other medications. On exam, the patient is distressed but alert, oriented, and no longer vomiting. Initial vital signs reveal tachycardia with a pulse of 115 bpm and blood pressure of 100/70 mm Hg. He has mild discomfort with deep palpation in the epigastrium; the remainder of his exam is unremarkable.

● DIFFERENTIAL DIAGNOSIS

For patients presenting with upper gastrointestinal (GI) bleeding, the source may be located in any portion of the GI tract, from the oropharynx through the ligament of Treitz (Figure 30-1). Gastroduodenal ulcers are the most common cause of upper GI hemorrhage, representing approximately 25% to 30% of all cases. Other causes of nonvariceal upper GI hemorrhage such as Mallory-Weiss tears and erosive diseases each account for an additional 10%. In addition, complications of portal hypertension such as esophagogastric varices or gastropathies comprise an additional 10% to

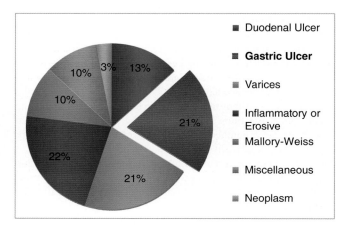

- Duodenal Ulcer
- **Gastric Ulcer**
- Varices
- Inflammatory or Erosive
- Mallory-Weiss
- Miscellaneous
- Neoplasm

FIGURE 30-1. Sources of upper gastrointestinal bleeding.

15% of all cases. While neoplasms such as adenocarcinoma or gastrointestinal stromal tumor (GIST) are less common sources of bleeding, their accurate identification is particularly important for treatment planning. Rare causes of GI hemorrhage include Dieulafoy's lesions, vascular ectasias, hemobilia, and iatrogenic bleeding following endoscopy.

The differential diagnosis of upper GI bleeding is broad. Early recognition of individual patient risk factors is critical and may assist in identification of underlying etiology. For example, patients with portal hypertension are at particular risk of variceal bleeding. In anyone who has had an aortic aneurysm repair, aortoenteric fistula must be immediately considered as a potentially lethal source of GI hemorrhage. This patient's ulcer history makes a recurrent gastric ulcer the most probable source of hematemesis.

● WORKUP

Upper GI bleeding secondary to gastroduodenal ulcers places a significant burden on health care with morality rate of 8.5%. Early goal-directed, intensive hemodynamic resuscitation is important to correct intravascular hypovolemia, to adequately maintain tissue perfusion, and to ultimately decrease mortality. Immediate management of upper GI bleeding is dictated by the patient's clinical condition. Prompt establishment of adequate intravenous access is critical, with administration of crystalloid or blood products (target hemoglobin >7 to 9 g/dL based on patient's comorbidities) as appropriate for the patient's vital signs and rate of blood loss. Poor prognostic indicators of patients presenting with GI bleeding include elevated serum blood urea nitrogen and creatinine levels and lower mean arterial blood pressure and oxygen saturation. These factors are suggestive of intravascular depletion secondary to ongoing hemorrhage. Patients taking warfarin or antiplatelet agents are likely to require reversal of anticoagulation. If the airway may be compromised by active hematemesis, encephalopathy, or agitation, the patient should be intubated. Nasogastric (NG) tube placement can be diagnostic of an upper GI bleed if bright red blood is aspirated, with specificity approaching 95%. NG tube placement also allows for evacuation of gastric contents and a rough estimation of the rate of bleeding. However, NG tube placement is not an absolute prerequisite for diagnosis of upper GI bleed and should not delay further treatment.

History and physical exam are rarely diagnostic for a bleeding ulcer but may provide information useful in its management. Most patients with gastric ulcer report symptoms of gnawing or burning epigastric pain with a waxing and waning course. Classically, discomfort from gastric ulcers is exacerbated by oral intake. Slow, chronic blood loss may cause melena and lead to symptoms of anemia. Identification of risk factors for ulcer development such as nonsteroidal anti-inflammatory drug (NSAID) use, smoking, or multiple endocrine neoplasia type I syndrome (MEN I) lends insight into the underlying etiology of the ulcer. Knowledge of any anticoagulant or antiplatelet agents taken by the patient allows for appropriate management of the associated coagulopathy. Physical exam is often unremarkable in ulcer patients, but some will exhibit epigastric tenderness. Peritoneal signs raise concern for perforation that infrequently accompanies hemorrhage. In the acutely bleeding patient, the main utility of physical exam is to identify signs of hemodynamic instability and estimate the degree of blood loss.

In parallel with the initial resuscitation, diagnostic studies are undertaken. Complete blood count (hematocrit is followed serially), coagulation profile, basic metabolic panel, and blood type and screen are obtained. Peritoneal signs should prompt an upright chest x-ray to evaluate for pneumoperitoneum. In the absence of peritonitis, no imaging studies are necessary. Esophagogastroduodenoscopy (EGD) is the most effective means of locating the source of upper GI bleeding, with successful identification of the responsible lesion in 95% of patients. In rare cases where the source of bleeding is not localized, repeat EGD, angiography, or technetium-99m–labeled red blood cell scan may be successful.

● DIAGNOSIS AND TREATMENT

Once a gastric ulcer is identified, endoscopic therapy is guided by the risk of recurrent hemorrhage and the patient's clinical stability. Although bleeding frequently resolves spontaneously, specific stigmata of hemorrhage predict continued or recurrent bleeding and the need for intervention (Table 30-1). Ulcers with evidence of active bleeding or a

Table 30-2 Etiology of Gastric Ulcer

NSAIDS
H. pylori
Zollinger-Ellison
Neoplasm

visible vessel within the lesion (Forrest grade 1a, 1b, and 2a) are at highest risk. Ulcers with an adherent clot and underlying oozing are also prone to recurrent bleeding. Endoscopic intervention is indicated for each of these high-risk lesions. Options include the application of clips, thermal coagulation, or injection of a vasoconstricting or sclerosing agent. When feasible, biopsy of the ulcer is important to identify any associated malignancy. Antral biopsies are used to establish a histologic diagnosis of *Helicobacter pylori*. For patients with a bleeding ulcer, endoscopic interventions carry a 90% success rate in achieving initial hemostasis. If a patient rebleeds after endoscopic intervention, a second endoscopic attempt at hemostasis is performed. Repeat EGD was demonstrated in a randomized trial to be safer than proceeding to surgery. However, for bleeding that cannot be controlled endoscopically (after two attempts), or for patients with hemorrhagic shock, surgery may be lifesaving.

Following initial hemostasis, the etiology of the ulcer must be identified and addressed. *H. pylori* and NSAIDs are the two most important factors contributing to the development of gastric ulcers (Table 30-2). Each is implicated in over 50% of cases, with additive effects. Tobacco use is also contributory. Four percent of gastric ulcers harbor an underlying malignancy, most commonly gastric adenocarcinoma. In rare cases, Zollinger-Ellison syndrome, either sporadic or hereditary (MEN I syndrome), may be underlying pathology. Ulcer location may also offer insight into etiology. Prepyloric and duodenal ulcers are typically related to acid hypersecretion, whereas NSAID-induced ulcers may be located anywhere in the stomach (Table 30-3).

Medical therapy directed at ulcer etiology is an important adjunct to endoscopic and surgical interventions.

Table 30-1 Forrest Classification of Peptic Ulcers

Grade	Stigmata		30-Day Risk of Rebleeding After Endoscopic Therapy (%)
1a	Actively bleeding	Pulsatile	20
1b	Ulcer	Nonpulsatile	<10
2a	Nonbleeding ulcer	Visible vessel	15
2b		Adherent clot	<5
2c		Hematin-covered base	7
3	Nonbleeding ulcer	Clean base	3

Table 30-3	Modified Johnson Classification of Gastric Ulcers	
Type	Location	Etiology
I	Lesser curve	Varies, not related to acid hypersecretion
II	Two ulcers, stomach body and duodenum	Acid hypersecretion
III	Prepyloric	Acid hypersecretion
IV	GE junction	Varies, not related to acid hypersecretion
V	Any location	NSAIDs

Acid suppression with a proton pump inhibitor (PPI) decreases the risk of rebleeding after endoscopic hemostasis, aids in ulcer healing, and prevents ulcer recurrence. Current guidelines based on randomized trials recommend an intravenous bolus (80 mg) followed by a high continuous infusion (8 mg per hour) for 72 hours postintervention. NSAIDs should be withheld if medically possible. If NSAIDs are to be continued, it is imperative to utilize a COX-2 selective NSAID at lowest effective dose together with daily PPI. Smoking cessation is strongly encouraged. For patients with *H. pylori*, eradication of the bacteria results in a decreased incidence of rebleeding as low as 0.15% per patient year. In 98.5% of colonized patients, this can be accomplished with a single course of "triple therapy"—two antibiotics active against *H. pylori* and a PPI. Following confirmation of eradication, maintenance PPI therapy is not warranted unless the patient requires NSAIDs or other antithrombotics. Almost uniformly, recurrence is related to *H. pylori* reinfection or NSAID use.

● SURGICAL APPROACH

While surgery remains the primary means of managing anatomic complications of ulcer disease, the development of effective pharmacotherapy for acid suppression and *H. pylori* clearance has reduced the role of surgery. Surgery should be considered in patients who are intolerant or noncompliant with medical management, are at high risk of recurrence, or failed previous treatment. When treating for anatomic complications, the operation should be carefully tailored to the patient's clinical scenario. The appropriate surgical procedure for a bleeding gastric ulcer is also dependent upon the patient's condition (Figure 30-2). For unstable patients, midline laparotomy is followed by anterior gastrotomy. Once the lesion is identified, the ulcer is oversewn, biopsied (if possible), and the gastrotomy repaired. For stable patients with a history of refractory ulcer disease, an antisecretory procedure such as truncal vagotomy or distal gastrectomy should be considered.

Algorithm for Management of Bleeding Gastric Ulcer

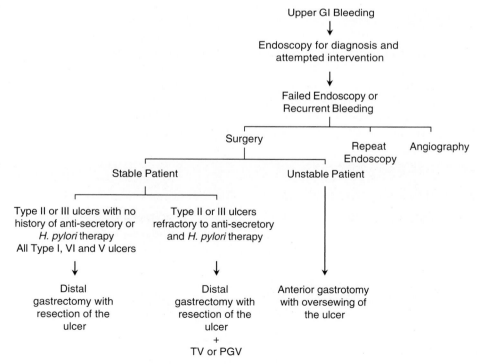

FIGURE 30-2. Algorithm for management of bleeding gastric ulcer.

TRUNCAL VAGOTOMY

In patients with bleeding gastric ulcers, truncal vagotomy is indicated for those who have failed previous medical therapy. These patients usually have a long-standing history of ulcer disease and have proven refractory to (or serially noncompliant with) PPIs and *H. pylori* eradication. Vagotomy markedly reduces cholinergic stimulation of gastric acid secretion. Because vagotomy also results in pyloric denervation, a concurrent procedure such as pyloroplasty or antrectomy is thus necessary to ensure gastric drainage.

To perform a truncal vagotomy, the left hepatic lobe is retracted cephalad and laterally with division of the triangular ligament as needed to expose the hiatus. The overlying peritoneum is incised and the esophagus dissected circumferentially for several centimeters about the gastroesophageal (GE) junction. Anteriorly, the vagal trunk is found closely applied to the esophageal wall. In contrast, the posterior vagus may reside 1 cm or more posterolateral to the esophagus. Palpation may aid in initial identification of the nerves. Once both trunks are located, proximal and distal clips are placed to allow for resection of a 2-cm intervening segment of nerve. These specimens are sent to pathology for histologic confirmation. There may be several divisions of each vagal trunk, so the area of the GE junction is carefully inspected to determine that all vagal fibers have been divided. Prior to closure, cruroplasty may be required to prevent development of a hiatal hernia.

DISTAL GASTRECTOMY

If a patient with bleeding gastric ulcer is stable, there are a few scenarios in which a distal gastrectomy can be considered. As with truncal vagotomy, patients are usually only considered candidates for distal gastrectomy if they have a history of failed medical management, especially patients with large antral ulcers that cannot be easily oversewn or patients with ulcers suspicious for cancer. Risks of operative death and complications are much higher for distal gastrectomy than simple oversewing or vagotomy, so this procedure should only be undertaken when clear indications exist.

To perform distal gastrectomy, a vertical incision in the supraumbilical midline affords adequate exposure in most cases. Following exploration of the abdomen, a Kocher maneuver is performed to mobilize the duodenum. Mobilization of the distal stomach begins with division of the gastrocolic ligament. Entry into the lesser sac permits examination of the posterior gastric wall. The omentum is then divided along the greater curvature, from the duodenum halfway to the GE junction. The right gastroepiploic vessels are ligated and divided near the gastroduodenal artery (GDA). The gastrohepatic ligament is then incised. The right gastric artery is identified, ligated, and divided near the superior border of the duodenum. Branches of the left gastric artery are divided along the lesser curve in preparation for resection and anastomosis. An area of healthy proximal duodenum is chosen and transected with a stapling device. The proximal extent of the resection is determined by the location of the ulcer and the condition of the gastric wall. The stomach is also divided with a stapling device, and all staple lines are oversewn. Continuity of the GI tract can be reestablished via either Billroth I or II reconstruction, depending upon the length and health of the duodenal stump.

SPECIAL INTRAOPERATIVE CONSIDERATIONS

Type IV gastric ulcers can be particularly challenging to manage due to their proximity to the GE junction. In most cases, the ulcer can be resected as part of the distal gastrectomy with an extension along the lesser curve. Traditional Billroth I or II reconstruction is avoided as it is likely to result in narrowing of the GE junction. Instead, roux-en-Y gastrojejunostomy permits construction of a wide anastomosis, incorporating the distal GE junction and the entirety of the gastrotomy. In rare circumstances, the ulcer may be oversewn and left in situ. A concurrent antisecretory procedure with *H. pylori* eradication, PPI, and cessation of NSAIDs results in satisfactory ulcer healing in most patients (Table 30-4).

POSTOPERATIVE MANAGEMENT

Following surgery for a bleeding gastric ulcer, patients remain on bowel rest with NG decompression. These measures may be discontinued as gastric emptying resumes. Patients should be observed for potential postoperative complications such as surgical site infection (SSI), hemorrhage, or anastomotic leak. For those with a Billroth II reconstruction, duodenal stump leak is a particularly morbid complication.

With initiation of oral intake, patients who undergo gastrectomy should also be monitored for postgastrectomy dumping syndrome. This is characterized by postprandial GI and vasomotor symptoms, such as nausea, abdominal pain, dizziness, and even syncope. In most patients, these symptoms are temporary and easily managed with frequent small meals. In a small minority of patients, however, dumping symptoms can become debilitating. Octreotide may be helpful in this circumstance. At discharge, all patients are counseled to avoid tobacco and NSAIDs as well as to continue PPI therapy. Those colonized with *H. pylori* receive triple therapy, and eradication is confirmed at follow-up.

Table 30-4   Distal Gastrectomy and Truncal Vagotomy

Key Technical Steps

1. General anesthesia, supine position, NG decompression.
2. Supraumbilical vertical midline incision.

Distal Gastrectomy

3. Kocher maneuver.
4. Divide the gastrocolic ligament to enter the lesser sac.
5. Examine the stomach and identify the region of the ulcer to determine the appropriate extent of resection.
6. Divide the greater omentum along the greater curve from duodenum halfway to the GE junction.
7. Ligate and divide the right gastroepiploic vessels near the GDA.
8. Incise the gastrohepatic ligament.
9. Ligate and divide the right gastric artery proximally.
10. Divide the duodenum and stomach with a stapling device.
11. Oversew both staple lines, leaving a portion of the gastrotomy closure available for reconstruction.
12. Reestablish GI tract continuity via either Billroth I or II reconstruction.

Truncal Vagotomy

13. Retract the left hepatic lobe laterally, with division of the triangular ligament as needed to expose the esophageal hiatus.
14. Incise the peritoneum and dissect the esophagus circumferentially.
15. Identify and dissect the anterior and posterior trunks of the vagus nerves.
16. Place proximal and distal clips ~2 cm apart on each trunk and then resect the intervening nerve segments.
17. Inspect the esophagus to ensure that all portions of the vagus nerves have been divided.
18. As needed, perform a cruroplasty to prevent hiatal hernia.
19. Confirm NG tube placement and then close the abdomen.

Potential Pitfalls

- Failure to identify an associated neoplasm.
- Injury to the porta or inferior vena cava with Kocher maneuver and duodenal dissection.
- Injury to the middle colic vessels with division of the gastrocolic ligament.
- Billroth I reconstruction under tension or with inflamed duodenum.
- Failure to divide all vagal branches.

Case Conclusion

The patient's immediate management included placement of two large-bore IVs, crystalloid resuscitation, and a pantoprazole infusion. His initial hematocrit was 28%, with normal coagulation studies. Endoscopy performed while the patient was still in the emergency room revealed a 2-cm gastric ulcer in the prepyloric region (type III) with a nonbleeding visible vessel. Clips were applied and biopsies performed endoscopically. He was then admitted to the hospital for observation. The following day, he had another episode of hematemesis. Endoscopy was again attempted, but unsuccessful in controlling the bleeding. He required two units of packed red blood cells but remained hemodynamically stable. He was taken to the operating room emergently for surgical intervention. Given the history of recurrent type III gastric ulcer following *H. pylori* eradication and long-term acid suppression, an antisecretory procedure was deemed appropriate. Truncal vagotomy was performed in conjunction with distal gastrectomy. The patient tolerated the procedure well, and recovered without recurrent bleeding or serious complication. Final surgical pathology confirmed a benign gastric ulcer.

TAKE HOME POINTS

- Although decreasing in incidence, peptic ulcer remains the most common cause of upper GI bleeding, with significant associated mortality.
- *H. pylori* infection and NSAID use are the most frequent inciting factors in bleeding gastric ulcers.
- Endoscopy is the first-line diagnostic intervention and is therapeutically effective in a majority of patients.
- Surgery is indicated in patients with massive bleeding, failure of endoscopic therapy, recurrent hemorrhage, or neoplasm.
- Anterior gastrotomy, ulcer oversewing, and biopsy is the procedure of choice for patients without a history of refractory ulcer disease.
- Truncal vagotomy is indicated only for patients with ulcers refractory to adequate PPI therapy and *H. pylori* eradication.
- Distal gastrectomy with inclusion of the ulcer in the specimen is the procedure of choice in stable patients with refractory ulcer disease who have large antral ulcers.
- *H. pylori* eradication significantly decreases the risk of recurrent bleeding gastric ulcer.

SUGGESTED READINGS

Enestvedt BK, Gralnek IM, Mattek N, et al. An evaluation of endoscopic indications and findings related to nonvariceal upper-GI hemorrhage in a large multicenter consortium. *Gastrointest Endosc.* 2008;67(3):422-429.

Gisbert, JP, Calvet X, Cosme A, et al. Long-term follow-up of 1,000 patients cured of *Helicobacter pylori* infection following an episode of peptic ulcer bleeding. *Am J Gastroenterol.* 2012;107:1197-1204.

Gralnek IM, Dumonceau JM, Kuipers EJ, et al. Diagnosis and management of nonvariceal upper gastrointestinal hemorrhage: European Society of Gastrointestinal Endoscopy (ESGE) Guideline. *Endoscopy.* 2015;47:1-46.

Gurusamy KS, Pallari E. Medical versus surgical treatment for refractory or recurrent peptic ulcer. *Cochrane Database Syst Rev.* 2016;3:CD011523.

Laine L, Jensen DM. Management of patients with ulcer bleeding. *Am J Gastroenterol.* 2012;107:345-360.

Quan S, Frolkis A, Milne K, et al. Upper-gastrointestinal bleeding secondary to peptic ulcer disease: incidence and outcomes. *World J Gastroenterol.* 2014;20(46):17568-17577.

Bleeding Duodenal Ulcer

CHRISTIAN PEREZ, NIRAV C. THOSANI, PETER A. WALKER, AND SHINIL K. SHAH

31

Based on the previous edition chapter "Bleeding Duodenal Ulcer" by Wendy L. Wahl

Presentation

A 70-year-old male with a history of coronary artery disease (on aspirin) and uncontrolled diabetes mellitus presents to the emergency room with sudden onset of hematemesis and melena. On admission, the patient is tachycardic and hypotensive. Physical exam demonstrates a soft and nontender abdomen. Rectal exam shows dark stool that is guaiac positive.

● DIFFERENTIAL DIAGNOSIS

The patient is presenting with signs of upper gastrointestinal (UGI) bleeding. He is a high-risk patient as he is older (>65 years) and taking aspirin and may have gastroparesis related to his uncontrolled diabetes. He has no evidence of current use of proton pump inhibitors.

The most common cause of UGI bleeding is peptic ulcer disease. The differential diagnosis for UGI bleeding is extensive, with other causes including variceal bleeding (in patients with cirrhosis), Dieulafoy lesion, arteriovenous (AV) malformations, and Mallory-Weiss tears in patients with history of persistent emesis. History can be very helpful in narrowing the diagnostic possibilities.

● WORKUP

The initial management of this patient consists of ensuring a secure airway, especially if there is massive hematemesis. Initial lab studies, including blood counts, metabolic profiles, blood gas, coagulation parameters, as well as a type and cross, should be drawn and sent. Two large bore intravenous lines should be placed with initial fluid resuscitation consisting of crystalloids and switching early to balanced resuscitation with blood products (packed red blood cells, fresh frozen plasma [FFP], and platelets) with persistent massive bleeding as well as if the patient does not respond to initial fluid management. Coagulopathy should be aggressively treated, especially with a history of anticoagulation, and in patients on the newer Factor Xa inhibitor class of medications (apixaban, rivaroxaban, and dabigatran).

Nasogastric tube placement (NGT) will help differentiate the origin of the bleeding and may assist with irrigation of the stomach for better visualization of the source of the bleeding. High-dose proton pump inhibitors (PPIs) should be initiated.

● DIAGNOSIS AND TREATMENT

The next step will be an esophagogastroduodenoscopy (EGD) for diagnosis and treatment. Early endoscopy (within 24 hours) has been shown to decrease morbidity, transfusion requirements, and surgical interventions. Use of prokinetic medications (erythromycin or metoclopramide) should be considered as it improves visibility and may lead to less need of repeat endoscopy for poor visualization. Biopsies with studies for *H. pylori* should be obtained at the time of endoscopy if feasible. Sample endoscopic images of duodenal ulcers are noted in Figure 31-1.

Presentation Continued

The patient initially stabilizes with transfusion of 2 units of packed red blood cells and 2 units of FFP. Platelets were additionally transfused secondary to his history of aspirin intake. He is taken to the endoscopy suite. EGD demonstrates a 2.5 cm duodenal ulcer in the posterior wall of the duodenum with a visible vessel.

The next step in the management of this patient is endoscopic therapy, preferably with two different methods, the most common being a combination of epinephrine injection, mechanical (endoscopic clips), and thermal (cautery, gold probe, and/or argon plasma coagulation) methods.

It is also important to identify the risk factors for recurrent bleeding on this patient. This is typically based on the endoscopic appearance according to the Forrest Classification (Table 31-1). This patient has a high-risk appearance for recurrent bleeding (visible vessel, IIA). Additional risk factors for recurrent bleeding include his age, aspirin use, and posterior duodenal ulcer >2 cm. The majority of recurrent episodes of bleeding occur within 72 hours of the initial event. The patient should be kept on high-dose PPI with close monitoring. Anticoagulation should be held.

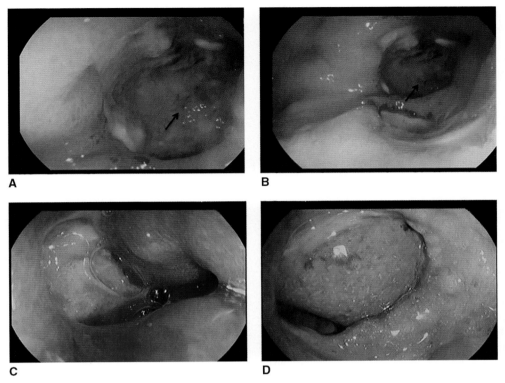

FIGURE 31-1. Sample endoscopic appearance of duodenal ulcers. Large anterior/superior duodenal ulcer **(A)** with smaller posterior/inferior ulcer **(B)** with visible vessels but no active bleeding (*arrow*). Non bleeding posterior **(C)** and anterior **(D)** duodenal ulcers.

Presentation Continued

Our patient underwent epinephrine injection and hemoclip placement with satisfactory control of the bleeding. The PPI drip was continued and he was transferred to the ICU for close monitoring. The patient stabilized over the next 24 hours. The following day, he presented with a new episode of hematemesis and melena, tachycardia (110 bpm), and hypotension (systolic blood pressure of 85 mm Hg). He responded to a repeat blood transfusion. A second endoscopy was performed demonstrating persistent bleeding at the site of the posterior duodenal ulcer with poor hemostasis. His tachycardia and hypotension persisted. Interventional radiology was notified to consider angioembolization, but they were not present at the hospital. Given his deteriorating clinical status, the patient was taken emergently to the operating room.

In this case, our patient with multiple risk factors had an episode of recurrent UGI bleeding. A second endoscopy was indicated as he was relatively stable. Multiple studies have shown a second endoscopy is 75% to 85% effective in stopping bleeding with a lower complication rate than surgery. If bleeding persists after a second endoscopy or the patient becomes clinically unstable, the patient should proceed to more definitive intervention.

The indications for surgery for peptic ulcer hemorrhage include:

1. Hemodynamic instability despite vigorous resuscitation (>4 to 6 units of blood).
2. Failure of endoscopic techniques to stop hemorrhage.
3. Recurrent hemorrhage after initial stabilization (with up to two attempts at obtaining endoscopic hemostasis).
4. Shock associated with recurrent hemorrhage.
5. Continued slow bleeding with transfusion requirement exceeding 3 units of blood per day.

Angioembolization may have been a reasonable option if the patient had not been clinically deteriorating and/or an

Table 31-1	Forrest Classification of Endoscopic Appearance of Bleeding Ulcers
Ia	Spurting bleeding
Ib	Nonspurting, active bleeding
IIa	Visible vessel
IIb	Nonbleeding ulcer with overlying clot
IIc	Ulcer with hematin-covered (black) base
III	Clean ulcer base

Reprinted by permission from Springer: Laporte JR, Ibanez L, Vidal X, et al. Upper gastrointestinal bleeding associated with the use of NSAIDs: newer versus older agents. *Drug Safety*. 2004;27(6):411-420. Copyright © 2004 Adis Data Information BV.

interventional radiology team was available. Studies show a technical success rate of 90% to 100% and a clinical success rate of 50% to 83%. Angioembolization should also be considered if the patient presents with recurrent bleeding after satisfactory surgical intervention.

Presentation Continued

The patient underwent exploratory laparotomy for hemostasis. Since the patient was naïve to PPI and was positive for *H. pylori* test, an acid-reducing procedure was not performed.

● SURGICAL APPROACH

The open surgical approach starts with a midline laparotomy. Once the peritoneal cavity is accessed, we recommend performing a generous Kocher maneuver to obtain better mobilization and digital control of the duodenum. It will also help relieve possible tension on the suture line at the time of repair.

A longitudinal pyloroduodenotomy is then performed followed by careful inspection of the duodenal mucosa with localization of the bleeding (endoscopic placed clips will provide some guidance). With posterior ulcers, the gastroduodenal artery (GDA) is usually the source of bleeding. Three-point ligation should be performed to achieve complete hemostasis. Sutures should be placed superiorly, inferiorly and medially to ligate the transverse pancreatic branches (Figure 31-2). Beware of the common bile duct in posterior ulcers. If there is a large amount of inflammation and difficulty identifying structures, placement of a biliary catheter should be considered for better identification of the duct.

Once satisfactory hemostasis has been achieved, closure of the duodenal ulcer or approximation should be done when possible.

The pyloroduodenotomy is then closed transversely (Heineke-Mikulicz pyloroplasty) in one or two layers (Figure 31-3). It is imperative to know a second way to complete a pyloroplasty. If there is a lot of tension or the borders will not come together easily, consider a Finney or Jaboulay pyloroplasty (gastroduodenostomies). These two techniques differ in whether the pylorus is incised (Finney, Figure 31-4A–D) or not (Jaboulay, Figure 31-5; Table 31-2).

● POSTOPERATIVE MANAGEMENT

In most cases, hemostasis and postoperative treatment with PPIs with treatment of *H. pylori* is sufficient. In cases where patients present with recurrent ulcer disease on PPI and those that are *H. pylori* negative, acid-reducing procedures should be consider if the patient is hemodynamically stable.

The most expedient acid-reducing procedure with reasonable morbidity and outcomes (70% to 80% acid suppression) is a truncal vagotomy (TV) with a drainage procedure (pyloroplasty). For vagotomy, the phrenoesophagic ligament should be opened and the esophagus encircled with a Penrose. The anterior and posterior vagus nerves should be identified. The anterior vagus nerve is usually adherent to the esophagus. The posterior one is usually further away. Once identified, the vagus nerves should be clipped proximally and distally and 2 to 3 cm of the vagus nerve should be excised and sent for histologic confirmation. The vagotomy should be performed 4 to 6 cm proximal to the gastroesophageal junction to make

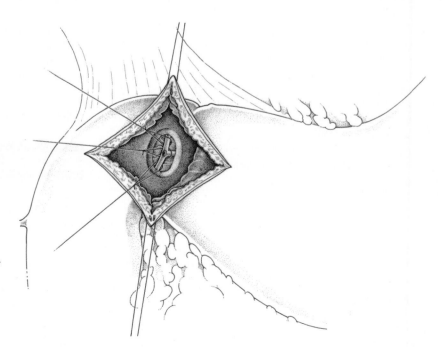

FIGURE 31-2. Technique of three-point suture ligation of a bleeding posterior duodenal ulcer (gastroduodenal artery). (From Schirmer BD. Chapter 88: bleeding duodenal ulcer. In: Fischer JE, ed. *Fischer's Mastery of Surgery*. Lippincott Williams & Wilkins, 2012:1023.)

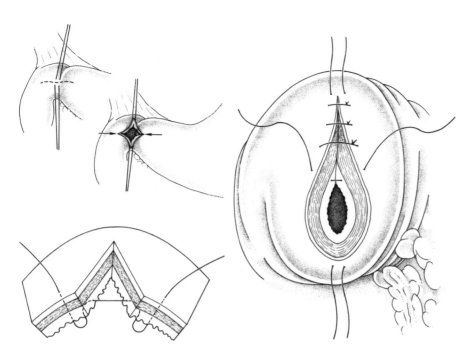

FIGURE 31-3. Technique of Heineke-Mikulicz pyloroplasty. Demonstrated is a single layered technique. Closure of the initial longitudinal incision is closed transversely. (From Schirmer BD. Chapter 88: bleeding duodenal ulcer. In: Fischer JE, ed. *Fischer's Mastery of Surgery.* Lippincott Williams & Wilkins, 2012:1024.)

sure the criminal nerve of Grassi is addressed; otherwise, the recurrence rates can be high (Figure 31-6; Table 31-3).

Selective and highly selective vagotomies are time-consuming and not recommended to be performed on patients taken to the operating room for active bleeding. Gastric resection procedures (antrectomy + vagotomy) require longer surgical times and are not advised on patients that had major episodes of bleeding and are overall clinically unstable.

Complications of these procedures include gastrointestinal leak, recurrent bleeding episodes, common bile duct ligation, and wound infection. Gastrointestinal leaks can be managed with drains and/or surgical intervention depending on the situation. If there is a leak from the pyloroplasty, resectional procedures should be considered. Recurrent bleeding after a fresh duodenal repair can be managed with angioembolization. Escalating treatment with a gastric resection procedure carries high risk of complications. Common bile duct ligation should be prevented with appropriate identification of anatomy during the surgery.

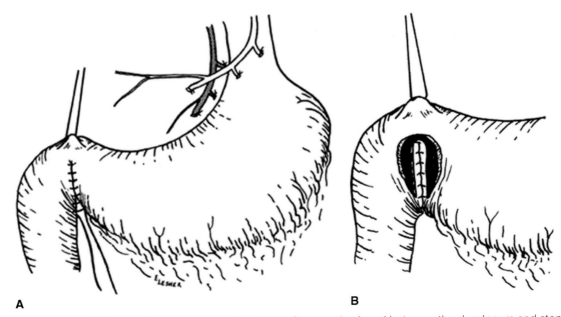

A   **B**

FIGURE 31-4. Technique of Finney pyloroplasty. A posterior row of sutures is placed between the duodenum and stomach **(A)**, followed by a U incision across the pylorus **(B)**, followed by completion of the two layer anastomosis

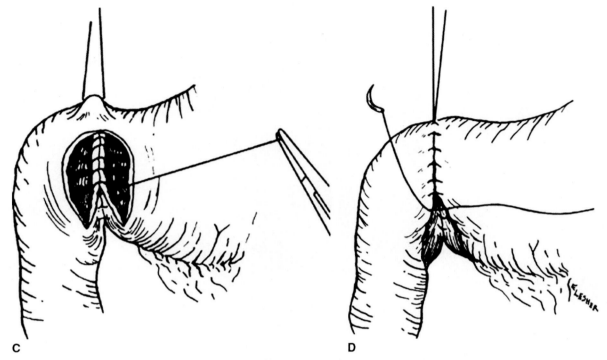

C   D

FIGURE 31-4. (*Continued*) **(C** and **D).** (From Schwaitzberg SD, Sawyers JL, Richards WO. Chapter 86: selective vagotomy and pyloroplasty. In: Fischer JE, ed. *Fischer's Mastery of Surgery.* Lippincott Williams & Wilkins, 2012:e18.)

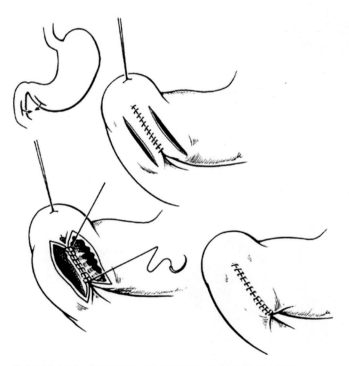

FIGURE 31-5. Technique of Jaboulay pyloroplasty. The technique is similar to that of the Finney pyloroplasty with the exception that the incision does not cross the pylorus. (From Schwaitzberg SD, Sawyers JL, Richards WO. Chapter 86: selective vagotomy and pyloroplasty. In: Fischer JE, ed. *Fischer's Mastery of Surgery.* Lippincott Williams & Wilkins, 2012:e18.)

Table 31-2	Duodenal Ulcer Hemostasis

Key Technical Steps

1. Exploratory laparotomy through an upper midline incision.
2. Localization of the pylorus and duodenum.
3. Generous Kocher maneuver.
4. Longitudinal pyloroduodenotomy.
5. Biopsies of the ulcer bed (if not performed endoscopically previously).
6. Three-point ligation of the gastroduodenal artery. Assure complete hemostasis. Beware of the common bile duct posteriorly.
7. Approximation of the ulcer.
8. Transverse closure of the gastroduodenostomy (Heineke-Mikulicz pyloroplasty) in one or two layers.

Potential Pitfalls

- Persistent bleeding after ligation of the bleeding vessel. Remember to complete three-point ligation of the gastroduodenal artery.
- Injury to or ligation of the common bile duct located posteriorly. If there are any questions, the duct should be probed for better identification.
- Inability to close the gastroduodenotomy. Perform Finney or Jaboulay pyloroplasty.

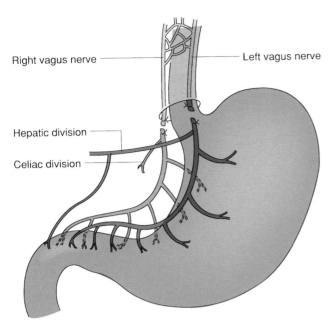

Right vagus nerve — Left vagus nerve

Hepatic division

Celiac division

FIGURE 31-6. Truncal vagotomy. (From Simeone DM, Doherty GM, Upchurch GR Jr, Lillemoe KD, Mulholland MW, Maier RV, eds. *Greenfield's Surgery: Scientific Principles and Practice.* Lippincott Williams & Wilkins, 2011.)

Table 31-3	Truncal Vagotomy

Key Technical Steps

1. Localize the hiatus.
2. Open phrenoesophageal ligament.
3. Encircle esophagus with Penrose.
4. Identify and dissect anterior and posterior vagus; beware of the criminal nerve of Grassi.
5. Clip the vagus nerves proximally and distally about 4–6 cm proximal to GE junction. Excise 2–3 cm of the vagus nerve and send for histologic confirmation.

Potential Pitfalls

- Vagotomy performed too distal with preservation of criminal nerve of Grassi. This can lead to high recurrence rates. Ligate the vagus at least 4 cm proximal to the GE junction.
- Transection of areolar tissue but not the vagus nerve. Excise 2–3 cm of the nerve and send for histologic confirmation.

Presentation Continued

The patient underwent three-point suture ligation and Heineke-Mikulicz pyloroplasty. He did well after the procedure without any further bleeding episodes. At discharge, the patient was sent home with treatment for *H. pylori* and long-term PPI therapy. Aspirin was restarted 5 days after discharge.

During the postoperative period, it is important monitor for complications from massive transfusion and the systemic response. This tends to be main causes of mortality in these patients. In patients with *H. pylori*, treatment should be provided as well as long term PPI therapy. Patient that test negative for *H. pylori* during the acute bleeding episodes should be tested again at a later time since there are studies that report high false negatives during an acute bleeding event. *H. pylori* is involved in about 90% of duodenal ulcers.

TAKE HOME POINTS

- If the patient presents with an UGI bleed and is unstable, initial management should include securing the airway and initiation of resuscitation.
- Aggressively correct coagulopathy with balanced resuscitation and adjuncts if necessary.

- EGD is the preferred initial test as it can be both diagnostic and therapeutic.
- Use two methods to achieve endoscopic hemostasis. Obtain biopsies to determine *H. pylori* status.
- Start high-dose PPI.
- Repeat EGD is the next step for recurrent bleeding in the stable patient. Angioembolization is an option in very high-risk patients.
- Take the patient to the OR without delay when patients presents with any indication for surgery. Delayed therapy is associated with worst outcomes.
- If surgery is required, the goal is to stop the bleeding. If the patient is stable and has a history of previously treated *H. pylori* and current PPI use, consider TV in addition to drainage procedure.

SUGGESTED READINGS

Beaulieu R, Eckhauser F. The management of duodenal ulcers. In: Cameron JL, Cameron AM, eds. *Current Surgical Therapy.* 11th ed. Philadelphia, PA: Elsevier-Saunders, 2014.

Cheung F, Lau J. Management of massive peptic ulcer bleeding. *Gastroenterol Clin N Am.* 2009;38:231-243.

Craenen EM, Hofker HS, Peters FT, Kater GM, Glatman KR, Zijstra JG. An upper gastrointestinal ulcer still bleeding after endoscopy: what comes next?. *Neth J Med*;71:355-358.

Feinman M, Elliot H. Upper gastrointestinal bleeding. *Surg Clin N Am.* 2014;94:43-54.

Laine L. Upper gastrointestinal bleeding due to a peptic ulcer. *N Engl J Med.* 2016;374:2367-2376.

Lee C, Sarosi G. Emergency ulcer surgery. *Surg Clin N Am.* 2011;91:1001-1013.

Lu Y, Chen Y, Barkun A. Endoscopic management of acute peptic ulcer bleeding. *Gastroenterol Clin N Am.* 2014;43:677-705.

Lundell L. Upper gastrointestinal hemorrhage—surgical aspects. *Dig Dis.* 2003;21:16-18.

Millat B, Fingerhut A, Borie F. Surgical treatment of complicated duodenal ulcers: controlled trials. *World J Surg.* 2000;24:299-306.

Rotondano G. Epidemiology and diagnosis of acute nonvariceal upper gastrointestinal bleeding. *Gastroenterol Clin N Am.* 2014;43:643-663.

Tavakkolizadeh A, Stanley A. Operations for peptic ulcer. In: Yeo CJ, Matthews JB, McFadden DW, Pemberton JH, Peters JH, eds. *Shackelford's Surgery of The Alimentary Tract.* 7th ed. Philadelphia, PA: Elsevier-Saunders; 2013.

Lower Gastrointestinal Bleeding

SCOTT E. REGENBOGEN

Based on the previous edition chapter "Lower Gastrointestinal Bleeding" by Scott E. Regenbogen

Case Presentation

A 53-year-old man presents to the emergency room with painless, bright red bleeding from the rectum. The bleeding is described as large volume, occurring three times in the preceding 8 hours. His medical history includes hypertension and obesity. He takes a daily aspirin and occasional ibuprofen for back pain. He has never had a colonoscopy. He has no family history of colorectal cancer. His blood pressure is 90/55, and heart rate is 120 per minute. Abdominal exam is normal. There is blood in the rectal vault, but no palpable mass.

● DIFFERENTIAL DIAGNOSIS

Bright red rectal bleeding typically comes from the colon or rectum, though in 10% to 15% of patients, brisk hematochezia results from upper gastrointestinal bleeding (UGIB), and another 10% to 15% originate in the small bowel. Diverticular hemorrhage is the most commonly identified source of major lower gastrointestinal bleeding (LGIB) in adults. Other common causes include inflammatory bowel disease and neoplasms, and in older adults, colonic angiodysplasia. In children and young adults, LGIB is most commonly caused by inflammatory bowel disease, Meckel's diverticula, or benign polyps. Minor intermittent bleeding in any age group may be related to anorectal disease, such as hemorrhoids or fissures. Ischemic colitis should be considered in patients with atherosclerotic disease, dehydration, or other causes of restricted mesenteric perfusion.

● WORKUP

After obtaining large-bore venous access, a sample for blood type and crossmatch is sent. Hematocrit is 18%; coagulation studies are normal. Nasogastric tube aspirate is bilious, without blood. Anoscopy reveals small, nonbleeding hemorrhoids. He is admitted to the intensive care unit and resuscitated with packed red blood cells. His blood pressure normalizes, and the bleeding seems to subside.

A bowel preparation is administered, and colonoscopy of the following day reveals extensive diverticulosis (Figure 32-1) and dark blood in the descending and transverse colon. Later that evening, he has another large bloody bowel movement

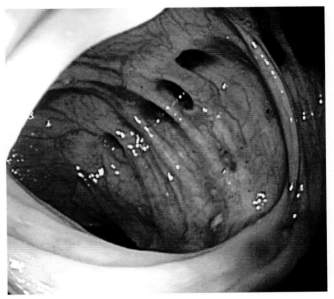

FIGURE 32-1. Colonoscopy in patient with lower gastrointestinal bleeding, revealing diverticulosis, but no source of active bleeding.

and becomes hypotensive. Again, his blood pressure improves after transfusion. Urgent mesenteric angiography is performed. There is evidence of atherosclerotic disease, but no active bleeding is identified (Figure 32-2A and B).

● DIAGNOSIS AND TREATMENT

Diverticular bleeding accounts for about half of acute LGIB hospitalizations in the United States and an even greater share of cases among older adults. Risk factors for bleeding among individuals with diverticulosis include systemic anticoagulation, hypertension, and use of nonsteroidal anti-inflammatory drugs (NSAIDs) or steroids. The bleeding can be massive and even life threatening, but it is often a diagnosis of exclusion, as the bleeding will cease spontaneously in 80% of cases, usually before the source can be identified. Recurrent bleeding will, however, occur in 15% to 30% of these patients.

Initial management is supportive, including close hemodynamic monitoring, and, in appropriate cases, blood transfusion. Surgery is rarely required for management, except in cases with hemodynamic instability refractory

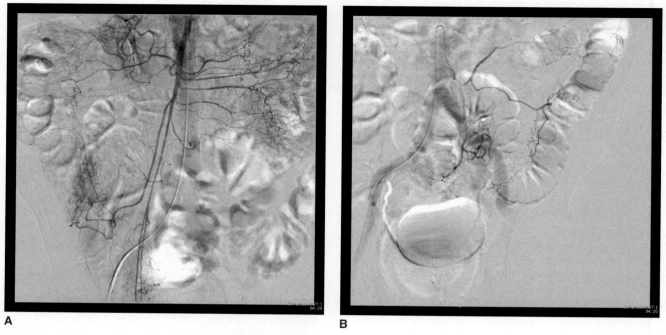

A **B**

FIGURE 32-2. Images from selective mesenteric angiogram revealing normal anatomy without evidence of active bleeding from the **(A)** superior mesenteric artery distribution and **(B)** inferior artery distribution.

to resuscitation and transfusion, or recurrent or ongoing bleeding that cannot be controlled by other means. When bleeding persists, all efforts should be made to localize the source, in an attempt to focus surgical resection and ensure that bleeding is indeed arising from the colon. A suggested algorithm for the evaluation of presumed diverticular LGIB is shown in Figure 32-3. Those with suspicion of UGIB (bloody nasogastric aspirate, history of peptic ulcer disease, recent

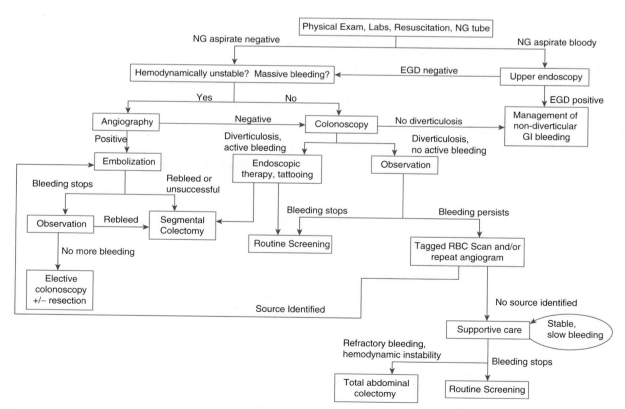

FIGURE 32-3. A suggested algorithm for the evaluation and management of patients with acute LGIB presumed to be from bleeding colonic diverticula.

NSAID use, cirrhosis, etc.) should undergo urgent upper endoscopy. Once an upper tract source has been excluded, the next test of choice may be either colonoscopy or angiography, depending on the patient's condition and institutional preference.

For patients with brisk ongoing bleeding, many advocate urgent angiography for localization and embolization. In some institutions, tagged red blood cell scan is used as a screening test, because of its higher sensitivity, to decide which patients will undergo angiography. If a bleeding source is found on angiography, selective therapeutic embolization is attempted. If successful, patients can undergo elective colonoscopy after the bleeding episode has resolved. Colon resection in this setting is not obligatory, because <20% of embolization patients will develop mucosal ischemia in the devascularized colon. If bleeding cannot be controlled with embolization, the angiographer can leave a catheter in the bleeding vessel, to facilitate localization at the time of surgery. In patients with recurrent intermittent bleeding and repeatedly negative angiograms, "provocative" angiography may be considered, using catheter-directed vasodilators, anticoagulants, or thrombolytics to reactivate a quiescent bleeding source. Provocative procedures should be performed only if urgent surgical intervention can be performed when needed.

Others advocate urgent colonoscopy for patients with ongoing bleeding, either with a "rapid-purge" bowel preparation with polyethylene glycol or preparation by enema only. Rates of colonoscopy completion and of successful localization of bleeding in this setting vary widely in the literature. Some nonrandomized studies have suggested that urgent colonoscopy with endoscopic epinephrine injection, coagulation, and/or clipping reduces rates of rebleeding, as compared with delayed colonoscopy. The only randomized study on the topic (Green et al., see Suggested Readings), however, found that urgent colonoscopy increased rates of localization, without reduction in mortality, length of stay, or need for surgical resection. In a hemodynamically stable patient, it is reasonable, therefore, to perform colonoscopy either promptly during the acute hospitalization or electively after resolution of the bleeding episode. Regardless of timing, all patients with acute LGIB who have not had a recent complete colon evaluation should undergo colonoscopy to exclude neoplasm.

Despite all attempts, bleeding can be difficult to localize in patients with intermittent diverticular bleeding. Some patients may require surgery even in the absence of localization, due to repeated episodes of bleeding or acute hemodynamic instability. Because diverticulosis is most common in the sigmoid and descending colon, empiric left-sided resections were once advocated for such nonlocalized LGIB. However, segmental resection in the absence of a demonstrated source carries significantly greater risk of recurrent bleeding than total colectomy in this setting and has fallen out of favor. Instead, when resection is required for unlocalized LGIB, total abdominal colectomy is recommended.

Presentation Continued

After angiography, the bleeding stops, and the patient is transferred out of the intensive care unit. Two days later, he has severe abdominal cramping, becomes hypotensive, and has a very large bloody bowel movement, associated with a 10% drop in hematocrit. Repeat angiography again fails to demonstrate a definite source of bleeding. He is persistently hypotensive, so with resuscitation ongoing, he is taken urgently to the operating room. Colonoscopy in the operating room reveals bright blood throughout the colon, but a discrete source cannot be identified.

● SURGICAL APPROACH FOR TOTAL ABDOMINAL COLECTOMY

Patients with persistent unlocalized bleeding may require operation (Table 32-1). After adequate resuscitation and correction of coagulopathy, all efforts should again be made to

Table 32-1 Total Abdominal Colectomy

Key Technical Steps

1. Lithotomy position or supine with split-leg position
2. Exploration for source of bleeding (colonoscopy, enteroscopy, bimanual palpation)
3. Mobilize ascending colon and hepatic flexure, ligate ileocolic vascular pedicle, divide ileum
4. If preserving omentum, separate from transverse colon; if resecting omentum, divide and ligate outside the gastroepiploic arcade
5. Mobilize sigmoid and descending colon, take down splenic flexure, ligate inferior mesenteric and middle colic vascular pedicles
6. Mobilize and ligate upper mesorectum, and divide across upper rectum
7. Construct ileorectal anastomosis or ileostomy

Potential Pitfalls

- Failure to identify an upper GI or small bowel source of bleeding
- Ureteral injury, typically due to dissection into the retroperitoneum, or during ligation of the inferior mesenteric artery pedicle
- Duodenal injury, due to dissection too far posteriorly on approach to the hepatic flexure
- Avulsion of a middle colic vein due to excessive traction on the hepatic flexure
- Splenic capsule laceration due to excessive traction on attachments to the splenic flexure
- Hypogastric nerve injury during mobilization of the upper mesorectum

localize bleeding in the operating room before undertaking resection. The patient should be positioned in the lithotomy or split-leg position to permit access to the anus for colonoscopy and/or anastomotic leak testing. Exploration and resection are typically performed through a midline laparotomy, but in a hemodynamically stable patient without prohibitive intra-abdominal adhesions, may be performed laparoscopically with or without hand assistance by surgeons with expertise in laparoscopic colon surgery. Trocar arrangements for total colectomy vary, but we favor the use of an umbilical trocar for the camera and dissecting ports in all four quadrants. When using a hand-assist technique, a hand port is placed in the suprapubic position, through a Pfannenstiel or lower midline incision. The specimen can be extracted through the hand port incision, or through a suprapubic, periumbilical, or stoma incision, depending on approach and anatomy. On-table colonoscopy, ideally with carbon dioxide insufflation can be used to evaluate the colon intraoperatively. A colonoscope passed orally can often traverse the entire small intestine if the bowel is manually reduced over the scope. Bimanual palpation and transillumination of the intestine can identify mass lesions. If no convincing source can be identified, but bleeding is absent proximal to the ileocecal valve, total abdominal colectomy is recommended.

The colon is mobilized from the retroperitoneum by incision along the line of Toldt. On the right, the ureter and gonadal vessels are identified and protected within the retroperitoneum, and the duodenum is swept posteriorly as dissection approaches the hepatic flexure. Care must be taken to avoid avulsing venous tributaries of the superior mesenteric vein as the flexure is elevated medially. The gastrocolic omentum can be preserved, by separating it from the transverse colon, or resected with the specimen by dividing it outside the gastroepiploic arcade. The transverse mesocolon is separated from the omentum, then mobilized from the retroperitoneum through dissection in the lesser sac. At this point, division of the ileum and ileocolic pedicle facilitates exposure for mobilization of the left and sigmoid colon. On the left, care is taken to avoid injury to the splenic capsule when taking down the flexure, and the ureter and gonadal vessels must be identified and protected in the retroperitoneum during mobilization of the sigmoid colon and ligation of the inferior mesenteric artery pedicle. As dissection continues behind the upper rectum in the presacral space, the hypogastric nerves, which contribute to sexual function, are preserved by sweeping them down off the mesorectum. After ligating the remaining mesenteric vasculature, the bowel is divided across the upper rectum, either with a linear stapler or between bowel clamps, and the specimen is passed off the field. Intestinal continuity can be restored with an ileorectal anastomosis, or end ileostomy can be constructed and the rectal stump turned in and left closed.

● SPECIAL INTRAOPERATIVE CONSIDERATIONS

Because most LGIBs are managed without surgery, those patients who require total abdominal colectomy in this setting typically will be either acutely unstable or debilitated from protracted preoperative manipulations. In the presence of hemodynamic instability, malnutrition, major comorbidity, inflammatory disease of the terminal ileum or rectum, or poor anal sphincter function and fecal incontinence, ileorectal anastomosis should be avoided and end ileostomy performed. Ileostomy and mucous fistula is also an option, but the divided rectum typically will not reach the abdominal wall, so the distal transection must occur above the rectosigmoid junction if mucous fistula is planned. The finding of an unexpected malignancy requires careful attention to an oncologically appropriate mesenteric lymphadenectomy. Other unexpected findings, such as inflammatory bowel disease, Meckel's diverticulum, arterial–intestinal fistula, or others, would require alteration of the operative plan and a focus on the source of bleeding.

● POSTOPERATIVE MANAGEMENT

Because of the extensive abdominal dissection, postoperative ileus after total abdominal colectomy is common. Total parenteral nutrition is often required, because patients who require surgery for LGIB may have suffered through extensive preoperative workup with prolonged restriction of oral nutrition. Routine prophylaxis for deep venous thrombosis should be used. Postoperative antibiotics are not typically necessary. After return of bowel function, stool output may be liquid and high volume, and the use of bulking agents plus antidiarrheal medications such as loperamide or diphenoxylate/atropine are often required to avoid dehydration. After the initial recovery period, most patients will continue permanently with several stools per day. Patients with good preoperative anal sphincter function will typically not suffer major deterioration in their continence.

Anastomotic leak rates after ileorectal anastomosis range from 2% to 5%. Leak can present as fever, pain, ileus, diarrhea, tenesmus, urinary retention, or fistula. Depending on patient condition and the location, size, and spread of the leak, management might involve simple observation, percutaneous drainage, transanal repair, or reoperation with repair or resection of anastomosis and fecal diversion.

TAKE HOME POINTS

- Diverticular bleeding accounts for a majority of LGIB requiring hospitalization in adults.
- Diverticular bleeding is self-limited in 80% of cases, but 15% to 30% will have recurrent bleeding.
- Options for localization of LGIB include angiography, flexible endoscopy, capsule endoscopy, and nuclear scintigraphy.
- Indications for surgery in LGIB include recurrent refractory bleeding or hemodynamic instability.
- The operation of choice for unlocalized LGIB distal to the ileocecal valve is total abdominal colectomy, with ileorectal anastomosis or end ileostomy.

SUGGESTED READINGS

ASGE Standards of Practice Committee. An annotated algorithmic approach to acute lower gastrointestinal bleeding. *Gastrointest Endosc.* 2001;53:859-863.

ASGE Standards of Practice Committee. The role of endoscopy in the patient with lower-GI bleeding. *Gastrointest Endosc.* 2005; 62:656-660.

Green BT, Rockey DC, Portwood G, et al. Urgent colonoscopy for evaluation and management of acute lower gastrointestinal hemorrhage: a randomized controlled trial. *Am J Gastroenterol.* 2005;100:2395-2402.

Hoedema RE, Luchtefeld MA. The management of lower gastrointestinal hemorrhage. *Dis Colon Rectum.* 2005;48:2010-2024.

Jensen DM, Machicado GA, Jutabha R, Kovacs TOG. Urgent colonoscopy for the diagnosis and treatment of severe diverticular hemorrhage. *N Engl J Med.* 2000;342:78-82.

Khanna A, Ognibene SJ, Koniaris LG. Embolization as first-line therapy for diverticulosis-related massive lower gastrointestinal bleeding: evidence from a meta-analysis. *J Gastrointest Surg.* 2005;9:343-352.

Hepatobiliary

Bile Duct Injury

EMILY R. WINSLOW AND CHRISTOPHER J. SONNENDAY

Based on the previous edition chapter "Bile Duct Injury" by Christopher J. Sonnenday

Presentation

A 57-year-old woman underwent an outpatient laparoscopic cholecystectomy for biliary colic. She notes anorexia, nausea, and vomiting beginning 2 days postoperatively and by 7 days post-op becomes jaundiced. Past medical history is notable for obesity, asthma, and fibromyalgia.

On physical exam, the patient appears uncomfortable and tired. Vital signs are notable for a temperature of 36.8°C, pulse of 84 beats per minute, blood pressure of 176/86, respiratory rate of 18, and an oxygen saturation of 96%. Her sclera and skin are icteric. The abdomen is mildly distended with RUQ tenderness but no peritonitis. Her laparoscopic port site incisions are dry and intact without erythema or induration.

● DIFFERENTIAL DIAGNOSIS

Abdominal pain following laparoscopic cholecystectomy, particularly pain significant enough to require an emergency room evaluation, should immediately prompt evaluation for technical complications of the procedure. Postoperative pain following laparoscopic cholecystectomy, now often accomplished as an outpatient operation, is generally moderate and should improve each subsequent postoperative day. It is unusual for otherwise healthy patients to require narcotic analgesics after the first 3 to 5 postoperative days, if at all. Patients who do not follow this expected course should be evaluated thoroughly, as early recognition and treatment of complications of cholecystectomy are paramount to limiting the impact of these events on the patient.

Complications common to any laparoscopic procedure should always be considered when evaluating the patient with abdominal pain following laparoscopic cholecystectomy. Inadvertent injury to the bowel from trocar placement or instrument passing may present with peritonitis and postoperative sepsis. Evidence of urinary tract or surgical site infection should be queried. Constipation or ileus may also be seen in some patients, but lack of return of bowel function should lead to consideration of a more serious underlying complication.

The major complications specific to laparoscopic cholecystectomy include postoperative hemorrhage, a retained common bile duct stone, and bile duct injury. Bleeding complications following cholecystectomy are rare and often present in the first 24 to 48 hours postoperatively. Common etiologies include hemorrhage from the cystic artery stump or liver parenchyma along the gallbladder fossa. A retained common bile duct stone may present days to weeks following cholecystectomy and is typically associated with signs and symptoms of obstructive jaundice, cholangitis, and/or pancreatitis. Other rare but important complications to consider include duodenal injury or postoperative pancreatitis. The former is related to the difficulty of the dissection and degree of preoperative inflammation; the latter can be the result of either endoscopic retrograde cholangiopancreatography (ERCP) performed just prior to surgery, the use of intraoperative cholangiography, or the presence of intraductal stones or sludge.

There is a spectrum of severity in patients with bile duct injury. Many patients have a biliary leak that is not due to complete transection of the hepatic duct but instead to an incompletely occluded cystic duct, biliary leak from biliary radicals in the hepatic parenchyma just deep to the cystic plate, or more rarely to a lateral injury to the main or sectional bile ducts. However, transection of the bile duct represents the most feared technical complication of cholecystectomy. It can present in protean ways dependent on whether the primary injury results in obstruction of the main duct or rather with free bile spillage from the hepatic duct or its tributaries. Maintaining a high index of suspicion for bile duct injury in patients with unexpected problems following cholecystectomy is essential to making an early and definitive diagnosis. Sending a patient with unusual postoperative pain home from the clinic or emergency room without proper assessment can have catastrophic consequences if underlying intra-abdominal sepsis or biliary obstruction is unaddressed.

● WORKUP

Evaluation of the postcholecystectomy patient with suspected complications should proceed in a methodical manner. Initial maneuvers include administration of appropriate analgesia and fluid resuscitation as indicated. Laboratory evaluation should include a complete blood count, metabolic panel, liver profile, amylase, lipase, coagulation profile, and urinalysis. The initial laboratory results can be helpful in guiding the selection of appropriate imaging procedures and other interventions. Laboratory evaluation may initially be underwhelming, though a leukocytosis may be present. When only a sectional duct is obstructed, the laboratory evaluation may be completely normal. The total bilirubin may be normal or only slightly elevated (2 to 4 mg/dL) in the case of a complete biliary transection with free leak. Reabsorption of bile from the peritoneum may elevate the bilirubin slightly. Marked elevation of the transaminases is not typical and should raise concern of an associated vascular injury when present. Biliary injuries are typically not associated with abnormalities of the serum amylase and lipase. When associated with an obstructive pattern to the liver profile, biochemical evidence of pancreatitis may indicate a retained common bile duct stone rather than a bile duct injury.

Initial diagnostic imaging may include ultrasound, to assess for perihepatic fluid collections and biliary ductal dilation, or computed tomography (CT) in select patients. If identified, significant perihepatic collections or generalized ascites may be percutaneously drained. If the fluid is bilious, a biliary injury of some type is definitely diagnosed, and the evaluation should proceed with direct cholangiography either by endoscopic retrograde cholangiography (ERC) or by percutaneous transhepatic cholangiography (PTC) in order to clarify the etiology of the leak and allow control. It is important to emphasize however that the priority in the initial stages of the patient's evaluation is control of the biliary leak, treatment of associated infectious sequelae, and management of the patient's symptoms. It is important to remember that it is not essential to understand the anatomic details of the leak at the outset.

Role of HIDA Scan

If the fluid visualized on ultrasound or CT is not easily drained, or if the question of a biliary injury is still unanswered, a hepatobiliary iminodiacetic acid (HIDA) nuclear medicine scan may be performed. HIDA scans can detect extravasation

of biliary drainage and may also demonstrate failure of bile excreted from the liver to enter the duodenum. Further anatomic detail is not available from HIDA scans, but the test may be sufficient to confirm a suspicion of biliary injury before proceeding to more invasive means of cholangiography. If a bile leak is already confirmed with aspiration of abdominal fluid or placement of a percutaneous drain, a HIDA scan will almost never add additional useful clinical information.

Role of Axial Imaging

CT imaging is most useful in patients with biliary injury to demonstrate the extent and location of intra-abdominal bilious collections and to later document control of those. CT angiography is probably the best way to evaluate the patency of the right hepatic artery, which should always be assessed before making a decision about the timing of reconstruction. Magnetic resonance cholangiopancreatography (MRCP) is an attractive noninvasive imaging option before direct cholangiography and is particularly useful when trying to distinguish between a biliary leak and a biliary transection. MR cholangiography with biliary-specific contrast agents (e.g., Eovist) can add complementary information to direct cholangiography about the patient's specific biliary anatomy as well. An important limitation of MR imaging is that it can be difficult for patients with significant abdominal discomfort to tolerate the lengthy exam and cooperate fully with breath-holding maneuvers. Additionally, either CT or MR imaging is essential in understanding the anatomic details in cases with more complicated patterns of vasculobiliary injury (Figure 33-1A and B).

Role of Cholangiography

The decision to proceed first with endoscopic (ERC) or percutaneous (PTC) cholangiography can be challenging. In cases

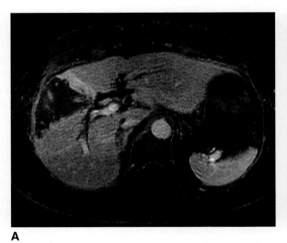 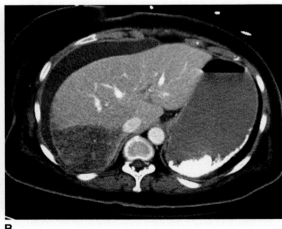

A   **B**

FIGURE 33-1. Vasculobiliary injury with hepatic infarction after cholecystectomy with associated ductal injuries. **A:** MR image with injury to the right anterior sectional portal vein and artery and subsequent infarction of segments 5 and 8. In this case, there was no ductal occlusion, and the injury at the biliary confluence was draining into an operatively placed subhepatic drain. **B:** CT image with injury to the right posterior sectional portal vein and artery and subsequent infarction of segments 6 and 7. The fluid around the liver is undrained bile from the associated injury to the hepatic confluence, and at this point post injury, it was not yet well drained.

where it is clear intraoperatively that there has been complete transection of the bile duct, there is no role for ERC, and proceeding directly to PTC is most effective. In cases where there is little concern for injury to the main duct and the clinical suspicion is that of a cystic duct or hepatic bed leak, ERC is clearly both diagnostic and therapeutic. In cases that are less clear cut, the usual choice is to start with ERC and, if a complete transection is found, then proceed to PTC.

In injuries in which the continuity of the extrahepatic biliary tree is preserved, ERC is both diagnostic and therapeutic. Endoscopic sphincterotomy and placement of an endobiliary stent is often sufficient to treat biliary leaks from the cystic duct stump or small accessory ducts (Figure 33-2). Incomplete transections may be bridged by endobiliary stents, with the need for subsequent operative intervention determined over time. In cases of common bile duct ligation, or in instances where a segment of the extrahepatic duct is excised with the gallbladder leaving an open proximal and distal extrahepatic bile duct, ERC will be diagnostic but not therapeutic. In these cases, PTC with placement of transhepatic biliary drains is typically necessary and should be performed in all patients with suspected bile duct injury in whom ERC was either not technically feasible or not definitive.

PTC in a patient without biliary ductal dilation is technically challenging and requires sophisticated interventional radiology resources and expertise. It is often necessary to place additional percutaneous drains to control bile leakage and drain infected bilomas and delay definitive source control until there are more favorable conditions. This can require a period of time to elapse so that either a percutaneous drain can be used to opacify the intrahepatic ductal system or the intrahepatic biliary ducts begin to dilate.

These patients truly require multidisciplinary management to ensure that procedures are coordinated with the goals of improving the patient's condition, defining the relevant anatomy, and facilitating eventual definitive repair. For this reason, the hepatobiliary surgeon and interventional radiologist need to work together in all decisions about placement of drains and transhepatic catheters and the timing of these procedures.

● CLASSIFICATION OF BILIARY INJURIES

Direct cholangiography allows classification of the type of biliary injury (Figure 33-3) according to the Bismuth-Strasberg classification. Type A injuries occur due to

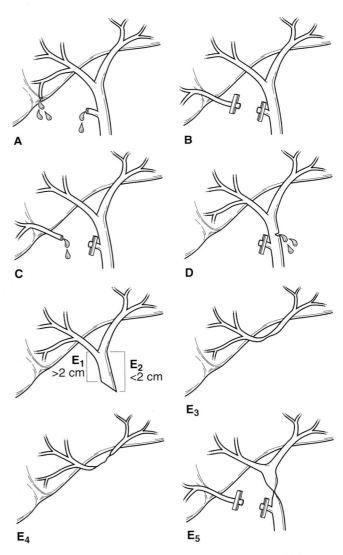

FIGURE 33-3. The Bismuth-Strasberg classification of biliary injuries following laparoscopic cholecystectomy. (Reprinted with permission from Winslow ER, Fialkowski EA, Linehan DC, et al. "Sideways": results of repair of biliary injuries using a policy of side-to-side hepatico-jejunostomy. *Ann Surg.* 2009;249(3):426-434.)

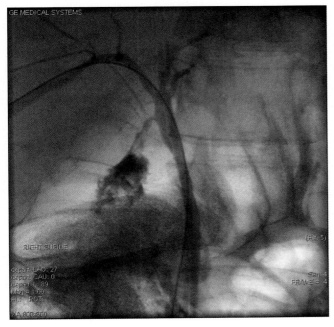

FIGURE 33-2. A lateral injury (Strasberg D) to the insertion of a right posterior duct without transection. The wire seen was placed endoscopically and a sphincterotomy performed prior to biliary stent placement.

leakage from the cystic duct stump or accessory ducts draining directly into the gallbladder (ducts of Luschka) and present as a biliary leak and/or subhepatic biloma. Type B injuries are defined as ligation and division of an anomalous right-sided segmental hepatic duct, typically the duct draining segment 6 (±segment 7). This injury is often facilitated by the associated anomaly where the anterior and posterior sectional duct drain separately into the common duct or more rarely by a cystic duct that drains into the right posterior duct. The proximal and distal ends of the anomalous segmental duct are clipped and divided during control of the cystic duct. Type B injuries are often asymptomatic or may present late with abdominal pain or cholangitis involving the occluded liver segment. Normally, the liver behind a type B injury will indolently atrophy over time, but some patients may have pain associated with the occlusion. Type C injuries occur in the same anatomic setting as type B injuries, though the proximal ductal segment is not ligated and leaks freely into the peritoneal cavity. This injury results in the symptoms associated with bile peritonitis. The difficulty in isolated right-sided injuries lies in their diagnosis, as ERC will not demonstrate a leak and often does not bring to attention the "missing" sectional or segmental ducts (Figure 33-4A and B). This is a perfect illustration of the importance of careful inspection of all cholangiograms for visualization of all sectional (and preferably segmental) ducts.

In type D injuries, a lateral injury to the extrahepatic bile duct occurs, either sharply or by thermal injury. The biliary tree remains in continuity, and the injury may manifest with a leak initially or a stricture in a delayed presentation. These injuries may be diagnosed accurately by ERC, which can also provide definitive treatment via endobiliary stenting.

Type E injuries are defined by complete disruption of biliary–enteric continuity due to transection, excision, and/or ligation of the extrahepatic biliary tree. Injuries that include a free biliary leak will present early with bile peritonitis and sepsis. Injuries with occlusion of the proximal hepatic drainage may present in a more delayed fashion with jaundice and/or cholangitis but still typically within 2 weeks of cholecystectomy as all biliary drainage is occluded. Type E injuries are further described according to the Bismuth classification (E1 to E5, as depicted in Figure 33-3), with important implications about the complexity of definitive repair. Type E injuries will require PTC to definitively characterize the anatomic extent of the injury and to establish stable biliary drainage.

In the present case, CT demonstrates the patient to have intrahepatic biliary ductal dilation without ascites or peritoneal collections. There is also a large abscess in the right anterior section with evidence of right hepatic artery occlusion. Magnetic resonance imaging (MRI) examination confirms an E4 injury (Figure 33-5A). PTC is performed demonstrating separation of the right and left hepatic ducts without biliary leak. Percutaneous biliary tubes are left bilaterally, and a pigtail catheter is placed in the hepatic abscess (Figure 33-5B and C). Antimicrobial therapy and general supportive care are initiated.

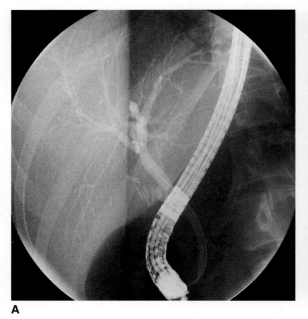

A

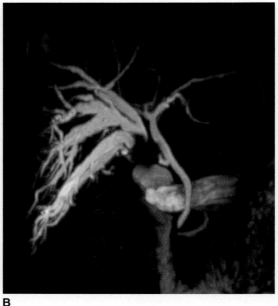

B

FIGURE 33-4. This patient had a laparoscopic cholecystectomy without obvious immediate complication but had persistent right upper quadrant pain for months. She underwent an ERCP **(A)**, which was interpreted as normal given that the common duct, right and left hepatic ducts, can be seen. She continued to have pain and several months later got an MRCP **(B)**, which demonstrated an occluded right posterior sectional duct with separation of the ducts to segments 6 and 7. The R anterior duct joins the left hepatic duct normally as shown on the fluoroscopic images.

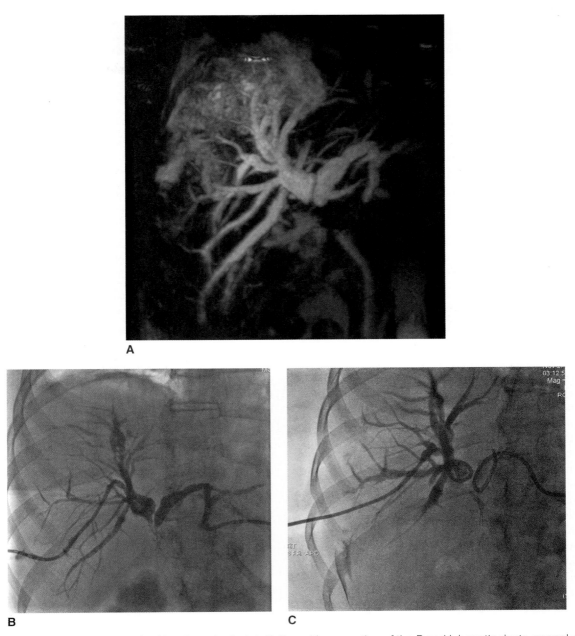

FIGURE 33-5. A: demonstrates marked intrahepatic ductal dilation with separation of the R and L hepatic ducts, normal decompressed common bile duct, and a large right hepatic abscess. Percutaneous cholangiography **(B)** confirms that finding and clearly demonstrates an E4 injury. Bilateral biliary tubes are placed **(C)**.

● DIAGNOSIS AND TREATMENT

The management of bile duct injuries should be catered to the condition of the patient, timing of the injury, and anatomic details according to the Bismuth-Strasberg classification. Principles that apply in all cases include control of sepsis, drainage of all intra-abdominal collections, and establishment of secure biliary drainage. Ongoing reassessment of the patient's clinical condition, with reimaging as clinically indicated to detect undrained bilomas, will get even the frailest patients through what can be tenuous early stages of their injury, allowing definitive repair to be performed in an

elective fashion with the patient in better condition. Timing of definitive repair for those patients that require biliary reconstruction is an individualized decision that requires careful surgical judgment.

Specific treatment strategies for bile duct injuries can be determined according to the Bismuth-Strasberg classification, as summarized in Table 33-1. The decision-making about the urgency of intervention and the need for surgical reconstruction varies based upon the timing of the patient's presentation and the patient's clinical condition. In the case of an injury recognized intraoperatively at the time of cholecystectomy, immediate repair should only be performed

Table 33-1	The Bismuth-Strasberg Classification of Biliary Injuries Following Laparoscopic Cholecystectomy		
Bismuth-Strasberg Classification	**Description**	**Extrahepatic Bile Duct in Continuity**	**Treatment**
Type A	Bile leak from cystic duct or accessory hepatic duct (duct of Luschka)	Yes	Endoscopic sphincterotomy and endobiliary stent placement
Type B	Ligation of posterior segment hepatic duct	Partially (posterior segment[s] excluded)	Hepaticojejunostomy in symptomatic patients
Type C	Bile leak from injured posterior hepatic duct	Partially (posterior segment[s] excluded)	Percutaneous transhepatic biliary drainage, followed by hepaticojejunostomy
Type D	Lateral injury with incomplete transection of the extrahepatic bile duct	Yes	Endoscopic sphincterotomy and endobiliary stent placement; hepaticojejunostomy if refractory stricture develops
Type E	Circumferential injury (ligation and/or transection) to hepatic duct(s)	No	Percutaneous transhepatic biliary drainage, followed by hepaticojejunostomy

when adequate surgical experience and expertise are available and the extent of the injury and sectional biliary ductal anatomy are completely understood. The inability to perform good quality cholangiography and the lack of surgical experience with biliary–enteric anastomoses are examples of contraindications to immediate repair. Other contraindications to early repair include a major vascular injury, hemodynamic instability, excessive blood loss, and a thermal injury to the duct with extensive devitalized tissue. The surgeon considering early repair needs to carefully consider if the inflammatory condition, which led to the injury, also will pose similar challenges for biliary reconstruction.

In the case of patients who present early after cholecystectomy (within the first 72 hours), early repair may be considered if the patient is clinically well without signs of sepsis or hepatic dysfunction and the anatomic details of the injury are well understood with cholangiography. Contraindications to early repair include associated vascular injury, thermal injury with extensive devitalized tissue, and E3 or greater injuries where achieving a quality repair to healthy tissue can be difficult in the acute setting. In the reconstruction of a biliary injury, it is important to emphasize that a successful outcome is only appropriately measured over the course of a patient's lifetime. The best chance of long-term stricture-free biliary patency is to optimize the conditions associated with the initial restoration at biliary–enteric continuity, as subsequent revisions and interventions are much more challenging.

In patients presenting beyond 72 hours from cholecystectomy, and/or with signs of intra-abdominal sepsis, the initial priorities should be appropriate resuscitation, broad-spectrum antibiotics, cross-sectional imaging, and percutaneous drainage of all significant fluid collections. Direct cholangiography via ERC or PTC is the next step, with an attempt to obtain definitive internal or external biliary

drainage. Once biliary drainage is established, the pressure of time is removed and the patient should be allowed to recover from the cholecystectomy and any associated sepsis. Most hepatobiliary surgeons will wait 6 to 8 weeks or more before proceeding with biliary reconstruction. This delay allows for the resolution of any associated peritonitis, provides time for the ischemic portion of the duct to die back and for collateralized biliary blood flow to be established, and allows the patient to rehabilitate physically.

● SURGICAL APPROACH

Preoperative Preparation

An important component to the operative approach for patients with biliary injury is ensuring the patient is adequately prepared preoperatively. Preoperative preparation can be classified into three areas—physiologically, anatomically, and emotionally. The most important physiologic consideration for patients whose repair is delayed is the management of fluid status during the period of external biliary drainage. Because most patients with diversion of all biliary outputs into drains will lose between 800 and 1500 mL of bile a day, careful attention must be paid to avoid volume depletion. The most physiologic way to replace the loss of fluid and electrolytes is to return the output to the gastrointestinal (GI) tract, which can be done via a feeding tube (e.g., nasojejunal or percutaneous gastrojejunal tubes) or simply by mouth. Additionally, patients may need additional intravenous fluids during this time. Weekly laboratory testing can help detect electrolyte imbalance or volume depletion before it becomes clinically apparent and when it can still be treated on an ambulatory basis. A related consideration is the development of depletion of the fat-soluble vitamins, particularly vitamin K. Many patients will require parenteral supplementation of vitamin K, even with bile refeeding, to maintain a normal coagulation profile. For obvious reasons, patients on warfarin preinjury will need to be transitioned to an alternative method of anticoagulation until biliary enteric continuity and hence reliable vitamin K absorption are restored. Because biliary diversion from the GI tract is an ulcerogenic state physiologically, many surgeons will treat patients with acid-suppressive therapy until after reconstruction. Finally, a thoughtful assessment of the patient's preoperative nutritional state is essential. For many reasons, most patients with biliary diversion have limited appetite and need to be encouraged and monitored to avoid being in a catabolic state at the time of operative repair. A home food journal, daily weights, use of nutritional supplements, and support of a nutritionist are all important adjuncts to help optimize nutritional reserves preoperatively.

A second area of preoperative preparation that is critical is to ensure complete ductal "accounting." The surgeon should have a full understanding of the biliary anatomy by rectifying all the imagings completed, including any preoperative studies available. Carefully comparing the axial imaging to the fluoroscopic imaging in order to have an appreciation of the drainage of each segmental duct before undertaking repair is critical. This fact cannot be overemphasized particularly in the case of complex injuries, such as E4 and E5 injuries where separation of the right anterior and posterior ductal systems can be difficult to repair without percutaneous tube placement preoperatively.

A third and final area of preoperative preparation is the patient's and family's emotional state. The very fact that the patient experienced a major surgical complication at the time of their cholecystectomy cannot simply be ignored at the time of the repair. Concerns about the potential for postrepair complications need to be thoroughly heard and addressed in advance. Spending time reviewing the postoperative recovery and what may be needed in the event of anastomotic leak or other complications is an important part of the comprehensive preparation of patients with Beck depression inventory (BDI).

Operative Approach

The preferred method for repairing most injuries is a Roux-en-Y hepaticojejunostomy (Table 33-2), and the key principles include creation of a large tension-free side-to-side anastomosis to healthy hepatic ducts that drain all biliary segments. Direct end-to-end repair of the extrahepatic bile duct is often unsatisfactory when a significant section of the duct has been devitalized or removed and is associated with a high rate of additional complications especially stricture.

Care should be taken to choose a part of the proximal jejunum that reaches easily to the right upper quadrant. The small bowel should be divided at an appropriate place

| Table 33-2 | Roux-en-Y Hepaticojejunostomy Procedure |

Key Technical Steps

1. Right subcostal incision, meticulous lysis of adhesions.
2. Careful portal dissection—mobilizing duodenum, omentum, hepatic flexure away from porta. Identify right and left lateral aspects of porta for proper orientation.
3. "Anterior-only" dissection of the hepatic duct.
4. Lowering of the hilar plate to allow exposure of the anterior aspect of the hepatic duct confluence.
5. Identify the long extrahepatic portion of the left hepatic duct to facilitate exposure of hepatic duct confluence.
6. Creation of tension-free Roux-en-Y limb, brought up to right upper quadrant via defect in transverse mesocolon to the right of the middle colic vessels.
7. Inspect biliary mucosa and seek an area for anastomosis where it is normal and not fibrotic appearing.
8. Reconcile the preoperative understanding of ductal anatomy with intraoperative findings and confirm all ductal orifices are included and adequately drained via the planned anastomosis.
9. Broad (2 cm) side-to-side biliary–enteric anastomosis using absorbable monofilament suture.
10. Closed suction drainage.

Potential Pitfalls

- Electing to perform repair too early, when peritonitis and adhesions from time of injury have not improved.
- Failure to account for all bile ducts preoperatively, risking exclusion of a duct from the anastomosis or including an injured duct but with inadequate mucosal exposure.
- Creation of the biliary–enteric anastomosis at the site of injury, to devitalized biliary tissue.
- Circumferential dissection of the hepatic duct, interrupting important collateral blood supply.
- Tension on the biliary–enteric anastomosis, caused by either failure to adequately mobilize the jejunum or placing the Roux limb in an antecolic position.

with a GIA stapler, and the mesentery divided to allow the Roux limb maximum mobility. Division of the first vascular arcade of the small bowel mesentery can usually be done safely, though the end of the Roux limb should always be inspected for sufficient perfusion. A retrocolic Roux-en-Y hepaticojejunostomy, brought to the right upper quadrant through a defect made in the mesocolon to the right of the middle colic vessels and above the duodenum, provides the most direct route to the porta and can avoid any undue tension created by draping the Roux limb over the colon. Alternatively, placing the Roux limb in a retrogastric retrocolic position allows similar advantages and puts the bowel in the least accessible position for injury during future unrelated operative interventions (e.g., right colectomy).

In patients with previous abdominal surgery, time should be taken to meticulously lyse any adhesions that tether the small bowel mesentery. In cases where patients have a foreshortened mesentery, due to previous surgery, radiation, or other conditions, a medial visceral rotation of the right colon will expose the root of the small bowel mesentery that can be mobilized up to the level of the duodenum and neck of the pancreas.

A few important principles apply to the dissection of the porta in the setting of a biliary injury. The mechanism of bile duct injury in these cases often arises from unintentional dissection of a long segment of the bile duct, which can strip the duct of its blood supply that runs through the periductal adventitial tissue. In early repair cases, it is therefore important to identify a portion of the duct that has not been completely dissected and carefully expose or shorten the hepatic duct in a location that is amenable to construction of the biliary anastomosis. In E1 injuries, it may be possible therefore to stay below the true hepatic duct bifurcation, but care should be taken not to sew to a traumatized end of the hepatic duct. Opening the duct on its anterior surface, with a ductotomy extended toward the long extrahepatic portion of the left hepatic duct, can expose healthy tissue and avoid dissection behind the duct, which can further compromise ductal blood supply. In later repair cases, avoiding dissection behind the hepatic duct is really essential, as this allows preservation of any collateralized blood supply that has been created at the site of the injury. This principle of "anterior-only" dissection also avoids creating additional vascular injury, as the right hepatic artery is often directly behind the hepatic duct at this level and can be obscured or difficult to identify in a chronically inflamed or scarred field. Several techniques can help facilitate the definitive identification of the biliary ducts when difficult conditions are present. Injection of the percutaneous biliary tubes with saline followed by needle aspiration in the location of the putative duct can be useful. Other strategies include the use of manual palpation of the stent, use of intraoperative ultrasound, or intraoperative cholangiography with use of orienting clamps or clips in the field.

All biliary anastomoses should be performed under loupe magnification, using fine monofilament absorbable suture, typically in an interrupted fashion. It is essential that the mucosa of the bile duct is carefully inspected and is normal appearing at the level of the anastomosis. If the anastomosis is fashioned to an area where the biliary mucosa is replaced by fibrosis, the likelihood of long-term patency is lessened. The stricture rate is also thought to be related to the size of the anastomosis, and it is therefore generally recommended that the ductotomy measures 2.0 to 2.5 cm in length.

Placement of subhepatic drains to monitor for biliary leak is typically performed. After completion of the biliary anastomosis, the Roux limb can be further anchored to relieve tension by taking seromuscular bites of the jejunum and tacking it to the former gallbladder fossa, portal plate, or umbilical fissure.

● SPECIAL INTRAOPERATIVE CONSIDERATIONS

For E2 injuries or higher, the hepatic duct bifurcation needs to be exposed by lowering the hilar plate. This involves incising into the liver parenchyma at the base of segment 4B to get above the hepatic duct bifurcation, beginning above the long extrahepatic course of the left hepatic duct. This can often be done with a blunt technique and judicious use of electrocautery but can be facilitated in difficult cases by the use of an ultrasonic or hydrojet dissector. Bleeding may be encountered during this technique, but can be stopped by packing gauze or other hemostatic material into the hepatotomy for a period of time. Returning to this area after completing other tasks, such as creating the enteroenterostomy of the Roux limb, allows performance of the biliary anastomosis in a dry and controlled field. In some cases, if there is a significant amount of overhanging liver in segment 4B, this may need to be resected to facilitate exposure and to allow room for the Roux limb to sit.

For injuries that result in an isolated right-sided system (B, C, E4, and E5), the approach to operative repair is more challenging. Important principles in these cases include opening up the lips of the gallbladder fossa, dividing the fibrous band at the base of the cystic plate, and coring the liver at the base of segment 5 to expose the anterior surface of the right portal pedicle. For reconstruction of isolated right-sided ducts, there length available for anastomosis is more limited. In this situation, the surgeon must decide if two separate anastomoses should be fashioned or if ductoplasty can allow for a more secure and wider "cloacal" anastomosis.

Controversy exists over the need for transhepatic biliary catheters to serve as a stent across a fresh biliary–enteric anastomosis. In the case of early repairs, many surgeons will go to the operating room without transhepatic catheters. Intraoperative placement of retrograde transhepatic biliary catheters is difficult and potentially adds additional trauma to the liver. Therefore in these cases, routine postoperative stenting is not possible or advised. In the case of delayed repairs, a transhepatic biliary catheter is typically in place at the time of repair and may be passed across the new biliary–enteric anastomosis. These tubes typically can be capped off ("internalized") in the immediate postoperative period if no evidence of anastomotic leak, used for postoperative cholangiography to interrogate the new anastomosis, and removed 3 to 6 weeks after repair.

● POSTOPERATIVE MANAGEMENT

The postoperative period in patients undergoing a biliary–enteric anastomosis is typical of other major upper abdominal operations. Appropriate analgesia, early mobilization, and sequential advancement in diet should occur in all patients. Wounds should be monitored for signs of infection, especially in patients with indwelling percutaneous biliary drains, which predispose to surgical site infection. Patients should be monitored for biliary leak or other signs of intra-abdominal infection. In cases where a closed suction drain is left at the time of operation, the output should be monitored for bilious fluid. Typically, the drain(s) can be removed in 3 to 4 days once the patient has resumed a diet if the output is not bilious. In the case of a low-volume biliary leak, observation with continued external drainage may be the only necessary intervention, as such leaks will resolve. In the case of a more significant leak, or a leak associated with signs of sepsis, percutaneous biliary drainage may be necessary if not already in place. Reoperation is typically not necessary for management of a biliary leak, but may be considered in select patients with high-volume biliary leaks in the first 24 to 48 hours postoperatively.

In the intermediate and long term, biliary stricture is the most significant potential postoperative event. As many as 15% of patients undergoing biliary reconstruction may develop an anastomotic stricture, with the majority of those patients able to be managed by percutaneous transhepatic dilation and stenting without the need for operative revision. Access to the hepaticojejunostomy for dilation and stenting may also be achieved via double-balloon enteroscopy in centers with that expertise available. The data suggest that as many as 5% of patients will require revision of the anastomosis over a 5-year follow-up period. As most biliary strictures may present indolently, a liver profile should be followed for signs of cholestasis. Often, an isolated rise in the alkaline phosphatase is the initial sign of a biliary stricture. A liver profile should be checked every 3 to 6 months for the first 2 years and then annually thereafter. The majority of anastomotic strictures will present in the first 2 years postoperatively, though some may present even in a markedly delayed fashion 1 to 2 decades postoperatively.

Case Conclusion

With percutaneous biliary drainage, drainage of the abscess, and antibiotics, the patient improves and is sent home. She is readmitted on two subsequent occasions for volume depletion and incomplete abscess drainage. After a 12-week delay, she is sufficiently improved and biliary reconstruction is performed with a Roux-en-Y hepaticojejunostomy with a ductoplasty to facilitate a single anastomosis. The left-sided biliary catheter is passed across the new biliary enteric anastomosis and removed after a follow-up cholangiogram at 3 weeks postoperatively revealing a widely patent anastomosis (Figure 33-6). At 8-year follow-up, the patient is clinically well with a normal liver profile.

TAKE HOME POINTS

- Patients who present following cholecystectomy with unusual pain or signs of infection should be considered to have a bile duct injury until proven otherwise.
- Initial diagnostic imaging of a patient with a suspected bile duct injury should include liver chemistries, ultrasound, and/or CT to assess for perihepatic fluid collections.

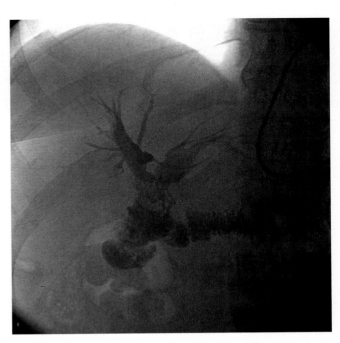

FIGURE 33-6. Postoperative injection of the biliary tube demonstrating patency of the hepaticojejunostomy. Contrast fills the right and left ductal systems and opacifies the Roux limb with prompt emptying. The tube was therefore removed.

- Initial management of bile duct injury should include control of sepsis, drainage of all bilomas, and establishment of secure internal or external biliary drainage.
- Patients who present beyond 48 to 72 hours from the time of their injury, and/or who show signs of intra-abdominal sepsis, are best managed with a delayed operative repair.
- A broad, side-to-side tension-free anastomosis using absorbable suture to healthy biliary mucosa is the preferred method for re-establishing biliary–enteric continuity.
- Biliary stricture is the primary significant long-term complication of hepaticojejunostomy; serial liver profile monitoring may detect an indolent stricture before it becomes clinically apparent.

SUGGESTED READINGS

AbdelRafee A, et al. Long-term followup of 120 patients after hepaticojejunostomy for treatment of post-cholecystectomy bile duct injuries: a retrospective cohort study. *Int Surg.* 2015;18:205-210.

Couinaud C. Exposure of the left hepatic duct through the hilum or in the umbilical of the liver: anatomic limitations. *Surgery.* 1989;105(1):21-27.

Fong ZV, et al. Diminished survival in patients with bile leaks and ductal injuries: management strategy influences outcomes. *J Am Coll Surg.* 2018;226:568. doi: 10.1016/j.jamcollsurg.2017.12.023.

Strasberg SM, et al. An analytical review of vasculobiliary injury in laparoscopic and open cholecystectomy. *HPB.* 2011;13:1-14.

Winslow ER, et al. "Sideways": results of repair of biliary injuries using a policy of side-to-side hepatico-jejunostomy. *Ann Surg.* 2009;249(3):426-434.

Severe Acute Pancreatitis

34

STEPHANIE NITZSCHKE AND STANLEY W. ASHLEY

Based on the previous edition chapter "Severe Acute Pancreatitis" by Marisa Cevasco, Stanley W. Ashley, and Amy L. Rezak

Presentation

A 39-year-old male with a history of alcohol abuse presents to the emergency department complaining of epigastric abdominal pain for the past 36 hours. He describes the pain as constant and radiating to his back. He also complains of nausea and has vomited several times. He had a normal bowel movement 1 day prior to presentation and denies melena. The patient is currently unemployed and recently divorced from his wife. He admits to drinking a case of beer each day for the past week. He denies smoking and illicit drug use. His family history is significant for hypertriglyceridemia.

Physical exam reveals abdominal distension and diffuse tenderness to palpation, worse over the epigastrium, but no guarding or rigidity. He is not jaundiced and has no Grey Turner's or Cullen's signs. His vital signs are notable for a temperature of 101°F, sinus tachycardia, and hypotension with a blood pressure of 90/60 mm Hg. He has palpable distal pulses and no pretibial edema.

● DIFFERENTIAL DIAGNOSIS

Epigastric abdominal pain radiating to the back, in a patient with a history of heavy alcohol consumption and a family history of hypertriglyceridemia, suggests acute pancreatitis. However, in a patient who is tachycardic, hypotensive, and vomiting, the differential diagnosis would also include perforated gastroduodenal ulcer and esophageal rupture (Boerhaave's syndrome). Cholecystitis and cholangitis are other important considerations, as these patients may present with fever, tachycardia, hypotension, and abdominal pain.

Presentation Continued

The patient has been hospitalized in the past for acute pancreatitis. He has no history of gallstone disease. Laboratory tests were notable for lipase of 18,200 U/L, amylase of 7,800 U/L, and mildly elevated transaminases (AST of 124 IU/L and ALT of 79 IU/L). Alkaline phosphatase, total bilirubin, and creatinine were within normal limits. Serum glucose was elevated at 230 mg/dL, and lactate

dehydrogenase (LDH) was 411 IU/L. He had a hematocrit of 48% and an elevated white blood cell (WBC) count of 16,400 cells/cm³. Triglycerides were 1,100 mg/dL. His respiratory rate was 16, and an arterial blood gas was notable for a pH of 7.31 and a P_aO_2 of 72 mm Hg. A Ranson score of 3 was calculated upon admission (Table 34-1).

A contrast-enhanced computerized tomographic (CT) scan of the abdomen and pelvis reveals stranding, inflammation, and edema within the peripancreatic area and extending inferiorly along the paracolic gutters to the pelvis (Figure 34-1). The low-attenuation area in the tail of the pancreas is consistent with necrosis and represents approximately 30% of the pancreatic parenchyma (Figure 34-2). Bowel wall thickening was also seen at the hepatic flexure of the transverse colon. There was no free air or evidence of biliary disease and no occlusion or thrombosis of the peripancreatic vasculature.

● WORKUP

This patient presents with severe acute necrotizing pancreatitis. The most common etiology of acute pancreatitis is obstructive biliary tract disease, responsible for up to 40% of cases. Excessive alcohol use is the second most common

Table 34-1	Ranson Criteria	
On Admission		**After 48 h**
Age > 55 y		Calcium < 8.0 mg/dL
WBC count > 16,000 cells/mm³		Hematocrit decreased > 10%
Blood glucose > 200 g/dL		Hypoxemia (P_aO_2 < 60 mm Hg)
AST > 250 IU/L		BUN increased by > 5 mg/dL
LDH > 350 IU/L		Base deficit > 4 mEq/L
		Sequestration of fluids > 6 L
Ranson score of:		
1–2:	1% mortality	
3–4:	15% mortality	
5–6:	40% mortality	

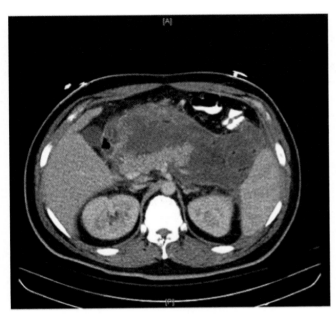

FIGURE 34-1. CT scan of the abdomen with IV and oral contrast reveals stranding, inflammation, and edema within the peripancreatic area.

cause of pancreatitis, responsible for approximately 35% of cases. Other causes include hypertriglyceridemia, endoscopic retrograde pancreatography (ERCP), anatomic abnormalities (e.g., pancreatic divisum), idiopathic, and abdominal trauma.

Nearly 20% to 30% of patients with acute pancreatitis have pancreatic necrosis; therefore, it is vital to determine the severity of pancreatitis. The Ranson criteria, based on the presence of 11 clinical signs (five measured at the time of admission and six measured 48 hours after admission), indicates the severity

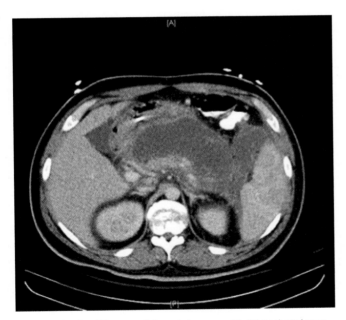

FIGURE 34-2. CT scan of the abdomen with IV and oral contrast reveals low attenuation of the tail of the pancreas. This is consistent with necrosis and represents approximately 30% of the pancreatic parenchyma.

of acute pancreatitis and the risk of associated mortality (Table 34-1). The presence of three or more Ranson criteria (or if the patient is in shock, renal insufficiency, or pulmonary insufficiency) indicates severe pancreatitis and a greater likelihood of necrosis. There are other scoring systems, but none has proven to be significantly better than the Ranson criteria. Severe pancreatitis is associated with multiple organ dysfunction syndrome (MODS) and mortality rates that exceed 15% in some series. In contrast, patients with mild disease generally recover completely with conservative management.

Contrast-enhanced abdominal CT is the gold standard for noninvasive diagnosis of pancreatic necrosis. CT is >90% accurate in diagnosing necrosis if more than 30% of the gland is affected. There are several CT-based classification schemes that predict disease severity and mortality. However, several recent studies revealed that the associated radiation exposure was significant and that, after CT imaging, changes in clinical management were infrequent. Subsequently, it is recommended that the use of CT be restricted to patients with severe pancreatitis.

● DIAGNOSIS AND TREATMENT

Initial treatment of the patient with severe pancreatitis includes monitoring, fluid resuscitation, and pain control with patient-administered or epidural analgesia (PCA). A Foley catheter to measure urine output should be considered. Oxygenation should be monitored closely and early intubation should be considered in the patient whose respiratory function is deteriorating. Caloric support should be initiated early in the hospital course, and enteral feeding via a nasojejunal tube is preferred, but gastric feeding can be initiated as well if the patient's ileus is not too severe.

In patients who are appropriately resuscitated, infectious complications are the main cause of mortality in severe pancreatitis. Multiple trials have examined the value of prophylactic antibiotics and this remains controversial; selection for resistant organisms and *Candida* species may be associated with even worse outcomes, and therefore prophylactic antibiotics are reserved for patients who are in severe refractory shock.

For patients with multisystem organ failure (MSOF) and signs of sepsis, CT-guided FNA of the necrotic areas should be performed to determine the presence of bacterial contamination. Although these developments may be the result of infection, MODS and the systemic inflammatory response syndrome can result from pancreatic necrosis alone. Infected pancreatic necrosis is an indication for intervention with either surgical or radiologic drainage. In extremely ill patients, a percutaneous drain placed at the time of the FNA can help stabilize the patient, and may be used to temporize or even definitively treat infected necrosis. If possible, waiting at least 4 weeks prior to necrosectomy will allow demarcation of necrosis, thereby minimizing resection of viable pancreas and the accompanying morbidity. Sterile necrotizing pancreatitis, on the other hand, has not been shown to benefit from drainage or debridement and may be managed nonoperatively. In patients who develop abdominal compartment syndrome, surgical decompression may improve respiratory, cardiovascular, and renal parameters, but it is unclear if this is associated with an improvement in mortality.

Presentation Continued

The patient was admitted to the intensive care unit. His pain was controlled with a patient controlled analgesia (PCA), and his electrolytes were closely monitored. A postpyloric feeding tube was placed under endoscopic guidance. Although he initially stabilized, on the eighth hospital day, the patient became tachycardic and hypotensive. His WBC count continued to rise, and his creatinine became elevated. An intra-abdominal pressure was measured at 15 mm Hg. He became increasingly dyspneic and required intubation. CT-guided FNA of a peripancreatic fluid collection revealed gram-negative rods, and a percutaneous drain was placed. After some improvement for 2 days, the patient deteriorated again and the GI service was consulted for endoscopic pancreatic necrosectomy. This was repeated twice with some improvement after each procedure. However, due to continued multi-organ failure despite these interventions, the patient was taken to surgery.

MINIMALLY INVASIVE APPROACHES

Due to the high mortality associated with open necrosectomy, minimally invasive strategies can be utilized in a step-up approach starting with the least invasive procedures first. Minimally invasive strategies include percutaneous catheter drainage and endoscopic, laparoscopic, and retroperitoneal necrosectomy. The step-up approach is associated with a lower mortality rate with approximately one-third of patients requiring percutaneous drainage only. If debridement is required, endoscopic debridement is another minimally invasive strategy that can be preformed. This method creates several small fistulous connections between the gastrointestinal tract, usually between the stomach and the necrotic pancreas. Serial debridements can be performed through the tract; however, these are prone to occlusion and often require frequent interventions. Another minimally invasive approach is videoscopic assisted retroperitneal debridement (VARD) which follows a fistulous tract from a prior placed IR drain into the retroperitoneal space with a laparscope to allow surgical debridement of the pancreas under direct visualization. Other minimally invasive approaches include the laparoscopic surgical debridement or perhaps even accessing the pancreas through the posterior lumbar space. These minimally invasive procedures have been shown to be safe in the literature but are not the procedure of choice for a patient with severe acute pancreatitis who is in MOSF with clinical deterioration. For patients who require surgical intervention for pancreatic necrosis outcomes are improved

if the procedure can be delayed which is why it is preferable to attempt minimally invasive techniques first. However, early surgical intervention is required in patients with clinically worsening sepsis despite these other interventions.

SURGICAL APPROACH

The approach to pancreatic debridement is determined by the interval to operation. Over time, the pancreatic necrosis becomes increasingly organized, permitting a more focused and even minimally invasive approach. In patients undergoing operation prior to a month after onset, open pancreatic necrosectomy is often required.

Open pancreatic necrosectomy (Table 34-2). Preoperative imaging should be used to guide placement of the incision. A vertical midline or Chevron incision may be employed. The greater omentum is usually separated from the middle of the transverse colon for a distance sufficient to expose the pancreas. When the collection extends into the mesocolon and the small bowel mesentery, a direct approach from below the transverse colon may be more appropriate. Once the pancreas is exposed, the capsule is opened and all purulent material and necrotic tissue is removed from the pancreatic bed, being careful to preserve viable pancreatic tissue. Sharp dissection is usually avoided; it is typically sufficient to remove tissue that comes easily with ring forceps or irrigation. The transverse colon should be inspected for viability; if the colon is compromised, a colectomy should be performed. Care should be taken to minimize intraoperative hemorrhage. Depending on the organization of the necrosis, the anticipated need for further debridement, and the degree

Table 34-2	Open Pancreatic Necrosectomy

Key Technical Steps

1. Midline vertical or Chevron incision and full exploration
2. Access to the lesser sac obtained through the gastrocolic ligament or mesocolon
3. Drainage of purulent material
4. Debridement of necrotic tissue
5. Placement of feeding jejunostomy
6. JP drains placed into the lesser sac for postoperative irrigation and drainage

Potential Pitfalls

- Generalized venous bleeding requiring intra-abdominal packing
- Recurrent necrosis after initial operative debridement requiring return to the operating room
- Enzymatic damage to the bowel or vasculature resulting in hemorrhage
- Bowel wall edema caused by generous resuscitation resulting in an open abdomen

of hemorrhage, it may be appropriate to pack the pancreatic bed and plan reoperation. In cases where the laparotomy incision will be closed, Jackson-Pratt (JP) drains should be placed to maximize postoperative drainage of debris. Closed continuous lavage of the retroperitoneum may be appropriate in patients in whom ongoing necrosis is anticipated.

Laparoscopic pancreatic necrosectomy. For critically ill, hemodynamically unstable patients or if the necrosis is not yet organized, laparoscopic intervention may be contraindicated. However, some case series suggest that laparoscopic necrosectomy is appropriate in patients who have undergone prior percutaneous drainage and/or have limited areas of necrosis that will benefit from a single-stage procedure. Full laparoscopic procedures with carbon dioxide pneumoperitoneum and modified laparoscopic procedures aided by a hand port have been described. Postoperative drainage is recommended with both techniques. Other minimally invasive techniques, such as endoscopic transgastric or transduodenal necrosectomy or retroperitoneal percutaneous necrosectomy, may be alternatives to surgical intervention, but a full description of these techniques and their indication is beyond the scope of this text.

SPECIAL INTRAOPERATIVE CONSIDERATIONS

Pancreatic necrosectomy may be combined with cholecystectomy if exposure is simple and mobilization is thought to be safe. However, in the patient with severe pancreatitis, even if secondary to gallstones, cholecystectomy should be deferred to a later date if the gallbladder is not easily accessible.

A subcostal incision can be performed if focal areas of necrosis are in the tail or in the head of the gland. Formal mobilization of the gastrocolic gutters is typically not performed but all areas of necrosis, identified by preoperative CT, need to be addressed. Postoperative closed irrigation with JP drains placed into the lesser sac through separate small incisions should be considered in patients with ongoing necrosis.

POSTOPERATIVE MANAGEMENT

Postoperative complications are common and significant. They include organ failure, retroperitoneal and intra-abdominal hemorrhage, endocrine dysfunction, and secondary fungal infections. Fistulae from the pancreatic duct and gastrointestinal tract, pseudocyst formation, pancreatic abscess, and vascular complications (e.g., mesenteric or splenic venous thrombosis and arterial pseudoaneurysms) are also late complications of acute pancreatitis. Follow-up with repeat imaging is required to identify and manage these sequelae of pancreatic necrosectomy. These patients are at high risk for endocrine and exocrine dysfunction and will need on-going evaluation in the future.

Case Conclusion

The patient underwent pancreatic necrosectomy via a vertical midline incision after failure of minimally invasive approaches. His abdomen was left open and he returned to the operating room for two additional irrigation and debridement procedures. He tolerated these procedures well. During the second take-back, he underwent placement of a feeding jejunostomy, and his abdomen was closed. Postoperatively, he remained hemodynamically stable and was successfully weaned from the ventilator. Follow-up imaging was notable for the development of a pancreatic pseudocyst, which was managed via endoscopic cystogastrostomy. He was ultimately discharged from the hospital to a subacute care facility, on tube feeds, and starting to tolerate a small amount of oral intake.

TAKE HOME POINTS

- Postpyloric enteral feeding is the preferred method of nutritional support.
- Patients with acute necrotizing pancreatitis and a question of infection should undergo CT-guided FNA of necrotic regions of the pancreas to differentiate between sterile and infected pancreatic necrosis.
- Infected pancreatic necrosis in patients is an indication for intervention, including radiologic drainage and/or surgery.
- A step-up approach leads to improved outcomes when minimally invasive strategies are employed first.
- Surgical intervention should favor an organ-preserving approach. Resection procedures such as partial or total pancreatectomy that remove vital pancreatic tissue are associated with postoperative exocrine and endocrine insufficiency and high mortality rates.
- Cholecystectomy should be performed when safe to avoid recurrence of gallstone-associated pancreatitis.

SUGGESTED READINGS

Ashley SW, Perez A, Pierce EA, et al. Necrotizing pancreatitis: a contemporary analysis of 99 consecutive cases. *Ann Surg.* 2001; 234:572-580.

Baron TH, Morgan DE. Acute necrotizing pancreatitis. *N Engl J Med.* 1999;340:1412-1417.

Clancy TE, Benoit EP, Ashley SW. Current management of acute pancreatitis. *J Gastrointest Surg.* 2005;9:440-452.

Connor S, Alexakis N, Raraty GT, et al. Early and late complications after pancreatic necrosectomy. *Surgery.* 2005;137:499-505.

Dellinger EP, Tellado JM, Soto NE, et al. Early antibiotic treatment for severe acute necrotizing pancreatitis: a randomized, double blind, placebo-controlled study. *Ann Surg.* 2007;245:674-683.

Santvoort HC, Besselink MG, Bakker OJ, et al. A step-up approach or open necrosectomy for necrotizing pancreatitis. *N Engl J Med.* 2010;362:1491-1502.

Incidental Liver Mass

CECILIA G. ETHUN AND SHISHIR K. MAITHEL

Based on the previous edition chapter "Incidental Liver Mass" by Shawn J. Pelletier

Presentation

A previously healthy 56-year-old woman is brought to the emergency room by EMS following a motor vehicle collision. A noncontrast CT scan performed on admission shows no major abdominal injuries but incidentally reveals a 4.5-cm solitary mass in the right hemiliver. She has no significant past medical history, is asymptomatic, and her exam is benign, without jaundice or abdominal pain.

● DIFFERENTIAL DIAGNOSIS

The potential differential diagnoses are listed in Table 35-1. Most incidental liver masses in otherwise healthy individuals are benign. These most commonly include cavernous hemangiomas, focal nodular hyperplasia (FNH), simple cysts, and hepatocellular adenomas. Cavernous hemangiomas are benign vascular lesions of unclear etiology. They are the most common benign liver tumor and can be found in all age groups. Despite being relatively large in some cases,

Table 35-1	Differential Diagnosis of Incidental Liver Mass

Primary Liver Malignancies
  Hepatocellular carcinoma
  Intrahepatic cholangiocarcinoma
  Hilar cholangiocarcinoma
  Gallbladder cancer

Metastatic Liver Malignancies
  Colorectal cancer
  Neuroendocrine tumors
  Other (breast cancer, reproductive tract cancers, melanoma, adrenocortical carcinoma, renal cell carcinoma, sarcoma)

Benign Liver Tumors
  Cavernous hemangioma
  Focal nodular hyperplasia
  Hepatocellular adenoma
  Hepatic cyst
  Intrahepatic abscess
  Focal fat sparing

most patients are asymptomatic and face no risk of spontaneous rupture and hemorrhage. FNH is the second most common benign lesion and is typically found in women between the ages of 30 and 50 years. In general, FNH is viewed as a hyperplastic and not neoplastic lesion and do not have malignant potential. Hepatocellular adenomas are typically found in women between 30 and 50 years and can enlarge, especially under the stimulation of circulating estrogens (including with the use of oral contraceptives or during pregnancy).

Although the majority of incidental liver masses are benign, the possibility of a malignant etiology should always be considered. These include both primary tumors—hepatocellular carcinoma (HCC) and intrahepatic cholangiocarcinoma (IHC)—and metastatic tumors of the liver. HCC is the most common primary liver tumor and third most common cause of cancer-related death worldwide. Cirrhosis underlies the development of HCC in nearly 90% of cases, with a mean annual HCC incidence of 3% to 4% in cirrhotic patients. Of those with cirrhosis, chronic infections from hepatitis B and hepatitis C viruses contribute to HCC development 80% of the time. Alcohol consumption is frequently a cofactor in cirrhosis-related HCC, and nonalcoholic fatty liver disease is increasingly becoming a recognized risk factor. Other risk factors for HCC include male gender and advanced age. Patients with human immunodeficiency virus (HIV) experience a higher rate of HCC, which tends to appear at younger ages, is more frequently symptomatic, and is associated with worse outcomes compared to HCC in non-HIV patients.

Intrahepatic cholangiocarcinoma (IHC) is the second most common primary liver tumor, and its incidence has been steadily rising in European and North American countries over the last 30 years from 0.1 to 0.6 cases per 100,000. The majority of patients who present with IHC are asymptomatic and have no known risk factors. However, specific risk factors have been identified, with chronic inflammation of the biliary epithelia being the final common pathway among them. These include primary sclerosing cholangitis, parasitic hepatic infections, hepatolithiasis, congenital biliary cystic disease, and cirrhosis. Other more general risk factors for IHC include diabetes, obesity, biliary-enteric bypass, and tobacco use.

Metastatic liver tumors represent a heterogeneous group of malignancies and should always be considered when evaluating an incidental liver mass. The most common metastatic liver tumor originates from primary colorectal cancer (CRC). The liver is the most common site for hematogenous spread from CRC. Roughly 25% of CRC patients present with synchronous liver metastases, and nearly 50% of CRC patients develop metachronous liver metastases after resection of their primary tumor. Neuroendocrine tumors (NETs) also commonly metastasize to the liver and are the second most common source of metastatic liver tumors. Over 80% of patients with metastatic NETs have liver involvement. Although liver metastases can be seen with any primary NET site, they most commonly originate from small bowel (midgut) NETs. Noncolorectal, non-NET liver metastases represent a small, but important, group of liver tumors. These most commonly include primary breast cancer, reproductive tract cancers, melanoma, adrenocortical carcinoma, renal cell carcinoma, and sarcoma.

● WORKUP

The algorithm for the evaluation of a patient with a liver mass is depicted in Figure 35-1. Laboratory evaluation includes a complete blood count, coagulation studies, hepatitis panel, liver function tests, and tumor markers (CEA, AFP, CA-19-9).

Imaging is a critical part of the workup for incidental liver masses, and various modalities may be used to rule-in or rule-out specific etiologies. These include right upper quadrant ultrasound (US), computed tomography (CT) scan, magnetic resonance imaging (MRI), positron emission tomography (PET) scan, and somatostatin receptor (SSR) scintigraphy. Although US is often the first test to be ordered and can be useful in detecting the presence of a cystic or solid liver lesion, it is rarely sufficient in isolation to accurately characterize the lesion and make a diagnosis. CT scan can identify the majority of liver lesions but is most useful when using a triple-phase protocol that generates precontrast, arterial, and early and delayed venous images.

A comprehensive MRI is the most sensitive and specific imaging modality for characterizing liver lesions and should incorporate multiple series, including fat-suppressed T1 pre- and postcontrast (arterial, portal venous, and 3- to 5-minute delay), T2 with and without fat suppression, MRCP, balanced-gradient sequence, dual-gradient echo in-phase and opposed-phase sequences, and diffusion-weighted images with a high B value of approximately 800. The sensitivity for detecting small lesions on MRI can be enhanced by using hepatobiliary-specific contrast agents, such as gadoxetate sodium, and the specificity of MRI can be optimized with

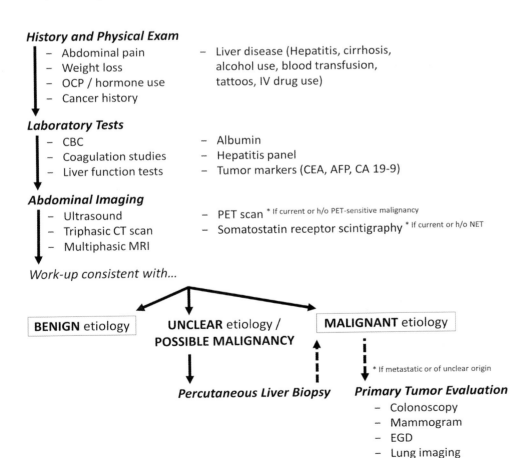

History and Physical Exam
- Abdominal pain
- Weight loss
- OCP / hormone use
- Cancer history

– Liver disease (Hepatitis, cirrhosis, alcohol use, blood transfusion, tattoos, IV drug use)

Laboratory Tests
- CBC
- Coagulation studies
- Liver function tests

– Albumin
– Hepatitis panel
– Tumor markers (CEA, AFP, CA 19-9)

Abdominal Imaging
- Ultrasound
- Triphasic CT scan
- Multiphasic MRI

– PET scan * If current or h/o PET-sensitive malignancy
– Somatostatin receptor scintigraphy * If current or h/o NET

Work-up consistent with...

BENIGN etiology   **UNCLEAR etiology / POSSIBLE MALIGNANCY**   **MALIGNANT etiology**

* If metastatic or of unclear origin

Percutaneous Liver Biopsy   **Primary Tumor Evaluation**
- Colonoscopy
- Mammogram
- EGD
- Lung imaging

FIGURE 35-1. Workup algorithm for an incidental liver mass.

an extracellular agent. PET scan and SSR scintigraphy have limited use in the initial workup of incidental liver masses and are most helpful for assessing tumor burden when metastases from PET-sensitive primary tumors and/or NETs are suspected.

If the diagnosis is uncertain after adequate imaging, consideration can be given to obtaining a percutaneous core liver biopsy. Biopsy should be performed only when the results will change management and should be avoided if HCC is suspected based on patient history and imaging characteristics. If a non-HCC malignancy (such as adenocarcinoma) is detected on biopsy, it is important to try to identify the primary tumor site, as prognosis and the role of liver resection can vary greatly depending on tumor origin.

Presentation Continued

Further evaluation of the patient reveals a slightly elevated alkaline phosphatase, but otherwise normal LFTs, an elevated CA 19-9, a borderline elevated CEA, and a normal AFP. A multiphasic liver MRI demonstrates a 4.5-cm solitary mass with delayed venous enhancement that involves segments 5, 6, 7, and 8 along the path of the right hepatic vein. No extrahepatic disease is noted. A percutaneous core biopsy reveals adenocarcinoma. The patient states that she had a mammogram and colonoscopy 6 months prior, which were both negative.

● DIAGNOSIS AND TREATMENT

Once adequate imaging is obtained, thorough review of all diagnostic studies should be performed in order to best elucidate the most likely diagnosis and determine resectability. Benign lesions are most often associated with normal lab values and low serum tumor markers. Lab derangements, such as elevated bilirubin, LFTs, and INR, as well as a low platelet count, are more suggestive of primary liver tumors, which often develop in the background of underlying liver dysfunction and are more likely to cause biliary obstruction. Similarly, both primary and metastatic liver tumors can be associated with elevated tumor markers. However, laboratory studies and tumor markers primarily play a supportive role in the diagnosis of incidental liver masses, and normal values do not exclude the possibility of a malignancy.

General imaging characteristics of liver tumors are shown in Table 35-2. Imaging is an important part of the evaluation of incidental liver masses, as the combination of radiologic characteristics and clinical features can often identify the etiology, without the need for percutaneous biopsy (Figure 35-2). Specific histopathologies, such as HCC or melanoma, detected on biopsy may both provide a clear

Table 35-2	General Radiographic Features of Solid Liver Tumors on Cross-Sectional Imaging

Precontrast Hypoattenuation
  Cavernous hemangioma
  Hepatocellular adenoma
Arterial Enhancement
  Hepatocellular carcinoma
  Neuroendocrine tumors
  Melanoma
  Renal cell carcinoma
  Focal nodular hyperplasia
  Colorectal cancer (slight)
  +/− Hepatocellular adenoma
Early Venous Enhancement
  Cavernous hemangioma (peripheral > central)
  Colorectal cancer (slight)
Delayed Venous Enhancement
  Cholangiocarcinoma
  Cavernous hemangioma (diffuse)
  Colorectal cancer (increasing)
Other Features
  Central scar—Focal nodular hyperplasia
  Telangiectatic components—hepatocellular adenoma (some)

diagnosis and guide treatment strategy. Alternatively, if adenocarcinoma is detected on biopsy, further staining for specific markers, including TTF-1 (lung), ER/PR (breast), CK-20 (colon), and CK-7 (pancreatobiliary), can help identify the likely site of origin, which may influence management decisions. If the diagnosis still remains indeterminate after high-quality imaging and biopsy, excisional biopsy with resection may be necessary.

Once a likely diagnosis is obtained, an appropriate treatment plan should be developed. When determining the resectability of hepatic lesions, several key considerations must be addressed: the operative indication, the surgical fitness of the patient, and the technical resectability of the tumor. In asymptomatic individuals, most benign lesions require no therapy, as the risks for rupture and hemorrhage or malignant transformation are minimal. If pain is the only symptom from a benign liver tumor, a thorough investigation for alternative causes of pain and careful patient selection are critical before proceeding with resection for this unusual indication. The management of adenomas, however, is generally more aggressive than other benign lesions because rupture and hemorrhage have been reported to occur between 11% and 29% and malignant transformation into HCC in up to 10% of lesions.

For malignant liver tumors, the operative indication refers to the oncologic appropriateness of resection, which largely dictates some survival benefit from surgery and is

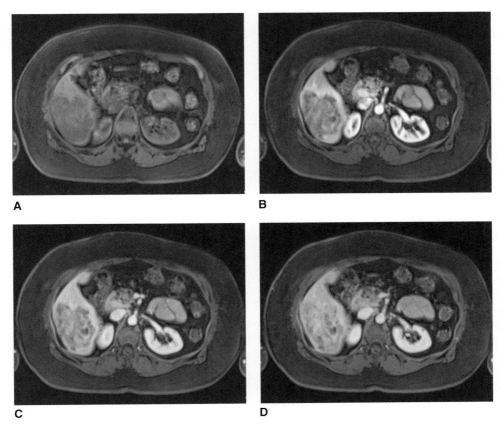

FIGURE 35-2. Comprehensive, multiphasic MRI showing intrahepatic cholangiocarcinoma in **(A)** precontrast phase, **(B)** arterial phase, **(C)** early venous phase, and **(D)** delayed venous phase. Cholangiocarcinomas typically display delayed venous enhancement on CT and MRI.

ultimately governed by tumor biology. For HCC and IHC, tumor size, multifocality, and vascular invasion should be considered when determining resectability, although specific cutoffs are inconsistent and guidelines variable. Unresectable HCC, particularly in the background of cirrhosis, that meet Milan's criteria should be considered for transplant evaluation. For colorectal liver metastases, hepatic resection has largely become the optimal treatment modality; however, considerations for synchronous liver disease, primary tumor node status and histology, number and size of liver tumors, CEA level, and disease-free interval should guide decisions about the appropriateness of resection. Liver resection for NETs in select patients may be associated with symptom improvement and prolonged progression-free survival. The role of liver resection for other metastatic tumors, such as breast cancer, melanoma, and sarcoma, is unclear and should be individualized to each clinical scenario. Regardless of the liver tumor being primary or metastatic, in general, the presence of extrahepatic disease is an indicator of aggressive tumor biology, and the value of resection should be questioned. In any case where the oncologic appropriateness of resection is in question, a trial of preoperative systemic or liver-directed therapy may help select more biologically favorable tumors prior to surgery.

Presentation Continued

The pathologist reports that on further staining, the tumor is negative for TTF-1, ER/PR, and CK-20, but positive for CK-7. The radiologic and pathologic findings are consistent with intrahepatic cholangiocarcinoma. An open, right hepatectomy is planned.

● SURGICAL APPROACH

Laparoscopic Resection

To perform laparoscopic liver resection safely, the surgeon must have extensive experience with both open liver surgery and advanced laparoscopic techniques. In general, experience can be accumulated by starting with peripheral lesions within the left lateral sector or on the inferior aspect of the liver. As skills develop, resection of lesions within segments five and six can be attempted. Resection of tumors within segments seven and eight are more difficult but can be performed safely with appropriate experience. As with any laparoscopic procedure, a surgeon should not hesitate to convert to an open procedure if there is inadequate exposure, hemorrhage, or concern for patient safety or obtaining an adequate surgical margin.

Laparoscopic liver resections can be performed using a straight laparoscopic, hybrid approach, or hand-assisted technique. The hand-assisted approach allows for palpation and direct examination of the liver and abdominal cavity, retraction of the relatively large liver, and the ability to manually control hemorrhage. The patient is placed in the supine position and adequately secured to the table to allow for steep reverse Trendelenburg and rotation of the operative table. If used, the hand-assist device is almost always placed in the midline near the umbilicus. For lesions in the superior aspect of the liver, the hand-assist device may be placed slightly higher on the abdomen. Positioning of the trocars depends on the location of the tumor for resection, but attention should be paid to placing 12-mm trocars strategically so that laparoscopic staplers can be utilized.

After the liver and the abdomen are visually inspected and palpated, ligamentous attachments are divided. An intraoperative liver US is performed, using either a probe introduced through the hand port or a laparoscopic US probe. Attention is first turned to a formal evaluation of the segmental anatomy of the liver with surveillance for lesions that were not identified on preoperative imaging. The known lesion is then evaluated and the vascular and biliary anatomy noted. The plane of transection can be marked on the capsule of the liver using electrocautery. For lesions that are very close to major vascular or biliary structures and the lesion is known to be benign, consideration can be given to enucleating the tumor near these areas. If the tumor is concerning for malignancy, a margin should be obtained. Intermittent inflow occlusion can be utilized by temporarily occluding the porta hepatis. The liver parenchyma is then divided using any number of different techniques, including energy devices or using ultrasonic dissection until major vascular structures are encountered. Small- to medium-sized vascular structures can be clipped and divided. Larger vascular structures are usually divided using an endovascular stapler. The specimen can then be removed via the hand port, or a periumbilical or Pfannenstiel incision. Hemostasis on the cut edge of the liver can be obtained using the argon beam coagulation or hemostatic agents with manual pressure. The cut edge of the liver is also carefully inspected for potential bile leaks that can be oversewn. The use of a sealant agent can be considered to minimize postoperative biliary leaks. Placement of a drain near the cut edge of the liver is usually not necessary unless specific circumstances dictate its use (Table 35-3).

Open Resection

In general, the technique used for open resection is like that of a laparoscopic resection. With the patient in the supine position, an upper midline or a right subcostal incision with upper midline extension is made. This allows adequate exposure to the left and right lobes of the liver as well as exposure to the suprahepatic vena cava and the lower abdomen if a Roux-en-Y hepaticojejunostomy needs to be constructed. Prior to placing a fixed retractor, the round and falciform ligament should be divided and any adhesions of the liver to the anterior abdominal wall should be mobilized to avoid tearing of the hepatic

Table 35-3   **Laparoscopic Liver Resection**

Key Technical Steps

1. Placement of trocar or hand-assisted device and induction of pneumoperitoneum
2. Laparoscopic evaluation of abdomen and liver
3. Placement of additional trocars
4. Mobilization of liver as necessary
5. Intraoperative liver ultrasound
6. Resection of liver mass/segment(s)/lobe
7. Insure adequate hemostasis
8. Evaluate adequate perfusion of the liver remnant and look for potential bile leaks
9. Placement of drain as indicated
10. Close abdomen

Potential Pitfalls

- Central lesions and large bulky tumors can compromise laparoscopic working space and be difficult to resect laparoscopically
- Control of potential hemorrhage
- Risk of air embolism related to pneumoperitoneum
- Skills in open and laparoscopic liver surgery are required

capsule leading to bleeding. As described in the laparoscopic approach, the abdomen and the liver are inspected, the part of the liver to be resected is mobilized, and an intraoperative liver US is performed. The liver resection itself is performed using similar techniques to divide the liver parenchyma. Inspection of the cut edge of the liver is also carefully performed to help avoid postoperative bile leaks. The abdomen is closed in the standard fashion (Table 35-4).

● SPECIAL INTRAOPERATIVE CONSIDERATIONS

Several unexpected findings or complications may be encountered. Although initially believed to be a primary liver tumor, the mass may intraoperatively be identified as a metastasis from an extrahepatic primary source. In this setting, biopsies to obtain an accurate diagnosis should be obtained and intraoperative staging should be performed. If appropriate, proceeding with resection of the liver tumor along with the primary tumor can be considered. Additional hepatic lesions may also be identified that were not identified on preoperative imaging. If possible, consideration can be given to resection of these lesions as well. If there is concern for leaving an inadequate remnant, these lesions may also be treated using radiofrequency or microwave ablation.

During resection, preparation should always be made for unexpected hemorrhage. This includes preoperative communication with the anesthesia team to ensure that adequate vascular access is present. Depending on the location of bleeding, control can often be obtained with manual compression or packing. Pringle's maneuver can also be used. In cases of extreme bleeding, total vascular isolation of the liver can be obtained by performing Pringle's maneuver as well as clamping the vena cava in a supra- and infrahepatic position. The best treatment for hemorrhage during parenchymal transection is prevention with employing low central venous pressure anesthesia techniques.

Finally, the hepatic vascular and biliary anatomy may have substantial anatomic variation. Up to 40% of patients have aberrant biliary anatomy, which increases to nearly 70% when vascular variations are considered. Thus, detailed knowledge of the portal anatomy, including the common variants and anomalies, is essential to perform safe and successful liver resections.

● POSTOPERATIVE MANAGEMENT

While most patients undergoing hepatic resection do not require treatment in an ICU, a low threshold for ICU care should be maintained if there is any concern for bleeding, hepatic insufficiency, need for observation of renal function, or other concerns based on the patient's comorbidities. The patient's volume status, hepatic, and renal function should be closely monitored and managed in the postoperative period. Pain can be controlled with either patient-controlled analgesia using intravenous opioids or an epidural, although other nonnarcotic pain control strategies are often sufficient. Perioperative nasogastric drainage is typically not indicated, and oral intake can be advanced relatively quickly. If a drain is placed at the time of operation and bile is not pres-

ent within the first few postoperative days, the drain can be removed. If bile is present within the drain and is at a relatively low volume, the drain should be left in place and can be removed as an outpatient once the bile leak has resolved. If a high-volume leak is present, ERCP with sphincterotomy and placement of an endobiliary stent to decompress the biliary tree may be necessary.

Case Conclusion

The patient successfully undergoes an open right hepatectomy and portal lymph node dissection and is discharged home from the hospital without complications on postoperative day 4. Final pathology report returns as intrahepatic cholangiocarcinoma, with negative margins and no lymph node involvement. One year following resection, she remains disease free.

TAKE HOME POINTS

- Modern imaging practices and technology have led to increased detection of incidental liver masses.
- In otherwise healthy individuals, most incidental masses are benign; however, a malignant etiology must be considered.
- Better definition of radiologic characteristics and clinical features has led to improved radiologic diagnosis with a reduced need for biopsy.
  - A good-quality, comprehensive MRI is the single best imaging modality for a liver lesion.
- The workup of a liver mass is dictated by benign versus malignant etiology and primary versus metastatic origin. Oncologic appropriateness, technical feasibility, and patient fitness must all be considered prior to performing resection.

Table 35-4	Open Liver Resection

Key Technical Steps

1. Upper midline incision or subcostal incision with upper midline extension
2. Evaluation of abdomen and liver
3. Mobilization of liver as necessary
4. Intraoperative liver ultrasound
5. Resection of liver mass/segment(s)/lobe
6. Insure adequate hemostasis
7. Evaluate adequate perfusion of the liver remnant and look for potential bile leaks
8. Placement of drain as indicated
9. Close abdomen

Potential Pitfalls

- Central lesions and large bulky tumors can be difficult to resect
- Control of potential hemorrhage
- Risk of air embolism if large inadvertent venotomy occurs

SUGGESTED READINGS

Clavien PA, Petrowsky H, DeOliveira ML, et al. Strategies for safer liver surgery and partial liver transplantation. *N Engl J Med.* 2007;356:1545-1559.

Jarnagin WR, Gonen M, Fong Y, et al. Improvement in perioperative outcome after hepatic resection: analysis of 1,803 consecutive cases over the past decade. *Ann Surg.* 2002;236:397-406; discussion 406-407.

Koffron AJ, Auffenberg G, Kung R, et al. Evaluation of 300 minimally invasive liver resections at a single institution: less is more. *Ann Surg.* 2007;246:385–392; discussion 392-394.

Maithel SK, Gamblin TC, Kamel I, Corona-Villalobos CP, Thomas M, Pawlik TM. Multidisciplinary approaches to intrahepatic cholangiocarcinoma. *Cancer.* 2013;119(22):3929-3942.

Maithel SK, Jarnagin WR, Belghiti J. Hepatic resection for benign disease and for liver and biliary tumors. In: Jarnagin WR, ed. *Blumgart's Surgery of the Liver, Biliary Tract, and Pancreas.* Vol. 1. 5th ed. Philadelphia, PA: Elsevier; 2012:1461-1511.

Yoon SS, Charny CK, Fong Y, et al. Diagnosis, management, and outcomes of 115 patients with hepatic hemangioma. *J Am Coll Surg.* 2003;197:392–402.

Liver Mass in Chronic Liver Disease

36

NICOLE NEVAREZ AND CHRISTOPHER J. SONNENDAY

Based on the previous edition chapter "Liver Mass in Chronic Liver Disease" by Christopher J. Sonnenday

Presentation

A 59-year-old man with cirrhosis secondary to chronic hepatitis C infection undergoes an annual screening liver ultrasound. A 2.5-cm solid, well-circumscribed mass in the posterior aspect of the right hepatic lobe is identified. The liver is noted to be nodular in appearance.

● DIFFERENTIAL DIAGNOSIS

While the differential diagnosis of a liver mass is broad and includes infectious lesions as well as both benign and malignant lesions, a new mass detected in a patient with chronic liver disease should be presumed to be a primary hepatic malignancy until proven otherwise. Hepatocellular carcinoma (HCC) is the leading cause of death in clinically compensated cirrhotics, and individuals with cirrhosis secondary to viral hepatitis have a 10% to 20% 5-year cumulative risk of developing HCC. Additionally, with the rise of obesity in Western countries, the incidence of HCC related to nonalcoholic fatty liver disease (NAFLD) is a growing problem. For these reasons, HCC screening has been shown to have a profound impact on HCC-related mortality among cirrhotics. The American Association for the Study of Liver Disease currently recommends screening at-risk populations (e.g., patients with cirrhosis of any etiology) with liver ultrasound and serum alpha-fetoprotein (AFP) every 6 to 12 months.

Although the evaluation of a liver mass in a patient with cirrhosis is aimed at diagnosing HCC, other diagnoses may be considered. Regenerative nodules may appear masslike and may represent an early stage in the development of hepatocellular neoplasms. Similarly, adenomas may be diagnosed in patients with chronic liver disease. These lesions are at high risk for malignant transformation, especially in this population, and imaging characteristics alone may be insufficient to distinguish hepatic adenomas from well-differentiated HCC. Other benign lesions that typically do not require surgical resection include focal nodular hyperplasia (FNH) and hemangioma.

Patients with chronic liver disease and cirrhosis are also at increased risk for developing intrahepatic cholangiocarcinoma. While classically described in patients with cholestatic liver disease (e.g., primary sclerosing cholangitis), patients with cirrhosis are also at increased risk of developing intrahepatic cholangiocarcinoma and mixed tumors that include both HCC and cholangiocarcinoma cell types, though these primary hepatic malignancies are much less common than HCC.

● WORKUP AND DIAGNOSIS

Any mass lesion seen or suspected on screening hepatic ultrasound should be further investigated with contrast-enhanced cross-sectional imaging, either computed tomography (CT) or magnetic resonance imaging (MRI) of the abdomen. MRI appears to be slightly more sensitive and specific than CT particularly in patients with chronic liver disease, and specific imaging characteristics—arterial phase enhancement with early washout of contrast on the venous or delayed phases of the scan—are considered diagnostic for HCC (Figure 36-1). Contrast-enhanced MRI may provide definitive diagnosis of FNH and hemangioma as well. Further characterization via image-guided percutaneous biopsy is reserved for cases in which the diagnosis in still in doubt following adequate imaging or in cases where further characterization would change management based on clinical suspicion (e.g., intrahepatic cholangiocarcinoma or a metastatic lesion).

Once the diagnosis of HCC is established by imaging and/or biopsy, the choice of appropriate therapy is made based upon tumor burden, severity of underlying liver disease, and patient performance status. Staging evaluation to assess metastatic tumor involvement should include measurement of serum AFP and chest CT. Bone scan may be appropriate when clinically indicated by symptoms or suspicion on cross-sectional imaging of the abdomen or chest.

Evaluation of underlying liver function and synthetic reserve is critical to providing safe treatment for HCC in patients with cirrhosis. There are multiple clinical classification systems that exist to predict severity of liver disease such as the Model for End-Stage Liver Disease (MELD) and the Child-Turcotte-Pugh (CTP) classification (Table 36-1). Consensus exists that CTP class C patients are not suitable to undergo hepatic resection due to excessive perioperative mortality, and CTP class B patients should only be considered for minor hepatic resections (resection of two or fewer Couinaud's segments) when they have excellent performance status. The evaluation of CTP class A patients for hepatic resection is more difficult, as these patients can vary substantially in their risk of perioperative mortality and postoperative liver failure.

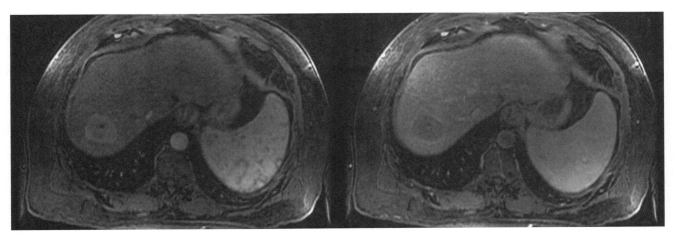

FIGURE 36-1. MRI of hepatocellular carcinoma, demonstrating characteristic enhancement on arterial phase imaging **(left panel)** with washout of contrast on delayed-phase imaging **(right panel)**.

CTP class A patients with overt evidence of portal hypertension are generally considered suboptimal candidates for hepatic resection. Clinical or radiologic signs of portal hypertension, such as a history of variceal hemorrhage, esophageal or gastric varices on upper endoscopy, visible upper abdominal varices on cross-sectional imaging, or grossly apparent ascites are all contraindications to resection. Thrombocytopenia is another critical clinical indicator of surgical risk with hepatic resection, reflecting the hypersplenism of advanced cirrhosis and portal hypertension. A platelet count under 100,000 is considered a relative contraindication to major hepatectomy. CTP class A patients with evidence of portal hypertension or thrombocytopenia should not undergo hepatic resection but may be considered for transplantation.

A number of quantitative liver function tests have been investigated to assess hepatic reserve prior to hepatic resection, including indocyanine green (ICG) clearance, galactose elimination capacity, and technetium-99m galactosyl human serum albumin scan, among others. The ICG clearance study is the most commonly used internationally, though it is not commonly used or available in the United States. Many surgeons use volumetric assessment as a proxy for hepatic reserve. This technique relies on the use of manual or automated serial measurement of cross-sectional liver volumes produced from a thin-section helical CT or MRI. The volume of the liver segments to be preserved following resection is then divided by the total estimated liver volume, which produces a percentage of future liver remnant (FLR) volume. In patients with normal liver parenchyma and function, an FLR of 25% to 30% is considered adequate, if two contiguous Couinaud's segments are preserved. However, in patients with cirrhosis, an FLR of at least 40% to 50% is desired.

Table 36-1	The CTP Classification of Liver Disease Severity		
Clinical Criteria	**Points**		
	1	2	3
Albumin (g/dL)	>3.5	2.8–3.5	<2.8
Bilirubin (mg/dL)	<2.0	2.0–3.0	>3.0
International normalized ratio	<1.7	1.7–2.3	>2.3
Ascites	None	Moderate (or suppressed by diuretics, not requiring regular paracentesis)	Severe (tense ascites, refractory to medication, or requiring regular paracentesis)
Encephalopathy	None	Grade I–II (or controlled with medication)	Grade III–IV (or refractory to medication)
CTP class A	**5–6 points**		
CTP class B	**7–9 points**		
CTP class C	**10–15 points**		

Presentation Continued

On contrast-enhanced MRI, the 2.5-cm solitary lesion demonstrates arterial phase enhancement with delayed phase contrast washout and is located in segment 6 of the right hepatic lobe. Chest CT shows no evidence of metastasis. The patient is active and independent in his activities of daily living and works full time. He has no history of ascites or hepatic encephalopathy. Upper endoscopy shows no esophageal or gastric varices. Laboratory evaluation reveals an albumin of 4.1 g/dL, total bilirubin of 1.1 mg/dL, INR of 1.0, and a platelet count of 148,000. CT volumetry suggests that resection of the posterior sector (segments 6 and 7) would leave an FLR of 65%.

● DIAGNOSIS AND TREATMENT

Treatment options for HCC are diverse and require careful consideration of both tumor stage and liver disease severity (Figure 36-2). Resection offers the best likelihood of survival in select patients with resectable disease, superior to nonsurgical therapies with 30% to 70% 5-year survival. In patients with CTP class B or C liver disease, liver transplantation may be the more appropriate choice of therapy as it treats both the malignancy and decompensated cirrhosis. Posttransplant survival has been shown to be excellent (65% to 80% 5-year survival) when patients are selected for transplant according to strict selection criteria, known as the Milan criteria

(solitary tumor under 5 cm, or 3 or fewer tumors each under 3 cm with no vascular invasion or extrahepatic involvement). Obviously, donor organ availability and the significant medical risks and costs associated with liver transplantation limit its expansion to all patients with HCC.

Among patients with more extensive tumor burden and/or decompensated liver disease, ablative therapies may be considered. Thermal ablation (radiofrequency or microwave) may offer prolonged survival and local tumor control, particularly in small solitary lesions (<3 to 4 cm) for those patients not suitable for hepatic resection or transplantation. Transarterial therapies (chemoembolization or radioembolization) have been shown to extend survival in select patients with unresectable disease, though the procedure may also precipitate hepatic decompensation and is best applied to CTP class A or select CTP class B patients. In patients with metastatic or recurrent disease, systemic chemotherapy with the multikinase inhibitor, sorafenib, may provide additional months of survival in patients not eligible for other therapies. In patients with late-stage HCC, best supportive care should be utilized.

In cirrhotic patients without an adequate predicted FLR who are otherwise good candidates for surgical therapy, portal vein embolization (PVE) may be considered as a way to augment the size of the remnant liver. PVE takes advantage of the contralateral hypertrophy and ipsilateral atrophy that takes place in response to selective portal vein occlusion. Repeat cross-sectional imaging is typically performed 3 to 6 weeks following embolization, with repeat liver volume estimates. Failure to respond to PVE portends a poor outcome

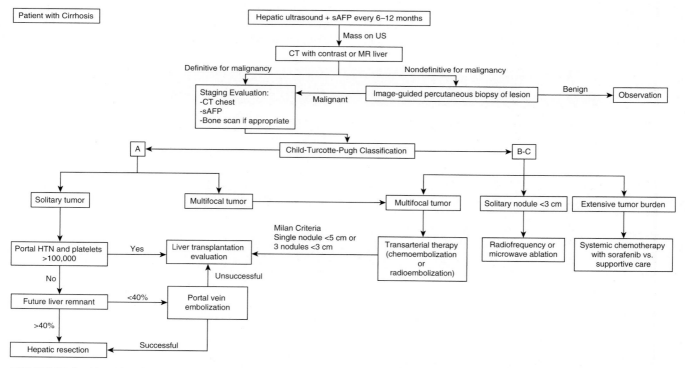

FIGURE 36-2. Algorithm for the diagnosis and treatment of hepatocellular carcinoma among patients with cirrhosis.

following resection. This should be considered a contraindication to proceeding with surgical therapy and transplantation may need to be considered. Most centers will aim to operate on patients with an appropriate response at 21 to 30 days following PVE, capitalizing on the peak hypertrophic response at this time period. However, longer waiting periods may be associated with additional hypertrophy in some patients.

● SURGICAL APPROACH

While hepatic resection can be accomplished safely by both open and minimally invasive techniques, cirrhotic patients present particular challenges in terms of transection of the fibrotic hepatic parenchyma and risk of blood loss. Therefore, only experienced laparoscopic liver surgeons should take on minimally invasive hepatic resections in cirrhotic patients. Laparoscopic liver surgery is discussed elsewhere in this text; this section describes open hepatic resection (Table 36-2).

Perioperative management of the hepatic resection patient can have a profound influence on outcomes, with maintenance of a low central venous pressure (CVP) as a central

Table 36-2	Open Hepatic Resection

Key Technical Steps

1. Right subcostal incision with midline extension.
2. Thorough laparotomy to assess for metastatic disease.
3. Limited mobilization of the liver to allow exposure for ultrasound.
4. Intraoperative ultrasound (IOUS):
    a. Define segments by portal and hepatic venous anatomy.
    b. Scan liver for all visible lesions.
    c. Plan resection, with marking of capsule along line of transection.
5. Portal dissection—encircle porta with tape to allow Pringle maneuver.
6. Extrahepatic ligation of segmental portal structures when indicated.
7. Parenchymal transection.
8. Obtain meticulous hemostasis and observe for biliary leaks.
9. Completion IOUS to document adequate inflow and outflow to liver remnant.

Potential Pitfalls

- Failure to leave an adequate liver remnant (≥40%–50% total liver volume in cirrhotic).
- Missing additional lesions due to inadequate IOUS.
- Excessive blood loss due to failure to control inflow and outflow vascular pedicles.
- Compromise of the surgical margin due to failure to reassess margin by IOUS during parenchymal transection.

tenet in intraoperative management. Establishment of large-bore venous access is essential, and arterial line placement for continuous systemic blood pressure monitoring is also advised. Central venous access, which has been advocated both for large-volume resuscitation and for CVP monitoring, can be helpful in the most complex cases but is probably not necessary in limited resection cases. Use of large-bore peripheral intravenous catheters (14 or 16 gauge) and conservative volume resuscitation can achieve similar goals.

Incision choice is critical to exposure and efficiency. Left-sided hepatic lesions can be approached from an upper midline incision, but typically a right subcostal incision is preferred. A right subcostal incision with midline extension is a very versatile incision, allowing exposure to the suprahepatic vena cava, making a bilateral subcostal or Chevron incision necessary only for cases with difficult exposure due to body habitus or large tumors. The abdomen should be carefully explored to assess for metastatic disease. Limited mobilization of the liver is performed to allow access for intraoperative ultrasound (IOUS).

Careful IOUS should follow a consistent three-step sequence, beginning with definition of Couinaud's segments based on the portal and hepatic venous anatomy. Attention is paid to important anatomic variants such as early or late division of the right portal pedicle or large accessory hepatic veins. The second phase of the IOUS exam should be a methodical scan through the entire liver parenchyma, with identification and measurement of all lesions, including those that have been identified on previous imaging and those found at the time of IOUS. The final step in an IOUS exam is planning of intended resection with note taken of the important critical vasculature to be included or avoided in a segmental resection.

The dissection phase of the operation begins with isolation of the portal structures by opening the pars flaccida (gastrohepatic ligament) and passing a finger through the foramen of Winslow such that the porta can be encircled with a tape. This maneuver facilitates quick access to the porta when necessary and can facilitate episodic inflow occlusion (Pringle maneuver). The amount of portal dissection necessary is then determined by the extent of hepatectomy planned. A peripheral nonanatomic or segmental resection will not require much additional portal dissection. A formal or extended lobectomy may be approached with a formal portal dissection and pedicle control prior to parenchymal transection.

Parenchymal transection may be performed by multiple techniques, with use of surgical energy devices, clips, or ligatures to control small vessels. Stapling devices may be used to control larger pedicles, including the hepatic veins. The role of inflow occlusion (Pringle maneuver) during parenchymal transection may be utilized to limit excessive blood loss when appropriate. While some surgeons use this technique routinely, others try to limit any potential ischemic injury to the liver remnant, preferring selective pedicle isolation and ligation. When inflow occlusion is utilized, it appears that intermittent periods of clamping followed by periods of reperfusion can limit the ischemic injury to the liver remnant.

Once the parenchymal transection is completed, achieving final hemostasis is critical. Significant bleeding vessels should be controlled with nonabsorbable fine sutures or clips. The argon beam coagulator is effective for small vessels and raw surfaces. Application of additional hemostatic agents such as fibrin- and thrombin-based agents can also be helpful. Care should be taken to identify occult biliary leaks from the parenchymal surface, which should be controlled with fine sutures when identified. Leaving a surgical drain after hepatectomy is a controversial practice and appears to be only partially successful in allowing diagnosis and adequate drainage of a postoperative biliary leak. Selective use of drains for cases with concomitant biliary reconstruction and/or difficult perihilar dissection is a reasonable strategy.

SPECIAL INTRAOPERATIVE CONSIDERATIONS

IOUS should be used throughout the hepatectomy operation, not just at the stage of planning the resection. Surgeons should use IOUS to reassess margin status throughout the parenchymal transection. Furthermore, IOUS can be used to identify large vascular pedicles that will need to be controlled in the parenchymal division. Finally, a completion IOUS with Doppler exam can assess the preserved inflow and outflow to the liver remnant, especially in larger segmental resections.

While obtaining a clear surgical margin has obvious oncologic applications, preservation of hepatic parenchyma is of particular concern in patients with cirrhosis. Thus, resection should be planned by IOUS to include an adequate but not excessive margin, with preservation of inflow and outflow to adjacent segments. In the case of hepatic surgery, it appears that the size of the margin is not oncologically relevant, as long as it proves to be histologically negative.

Improved outcomes with hepatic resection have allowed the cautious expansion of advanced hepatobiliary techniques to allow resection of more locally advanced tumors, including those with vascular involvement. Total vascular isolation of the liver may allow resection of tumors involving the vena cava, hepatic veins, or portal structures and subsequent reconstruction of these vascular structures. However, given the increased risk of postoperative hepatic dysfunction in patients with cirrhosis, these techniques are not advisable in these patients.

POSTOPERATIVE MANAGEMENT

Perioperative monitoring should include observation for evidence of hemorrhage, particularly in thrombocytopenic or coagulopathic patients. While surgical site infections in hepatectomy patients are relatively rare when compared to patients undergoing gastrointestinal operations, biliary leaks from the cut surface of the liver may predispose to biloma and abscess formation. Typically low-volume leaks

can be controlled with adequate percutaneous drainage and observation, but larger, more central leaks may benefit from endoscopic sphincterotomy and endobiliary stent placement to divert bile flow away from the site of leak.

Obviously in the cirrhotic patient, monitoring for signs of hepatic dysfunction is the most important postoperative concern. Mild hepatic dysfunction can present with progressive jaundice or ascites. If the patient remains otherwise clinically well and free of infection, these clinical problems will often resolve over the first 1 to 2 postoperative weeks. More ominous signs of liver failure include progressive coagulopathy, lactic acidosis, renal dysfunction, vasodilatation, and encephalopathy. Evaluation of a patient with progressive liver dysfunction should include liver duplex to establish patent hepatic vascular inflow and outflow. Renal replacement therapy should be considered in more severe cases to address volume overload and more hepatic injury from congestion. Supportive care is the only intervention in most cases, although salvage liver transplantation may be considered in patients who are otherwise appropriate candidates who have surgical pathology revealing tumors within Milan criteria and without vascular invasion.

Case Conclusion

The patient undergoes an open segment 6/7 resection with IOUS. The liver is stiff and cirrhotic, making division of the hepatic parenchyma challenging. Estimated blood loss is 800 mL.

Postoperatively, the patient develops mild ascites and lower extremity edema, and his bilirubin rises to 3.1 mg/dL by postoperative day 5. Over the ensuing week, the ascites resolves with gentle diuresis, and the bilirubin returns to normal.

Final pathology from the resection specimen reveals a 2.3-cm moderately differentiated HCC with negative margins and no vascular invasion.

At 18 months postoperatively, the patient remains free of disease with stable liver function.

TAKE HOME POINTS

- A liver mass identified in a patient with cirrhosis should be considered a primary hepatic malignancy until proven otherwise.
- Contrast-enhanced MRI is the preferred confirmatory diagnostic study for investigation of a liver mass in a cirrhotic patient.
- Arterial phase enhancement with delayed phase washout is diagnostic for HCC on cross-sectional imaging.
- Evaluation of a cirrhotic patient for hepatic resection includes careful assessment of both tumor burden and severity of underlying liver disease.
- CTP class B and C patients and CTP class A patients with obvious portal hypertension or thrombocytopenia are not appropriate candidates for hepatic resection.

SUGGESTED READINGS

Bruix J, Sherman M. Management of hepatocellular carcinoma: an update. *Hepatology.* 2011;53(3):1020-1022.

Heimbach JK, Kulik LM, Finn RS, et al. AASLD guidelines for the treatment of hepatocellular carcinoma. *Hepatology.* 2018;67: 358-380.

Khan AS, Hussain HK, Johnson TD, Weadock WJ, Pelletier SJ, Marrero JA. Value of delayed hypointensity and delayed enhancing rim in magnetic resonance imaging diagnosis of small hepatocellular carcinoma in the cirrhotic liver. *J Magn Reson Imaging.* 2010;32:360-366.

Metastatic Colorectal Cancer

37

RICHARD A. BURKHART AND TIMOTHY M. PAWLIK

Based on the previous edition chapter "Metastatic Colorectal Cancer" by Peter D. Pengand Timothy M. Pawlik

Presentation

A 62-year-old man is referred to your office 2 years after a right hemicolectomy for colon cancer (T3N1M0) detected on screening colonoscopy. Following surgery, the patient received adjuvant chemotherapy with 5-fluorouracil, leucovorin, and oxaliplatin (FOLFOX). He now presents with an elevated carcinoembryonic antigen (CEA) of 80 ng/mL and cross-sectional imaging demonstrating new masses in the right hemiliver and a solitary lung lesion.

● DIFFERENTIAL DIAGNOSIS

The differential diagnosis of a liver mass includes both benign (cyst, hemangioma, focal nodular hyperplasia, hepatic adenoma) and malignant (metastatic disease, primary hepatocellular carcinoma, intrahepatic cholangiocarcinoma, gallbladder cancer) disease processes. In a patient with a history of colon cancer and a rising CEA, metastatic colon cancer is the most likely diagnosis. Approximately half of all patients diagnosed with colon cancer will experience disease spread to the liver at some point in their lifetime. Patients with colorectal liver metastasis can be grouped according to the time interval between the primary diagnosis and development of metastatic disease. The term synchronous hepatic metastasis is used when the diagnosis of liver involvement is concurrent or within 6 months of the initial colon lesion. Metachronous disease typically describes disease in the liver that is identified after 6 months following the primary diagnosis. Approximately 15% to 25% of patients will present with synchronous disease, while 20% to 25% will develop metachronous colorectal liver metastasis. Patients with liver only disease, as well as those with limited extrahepatic metastasis (especially oligometastatic disease of the lung), should be considered for surgery when resection is technically feasible and an R0 (microscopically negative) margin can be achieved.

● WORKUP

High-quality cross-sectional imaging should be obtained to evaluate patients who appear to have liver-only metastatic disease. Imaging can include triphasic computed tomography (CT) scan or contrasted enhanced magnetic resonance imaging (MRI). On CT, colorectal liver metastasis are typically best visualized in the venous phase, appearing as hypointense, low-attenuating masses within the liver (Figure 37-1). With multidetector CT, the sensitivity of identifying liver metastasis is about 80% to 90%. On contrast-enhanced MRI, colorectal liver metastases are often best seen on the T2-weighted images. Overall sensitivity of MRI to detect colorectal liver metastasis is approximately 80% to 90%, which is similar to CT. Imaging to rule out sites of extrahepatic spread should be used liberally to define thoroughly the exact extent of disease. Chest imaging (often with CT at the time of abdominal imaging) should be routinely used before resection of colorectal liver metastasis to rule out pulmonary metastasis. The use of positron emission tomography (PET), either alone or in combination with CT (PET/CT), can also be considered to assess more broadly for the presence of metastatic disease. Some studies have reported that PET may change clinical management in up to 20% of patients with colorectal liver metastasis who are being considered for surgical resection. While extrahepatic metastases can be a relative contraindication to hepatic resection, resection of oligometastatic lesions (especially in the presence of solitary extrahepatic pulmonary) may still be considered. The use of preoperative systemic chemotherapy should be strongly considered in patients with extrahepatic disease, as patient selection in this clinical situation is critical.

Biopsies of suspected metastatic lesions should not be routinely performed in isolated and resectable hepatic disease. In the appropriate clinical context, such as pathognomonic radiologic features on cross-sectional imaging associated with elevation of serum CEA, a biopsy is unnecessary to make the diagnosis (Figure 37-2). Although the risk is small, biopsy does carry some periprocedural risk and can result in tumor dissemination. Furthermore, in the setting of a history of colon cancer and a suspicious liver lesion on cross-sectional imaging, a "negative" biopsy would not preclude recommendation for surgery. Therefore, biopsy should be reserved only for those situations when there is diagnostic uncertainty or when nonsurgical treatment options are being considered.

Finally, a repeat colonoscopy should be considered on a case-by-case basis. Whether to obtain a repeat colonoscopy depends on the timing of the liver lesion relative to the primary tumor resection, the disease-free interval, and the date of the most recent colonoscopy following the index colectomy.

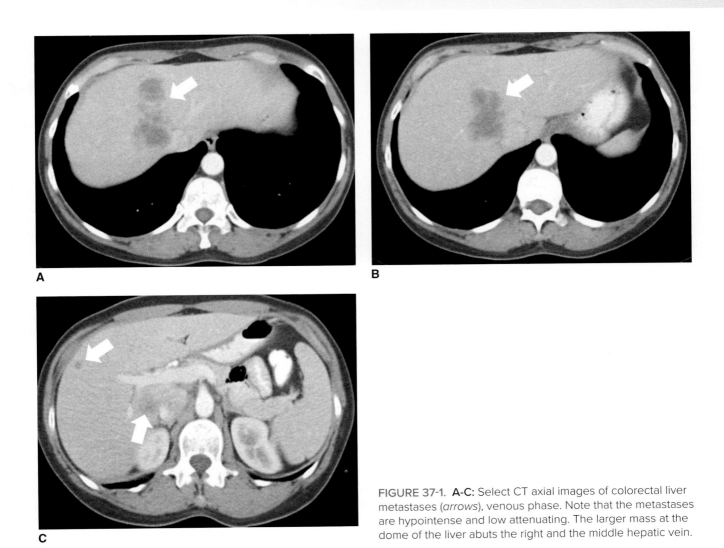

FIGURE 37-1. A-C: Select CT axial images of colorectal liver metastases (*arrows*), venous phase. Note that the metastases are hypointense and low attenuating. The larger mass at the dome of the liver abuts the right and the middle hepatic vein.

FIGURE 37-2. A,B: PET scan demonstrating multiple FDG-avid lesions (*arrows*) in the liver that correlate with the metastases identified on cross-sectional CT imaging.

● DIAGNOSIS AND TREATMENT

Surgical therapy for colorectal liver metastasis is typically the best management option for intrahepatic disease control, as well as long-term hope of cure. While reported 5-year overall survival following resection approaches 45% to 60%, up to two-thirds of patients will experience a recurrence at some point. Liver resection may provide, however, a survival benefit even among patients who experience a recurrence, due to improved control rates of intrahepatic disease. Over the last two decades, there has been a dramatic shift in the paradigm of how resectable disease is defined among patients with colorectal liver metastasis. For example, factors such as tumor number ≥4, bilobar disease, metastasis within 1 cm of the planned transection margin, or extrahepatic disease were traditionally considered contraindications to hepatic resection. With improvements in operative technique and—more importantly—systemic chemotherapy, these factors are no longer considered strict criteria to define whether or not a patient is a candidate for hepatic resection. Rather, clinical decisions should focus on whether all the disease can be removed (both intra- and extrahepatic) with a negative margin while preserving an adequate liver volume that has preserved vasculature inflow and outflow and biliary drainage. Regarding the extent of disease in the liver, when considering liver resection, the surgeon must ensure that an adequate liver remnant remains following hepatectomy. In general, following liver resection, at least two contiguous hepatic segments with adequate inflow, outflow, and biliary drainage need to be preserved. Additionally, a functional liver remnant (FLR) volume of roughly 20% to 30% should be maintained to avoid postoperative liver insufficiency or failure. For patients with underlying liver injury (e.g., steatosis, steatohepatitis), a larger FLR is required (i.e., 30% to 40%). When the FLR is too small, preoperative portal vein embolization can be used in an effort to increase the FLR and allow for safe hepatectomy. In these cases, the portal vein flowing to the tumor-bearing side of the liver is embolized, which induces hypertrophy of the contralateral liver (i.e., the FLR). Another emerging technique being utilized in select cases of patients with extensive colorectal liver metastasis is the associating liver partition and portal vein ligation for staged hepatectomy (ALPPS) approach. In this two-staged operation, one side of the liver is cleared of tumor and then the hilum is dissected to ligate the portal vein on the more heavily diseased side; the liver is then partially transected in the plane to be used at the second operation. Rather than completing the hepatectomy, the patient is closed and the liver is allowed to hypertrophy for a period of time. Subsequently, upon re-exploration, the portal dissection is completed, taking the arterial and biliary structures to the diseased liver, and the hepatectomy is completed in the plane begun at the first operation. Proponents of this technique highlight the rapid liver hypertrophy that the first stage of the procedure induces. The ALPPS approach may, however, be associated with higher morbidity and mortality and therefore remains utilized only in select centers. The final technical point that is important to remember is, when feasible, that colorectal liver metastasis should be extirpated using a parenchymal sparing approach, as the width of the surgical margin does not impact long-term outcomes.

While extrahepatic disease was traditionally a relative contraindication to resection of concomitant liver metastasis, current data would support an approach in which some patients with extrahepatic disease are offered surgery. Typically, individuals with extrahepatic disease who might be surgical candidates are those who have had a long disease-free interval, the presence of isolated or oligometastasis located in the lung, as well as those patients who have been treated with preoperative chemotherapy and have had either stable or responsive disease.

When patients present with extensive liver disease or concurrent extrahepatic metastasis, typically preoperative chemotherapy should be employed. Preoperative chemotherapy is usually given for either a set period of time (e.g., 3 to 6 months) or until the disease has responded such that surgical resection is feasible. The improved efficacy of chemotherapy for colorectal liver metastasis has allowed a subset of previously unresectable patients to undergo potentially curative liver surgery after tumor downsizing. When patients do not need to be downstaged (i.e., hepatic disease is resectable upon presentation), the use of neoadjuvant chemotherapy is also an option; however, its routine use is more controversial. For multifocal disease, the rationale for using neoadjuvant chemotherapy prior to hepatectomy is supported, in part, by limited data demonstrating improved prognosis compared with immediate surgery alone. The use of chemotherapy in the preoperative setting for patients with isolated and resectable colorectal liver metastasis is more debated, with many experts advocating for a hepatectomy-first approach in these patients. Some critics of this sequence caution that patients who experience postoperative complications may fail to receive adjuvant chemotherapy. In all cases, the decision to give chemotherapy before or after surgery should be individualized, based on the specific clinical situation, and discussed in a multidisciplinary setting of experts (Figure 37-3). Excessively prolonged periods of preoperative chemotherapy should, however, typically be avoided among patients being considered for hepatic resection as chemotherapy-induced liver toxicity has been reported, which may lead to increased perioperative complications (Figure 37-4).

● SURGICAL APPROACH

With the goal being complete surgical extirpation of metastatic disease and maintenance of patient safety, hepatectomy can be performed using either an open or a laparoscopic approach (Table 37-1). While there are increasing data emerging about the use of laparoscopic liver resection to treat malignancies, most major hepatectomies are still performed using an open technique. There are several incisions

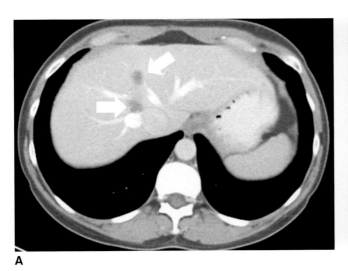
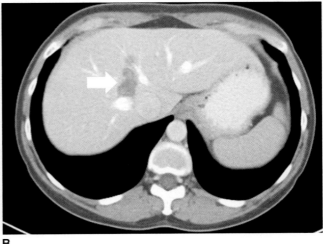

A   **B**

FIGURE 37-3. Repeat CT axial imaging following treatment with neoadjuvant treatment with four cycles of FOLFOX plus bevacizumab chemotherapy. Note the reduction in the size of the liver metastases (*arrows*).

that may facilitate the safe performance of a hepatectomy. Common choices include midline, Kocher (right subcostal), modified Kocher (right subcostal with midline superior extension), and the chevron (bilateral, often asymmetric subcostal). Upon entering the abdomen, the ligamentum teres and falciform ligament are taken down and a full evaluation of the liver is performed visually, by palpation, and with intraoperative ultrasound (IOUS). IOUS is an important tool for accurately staging liver tumors, assessing the true extent of disease, and making intraoperative decisions. IOUS is usually performed using a midfrequency (5.0 and 7.5 MHz) transducer probe, with the 7.5-MHz probe able to penetrate 6 to 8 cm. IOUS needs to be performed in a systematic manner in both the transverse and the sagittal planes to avoid missing any small occult lesions. The hepatic vasculature should also be examined with IOUS to identify possible anatomic variants and to aid in the planning of the resection.

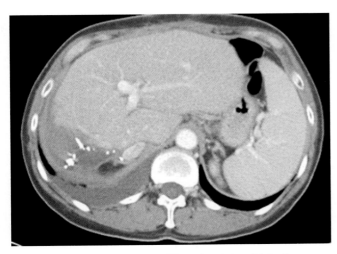

FIGURE 37-4. Postoperative CT axial imaging. Note the hypertrophy of the remnant left hemiliver, especially segments 2 and 3.

Inflow control through an intermittent Pringle's maneuver of the porta hepatis can be utilized to help reduce blood loss during the parenchymal transection. In the case of a formal hemihepatectomy, the hepatic inflow pedicle is often dissected at the level of the hilum. In many cases, the ipsilateral hepatic artery and portal vein can be divided outside the substance of the liver after lowering the hilar plate. Following division of the hepatic artery and the portal vein, the liver usually demarcates along the principal plane of the liver. Depending on the location of the lesion (i.e., for those lesions not near the hilum), an intrahepatic technique can alternatively be utilized to obtain control of the inflow as it enters the substance of the liver.

The need for liver mobilization is dictated by the extent and type of procedure planned. The coronary ligament is taken down with a combination of electrocautery and sharp dissection to expose the suprahepatic vena cava and hepatic veins. In the case of a right hemihepatectomy, the right hemiliver is mobilized by taking down the right triangular ligament and exposing the bare area of the liver along the right diaphragm. Complete mobilization is accomplished by taking down the retroperitoneal attachments along the inferior aspect of the right liver and dissecting the posterior liver away from the right adrenal gland. With the right liver rotated medially and superiorly, the retrohepatic vena cava is exposed and small venous branches traveling directly from the cava to the right hemiliver can be ligated and divided. The hepatocaval ligament is dissected free and divided, often with an endovascular stapling device. The right hepatic vein is circumferentially dissected free and can be divided between clamps or with an endovascular stapling device. For a left hemihepatectomy, the left hemiliver is mobilized by taking down the left triangular ligament. The ligamentum venosum is dissected free and divided to better expose the left hepatic vein. For a left hepatectomy, the left hepatic vein is often not dissected along its extrahepatic course but instead is typically divided within the substance of the liver

Table 37-1	Open Major Hepatectomy

Key Technical Steps

1. Midline or subcostal incision.
2. Exploration to rule out extrahepatic disease.
3. Exposure with self-retaining retractor (Thompson, Bookwalter, "Upper-Hand," etc.).
4. Liver mobilization (taking down ligamentous attachments of the liver, exposing retrohepatic cava for right hepatectomy, etc.).
5. Intraoperative ultrasound.
6. Inflow control (Pringle's maneuver).
7. Extra- or intrahepatic control of ipsilateral hepatic pedicle with division of the hepatic artery and the portal vein.
8. Extrahepatic division of the right hepatic vein when performing right hepatectomy; in general, when performing a left hepatectomy, the left hepatic vein is divided within the substance of the liver during the parenchymal transection (depending on location of lesion in left hemiliver).
9. Parenchymal transection while maintaining a low CVP.
10. Hemostasis. Larger bleeding structures are controlled surgically with sutures, while smaller parenchymal bleeding is controlled with selected use of electrocautery or topical hemostatic agents.
11. Examination for bile leak and oversewing of any sites of leak.
12. Selective use of closed suction drains (drains are not needed routinely for major hepatectomy).
13. Abdominal closure.

Potential Pitfalls

- Failure to mobilize the liver adequately prior to initiation of hepatic transection.
- Failure to identify all hepatic disease. Preoperatively, this may be due to suboptimal imaging. Intraoperatively, this may be due to failures during IOUS.
- Injury or stricture of the bile duct in remnant liver due to injury caused to the bile duct during the hilar or parenchymal dissection.
- Injury or stricture of bile duct in remnant liver due to inappropriate use of ablation technology in the setting of a lesion too close to hilum.
- Bleeding from middle hepatic vein during division along principle plane.
- Failure to obtain negative surgical margin due to poor planning of parenchymal transection.

during the hepatic parenchymal transection. The specifics of the dissection are, however, dictated by the size and location of the lesion relative to the hepatic vein.

A number of techniques can be utilized for parenchymal transection. Options include crush-clamp, bipolar or monopolar cautery, radiofrequency ablation (Habib device), harmonic scalpel, ultrasonic aspirator, or hydrojet devices. While different surgeons prefer different transection techniques, none have demonstrated clear superiority over the others. As such, the most important factor in choosing a method of liver transection should be the surgeon's comfort and familiarity with the technique. Emphasis should remain on patient safety throughout the operation with a controlled parenchymal transection to minimize blood loss and achieve complete tumor extirpation. An experienced anesthesia team should be present during all major liver surgery as safety is enhanced by maintaining a low central venous pressure (CVP) (<5 mm Hg) before and during parenchymal transection. While energy devices are a helpful adjunct to the efficient completion of a hepatectomy, larger structures are best controlled with ties and sutures. Hemostasis of the transected liver margin may also require topical hemostatic

agents such as methylcellulose, collagen sponges, and thrombin sealants. Following transection, the liver margin should be carefully inspected for bile leakage and identified sites can be oversewn.

The goal of any hepatic resection should be to achieve R0 status. Typically, intraoperative pathologic confirmation of an R0 margin is obtained after removal of the specimen. While attaining an R0-negative margin is important, the width of the negative margin has not been demonstrated to correlate with recurrence. Routine placement of closed suction drains is unnecessary following major liver resections. Selective use of drains is encouraged when concurrent diaphragmatic resection, biliary-enteric anastomosis, or multivisceral resections are required.

SPECIAL INTRAOPERATIVE CONSIDERATIONS

The identification of aberrant arterial and biliary anatomy is critical to successful liver surgery. Hepatic artery variants should be identified before beginning the parenchymal transection. Often vascular variants can be detected on high-quality preoperative imaging. In the operating room, the lesser omentum should be examined to identify a replaced/accessory left hepatic artery coursing toward the base of the umbilical fissure. Similarly, the lateral aspect of the porta hepatis should be palpated to detect a replaced/accessory right hepatic artery originating from the superior mesenteric artery.

Not infrequently, IOUS may identify disease not recognized on preoperative imaging. New findings may necessitate a change in the operative plan, including either a revision in the type of planned hepatic resection or the addition of ablation. When unsuspected extrahepatic disease is encountered, in general, hepatic resection is not warranted. Patients with unsuspected peritoneal disease or gross hilar adenopathy probably do not derive long-term survival benefit from hepatic resection. Rather, this subset of patients is probably best treated with systemic chemotherapy and should only be considered for liver-directed surgery after restaging and careful multidisciplinary consideration.

● POSTOPERATIVE MANAGEMENT

Following major hepatic resection, most patients are monitored in the intensive or intermediate care unit overnight. During this time, goal-directed crystalloid resuscitation and postoperative care is instituted. Following a major hepatectomy, the ability of the liver to clear lactate may be diminished. As such, blood lactate levels may not be appropriate to use as a marker of adequate resuscitation and should not routinely be followed as a guide for goal-directed resuscitation. Rather, the use of alternative markers of resuscitation, such as urine output or CVP, should be encouraged. Electrolytes, liver function tests, hemoglobin, and prothrombin (PT) are checked immediately following the operation and daily thereafter. Hypophosphatemia is common after a major hepatic resection; phosphate levels should therefore be checked and repleted as necessary. Following an extended hepatic resection (removal of 70% to 80%), liver insufficiency/failure can sometimes occur. In these circumstances, the coagulation profile may be impaired and can be treated at the discretion of the surgeon with vitamin K administration and/or fresh frozen plasma infusion. Although uncommon, another possible complication following hepatic resection is a bile leak. This complication can manifest itself with fever and an elevated bilirubin level in the setting of a normal alkaline phosphatase. Cross-sectional imaging can be obtained to identify a biloma. When large and symptomatic, bilomas can usually be adequately drained using percutaneous techniques. Most bilomas will subsequently resolve following drainage and expectant management. Rarely, endoscopic sphincterotomy can be required to help make it easier for the bile to drain from the liver via the distal common bile duct and into the duodenum. When no complications arise, a regular diet can usually be started on postoperative day 2 or 3, with an anticipated discharge on day 4 or 5. Laparoscopic approaches may shorten length of stay in experienced centers.

Case Conclusion

The patient received four cycles of FOLFOX plus bevacizumab with a measureable decrease in the size of the intrahepatic metastases and lung nodule. After 6 weeks off bevacizumab and 4 weeks off of FOLFOX, the patient underwent a right hemihepatectomy with complete extirpation of all intrahepatic disease and a concurrent video-assisted thoracoscopic surgery (VATS) to resect the lung metastasis. Postoperatively, the patient received adjuvant chemotherapy and remains disease free.

TAKE HOME POINTS

- Resection of solitary colorectal hepatic metastasis is associated with approximately 50% 5-year survival.
- The criteria for resectability have changed over the past decade. Hepatic resection for colorectal liver metastasis should be considered when complete tumor extirpation can be achieved while preserving two or more contiguous segments with vascular inflow, outflow, and biliary drainage.
- Limited extrahepatic disease, especially an isolated lung metastasis, does not preclude surgical consideration.
- Combination cytotoxic chemotherapy can result in excellent response in nearly half of patients with metastatic disease. Systemic chemotherapy regimens should be integrated into the overall therapeutic plan (i.e., neoadjuvant, conversion, or adjuvant depending on the situation). A multidisciplinary tumor board is integral in the treatment of patients with colorectal liver metastasis.
- Overall goals for resection include the maintenance of patient safety, complete tumor extirpation, parenchymal preservation as able, and the integration of surgical care into a broader multidisciplinary treatment regimen.

SUGGESTED READINGS

Charnsangavej C, Clary B, et al. Selection of patients for resection of hepatic colorectal metastasis: expert consensus statement. *Ann Surg Oncol.* 2006;13(10):1261-1268.

Nordlinger B, Sorbye H, et al. Perioperative FOLFOX4 chemotherapy and surgery versus surgery alone for resectable liver metastases from colorectal cancer (EORTC 40983): long-term results of a randomized, controlled, phase 3 trial. *Lancet Oncol.* 2013;14(12):1208-1215.

Pawlik TM, Choti MA. Surgical therapy for colorectal metastases to the liver. *J Gastrointest Surg.* 2007;11(8):1057-1077.

Pawlik TM, Scoggins CR, et al. Effect of surgical margin status on survival and site of recurrence after hepatic resection for colorectal metastasis. *Ann Surg.* 2005;241(5):715-724.

Reddy SK, Pawlik TM, et al. Simultaneous resections of colorectal cancer and synchronous liver metastasis: a multi-institutional analysis. *Ann Surg Oncol.* 2007;14(12):3481-3491.

Sadot E, Koerkamp BG, et al. Resection margin and survival in 2368 patients undergoing hepatic resection for metastatic colorectal cancer: surgical technique or biologic surrogate? *Ann Surg.* 2015;262 (3):476-485.

Schadde E, Ardiles V, et al. Early survival and safety of ALPPS: first report of the International ALPPS Registry. *Ann Surg.* 2014;260(5):829-838.

Schüle S, Dittmar Y, et al. Long-term results and prognostic factors after resection of hepatic and pulmonary metastases of colorectal cancer. *Int J Colorectal Dis.* 2013;28(4):537-545.

Vauthey JN, Pawlik TM, et al. Chemotherapy regimen predicts steatohepatitis and an increase in 90 day mortality after surgery for hepatic colorectal metastasis. *J Clin Oncol.* 2006;24(13): 2065-2072.

Obstructive Jaundice

ERIN A. STRONG AND SUSAN TSAI

Based on the previous edition chapter "Obstructive Jaundice" by Timothy L. Frankel and Christopher J. Sonnenday

Presentation

A 63-year-old African American woman who was recently diagnosed with diabetes presents with "yellowing" of her eyes, gums, nail beds for the last month. She experiences mild abdominal discomfort but denies abdominal pain. She reports frequent episodes of diarrhea and a 20-lb unintentional weight loss over the last 6 months. She denies any family history of cancer.

● DIFFERENTIAL DIAGNOSIS

In a patient who presents with new-onset jaundice, the cause of jaundice can be broadly classified as prehepatic, intrahepatic, or posthepatic causes (summarized in Table 38-1). Obstructive jaundice is usually related to posthepatic biliary obstruction due to either intraluminal obstruction or extraluminal compression. The most common cause of intraluminal obstruction is cholelithiasis, which frequently presents with an acute onset abdominal pain, jaundice, and fevers. The

location of the intraluminal obstruction can be confirmed by radiographic studies demonstrating a filling defect of the common bile duct (CBD), usually in the presence of a normal caliber pancreatic duct. In contrast, extraluminal compression of the distal biliary tree is usually painless and can be the result of either a chronic inflammatory process (chronic pancreatitis) or a periampullary malignancy. These patients often present with unintentional weight loss, worsening exocrine function (steatorrhea), or endocrine function (diabetes) but rarely have fevers or cholangitis. The double duct sign is the classic radiographic finding in these patients, where the extrinsic compression of the mass obstructs both the CBD as well as the pancreatic duct. Patients with chronic pancreatitis usually have radiographic features notable for a smooth tapered narrowing of the CBD, absence of a discrete pancreatic head mass, and pancreatic calcifications. In contrast, biliary obstruction related to neoplastic growth is usually associated with a mass, which causes a Shelf-like cutoff of the CBD. Since pancreatic cancer is the most common periampullary neoplasm, the remainder of this chapter will focus on the diagnosis and management of pancreatic cancer.

Table 38-1	Differential Diagnosis of Jaundice	
Classification	**Etiology**	**Common Laboratory Findings**
Prehepatic	• Hemolysis • Hematoma resorption • Inherited disorders of unconjugated hyperbilirubinemia	• Primarily unconjugated hyperbilirubinemia • Normal alkaline phosphatase and aminotransferases
Intrahepatic	• Hepatitis (viral or inflammatory) • Intrinsic liver dysfunction (cirrhosis)	• Both conjugated and unconjugated hyperbilirubinemia • Aminotransferases significantly more elevated than alkaline phosphatase

Posthepatic	• Choledocholithiasis
	• Chronic pancreatitis
	• Periampullary tumor
	  • Pancreatic cancer
	  • Ampullary cancer
	  • Duodenal cancer
	  • Distal cholangiocarcinoma
		• Primarily conjugated hyperbilirubinemia
		• Alkaline phosphatase significantly more elevated than aminotransferases

● WORKUP

Initial evaluation should include a detailed history and physical exam. A review of systems should focus on signs and symptoms of endocrine or exocrine insufficiency, specifically new or worsening diabetes, weight loss, or steatorrhea. Many patients will complain of vague abdominal discomfort. When present, pain is often epigastric in nature with radiation to the back, which may be indicative of tumor invasion into the celiac ganglion. On physical exam, jaundice may be less apparent in patients of color, and mucosal surfaces including the gums, tongue, nail bed, palms, and soles should be examined. Careful inspection for clinical signs of metastatic disease such as peritoneal metastases involving the abdominal wall (Sister Mary Joseph node) or distant metastases, such as supraclavicular lymphadenopathy (Virchow's node), is essential.

Lab testing should include complete blood count, comprehensive metabolic panel, and coagulation studies. Carbohydrate antigen 19-9 (CA19-9) is a cell surface glycoprotein, which is a valuable prognostic biomarker in pancreatic cancer but can be falsely elevated in the setting of jaundice and should be measured only when the total bilirubin is <2 mg/dL to avoid false elevations. In addition, careful assessment of diabetic control (glycosylated hemoglobin), nutritional status, and performance status should be performed.

Diagnosis

An abdominal ultrasound may be ordered early in the workup of a jaundiced patient but offers limited information for staging purposes. The preferred imaging modality for staging is a dual-phase (late arterial and portovenous phase) computed tomography (CT) scan of the abdomen and pelvis with acquisition of images at 1-mm slices. Since the staging of pancreatic cancer is determined by radiographic criteria, high-quality imaging is critical. Importantly, acute inflammation can distort tumor–vessel relationships and result in misclassification of the true tumor–vessel relationship. For this reason, high-quality CT imaging should be performed prior to any endoscopic intervention (endoscopic retrograde cholangiopancreatography (ERCP)), which could inadvertently result in a procedure-related complication, such as pancreatitis. Although patients with pancreatic cancer may present with profound jaundice, this is rarely associated with cholangitis, and therefore, emergent biliary decompression is rarely necessary. To complete a staging workup, chest x-ray or chest CT is recommended at the time of diagnosis.

Determination of Clinical Stage

The four clinical stages of pancreatic cancer are summarized in Table 38-2. There are two operable (resectable and borderline resectable disease) and two inoperable (locally advanced and metastatic disease) disease stages, as defined by the relationship of the tumor to critical vascular structures. Key nomenclature used to describe the tumor–vessel relationship includes tumor "abutment" of any vascular structure, defined as up to 180° contact of the circumference of the vessel wall, or "encasement," defined as tumor contact of the vessel wall, which exceeds 180° circumference. Resectable pancreatic cancers (Figure 38-1A) have no abutment of arterial and minor or no venous involvement. The distinction between borderline resectable and locally advanced pancreatic cancer is determined by the degree of tumor–vessel interface. Borderline resectable pancreatic cancers are defined as having (1) tumor abutment of the superior mesenteric artery (SMA) or celiac artery (Figure 38-1B), (2) short segment common hepatic artery (CHA) encasement amenable to resection and reconstruction, and/or (3) involvement of the superior mesenteric vein (SMV) or portal vein (PV) amenable to resection and reconstruction. In contrast, locally advanced pancreatic cancers have >180° encasement of the SMA (Figure 38-1C) or celiac artery and/or occlusion of the SMV/PV without option for reconstruction. Metastatic disease includes evidence of peritoneal or distant metastases.

Following radiographic imaging, histologic confirmation of malignancy is recommended. In rare cases, when a mass cannot be visualized on radiographic imaging or by endoscopic ultrasound (EUS) and tissue diagnosis cannot be obtained, patients should be taken to the operating room for resection when a high clinical index of suspicion for malignancy exists. For patients in whom a mass can be identified, endoscopic ultrasound and fine needle aspiration (FNA) of the pancreatic mass is preferred over percutaneous biopsy to prevent peritoneal tumor dissemination. At high-volume institutions, a cytopathologist may be present in the endoscopy suite to confirm a cytologic diagnosis, after which the advanced endoscopist can perform an ERCP to decompress the biliary system. Durable biliary drainage with uncovered metal stents placed below the insertion of the cystic duct is preferred if neoadjuvant therapy is planned, as silastic stents may need to be changed every 6 to 8 weeks to maintain patency.

Presentation Continued

Her labs were remarkable for a total bilirubin of 12.0, alkaline phosphatase of 329, and CA19-9 of 995 mg/dL. Pancreas protocol CT demonstrated a 2-cm head of pancreas mass with 180° abutment of the SMA and no evidence of distant metastases. Pathology on tissue specimen from EUS-FNA was consistent with adenocarcinoma. Based on these findings, she was classified as a borderline resectable pancreatic cancer. A short metal, endobiliary stent was placed at the time of EUS/FNA, and after normalization of her bilirubin, her CA19-9 was 550 mg/dL.

Table 38-2	Radiographic Definitions of Pancreatic Cancer Clinical Stage

	MCW Stage	Anatomic Structure	Relationship with the Tumor
Operable	**Resectable**	SMA, celiac	No abutment
		CHA	No abutment
		SMV-PV	No tumor contact or ≤180° contact without vein contour irregularity
	Borderline resectable	Pancreatic Head/Uncinate Process	
		SMA	≤180° (abutment)
		Celiac	≤180° (abutment)
		CHA	Short segment encasement without extension to celiac or CHA bifurcation amenable to resection and reconstruction
		Pancreatic Body/Tail	
		Celiac	≤180° (abutment)
		SMV-PV	Contact >180° or contour irregularity or thrombosis and amenable to resection and reconstruction
Inoperable	**Locally advanced**	Pancreatic Head/Uncinate Process	
		SMA, celiac	>180° (encasement) of the SMA >180° abutment/encasement of the celiac origin without involvement of the aorta and amenable to resection and/or reconstruction
		SMV-PV	Unreconstructible SMV/PV
		Pancreatic Body/Tail	
		SMA, celiac	>180° (encasement) of the SMA >180° abutment/encasement of the celiac origin without involvement of the aorta and amenable to resection and/or reconstruction
		Aorta	Abutment of the aorta and celiac

MCW, Medical College of Wisconsin; SMA, superior mesenteric artery; CHA, common hepatic artery; Celiac, celiac axis; SMV, superior mesenteric vein; PV, portal vein.

● TREATMENT SEQUENCING

Historically, upfront surgery has been recommended for patients who presented with a pancreatic mass suspicious for malignancy, even in the absence of a tissue diagnosis. Surgery provided an opportunity for simultaneous diagnosis, staging, and treatment of the cancer. Over the last 30 years, several high-volume institutions have published the outcomes of the surgery-first approach for pancreatic cancer and have consistently reported a median overall survival of 24 months. Unfortunately, the majority of patients will experience disease recurrence with a 7-month median disease-free survival following pancreatectomy in the absence of postoperative (adjuvant) therapy. Given the high probability of disease relapse, adjuvant therapy is recommended for all patients with pancreatic cancer regardless of stage. However, the feasibility of delivering adjuvant therapy after

pancreatectomy remains problematic. In an analysis of the SEER database, approximately 50% of patients who undergo upfront surgical resection were unable to receive adjuvant therapy, likely due to perioperative complications or failure to adequately recover from surgery. Since surgical therapy is necessary but not sufficient for long-term survival and the delivery of salvage adjuvant is unpredictable, there has been a growing interest in preoperative (neoadjuvant) therapy for patients with both resectable and borderline resectable pancreatic cancer.

Neoadjuvant Therapy

The initial goal of neoadjuvant therapy for pancreatic cancer was to minimize unnecessary operations in patients who had micrometastatic disease at the time of diagnosis. In initial neoadjuvant trials, ~30% of patients with resectable

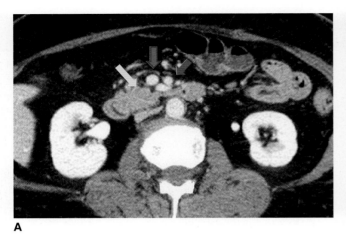

A

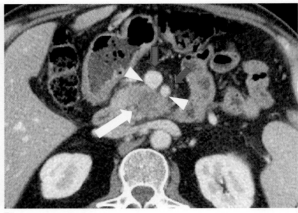

B

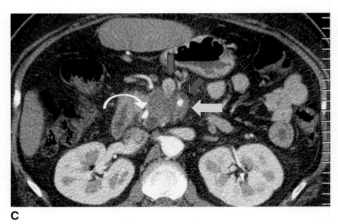

C

FIGURE 38-1. Radiographic examples of localized pancreatic cancer. *White arrows* denote pancreatic tumor, *blue arrows* denote superior mesenteric vein (SMV), and *red arrows* denote superior mesenteric artery (SMA). **A:** Resectable disease: fat plane is present between tumor and the SMV and SMA. **B:** Borderline resectable disease: tumor abut both SMV and SMA for <180°. **C:** Locally advanced disease: tumor abuts the SMV for <180° but encases SMA for >180°.

pancreatic cancer demonstrated metastatic disease progression prior to potential surgery. These patients experienced a median overall survival (~12 month) similar to patients with advanced inoperable disease and were spared the morbidity and mortality of an operation, which would have no oncologic benefit. Unexpectedly, among patients who received neoadjuvant therapy and surgery, the median overall survivals have exceeded that of patients treated with a surgery-first approach (34 vs. 24 months). Furthermore, the patients who completed all neoadjuvant therapy and surgery had lower rates of nodal metastases (30% vs. 70%) and lower rates of positive margins (10% vs. 40%) suggesting a downstaging effect of the therapy. Initial concerns with the use of neoadjuvant therapy were that patients with potentially operable pancreatic cancer may develop local disease progression, which would prevent potentially curative surgical resection. However, <2% of patients have been found to have isolated local disease progression during neoadjuvant therapy, which would preclude surgery. In addition, early concerns over the toxicity of neoadjuvant therapy and the impact of treatment-related side effects on operative morbidity and mortality were not realized. In particular, the rates of pancreatic fistula are lower in patients who have received neoadjuvant therapy as compared to patients who undergo surgery first.

Patients with borderline resectable pancreatic cancer are at the highest possible risk for distant disease progression and for positive surgical margins, and current societal and practice guidelines universally recommend neoadjuvant therapy for these patients. In general, patients with locally advanced tumors are not considered for operation. Pancreatic cancers are neurotropic and tumor encasement of the celiac axis, and SMA represents tumor infiltration of the substantial neural plexus surrounding these structures. Once the tumor has encased the neural tissues, it is unlikely that a negative margin can be achieved without resection of the arterial structure. Current practice guidelines suggest upfront surgical therapy for patients with resectable pancreatic cancer, although at some institutions, neoadjuvant therapy has become standard for patients with resectable pancreatic cancer.

Presentation Continued

The patient underwent neoadjuvant therapy with sequential chemotherapy and chemoradiation. Her restaging imaging after neoadjuvant therapy demonstrated a stable 2-cm mass in the head of the pancreas with no evidence of metastatic disease and her CA19-9 decreased to 76 mg/dL.

● SURGICAL APPROACH

Preoperative Planning

High-quality CT imaging is essential and should be obtained within 30 days of any planned surgery. Careful assessment of the tumor's relationship to the SMA, celiac axis, and hepatic arteries is critical as surgical resection of tumors with clear arterial encasement is not recommended. To avoid unanticipated intraoperative complications, a systematic approach should be utilized to review the tumor–vessel relationships preoperatively, including (1) identification of anomalous arterial variants (replaced/accessory right or left hepatic arteries); (2) loss of the normal tissue plane between the tumor and SMV/PV, which should alert the surgeon to potential direct tumor invasion of the vessel wall and need for venous resection and reconstruction; and (3) identification of venous aberrations, such as drainage of the inferior mesenteric vein into the SMV or a first jejunal branch draining anterior to the SMA. The operation for pancreatic cancers is dictated by the anatomic location of the tumor. Head/uncinate tumors are removed with a pancreaticoduodenectomy and are the focus of this chapter. Body/tail tumors are removed with a distal pancreatectomy and splenectomy. Tumors involving the neck of the pancreas are generally the most challenging, as they may abut the celiac axis or SMA and also involve the SMV/PV. These tumors can be removed with extended pancreaticoduodenectomies or distal pancreatectomies but may occasionally require a total pancreatectomy.

Pancreaticoduodenectomy

Appropriate positioning and draping of the patient facilitates an expedient surgical procedure. If vascular reconstruction is anticipated, the patient's groin and/or neck is included in the operative field in the event that a saphenous vein or internal jugular vein is needed. Approximately 10% of patients will have radiographically occult metastatic disease at the time of surgery, and therefore, diagnostic laparoscopy is often performed prior to laparotomy. In the absence of metastatic disease, the abdomen is explored through a midline laparotomy. Upon entry to the abdomen, the round ligament can be preserved as a pedicled flap to cover the stump of the gastroduodenal artery (GDA) at the end of the case. Once the abdomen is exposed, bimanual palpation of the liver and a thorough inspection of the small bowel and peritoneal surfaces should be performed.

There are six steps in resection portion of a pancreaticoduodenectomy (Figure 38-2). First, the infrapancreatic border of the pancreas and the infrapancreatic SMV are defined. This is performed by entering the lesser sac by removing the greater omentum from the transverse mesocolon. A limited mobilization of the hepatic flexure of the colon facilitates the exposure of the proximal third portion of the duodenum. The inferior border of the pancreas can usually be palpated at the base of the transverse mesocolon. Incising the visceral peritoneum at the inferior border of the pancreas will reveal an alveolar plane, which can be followed to the patient's right and will terminate in the identification of the infrapancreatic SMV. The middle colic vein may enter directly into the anterior surface of the SMV or arise as a common trunk with the gastroepiploic vein (gastrocolic trunk). When possible, the middle colic vein should be preserved, but in patients with large tumors of the uncinate process or significant visceral obesity, it may be preferable to ligate the middle colic vein to prevent inadvertent traction injury. If a large uncinate tumor is present or infrapancreatic SMV venous resection is anticipated, then a full mobilization of the retroperitoneal attachments (Cattell-Braasch maneuver) should be performed to allow for the complete exposure of the third and fourth portions of the duodenum. With SMV exposed, careful dissection under the inferior border of the pancreatic neck will expose an avascular plane beneath the neck of the pancreas.

The second step requires an extensive Kocher's maneuver to expose the underlying inferior vena cava. Kocher's maneuver should extend superiorly to the foramen of Winslow and inferiorly to allow the mobilization of the third portion of the duodenum off the transverse mesocolon. The third step involves the portal dissection. Aberrant arterial anatomy should be identified on preoperative imaging, but palpation

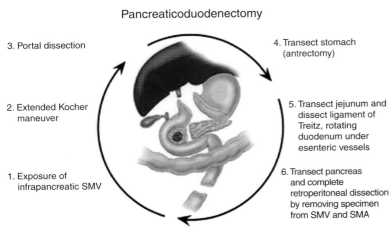

Pancreaticoduodenectomy

3. Portal dissection

2. Extended Kocher maneuver

1. Exposure of infrapancreatic SMV

4. Transect stomach (antrectomy)

5. Transect jejunum and dissect ligament of Treitz, rotating duodenum under esenteric vessels

6. Transect pancreas and complete retroperitoneal dissection by removing specimen from SMV and SMA

FIGURE 38-2. Critical steps of a pancreaticoduodenectomy.

of the portal structures is a useful intraoperative adjunct to identify anomalous arterial anatomy. In general, the CHA is the most medial structure in the portal trial; therefore, a pulsation along the lateral aspect of the portal triad would suggest aberrant arterial anatomy. Careful dissection of the CHA is critical to avoid inadvertent injury. There is a large lymph node invariably situated over the CHA, and removal of this lymph node facilitates a clear identification of the CHA and allows the surgeon to identify the takeoff of the gastroduodenal artery. Further dissection of the proper hepatic artery as it branches into right and left hepatic arteries is helpful. Once the GDA is divided, the common and proper hepatic arteries can be fully mobilized from the underlying PV. If the gallbladder is present, a retrograde cholecystectomy is performed to isolate the cystic duct and its insertion into the CBD. The CBD is usually divided at the level of the common hepatic duct. If an endobiliary stent is in place, intraoperative bile cultures may be sent to help guide postoperative antibiotic therapy in the event of an intra-abdominal abscess. The distal CBD margin can be sent and then the distal bile duct is oversewn. Division of the CBD and GDA allows complete exposure of the anterior surface of the PV along the superior border of the pancreas. Using gentle blunt dissection, a tunnel can be made to develop the avascular space between the superior and inferior borders of the neck of the pancreas and the underlying PV. Importantly, if this space cannot be easily established with gentle dissection, it should not be attempted forcibly. Rather vessel loops should be place to ensure distal control of the PV and proximal control of the SMV, and the pancreatic neck should be slowly divided down to the level of the PV at step 6.

The fourth step requires dividing the stomach, which begins with the division of the greater omentum and the gastroepiploic vessels along the greater curvature of the stomach. Similarly, the pars flaccida is divided with careful attention to the potential presence of an accessory or replaced left hepatic artery. The stomach is then divided approximately 3 to 4 cm proximal to the pylorus. Alternatively, pylorus-preserving pancreaticoduodenectomy can be performed in patients with small periampullary neoplasms who have not received neoadjuvant radiation. If pylorus preservation is attempted, at least 2 cm of duodenum should be preserved distal to the pylorus and if possible the right gastroepiploic vessels should be preserved.

The fifth step involves the mobilization of the ligament of Treitz. The jejunum may be divided approximately 10 cm distal to the ligament of Treitz, and the small bowel mesentery may be taken down using the LigaSure (Valleylab, Boulder, CO) device. The small bowel is then mobilized from the retroperitoneal attachments, and once the duodenal mesentery is sufficiently mobilized, the jejunum can be passed beneath the transverse colon mesentery into the right upper quadrant.

During a pancreaticoduodenectomy, the greatest risk for a positive margin is in the anatomic region between the pancreatic head and superior mesenteric vessels. Therefore, the final step, which involves dividing the neck of the pancreas and separating the head of the pancreas from the SMV/PV and SMA, is considered the most important oncologic step. To begin, hemostatic sutures are placed on the inferior and superior borders of the pancreatic neck both medial and lateral to the planned transection. Using the tunnel established between the pancreatic neck and SMV/PV (Step 3), the neck can be divided to expose the full length of the PV and SMV. At this point, the pancreatic neck margin can be sent for frozen section. Complete mobilization of the SMV/PV facilitates the safe dissection of the uncinate process from the SMA. Small venous tributaries to the uncinate process will need to be ligated to achieve complete mobilization of the SMV/PV. During the inferior mobilization of the SMV, the first jejunal branch of the SMV is generally encountered travelling posterior to the SMA. If possible, the jejunal branch should be preserved by ligating individual small tributary branches from the vein to the uncinate process. Once the jejunal branch is separated from the uncinate process, the SMA can be more easily exposed and identified. Most patients have one or two IPDAs, which are best managed with direct suture ligation.

After confirming hemostasis, the reconstruction classically begins with the pancreaticojejunostomy. To facilitate the pancreatic reconstruction, mobilization of approximately 2 cm of the pancreatic remnant facilitates suture placement and prevents inadvertent injury to the adjacent splenic artery or vein. A two layer, end-to-side, duct-to-mucosa anastomosis is performed with 4-0 or 5-0 monofilament sutures. A small silastic stent can be placed across the anastomosis if the pancreatic duct is small. A single layer biliary anastomosis is then performed approximately 10 to 15 cm from the pancreaticojejunostomy, using 4-0 or 5-0 absorbable monofilament suture. Finally, an antecolic, end-to-side gastrojejunostomy is performed at least 50 cm from the hepaticojejunostomy. Closed suction drains are variably used but can be helpful in controlling postoperative pancreatic fistula. When utilized, it is important that the drain is placed adjacent to but not in contact with an anastomosis, and early drain removal guided by biochemical testing of the drain fluid is preferred.

Special Intraoperative Considerations

As with other solid organ tumors, the goal of the operation should be to achieve a margin-negative resection. Resection and reconstruction of vascular structures during pancreaticoduodenectomy may be necessary to achieve a negative margin but should only be performed in the context of prior neoadjuvant therapy and should be performed by surgeons experienced in these procedures. If the neck of the pancreas cannot be separated from the SMV/PV, a more medial transection margin away from the involved vascular involvement should be created. After the pancreatic parenchyma has been transected, dissection of the tumor from the SMV/PV confluence can then be more safely performed under direct visualization and en bloc venous resection can be performed if needed. Venous reconstruction can include (1) primary repair, (2) patch venorrhaphy, (3) segmental resection and primary anastomosis, or (4) resection with interposition graft. In situations where the SMV/PV cannot be separated from the tumor, an "SMA-first" can be performed, approach in which the head and uncinate process are first separated from the SMA prior to the SMV. In general, the SMA can be located approximately 1 cm medial to the infrapancreatic SMV and 1 cm inferior to the inferior border of the pancreas. If the SMA can be identified in this area, dissection of the uncinate process from the SMA may be possible with or without division of the splenic vein. Dividing the splenic vein often improves exposure and facilitates mobilization of the SMV/PV if primary repair is planned. Whenever possible, splenic vein preservation is preferred; however, tumors that involve the SMV/PV confluence will require splenic vein division. In general, for venous reconstruction, if the involved segment is <2 cm, then primary repair can usually be achieved. Larger resections may require an interposition graft, and generally, the internal jugular vein has been favored due to an appropriate size match to the SMV/PV.

Postoperative Complications

The most common procedure-related complications after pancreatectomy include pancreatic fistula, delayed gastric emptying, and postpancreatectomy hemorrhage. Pancreatic fistulas are the most common complication and have been reported to occur in up to 30% of patient after surgery. Pancreatic fistula has been defined as drain output on or after postoperative day (POD) 3 with an amylase content greater than three times the upper normal serum value. Such output generally has cloudy or turbid yellowish appearance and may be associated with abdominal pain, delayed gastric emptying, fever, or leukocytosis. Importantly, pancreatic fistula can be associated with other postoperative complications, including intra-abdominal abscess, delayed gastric emptying, or postpancreatectomy hemorrhage. An isolated low output pancreatic fistula in the absence of a leukocytosis or other postoperative complications may be managed with a somatostatin inhibitor with or without antibiotics. However, in the setting of fevers, leukocytosis, ileus, or delayed gastric emptying, CT imaging is necessary to identify undrained intra-abdominal abscesses. Since anastomotic leaks from either a hepaticojejunostomy or gastrojejunostomy are uncommon, any intra-abdominal abscess is presumed to originate from a pancreatic fistula. It is important to have source control if there is any evidence of an intra-abdominal abscess related to a pancreatic fistula, as the proximity of amylase-rich fluid to adjacent vascular structures can lead to pseudoaneurysm formation.

Delayed gastric emptying occurs in approximately 15% of patients, and the cause is unclear and may be multifactorial. Delayed gastric emptying is defined by failure to remove a nasogastric tube by POD 4 or reinsertion of a nasogastric tube after POD 3. Although delayed gastric emptying results in prolonged hospital stays and patients discomfort, the natural history is self-limited and usually resolves with time.

In contrast, postpancreatectomy hemorrhage is a rare but life-threatening postoperative complication, which often requires emergent medical intervention. Postpancreatectomy hemorrhage is most commonly caused by bleeding from arterial pseudoaneurysms. Any frankly sanguineous drain output should immediately prompt a radiographic evaluation (CT angiogram or selective visceral angiogram) due to concern for potential pseudoaneurysm of the GDA or IPDA. Pseudoaneurysms are best managed with endovascular techniques (hepatic artery embolization) as surgical exploration in the postoperative setting often in the setting of intra-abdominal abscess can be exceedingly difficult (Table 38-3).

Table 38-3	**Pancreaticoduodenectomy**

Key Technical Steps

Pancreatic resection

1. Isolation of the infrapancreatic SMV
2. Extensive Kocher's maneuver
3. Portal dissection, CHA exposure, cholecystectomy, and transection of the bile duct
4. Transection of the stomach or pylorus
5. Mobilization of the jejunum and takedown of the ligament of Treitz
6. Pancreatic transection, resection of the pancreatic head/uncinate process from SMV-PV and SMA margin dissection (critical oncologic Step)

Pancreatic, biliary, and gastrointestinal reconstruction

1. Pancreatic anastomosis (usually two layer)
2. Biliary anastomosis (usually single layer)
3. Gastrointestinal reconstruction (usually two layer)

Potential Pitfalls

- Inadequate preoperative imaging resulting in poor characterization of tumor–vessel anatomy and/or aberrant anatomy based on preoperative radiologic evaluation
- Misidentification of the hepatic arterial anatomy resulting in transection of common or proper hepatic artery
- Inadvertent injury to the SMV/PV due to forceful, blunt dissection of the pancreatic neck off the SMV/PV
- Inadequate early exposure of the SMA during the pancreatic transection resulting in injury to the SMA

SMA, superior mesenteric artery; CHA, common hepatic artery; SMV, superior mesenteric vein; PV, portal vein.

Case Conclusion

The patient was discharged on POD 7. Her pathology demonstrated a T3N0M0 pancreatic cancer with negative margins and her CA19-9 level normalized following surgery. Due to deconditioning, she was unable to receive additional adjuvant therapy, but remained disease-free at her last follow-up, 32 months from surgery.

TAKE HOME POINTS

- Dual-phase CT imaging is essential for the accurate staging of pancreatic cancer.
- Patients with resectable and borderline resectable disease are considered to have operable disease. Patients with locally advanced and metastatic disease are considered inoperable.
- Due to the high likelihood for recurrent disease, systemic therapy is recommended for all patients with pancreatic cancer. Neoadjuvant therapy should be performed in patients with borderline resectable disease and is increasingly utilized for patients with resectable disease.
- If neoadjuvant therapy is planned, uncovered metal stents provide more durable biliary decompression than silastic stents.

- CT imaging should be performed within 30 days of planned surgical resection and careful review of tumor vessel relationships is critical to avoid intraoperative vascular injuries.
- Pancreaticoduodenectomy can be organized into six steps, performed in counterclockwise direction. Venous resection and reconstruction can facilitate a margin-negative resection, but such cases should be identified preoperatively and should only be performed by experienced surgeons.

SUGGESTED READINGS

Appel BL, Tolat P, Evans DB, Tsai S. Current staging systems for pancreatic cancer. *Cancer J.* 2012;18(6):539-549.

Evans DB, Christians KK, Foley WD, eds. Pancreaticoduodenectomy (Whipple operation) and total pancreatectomy for cancer. In: Fischer JE, ed. *Fischer's Mastery of Surgery.* 6th ed. Philadelphia, PA: Lippincott Williams & Wilkins; 2012: Chapter 133.

Mayo SC, Gilson MM, Herman JM, et al. Management of patients with pancreatic adenocarcinoma: national trends in patient selection, operative management, and the use of adjuvant therapy. *J Am Coll Surg.* 2012;214(1):33-45.

Sohal DP, Walsh RM, Ramanathan RK, Khorana AA. Pancreatic adenocarcinoma: treating a systemic disease with systemic therapy. *J Natl Cancer Inst.* 2014;106(3):dju011.

Tsai S, Evans DB. Therapeutic advances in localized pancreatic cancer. *JAMA Surg.* 2016;151(9):862-868.

Management of Incidental Pancreatic Cysts

SONIA COHEN AND CRISTINA R. FERRONE

Based on the previous edition chapter "Incidental Pancreatic Cyst" by Joshua A. Waters and C. Max Schmidt

Presentation

A healthy 48-year-old female presents to your clinic for evaluation of an incidentally identified pancreatic mass. While visiting a friend abroad, she volunteered to undergo an abdominal ultrasound at a new radiology facility as a test subject. To her surprise, a pancreatic lesion was identified. Upon her return home, the patient saw her primary care physician who obtained a repeat abdominal ultrasound that revealed a complex heterogeneous solid and cystic pancreatic body lesion measuring up to 4 cm. She has remained entirely asymptomatic. She denies any history of abdominal pain, jaundice, or weight loss. She has no history of ethanol abuse or abdominal trauma. She appears well with an unremarkable physical examination.

● DIFFERENTIAL DIAGNOSIS OF THE INCIDENTALLY IDENTIFIED PANCREATIC CYST

The recent increase in incidentally identified pancreatic cysts has been attributed to the overall increased use of cross-sectional imaging. Several case series have demonstrated that the prevalence of incidental pancreatic cysts identified via computed tomography (CT) and magnetic resonance imaging (MRI) may be as high as 5%. The most common etiology of a cystic lesion of the pancreas is an inflammatory pseudocyst, which is typically associated with a history of pancreatitis. Risk factors such as a personal history of cholelithiasis, biliary pathology, ethanol abuse, and abdominal or spinal trauma may be associated with the presence of a pancreatic pseudocyst. These pseudocysts are collections of a fluid that is high in amylase and lack an epithelial lining; they emanate from the parenchyma of the pancreas at the site of a ductal disruption. There is no malignant potential associated with pancreatic pseudocysts. In contrast, approximately 15% to 20% of all pancreatic cysts represent cystic neoplasms arising from the exocrine pancreas (Table 39-1). Of these, over 75% are serous cystadenomas (SCAs), mucinous cystic neoplasms (MCNs), or intraductal papillary mucinous neoplasms (IPMNs).

SCAs account for approximately 20% of all pancreatic cystic neoplasms. These lesions are more common in women, with a peak incidence in patients 60 to 70 years old, and are associated with mutations in the von Hippel-Lindau gene. These tumors have an extremely low risk of malignant transformation but may arise anywhere within the pancreas, leading to symptoms associated with the location and size of the lesion.

MCNs account for an additional 30% of pancreatic cystic neoplasms. These tumors occur almost exclusively in women, with an average age at presentation of 45 to 50. Because MCNs most commonly arise in the tail of the pancreas, these lesions are often asymptomatic. However, MCNs do harbor a risk of malignancy, and approximately 20% have undergone malignant transformation by the time they are identified.

IPMNs are the most commonly identified cystic neoplasm. They are found in both men and women between 60 and 70 years of age, arising throughout the pancreas. All IPMNs communicate with the pancreatic duct: either the main pancreatic duct (MD-IPMN), one of its branches (BD-IPMN), or both (mixed type). All IPMNs are associated with a risk of malignant transformation, either arising in the IPMN lesion itself or elsewhere in the pancreas. Up to 50% of MD-IPMNs are associated with malignancy, with lower rates described for BD-IPMNs and mixed-type lesions.

Presentation Continued

Our patient presents with an incidentally identified pancreatic cystic lesion. Her history and CT scan suggest that this is less likely an inflammatory pseudocyst despite the relative predominance of these lesions. Of the most common cystic neoplasms discussed above, both MCNs and IPMNs carry a significant risk of malignant transformation. Cystic variants of solid neoplasms, such as ductal adenocarcinoma, can also present as incidentally identified findings on imaging studies. As a result, accurate assessment is essential because not all pancreatic cysts require surgical intervention, but those with malignant potential should be identified and resected when appropriate.

● WORKUP

Once a cystic pancreatic lesion is identified, pancreatic-specific imaging and cyst fluid samples are obtained in order to narrow the differential diagnosis. High-quality cross-sectional imaging—either CT with thin sections through the

Table 39-1	Classification of Pancreatic Cysts

Cyst	Characteristics
Pancreatic pseudocyst	Associated with pancreatitis Lack epithelial lining Fluid is high in amylase No malignant potential
Serous cystadenoma	Occur more frequently in females than males Mean age at diagnosis is 60 Microcystic: honeycomb appearance with central calcifications or scar Macrocystic: unilocular or bilocular cysts with central calcification Arise throughout the pancreas Low risk of malignancy
Mucinous cystic neoplasm	Occur almost exclusively in females Median age at diagnosis mid- to late 40s Solitary cyst with septations, peripheral calcifications, mural nodules Located within body or tail of pancreas Harbor risk of malignancy Resection recommended
Intraductal papillary mucinous neoplasm	Found in both males and females Most common in sixth and seventh decade of life BD-IPMN more common than MD-IPMN MD-IPMN more likely to be symptomatic at presentation Ductal involvement seen on dedicated pancreatic imaging Large size, thick septations, or solid components are concerning features All harbor risk of malignancy (MD-IPMN less than BD-IPMN) Resect MD-IPMN and BD-IPMN with worrisome features

pancreas or magnetic resonance cholangiopancreatography (MRCP)—can often provide sufficient information to distinguish between pancreatic cystic neoplasms. Imaging features allow SCAs to be classified as either microcystic or macrocystic. Microcystic SCAs have a characteristic appearance with multiple <2 cm cysts arranged in a "honeycomb" pattern and associated with a stellate-shaped central scar. Macrocystic SCAs are typically unilocular or bilocular cysts >2 cm in size and can be difficult to distinguish from inflammatory pseudocysts or MCNs. However, while macrocystic SCAs often show central calcification on imaging, MCNs more typically have peripheral calcifications. Neither SCAs nor MCNs communicate with the pancreatic duct, while IPMNs invariably show ductal involvement. MRCP is the most useful imaging modality for demonstrating ductal involvement and can reliably distinguish between a MD-IPMN and BD-IPMN. In addition to providing clues as to the type of a pancreatic cystic neoplasm, concerning radiographic features can also predict the malignant behavior of individual lesions. These features include the size of the lesion, the thickness of septations within the lesion, and the presence or absence of mural nodules or other solid components. As a result, cross-sectional imaging may provide enough information about an individual's pancreatic cystic neoplasm to drive management decisions. Otherwise, further diagnostic information can be obtained via cyst fluid analysis.

Endoscopic ultrasound (EUS) can be used to further evaluate radiographically indeterminate lesions and obtain cyst fluid samples via aspiration. EUS allows sampling of the pancreatic lesion of interest under direct visualization across the gastric or duodenal wall. Cyst fluid cytology, viscosity, amylase levels, and the tumor marker carcinoembryonic antigen (CEA) can be used to distinguish between pancreatic cystic neoplasms (Table 39-2). While SCAs contain thin, glycogen-rich fluid and demonstrate low CEA levels, both MCNs and IPMNs are composed of thick, mucinous fluid, and their CEA levels are relatively high. MCNs and IPMNs can be distinguished by the cyst fluid amylase level: low in IPMNs and elevated in MCNs. Together with radiologic features, these cyst fluid characteristics allow for the appropriate diagnosis and treatment of an individual pancreatic cystic neoplasm.

Table 39-2 **Pancreatic Cystic Fluid Analysis**

	Cytology	Viscosity	Amylase	CEA
SCA	Cuboidal cells Glycogen+	Thin		Low
MCN	Columnar cells Mucin+	Viscous	Low	High
MD-IPMN	Columnar cells Mucin+	Viscous	High	High
BD-IPMN	Columnar cells Mucin+		High	High

Presentation Continued

You recommend that our patient undergo an MRCP to better characterize her pancreatic lesion and its relationship to the pancreatic duct. This study demonstrated a septated cystic mass in the body of the pancreas with a question of association with the main pancreatic duct and some solid components. The main pancreatic duct is not dilated. Given your concern for a pancreatic cystic neoplasm, in particular a BD-IPMN with solid components, which would require surgical resection given the risk of malignant transformation, you refer her for EUS and fine needle aspiration (FNA). EUS again demonstrates a large, complex, multicystic mass, and transgastric aspiration is used to obtain a 6-cc sample of clear, slightly viscous fluid. Analysis of this fluid demonstrates an undetectable CEA level, an amylase level of 41,525, and cytology negative for any malignant cells. While your patient's imaging is most consistent with an IPMN or MCN with solid component, her fluid analysis is atypical. You ask her to return to your clinic to discuss management options.

● DIAGNOSIS AND TREATMENT

Not all pancreatic cystic neoplasms require surgical intervention. Lesions with a clear diagnosis based on initial imaging and cyst fluid studies can either be observed or offered immediate surgical resection based on malignant potential and individual patient risk factors. For example, SCAs have essentially no malignant potential: if they are asymptomatic, nonoperative management should be offered. The need for further imaging is debated, since there is essentially no risk of malignancy. Further follow-up imaging upon development of symptoms would be acceptable. The location of the lesion within the pancreas should also be considered during this decision as a pancreatic head lesion may require Whipple's procedure rather than a distal pancreatectomy. Along these lines, the possibility of continued interval growth of a lesion and a future need for more extensive resection should also be considered when advising a patient to continue observation.

Patients with BD-IPMNs, if small in size (<3 cm), asymptomatic, and without worrisome radiographic features, such as mural nodules, can also be offered observation with serial imaging. In contrast to BD-IPMNs, all MCNs and MD-IPMNs should be managed operatively based on their more aggressive malignant potential. Similarly, patients without a definitive preoperative diagnosis for whom the likelihood of an MCN or MD-IPMN is felt to be high should be offered operative management, especially if the patient is a low-risk surgical candidate.

Presentation Continued

Your patient returns to the clinic to discuss management of her incidentally identified pancreatic cystic neoplasm. Her workup suggests that she may have a BD-IPMN with a mural nodule or MCN with features concerning for malignant transformation. Given her young age and relative health, you recommend resection of the lesion for definitive diagnosis and treatment.

● SURGICAL APPROACH

The approach to resection of any pancreatic lesion depends on the lesion size, its location within the pancreas, and the relationship to the main pancreatic duct and portal vein. Lesions located in the body or tail of the pancreas can be resected via distal or middle pancreatectomy with resection of the lesion and surrounding pancreatic tissue. Lesions in the head, neck, or uncinate process of the pancreas require a pancreaticoduodenectomy. Review of preoperative imaging can help to guide operative planning, but the ultimate approach for resection will rely on intraoperative findings and the surgeon's determination of which operation can safely facilitate complete resection.

If distal pancreatectomy is anticipated for resection of a cyst in the body or tail of the pancreas, the patient should undergo preoperative vaccination against encapsulated bacterial pathogens in preparation for possible splenectomy. We recommend a laparoscopic approach to these lesions. A 15-mm port is placed at the umbilicus, 5 mm in the right upper quadrant to help retract the stomach cephalad, a 5-mm port in the midclavicular line in the left upper quadrant, and a 5-mm port in the left anterior axillary line. The laparoscopic approach provides excellent visualization of the pancreas and its blood supply, as well as the splenic hilum. In this approach, the pancreas is dissected from medial to lateral, allowing for division of the pancreas proximal to the cystic lesion with the distal extent of the dissection at the splenic hilum. If laparotomy is performed, a vertical midline incision is used to enter the abdominal cavity. The lesser sac is opened by separating the greater omentum from the transverse colon. The stomach is reflected caudally to expose the body and tail of the pancreas, and the location of the cystic lesion is verified. Intraoperative ultrasound can be utilized to identify the cyst. If a splenic preservation via Warshaw's technique is performed, the short gastrics must remain intact. The splenic artery and vein are taken with a stapler or via suture ligation. Once the cyst is clearly identified, a stapler can be utilized to transect the pancreatic parenchyma. If the parenchyma is too thick for a stapler, the end of the pancreas can be fish mouthed and the edges approximated. If the spleen is removed, all the short gastrics need to be divided before dividing the lateral attachments of the spleen and mobilizing it medially. A surgical drain is placed near the pancreatic stump prior to closure of the abdomen.

Alternatively, a middle pancreatectomy will allow for resection of a cystic lesion within the body of the pancreas with preservation of both the spleen and the tail of the pancreas, which may help to prevent postoperative endocrine or exocrine insufficiency. In this case, the pancreatic parenchyma on either side of the cystic lesion is divided. The proximal pancreas is oversewn, while a pancreaticojejunostomy or pancreaticogastrostomy is performed with the distal remnant of the pancreas.

Patients with cystic lesions of the head or neck of the pancreas that require resection will need to undergo a pancreaticoduodenectomy or Whipple's procedure. After entering the abdomen, a cholecystectomy is performed, and then the lesser sac is entered to examine the pancreas. The right colon is mobilized and a generous Kocher maneuver performed to mobilize the duodenum and the head of the pancreas. The stomach, or proximal duodenum in the case of a pyloric-sparing procedure, is divided. A portal dissection is performed using the cystic duct stump to identify the common bile duct, which is divided. The gastroduodenal artery is then divided, with care taken to ensure that the patient has standard anatomy and that the vessel divided is not a recurrent right hepatic artery. The neck of the pancreas distal to the cystic lesion is then divided, followed by the proximal jejunum. The uncinate process is dissected from the superior mesenteric vessels, and then the specimen containing the cyst is removed. Gastrointestinal continuity is then restored by performing a gastrojejunostomy, pancreaticojejunostomy, and choledochojejunostomy, often with creation of a Roux-en-Y limb.

● POSTOPERATIVE MANAGEMENT

Postoperatively, patients who undergo a distal pancreatectomy have their nasogastric tube removed on postoperative day 0 or 1. They are advanced to liquids on day 1. Return of bowel function and advancement of diet range between 2 and 5 days. Most laparoscopic patients are discharged on postoperative day 3 or 4. Patients who have undergone a laparotomy are discharged in 5 to 6 days. Drain amylase is checked between 2 and 5 days postoperatively to assess for pancreatic leak.

Whipple's patients are typically discharged 6 to 7 days after their operation. Similarly, the nasogastric tube is removed on postoperative day 1. As bowel function returns, patients are advanced from a liquid to a solid diet. Drain amylase is checked between 3 and 5 days postoperatively.

Middle pancreatectomy has the advantage of sparing the most pancreatic parenchyma, especially if the lesion is in the neck or body. The disadvantage is that the pancreatic fistula rate is high due to the presence of two pancreatic transection sites.

In addition to monitoring for pancreatic fistula, which may require prolonged bowel rest and drainage if high output, all patients who have undergone pancreatectomy require monitoring for the development of endocrine or exocrine pancreatic insufficiency. Treatment with insulin or enzymatic supplementation may be required.

Laparoscopic Distal Pancreatectomy for Lesions in Body or Tail of Pancreas

Key Technical Steps

1. A 15-mm port is placed at the umbilicus, 5 mm in the right upper quadrant to help retract the stomach cephalad, a 5-mm port in the midclavicular line in the left upper quadrant, and a 5-mm port in the left anterior axillary line.
2. Enter the lesser sac by separating the greater omentum from the transverse colon and lifting the posterior gastric wall away from the pancreas.
3. Examine the pancreas from the duodenum to splenic hilum to verify location of lesion and relationship to the main pancreatic duct and vessels.
4. Intraoperative ultrasound through the 15-mm umbilical port can be very helpful.
5. Leave short gastric vessels intact to attempt splenic preservation via Warshaw's technique.
6. Dissect out splenic artery and divide it with a stapler.
7. Utilize a second stapler to transect the splenic artery and vein in the splenic hilum.
8. If the spleen does not appear viable, mobilize the spleen by ligating the short gastrics and the splenorenal ligament.
9. Medialize the spleen and free pancreatic tail.
10. The splenic vein can be taken separately or with the pancreatic parenchymal division utilizing a stapler.
11. If possible, preserve the inferior mesenteric vein at inferior border of the pancreas.
12. If the stapler is too thick to be stapled, divide the pancreas proximal to the cystic lesion using cautery and oversew the pancreatic duct end and cut surface of the pancreas in the fish-mouth technique.
13. Place drain at resection bed.
14. Close the abdomen.

Whipple's Procedure for Lesions in Head or Neck of Pancreas

Key Technical Steps

1. Vertical midline incision vs. R subcostal incision that crosses the midline with exploration of the peritoneal cavity.
2. Cholecystectomy.
3. Enter the lesser sac by separating the greater omentum from the transverse colon and lifting the posterior gastric wall away from the pancreas.
4. Kocher maneuver and mobilization of the duodenum and head of the pancreas from underlying vessels.
5. Division of the stomach or proximal duodenum with a stapler.
6. Perform portal dissection and division of GDA and bile duct.
7. Division of neck of pancreas, dissection of portal and superior mesenteric veins and SMA from the uncinate process, and division of proximal jejunum.
8. Removal of Whipple's specimen including cyst.
9. End-to-side duct-to-mucosa pancreaticojejunostomy with placement of pancreatic duct stent, hepaticojejunostomy, and gastrojejunostomy.
10. Place two drains above and below the pancreatic and biliary anastomoses.
11. Close the abdomen.

Potential Pitfalls

- Mistaking a replaced right hepatic artery for the GDA during Whipple's.
- Utilizing an inadequate sized stapler for the thickness of the pancreas when dividing pancreatic parenchyma.

Case Conclusion

Our patient is taken to the operating room, and a cystic lesion is identified in the proximal body of the pancreas. She undergoes an uncomplicated middle pancreatectomy with anastomosis between her remnant distal pancreatic duct and stomach. Her postoperative course was uncomplicated, and she was discharged home on postoperative day 5. Her final pathology revealed a 2.3-cm serous cystadenoma, which was completely excised and therefore carries no risk of recurrence or malignancy. She requires no further treatment or follow-up for her incidentally identified pancreatic cyst.

TAKE HOME POINTS

- Categorization of incidentally identified pancreatic cysts is important as nonneoplastic cysts require treatment only if symptomatic, while those with malignant potential require resection.
- Categorization can be accomplished by cross-sectional imaging and EUS-FNA to assess the composition of the cystic fluid.
- Serous cystadenomas have a low risk of malignant transformation and may arise anywhere within the pancreas.
- Mucinous cystic neoplasms most commonly arise in the tail of the pancreas and have the potential to undergo malignant transformation.

- Intraductal papillary mucinous neoplasms arise throughout the pancreas and communicate either with the main pancreatic duct or one of its branches. All IPMNs are associated with a risk of malignant transformation.
- For cysts that require surgical resection, the location within the pancreas determines the operative approach: pancreaticoduodenectomy (Whipple's procedure), middle pancreatectomy, or distal pancreatectomy.

SUGGESTED READINGS

Attiyeh MA, et al. Development and validation of a multi-institutional preoperative nomogram for predicting grade of dysplasia in IPMNs of the pancreas. *Ann Surg.* 2018;267:157.

Greer JB, Ferrone CR. Spectrum and classification of cystic neoplasms of the pancreas. *Surg Oncol Clin North Am.* 2016;25:339.

Shi N, et al. Splenic preservation versus splenectomy during distal pancreatectomy: a systemic review and meta-analysis. *Ann Surg Oncol.* 2016;23:365.

Tanaka M, et al. International consensus guidelines 2012 for management of IPMN and MCN of the pancreas. *Pancreatology.* 2012;12:183.

Refractory Pain from Chronic Pancreatitis

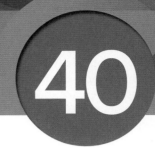

ANDREW B. SCHNEIDER AND JEFFREY B. MATTHEWS

Based on the previous edition chapter "Refractory Pain from Chronic Pancreatitis" by
Sajid A. Khan and Jeffrey B. Matthews

Presentation

A 57-year-old male presents with a 4-year history of abdominal and back pain, steatorrhea, and insulin-dependent diabetes mellitus. He carries the diagnosis of chronic pancreatitis, which has been attributed to significant ethanol and tobacco abuse in his past. Steatorrhea has been controlled by pancreatic enzyme supplementation. The pain interferes with his activities of daily life including the ability to work, and he became increasingly dependent on oral oxycodone for relief. There is no family history of pancreatic disease. The physical examination is without significant findings.

● DIFFERENTIAL DIAGNOSIS

The differential diagnosis of chronic abdominal pain is extensive. However, in this setting, the association with symptoms of steatorrhea combined with a history of ethanol abuse significantly narrows the possibilities. Other entities to consider include peptic ulcer disease, biliary tract dysfunction, thoracic/lumbar spine disorders, and retroperitoneal fibrosis. Pancreatic carcinoma can produce symptoms similar to chronic pancreatitis when the tumor obstructs the pancreatic duct and produces pain due to neurovascular invasion. Finally, complications of chronic pancreatitis may also contribute to the progression of symptoms, including pseudocyst formation and biliary or duodenal obstruction.

● WORKUP

Chronic pancreatitis is an inflammatory and fibrosing disease of the pancreas characterized by irreversible morphologic changes and permanent loss of exocrine function.

The most common risk factor for chronic pancreatitis is excessive alcohol. Tobacco appears to increase the risk independent of alcohol usage. Elicitation of modifiable risk factors is an important first step in the evaluation.

However, chronic pancreatitis occurs in patients without any significant toxic exposures. A careful family history is important, as an increasing number of variations of specific genes have been found to be associated with acute and chronic pancreatitis in recent decades. The genes demonstrate both autosomal dominant and recessive patterns of inheritance as well as variable degrees of penetrance. Mutations in the cationic trypsinogen gene PRSS1 are associated with hereditary pancreatitis in an autosomal dominant fashion. The most common pancreatitis-associated PRSS1 mutation is R122H, which leads to an unusually stable trypsin that is resistant to autolytic inactivation and may be associated with premature activation of trypsin within pancreatic acinar cells. The risk of pancreatic cancer is increased in hereditary pancreatitis, particularly in smokers. A number of splice variations and mutations in the gene that encodes the cystic fibrosis transmembrane conductance regulator (CFTR) have also been associated with a pancreas-specific phenotype characterized by recurrent acute and chronic pancreatitis in the absence of pulmonary or other organ system manifestations of cystic fibrosis. Recently, other genes have been implicated in predisposing an individual to chronic pancreatitis such as anionic trypsinogen (PRSS2), calcium-sensing receptor (CASR), and serine protease inhibitor Kazal type 1 (SPINK1).

Patients usually report epigastric abdominal pain that may radiate through or around to the back. The pattern of pain varies among patients. Some describe cyclic episodes of severe pain followed by quiescence. Others have unrelenting persistent pain that can limit activities of daily living. Details of prior treatment of pain, particularly the use and potentially dependence on narcotic analgesics should be documented. Patients who develop significant exocrine insufficiency may experience steatorrhea with consequent weight loss, malnutrition, and fat-soluble vitamin deficiencies. These patients may also experience postprandial pain and bloating that should be addressed by pancreatic enzyme replacement therapy. Unfortunately, the potential contribution of exocrine insufficiency to patient-reported symptoms are often underappreciated by inexperienced clinicians leading to inappropriate prescription of opioid analgesics. Endocrine insufficiency usually develops later in the disease process, typically several years after exocrine insufficiency. The pattern of abdominal pain, degree of impairment with quality of life, and the response to prior therapies including medication can assist in determining the appropriateness of surgical options.

Blood tests including amylase and lipase are of limited value, particularly in later stages of disease characterized by parenchymal fibrosis and exocrine atrophy.

Axial imaging by computed tomography (CT) can confirm the diagnosis of chronic pancreatitis by providing evidence of calcifications (ductal or parenchymal), focal inflammatory enlargement or masses, ductal dilation, and the presence of complications such as pseudocysts. Extrapancreatic complications including splenomesenteric vein thrombosis and biliary or duodenal obstruction may also be present. Additional diagnostic imaging may be useful for therapeutic decision-making.

Pancreatic duct visualization is important in the assessment of treatment options and can be achieved by endoscopic retrograde or magnetic resonance cholangiopancreatography (ERCP or MRCP). These imaging approaches can provide information regarding anatomic ductal anomalies including pancreatic divisum and focal duct strictures. MRCP is preferred to ERCP secondary to higher image resolution, lack of ionizing radiation, and its noninvasive nature. ERCP is useful for endotherapy options including sphincterotomy, lithotripsy, stone extraction, stricture dilation, and stent placement. The addition of endoscopic ultrasound (EUS) may be useful in diagnosis of early-stage chronic pancreatitis. Furthermore, EUS can be used to guide needle biopsy of suspicious mass lesions of the pancreas to rule out underlying malignancy.

An important goal of the workup of the patient with refractory pain in chronic pancreatitis is the identification of possible therapeutic targets for surgical (or occasionally endoscopic) intervention. This requires imaging of both pancreatic ductal as well as parenchymal changes associated with the disease, as this information may indicate which treatment options might be applicable. As a general rule, the choice of therapy should be directed at the presumed mechanism for the pain. However, it should be acknowledged that the precise mechanism of pain in chronic pancreatitis is incompletely understood and may reflect multiple factors. In some patients, obstruction of the pancreatic duct by stones and stricture leads to ductal dilation ("large duct" disease) and pain due to increased intraductal pressure. In other situations, it is postulated that parenchymal edema associated with chronic inflammation leads to organ hypertension and capsular stretch. Chronic exposure to local inflammatory mediators may lead to retroperitoneal sensory neural remodeling including up-regulation of nociceptors and altered neurostimulatory thresholds. An anatomic concentration of inflammation and parenchymal/intraductal calcifications within the pancreatic head may not only produce pain and local symptoms due to mass effect but may contribute to ongoing obstruction of the upstream dorsal pancreas. An inflammatory pancreatic head mass has been described as the "motor" of chronic pancreatitis and may be seen on axial imaging such as triple-phrase (pancreatic protocol) CT.

In the patient presented above, abdominal CT demonstrated diffuse parenchymal and ductal calcifications characteristic of large duct disease (Figure 40-1). The presence of an inflammatory pancreatic head mass raised suspicion of possible malignant transformation. EUS furthered revealed a 4-cm poorly defined relatively hypoechoic area in the head of the pancreas that was clinically suspicious, although fine needle biopsy yielded only nondiagnostic reactive cells.

● DIAGNOSIS AND TREATMENT

Medical therapy begins with elimination of alcohol and smoking, although the challenge of substance dependence often contributes both to the pathogenesis and the treatment of chronic pancreatitis. Exocrine insufficiency should be treated with pancreatic enzyme replacement therapy, typically enteric-coated preparations taken together with meals and spaced appropriately to optimize mixing with ingested protein and fat. Pharmacotherapy for analgesia should start with nonsteroidal anti-inflammatory medications with escalation to propoxyphene if required. Narcotics should be utilized sparingly and only in the setting of an acute exacerbation. Once narcotic dependence has occurred, further treatment becomes complicated by

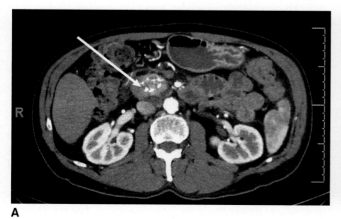

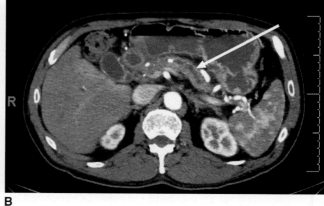

FIGURE 40-1. **A:** Diffuse calcifications in the head of the pancreas. **B:** Main duct dilation.

the stigma of opioid addiction, and the impact of interventions becomes difficult to assess. It can become challenging to distinguish disease exacerbation from narcotic withdrawal. Alternatives for chronic pain include gabapentin and related compounds. Neurolysis by celiac plexus block or thoracoscopic splanchnicectomy should be reserved for patients who have failed medical therapy and do not have favorable anatomy for surgical intervention. However, the impact of neurolysis is often disappointingly transient with a majority of patients developing recurrent pain within months.

Intractable pain is the most common indication for operation. Surgical intervention may alleviate pain by the combination of two mechanisms: (1) decompression of the main pancreatic duct in order to relieve obstruction and improve drainage and (2) resection of parenchyma to remove dominant foci of inflammation, calcifications, cystic changes, or malignant degeneration. A secondary goal is the preservation of pancreatic parenchyma to limit the loss of exocrine and endocrine function.

● SURGICAL APPROACH

The choice of surgical procedure should reflect the anatomy and distribution of the disease including involvement of adjacent organs (e.g., duodenal obstruction), the presence of pancreatic pseudocyst, and splenomesenteric vein thrombosis with associated venous collateralization and sinistral portal hypertension. Some patients have a pattern of disease termed large duct chronic pancreatitis, associated with dilation of the main pancreatic duct above 7 to 8 mm, with or without intervening strictures and stones. In the absence of clinically significant biliary obstruction or a dominant pancreatic head mass, large duct disease is amenable to simple pancreatic duct-enteric drainage (Roux-en-Y lateral pancreaticojejunostomy), also termed a Puestow-type procedure. With a significant inflammatory head mass, typically associated with a dense concentration of calcifications, the pancreatic head and uncinate process may be additionally cored out (Frey procedure). Patients with a dominant inflammatory head mass may be considered for pancreaticoduodenectomy or duodenum-sparing pancreatic head resection, whether or not the main (dorsal) pancreatic duct is dilated. Pancreaticoduodenectomy is preferred if there is suspicion of malignant transformation. Patients with hereditary pancreatitis (and concomitant increased cancer risk), small duct pancreatitis, or those who failed previous operative intervention may be candidates for total pancreatectomy with autologous islet transplantation (Table 40-1).

Lateral Pancreaticojejunostomy

A midline incision is preferred, although a generous left subcostal approach (usually with extension across the midline) may also be used. Exposure of the entire pancreas is achieved by elevating and fully freeing the greater omentum from the transverse mesocolon from the hepatic to the splenic flexure. Kocher maneuver performed to the level of the superior mesenteric vein (SMV) helps elevate the head and uncinate process of the pancreas. The main pancreatic duct is identified by palpation and/or intraoperative ultrasound and then entered with electrocautery. The entire length of the pancreatic duct is opened with electrocautery, first toward the tail and then toward the ampulla. Intraductal stones are removed and strictures unroofed during this process. The duct should be opened fully to within 2 cm of the tip of the tail and within 1 to 2 cm of the duodenal wall. Care should be taken to control with suture ligation the anterior superior and inferior pancreaticoduodenal arcade that parallels the duodenal sweep. Both the dorsal and ventral systems should be unroofed. A 60-cm jejunal conduit in retrocolic Roux-en-Y configuration is used for drainage of the main duct. The pancreaticojejunostomy is sewn with a 4-0 double-armed running polyglyconate suture in a side-to-side fashion (Figure 40-2).

The steps of the Frey procedure are essentially the same as a lateral pancreaticojejunostomy, with the addition of a coring-out of the pancreatic head. This is performed using electrocautery, and the resected pancreatic parenchyma is sent for pathologic evaluation. Control of the pancreaticoduodenal arteries and branches may require suture ligation. It is important to avoid violation of the posterior border of the pancreatic neck over the SMV and portal vein. The pancreaticojejunostomy at the level of the pancreatic head is sewn to the border of the parenchymal excavation in the head.

Pancreaticoduodenectomy (Whipple Procedure)

After an upper midline laparotomy incision, a generous Kocher maneuver is performed, and the hepatic flexure is taken down. Preliminary determination of feasibility of resection is accomplished by inspection of the root of the mesentery and, if necessary, exposure of the lower border of the pancreas and SMV via the lesser sac. Cholecystectomy is performed, and the common bile duct is encircled and controlled proximally by bulldog clamp. The bile duct is divided above or below the cystic duct junction depending upon its diameter. The gastroduodenal artery (GDA) is identified. Prior to it division, temporary compression of the GDA is performed, and the persistence of strong distal hepatic artery pulsations must be confirmed. The anterior aspect of the portal vein is cleared. The lesser sac is then entered by elevating the greater omentum from the transverse mesocolon. The SMV is identified, and its gastroepiploic tributary is divided. A tunnel is completed behind the neck of the pancreas, anterior to the SMV and portal vein, and a Penrose drain or umbilical tape is placed through this tunnel to expose and define the line of transection

Table 40-1   Refractory Pain from Chronic Pancreatitis

I. Lateral Pancreaticojejunostomy (Puestow-type)

Key Technical Steps

1. Enter lesser sac and expose pancreatic head with generous Kocher maneuver.
2. Identify and unroof main pancreatic duct.
3. Perform retrocolic Roux-en-Y conduit for main duct drainage.

Potential Pitfalls

- Hemorrhage from pancreaticoduodenal arterial arcades.
- Failure to remove large intraductal stones or to fully unroof pancreatic duct strictures.

II. Pancreaticoduodenectomy (Whipple)

Key Technical Steps

1. Exposure of lesser sac, pancreatic head, and infrapancreatic SMV.
2. Division of GDA.
3. Creation of tunnel behind neck of pancreas.
4. Cholecystectomy and division of bile duct.
5. Transection of stomach/proximal duodenum.
6. Takedown of ligament of Treitz with division of jejunum and mesentery.
7. Transection of pancreas.
8. Portal lymph node dissection.
9. Creation of pancreatico-, hepatico-, and gastro- or duodenojejunostomy.

Potential Pitfalls

- Failure to control portal venous tributaries.
- Failure to safely separate fibroinflammatory adhesions from major vessels.
- Failure to identify accessory and replaced arteries.

III. Duodenum-Sparing Pancreatic Head Resection

Key Technical Steps

A. Beger Procedure

   1. Exposure of lesser sac, pancreas head, and creation of tunnel behind pancreas neck.
   2. Spare GDA.
   3. Transection of pancreas.
   4. Resect pancreas head with 5 mm margin to duodenum.
   5. Creation of Roux-en-Y with pancreas body and remnant head to jejunum.

B. Frey Procedure

   1. Exposure of lesser sac and pancreas head.
   2. Core out pancreas head.
   3. Unroofing of pancreas duct from head to tail.
   4. Creation of longitudinal Roux-en-Y pancreaticojejunostomy.

Potential Pitfalls

- Duodenal ischemia.
- Hemorrhage from portal vein tributaries or pancreaticoduodenal arterial arcade.
- Stricture of common bile duct.

(Figure 40-3). In a standard Whipple procedure, the stomach is then divided by linear surgical stapler starting from the greater curve near the junction of the right and left gastroepiploic arcades and ending at the lesser curve just proximal to the *incisura angularis*. The lesser curvature staple line is imbricated with Lembert silk sutures. Next, the ligament of Treitz is taken down and fully mobilized. The jejunum is divided by linear stapler approximately 20 cm distal to the ligament of Treitz. The mesojejunum and mesoduodenum are divided, and the jejunum is then passed posterior to the superior mesenteric vessels into the supracolic compartment. The ligament of Treitz is then closed

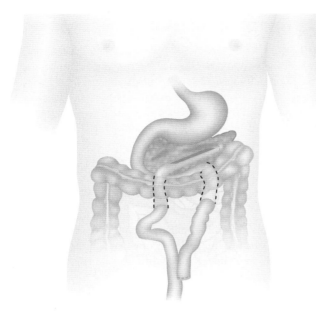

FIGURE 40-2. A lateral Roux-en-Y retrocolic pancreaticojejunostomy.

with interrupted sutures. After stay sutures are placed in the pancreas, the neck of the pancreas is divided with electrocautery (Figure 40-4). Retroperitoneal attachments including small tributaries to the portal vein and branches of the inferior pancreaticoduodenal artery are divided to complete the resection. The jejunum is then advanced through the mesocolon to the right of the middle colic vessels. There are a number of well-described techniques of pancreaticojejunostomy. The authors prefer a pancreatic duct-to-mucosa anastomosis performed over a transanastomotic 5F pediatric feeding tube that is exteriorized through the jejunal limb using a Witzel-type technique. A second, outer row of sutures is performed between the jejunum and pancreatic capsule with interrupted or continuous suture. Biliary-enteric continuity is reestablished with interrupted or

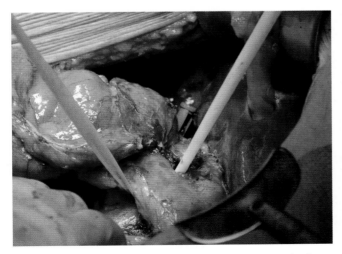

FIGURE 40-3. Penrose's drain tunneled between neck of pancreas and portal vein.

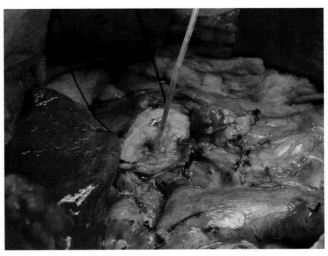

FIGURE 40-4. Transected pancreas with feeding tube inserted in the main pancreatic duct.

continuous suture technique in end-to-side configuration. Finally, the gastrojejunostomy is completed in a hand-sewn two-layer fashion to the greater curve staple line with the afferent limb oriented toward the lesser curvature.

Duodenum-Preserving Pancreatic Head Resection

The three variants of duodenum-preserving pancreatic head resection (DPPHR) are Beger, Frey, and Berne procedures. Each is performed via midline laparotomy, and the pancreas is exposed within the lesser sac. In the Beger procedure, a tunnel is created between the pancreatic neck and SMV and Penrose's drain passed as in the Whipple procedure. The neck is divided with electrocautery, and the head of the pancreas is then cored out leaving a small rim of pancreas along the duodenal wall with the intact bile duct. A two-sided Roux-en-Y pancreaticojejunostomy is then fashioned; a double-layer pancreaticojejunostomy to the body/tail is performed as in the Whipple procedure, whereas the anastomosis to the duodenum side may be performed as a continuous single layer between the jejunum and the remnant rim of the head of the pancreas. The Frey and Berne procedures both include a coring of the pancreas head and a Roux-en-Y pancreaticojejunostomy; in the Frey variant, this anastomosis is extended along the full length of an unroofed pancreatic duct as described above.

● OPERATIVE OUTCOMES

Few prospective trials exist directly comparing the outcomes of the different pancreatic operations. Durable pain relief is achieved in approximately 80% to 85% of appropriately selected patients at 5-year follow-up regardless of the choice of operation. Lateral pancreaticojejunostomy has a decreased perioperative morbidity and preserved exocrine and endocrine function compared to resection-type surgeries. Comparisons between DPPHR (Frey vs. Beger) show no significant differences; however, endocrine and digestive functions appear to be better preserved with DPPHR compared to pancreaticoduodenectomy. Studies comparing surgical intervention to endotherapy with extended follow-up clearly demonstrate significantly superior long-term pain relief in the surgical group.

● SPECIAL INTRAOPERATIVE CONSIDERATIONS

The extent of fibrosis, adherence to adjacent structures including vasculature, and the degree of venous collaterals may substantially increase the risk of procedures involving resection. For example, dense fibrosis around the SMV or portal vein may prohibitively increase the risk of pancreaticoduodenectomy, making a DPPHR a safer alternative. Chronic pancreatitis carries an increased risk of pancreatic adenocarcinoma. Intraoperative biopsy of suspicious masses by frozen section may change operative approach, for example, decompressive pancreaticojejunostomy or limited DPPHR to formal resection.

● POSTOPERATIVE MANAGEMENT

Postoperatively, resumption of oral intake parallels the return of bowel function. Most patients will require pancreatic enzyme replacement with meals. Delayed gastric emptying affects as many as one-third of patients after pancreaticoduodenectomy and may require prolonged nasogastric decompression and nutritional support. Pancreatic resection, combined with preexisting loss of islet mass due to progressive fibrosis, leads to type 3c diabetes mellitus, which is characterized by difficult and labile blood sugar associated with insulin hypersensitivity (a consequence of loss of counter-regulatory capacity). Deep space infections including anastomotic leak occur in approximately 15% of patients and may be recognized by fever, persistent leukocytosis, or failure to progress. The incidence of postoperative pancreatic fistula is much lower in the setting of chronic pancreatitis than other indications for pancreatic resection

Patients should refrain from ethanol and tobacco and maintain close follow-up with longitudinal medical providers to optimize pancreatic enzyme supplementation, insulin therapy, and nutritional sequelae.

Case Conclusion

The patient underwent a pancreaticoduodenectomy, which was selected because of the presence of an inflammatory pancreatic mass with suspicion of malignancy. He had an uneventful postoperative course and was discharged on postoperative day 6. Pathology revealed no evidence of malignancy. Three month after his operation, he is pain free, discontinued all narcotics, and taking minimal pancreatic enzyme supplementation with meals.

TAKE HOME POINTS

- Intractable abdominal pain is the most common indication for surgical intervention of chronic pancreatitis.
- Amylase and lipase offer little value in diagnosing chronic pancreatitis.
- CT scan of the abdomen with intravenous contrast is helpful to define the extent of the disease and sequelae of chronic pancreatitis.
- MRCP provides a noninvasive modality to obtain ductography to identify ductal anatomy (dilation, stones, strictures) that may be relevant to interventional decisions.
- Surgical intervention affords better pain relief than endotherapy.
- The goal of surgery is to relieve pain while maximizing postoperative pancreatic exocrine and endocrine function.
- The choice of operation should be tailored to the patient's anatomy, ductal dilation, presence of an inflammatory mass, and surgeon experience.
- Eighty to eighty-five percent of patients have long-term pain relief after undergoing surgery for chronic pancreatitis.

SUGGESTED READINGS

Chinnakotla S, et al. Factors Predicting Outcomes After a Total Pancreatectomy and Islet Autotransplantation Lessons Learned From Over 500 Cases. *Ann Surg.* 2015;262(4):610-622.

McClaine RJ, et al. A comparison of pancreaticoduodenectomy and duodenum-preserving head resection for the treatment of chronic pancreatitis. *HPB (Oxford).* 2009;11(8):677-683.

Morrison CP, et al. Surgical management of intractable pain in chronic pancreatitis: past and present. *J Hepatobiliary Pancreat Surg.* 2002;9(6):675-682.

Schnelldorfer T, Lewin DN, Adams DB. Operative management of chronic pancreatitis: longterm results in 372 patients. *J Am Coll Surg.* 2007;204(5):1039-1045; discussion 1045-1047.

Steer ML, Waxman I, Freedman S. Chronic pancreatitis. *N Engl J Med.* 1995;332(22):1482-1490.

Symptomatic Pancreatic Pseudocyst

41

MICHAEL G. HOUSE AND SHILPA S. MURTHY

Based on the previous edition chapter "Symptomatic Pancreatic Pseudocyst" by Michael G. House

Presentation

A 62-year-old woman presented with progressively worsening upper abdominal pain and nausea over 2 days. Initial lab studies were notable for severe hyperlipasemia with normal transaminase and bilirubin levels. A right upper quadrant ultrasound demonstrated cholelithiasis. She was admitted to the hospital with biliary-type acute pancreatitis and managed with intravenous fluids and gut rest. Two days later, her abdominal pain and nausea improved, and she was introduced to a clear liquid diet. A laparoscopic cholecystectomy was performed uneventfully, and she was advanced to a low-fat diet prior to hospital discharge. Approximately 4 weeks later, she again developed upper abdominal pain with nausea and early satiety. Cross-sectional imaging with intravenous contrast was ordered and demonstrated a large amount of necrosis within the central compartment of the retroperitoneum (Figure 41-1). A nasojejunal feeding tube was placed for enteral nutrition support. Multidisciplinary team discussions were held to consider management of the walled-off pancreatic necrosis (WON) with endoscopic or operative intervention. Postcholecystectomy status favored endoscopic intervention. Endoscopic ultrasound (EUS)-guided placement of a lumen-apposing metal stent facilitated transgastric drainage and complete debridement of the WON during two endoscopic sessions. A surveillance computed tomography (CT) scan 3 months later revealed no residual necrosis, and the transgastric stent was removed endoscopically. Approximately 6 months later, she began to experience abdominal pain and early satiety associated with weight loss. Imaging demonstrated a large pancreatic pseudocyst arising from a disconnected distal pancreatic segment (Figure 41-2). Open distal pancreatectomy with splenectomy was recommended as definitive treatment.

● DIFFERENTIAL DIAGNOSIS

The differential diagnosis of a pancreatic fluid collection in the setting of acute pancreatitis is based on the Atlanta classification system (Table 41-1). Acute peripancreatic fluid collections (APFC) and acute necrotic collections (ANC) are pancreatic fluid collections that have been present <4 weeks after an initial diagnosis of acute pancreatitis. Pancreatic pseudocyst and walled-off pancreatic necrosis (WON) are chronic collections that have been present for longer than 4 weeks and have a well-defined enhancing wall on radiologic imaging. The difference between APFC and pancreatic pseudocyst versus ANC and WON is a clinical history of necrotizing pancreatitis and the presence of necrosis on radiologic imaging. All of these pancreatic fluid collections can be classified further as sterile or infected. Pancreatic cysts are included in the differential diagnosis, particularly when an antecedent history of acute pancreatitis is not established. Cystic lesions of the pancreas include mucinous cystic neoplasm (e.g., mucinous cystadenoma, intraductal papillary mucinous neoplasm, mucinous cystadenocarcinoma), serous cystic tumors (e.g., serous cystadenoma), lymphoepithelial cyst, cystic neuroendocrine tumor, congenital pancreatic retention cyst, lymphangioma, and visceral artery aneurysm.

● WORKUP

Acute pancreatitis is diagnosed in any patient experiencing upper abdominal pain with a serum amylase or lipase level that is three times above normal limits. The early phase of acute pancreatitis occurs within 2 weeks of the onset of symptoms, and clinical severity can be established by applying

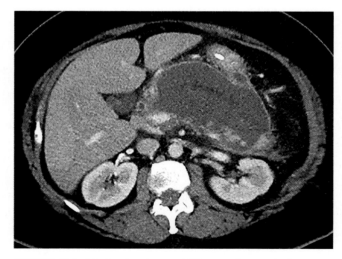

FIGURE 41-1. Contrast-enhanced CT scan demonstrates walled-off necrosis (WON) involving the body and tail of the pancreas.

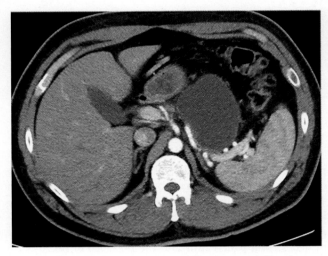

FIGURE 41-2. Contrast-enhanced CT with a centralized pseudocyst within the lesser sac arising from a disconnected left pancreas.

Table 41-2	Laparoscopic or Open Cystogastrostomy

Key Technical Steps

1. Cholecystectomy with intraoperative cholangiography for biliary pancreatitis.
2. Intraoperative ultrasound to define the necrotic collection.
3. Anterior gastrotomy (at least 5 cm) to expose posterior gastric wall.
4. Aspiration of pseudocyst/WON fluid for microbiology cultures.
5. Electrocautery for entry into the pseudocyst/WON cavity.
6. Biopsy pseudocyst wall to exclude epithelial-lined cyst.
7. Explore pseudocyst/WON cavity and debride necrosis.
8. Anastomosis (at least 5 cm) completed with locking PDS suture.

Potential Pitfalls

- Bleeding from pseudocyst/WON cavity walls.
- Bleeding from splenic, portal, or SMV vessels during necrosectomy.
- Dehiscence of the gastric and pseudocyst walls.
- Loss of necrosis containment and spillage into the peritoneum.

any one of several scoring systems (e.g., APACHE II, SIRS, Marshall, or Ranson Criteria). Balthazar Radiographic Severity Scoring System designates findings on CT imaging performed with portal phase intravenous contrast. Acute edematous interstitial pancreatitis does not involve pancreatic necrosis but may result in pseudocyst formation if ductal disruption occurs. Acute necrotizing pancreatitis results in necrosis of the gland and peripancreatic tissues. Fluid collections and later pancreatic pseudocysts arise from disruption of the main pancreatic duct or its branches. A disconnected left pancreas with pseudocyst formation is often a consequence of extensive pancreatic necrosis involving the neck of the pancreas.

Depending on the severity of acute pancreatitis with or without progression toward chronic pancreatitis, patients may manifest signs of pancreatic endocrine and/or exocrine insufficiency including diabetes mellitus, steatorrhea, and weight loss. Any clinical history of steatorrhea should be evaluated with formal fecal fat content studies. Daily fecal

excretion of >7 g of total fat is considered abnormal in the context of a regularly balanced diet. Patients with moderate or severe pancreatitis will experience some degree of malnutrition. Nutritional status should be evaluated with serial body mass index measurements, serum albumin, transferrin, and prealbumin levels.

Pseudocysts arising from duct disruptions within the head or neck of the pancreas may cause biliary and/or gastric outlet obstruction. Cross-sectional imaging with dual phase intravenous contrast (i.e., CT or MRI/MRCP)

Table 41-1	Defining Features of Pancreatic Fluid Collections	
Type of Pancreatic Fluid Collection	**Timing after Pancreatitis Onset**	**Radiographic Features**
APFC	<4 wks	Extrapancreatic homogeneous fluid without encapsulation. Lacks necrosis
Pseudocyst	>4 wks	Usually extrapancreatic but with ductal communication. Encapsulated homogeneous fluid density
ANC	<4 wks	Necrosis of the pancreas and extrapancreatic tissues. Lacks a well-defined wall/capsule
WON	>4 wks	Heterogeneous solid and liquid collection contained by a well-defined wall

can assess for these and other secondary complications of pseudocysts. Radiologic studies permit reliable assessment of peripancreatic structures, anatomical status of the pancreatic duct (e.g., stricture, dilation, disruption), residual necrosis, size and number of pancreatic pseudocysts, portal or splenic vein thrombosis, and visceral artery pseudoaneurysms. Endoscopic retrograde cholangiopancreatography (ERCP) can achieve biliary drainage in patients with obstructive jaundice. ERCP may also be helpful in treating a short disruption of the main pancreatic duct that is contributing to an enlarging pseudocyst or uncontained pancreatic leak.

Distinguishing between a pseudocyst and cystic neoplasm of the pancreas is especially important in patients who are being considered for internal drainage procedures but have no established history of acute pancreatitis. EUS characterization for internal cyst septations and EUS-guided aspiration for cyst fluid analysis measuring mucin, amylase, and carcinoembryonic antigen levels should provide an accurate diagnosis.

● DIAGNOSIS AND TREATMENT

Patients with symptomatic pancreatic pseudocysts should be considered for treatment. Several treatment interventions are available depending on pseudocyst location. Options include EUS-guided transgastric drainage, ERCP with transpapillary drainage, EUS-guided drainage with nasocystic drainage, operative cystogastrostomy or cystojejunostomy, and percutaneous pseudocyst drainage.

Percutaneous external drainage is not ideal for pseudocyst drainage in the absence of infected necrosis. ERCP-guided transpapillary drainage involves partial stenting of the ampulla and main pancreatic duct. This technique is best suited for patients with mature pseudocysts of the head and neck of the pancreas that communicate directly with the main pancreatic duct. EUS-guided transgastric internal drainage results effectively as a cystogastrostomy. This procedure is most appropriate for pseudocysts arising from the body of the pancreas that abut the posterior gastric wall and may include placement of a double pigtail stent or lumen-apposing metal stent depending on the amount of solid necrosis within the WON or pseudocyst cavity. EUS-guided transduodenal drainage can be accomplished in a similar manner for pseudocysts or WON cavities that arise from the head or neck of the pancreas. WON may require repeated endoscopic debridements through the established transgastric orifice over several weeks.

Relative contraindications for endoscopic drainage include transmural distances between the visceral lumen and WON or pseudocyst cavity that exceed 1 cm. Intervening varices, often observed in patients with splenic or portal vein thrombosis, increase the risk for procedure-related hemorrhage. Operative therapies, described below, are recommended for patients who are not candidates for endoscopic drainage procedures and those who have failed initial attempts at endoscopic intervention.

● SURGICAL APPROACH

The most common operations to achieve internal drainage of a pancreatic pseudocyst include direct cystogastrostomy or Roux-en-Y cystojejunostomy. Direct cystoduodenostomy is not commonly performed but may be considered for pseudocysts arising from the head of the pancreas. Cholecystectomy at the time of drainage operation should be performed for all patients with gallstones and especially for patients diagnosed with biliary pancreatitis. Distal pancreatectomy with or without splenectomy is applied to patients with pseudocysts arising from a disconnected left pancreas. Pseudocysts associated with endoscopically untreatable strictures of the distal common bile duct or duodenum require pancreatoduodenectomy. Even after thorough evaluation, some pseudocysts cannot be discriminated from cystic neoplasms of the pancreas. Regional pancreatectomy may be necessary in this unusual situation.

Depending on the location of the pseudocyst, open, laparoscopic, and robotic surgical techniques can accomplish successful internal drainage into the stomach, duodenum, or jejunum. Cystogastrostomy is the preferred operation for pseudocysts arising from the pancreatic body that abut and deform the posterior gastric wall on cross-sectional imaging. The classic open approach to cystogastrostomy is performed through an upper midline incision. The anterior wall of the stomach is open longitudinally in the widest portion of the gastric fundus, exposing the posterior wall. Ultrasound and aspiration may be utilized to identify where the pseudocyst is best opposed to the posterior gastric wall, for creation of the cystogastrostomy. The posterior wall is then incised with electrocautery, and often a small round or elliptical portion of the gastric wall may be excised to provide a broad aperture for drainage of the pseudocyst. A full-thickness running absorbable suture may be used around the aperture to provide hemostasis. Opening the gastric wall with bipolar or ultrasonic energy device may accomplish the same objective. Any solid debris within the pseudocyst cavity should be bluntly removed. The anterior wall of the stomach is then closed transversely, either in a standard two-layer closure or using a GIA stapler. Closed suction drains are not typically placed. Nasogastric suction may be maintained for 24 to 48 hours postoperatively.

Pseudocysts that lie along the head of the pancreas and do not compress the ampulla or common bile duct can be approached with a direct cystoduodenostomy or Roux-en-Y cystojejunostomy. In most situations, Roux-en-Y cystojejunostomy is a straightforward procedure for head of the pancreas pseudocysts and for pseudocysts that project through the transverse mesocolon.

● POSTOPERATIVE MANAGEMENT

Patients should be initiated on nutritional therapy within 48 hours after operation. A liquid diet can be introduced very early in the postoperative course and advanced according to patient tolerance. Rapid goal enteral nutrition is particularly important for patients with preoperative malnutrition. This can be accomplished easily with a nasojejunal tube or a direct jejunostomy tube placed at the time of operation. Enteral nutrition is always preferred over parenteral nutrition.

Antibiotic therapy is discontinued after the perioperative period unless infected necrosis is present at the time of drainage of WON. Antibiotics should be prescribed according to the microbiology of the necrosis specimen obtained at the time of drainage. Chronic pancreatitis and necrotizing pancreatitis are associated frequently with venous thromboembolism; thus, appropriate prophylaxis for deep venous thrombosis should continue for 4 weeks into the postoperative period. Postoperative complications after cystogastrostomy or cystojejunostomy occur in approximately 30% of patients and include surgical site and deep organ space infection, anastomotic bleeding, venous thromboembolism, ileus, and visceral artery pseudoaneurysm.

TAKE HOME POINTS

- Internal drainage procedures for pancreatic pseudocysts and walled-off necrosis should be considered in symptomatic patients.
- Pancreatic pseudocysts and walled-off necrosis can become complicated by infection and bleeding.
- EUS can help secure a diagnosis of pancreatic pseudocyst over cystic neoplasm in patients without a clear history of pancreatitis.

- Magnetic resonance cholangiopancreatography (MRCP) and ERCP can characterize pancreatic ductal anatomy and communication with pseudocysts.
- Endoscopic internal drainage procedures are first-line therapy for patients with chronic symptomatic pseudocysts.
- Surgical cystogastrostomy and cystojejunostomy are indicated for symptomatic patients who are not candidates for endoscopic drainage procedures.
- Operative procedures and techniques are selected on the basis of pseudocyst location and adjacent anatomic relationships.

SUGGESTED READINGS

Cahen D, Rauws E, Fockens P, et al. Endoscopic drainage of pancreatic pseudocysts: long-term outcome and procedural factors associated with safe and successful treatment. *Endoscopy.* 2005;37:977-983.

Gurusamy KS, Pallari E, Hawkins N, Pereira SP, Davidson BR. Management strategies for pancreatic pseudocysts. *Cochrane Database Syst Rev.* 2016;(4):CD011392. doi: 10.1002/14651858.

Jester A, House M, Nakeeb A, et al. Transgastric pancreatic necrosectomy: How I Do It. *J Gastrointest Surg.* 2016;20:445-449.

Murage K, Ball C, Zyromski N, et al. Clinical framework to guide operative decision making in disconnected left pancreatic remnant (DLPR) following acute or chronic pancreatitis. *Surgery.* 2010;148:847-857.

Nealon W, Walser E. Main pancreatic ductal anatomy can direct choice of modality for treating pancreatic pseudocysts. *Ann Surg.* 2002;235:751-758.

Siddiqui A, Kowalski T, Loren D, et al. Fully covered self-expanding metal stents versus lumen-apposing fully covered self-expanding metal stent versus plastic stents for endoscopic drainage of pancreatic walled-off necrosis: clinical outcomes and success. *Gastrointest Endosc.* 2017;85(4):758-765.

Theoni R. The revised atlanta classification of acute pancreatitis: its importance for the radiologist and its effect on treatment. *Radiology.* 2012;262(3):751-764.

Gallstone Ileus

JOANNA L. HUNTER-SQUIRES AND EUGENE P. CEPPA

42

Presentation

A 65-year-old woman with a history of hypertension and poorly controlled diabetes mellitus presents to the emergency room complaining of 5 days of intermittent abdominal pain and emesis. The pain, which was initially epigastric, is now diffuse and crampy. She has had several episodes of emesis, initially coffee ground and now bilious. She is passing flatus but is uncertain of her last bowel movement. Her only surgical history is a cesarean section performed 32 years ago.

On exam, her heart rate is 96 bpm. Her blood pressure is 99/55 mm Hg. Her abdomen is moderately distended, and there is no evidence of peritonitis. She does have mild focal tenderness to palpation in the right upper quadrant.

● DIFFERENTIAL DIAGNOSIS

While the differential diagnosis for abdominal pain is broad, and in this patient may include such diverse entities as pancreatic and biliary disease, urinary tract infection, peptic ulcer disease, and metabolic derangements associated with diabetes mellitus, the constellation of nausea, vomiting and abdominal pain should raise concern for intestinal obstruction (Table 42-1).

Gallstone ileus is a rare cause of intestinal obstruction, occurring in <0.5% of patients presenting with intestinal obstruction and disproportionately in elderly and female patients with multiple comorbid conditions. The classic

Table 42-1	Differential Diagnosis for Intestinal Obstruction

Surgical adhesions

Hernia

Malignancy—metastasis or primary bowel malignancy

Inflammatory bowel disease—active disease, chronic
   strictures

Intussusception

Volvulus

Gallstone ileus

Infection—tuberculosis/typhoid/abscess

Bezoar

presentation is that of subacute small bowel obstruction, with intermittent symptoms as a large gallstone, typically 2.5 cm or greater, makes its way through the bowel often becoming lodged in the distal ileum. The average duration of symptoms is 5 days prior to presentation. Only half of patients report prior gallbladder disease, and episodes of right upper quadrant pain typically subside when the gallbladder is decompressed through the formation of a cholecystoenteric fistula. Occasionally, patients may present with hematemesis due to hemorrhage at the site of bilioenteric fistula.

● WORKUP

Following a history and physical examination, workup includes a complete blood count and comprehensive metabolic panel. Imaging may begin with plain abdominal radiographs, but Rigler's triad—pneumobilia secondary to the bilioenteric fistula, evidence of bowel obstruction with dilated bowel loops and air fluid levels, and ectopic gallstone—is often absent as gallstones may not be radiopaque. Consequently, cross-sectional imaging with computed tomography of the abdomen and pelvis is the diagnostic study of choice in workup of gallstone ileus. This has the advantage of frequently pinpointing the level of obstruction and allowing visualization of a greater proportion of gallstones. CT scan may also show evidence of gallbladder wall thickening and pericholecystic inflammation.

Presentation Continued

Laboratory investigations demonstrate significant metabolic derangements with blood glucose of 836, severe dehydration, metabolic acidosis, and acute renal failure. She has mild leukocytosis and mild anemia. Urinalysis shows ketones, glucose, and pyuria without nitrites. Liver function tests and bilirubin are within normal limits. Lipase is mildly elevated and troponins are normal.

CT scan demonstrates a 3.5-cm gallstone seen within the small bowel in the right lower quadrant and resultant upstream small bowel dilatation. There is inflammatory stranding surrounding the gallbladder and duodenum as well as pneumobilia and a 5-cm gallstone within the gallbladder lumen (Figure 42-1).

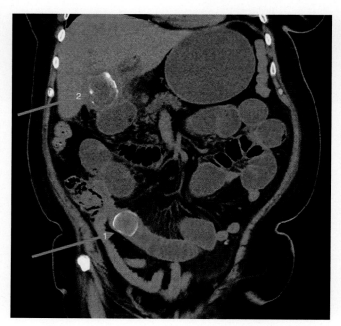

FIGURE 42-1. CT scan demonstrating gallstone ileus with a 3-cm calcified gallstone (*arrow 1*) within the terminal ileum and proximal dilation of the bowel. RUQ inflammatory stranding is also visible, as is pneumobilia, and a second 5-cm gallstone (*arrow 2*) within the gallbladder.

Table 42-2	Enterolithotomy

Key Technical Steps

1. Midline laparotomy.
2. Evaluate bowel to identify point of obstruction.
3. Place stay sutures prior to enterotomy.
4. Perform longitudinal enterotomy along the antimesenteric border of the bowel proximal to the site of obstruction.
5. Extract gallstone by retrograde approach through the enterotomy.
6. Milk forward any additional stones and extract them through the same enterotomy.
7. Close the enterotomy transversely to prevent stricture.

Potential Pitfalls

- Additional stones may be present in 15% of patients, and the gallbladder and entire bowel should be carefully inspected and stones removed to prevent recurrent episodes of obstruction (Figure 42-2).
- Attempting to milk the stone past the ileocecal valve may lead to unrecognized mucosal and serosal injuries and should be avoided.
- Typically, cholecystectomy and takedown of cholecystoenteric fistula should NOT be attempted at initial laparotomy.

● DIAGNOSIS AND TREATMENT

Initial management involves fluid resuscitation, stabilization of the patient and medical optimization. A nasogastric tube should be placed, and electrolyte derangements should be corrected. A Foley catheter should be placed to monitor resuscitation. Patients are frequently malnourished given the subacute time course of the obstruction and perioperative nutritional support with parenteral nutrition should be considered. Any modifiable chronic conditions should be rapidly evaluated and addressed. Once the patient is stabilized, proceed to the operating room. Ongoing obstruction and pressure from the gallstone being lodged in the bowel results in risk for ischemia.

● SURGICAL APPROACH

Most patients with gallstone ileus are American Society of Anesthesiology (ASA) Class III to IV. The initial goal in management is to safely relieve the patient's bowel obstruction and minimize anesthetic time. We favor enterolithotomy via open approach as this will allow for complete manual evaluation of the GI tract for stones.

The surgery begins with abdominal exploration via a midline laparotomy and running the bowel in order to identify the point of obstruction and any additional gallstones

within the gastrointestinal tract. After identifying the point of obstruction, a longitudinal enterotomy is made on the antimesenteric side of the bowel just proximally. The stone is removed through the enterotomy, any additional stones are milked down the bowel and extracted through this same site. The enterotomy is closed transversely to avoid narrowing of the intestinal lumen and the patient is closed. A minority of patients will require formal bowel resection for prolonged obstruction resulting in intestinal ischemia (Table 42-2).

● SPECIAL OPERATIVE CONSIDERATION

Historically, cholecystectomy and takedown of the bilioenteric fistula were performed at the time of initial operation. This is now the exception and reserved for medically fit patients, ASA Class I to II who are clinically stable. The majority of patients should be treated with enterolithotomy alone at initial laparotomy. Postoperatively, they should undergo a period of observation with optimization of their chronic medical conditions and nutritional status. At 6 to 8 weeks postoperatively, a second stage procedure may be considered to address the bilioenteric fistula. Patients who are

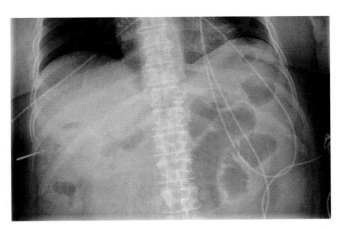

FIGURE 42-2. Abdominal radiograph demonstrating retained gallstone (*arrow*) and pneumobilia.

not elective surgical candidates may be observed indefinitely but do have moderately higher rates of recurrent gallstone ileus and cholangitis.

Some degree of Mirizzi's syndrome may coexist with bilioenteric fistulization, and care should be taken to evaluate for common bile duct involvement, either preoperatively with MRCP or intraoperatively with cholangiography, prior

to attempting cholecystectomy. Following cholecystectomy, the enteric side of the fistula is addressed. In cases of cholecystoduodenal fistula, the fistula track is resected back to fresh, viable edge of duodenum, which, in the majority of cases, can be closed in Heineke-Mikulicz fashion followed by omental patch reinforcement. Duodenal exclusion may rarely be considered in cases with large duodenal defects. Fistulas to the colon or stomach are typically amenable to layered primary closure following debridement to healthy tissue as well.

● POSTOPERATIVE MANAGEMENT

Complications following initial laparotomy and enterolithotomy are significantly less common than following formal cholecystectomy and bilioenteric fistula takedown. Gallstone ileus recurrence rate is reported to be as high as 10%, and this may be avoided by careful evaluation of the gallbladder and gastrointestinal tract at the time of initial laparotomy (Figure 42-3). The comorbid conditions and malnutrition present in these patients place them at high risk for routine postoperative complications, and a high suspicion for leak from enterotomy closure or anastomosis should be maintained.

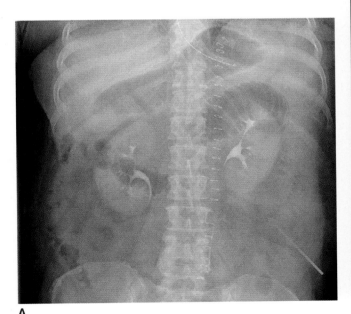

A

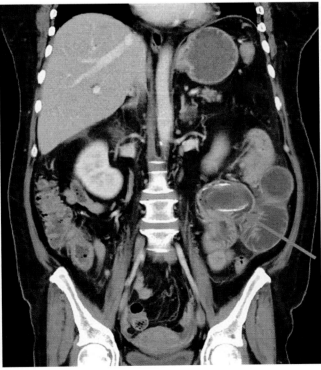

B

FIGURE 42-3. Radiograph (**A**) shows the previously described 5-cm gallstone (*arrow*) now projecting over the left midabdomen with Rigler's triad (pneumobilia, evidence of bowel obstruction, ectopic gallstone). **B:** Recurrent gallstone ileus more clearly demonstrated on CT.

Case Conclusion

Following placement of a nasogastric tube and urinary catheter, fluid resuscitation, correction of hyperglycemia, and electrolyte repletion, the patient is taken to the operating room. The point of obstruction is identified in the distal ileum, and enterolithotomy is performed. An additional large stone is identified within the gallbladder and milked forward and extracted from the bowel. The intestine is all viable. Following the operation, the patient has a slow return of bowel function and is maintained on parenteral nutrition in the perioperative period until tolerating a regular diet. She is eventually discharged to a nursing facility and then home. She has no further documented episodes of right upper quadrant pain.

TAKE HOME POINTS

- Gallstone ileus should be considered within the differential diagnosis of intestinal obstruction, particularly in elderly patients and those with subacute presentations.
- Absence of known gallstone disease does not exclude the diagnosis of gallstone ileus.

- The majority of patients presenting with gallstone ileus are frail and have other significant medical conditions contributing to high morbidity and mortality.
- Patients frequently present with significant metabolic derangements and require stabilization prior to operative intervention.
- The goal with initial operative management is to safely and rapidly relieve obstruction.
- Enterolithotomy is the operation of choice.
- The entire gastrointestinal tract should be evaluated to avoid recurrence due to retained gallstones.
- Consider second laparotomy at 6 to 8 weeks postoperatively for cholecystectomy and bilioenteric fistula takedown in patients who are surgical candidates.

SUGGESTED READINGS

Berry SM, Fischer JE. Biliary and gastrointestinal fistulas. *Maingot's Abdominal Operations.* 10th ed. Appleton & Lange; 1997:581-625.

Halabi WJ, Kang CY, Ketana N, et al. Surgery for gallstone ileus: a nationwide comparison of trends and outcomes. *Ann Surg.* 2014; 259:329.

Rodriguez-Sanjuan JC, Casado F, Fernandez MJ, et al. Cholecystectomy and fistula closure versus enterolithotomy alone in gallstone ileus. *Br J Surg.* 1997;84:634-637.

Colorectal

Splenic Flexure Colon Cancer

43

DANIEL ALBO

Presentation

An 83-year-old patient with known history of diabetes mellitus, hypertension, chronic renal failure, and congestive heart failure presents with a 2-week history of crampy abdominal pain following meals with thin-caliber bowel movements but no nausea and vomiting. His vital signs were normal. On physical exam, his abdomen was nontender, somewhat distended, with a palpable mass in the left upper quadrant of his abdomen. His rectal exam revealed guaiac-positive brown stool. His laboratory exams were significant for a hemoglobin of 10, a white cell blood count of 9, a creatinine of 2.9, and an albumin of 2.9.

● DIFFERENTIAL DIAGNOSIS

An elderly patient presenting with symptomatic anemia, a high-grade partial bowel obstruction, and a palpable left upper quadrant mass is highly suggestive of a distal colon cancer. However, the differential diagnosis is relatively broad and includes inflammatory conditions such as diverticulitis (less likely in this patient due to the lack of a fever and of left-sided abdominal tenderness on exam and with a normal white cell blood count), ischemic colitis (although he has risk factors for vascular disease, he did not present with bloody diarrhea, and he had a palpable left upper quadrant mass), an enlarged spleen (such as seen in hematologic malignancies), and other neoplastic processes involving the left upper quadrant (gastric, pancreatic tail, adrenal or kidney cancer as well as retroperitoneal sarcomas).

● WORKUP

The patient underwent a computed tomography (CT) scan of the abdomen and the pelvis (with oral contrast only due to his elevated creatinine), which revealed a large, obstructing mass in the splenic flexure of the colon (Figure 43-1), with a moderately distended cecum (<10 cm) and small bowel, with no evidence of liver metastases or carcinomatosis. A colonoscopy revealed a nearly completely obstructing mass at the level of the splenic flexure of the colon (Figure 43-2). The mass could not be traversed, and they were unable to evaluate the proximal colon. A biopsy was obtained that showed a moderately to poorly differentiated adenocarcinoma. A carcinoembryonic antigen (CEA) level was obtained and it was 34.6. This workup confirmed the diagnosis of an obstructing splenic flexure colon cancer.

● DISCUSSION

Carcinoma of the transverse colon (of which splenic flexure colon cancer is a subset) accounts for 10% of all colorectal cancers. Diagnosis is often delayed and complicated forms (perforation, fistulization, obstruction) occur in 30% to 50% of cases. The progression of symptoms is often insidious, and tumors may be quite large by the time of diagnosis. These tumors can also extend or fistulize into adjacent organs. Distal transverse cancers may be small annular lesions, which are prone to obstruction.

From a surgeon's perspective, it is important to consider two types of complete colonic obstructions, those with a competent or with an incompetent ileocecal valve. In patients with an incompetent ileocecal valve, the pressure that builds up proximal to the splenic flexure tumor partially decompresses into the small bowel, allowing for preoperative stabilization of the patient (by nasogastric tube decompression, rehydration, and correction of underlying electrolyte disorders)

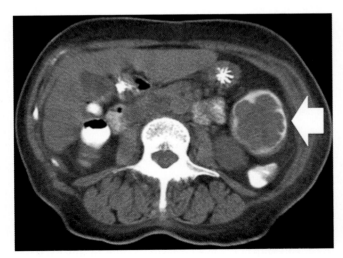

FIGURE 43-1. CT scan of the abdomen showing a large, obstructing splenic flexure colon cancer (*arrow*). This CT scan was obtained with oral contrast only due to the patient's impaired kidney function.

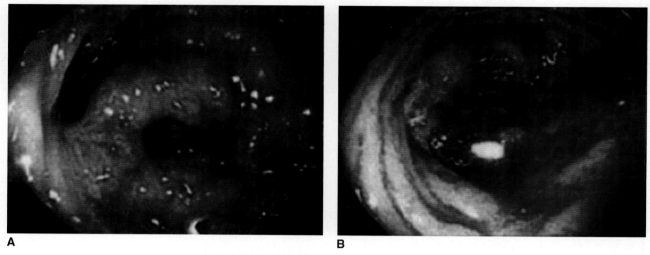

A   **B**

FIGURE 43-2. Colonoscopy. **A:** Splenic flexure of the colon showing a large, fungating circumferential mass that is obstructing the lumen of colon. **B:** Descending colon, showing a normal colonic lumen distal to the splenic flexure mass and some evidence of bleeding from the tumor.

and performance of a full workup, including a colonoscopy. Patients that present with a complete large bowel obstruction with a competent ileocecal valve, on the other hand, represent a true surgical emergency. In these patients, the pressure that builds up proximal to the splenic flexure tumor cannot decompress into the small bowel due to the competency of the ileocecal valve. In this situation, the proximal colon will progressively get more dilated and the tension on the proximal colonic wall will increase. According to Laplace's law, the increase in tension on the wall of the cavity will be directly proportional to the fourth potency of radius of the cavity. Therefore, the part of the proximal colon with the largest radius, the cecum, will suffer the greatest increase in colonic wall tension. This increase in wall tension will lead to collapse of the intramural capillaries and ischemia, eventually producing a catastrophic cecal perforation. Patients with a complete colonic obstruction that present with right lower quadrant abdominal pain should be operated on emergently, since this likely represent a sign of an impending cecal rupture. Colonoscopy in these patients is formally contraindicated, since it could lead to a critical delay before surgery, and the increase in intraluminal pressure due to insufflation during the colonoscopy could lead to a full-blown cecal perforation.

● WORKUP

Clinical presentation permitting, the preoperative staging workup should include a CT scan of the abdomen and the pelvis with oral and intravenous contrast, a chest x-ray or a CT scan of the chest, a CEA blood level, and a full colonoscopy. In patients with bulky splenic flexure tumors in which it is not possible to evaluate the proximal colon by colonoscopy, a barium enema is indicated to rule out synchronous colon cancer in the proximal colon, although it frequently is either not feasible or reliable. Although the use of on-table colonoscopy

through the appendiceal orifice has been described, this is often not practical. The incidence of a synchronous proximal colon cancer, though, is only about 5%, and only a subset of these synchronous tumors will not be detected by either preoperative CT scan or intraoperative palpation of the colon. Therefore, although evaluation of the full colon preoperatively by colonoscopy is preferred, in patients in whom evaluation of the proximal colon is just not possible, it is acceptable to perform surgery for the splenic flexure tumor and perform a short-interval colonoscopy postoperatively (6 months after surgery) to fully evaluate the reminder of the colon.

● SURGICAL APPROACH

Colonic stenting is the best option either for palliation or as a bridge to surgery in patients with a complete bowel obstruction due to a splenic flexure colon cancer with a competent ileocecal valve. This approach reduces morbidity and mortality rate, and it eliminates the need for temporary colostomy. Nevertheless, surgical management remains relevant as colonic stenting has a small rate of failure, and it is not always available. There are various surgical options for dealing with patients with obstructing splenic flexure colon cancer. One-stage primary resection and anastomosis is the preferred choice for low-risk patients. It is paramount not only to resect the bowel segment involving the splenic flexure of the colon with negative margins of resection but also to include the entire lymphovascular pedicles associated with the splenic flexure of the colon (a minimum of 12 lymph nodes should be obtained). These include the left colic vessels, the left branches of the middle colic vessels, and the inferior mesenteric vein. Subtotal colectomy is useful in cases of proximal bowel damage (i.e., cecal perforation) or synchronous tumors. A two-stage procedure, with a resection and colostomy as a first step and colostomy

Table 43-1	Advantages of Minimally Invasive Surgery for Colon Cancer

- Smaller incisions
- Less pain
- Less use of narcotics
- Faster return to bowel function
- Shorter hospital stays
- Lower incidence of wound complications:
  - Wound infections
  - Incisional hernias
- Lower incidence of cardiopulmonary complications
- Faster recovery
- Potential decrease in overall cost of care

takedown as a second step, should be reserved for high-risk patients. A three-stage procedure, with the creation of simple colostomy as a first stage, has no role other than for use in very ill patients who are not fit for any other procedure. The multistage approach is marred by a higher cumulative rate of perioperative morbidity and mortality and frequent failure to complete the planned sequence of operations and a resulting high permanent stoma rate (up to 40% of patients).

One of the most significant changes in colon surgery over the last decade has been the increased application of minimally invasive surgery (MIS) techniques. MIS offers several key short-term patient advantages to open surgery (Table 43-1), including less perioperative pain, smaller incisions

(Figure 43-3B), shorter hospital stays, faster recovery, and lower wound morbidity (including wound infections and incisional hernias). In elderly patients, and in patients with significant comorbidities, it may also reduce the incidence of postoperative pulmonary and cardiac complications. In addition, we believe that laparoscopic surgery offers a superior visualization in the left upper quadrant of the abdomen and an easier, more controlled mobilization of the splenic flexure versus open surgery (Figure 43-3A). Due to these advantages, for surgeons with the requisite skill and experience, we feel strongly that MIS should be considered the preferred approach to patients with colon cancer, including those with splenic flexure tumors.

Patients with large splenic flexure tumors can be particularly challenging even for advanced laparoscopic surgeons. The position of these tumors deep in the left upper quadrant and the close proximity to the spleen, the pancreas, and the stomach can make these cases extremely complex. As a result, surgeons tend to shy away from laparoscopic surgery in the management of these tumors. An alternative to conventional laparoscopic surgery is hand-assisted laparoscopic surgery (HALS). In this technique, the surgeon has the option of introducing a hand in the abdomen during surgery through a special port (called a GelPort) that can be inserted in the expected extraction site. This provides the surgeon with tactile feedback and allows for greater versatility during surgery. While preserving all the known short-term advantages of conventional laparoscopic surgery versus open surgery, HALS offers several key advantages over conventional laparoscopic surgery (Table 43-2),

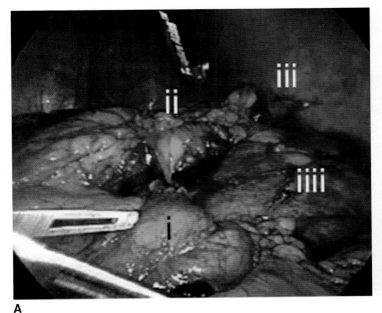

A

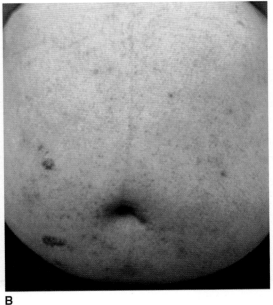

B

FIGURE 43-3. HALS for colon cancer of the splenic flexure. **A:** Full mobilization of the splenic flexure showing the splenic flexure of the colon (*i*) fully mobilized to the midline, the tail of the pancreas (*ii*), the spleen (*iii*), and Gerota's fascia (*iv*). **B:** Ten days postoperatively, the extraction site (placed as small transverse suprapubic incision hiding in a skin crease) and the 5-mm umbilical port site are no longer visible. The 5-mm and the 12-mm right-sided port sites are noticeable only due to the Dermabond that we use to seal the incisions; after the Dermabond falls off, these ports will be barely noticeable.

Table 43-2	Advantages of HALS Over Conventional Laparoscopy in the Management of Splenic Flexure Tumors

- Increased utilization of MIS
- Shorter operative times
- Lower conversion to open surgery rates
- Lower estimated blood loss
- Same short-term advantages over open surgery than conventional laparoscopy

including higher percentage of utilization of MIS, lower conversion to open rates, shorter operating times, and lower estimated blood loss rates. Key operative principles of MIS for the surgical management of splenic flexure colon cancer are summarized in Table 43-3.

● ADJUVANT THERAPY

Adjuvant chemotherapy is reserved for patients with stage III (positive lymph nodes) and stage IV (distant metastases) disease. Node-negative patients that may be considered for adjuvant chemotherapy include patient with high-risk characteristics, including lymphovascular invasion, perineural invasion, and lack of microsatellite instability. For patients with borderline lesions, genetic testing (such as Oncotype evaluation) is rapidly emerging as a potentially useful tool in determining which node-negative patients may benefit from additional therapy. Current adjuvant therapy protocols often times include oxaliplatin and 5-fluorouracil (FOLFOX) chemotherapy. The use of

Table 43-3	HALS for Splenic Flexure Colon Cancer (HALS left hemicolectomy)

Key Technical Steps

1. Port placement: GelPort at extraction site (6-cm Pfannenstiel incision), 5-mm camera port (umbilicus), and two working ports, a 5-mm port in the right upper quadrant and a 12-mm port in the right lower quadrant of the abdomen.
2. Step 1: Transect inferior mesenteric vein at the level of the ligament of Treitz.
3. Step 2: Transect the left colic artery at the level of its origin from the inferior mesenteric artery.
4. Step 3: Complete medial to lateral mobilization of the splenic flexure of the colon.
5. Step 4: Transect the white line of Toldt.
6. Step 5: Transect splenocolic and gastrocolic ligaments.
7. Step 6: Intracorporeal transection of the colon.
8. Step 7: Intracorporeal colo-colonic anastomosis.

biologic cancer therapy (such as Avastin) is also emerging as a potential treatment option in addition to more standard chemotherapy regimens.

● SURVEILLANCE

Eighty-five percent of colon cancer recurrences occur within 3 years of surgery, with the majority of the remaining recurrences occurring between years 3 and 5. The 2005 American Society of Clinical Oncology surveillance recommendations for colon cancer include an annual CT scan of the chest and abdomen for 3 years, a colonoscopy at 3 years, a history and physical examination and risk assessment every 3 to 6 months for the first 3 years and then every 6 months during years 4 and 5, and a CEA level checked every 3 months for at least 3 years after surgery.

Case Conclusion

The patient underwent a hand-assisted laparoscopic left hemicolectomy with a primary stapled midtransverse colon–sigmoid anastomosis. During surgery, we found a very large mass in the splenic flexure of the colon, with no direct extension into contiguous organs, and no evidence of synchronous colonic lesions in the right colon, liver metastases, or carcinomatosis. The estimated blood loss was <50 mL, and the operative time was 120 minutes. The patient recovered uneventfully and was discharged home on postoperative day 4, tolerating a regular diet, ambulating, with minimal incisional pain, and having bowel movements. The final pathology revealed an ulcerated, moderately differentiated adenocarcinoma involving the entire lumen of the colon that extended through the colonic wall and into the pericolonic adipose tissue with negative proximal, distal, and radial margins. There were 26 lymph nodes with no evidence of malignancy. There was no evidence of lymphovascular or perineural invasion. The tumor was positive for MLH-1, MSH-2, MSH-6, and PMS-2 by immunoperoxidase staining (microsatellite instability).

Due to the patient's advanced age, adequate lymphadenectomy negative for cancer, and lack of lymphovascular and perineural invasion, and the presence of microsatellite instability in the primary tumor, the medical oncologist decided that chemotherapy was not indicated in this patient.

TAKE HOME POINTS

- Diagnosis of transverse colon cancer is often delayed, and complicated forms (perforation, fistulization, obstruction) occur in 30% to 50% of cases.
- Patients that present with a complete large bowel obstruction with a competent ileocecal valve represent a true surgical emergency.

- Clinical presentation permitting, the preoperative staging workup should include a CT scan of the abdomen and the pelvis with oral and intravenous contrast, a chest x-ray or a CT scan of the chest, a CEA blood level, and a full colonoscopy.
- Colonic stenting is the best option either for palliation or as a bridge to surgery in high-risk patients with a complete bowel obstruction due to a splenic flexure colon cancer with a competent ileocecal valve.
- In patients undergoing surgery, it is paramount not only to resect the bowel segment involving the splenic flexure of the colon with negative margins of resection but also to include the entire lymphovascular pedicles associated with the splenic flexure of the colon (a minimum of 12 lymph nodes should be obtained). This should include high ligation of the left colic vessels, the left branches of the middle colic vessels, and the inferior mesenteric vein.
- Subtotal colectomy is useful in cases of proximal bowel damage (i.e., cecal perforation) or synchronous tumors.

SUGGESTED READINGS

Guo MG, Feng Y, Zheng Q, et al. Comparison of self-expanding metal stents and urgent surgery for left-sided malignant colonic obstruction in elderly patients. *Dig Dis Sci.* 2011;56:2706-2710.

Guo MG, Feng Y, Zheng Q, et al. NCCN Clinical Practice Guidelines in Oncology: colon cancer. National Comprehensive Cancer Network. *J Natl Compr Canc Netw.* 2009;7(8):778-831.

Stipa F, Pigazzi A, Bascone B, et al. Management of obstructive colorectal cancer with endoscopic stenting followed by single-stage surgery: open or laparoscopic resection? *Surg Endosc.* 2008;22:1477-1481.

Anastomotic Leak After Colectomy

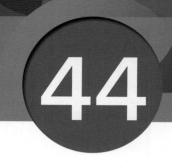

SARA AMELIA GAINES AND NEIL HYMAN

Based on the previous edition chapter "Anastomotic Leak After Colectomy" by Neil Hyman

Presentation

A 64-year-old man with hypertension and mild chronic obstructive pulmonary disease is now 6 days after an elective sigmoid colectomy for recurrent diverticulitis. His initial postoperative course was unremarkable, but he developed confusion and agitation on the evening of postoperative day 4. His abdomen became more distended, but he did not have evidence of peritonitis. His morphine was stopped, and a nasogastric tube was inserted. He seemed to improve somewhat initially but then developed progressive tachypnea and a low-grade fever over the next 24 hours. He remained hemodynamically stable but required two fluid boluses to maintain adequate urine output. On postoperative day 6, his clinical status acutely worsened. At this point, he developed respiratory distress and tachycardia with a heart rate of 130. His lungs were clear with decreased breath sounds at the bases. He had marked abdominal distention and was tender across his lower abdomen with diffuse peritoneal signs.

● DIFFERENTIAL DIAGNOSIS

Anastomotic leaks are perhaps the most dreaded complication of bowel resection. The reported incidence varies greatly based on definitions, indication for surgery, and anastomotic site. For a sigmoid colon resection, the anastomotic leak rate should be approximately 5%. Early postoperative leaks classically present in a dramatic fashion with severe abdominal pain, tachycardia, high fevers, and a rigid abdomen, often with hemodynamic instability. But leaks manifesting further along the postoperative course usually present far more insidiously, often with low-grade fever, ileus, and failure to progress. To complicate matters, a low-grade fever and leukocytosis are relatively common after a colectomy, and the positive predictive value of abnormal vital signs in this situation is only 4% to 11%. These nonspecific signs and symptoms can also mimic other infectious complications, such as pneumonia or urinary tract infection, or an early postoperative small bowel obstruction. Mental status changes and tachypnea are often the earliest signs of anastomotic leak, but again, these signs are nonspecific and could also suggest pulmonary embolism, pneumonia, atelectasis, or an adverse drug reaction.

In our clinical scenario, the patient presents with symptoms that were initially nonspecific (fever, tachypnea, and tachycardia), and the differential diagnosis includes leak as well as other infectious complications. This patient, however, eventually progresses to having a distended abdomen with peritonitis, which makes anastomotic leak the clear working diagnosis.

● WORKUP

Patients with an early postoperative leak often have signs and symptoms of peritonitis and sepsis. In many circumstances, the diagnosis is clinically evident, and prompt return to the operating room is warranted. Too often, radiologic studies are wishfully obtained, when the indication for reexploration is clear. However, these studies are appropriate in cases where there is some clinical uncertainty about the diagnosis. A water-soluble contrast enema will often rapidly confirm the presence of a leak in equivocal cases in the first few days after surgery (Figure 44-1). This study is particularly useful with colorectal anastomoses as it has a higher positive predictive value than when used to examine more proximal anastomoses. Later in the postoperative period, however, when the leaks that manifest themselves tend to be smaller and contained, a water-soluble contrast enema becomes less reliable, and a CT scan is preferable. In our experience, contrast enema failed to show a proven leak 60% of the time.

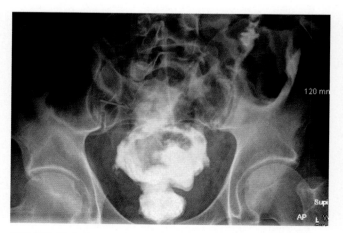

FIGURE 44-1. Anastomotic leak: contrast enema. *Arrow* indicates extravasation of water-soluble contrast from the colorectal anastomosis.

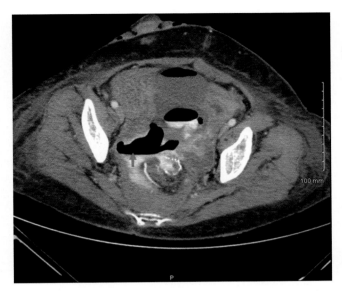

FIGURE 44-2. Anastomotic leak: CT scan. *Arrow* denotes the interface between extraluminal air and extravasated rectal contrast.

As described above, most leaks occurring later in the postoperative course are associated with a nonspecific presentation, and the diagnosis can actually be quite difficult to make. It must be recognized that a clouded sensorium or respiratory symptoms are often the presenting signs of a leak.

A chest x-ray and PE protocol chest CT scan may demonstrate pneumonia, lobar collapse, or pulmonary embolism. However, caution must be exercised in ascribing a downhill clinical course to subtle or minor abnormalities on these studies. Laboratory evaluation is generally nonspecific and often indicative of early multiorgan dysfunction. Plain abdominal films are usually not specific enough to make the diagnosis, but a large or an increasing amount of free intraperitoneal air noted on up-right chest x-ray is suggestive of a leak. The most helpful study in the setting of an occult leak is usually a CT scan of the abdomen and the pelvis with rectal contrast (Figure 44-2). We have found that CT demonstrates the diagnosis almost 90% of the time, but it must be acknowledged that there is broad overlap in CT findings in postoperative patients with or without a leak. Free air may be present up to 10 days in patients without a leak and loculated air up to 30 days after surgery.

● DIAGNOSIS AND TREATMENT

Leaks occurring within the first few days after surgery almost invariably require operative exploration. Patients should be properly prepared for surgery with fluid resuscitation, administration of broad-spectrum antibiotics, and adequate intravenous access. A Foley catheter should be inserted as well as appropriate monitors such as a central line and an arterial line as needed. Of particular importance, patients

should usually be marked for an intestinal stoma as this will often be required. Many ostomies created in the setting of a leak turn out to be permanent. Poor stoma siting (e.g., in a skin crease) can be a nightmare for the patient and be the difference in whether the patient can reassume self-care once they recover from surgery.

Contained leaks manifesting later on in the postoperative period in stable patients can often be managed nonoperatively with patience, antibiotics, and percutaneous drainage. Reoperation beyond 7 to 10 days after the initial procedure can be hazardous and may make the situation worse. Minor anastomotic disruptions may heal over time and obviate the need for any further operative treatment and an intestinal stoma.

● SURGICAL APPROACH

The value and the importance of surgical planning when it comes to the management of an anastomotic leak cannot be overemphasized. Both the patient's physiologic condition and the nature of the leak are crucial to medical decision-making. As a rule of thumb, the longer the interval between reoperation and the initial surgery, the more difficult the procedure is likely to be. Surrounding viscera will attempt to seal the leak off, incorporating the anastomosis into an inflammatory mass surrounded by friable bowel with serositis. There is usually an associated ileus making the bowel distended and tense. As such, mobilizing the anastomosis without tearing the bowel or extending the anastomotic defect can be a challenge. In this setting, precision of purpose (e.g., having a clearly defined plan) and technical efficiency (e.g., avoiding unnecessary dissection) are the key elements to success.

The patient is usually positioned supine, but the lithotomy position is preferred in patients who have a colorectal anastomosis, so it can be tested with betadine or inspected endoscopically. The previous incision is utilized and extended as necessary. Using primarily gentle blunt maneuvers, the bowel is pinched off the abdominal wall to facilitate access and exposure. The peritoneal cavity is irrigated and suctioned to clear as needed and a specimen obtained for Gram stain and culture. The anastomosis is gently exposed and inspected. In a hemodynamically stable patient, right-sided anastomoses (e.g., ileocolic) can be resected and redone as long as the ends are not ischemic. In patients with extensive local sepsis and hemodynamic instability, an end-loop stoma should be created whenever possible (Figure 44-3). Although the surgeon's primary goal is control of sepsis, exteriorizing the distal end of the bowel will save the patient another major laparotomy down the line to restore gastrointestinal continuity. Resection with anastomosis and proximal loop ileostomy is another alternative.

Left-sided anastomotic leaks usually require fecal diversion. Again, preoperative stoma marking is vital, especially in obese patients. The anastomosis is inspected and

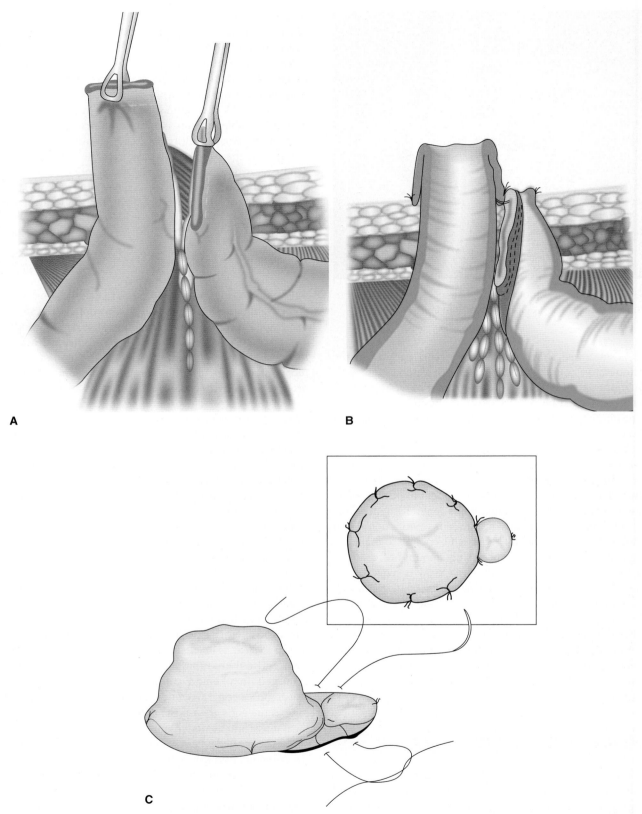

FIGURE 44-3. End-loop stoma. The ileum and the proximal colon are exteriorized through the same hole to facilitate later closure without the need for laparotomy. **A:** The stapled ileum and the colon are delivered through the stoma site. **B:** A standard Brooke ileostomy is created. The antimesenteric edge of the colonic staple line is excised and sutured to the skin. **C:** The end-loop stoma is completed.

the patient's hemodynamic status reviewed. Stable patients with a small leak in an otherwise intact anastomosis, without evidence of ischemia or overt local contamination, can be treated with repair, omentoplasty, and loop ileostomy. Otherwise, ischemic anastomoses, major disruptions, or those associated with severe systemic sepsis should usually have the anastomosis resected and a Hartmann procedure performed. Resection with anastomosis and loop ileostomy is another option for stable patients. Most patients with leaking low colorectal anastomoses are best treated with fecal diversion and drainage. The anastomosis is usually deep in the pelvis, and attempts at exposure will usually worsen the defect. Endoscopic visualization to assure the anastomosis is not ischemic and to visualize the defect can provide the needed information for decision-making without worsening the problem. A presacral drain is placed, and the omentum is mobilized for placement over the anastomosis (or at least into the pelvis).

Common pitfalls are doing too much or too little at surgery. As noted above, the dissection should be restricted and focused to only what is needed to examine the anastomosis and washout the contaminated fluids. On the other hand, the surgeon must acknowledge the nature of the problem and treat the leak adequately. An anastomotic leak has a major emotional toll on the patient, their family, and the operating surgeon. It can be tempting just to suture the hole closed and hope, in lieu of creating an intestinal stoma ("perfuming the pig"). But if the patient had a leak under "ideal" or elective conditions, it is even more likely they will develop another leak in an emergency situation with local and systemic signs of sepsis. Patients who have suffered a leak often cannot readily tolerate another septic insult. When in doubt, it is a good time to "phone a friend" and speak with a trusted and experienced colleague (Table 44-1).

SPECIAL INTRAOPERATIVE CONSIDERATIONS

Special mention is made of the obese patient with a leak. Although the principles of management are the same, there are a few additional considerations. First, most obese patients have a much thinner upper than lower abdomen wall, where most of the pannus resides. Bringing out an ostomy in the lower abdomen without undue tension or ischemia may be difficult or impossible. As such, strong consideration should be given to placing the stoma in the right (or left) upper quadrant. Further, a loop ileostomy is possible in almost any patient, whereas creating a colostomy in an obese patient with a leak may be a nightmare. The bowel is friable; there is marked distension from the associated ileus; and the mesentery may be rigid, inflamed, and unyielding. This is one scenario where either repair with diverting loop ileostomy or resection with anastomosis and proximal loop ileostomy may be the only option.

POSTOPERATIVE MANAGEMENT

An anastomotic leak is associated with a mortality rate of 10% to 15%. The first step in postoperative management is to support the patient through the sepsis as needed with inotropes, ventilatory support, and modern intensive care. Unfortunately, patients who leak commonly require prolonged hospitalization, further reoperations, and aggressive rehabilitation. Antibiotics should be administered in a goal-directed manner (e.g., until afebrile with a normal white blood cell count and resolved ileus) instead of continued indefinitely. Nutritional support, good enterostomal therapy, and careful wound management are usually cornerstones of supportive care. Patients who have been reoperated on for a leak are at high risk for further complications such as wound infection or intra-abdominal abscess. These patients often require postoperative imaging studies and percutaneous drainage of residual infected collections.

Table 44-1	Surgical Management of an Anastomotic Leak

Key Technical Steps

1. Adequate resuscitation and stoma marking.
2. Clear and well-delineated preop plan.
3. Careful blunt dissection.
4. Gentle exposure of the anastomosis when accessible.
5. Assessment of the patient's hemodynamic status.
6. Resect and redo it on the right if stable.
7. End-loop stoma on the right if unstable.
8. Repair/redo and proximal diversion on the left if stable.
9. Resect and stoma on the left if unstable.

Potential Pitfalls

- Have a plan.
- Do not "perfume the pig."
- Phone a friend as needed.

Case Conclusion

In our patient, he was taken to the operating room without radiographic studies, since he had a clear clinical presentation of an anastomotic leak and was severely ill. He was given additional intravenous fluid and broad-spectrum antibiotics while readying an operating room. He was placed in lithotomy position, and his midline incision was reopened. After exposing the pelvis and irrigating the abdomen, a small disruption in the lateral colorectal anastomosis was found. The colon and the rectum appeared healthy and viable. The area of anastomotic dehiscence was reinforced with lembert sutures, and omentum was placed over the reinforced area. A diverting loop ileostomy was performed to allow healing of the anastomosis. The patient recovered well and was discharged home after 10 days. At 2 months, a contrast enema showed healing of his anastomosis without leak or stricture. His ileostomy was taken down electively 3 months after his initial surgery.

TAKE HOME POINTS

- Anastomotic leaks are a devastating complication of intestinal surgery.
- Many early leaks are readily diagnosed clinically (not radiographically) and require prompt reoperation and treatment.
- Most leaks actually occur 6 days or more after surgery, and the diagnosis can be very challenging as signs and symptoms are nonspecific.
- CT scan is usually the imaging modality of choice for late leaks.
- Reoperation requires thoughtful planning and a goal-directed approach.

SUGGESTED READINGS

Bruce J, Krukowski ZH, Al-Khairy G, et al. Systematic review of the definition and management of anastomotic leak after gastrointestinal surgery. *Br J Surg.* 2001;88:1157-1168.

Erb L, Hyman NH, Osler T. Abnormal vital signs are common after bowel resection and do not predict anastomotic leak. *J Am Coll Surg.* 2014;218(6):1195-1199.

Hyman N, Manchester TL, Osler T, et al. Anastomotic leaks after intestinal anastomosis: its later than you think. *Ann Surg.* 2007;245:254-258.

Hyman N, Osler T, Cataldo P, et al. Anastomotic leaks after bowel resection: what does peer review teach us about the relationship to postoperative mortality? *J Am Coll Surg.* 2009:208:48-52.

Power N, Atri M, Ryan S, et al. CT assessment of anastomotic bowel leak. *Clin Radiol.* 2007;62:37-42.

Large Bowel Obstruction from Colon Cancer

NOELLE L. BERTELSON AND DAVID A. ETZIONI

45

Based on the previous edition chapter "Large Bowel Obstruction from Colon Cancer" by Noelle L. Bertelson and David A. Etzioni

Presentation

A 78-year-old female is evaluated in the emergency department with a 2-day history of worsening nausea/anorexia, abdominal pain, and distention. Her last bowel movement and flatus were 36 hours ago. She has no significant medical history and no prior abdominal or pelvic surgical procedures; her vital signs are normal. On examination, her abdomen is soft and nontender; there is significant tympany, however, especially on the right side. Her white blood cell count is 10.3. Initial workup proceeds with a supine x-ray, demonstrating gaseous distention of the right and proximal transverse colon, with a paucity of gas in the distal colon and rectum (Figure 45-1).

● DIFFERENTIAL DIAGNOSIS

This patient presents with signs, symptoms, and radiographic evidence of a large bowel obstruction. Generally speaking, the differential diagnosis of a large bowel obstruction can be broadly classified as being infectious, inflammatory, or neoplastic in origin. One of the key elements of this patient's

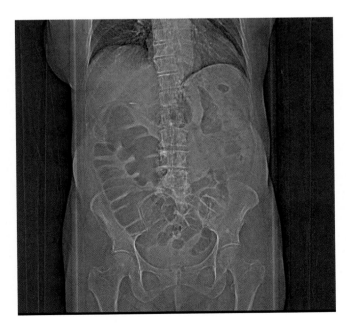

FIGURE 45-1. Supine x-ray.

history is the absence of prior abdominal or pelvic operations. The most likely cause of this type of presentation varies widely depending on the population from which the patient emerges. In most developed countries, this patient should be considered to have a gastrointestinal malignancy—most commonly colorectal cancer—until proven otherwise.

Infectious causes may be related to a wide variety of organisms, none of which occur with great prevalence in the United States, but include *Ascaris* species, *Taenia* species, tuberculosis, and *Yersinia*. Diverticulitis and inflammatory bowel disease (including Crohn's, ulcerative colitis, and sarcoidosis) can present with acute/subacute colonic obstruction. On radiologic investigation, these disease processes can be indistinguishable from colorectal cancer. The most common neoplastic disorders of the colon are benign adenomas and their malignant counterpart, adenocarcinoma. Noncolonic carcinoma, either metastatic or extrinsically compressing, may also involve the colon. Other, less common neoplastic disease entities, including lymphoma and carcinoid, followed by sarcoma, plasmacytoma, melanoma, leukemic infiltration, neuroendocrine tumor, medullary carcinoma, and Schwannoma are also potential causes of colonic obstruction. Nonneoplastic/noninfectious processes, most notably volvulus and intussusception, can cause acute large bowel obstruction, with volvulus causing 10% of colonic obstructions and intussusception occurring in 1% of all bowel obstructions.

● INITIAL WORKUP

In reviewing the initial x-ray study (Figure 45-1), it is worth noting that the small bowel loops are not prominent and that there is no significant bubble of gastric air. Based on this plain film, a computed tomography (CT) of the abdomen/pelvis with oral and intravenous contrast is ordered (Figure 45-2). This scan shows an obstructing mass in/around the midportion of the transverse colon. Of note, the right colon is significantly distended (maximum dimension 10 cm). The patient's liver and intraperitoneal structures (omentum, etc) do not show any evidence of metastatic disease or ascites.

Although this study is performed less commonly now than in the past, a contrast enema (with water-soluble contrast) can be informative about the location and patency of an obstructing or partially obstructing mass. Another useful

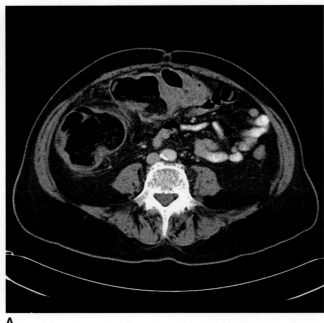
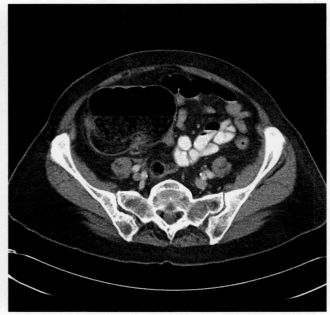

A   **B**

FIGURE 45-2. **A-B:** CT scan of abdomen/pelvis.

option for investigation in this circumstance is a CT scan with the instillation of rectal contrast.

● DISCUSSION

Colon cancer is diagnosed in over 130,000 individuals in the United States per year, resulting in over 90,000 colectomies. While the vast majority of these undergo surgical treatment on an elective basis, a distinct proportion is discovered during evaluation for an acute bowel obstruction (Table 45-1).

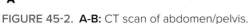

Table 45-1	Extended Right Colectomy in the Presence of Transverse Colon Obstruction

Key Technical Steps

1. Lithotomy positioning.
2. Midline incision, exploratory laparotomy (examine peritoneal surfaces, liver).
3. Decompressive enterotomy in right colon (if necessary).
4. Mobilize the right colon from lateral to medial.
5. Enter lesser sac at hepatic flexure.
6. Remove greater omentum from stomach.
7. Mobilize splenic flexure.
8. Divide mesentery.
   - Ligate ileocolic vascular pedicle.
   - Ligate middle colic pedicle.
   - Ligate ascending branch of left colic artery.
9. Construct ileocolic anastomosis.
10. Close mesenteric defect (surgeon preference).
11. Irrigate and close abdomen.

In the management of any patient with a bowel obstruction, the determinations that should guide intervention are the following: (1) likelihood of resolution of the current obstruction without intervention, (2) risks of urgent/emergent intervention, (3) need for intervention in the imminent future if the current process resolves, and (4) the impact of an urgent versus a delayed intervention on the patient's short/long-term health.

For this particular patient, a critical prognostic feature is the presence of a closed loop obstruction. Nondilated terminal ileum immediately proximal to a distended cecum indicates a *competent* ileocecal valve. The portion of colon between the ileocecal valve and the obstruction lesion in the transverse colon has no mechanism by which to decompress and is therefore a closed loop. Any closed loop intestinal obstruction is an indication for *urgent* decompression.

As surgeons, we all develop a level of comfort with the initial nonoperative treatment of bowel obstructions. However, without prompt intervention, the patient with a closed loop large bowel obstruction may progress quickly to right colon perforation. The absence of focal peritonitis or signs of significant systemic toxicity *are not reassuring*.

● DECISION-MAKING

Colon obstructions can be decompressed effectively using nonsurgical and surgical approaches.

The only reasonable nonsurgical options would involve the endoscopic placement of a self-expanding metallic stent (SEMS). Intuitively, this stent would be used as a "bridge" to surgery, potentially allowing for the operation to be performed electively with a preoperative bowel preparation. The choice of whether or not to use a stent in a patient with an obstructing left-sided lesion is complex and at least partially subjective. A recent multicenter randomized trial examining stenting versus surgery for stage IV left-sided colorectal cancer was closed due to a high rate of serious complications in the stenting arm. The use of stents in patients with left-sided malignant obstruction is controversial in current professional guidelines.

In making a decision to operate versus stenting, several factors should be considered. For a stent to have a good likelihood of success, a retrograde contrast study showing some extent of luminal patency is required. Patients with advanced metastatic disease and limited prognosis may do better with a stent than with a major operation (with or without colostomy formation). The severity of the obstruction is also relevant—impending perforation strongly favors a definitive operative approach.

In this particular patient, however, the decision is made easier by the fact that the lesion is proximal to the splenic flexure. The operation of choice in this situation is an extended right colectomy with ileocolic anastomosis. Ileocolic anastomoses are robust, with leak rates routinely reported at <2%. In this patient, the risks of a procedural complication from stent placement are almost certainly greater than any potential gains from converting the operation from an urgent to a planned procedure.

What about problems related to the absence of a mechanical bowel preparation? The utility of a mechanical bowel preparation in elective colorectal surgery has been studied extensively. While the majority of the literature in this topic is of poor quality, the overall synthesis (including two large, well-conducted trials) of existing knowledge is that these efforts provide little, if any benefit. Placing a stent with the goal of being able to prevent operating on unprepared bowel would not be justified. Furthermore, in this patient, the two portions of bowel (terminal ileum and descending colon) are spared of fecal loading, thereby obviating any benefit of the preparation.

An important issue in planning for this patient is what efforts should be made to ensure that the portion of colorectum that will remain after the resection is free of neoplasia. Case series have documented a 6% to 10% rate of synchronous carcinoma in patients presenting with obstructing colonic tumors. While the proximal dilated portion will necessarily be removed with surgical resection, an intraoperative colonoscopy with minimal insufflation performed to the level of the tumor is a useful and important test. Carbon dioxide colonoscopy, if available, may minimize resulting distention of the distal colon. No mechanical bowel preparation is necessary except for a couple of enemas.

The best treatment plan for the patient in the case described above is to be taken to the operating room for intraoperative colonoscopy and extended right colectomy.

● TECHNICAL ASPECTS OF SURGERY

The usual administration of preoperative antibiotics and subcutaneous heparin should be performed. Colonoscopy, if performed, is easiest with the patient in left lateral decubitus position on the transport gurney. During the operation, a low lithotomy position will facilitate the planned operation, particularly the splenic flexure mobilization. While there has been a small case series of laparoscopically managed large bowel obstructions, the extent of distention of the proximal bowel generally precludes safe laparoscopic mobilization of the right colon and should not be performed.

Once the abdomen has been explored through a generous midline incision, the right colon will be easily identified, usually tensely distended and potentially demonstrating early signs of impending perforation (discoloration, deserosalization, etc). After placing a purse-string suture, a decompressive enterotomy in the anterior surface of the proximal right colon will greatly facilitate the procedure. Careful attention to avoiding unnecessary stool spillage will minimize the potential risks from this maneuver.

With the right colon decompressed, dissection proceeds along the right paracolic gutter, moving toward the hepatic flexure. The dissection is carried medially to the level of the anterior surface of the second portion of the duodenum. Great care should be taken in retracting the colon to avoid avulsion of the pancreaticoduodenal veins in this region.

It is a generally accepted oncologic principle that the omentum is resected en bloc with any transverse colon carcinoma, so the omentum should be removed from the greater curvature of the stomach. This exposes the lesser sac and the transverse mesocolon. Continuing distally, the splenic flexure should be mobilized in order to facilitate an anastomosis between the descending colon and the terminal ileum.

The distal extent of the resection is controversial, but for tumors distal to the midtransverse colon, a resection which encompasses the ascending branch of the left colic artery is prudent. An anastomosis into the splenic flexure of the colon is potentially risky because of potential problems with blood supply in this watershed area, especially in older patients or those with known vascular disease. The descending colon is a preferred location for the ileocolic anastomosis.

Once the colon is mobilized, the mesentery is divided, and a high ligation is performed for all feeding vessels (ileocolic, middle colic, ascending branch of left colic). An anastomosis is then constructed between terminal ileum and descending colon. There are several options for reconstruction. A hand-sewn end-to-end anastomosis with an inner layer of running absorbable 3-0 suture and an outer layer of 3-0 interrupted silk sutures is a commonly employed technique. In order to manage the size discrepancy between small and large bowel, the small bowel can be "beveled", enlarging the small bowel aperture along the antimesenteric side of the intestine. A stapled side-to-side/functional end-to-end anastomosis may also be performed.

There are no good data to support one technique over the other at this time. Though there is some evidence that leak rates are lower in stapled ileotransverse anastomoses after right colectomy, it is uncertain whether this finding can be applied to ileodescending anastomoses.

After anastomosis is performed, the mesenteric defect may be approximated (or not, based on surgeon preference), and the abdomen is irrigated and the fascia and skin closed.

● SPECIAL CONSIDERATIONS

Perforation

In the setting of cecal perforation, resection of the ischemic segment of bowel as well as the tumor is mandatory. In these cases, an extended right versus subtotal colectomy is the preferred operation. If the patient is unstable secondary to intra-abdominal sepsis from the perforation, judgment must be exercised in deciding whether to construct an anastomosis. A double-barreled stoma, incorporating the terminal ileum and a corner of the proximal colon (Prasad ileostomy), will avoid the risk of anastomotic leakage and allow for stoma reversal in the future without a formal laparotomy.

Duodenal/Pancreatic Invasion

Rarely, a transverse colon carcinoma may involve the duodenum or head of the pancreas. Intraoperatively, any points of adherence between a known carcinoma and adjacent structures should be considered invasion and mandate consideration for en bloc resection. The magnitude of benefit compared with risk of such a resection needs to be considered on a case-by-case basis. Pancreaticoduodenectomy can be performed in the setting of invasion into the pancreatic head, and there does appear to be some long-term survival in some patients with small case series quoting up to 55% 5-year survival. Duodenal invasion usually does not require a pancreaticoduodenectomy. When feasible, resection with primary should be performed. In cases of more extensive resection, a serosal or mucosal patch using proximal jejunum may be required. In unusual situations, a Roux-en-Y reconstruction with duodenojejunostomy may be required.

Unsuspected Metastatic Disease

At the time of surgery, it is not uncommon to discover metastatic disease that was not clearly detected on preoperative imaging studies. Metastatic disease should not be considered a contraindication to a palliative resection, though the presence of gross peritoneal disease or a significant burden of hepatic disease may prompt the use of a stoma or intestinal bypass over a high-risk anastomosis. In the setting of unexpected hepatic disease, intraoperative ultrasound can assist in further characterizing and identifying lesions. In an otherwise stable patient, isolated metastases amenable to simple wedge resection can reasonably be addressed at the time of the initial operation. However, in an unstable patient, metastatic disease should be noted, confirmed with biopsy, and addressed at a later date.

A guiding principle in these situations is to weigh the risks versus benefits of metastasectomy. Over time, surgeons have developed a greater comfort with synchronous resection of the colon and liver metastases. In an urgent situation, a major liver resection of multiple segments or a lobectomy may be too great of a physiologic stressor.

● POSTOPERATIVE MANAGEMENT

Patients who demonstrate hemodynamic instability in the operating room or who experience unexpected massive fluid shifts/blood loss may require an intermediate level of care; most other patients should not need elevated levels of care. Nasogastric decompression is unnecessary. While early feeding has been associated with some improved outcomes and shorter hospital stays in elective cases, the obstructed patient may have a prolonged ileus, such that feeding should be delayed until the abdomen is flat and the patient is without nausea or emesis. There is no role for routine postoperative antibiotics beyond a 24-hour perioperative period. Prophylaxis for deep venous thromboembolism should be employed routinely, including subcutaneous heparin injections and sequential compression devices for the legs. Discharge can be expected when the patient is tolerating oral feeding and has had a bowel movement. Inpatient oncology consultation and outpatient surveillance are elements of care, which are also part of the standard of care for these patients.

Case Conclusion

The patient was taken to the OR based on the clinical presentation and imaging studies described. Her preoperative informed consent process included discussion of intraoperative carbon dioxide colonoscopy, exploratory laparotomy, bowel resection, and possible ostomy formation. At the time of surgery, her right colon was tensely distended and a 14-gauge IV catheter was inserted through a purse-string suture in order to decompress the bowel and avoid uncontrolled rupture. Following this, the right colon, hepatic flexure, and splenic flexure were mobilized completely. The resection specimen encompassed the entire right colon, transverse colon, splenic flexure, and omentum. An ileo-descending anastomosis was constructed using a GIA-80 mm and TA-60 mm stapler, with suture reinforcement. The patient's recovery was complicated by ileus requiring nasogastric decompression and urinary tract infection, but she was discharged on postoperative day #9. Her pathologic stage was IIIb (T3N1, 1/28 lymph nodes positive), and she completed an adjuvant therapy regimen including capecitabine and oxaliplatin. Surveillance examinations including colonoscopy and CT studies are negative at 2 years postoperative.

TAKE HOME POINTS

- Obstructing colon cancer is a surgical emergency, especially in the presence of a competent ileocecal valve (closed loop obstruction); clinical findings of focal peritonitis and/or systemic toxicity are late findings.
- Colonic obstruction is most often secondary to malignancy.
- Self-expanding metallic stents have no role in the treatment of tumors that are within the scope of an extended right colectomy (tumors proximal to splenic flexure). Their role in left-sided lesions is controversial.
- Intraoperative colonoscopy is an important exam in the stable patient and may lead to changes in the operative plan.
- Primary ileocolic anastomosis should be performed except in cases of hemodynamic instability and gross feculent peritonitis. In these cases, a double-barreled stoma is preferred.

SUGGESTED READINGS

Bat L, Neumann G, Shemesh E. The association of synchronous neoplasms with occluding colorectal cancer. *Dis Colon Rectum.* 1985;28(3):149-151.

Choy PY, Bissett IP, Docherty JG, et al. Stapled versus handsewn methods for ileocolic anastomoses. *Cochrane Database Syst Rev.* 2007(3):CD004320.

Contant CM, Hop WC, van't Sant HP, et al. Mechanical bowel preparation for elective colorectal surgery: a multicentre randomised trial. *Lancet.* 2007;370(9605):2112-2117.

Gordon PH, Nivatvongs S. *Principles and Practice of Surgery for the Colon, Rectum, and Anus.* 3rd ed. CRC Press; 2007.

Jung B, Pahlman L, Nystrom PO, et al. Multicentre randomized clinical trial of mechanical bowel preparation in elective colonic resection. *Br J Surg.* 2007;94(6):689-695.

Siegel RL, Miller KD, Jemal A. Cancer statistics, 2016. *CA Cancer J Clin.* 2016;66(1):7-30.

Slim K, Vicaut E, Launay-Savary MV, et al. Updated systematic review and meta-analysis of randomized clinical trials on the role of mechanical bowel preparation before colorectal surgery. *Ann Surg.* 2009;249(2):203-209.

van Hooft JE, Bemelman WA, Oldenburg B, et al. Colonic stenting versus emergency surgery for acute left-sided malignant colonic obstruction: a multicentre randomised trial. *Lancet Oncol.* 2011; 12(4):344-352.

van Hooft JE, van Halsema EE, Vanbiervliet G, et al. Self-expandable metal stents for obstructing colonic and extracolonic cancer: European Society of Gastrointestinal Endoscopy (ESGE) Clinical Guideline. *Endoscopy.* 2014;46(11):990-1002.

Recurrent Uncomplicated (Sigmoid) Diverticulitis

JOHN C. BYRN

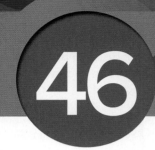

Presentation

A 48-year-old healthy female marathon runner presents to your outpatient surgical clinic office with a history of three distinct attacks of left lower quadrant pain. She is currently pain-free and training for an upcoming marathon. For the attacks, she sought medical attention at the local emergency room or her primary care provider. For the first attack, while in the emergency room, a CT scan was performed of the abdomen and pelvis, and the patient reported she was given a diagnosis of diverticulitis. She was admitted to the inpatient floor for 4 days prior to release. Her treatment course was antibiotics, initial bowel rest and hydration, and subsequent slow resumption of normal diet. The patient presents for discussion of options for elective sigmoid resection.

● DIFFERENTIAL DIAGNOSIS

The differential diagnosis for this patient includes colon cancer, ischemic colitis, Crohn's disease, ulcerative colitis, irritable bowel syndrome, and infectious colitis. Colon cancer, although potentially excluded by history and cross-sectional imaging, must be omnipresent in the surgeons mind and ruled out, to whatever extent possible, prior to surgical recommendation. Ischemic colitis can be managed surgically if chronic and recurring, while acute events are managed medically in the majority of patients. Segmental resections, akin to resection for diverticulitis, can be appropriate, but patient counseling and surgical planning is best accomplished after accurate preoperative diagnosis.

Crohn's disease and ulcerative colitis may clinically mask as diverticulitis in its episodic nature, and even radiographically, but has a myriad of medical management options, and the segmental colectomy is inappropriate for ulcerative colitis and rarely appropriate for Crohn's disease. Infectious colitis is less commonly segmental and is largely self-limited. It may be associated with travel or dietary indiscretion. In the case of *Clostridium difficile*, infectious colitis is associated with recent antibiotic treatment, hospitalization, and surgery. Lastly, irritable bowel syndrome is largely a diagnosis of exclusion and most appropriately diagnosed by the gastroenterologist. Typically, the symptoms are more chronic in nature and not associated with systemic signs of infection, inflammation, or radiographic abnormalities.

● WORKUP

A probing history should be performed assessing the symptoms of each attack, presence of fever or other systemic signs of infection, life-long history of diarrhea or episodic gastrointestinal upset, risk factors for ischemia, and response to medical management during the attacks.

Without current symptoms, a routine physical exam should be performed. During abdominal examination, the patient may be able to localize the left lower quadrant pain specifically and any radiating pain or associated tenderness. Surgical scars should be noted for surgical planning if so decided upon. Laparoscopic resection of uncomplicated diverticulitis is the typical surgical approach but may need to be considered more carefully in a patient with multiple previous abdominal surgeries.

When taking a focused history for a patient with uncomplicated diverticulitis, it is useful to begin by excluding competing diagnoses based on atypical diverticulitis narratives. For example, a surgeon could become suspicious of Crohn's disease in this patient if upon further questions, they reported a history of mucous-like and bloody diarrhea episodes over a period of years in their early 20s. To cover the breadth of the differential and historical cues, it may be helpful to focus on what the history chronic uncomplicated diverticulitis is, while trying to catalog the important historical anecdotes for competing diagnoses.

To that point, diverticulitis in this patient will present without remote history of gastrointestinal symptoms and will be isolated attacks associated with well-localized pain to the left lower quadrant. Associated signs of systemic infection will include fever, chills, and malaise. The patient's attack will uncommonly be self-limited and should respond almost exclusively to antibiotic therapy. Patients reporting an attack that they did not seek medical attention for, and whose symptoms improved without antibiotic treatment, may have not been having diverticulitis-associated symptoms. While some change in bowel habits is common with diverticulitis, the attacks will rarely be dominated by diarrhea with blood or mucous filled bowel movements, as would be typical of inflammatory bowel disease or ischemic colitis. Recent travel or treatment with antibiotics for other reasons preceding the attacks may raise suspicion of infectious colitis. Vague abdominal pain associated with eating or alternating diarrhea and constipation not responding to antibiotics

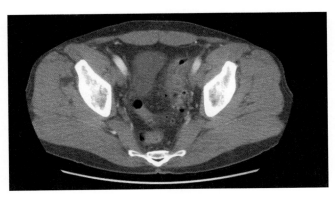

FIGURE 46-1. CT scan showing uncomplicated sigmoid diverticulitis.

treatments may lead the surgeon to consider irritable bowel syndrome in this patient. A family history of colorectal cancer or inflammatory bowel disease should be investigated, and gradual unexplained weight loss or blood in the patients' stool might importantly raise concern for colorectal cancer masking as diverticulitis.

The gold standard diagnosis of diverticulitis is the alignment in time of an attack of the symptomology with associated objective markers of inflammation such as leukocytosis or fever and a CT scan with radiographic diagnosis of the diverticulitis. Follow-up colonoscopy is mandatory to exclude mucosal inflammation (ischemic colitis, infectious colitis, Crohn's disease, or ulcerative colitis) and colorectal cancer. Colonoscopy and CT images should be reviewed by the surgeon whenever possible.

Upon further investigation of the patient in our case scenario, two of the attacks were managed in the inpatient or emergency room setting with records available showing leukocytosis and fever and CT imaging classic for acute uncomplicated diagnosis. Records reviewed and additional history show prompt resolution of the attack with antibiotics, and the patient reports feeling well and her normal self between attacks. A third attack was "caught early" by the patient, and her primary care physician saw her in the office and treated with oral antibiotics—again with prompt resolution of symptoms.

A complete colonoscopy was performed without evidence of mucosal disease. Diverticulosis was evident in the sigmoid colon with subjective edema in the distal sigmoid but without stricture or inflammation (Figure 46-1).

● DIAGNOSIS AND TREATMENT

The patient carries a diagnosis of uncomplicated recurring sigmoid diverticulitis. Competing diagnoses have been almost entirely ruled out by CT scan, endoscopy, and the episodic symptoms responding to antibiotics.

There are no reliable recommendations for the medical prevention of additional episodes of diverticulitis. Dietary recommendations subjected to study have largely shown that

the fiber content of the patients' diet does not impact recurrence of disease. Occasionally, patients will offer up dietary triggers for their attacks, and recommendation against these foods, although not backed by medical study, is at least commonsensical. Other studied medical therapies without conclusive impact on the natural history of the attacks include prophylactic antibiotics, antiinflammatory agents, and probiotics.

The role of elective sigmoid colectomy for chronic uncomplicated diverticulitis has been subject to a recent renaissance. Previously well-known recommendations of surgery based on number of attacks, and to some extent age, have fallen out of favor. Currently, more patient-specific recommendation should be made after discussions of the risks of surgery and the potential for recurrent attacks with the patient.

Retrospective studies with long-term follow-up on patients with recurrent uncomplicated diverticulitis not undergoing surgery have shown that a minority of patients will have life-threatening complications or complications requiring emergency surgery. The hard and fast rules of the number of attacks and patient age predicting recurrence have not necessarily been disproven, but the significance and frequency of these attacks has likely been over estimated in the past. Patients with recurrent uncomplicated diverticulitis have a definable risk of continued attacks; however, it is the assumption of the surgeon who does not recommend surgery that the patient understands this and that these attacks can confidently be predicted to be uncomplicated and not requiring emergency surgery or stoma formation. The risk of fecal peritonitis from free perforation of the sigmoid diverticulitis is assuredly low.

Patients opting for elective sigmoid resection should be counseled on surgical complication rates, realistic length-of-stay, and time off work or full activity. Importantly, major complication rates of <5%, depending on patient comorbidity, must be realistic in the surgeons practice to even consider the morbidity of resection over observation and treatment of recurrent uncomplicated attacks of diverticulitis.

Currently, this patient should be counseled that recurrent attacks are probable, and the severity is predictably similar to the previous episodes. The major complication rate of what would likely be a laparoscopic sigmoid colectomy is <5%. Surgery should only be performed, however, if the symptoms of the attacks crescendo or develop a late complication such as stricture. Unique circumstances such as a patient in an ultra-demanding profession or world travelers, who would be unsafe to have even an uncomplicated attack in an area of the world without medical care, may be considered relative indications for elective resection.

One year later, the patient returns to your office. The patient had another attack similar to her first episode requiring a trip to the emergency room and admission to the hospital for intravenous antibiotics. She recovered quickly and completely. CT scan from the admission confirmed recurrent uncomplicated diverticulitis. Unfortunately, the attack was on the eve a very important marathon race for the patient and she is seeking surgery as she cannot afford the risk of an attack interrupting future marathons. You and the patient agree to proceed with surgery.

● SURGICAL APPROACH

When approaching elective surgery for recurrent uncomplicated sigmoid diverticulitis, a laparoscopic approach is recommended. While previous surgery may preclude laparoscopy, initial laparoscopic approach is the standard of care for most patients. A medial to lateral approach with high ligation of the inferior mesenteric artery (IMA) is appropriate for most patients as the blood supply is handled in an area of less inflammation than may be encountered near the colon wall, adequate lymphadenectomy is performed in case a diagnosis of colon cancer is unexpectedly encountered, and mesentery mobilization for a colorectal anastomosis is more routinely achieved.

Adequate proximal mobilization of the remaining colon for creation of the anastomosis should be assessed intraoperatively. Mobilization of the splenic flexure and second ligation of the inferior mesenteric vein (IMV) at the level of Ligament of Treitz may not be necessary for all patients (Figures 46-2 **and** 46-3).

Midline extraction of the specimen should be avoided. Options include a muscle splitting extension of a lower quadrant trocar site or creation of a Pfannenstiel incision. The trocar extended extraction may be cumbersome in the obese patient and requires laparoscopic division of the rectosigmoid and laparoscopic vision during the end-to-end anastomosis (EEA). A Pfannenstiel extraction may be a more reproducible technique in the obese patient and can often allow for open stapling of the rectosigmoid, and direct vision of the EEA and leak test.

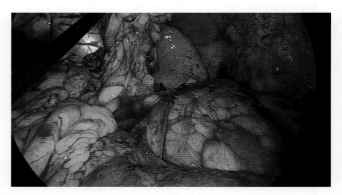

FIGURE 46-3. Fully mobilized splenic flexure with gastrocolic omentum retracted cephalad.

After establishing pneumoperitoneum, trocar placement can be individualized by the surgeon to the patient. In general, the camera port is at the umbilicus and an assistant port in the left abdomen can double as a working port for mobilization of the splenic flexure. For the main operating ports, right side ports are placed in a "diamond" configuration right lateral to the suprapubic region and the high right lower quadrant almost lateral to the umbilicus. A "quadrant" configuration in the right upper quadrant and right lower quadrant is also described (Figure 46-4).

Although not mandatory for benign disease, isolating and ligating the IMA first in a medial to lateral manner is recommended. Prior to ligation of the IMA, the left ureter should be identified and protected (Figure 46-5). Next perform the lateral mobilization of the sigmoid and descending colon to the level of splenic flexure. Identify soft colon proximal to the area of diverticulitis and determine its reach to the soft, top of the rectum (splaying of taenia is the traditional intraoperative anatomic landmark for the rectum). At the level of the rectum determined suitable for division and anastomosis, the rectal mesentery will need to be thinned with cautery or a ligating energy source. Once the mesentery is thinned, the rectum can be divided intracorporeally with a laparoscopic stapler or extracorporeally through a Pfannenstiel extraction site.

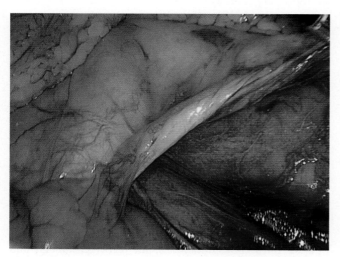

FIGURE 46-2. Inferior mesenteric vein at level of ligament Treitz.

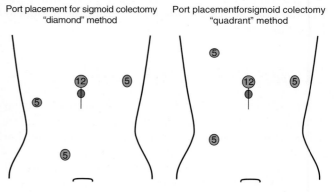

FIGURE 46-4. Trocar placement options.

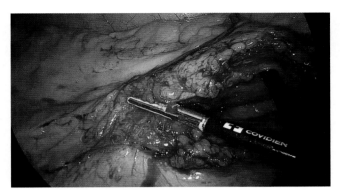

FIGURE 46-5. Inferior mesenteric artery being ligated with ureter in view in background.

Fashion an EEA either by laparoscopic vision or through the Pfannenstiel extraction site and perform a leak test with a flexible sigmoidoscopy. The colon proximal to the bowel should be occluded and the anastomosis submerged in irrigation saline for adequate leak testing.

Close fascia of extraction site and any laparoscopic trocar 10 mm or greater. The skin can be closed with a subcuticular suture.

Potential pitfalls of the operation include identification and protection of the left ureter while isolating and ligating the sigmoid mesentery (IMA), adequate mobilization for a tension-free colorectal anastomosis, and performing and leak testing the anastomosis. While not mandatory, high ligation of the IMA does allow for a reproducible technique that overlaps with the handling of a sigmoid colon cancer, known steps to identify and protect the ureter, and the handling of the major blood supply to the target organ in an uninflamed area that is likely to preserve collateral blood flow. If patient anatomy or inflammation makes handling the root of the mesentery treacherous, this approach can be abandoned for a lateral mobilization of the sigmoid and more distal mesenteric division.

Adequate mobilization of the colon for anastomosis and whether the splenic flexure and distal IMV must be taken down will likely require some degree of experience and judgment. If after the extraction of specimen, the anastomosis appears to be under tension that a return to laparoscopy for further mobilization is likely prudent. A well-perfused, tension-free anastomosis should still undergo leak test.

If the leak test is positive, a search for the defect should be undertaken. Options for repair include reresection and anastomosis to achieve a negative leak test, repair with leak test, or repair with leak test and proximal diversion. Abandonment of anastomosis and end colostomy may be necessary but only in the comorbid or extremely challenging case. Conversion to open and attempt and establishing continuity should likely precede end colostomy. The most time consuming and technically difficult option, resection and reanastomosis, is probably the best option as diversion of repaired, originally faulty anastomosis, has been associated with increased complications (Table 46-1).

Table 46-1	Laparoscopic Sigmoid Resection

Key Technical Steps

1. Establish pneumoperitoneum through preferred method, explore abdomen laparoscopically to identify stigmata of inflamed sigmoid colon, and rule out other unexpected findings.
2. Place inferior mesenteric artery (IMA) on stretch, incise peritoneum underlying it, and identify left ureter from medial perspective.
3. Ligate IMA with vessel sealer or vascular stapler.
4. Mobilize lateral attachments of sigmoid, descending colon, and splenic flexure if necessary to create a tension-free anastomosis (may ligate inferior mesenteric vein at level of ligament of Treitz (inferior border of pancreas)) for further mobilization.
5. Thin the rectal mesentery at top of rectum and divide with laparoscopic stapler or with open stapler through Pfannenstiel extraction site if applicable.
6. Identify soft, uninflamed sigmoid colon proximal to area of diverticulitis for area of proximal division and purse-string end-to-end anastomosis (EEA) stapler anvil into bowel edge.
7. Stapled EEA is preferred with leak test using flexible sigmoidoscopy after occluding lumen proximal to anastomosis with saline filled pelvis.
8. Closure of fascia of trocar incisions 10 mm or greater and Pfannenstiel incision.

Potential Pitfalls

- Failure to clearly identify and preserve left ureter when ligating IMA and while freeing inflammatory adhesions of sigmoid colon to pelvic brim.
- Failure to recognize need for splenic flexure mobilization and IMV ligation for a tension-free anastomosis.
- Failure to create a tension-free anastomosis with soft, well-perfused proximal sigmoid colon to uninflamed rectum with negative leak test.

● SPECIAL INTRAOPERATIVE CONSIDERATIONS

The most likely intraoperative finding that could require alteration of the operative plan is unexpectedly intense inflammation with or without accompanying fistula to the genitourinary system. Occasionally, despite a benign clinical course, the surgeon encounters an intense inflammatory process with tethering, if not subclinical fistula formation, of the inflamed sigmoid to the pelvic sidewall or genitourinary system. Inflammation of this nature may require conversion to open surgery or consideration of a colostomy formation or diverting loop ileostomy. Frank pus in the pelvis should trigger the consideration for stoma formation. Typically, a soft proximal sigmoid for anastomosis is easily achievable but intense reactive changes of the top of the rectum may make a healthy distal transection point more obscure. Takedown of a clinical fistula is technically a contaminated case, even without frank pus or feces, and measures to reduce surgical site infection, such as leaving a skin incision open for packing and to heal by secondary intention, may be considered. Careful dissection around the IMA and proximal sigmoid mesentery and pelvic brim must be performed to protect the left ureter.

● POSTOPERATIVE MANAGEMENT

The most common postoperative complications from elective sigmoid colectomy for diverticulitis are surgical site infections. Superficial surgical site infections are managed mainly by opening the incisions to drain pus or infected hematoma with antibiotic therapy reserved for cellulitis not responding to wound opening. Urinary tract infections also occur and uniformly respond to antibiotic therapy.

The most common major surgical complication is anastomotic leak or abdominal–pelvic abscess. Both require a significant convalescence and often reintervention, including laparotomy and Hartmann's procedure in some situations. The impact of leak or abscess on the patients' recovery, quality of life, and risk of occurrence should not be underestimated. Patients with abscess will present approximately 7 days postoperatively with fever, leukocytosis, possible ileus, and possible urinary retention. A spurious diagnosis of urinary tract infection occasionally masks postoperative abscess. Diagnosis is routinely made on CT scan in these patients and rectal contrast is optional, although sometimes helpful, in ruling out anastomotic leak. Treatment is via interventional radiographic drainage and intravenous antibiotics. In some instances, a small leak can present as an abscess and be treated as such. Weeks later when drain removal is being considered, a drain injection study may show communication with the anastomosis. Typically, however, anastomotic leak is accompanied by peritonitis and sepsis. Very few patients will tolerate an anastomotic leak without emergent laparotomy, washout, and diversion. While anastomotic repair with or without proximal diversion is an option, resection of the anastomosis and end colostomy (Hartmann's procedure) is the gold standard. Departure from this approach should be considered carefully as fecal peritonitis from an anastomotic leak carries a significant mortality rate.

TAKE HOME POINTS

- Accurate diagnosis of recurrent uncomplicated sigmoid diverticulitis requires CT confirmation, exclusion of mucosal disease by endoscopy, and the clinical symptoms of left lower quadrant pain, fever, and leukocytosis that respond to antibiotic therapy.
- Recommendation for elective resection of recurrent, uncomplicated sigmoid diverticulitis must be individualized to the patient based on a discussion of risks and benefits with each patient. Recommendations based on patient age and/or number of attacks is no longer valid.
- A laparoscopic approach is preferred with common pitfalls involving safe isolation and ligation of the inferior mesenteric artery, protection of the left ureter, and a leak proof, well-perfused, tension free colorectal anastomosis.
- Postoperative management is largely routine with common complications being infectious. Anastomotic leak and abdominal–pelvic abscess should be discussed with patient preoperatively and managed aggressively due to the significant sequela and mortality associated with fecal peritonitis.

SUGGESTED READINGS

Daniels L, Unlu C, de Wijkerslooth TR, Stockmann HB, Kuipers EJ, Boermeester MA, Dekker E. Yield of colonoscopy after recent CT-proven uncomplicated acute diverticulitis: a comparative cohort study. *Surg Endosc.* 2015;29:2605-2613.

Morris AM, Regenbogen, SE, Hardiman KM, Hendren S. Sigmoid diverticulitis: a systematic review. *JAMA.* 2014;311:287-297.

Pendlimari R, Touzios JG, Azodo IA, Chua HK, Dozois EJ, Cima RR, Larson DW. Short-term outcomes after elective minimally invasive colectomy for diverticulitis. *Br J Surg.* 2011;98:431-435.

Regenbogen SE, Hardiman KM, Hendren S, Morris AM. Surgery for diverticulitis in the 21st century: a systematic review. *JAMA Surg.* 2014;149:292-303.

Ricciardi R, Roberts PL, Marcello PW, Hall JF, Read TE, Schoetz DJ. Anastomotic leak testing after colorectal resection: what are the data? *Arch Surg.* 2009;144:407-411.

Samia H, Lawrence J, Nobel T, Stein S, Champagne BJ, Delaney CP. Extraction site location and incisional hernias after laparoscopic colorectal surgery: should we be avoiding the midline? *Am J Surg.* 2013;205:264-267.

Silva-Velazco J, Stocchi L, Costedio M, Gorgun E, Kessler, H, Remzi, FH. Is there anything we can modify among factors associated with morbidity following elective laparoscopic sigmoidectomy for diverticulitis. *Surg Endosc.* 2016;30:3541-3551.

Thaler K, Baig MK, Berho M, et al. Determinants of recurrence after sigmoid resection for uncomplicated diverticulitis. *Dis Colon Rectum.* 2003;46:385-388.

Ischemic Colitis

47

MUNEERA R. KAPADIA AND ANN C. LOWRY

Based on the previous edition chapter "Ischemic Colitis" by Muneera R. Kapadia and Ann C. Lowry

Presentation

A 75-year-old man with a history of diabetes and hypertension presents with sudden onset of left-sided abdominal pain. He complains of bloody diarrhea for the last few hours and anorexia without nausea or emesis. On examination, he is mildly tachycardic with a low-grade fever, but otherwise his vitals are normal. He is slightly distended and tender in the left lower quadrant of his abdomen but does not have diffuse peritoneal signs. Rectal examination is normal, but his stool is heme positive.

● DIFFERENTIAL DIAGNOSIS

Ischemic colitis should be considered when a patient presents with sudden-onset abdominal pain with associated bloody diarrhea. The most common entities in the differential diagnosis are infectious colitides, inflammatory bowel disease, radiation enteritis, diverticulitis, and malignancy; a more complete list can be found in Table 47-1.

Ischemic colitis typically develops in patients over 65 years but can occur in younger patients as well. Risk factors include cardiac or vascular comorbidities such as diabetes or hypertension. Typical presenting symptoms include crampy abdominal pain of sudden onset followed by bloody diarrhea. Some patients also experience fecal urgency as well as nausea and vomiting secondary to an ileus. The abdominal examination is usually significant for tenderness over the affected area of colon but can include peritoneal signs in more severe cases.

● WORKUP

In the patient presenting above, serum laboratory values reveal a hemoglobin of 14.2 g/dL, a white blood cell count of 15.5, and a lactic acid level of 0.8 mEq/L. A CT scan shows mild descending and sigmoid colonic thickening (Figure 47-1). Endoscopy demonstrates erythematous mucosa with superficial ulcerations in the area of the splenic flexure (Figure 47-2). Stool cultures are negative.

During the workup of ischemic colitis, blood tests and abdominal imaging are frequently obtained, but the findings are often nonspecific. The white blood cell count and the lactate level may be elevated, and metabolic acidosis may be present. Stool cultures and *Clostridium difficile* toxin studies should be obtained to rule out infectious colitides. Abdominal radiographs are generally not helpful unless severe ischemic colitis is present; in that case, plain films may demonstrate free air, pneumatosis, or portal venous gas. CT scans may demonstrate colonic wall thickening but are most useful for excluding other conditions. Barium enema may show the classic

Table 47-1	Differential Diagnosis of Sudden-Onset Abdominal Pain and Bloody Diarrhea

Ischemic colitis
Infectious colitis
Diverticulitis
Radiation enteritis or colitis
Inflammatory bowel disease
Solitary rectal ulcer
Malignancy
Microscopic colitis
Eosinophilic colitis
Neutropenic enterocolitis (Typhlitis)
Drug-induced colitis
Collagen vascular–associated colitis

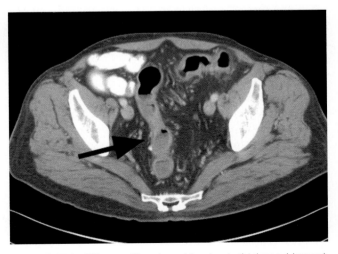

FIGURE 47-1. CT scan: The sigmoid colon is thickened (*arrow*).

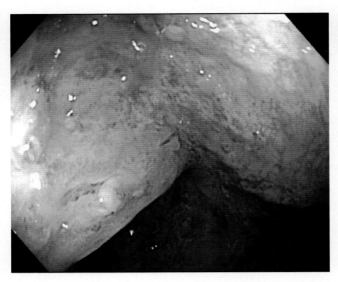

FIGURE 47-2. Endoscopic image of moderate ischemic colitis.

Table 47-2	Causes of Ischemic Colitis
Hypoperfusion	
Sepsis	
Cardiac failure	
Hypovolemia	
Occlusive Disease (Thrombotic or Embolic)	
Hypercoagulable states	
Cardiac embolus	
Small Vessel Disease	
Atherosclerosis	
Vasculitis	
Radiation	
Iatrogenic	
Abdominal aortic aneurysm repair	
Previous colon resection	
Drugs	

sign, "thumbprinting," which represents submucosal hemorrhagic nodules. Colonoscopy with biopsies of the affected area confirms the diagnosis. Angiography is rarely indicated unless acute small intestinal mesenteric ischemia is suspected.

The diagnostic test of choice is an unprepped colonoscopy unless there is evidence of peritonitis on examination. It allows for direct visualization of mucosal changes, and biopsies can be obtained. Ischemic colon can be fragile, and colonoscopy should be performed with care to avoid overdistension of the colon. The distribution of findings depends on the vascular insult sustained, and the mucosal changes can be variable. In mild to moderate ischemic colitis, the mucosa may appear erythematous and edematous with petechiae. Additionally, ulcerations and hemorrhagic nodules, which represent submucosal bleeding, may be seen. In severe ischemic colitis, the mucosa may appear gray or black, indicating transmural infarction. If this is encountered, the colonoscopy should be terminated due to significant risk of perforation. If peritonitis is present on physical examination, a colonoscopy should be avoided and laparotomy should be performed.

● DISCUSSION

Etiologic factors are numerous (Table 47-2); however, in most cases, a specific cause cannot be identified. Frequently the predisposing event, such as an episode of acute illness, has resolved by the time the patient presents.

Ischemic colitis can be divided into two categories: nongangrenous and gangrenous. Accounting for approximately 80% to 85% of cases, the nongangrenous type can be further subdivided into transient and chronic forms. Transient ischemic colitis involves the mucosa and submucosa and typically resolves in 1 to 2 weeks. The chronic nongangrenous form is characterized by injury to the deeper layers of the colonic wall. Healing may result in colonic fibrosis

and development of a stricture. The gangrenous form with acute severe transmural injury results in perforation and/or sepsis and requires surgical resection of the compromised colon.

Typically segmental, ischemic colitis may involve any area of the colon and rectum. The splenic flexure, descending colon, and sigmoid colon are most commonly affected, which can be explained by the vascular anatomy. The blood supply to the colon and rectum occurs through the superior mesenteric artery, the inferior mesenteric artery, and the superior hemorrhoidal artery. Watershed areas, regions dependent upon collaterals between the inferior and the superior mesenteric arteries (e.g., the splenic flexure and the descending colon), are especially susceptible to ischemic injury in low-flow states (Figure 47-3).

● DIAGNOSIS AND TREATMENT

Once the diagnosis is established, the treatment varies depending on the etiology and the severity of disease. Most patients can be managed expectantly with intravenous fluids, bowel rest, and broad-spectrum antibiotics. Restoration of adequate intravascular volume is important. If symptomatic ileus is present, the patient may benefit from nasogastric decompression. Additionally, any specific causal agent should be addressed. If a patient has peritonitis or evidence of perforation or deteriorates clinically with conservative medical management, laparotomy is warranted. Patients with right-sided ischemic colitis or ischemic colitis without hematochezia have been shown to need surgery more frequently and have worse outcomes. Additionally, if a patient develops a stricture or chronic colitis following ischemic colitis, colonic resection may be indicated.

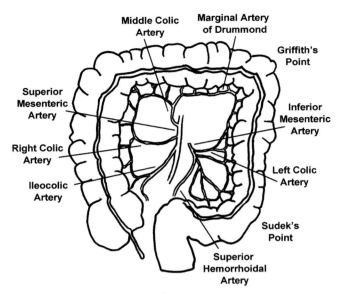

FIGURE 47-3. Colonic bloody supply is derived from the superior mesenteric (SMA), inferior mesenteric (IMA), and superior hemorrhoidal (SHA) arteries. "Watershed" areas lie between two of the arteries and are susceptible to ischemia. Griffith's point is located at the splenic flexure, between the SMA and IMA. Sudek's point is located at the rectosigmoid junction, between the IMA and SHA. While these two points are particularly susceptible to ischemia, any portion of the colon and rectum can be affected by ischemic colitis.

● SURGICAL APPROACH

In our clinical scenario above, after 48 hours of medical management, the patient becomes acutely febrile and tachycardic. On examination, his abdomen is diffusely tender. Given the patient's clinical decline, emergent laparotomy is undertaken.

When operative intervention is warranted, a laparotomy should be performed through a midline incision. The abdomen is explored, and the compromised segment of colon is identified. The extent of ischemic colon can usually be easily assessed by a visual inspection. If there is doubt, the combination of intraoperative colonoscopy, palpation, Doppler assessment of the colonic vessels, and intravenous fluorescein can be helpful. Once the involved region is determined, all nonviable colon should be resected. There should be brisk bleeding at the resection margins. If the remaining bowel appears viable and healthy and the patient is stable, it is reasonable to perform a primary anastomosis. If the patient is hypotensive or there is significant surrounding inflammation, a primary anastomosis should be avoided and instead an end stoma created. If there is a question about bowel viability, the resected colonic ends should be brought out as a stoma and mucous fistula. In an unstable patient, the ends may be stapled and left discontinuous, and a second-look laparotomy should be performed after 24 to 48 hours (Table 47-3).

Table 47-3	Operative Management of Ischemic Colitis

Key Technical Steps

1. Midline abdominal incision.
2. Determine extent of gangrenous colon.
3. Mobilize and resect nonviable colon.
4. Check for brisk bleeding at the resection margins.
5. Creation of anastomosis or stoma depending on patient and bowel status.
6. Close abdomen.

Potential Pitfalls

- Inadequate resection leaving nonviable bowel.
- Anastomosis should be avoided in hemodynamically unstable patients.

● SPECIAL CIRCUMSTANCE

Ischemic Colitis Following Aortic Surgery

Ischemic colitis is a well-described complication of aortic surgery. The overall incidence is about 2%; however, among patients requiring emergency surgery for ruptured aortic aneurysms the incidence is significantly higher. The underlying etiology is usually related to disruption of the inferior mesenteric artery, but additional contributory factors can include prolonged cross-clamping of the aorta and hemodynamic instability. Reimplantation of the inferior mesenteric artery may be necessary to prevent ischemic colitis if the superior mesenteric artery is stenotic and collateral bloody supply is inadequate to support the left colon. Symptoms of ischemic colitis develop in the first few days after aortic surgery and can include pain, fever, distension, and diarrhea. Diagnosis and treatment should proceed as previously discussed. If colonic resection is deemed necessary, a primary anastomosis should be avoided as an anastomotic leak risks graft contamination.

● POSTOPERATIVE MANAGEMENT

Depending on postoperative hemodynamic stability, patients may require a stay in the intensive care unit with close monitoring of urine output and volume status. A nasogastric tube is unnecessary unless the patient suffers a significant ileus. Dietary advancement should be as tolerated. If a primary anastomosis is created, patients should be monitored for evidence of an anastomotic leak. Return of bowel function should occur prior to discharge. If colonic diversion is deemed necessary at the initial operation, stoma takedown can be considered at 3 to 6 months following the initial operation, depending on the patient's overall health status.

TAKE HOME POINTS

- Sudden-onset abdominal pain followed by bloody diarrhea should prompt suspicion of ischemic colitis.
- Colonoscopy is the test of choice for diagnosis of ischemic colitis.
- Ischemic colitis most commonly involves the splenic flexure and descending and sigmoid colon.
- Most patients can be treated effectively with hydration, bowel rest, and broad-spectrum antibiotics.
- Peritonitis, evidence of perforation, or clinical deterioration should prompt immediate surgical intervention.
- Operative management should include resection of compromised colon, followed by either primary anastomosis or creation of a stoma depending on the overall status of the patient.

SUGGESTED READINGS

Brandt LJ, Boley SJ. Colonic ischemia. *Surg Clin North Am.* 1992;72:203-229.

Brandt LJ, Feuerstadt P, Blaszka MC. Anatomic patterns, patient characteristics, and clinical outcomes in ischemic colitis: a study of 313 cases supported by histology. *Am J Gastroenterol.* 2010;105: 2245-2252; quiz 53.

Montoro MA, Brandt LJ, Santolaria S, et al. Clinical patterns and outcomes of ischaemic colitis: results of the Working Group for the Study of Ischaemic Colitis in Spain (CIE study). *Scand J Gastroenterol.* 2011;46(2):236-246.

Mosele M, Cardin F, Inelmen EM, et al. Ischemic colitis in the elderly: predictors of the disease and prognostic factors to negative outcome. *Scand J Gastroenterol.* 2010;45:428-433.

Paterno F, McGillicuddy EA, Schuster KM, et al. Ischemic colitis: risk factors for eventual surgery. *Am J Surg.* 2010;200: 646-650.

Perry RJ, Martin MJ, Eckert MJ, et al. Colonic ischemia complicating open vs endovascular abdominal aortic aneurysm repair. *J Vasc Surg.* 2008;48:272-277.

Scowcroft CW, Sanowski RA, Kozarek RA. Colonoscopy in ischemic colitis. *Gastrointest Endosc.* 1981;27:156-161.

Steele SR. Ischemic colitis complicating major vascular surgery. *Surg Clin North Am.* 2007;87:1099-1114, ix.

Sun MY, Maykel JA. Ischemic colitis. *Clin Colon Rectal Surg.* 2007;20:5-12.

Sun D, Wang C, Yang L, Liu M, Chen F. The predictors of the severity of ischaemic colitis: a systematic review of 2823 patients from 22 studies. *Colorectal Dis.* 2016;10:949-958.

West BR, Ray JE, Gathright JB. Comparison of transient ischemic colitis with that requiring surgical treatment. *Surg Gynecol Obstet.* 1980;151:366-368.

Medically Refractory Ulcerative Colitis

48

ARIELLE E. KANTERS AND SAMANTHA HENDREN

Based on the previous edition chapter "Medically Refractory Ulcerative Colitis" by Samantha Hendren

Presentation

A 28-year-old man with a history of ulcerative colitis (UC) diagnosed 13 months ago presents to the emergency department with bloody diarrhea and abdominal pain. His symptoms worsened 2 weeks ago, and his outpatient gastroenterologist started him on Prednisone 40 mg daily, in addition to his usual medications, Pentasa and Azathioprine. He is now having about 12 to 15 bloody BM's every 24 hours. This is his third hospital admission since diagnosis, the most recent 3 months ago. Laboratory testing reveals hemoglobin of 9.8 g/dL, erythrocyte sedimentation rate (Westergren) of 43 mm/h, C-reactive protein of 12.06 mg/dL, and albumin of 2.8 g/dL.

● DIFFERENTIAL DIAGNOSIS

This patient presents with an exacerbation of UC, superimposed on a relatively aggressive disease course since diagnosis. While medically refractory disease is the most likely diagnosis, it is important to remember that superimposed infectious colitis including *Clostridium difficile* colitis affects up to 30% of UC patients presenting with acute exacerbations of their disease. As such, ruling out superimposed infection and optimizing medical therapy is an essential step prior to proceeding with surgical therapy. A misconception among surgeons is that surgical therapy is inevitable for severe UC. On the contrary, with improvements in biologic therapies, recent cohort analysis has shown colectomy rates as low as 10% in the first 5 years of UC diagnosis. Long term, about 15% to 30% of all UC patients undergo colectomy.

The consulting surgeon has a responsibility to recognize the severity of the colitis when considering emergent surgical intervention and offer immediate surgical treatment for toxic megacolon (Figure 48-1). This is characterized by the following signs and symptoms: abdominal distention, tenderness, fever, leukocytosis, more than 10 bowel movements per day, continuous bleeding, transfusion requirement, hypoalbuminemia, radiologic evidence of colonic wall thickening, and possible dilatation (not always present). Diagnosis of severe colitis is based on the Truelove and Witts criteria and is defined as ≥6 bloody stools per day and one or more of the following: temperature >37.5°C, pulse >90, Hgb <10.5, or ESR>30.

● WORKUP

The patient is admitted to the medicine service, and the gastroenterologists perform a computed tomography scan (CT scan) and a colonoscopy. The colonoscopy reveals pancolitis with ulcerations, granularity, and distorted vascular pattern.

Stool samples were sent for *Clostridium difficile* toxin and antigen, and biopsies for cytomegalovirus infection were obtained at colonoscopy; these were both negative. The patient was offered treatment with the anti-TNF agent, infliximab, and surgery was also consulted to introduce the principles of surgical treatment to the patient. He did not have signs or symptoms of toxic megacolon.

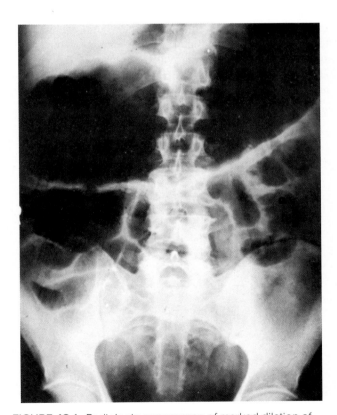

FIGURE 48-1. Radiologic appearance of marked dilation of transverse colon (toxic megacolon). (Reprinted with permission from Corman M, Nicholls RJ, Fazio VW, Bergamaschi R. *Corman's Colon and Rectal Surgery*. 6th ed. Philadelphia, PA: Lippincott Williams & Wilkins, a Wolters Kluwer Business: 2013.)

As the surgical consultant, important features of the history and physical examination include the following: reviewing documentation of all prior colonoscopy, pathology and radiologic testing to insure there is no evidence of Crohn's disease (such as small bowel disease), or dysplasia/malignancy that might alter the surgical approach. It is also essential to ask about any history of anorectal surgery or abscess–fistula disease, assessing continence (keeping in mind that some fecal incontinence during a severe flare is common), and quality of life related to disease activity and medical therapy. A patient who is unable to work due to frequent disease flares or toxic effects of medical treatments should be considered for surgery. Physical exam for signs of toxic colitis and for anal sphincter integrity and signs of any current or prior abscess-fistula disease are also essential.

● DIAGNOSIS AND TREATMENT

Based on the workup, this patient has medically refractory UC. The principles of treatment include consideration of salvage medical therapy versus surgical treatment. The decision-making between these two options should include a multidisciplinary approach, and the patient should always be introduced to the option of surgery at this point. The patient elected to proceed with infliximab treatment and was discharged after an improvement but not resolution of his symptoms on infliximab and high-dose steroids. Unfortunately, his symptoms persisted at home, with bloody bowel movements, abdominal pain, and malaise. His gastroenterologist calls you and asks you to consider surgical treatment at this point.

● SURGICAL APPROACH

The goal of surgery for UC is removal of the entire colon and rectum, which can be immediately performed, or performed in a staged fashion. Both a total proctocolectomy with end ileostomy and reconstructive surgery with a pelvic pouch provide good quality of life, but most patients prefer reconstructive surgery to avoid a permanent ostomy. Since the 1980's, the most popular operation for medically refractory UC has been the ileal pouch anal anastomosis operation (IPAA, also called restorative proctocolectomy), usually with a J-pouch. This operation is associated with high but acceptable complication rates, good quality of life, and an overall success rate of about 90% long-term (Figure 48-2).

A frank discussion with the patient is required, regarding postoperative expectations and possible complications. Important points include expected bowel function, pouchitis, pouch failure, infertility in women, or late discovery of Cohn's disease.

Bowel Function: Patients must be advised that frequent bowel movements are not a complication following IPAA, but rather the expected functional outcome. Reasonable function includes 5 to 7 loose bowel movements per day and one per night, along with possible nighttime leakage. Long-term incontinence has been reported at about 20%.

Pouchitis: This is the most common late complication following IPAA. In a recent study by Cleveland Clinic, 34% of patients were affected by pouchitis, and 16% went on to develop chronic pouchitis, which was defined as 3 attacks per year.

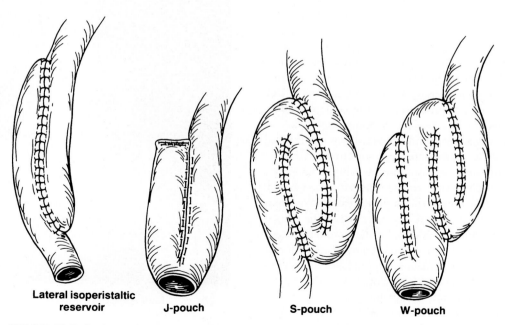

Lateral isoperistaltic reservoir   **J-pouch**   **S-pouch**   **W-pouch**

FIGURE 48-2. Ileal pouch configurations.

Pouch Failure: In experienced centers, pouch failure rates are as low as 5% to 10% and is often due to septic complications, chronic pouchitis, or other infectious processes such as fistula formation. Patients with pouch failure are typically treated with pouch excision and permanent end ileostomy.

Infertility in Women: There is an increased risk of infertility in women after IPAA. Studies have shown that it is about 10% above the average population (25% to 35%), though some report rates as high as 50%. IVF can be effective in these situations.

Late Diagnosis of Crohn's Disease: Evidence of Crohn's disease can occasionally be discovered at the time of surgery. With the exception of highly selected Crohn's colitis patients, small bowel or anal Crohn's disease is a contraindication to IPAA. Instead ileorectal anastomosis or ileostomy should be performed if discovered intraoperatively.

The decision of whether to perform UC surgery in 1-stage, 2-stages, or 3-stages is influenced by several factors: patient presentation, medications, nutritional status, comorbidities, and technical issues encountered at the time of surgery (such as the degree of tension on the pouch-anal anastomosis). For the patient in this scenario, a 2- or 3-stage approach beginning with a subtotal colectomy is probably the safest option, given recent administration of infliximab, malnutrition, and steroids—all of which may increase anastomotic leak rate if IPAA is performed immediately. Historically, anti-TNF agents and high-dose steroids have been associated with higher complication rates, such as anastomotic leak. However, some recent studies demonstrated no difference in complications in patients undergoing proctocolectomy with pouch construction when receiving anti-TNF agents, steroids, or in the urgent setting. Rather, surgeon experience was associated with perioperative complications. These data remain controversial but suggests that IPAA with diverting ileostomy may be appropriate in the acute setting, when performed by a high-volume IBD surgeon.

A subtotal colectomy for UC can be performed laparoscopically or open. The key technical features include preoperative marking of the ileostomy site with the patient sitting and supine (avoiding folds and scars), and avoiding pelvic dissection to maintain the virgin tissue planes for the next stage of surgery. For severe colitis in which rectal stump leak is a concern, consider a mucus fistula of the Hartmann's pouch, suturing the pouch to the abdominal wound so a leak can drain via the wound. In our practice we often staple, then oversew the rectal stump, as well as irrigate the rectal stump clear of all stool, leaving a large malincot drain in the rectum (transanal) overnight. Anecdotally, we have noted an increase in rectal stump leak in recent years, with devastating infection in some cases.

The steps of the routine IPAA procedure are outlined in Table 48-1. These include resection of the entire or remaining colon and rectum, mobilization of the small bowel and its mesentery, creation of a 15- to 20-cm long J-pouch, suturing or stapling the pouch to the anus, and performing a diverting loop ileostomy in most cases. In the case of a double-stapled

Table 48-1	Ileal Pouch Anal Anastomosis (IPAA)

Key Technical Steps

1. Patient is placed in the modified lithotomy position with access to the anus
2. Perform total proctocolectomy or completion proctectomy, dividing the mesentery near the bowel, unless cancer is a concern
3. Staple and divide the terminal ileum, preserving the ileocolic artery initially
4. For double-stapled technique, use a TA-30 or other suitable stapler to staple the anorectal junction at the level of the levator muscles
5. Mobilize the small bowel and its mesentery, including full lysis of adhesions and separation of the superior mesenteric artery pedicle from the duodenum
6. If reach is insufficient, perform lengthening procedures including divide peritoneum, selective vascular ligation, and or consideration of alternate pouch shape
7. Create a 15- to 20-cm long J-pouch by stapling the distal two limbs of ileum together with GIA stapler and inserting anvil of EEA stapler, if double-stapled technique planned
8. Perform stapled or hand-sewn anastomosis, with mucosectomy if hand-sutured technique chosen
9. Perform diverting loop ileostomy

Potential Pitfalls

- Injury to the small bowel mesentery during maneuvers to create length
- Failure to separate the anal cuff from the vagina/prostate can result in fistula

technique, the rectum is stapled and divided at the level of the levator ani muscles and then the pouch is stapled to the anal canal using the EEA stapler. In the case of the hand-sewn pouch-anal anastomosis, the distal rectum is divided, the mucosa above the dentate line is stripped transanally, and the pouch is pulled through the rectal cuff and hand sutured at the dentate line (Figure 48-3).

● SPECIAL INTRAOPERATIVE CONSIDERATIONS

The key intraoperative problem for which the surgeon must be prepared is the possibility that an ileal J-pouch will not reach to the anal canal for anastomosis. This is a particular problem for tall or obese male patients. In these cases, maneuvers to create length must be performed, including division of peritoneum overlying the mesentery and selective ligation of the mesenteric vessels with transillumination to ensure there are collateral pathways for blood flow to the entire small bowel. Usually, ileocolic artery ligation will result in sufficient length, but if not consider temporary occlusion

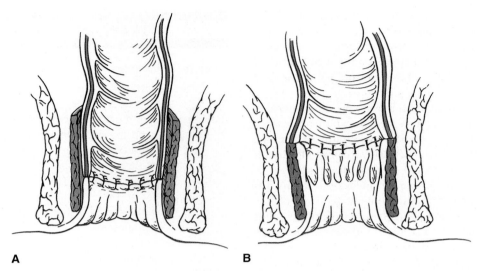

A   **B**

FIGURE 48-3. Ileal pouch-anal anastomosis. **A:** Sutured anastomosis at dentate line after mucosectomy. **B:** Double-stapled anastomosis. There is a residual 1- to 2-cm cuff of rectal mucosa.

of vessels (e.g., with a bulldog clamp) prior to selective ligation. If reach is still a problem, an S-shaped or W-shaped pouch may be considered, as these may reach better depending on the individual's mesenteric vascular anatomy.

● POSTOPERATIVE MANAGEMENT

Complications are common after IPAA. The ACS-NSQIP database shows that 24% of patients had major complications and 17% had minor complications within 30 days after IPAA, most commonly superficial and organ space surgical site infections. The most feared early complication is anastomotic leak, for which management depends on the severity of presentation and whether or not ileostomy was performed at the original operation. Some combination of broad-spectrum antibiotics, percutaneous drainage, diverting ileostomy, and open washout may be required depending on the situation. While there is controversy about the value of diverting ileostomy with IPAA, most procedures are performed with diversion due to concern for increased risk of pelvic sepsis without diversion, and possible poor functional outcome after pelvic sepsis. Long-term septic complications include anastomotic strictures and fistulas. Finally, endoscopic follow-up for dysplasia of the pouch-anal anastomosis is usually recommended beginning 8 to 10 years after onset of UC.

TAKE HOME POINTS

- Surgical treatment should be considered for medically refractory ulcerative colitis (UC), and decision-making is multidisciplinary.
- Prior to surgery, medical treatment should be optimized, including ruling-out superimposed infectious colitis.
- Evaluate for signs and symptoms of toxic colitis and Crohn's disease.

- Consider a 3-stage approach with initial subtotal colectomy for ill patients.
- Ileal pouch anal anastomosis is the most common surgical treatment for UC.
- Be prepared with lengthening procedures and alternative pouch configurations for cases in which the pouch will not reach the anus.
- Diverting ileostomy is usually performed.
- Complications are common after IPAA, but 90% long-term success rates

SUGGESTED READINGS

Andersson T, et al. Long-term functional outcome and quality of life after restorative proctocolectomy with ileo-anal anastomosis for colitis. *Colorectal Dis.* 2011;13:431-437.

Aratari A, et al. Colectomy rate in acute severe ulcerative colitis in the infliximab era. *Dig Liver Dis.* 2008;40(10):821-826.

Berndtsson I, et al. Long-term outcome after ileal pouch-anal anastomosis: function and health-related quality of life. *Dis Colon Rectum.* 2007;50(10):1545-1552.

Bret A, Lashner M, Aaron Brzezinski M. *Medical Treatment of Ulcerative Colitis and Other Colitides, in Current Therapy in Colon and Rectal Surgery,* 2nd ed. M. Victor W. Fazio, MS, MD (Hon), FRACS, FRACS (Hon), FACS, FRCS, FRCS (Ed), M. James M. Church, M Med Sci, FRACS, and M. Conor P. Delaney, MCh, PhD, FRSCI (Gen), FACS, Editors. Philadelphia: Elsevier Mosby; 2005.

Cottone M, et al. Clinical course of ulcerative colitis. *Dig Liver Dis.* 2008;40(suppl 2):S247-S252.

Devaraj B, Kaiser AM. Surgical management of ulcerative colitis in the era of biologicals. *Inflamm Bowel Dis.* 2015;21(1):208-220.

Dayan B, Turner D. Role of surgery in severe ulcerative colitis in the era of medical rescue therapy. *World J Gastroenterol.* 2012;18(29):3833-3838.

Farouk R, et al., Incidence and subsequent impact of pelvic abscess after ileal pouch-anal anastomosis for chronic ulcerative colitis. *Dis Colon Rectum.* 1998;41(10):1239-1243.

Fazio VW, et al. Long-term functional outcome and quality of life after stapled restorative proctocolectomy. *Ann Surg.* 1999;230(4):575-584; discussion 584-586.

Fleming FJ, et al. A laparoscopic approach does reduce short-term complications in patients undergoing ileal pouch-anal anastomosis. *Dis Colon Rectum.* 2011;54(2):176-182.

Hahnloser D, et al. Results at up to 20 years after ileal pouch-anal anastomosis for chronic ulcerative colitis. *Br J Surg.* 2007;94(3):333-340.

Hicks CW, Hodin RA, Bordeianou L. Possible overuse of 3-stage procedures for active ulcerative colitis. *JAMA Surg.* 2013;148(7):658-664.

McMurrick PJ., M.h., FRACS and M. R.R. Dozois, MS, FACS, FRCS(Glas) (Hon), DSC, Chronic Ulcerative Colitis: Surgical Options, in Current Therapy in Colon and Rectal Surgery, 2nd Edition, M. Victor W. Fazio, MS, MD (Hon), FRACS, FRACS (Hon), FACS, FRCS, FRCS (Ed), M. James M. Church, M Med Sci, FRACS, and M. Conor P. Delaney, MCh, PhD, FRSCI (Gen), FACS, Editors. 2005: Philadelphia.

Michelassi F, et al. Long-term functional results after ileal pouch anal restorative proctocolectomy for ulcerative colitis: a prospective observational study. *Ann Surg.* 2003;238(3):433-441; discussion 442-445.

Peyrin-Biroulet L, et al. Systematic review: outcomes and post-operative complications following colectomy for ulcerative colitis. *Aliment Pharmacol Ther.* 2016;44:807-816.

Ricciardi R, et al. Epidemiology of *Clostridium difficile* colitis in hospitalized patients with inflammatory bowel diseases. *Dis Colon Rectum.* 2009;52(1):40-45.

Ross H, et al. Practice parameters for the surgical treatment of ulcerative colitis. *Dis Colon Rectum.* 2014;57(1):5-22.

Tjandra JJ, et al. Omission of temporary diversion in restorative proctocolectomy-is it safe? *Dis Colon Rectum.* 1993;36(11):1007-1014.

Truelove SC, Witts LJ. Cortisone in ulcerative colitis; preliminary report on a therapeutic trial. *Br Med J.* 1954;2(4884):375-378.

Waljee A, et al., Threefold increased risk of infertility: a meta-analysis of infertility after ileal pouch anal anastomosis in ulcerative colitis. *Gut.* 2006;55(11):1575-1580.

Williet N, et al. Incidence of and impact of medications on colectomy in newly diagnosed ulcerative colitis in the era of biologics. *Inflamm Bowel Dis.* 2012;18(9):1641-1646.

Crohn's Disease with Small Bowel Stricture

49

YERANUI LEDESMA AND EMILY FINLAYSON

Based on the previous edition chapter "Crohn's Disease with Small Bowel Stricture" by Hueylan Chern and Emily Finlayson

Presentation

A 19-year-old otherwise healthy woman presents with abdominal pain and diarrhea. The abdominal pain is described as sharp and constant in the right lower quadrant. She denies melena or bloody diarrhea. She reports postprandial nausea and bloating without emesis. She denies recent travel history, and her family history is unremarkable. Her menstrual cycle has been regular. On abdominal examination, her right lower quadrant is tender to palpation.

● DIFFERENTIAL DIAGNOSIS

Differential diagnoses for right lower quadrant abdominal pain include irritable bowel syndrome, appendicitis, inflammatory bowel disease, Meckel's diverticulum, urinary tract infection, and infectious enterocolitis. *Campylobacter* and *Yersinia* infection from poor handling of food can affect the ileocolic region and mimic Crohn's ileocolic disease. In women, gynecologic causes such as ovarian torsion, tubal ovarian abscess, pelvic inflammatory disease, and ectopic pregnancy need to be considered as well.

● WORKUP

The patient undergoes computed tomography (CT) scan of the abdomen and pelvis with IV and oral contrast that reveals an inflamed, narrowed segment of terminal ileum (Figure 49-1). Serum laboratory values include hemoglobin of 11 g/dL, an albumin level of 3.3 g/dL, and a C-reactive protein level of 86 g/dL.

● DISCUSSION

Crohn's disease (CD) is a chronic inflammatory intestinal disease that can be unremitting and is incurable. It can affect any part of the gastrointestinal tract. The distribution is usually discontinuous with segments of uninvolved intestine. The inflammation in CD is transmural involving the full thickness of the bowel wall from the mucosa to serosa.

The etiology for CD remains uncertain. CD has a bimodal age distribution with the first peak occurring between the ages of 15 and 30 years and the second between 60 and 80 years. The most common anatomic pattern in patients with CD is ileocolic disease occurring in 40%, followed by small intestinal disease, isolated colonic disease, and gastroduodenal disease. The disease behavior is classified into three categories: inflammatory, stricturing, and fistulizing. However, the anatomic distribution and behavior can change in any given Crohn's patient over time.

The keys to evaluation of CD are determining extent and location of involved intestines and obtaining tissue for diagnosis. Several imaging modalities such as contrast studies, CT, and magnetic resonance imaging (MRI) have been used to evaluate CD. In the acute setting, CT of the abdomen and pelvic with contrast is a good choice to look for acute complication such as abscess, obstruction, or perforation and also to eliminate other causes for acute abdomen. CT is also helpful in looking for thickened intestine, stricture, adjacent organ involvement, fistulas, phlegmon, and abscess (Figure 49-2A). CD complicated by enterovesical or colovesical fistulas will present with air or oral contrast within the bladder (Figure 49-2B).

CT enterography, MRI enterography, and capsule endoscopy are other modalities used to diagnose proximal small bowel disease. MRI enterography has recently gained

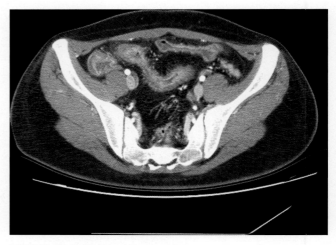

FIGURE 49-1. Terminal ileum stricture.

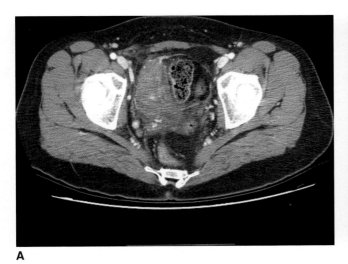 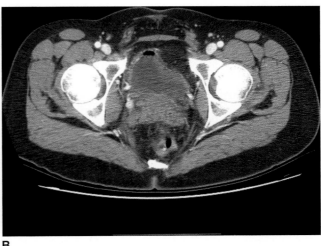

A   **B**

FIGURE 49-2. A: Right lower quadrant phlegmon. **B:** Air in the bladder indicating fistula to the gastrointestinal tract.

popularity because it avoids radiation exposure in a typically young patient requiring imaging over lifetime for follow-up or diagnosis. Furthermore, unlike contrast studies, it has the ability to demonstrate both extraluminal and intraluminal pathology.

Endoscopy is critical in workup, surveillance, and management of CD. Both colonoscopy and esophagogastroduodenoscopy are essential for demonstrating mucosal inflammation and obtaining tissue for diagnosis. The terminal ileum should be intubated and examined whenever possible during colonoscopy. The classic endoscopic findings for Crohn's include aphthous ulcers, patchy erythema, linear serpiginous ulcers, deep "bear claw" ulceration, and strictures. However, the risk of perforation from colonoscopy in acute inflammation is high. Therefore, colonoscopy is generally avoided in an acute setting. A limited endoscopy such as flexible sigmoidoscopy can be considered if results will alter management in the acute setting.

● DIAGNOSIS AND TREATMENT

Medical Therapy

In this patient with newly diagnosed CD and a stricture that is likely inflammatory in nature, medical therapy is the most appropriate initial approach. Very few patients will require surgery at initial disease presentation. Patients presenting with obstructive symptoms can be managed with bowel rest and nasogastric tube. The fact that this patient has an elevated C-reactive protein level suggests that her stricture is most likely inflammatory in nature (not fibrostenotic). Intravenous steroid can be used to treat the acute inflammation. Patients presenting with an associated intra-abdominal abscess can undergo percutaneous drainage. Surgery if indicated for persistent symptoms can then be delayed and performed in an elective setting when inflammation is not as severe and overall condition more stable. The goal of staged

resection is to avoid bleeding associated with acute inflammation and to preserve bowel length.

For medical treatment, there are two treatment phases, the induction phase followed by maintenance of remission.

Mild to Moderate Crohn's: Induction

The first-line induction treatment for mild to moderate ileocolonic CD is budesonide, a glucocorticoid. It is typically initiated at 9 mg daily followed by a taper. Once patient is successfully off budesonide, maintenance therapy can be initiated. If tapering of budesonide is difficult, escalation of treatment with a thiopurine or biologic medication should be started.

Alternative agents for induction include oral glucocorticoids and 5-aminosalicylates (5-ASA). Prednisone 40 mg per day for 7 days, followed by gradual tapering by 5 to 10 mg per week is the typical dose that has proven to have good response. Mesalamine tablets, such as Pentasa or Asacol, are the only 5-ASA agents known to be useful in ileal CD. This class can be used in patients who prefer to avoid steroids or where steroids are contraindicated.

Mild to Moderate Crohn's: Remission

For patients who achieved remission with either budesonide or prednisone, it is recommended to taper the drug off completely and follow the patient both clinically and endoscopically. Colonoscopy with evaluation of the terminal ileum should be performed at 6 and 12 months after remission. 5-ASA agents used for induction should be continued for long-term maintenance with similar endoscopic evaluations

Moderate to Severe Disease

Patients who cannot be weaned off budesonide or prednisone, who do not respond to treatment above, or have repeated relapse should be considered to have moderate to severe disease. The treatment options for this group include immunomodulators (i.e., azathioprine, 6-mercaptopurine) and biologic therapies (anti–tumor necrosis factor [TNF], monoclonal antibodies).

Surgical Therapy

If this patient has persistent pain and obstructive symptoms despite medical therapy, surgical resection is indicated. In general, surgical therapy is reserved for failed medical therapy or an acute, severe complication of CD (Table 49-1). Because CD is not curable, operative intervention is only intended to address complication and alleviate symptoms to improve quality of life.

The most common indication for operation is obstruction from stricture. Several options exist including resection with or without anastomosis, strictureplasty, and bypass. What operation to perform depends on factors such as nutritional status, number of prior bowel resections, the length and number of strictures, surrounding inflammation, and immunosuppression status. Resection, strictureplasty, and bypass techniques may be used in one operation to treat multiple strictures. In this patients with a long, isolated segment of strictured terminal ileum, ileocolic resection is the recommended option.

Surgical Approach for Ileocolic Crohn's Disease

Laparoscopic resection by experienced surgeons can be done safely in inflammatory bowel disease (Table 49-2). Preoperative imaging is essential to assess the entire gastrointestinal tract. If performed laparoscopically, one camera port and three working ports are typically necessary (Figure 49-3). The entire small bowel is examined to assess the full extent of disease. Nondiseased intestines may be drawn into the inflammatory process, and they should be freed and preserved. A medial to lateral approach can sometimes be difficult in ileocolic Crohn's because of associated inflammation, phlegmon, or abscess. However, if the duodenum can be identified and the ileocolic vessels can be appreciated, scoring underneath the ileocolic

Table 49-2	Ileocolic Resection

Key Technical Steps
1. Laparoscopic port placement (Figure 49-3).
2. Visual evaluation of entire small bowel.
3. Lateral to medial or medial to lateral mobilization of the ascending colon and mesentery.
4. Identification of the duodenum.
5. Ligation and division of the ileocolic vessels.
6. Division of the bowel proximal and distal to grossly diseased intestines.
7. Anastomosis of the ileum to the ascending colon.

Potential Pitfalls
- Bleeding from inflamed mesentery.
- Injury to the duodenum.
- Injury to the ureter.

vessels may allow entry into the avascular plane between the mesentery and the retroperitoneum. If not, a lateral to medial dissection can be started by dividing along the line of Toldt. The terminal ileum, the right colon, and the hepatic flexure need to completely mobilized. Once the ileocolic vessels are ligated and divided, grossly abnormal bowel is resected. The bowel is divided and an anastomosis is constructed ensuring correct orientation, without tension, and with good blood supply. The anastomosis can be performed with stapled technique, hand-sewn technique in a side-to-side or an end-to-end fashion. The abdomen cavity is washed out and the fascia closed.

Table 49-1	Indications for Surgery

- Medically refractory disease
- Medication-related complication
- Massive hemorrhage
- Free perforation
- Acute obstruction
- Neoplasia
- Abscess not amenable to percutaneous drainage
- Symptomatic fistula

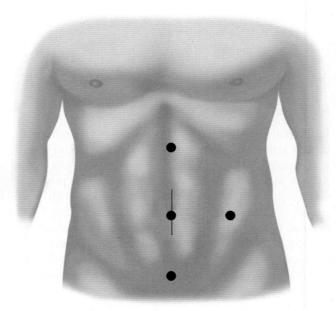

FIGURE 49-3. Common port placement for a laparoscopic ileocolic resection.

Intraoperative Considerations

When operating for CD, caution should be exercised in dividing the mesentery. Mesentery in CD is typically thickened with fat deposit and lymphadenopathy making division difficult. Rapid spread of mesenteric hematoma can result in further loss of intestinal length. Nondiseased intestine can also be drawn into the diseased process and involved in fistula formation or inflammatory adhesion. Care should be taken to preserve all normal intestines. Primary closure of the fistula after wedge resection in the unaffected intestine is usually sufficient. Wider margins do not decrease postoperative recurrence, and it is not necessary to achieve microscopic negative margins. Therefore, to preserve bowel length, the margins can be determined by resection to macroscopically normal intestine.

Risk of Recurrence, Postop Surveillance, and Treatment

After resection, endoscopic recurrence can be as high as 80% at 1 year. Twenty percent of the patients may experience clinical relapse at 1 year. The risk of developing disease complications requiring surgery approaches 50% at 10 years. Aminosalicylates, antibiotics, and thiopurines are only modestly effective in preventing disease recurrence. The anti-TNF agent has been shown to be most effective in preventing recurrence and therefore should be considered in patients at high risk for recurrence. Smoking is a well-known independent risk factor for recurrence. Therefore, smoking cessation is encouraged.

Case Conclusion

A CT of the abdomen and pelvis was done and showed inflamed terminal ileum. She, however, continued to have significant obstructive symptoms on maximal medical treatment and eventually required a laparoscopic ileocolic resection.

TAKE HOME POINTS

- Crohn's disease (CD) is a chronic inflammatory panintestinal disease that relies on medical treatment and surgery is not curable.
- Emergent surgery is rarely necessary because acute complication such as obstruction and abscess can often be managed nonoperatively.
- Preservation of healthy bowel is essential when operating on patients with CD.
- Surgery is intended to address complications and alleviate symptoms to improve quality of life.

SUGGESTED READINGS

Gomollón F, Dignass A, Annese V, et al. ECCO. 3rd European evidence-based consensus on the diagnosis and management of Crohn's disease 2016: part 1: diagnosis and medical management. *J Crohns Colitis.* 2017;11(1):3-25.

Strong SA, Steele SR, Boutrous M, et al. Clinical practice guideline for the surgical management of Crohn's disease. *Dis Colon Rectum.* 2015;58:1021-1036.

Yamamoto T, Fazio VW, Tekkis PP. Safety and efficacy of strictureplasty for Crohn's disease: a systematic review and meta-analysis. *Dis Colon Rectum.* 2007;50(11):1968-1986.

Neuroendocrine Tumor of the Appendix

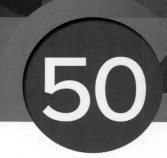

WOLFGANG B. GAERTNER AND GENEVIEVE B. MELTON-MEAUX

Based on the previous edition chapter "Appendiceal Carcinoid Tumor" by
Wolfgang B. Gaertner, Elizabeth C. Wick, and Genevieve Melton-Meaux

Presentation

A 44-year-old female presents with a 2-day history of right lower quadrant pain associated with anorexia and nausea. WBC is 12,000. An abdominal CT shows a thickened appendix with minimal free fluid in the right lower quadrant. The patient undergoes an uneventful laparoscopic appendectomy and is discharged to home on postoperative day 1. Pathology returns 2 days later and shows a 1.5-cm neuroendocrine tumor located at the midappendix with invasion of the mesoappendix.

● DIFFERENTIAL DIAGNOSIS

Appendiceal tumors are exceedingly rare with an age-adjusted incidence of 0.12 cases per 1,000,000 people per year. It is estimated that appendiceal cancer is found in 1% of all appendectomy specimens. In addition to being a rare form of cancer, the vast majority of appendiceal tumors are not diagnosed preoperatively; rather, they present with acute appendicitis or are detected as an incidental finding during a surgical procedure for an unrelated indication. Although neuroendocrine tumors (NETs, formerly known as carcinoids), were once considered the predominant type of appendiceal tumor, their reported incidence has decreased since the 1970s, and appendiceal adenocarcinoma is increasingly common.

● WORKUP

The patient is further evaluated with a computed tomography (CT) scan of the chest, abdomen, and pelvis that shows postoperative changes in the right lower quadrant, but no evidence of metastatic disease or enlarged lymph nodes. Further histologic evaluation reveals positive Ki67 staining and mitotic activity >2 cells/mm². The patient inquires if she needs further treatment.

● DISCUSSION

Neuroendocrine tumors of the appendix occur in 1 of 100 to 300 patients undergoing appendectomy. Autopsy series report an overall incidence ranging from 0.009% to 0.17%, suggesting a natural degeneration of small benign lesions during later life. NETs originate from subepithelial neuroendocrine cells, usually present in the fourth decade, and favor the female gender. Some authors have ascribed a higher incidence in females to higher rates of laparoscopy and appendectomy among women. Crohn's disease has also been identified as a risk factor for gastrointestinal (GI) NETs overall. NETs comprise 32% to 57% of all appendiceal tumors. They predominantly affect the small intestine (44.7%), followed by the rectum (19.6%), and the appendix (16.7%). Primary adenocarcinoma of the appendix, although also quite rare, has seen an increase in incidence over the past 20 years with reports of up to 26% of all appendiceal malignancies.

● DIAGNOSIS AND TREATMENT

Most appendiceal NETs are asymptomatic and are found incidentally. Patients usually present with nonspecific abdominal pain at the lower right abdomen that leads to appendectomy. Although most patients undergo some form of abdominal imaging, a CT scan of the abdomen and pelvis should be performed whenever an appendiceal mass is suspected (Figure 50-1). While CT is being increasingly used for the workup of abdominal pain, the routine application of this imaging technique for nonspecific abdominal pain is not warranted with respect to associated cost and diagnostic yield. Appendiceal NETs occur more frequently at the appendiceal tip (60% to 70%), followed by the body (5% to 21%), and base (7% to 10%). With regard to size, 60% to 76% are <1 cm, 4% to 27% are 1 to 2 cm, and 2% to 17% are >2 cm in diameter. NETs are histologically characterized as benign, borderline malignant, low-grade malignant, or high-grade malignant. The majority of reported metastasized appendiceal NETs have been graded as low-grade malignant. Assessing the mitotic activity (>2 cells/mm²) and percentage of proliferation marker Ki67 is helpful to assess the need for extended resection as well as prognosis.

Tumors < 1 cm in size require no staging unless identified as high-grade malignant. Patients with tumors between 1 and 2 cm may benefit from additional screening. Plasma chromogranin A is the most important tumor marker available, with 80% to 100% of patients with NETs having increased levels. Chromogranin A levels also correspond to tumor load and

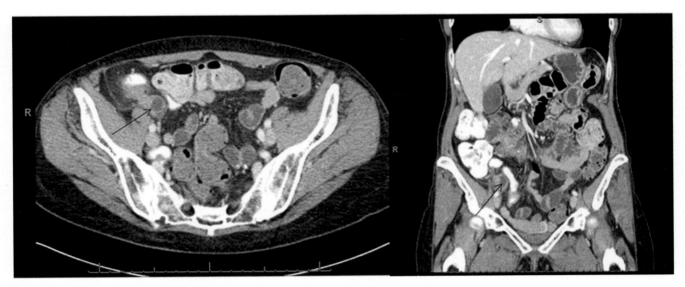

FIGURE 50-1. CT of a patient with an appendiceal mucinous cystadenoma.

levels >5,000 μg/L correlate with poor outcomes. Patients with elevated chromogranin A levels require further imaging. In these patients, ^{111}In-labeled octreotide scintigraphy, 18F-fluorodihydroxyphenylalanine (18F-FDOPA) positron emission tomography/CT (PET/CT), and 11C-5-hydroxy-tryptophan (11C-5-HTP) PET/CT are the most sensitive imaging modalities in the diagnosis and staging of metastatic disease and may further impact definitive management. Patients with tumors >2 cm, incomplete resections, evidence of metastatic disease, or goblet cell tumors warrant further investigation including determination of plasma chromogranin A levels, 24-hour urinary levels of 5-hydroxyindole-acetic acid; 18F-FDOPA PET/CT, 11C-5-HTP PET/CT, or ^{111}In-labeled octreotide scintigraphy. A significant number of coexistent malignant tumors can be found in patients with appendiceal NETs (7% to 48%), primarily throughout the GI tract. Therefore, high-risk or symptomatic patients should be evaluated endoscopically with colonoscopy and sometimes upper GI endoscopy, when indicated, to assess the remainder of the GI tract.

● OPERATIVE TREATMENT

The type of surgical intervention for NETs depends upon tumor, histopathology, location, and size. Although the size hypothesis is not well understood or validated, the risk of metastases is thought to increase with primary tumor size. The risk of metastases in tumors <1 cm is virtually zero; tumors between 1 and 2 cm metastasize in 0% to 1%, and tumors >2 cm metastasize in 20% to 85%. These findings give the rationale for the hypothesis that patients with tumors >2 cm in diameter may benefit from an oncologic resection of the right colon.

NETs <1 cm in size, located at the body or tip of the appendix, and with no unfavorable histology or evidence of metastatic disease are appropriately managed with appendectomy alone. On the other end of the spectrum, patients with NETs >2 cm, goblet cell adenocarcinoid tumors of any size, positive mesoappendix or vascular invasion, localization at the base of appendix, positive margins, or evidence of nodal metastasis should undergo right colectomy (Table 50-1). With regard to NETs between 1 and 2 cm in size, one must take in account the patient's operative risk and tumor biology. For patients with low risk and a NET between 1 and 2 cm with unfavorable histology (mitotic activity >2 cells/mm^2 or presence of proliferation marker Ki67), a right colectomy is indicated. For patients with high operative risk and a NET between 1 and 2 cm in size with favorable histology and located at the body or tip of the appendix, appendectomy is recommended.

With the widespread use of laparoscopic appendectomy, the question arises if this technique is adequate for the treatment of appendiceal malignancies. Laparoscopic appendectomy for NETs has not been associated with a significantly worse prognosis compared to the open approach. The level of available evidence at present for recommendations with respect to use of laparoscopy is generally low for NETs in large part because of their low prevalence and often incidental detection. Timing of a subsequent right colectomy should be within 3 months after appendectomy and can safely be performed laparoscopically. There are no data to support that a two-step approach may negatively affect prognosis. Adenocarcinoma of the appendix of any size should be treated with right colectomy due to the high rate of invasion and nodal metastases.

● SPECIAL CONSIDERATIONS

Certain histologic characteristics should receive particular attention when treating appendiceal NETs. Goblet cell or crypt cell (adenocarcinoid) NETs exhibit histologic features that differ from both ordinary NETs and adenocarcinoma and have

Table 50-1	Treatment Recommendations for Appendiceal NETs		
Tumor size	**Risk of lymphatic spread**	**Aggressive characteristics that may tailor therapy**	**Treatment**
<1 cm	0%	Serosal invasion	Appendectomy
1–2 cm	0%–1%	Mesoappendiceal or vascular invasion, mitotic activity (>2 cells/mm^2), proliferation markers (*i.e.*, Ki67), localization at base of appendix, positive margins.	Individual risk evaluation: appendectomy for high-risk (elderly) patient; right colectomy for low-risk (young) patient.
>2 cm	30%	None	Right colectomy
Goblet cell histology (any size)	10%–20%	None	Right colectomy

shown to be more aggressive (Figure 50-2). Patients with these tumors tend to present at a later age (fifth decade), often present with a diffusely inflamed appendix on CT scan, and treatment should involve right colectomy regardless of the size of the tumor. While the role of proliferation markers such as Ki67 and mitotic activity (>2 cells/mm^2) is not precisely defined for appendiceal NETs, these parameters seem to indicate metastatic potential for other NET locations and might justify more extensive resection when present. Serosal involvement is present in approximately 70% of all malignant NETs but has not been related to outcomes in the published literature.

A variety of terms have been used to describe appendiceal mucinous lesions that are not frankly malignant, including cystadenomas, mucinous tumor of uncertain potential, disseminated peritoneal adenomucinosis, and malignant mucocele. Most reports describe these lesions as low-grade mucinous neoplasms. They have the potential to spread to the peritoneal cavity producing mucinous intraperitoneal ascites, resulting in pseudomyxoma peritonei. The malignant potential of these tumors largely depends on the degree of cellular atypia. Perforated neoplasms or lesions ruptured intraoperatively may also result in pseudomyxoma peritonei. These patients require close surveillance with CT and second-look diagnostic laparoscopy at short intervals in order to assess for peritoneal involvement. Although we do not recommend prophylactic cytoreductive surgery with hyperthermic intraperitoneal chemotherapy (HIPEC) at our institution, if objective evidence of peritoneal disease is present, HIPEC is typically recommended.

Lesions confined to the appendix with benign histology should be treated by appendectomy. Involvement of the base of the appendix requires cecectomy with en bloc resection of the mesoappendix. Mucinous adenocarcinomas are more common in the appendix than the colon and account for 40% to 67% of all appendiceal adenocarcinomas. These tumors can also rupture and spread throughout the peritoneum causing pseudomyxoma peritonei and peritoneal carcinomatosis. Localized lesions should be treated with right colectomy, while selective ruptured lesions may benefit from cytoreductive surgery and HIPEC.

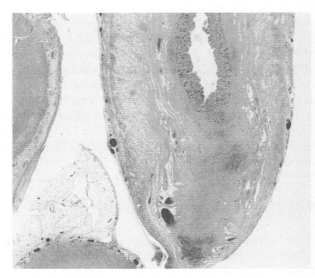 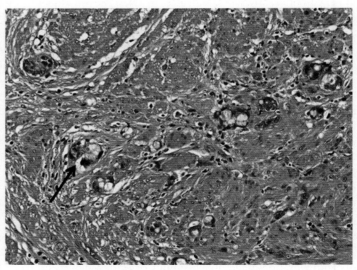

FIGURE 50-2. Microscopic view of a goblet cell NET. High-power view shows a typical goblet cell (*arrow*).

The current treatment algorithm for appendiceal cancer best relies on histopathologic tissue diagnosis NET *versus* other histology. However, this requires a frozen section in the operating room, which in many cases is unreliable and inconsistent with final pathology. Instead of relying on tissue diagnosis, a number of experts have proposed that all appendiceal malignancies should be treated with right colectomy. To further support this approach, reports have shown a decrease incidence of appendiceal NETs that would be appropriate for appendectomy alone, and an overall underutilization of right colectomy in the treatment of appendiceal tumors. Other more recent reports have shown no difference in survival rates between right colectomy *versus* appendectomy alone, suggesting that appendectomy may be a viable treatment option even for larger tumors, therefore questioning the benefit of right colectomy with the currently available data. When advanced disease is present, a palliative gastrostomy tube, diverting ostomy, or intestinal bypass may be helpful in selective cases. However, right colectomy or palliative resection in this setting are typically of little value and rarely prevent complications such as bowel obstruction or carcinoid syndrome. Although the role and impact of cytoreductive surgery and HIPEC is better defined in properly selected patients with appendiceal adenocarcinoma, specifically the mucinous and goblet cell subtypes, this form of therapy is not efficacious for appendiceal NETs.

● POSTOPERATIVE MANAGEMENT

Patients with appendiceal NETs >2 cm, incomplete resections, metastatic disease, or goblet cell histopathology require postoperative screening with serial plasma chromogranin A levels and CT of the chest, abdomen, and pelvis. ^{111}In-labeled octreotide scintigraphy or PET/CT should be performed to stage patients with evidence or suspicion of metastatic disease. Imaging in the postoperative setting is best performed at least 2 weeks after surgery.

The calculated risk of metastases from tumors <1 cm is near zero, and patients with tumors over 2 cm develop metastases in approximately 20% of cases. Appendiceal NETs usually metastasize to regional lymph nodes rather than to the liver. Five-year survival ranges from 80% to 89% for all stages. Patients with local disease have a 5-year survival rate ranging from 92% to 94%, those with regional metastases 81% to 84%, and those with distant metastases 31% to 33%. Although epidemiologic data on synchronous GI NETs and other GI malignancies are lacking, endoscopic surveillance for synchronous or metachronous tumors is warranted because of an increasingly reported elevated risk of a second primary malignancy in the GI tract.

In patients with metastatic disease, optimal management requires a multidisciplinary team with medical and surgical oncology expertise. Distant disease with carcinoid syndrome is most often treated with somatostatin analogs. Disease progression may also be delayed with long-acting release octreotide. In some cases, liver-directed ablation or debulking surgery may provide symptomatic improvement.

TAKE HOME POINTS

- NETs are common neoplasms of the appendix, occurring in 1 of 100 to 300 patients undergoing appendectomy.
- Patients with NETs >2 cm, unfavorable histology, incomplete resection, metastatic disease or goblet cell tumors warrant further oncologic staging and postoperative screening.
- Small appendiceal NETs (<1 cm) have an excellent prognosis after appendectomy.
- NETs >2 cm, goblet cell histology regardless of size, positive mesoappendix or cecal margins, or evidence of nodal metastasis require right colectomy. Right colectomy should also be considered in selective patients with NETs 1 to 2 cm in diameter or with unfavorable histology.

SUGGESTED READINGS

Boudreaux JP, Klimstra DS, Hassan MM, et al. The NANETS consensus guideline for the diagnosis and management of neuroendocrine tumors: well-differentiated neuroendocrine tumors of the jejunum, ileum, appendix, and cecum. *Pancreas.* 2010;39(6): 753-766.

Goede AC, Caplin ME, Winslet MC. Carcinoid tumour of the appendix. *Br J Surg.* 2003;90:1317-1322.

McGory ML, Maggard MA, Kang H, et al. Malignancies of the appendix: beyond case series reports. *Dis Colon Rectum.* 2005;48: 2264-2271.

Murphy EM, Farquharson SM, Moran BJ. Management of an unexpected appendiceal neoplasm. *Br J Surg.* 2006;93:783-792.

Rectal Cancer

CAMPBELL S. ROXBURGH AND MARTIN R. WEISER

51

Based on the previous edition chapter "Rectal Cancer" by Hyaehwan Kim and Martin R. Weiser

Presentation

A 65-year-old male presents with complaints of bright red blood per rectum and a change in caliber of stools over the past 3 to 4 months. He has never had a colonoscopy or upper endoscopy. His current medications include daily aspirin 81 mg and Lipitor 40 mg. He has no significant medical comorbidities, no previous surgical history, and no known allergies. He is an ex-smoker, having quit at the age of 35 years. He drinks alcohol only occasionally. His father died of metastatic prostate cancer at the age of 76 years, and his mother died of pneumonia in a hospital at the age of 88 years. He is overweight, with a body mass index of 35 kg/m². Abdominal examination is unremarkable, but rectal examination reveals a palpable mass, which bleeds on contact, at 6 cm from the anal verge. His hemoglobin is 9.7 g/dL.

DIFFERENTIAL DIAGNOSIS

The presence of a mass makes rectal cancer the likely diagnosis. A range of benign conditions (including diverticular disease, hemorrhoids, anal fissure, and inflammatory bowel disease) could be considered in the absence of a mass, but in a patient presenting with new lower gastrointestinal symptoms in this age group, the possibility of a malignancy must be excluded, and colonoscopy is warranted.

WORKUP

The patient undergoes colonoscopy, which is required to adequately visualize the lesion, obtain tissue for pathologic diagnosis, and exclude synchronous malignant lesions. Depending on the location of the pathology, tattoo marking can be placed just distal to the lesion on two opposite sides of the lumen to aid intraoperative localization. The colonoscopy was complete to the cecum. A circumferential, nonobstructing mass is identified between 6 and 10 cm from the anal verge. Clinically, the mass is 3 cm above the anorectal ring (top of the anal sphincter complex). Biopsies confirm moderately differentiated adenocarcinoma. Additionally, a 1-cm transverse colon pedunculated polyp is completely excised and confirmed as a tubular adenoma. A staging

computerized tomography (CT) of the chest, abdomen, and pelvis with oral and intravenous contrast is performed to assess for the presence of distant metastases. This scan demonstrates the known rectal mass, a 2-mm nonspecific right upper lobe lung nodule but no overt distant metastatic spread. Local staging of the primary tumor is performed using magnetic resonance imaging (MRI) to establish the site and involved structures, clinical T stage, nodal status, and possibility of a threatened circumferential radial margin (CRM). The tumor is staged clinically as cT3 N+, located 6 cm from the anal verge and extending to within 2 mm of the CRM. The baseline level of serum carcinoembryonic antigen (CEA) is within the normal range.

DIAGNOSIS AND TREATMENT

Rectal cancer accounts for almost 30% of colorectal cancer cases, with approximately 41,000 new diagnoses per year in the United States. Most rectal cancers present in the sixth or seventh decade of life. Complete colonoscopy is indicated prior to surgery, as synchronous adenomas and colorectal cancers are seen in 30% and 3% of cases, respectively. Rectal cancer specifically refers to extraperitoneal lesions (i.e., lesions below the peritoneal reflection). Generally, these lesions are located <15 cm from the anal verge (as found on proctoscopy). Lesions above the peritoneal reflection are usually treated as colon cancers.

Clinical examination can provide some early details on likely clinical staging of the tumor. The degree of tumor fixity in the pelvis relates to the depth of penetration of the primary lesion. Mobile lesions are often limited to the mucosa, submucosa (cT1), or muscularis propria (cT2), whereas tethered lesions suggest tumor extension into the perirectal fat or the mesorectum (cT3). Fixed tumors may extend into adjacent pelvic structures including the prostate, seminal vesicles, or vagina (cT4). Most patients present without pain, but when present, pain may indicate sphincter involvement by tumor. Endorectal ultrasound (Figure 51-1) is gradually being replaced by MRI (Figure 51-2) as the primary imaging modality for local staging of rectal cancer. MRI-based staging has a >90% accuracy for primary lesions and a 60% to 80% accuracy for locoregional lymph nodes. While endorectal ultrasound remains important and is slightly better than MRI in the staging of early lesions, MRI is superior for staging bulky and locally advanced lesions (T3-4 tumors). T2-weighted

294

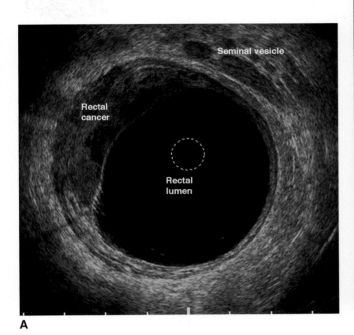

A

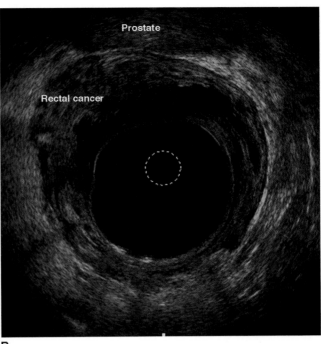

B

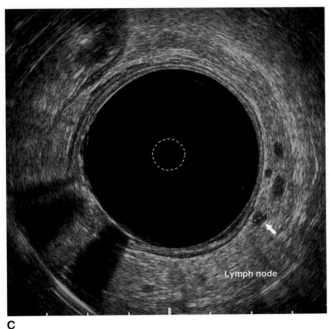

C

FIGURE 51-1. Endorectal ultrasound images of the hypoechoic primary rectal tumor at the level of the seminal vesicles (A) and the prostate (B), with invasion into the peri-rectal fat. Endorectal ultrasound image of a hypoechoic meso-rectal lymph node indicative of nodal metastasis (C).

advanced rectal cancers (cTNM stage II or III, cT3-4, or cN+) require multimodality treatment with a view to downstaging the tumor, optimizing local control, and minimizing risk of incomplete (R1) resection with positive CRM. This patient has a cT3N1 tumor and should be managed with combined modality therapy. In North America, standard management is neoadjuvant long-course chemoradiotherapy consisting of oral capecitabine or infusional fluorouracil in combination with 5,040 cGy administered in 25 to 28 fractions (Monday through Friday for 5.5 weeks). Following chemoradiotherapy, repeat staging is recommended prior to resection.

Surgery is performed 8 to 12 weeks following completion of chemoradiotherapy to optimize treatment response. Postoperative chemotherapy (capecitabine or 5-fluorouracil in combination with oxaliplatin) is recommended for locally advanced rectal cancer, although this remains a topic of ongoing debate, given the lack of randomized trials. In recent years, moving adjuvant chemotherapy to the preoperative period has been described, and this treatment option is now included in NCCN guidelines. Such a strategy is reported to optimize delivery of chemotherapy to reduce distant metastases but may also enhance treatment responses. There is also an emerging role for nonoperative, or watch-and-wait, management after complete clinical response

phased-array MRI provides high-resolution visualization of pelvic anatomy for accurate staging, but there is a developing role for diffusion-weighted MRI in addition to advanced functional sequences, which can be useful in quantification of responses to neoadjuvant therapy, that is, in determining whether biologically active tumor remains.

Accurate local staging is essential to ensure optimal treatment. Early tumors (cTNM stage I or cT1-2, N0) are generally treated with surgery alone. However, locally

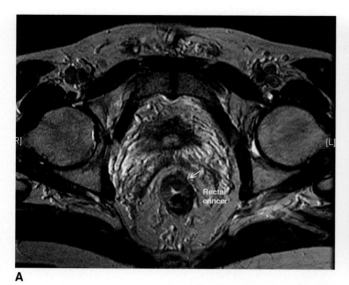

A

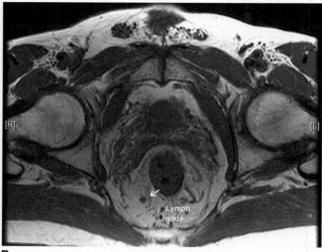

B

FIGURE 51-2. MRI axial views of the primary rectal tumor (**A**) and mesorectal adenopathy (**B**). MRI sagittal view of the tumor (**C**).

to neoadjuvant therapy. In many centers, watch-and-wait remains a nonstandard approach, and this strategy should ideally be followed within the confines of a local study protocol or registry.

Rectal resection should be performed in accordance with the principles of total mesorectal excision, which have been proven to reduce the likelihood of local recurrence. Furthermore, resection with an intact mesorectum, without fascial breach, is associated with better outcome, and the importance of high-quality surgery cannot be overstated. Sharp dissection along the embryonic planes between the visceral and the parietal layers of the endopelvic fascia ensures complete removal of the locoregional lymph nodes in the mesorectum, preserves autonomic nerve function, and minimizes blood loss.

Preoperative counseling should include a discussion regarding the possibility of a diverting stoma. Preoperative education and site marking by a stoma therapist improves postoperative patient satisfaction. The possibility of postoperative sexual and bladder dysfunction as well as low anterior resection syndrome (which includes stool frequency, urgency, and clustering) should be discussed. The patient should be aware that postoperative bowel function may take 12 to 24 months to plateau and may be permanently altered. Although the utility of bowel preparation has been questioned in regard to surgery for colon cancer, bowel preparation remains useful in rectal cancer surgery.

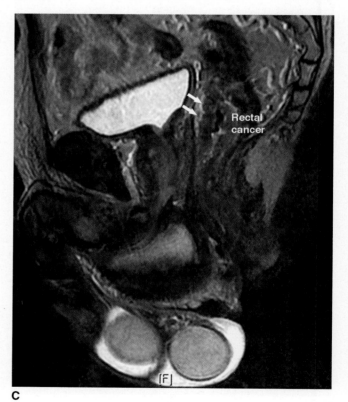

C

● NEOADJUVANT THERAPY

The patient's clinical staging with MRI (cT3 N+) merits treatment with neoadjuvant therapy, with the goal of curative

resection. After discussion with his oncologist, the patient elects to receive a total neoadjuvant therapy regimen with induction chemotherapy administered over 4 months prior to chemoradiotherapy. About 8 weeks after chemoradiotherapy, he undergoes repeat endoscopic and MRI assessments. Although the response to treatment is good, with significant tumor downsizing, residual tumor remains, and surgery is recommended. Other staging investigations demonstrate disappearance of the indeterminate lung nodule. The patient receives preoperative counseling on the risks and complications of surgery, adherence to enhanced recovery protocols, and stoma therapy.

● SURGICAL APPROACH

Surgery can be performed using an open or a minimally invasive (laparoscopic or robotic) approach, depending on local expertise, individual patient considerations, and most importantly, oncologic safety. For tumors in the mid or lower rectum, the key technical steps for open surgery and minimally invasive surgery are identical (Table 51-1). The authors' preference is to employ a minimally invasive approach using the robotic platform. The oncologic adequacy of the minimally invasive approach is evidenced by data from the COLOR-II and COREAN trials showing that long-term outcomes are comparable to those for open surgery, with long-term data from the ACASOG Z6051 and ALaCaRT trials still pending.

In the operating room, the patient is placed securely in a modified lithotomy position. Tilt positions are tested before surgery begins. A bladder catheter is introduced. Pneumatic compression stockings are applied, and deep vein thrombosis prophylaxis is administered. A digital rectal exam and irrigation are performed to again assess the location of the tumor and remove any remaining stool from the rectum.

Minimally Invasive Surgery

Although various approaches have been described, the authors place the patient with a left-side-up tilt. After the abdomen is explored for possible presence of metastatic disease in the liver or peritoneal surfaces, the small bowel is moved to the right abdomen, and the omentum is placed superiorly. The distal sigmoid colon is retracted anteriorly, and the peritoneum is scored medially 1 to 2 cm anterior to the landmark of the right iliac artery. A medial-to-lateral dissection is performed, and a plane immediately posterior to the superior rectal artery is developed, allowing the

---

Table 51-1   Low Anterior Resection

Key Technical Steps

1. Check for presence of metastatic disease during laparotomy/laparoscopy.
2. Identify ureter early in dissection.
3. Divide superior rectal artery or inferior mesenteric artery as appropriate to clear lymph nodes and provide length for tension-free pelvic anastomosis.
4. Mobilize left colon with takedown of splenic flexure and division of inferior mesenteric vein at the inferior border of pancreas if necessary to provide length for tension-free anastomosis.
5. Divide mesocolon onto the bowel at site selected for proximal transection.
6. Perform total mesorectal excision by entering plane between visceral and parietal layers of endopelvic fascia.
7. En bloc resection of adherent structures to provide adequate tumor clearance.
8. Identify distal point of transection and divide mesorectum onto rectal muscle tube.
9. Staple and transect distal rectum.
10. Transect bowel proximally and prepare proximal colonic conduit by inserting anvil, which is secured with purse-string suture.
11. Complete the double-stapled anastomosis under direct vision.
12. Perform air leak test.
13. Construct diverting ileostomy if necessary.

Potential Pitfalls

- Failure to adequately identify left ureter, risking potential injury.
- Capsular tears on spleen due to excessive retraction on tissues.
- Injury to autonomic nerves posterior to superior rectal artery at pelvic inlet and laterally during pelvic dissection.
- Breach of mesorectal fascia or coning in on resection specimen in vicinity of tumor.
- Injury to presacral veins during pelvic dissection.
- Failure to divert high-risk low anastomosis.

autonomic nerves to be reflected posteriorly. The left ureter is a key landmark that should be located in the initial dissection. Dissection continues cephalad to expose the inferior mesenteric artery pedicle, which once cleared, can be divided using an appropriate energy source or vascular clips. The inferior mesenteric artery can be taken selectively, as in the presence of bulky nodal disease, or alternatively preserved with division of the superior rectal artery. The authors generally prefer high ligation to clear nodal disease and provide length for a tension-free anastomosis.

As the medial-to-lateral dissection continues, retroperitoneal structures are reflected posteriorly. The authors generally prefer routine splenic flexure mobilization, again to allow the left colon to rotate into the pelvis for a tension-free anastomosis. The inferior mesenteric vein is identified at the duodenal–jejunal junction and divided with an appropriate energy source or vascular clips just distal to the pancreas. The flexure is mobilized using a medial-to-lateral approach, with elevation of the left colon mesentery off the retroperitoneum and reflection of the pancreas posteriorly with division of mesocolon adhesions. This dissection leads into the lesser sac. The omentum is mobilized free of the transverse colon, and attachments to the splenic flexure are divided. The remaining lateral attachments are divided, and the colon is mobilized from the middle colic vessels to the pelvic brim. The mesocolon is divided onto the bowel at a point deemed appropriate for proximal transection. Preferably, the left colon, or occasionally the sigmoid (if it is supple and well vascularized), is used for reconstruction.

The patient is then placed in the Trendelenburg position for the pelvic dissection. For tumors in the mid or lower rectum, sharp dissection is performed in the avascular plane between the visceral and the parietal layers of the endopelvic fascia onto the pelvic floor. Unlike in open surgery, the anterior dissection is performed early. The anterior and lateral peritoneum is scored, and the anterior dissection is developed. In male patients, the dissection is continued through or anterior to Denonvilliers fascia, and if possible, both layers are removed from the seminal vesicles and the upper prostate, especially in the case of anterior lesions.

Then, distal dissection continues sharply through Waldeyer's fascia (rectosacral fascia that extends from S4 to the rectum/mesorectum). Laterally, care is taken to avoid injury to the pelvic parasympathetic nerves. Pelvic sidewall dissection with en bloc removal of the parietal layer of the endopelvic fascia is performed, when necessary, to ensure clear circumferential margins. Once rectal mobilization is complete, a suitable point for rectal transection is identified to ensure adequate distal margin that can be verified endoscopically.

For tumors in the upper rectum, dissection continues 5 cm below the level of the mass. The mesorectum is then divided perpendicular to the intestine, to avoid "coning." This is referred to as a tumor-specific mesorectal excision. For tumors in the mid or lower rectum, dissection is completed to the pelvic floor, where the mesorectum ends. In the past, for a complete mesorectal excision, a 2-cm distal rectal margin was recommended. However, numerous reports have verified that a 1-cm, or even smaller, distal margin is sufficient, especially in patients who have undergone preoperative chemoradiotherapy. Once the distal resection line is identified, the bowel is occluded below the tumor and irrigated to remove exfoliated cells and debris.

The authors generally perform a double-stapled anastomotic technique. An articulating stapler is introduced and deployed at the desired level of the rectum (first staple line). Through a small incision, the rectum is delivered and the proximal bowel is divided. A circular stapler is then chosen, and the anvil is placed within the opened bowel with purse-string suture. After verification of hemostasis, the bowel is returned to the abdomen, and pneumoperitoneum is reestablished. Under direct vision, the anvil is brought down to the stapler and connected; the staple is closed, and anastomosis is created (second staple line). The tissues from the proximal and distal bowels are inspected to ensure that the two rings of tissue ("donuts") are intact. Further verification of intact anastomosis is performed using endoscopy, and while the rectum is insufflated, the pelvis is filled with saline to assess for leakage of air. If necessary, a diverting loop ileostomy can be brought out at a premarked site and matured after closure of the other incisions.

Open Surgery

A midline incision is made, extending from the pubis to above the umbilicus. Additional cephalad extension is usually necessary to mobilize the splenic flexure. The patient is placed in a slight Trendelenburg position. A lateral-to-medial approach is followed with mobilization of the sigmoid colon off the retroperitoneum by scoring the white line of Toldt. The left ureter and gonadal vessels are identified. The peritoneum is scored along the superior rectal artery to the base of the inferior mesenteric artery, preserving the sympathetic autonomic nerves. The pedicle is ligated just distal to the takeoff of the left colic pedicle, or alternatively, high ligation of the inferior mesenteric artery is performed. As noted above, the authors generally prefer high ligation of the inferior mesenteric artery to clear at-risk lymph nodes and facilitate a tension-free anastomosis.

The mesentery is divided up to the left colon, which is divided with a stapler. The peritoneum is then scored bilaterally into the pelvis and around the anterior peritoneal reflection. The sigmoid mesentery is raised off the retroperitoneum again, with care taken to avoid injury to the autonomic nerves. With the rectum retracted anteriorly, the avascular plane between the visceral and the parietal layers of the endopelvic fascia is developed, characterized by loose areolar tissue. Posterior dissection, facilitated by use of the St. Marks retractor, continues sharply through Waldeyer's fascia. Blunt dissection should be avoided, as Waldeyer's fascia can tear at the presacral fascia, causing bleeding into the mesorectum and resulting in an incomplete nodal dissection. The same principles as those described for minimally invasive surgery apply, and a suitable point for transection is identified before a double-stapled anastomosis is constructed. Anterior dissection is generally performed after posterior dissection. Splenic flexure mobilization is usually required to facilitate a tension-free anastomosis between the descending colon and distal rectum.

SPECIAL INTRAOPERATIVE CONSIDERATIONS

Patients with obstructing lesions may require colonic stenting or colostomy prior to beginning chemoradiotherapy. The decision to intervene surgically before starting chemoradiotherapy depends on the patient's symptoms as well as clinical examination.

For patients with bulky tumors and possible extension of the tumor into surrounding structures (small intestine, ovary, bladder, vagina, prostate, or seminal vesicle), en bloc resection should be performed. It is often not possible to identify a malignant fistula from a benign adhesion. Mere division, or "pinching," of a tumor is not an acceptable surgical technique, as it may reduce the chance of cure.

Following creation of an anastomosis, an air leak test is performed to search for incomplete stapling. If the air leak test is positive, the anastomosis should be carefully evaluated by proctoscopy. Anastomosis takedown should be considered if large anastomotic defects are noted. Small defects can be repaired with sutures. If the leak is small and cannot be identified, a diverting stoma should be strongly considered.

PATIENT'S LOW ANTERIOR RESECTION

At approximately 10 weeks after completion of chemoradiotherapy, a robot-assisted low anterior resection is performed with a low pelvic anastomosis and diverting ileostomy. The specimen is retrieved through the right lower quadrant port site, the site used for robotic stapling and for the diverting stoma. Local nerve block, nonsteroidal anti-inflammatory medication, and limited intravenous narcotics provide analgesia on postoperative days 0 and 1. Narcotics are discontinued beyond postoperative day 1. The patient resumes liquid diet on the day of surgery and regular diet on postoperative day 1. Ambulation on the day of surgery is encouraged. A pelvic drain and a Foley catheter are removed on postoperative day 3 due to the low pelvic dissection. An enhanced recovery protocol is employed, and the patient remains in the hospital for 4 days until ileostomy competence has been demonstrated.

POSTOPERATIVE MANAGEMENT

Where possible, enhanced recovery protocols should be employed to facilitate early return to function and discharge after surgery. The multimodality enhanced recovery approach includes preoperative counseling, minimization of the use of epidural or opiate-based analgesia with the aid of regional adjuncts (transverse abdominal plane blocks), early resumption of oral intake, and early mobilization. Nasogastric tubes should be avoided postoperatively. Foley catheters may be removed early or, in cases of low pelvic dissection, left in place for several days, as urinary retention (due to nerve edema associated with low dissection) can occur after early catheter removal. Anastomotic leak occurs in up to 15% of patients and usually presents with fever, tachycardia, arrhythmia, tachypnea, or diffuse peritonitis within 4 to 7 days postoperatively. The incidence is higher in low rectal anastomoses (<7 cm from the anal verge) and in patients who have received antiangiogenic therapy (i.e., bevacizumab). Fecal diversion is commonly utilized in order to avoid the potential sequelae of anastomotic leak. In a meta-analysis of data from four randomized controlled trials and 21 nonrandomized studies ($N = 11,429$), Tan et al. found that a lower clinical anastomotic leak rate (risk ratios, 0.39 and 0.74, respectively) and a lower reoperation rate (risk ratios, 0.29 and 0.23, respectively) were associated with the use of a diverting stoma in both randomized control trials and nonrandomized studies. Temporary fecal diversion should therefore be considered for patients thought to be at high risk for anastomotic leak.

Long-term complications include sexual and bladder dysfunction, associated with pelvic sidewall dissection, preoperative chemoradiotherapy, and abdominoperineal resection. Many patients opt for sphincter-sparing low anterior resection over a permanent stoma. Subsequent potential changes in bowel function, including increased stool frequency, urgency, clustering (stool fragmentation), and incontinence, are referred to as low anterior resection syndrome. The rate of low anterior resection syndrome approaches 70% to 80%, and this condition is particularly common in patients with ultra low colorectal anastomosis and those who received pelvic radiotherapy. Symptoms improve over 12 to 18 months, but long-term deficits remain common.

While preoperative combined modality therapy has been found to be beneficial, the role of adjuvant chemotherapy remains somewhat controversial. No randomized trials have been conducted to determine the necessity of postoperative adjuvant chemotherapy, but adjuvant chemotherapy remains the standard of care in the United States for Stage III colorectal cancer.

Long-term rectal cancer follow-up includes measurement of serum CEA and physical examination every 3 to 6 months for 2 years and then every 6 months for an additional 3 years. CT of the chest, abdomen, and pelvis is performed yearly for 3 years. Colonoscopy is performed 1 year from surgery and then 3 years later if no additional polyps are seen.

Case Conclusion

The patient returns to full function within 2 to 3 weeks. His pathologic staging is ypT2 N0. Because he received total neoadjuvant therapy with preoperative chemotherapy, no postoperative treatment is needed. A water soluble contrast enema and direct visualization with endoscopy demonstrate anastomotic integrity at 6 weeks after surgery. The patient undergoes ileostomy closure at 8 weeks after resection. Following a short hospital admission for ileostomy closure, he returns to full daily activities and enters a routine surveillance program. In the initial months following ileostomy closure, he experiences some frequency and clustering of bowel motions, which decrease with time and with the use of bulking agents (such as a psyllium supplement). His bladder and sexual function are not affected by the treatment.

TAKE HOME POINTS

- Rectal cancer often presents in asymptomatic patients in the sixth or seventh decade of life. When the disease is symptomatic, bright red blood per rectum, with or without a change in the pattern of bowel movements, is most common.
- Full colonoscopy is required to rule out synchronous lesions. If colonoscopy is not possible due to obstruction, preoperative virtual colonoscopy or early postoperative colonoscopy is recommended.
- Rectal cancer workup includes CT of the chest, abdomen, and pelvis to determine the extent of the disease. Primary lesions should be staged with MRI and evaluated endoscopically. Positron emission tomography is not used routinely.
- The standard treatment for tumors in the mid or lower rectum that extend into the mesorectum or involve locoregional lymph nodes (clinical Stage II or III) is chemoradiotherapy followed by mesorectal excision.
- Mesorectal excision involves dissection along the areolar plane between the visceral and the parietal layers of the endopelvic fascia. Sharp mesorectal excision reduces postoperative morbidity by preserving the superior and the inferior hypogastric nerve plexuses.
- Postoperative complications following rectal surgery include immediate postoperative leak and long-term sexual and urinary dysfunction as well as low anterior resection syndrome.
- A diverting ileostomy should be considered for low anastomosis, especially if chemoradiotherapy was administered preoperatively.
- Serum CEA is measured, and a physical exam is performed every 3 to 6 months for 2 years after surgery and then every 6 months for an additional 3 years. CT of the chest, abdomen, and pelvis is performed annually for 3 years. Colonoscopy is performed after the first year; if no additional polyps are seen, it can subsequently be performed 3 years later.

SUGGESTED READINGS

Cercek A, et al. Neoadjuvant chemotherapy first, followed by chemoradiation and then surgery, in the management of locally advanced rectal cancer. *J Natl Compr Canc Netw.* 2014;12(4): 513-519.

Emmertsen KJ, Laurberg S. Low anterior resection syndrome score: development and validation of a symptom-based scoring system for bowel dysfunction after low anterior resection for rectal cancer. *Ann Surg.* 2012;255(5):922-928.

Minsky BD. Chemoradiation for rectal cancer: rationale, approaches, and controversies. *Surg Oncol Clin N Am.* 2010;19(4):803-818.

National Comprehensive Cancer Network. *NCCN Guidelines*; 2015. Available from http://www.nccn.org

Nelson H, et al. Guidelines 2000 for colon and rectal cancer surgery. *J Natl Cancer Inst.* 2001;93(8):583-596.

Sauer R, et al. Preoperative versus postoperative chemoradiotherapy for rectal cancer. *N Engl J Med.* 2004;351(17):1731-1740.

Smith JJ, Garcia-Aguilar J. Advances and challenges in treatment of locally advanced rectal cancer. *J Clin Oncol.* 2015;33(16): 1797-1808.

Weiser MR, et al. Sphincter preservation in low rectal cancer is facilitated by preoperative chemoradiation and intersphincteric dissection. *Ann Surg.* 2009;249(2):236-242.

Anal Carcinoma

AMY L. HALVERSON

Based on the previous edition chapter "Anal Carcinoma" by A.V. Hayman and Amy L. Halverson

Presentation

Case subject is a 63-year-old female who presents to her primary care physician (PCP) with complaints of anal pain and spotting of blood on the toilet paper when wiping. Her past medical history is notable for a history of cervical dysplasia. Ten years prior, she underwent a hysterectomy for uterine fibroids. Her last colonoscopy was 13 years prior. Five months ago, the patient started experiencing anal pain with bowel movements and itching. Her primary care physician (PCP) diagnosed her with an anal fissure, and she was started on stool softeners and psyllium husk powder. A month later, the patient returned to her PCP with worsening symptoms, and she was then prescribed topical nifedipine cream. A month later, the patient returned with no relief. Her PCP then referred patient to a gastroenterologist for "chronic, nonhealing anal fissure."

● DIFFERENTIAL DIAGNOSIS

Anal pathology is common in the general population. A thorough history can help differentiate between the most common problems, such as internal or external hemorrhoids, anal fissure, anal fistula, and pruritus ani. Anal fissures present primarily with sharp pain during defecation and are often associated with spotting of bright red blood on the toilet paper. Internal hemorrhoids may cause painless rectal bleeding. Thrombosed external hemorrhoids cause a constant pain that persists for several days. Pruritus ani may be caused by rectal mucosal prolapse or irritation from external hemorrhoidal skin tags. Pruritus has also been attributed to dietary irritants, such as citrus, caffeine, spicy foods, tomatoes, or milk. In the absence of other contributing pathology, the treatment for pruritus ani is supportive and includes avoidance of exacerbating elements.

Anal symptoms are often attributed to "hemorrhoids" without further workup, potentially leading to a delay in therapy for an undiagnosed malignancy. Any anal complaint in a high-risk patient, that is, age 50 or older, man with male sexual partners, HIV seropositivity, chronic pharmacologic immunosuppression, history of anal or gynecologic human

papilloma virus (HPV) or colorectal adenomas, or a relevant family history should prompt endoscopic evaluation to rule out malignancy. For average-risk individuals, symptoms that persist more than 6 weeks with diet and/or medical therapy warrant endoscopic examination. Initial evaluation should include a complete history and physical exam, including digital rectal exam and anoscopy. Examination under anesthesia should be performed in individuals with persistent symptoms who are unable to tolerate anoscopy in the office.

Presentation Continued

For the patient in this scenario, during her appointment with the specialist, the gastroenterologist identified a 2-cm area of induration in the anal canal on digital rectal exam. Anoscopy identified ulceration overlying the area of induration. The ulcer was biopsied, and histology confirmed squamous cell carcinoma.

● WORKUP

The patient should undergo a thorough physical examination. Particular attention should be paid to inguinal lymph node evaluation. Any lymphadenopathy should prompt a fine needle aspiration to rule out regional lymph node involvement. Indications for colonoscopy should be based on established colorectal cancer screening guidelines, beginning at age 50 (or earlier if a first-degree relative has a history of colon cancer or polyps) or if the patient is symptomatic.

In order to assess for distant metastases, the patient should undergo abdominal/pelvic computed tomography (CT) (or MRI) and a chest CT, although it should be noted that most lymph node metastases are small and may not be able to be detected by cross-sectional imaging. In some cases, a positron emission tomography–computed tomography (PET–CT) may be obtained. HIV status should be ascertained. Evaluation for gynecologic dysplasia should be performed in females, since the same pathogen, the HPV, is implicated in both neoplastic processes (Table 52-1).

Table 52-1	Staging of Anal Canal Carcinoma		
Stage	T	N	M
	T1: <2 cm	N1: perirectal nodes	0: no distant mets
	T2: 2–4.9 cm	N2: unilateral internal iliac or inguinal nodes	1: distant mets
	T3: 5+ cm	N3: perirectal and inguinal nodes OR bilateral internal iliac or inguinal nodes	
	T4: invades adjacent organs		
I	T1	N0	M0
II	T2-3	N0	M0
IIIA	T1-3	N1	M0
IIIB	T4	N1	M0
	Tany	N2	M0
IV	Tany	Nany	M1

Reprinted from Amin MB, Edge S, Greene F, et al. eds. *AJCC Cancer Staging Manual.* 8th ed. Springer International: Switzerland; 2017, with permission.

Presentation Continued

The patient underwent computed tomography of the chest, abdomen and pelvis, which showed no evidence of regional or distant metastases. There was no inguinal lymphadenopathy detected on physical examination. Colonoscopy was otherwise normal.

● TREATMENT

Initial treatment for squamous cell carcinoma of the anal canal is nonsurgical and consists of combined chemotherapy and radiation. The standard radiation protocol consists of a minimum of 45 Gy administered in 25 fractions over 5 weeks to the primary cancer. 5-fluorouacil (5-FU) is infused on days 1 to 4 and 29 to 32 with mitomycin C bolus on days 1 and 29. Oral capecitabine may be substituted for 5-FU. Systemic treatment for metastatic disease consists of 5-FU and cisplatin.

In carefully selected patients with invasive lesions < 1 cm in the anal canal, local excision alone may be considered (Chai, 2017). It is important to distinguish between squamous cell carcinomas of the squamous epithelial-lined anal canal (proximal to the anal verge), which are approached as outlined above, as opposed to the epidermis-lined anal margin (distal to the anal verge). For anal margin cancers, superficial, localized lesions (T1) are treated initially by wide local excision with negative margins. If margins are positive, re-excision is recommended if anatomically feasible; otherwise, the patient should be referred for chemoradiation therapy as above. All other therapies follow the above guidelines.

Presentation Continued

Given the absence of distant metastases, the patient was referred for chemoradiation, which she successfully completed. The patient returned 8 weeks after completion of chemoradiation. The patient reported improved anal pain. Examination revealed persistent ulceration. The patient was told to return for repeat exam in 3 months.

Recent data have shown that clinical response of anal cancer to chemoradiation may continue for 26 weeks following the initiation of chemoradiation. Glynne-Jones and colleagues reported than 72% of individuals with residual tumor at 11 weeks following the initiation of chemoradiation demonstrated a complete clinical response at 26 weeks (Glynne-Jones, 2017).

Presentation Continued

The patient returns for repeat examination 3 months later. Residual cancer is confirmed by biopsy of a persistent mass. The patient is recommended to undergo an abdominoperineal resection.

● PREOPERATIVE CONSIDERATION

1. Stoma marking by a certified enterostomal therapist
2. Perioperative antibiotics
3. Venous thromboembolism prophylaxis

SURGICAL APPROACH

The procedure is commonly performed with the patient in the lithotomy position. Mobilization of the distal colon and rectum and division of the mesentery may be performed using an open technique or laparoscopically. The surgical approach should include careful dissection to maintain the anatomic planes and preserve the peritoneal envelope around the mesorectum. Careful dissection avoids nerve injury that may result in sexual dysfunction (Hojo, 1991). The mesentery should be divided at the proximal superior rectal artery branch off the inferior mesenteric artery. Once the pelvic floor is reached, dissection is performed from the perineal approach continuing cephalad to meet the intra-abdominal portion of the dissection. Care should be taken to maintain a wide dissection through the levator muscles. Grossly close margins may be sent for frozen section evaluation.

When performing an abdominoperineal resection in patients who have been treated with pelvic radiation, an omental or myocutaneous flap should be considered to facilitate wound healing. After resection of the specimen, the flap is placed into the pelvis. The perineal defect is closed in several layers with absorbable suture, including absorbable suture in the skin to avoid uncomfortable suture or staple removal postoperatively.

An alternative approach is to perform the abdominal portion of the procedure in the supine position. After creation of the colostomy and closure of the abdominal incision, the patient is turned prone for the completion of the perineal portion of the procedure. Inguinal node dissection should be considered for residual disease in the inguinal lymph nodes.

POSTOPERATIVE MANAGEMENT

All anal canal cancer patients should be examined every 3 to 6 months for 5 years. Surveillance examination should include inguinal node palpation and digital rectal examination. Anoscopy should be performed every 6 to 12 months for 3 years. Anoscopy with topical acetic acid should be considered to survey for recurrent HPV-related dysplasia. For T3+ or N1+ lesions, annual chest/abdominal/pelvis imaging is also recommended for the first 3 years (NCCN 2017).

Table 52-2	Abdominoperineal Resection for Recurrent Anal Cancer

Key Technical Steps

1. Maintain anatomic planes, that is, total mesorectal excision.
2. Continue wide dissection around the anal canal.
3. Consider myocutaneous or omental flap.

SPECIAL INTRAOPERATIVE CONSIDERATIONS

If metastatic disease is encountered at the time of surgery, proceeding with abdominoperineal resection (APR) may be appropriate for palliation of symptoms from local disease.

TAKE HOME POINTS

- Anal bleeding that does not respond to medical management should be assessed via anoscopy and/or colonoscopy.
- The first-line treatment for nonmetastatic anal canal carcinoma is chemotherapy and radiation.
- Allow up to 26 weeks from the start of chemoradiation for regression of lesion prior to proceeding with surgical resection.
- Abdominoperineal resection is indicated if combined chemoradiation fails.

SUGGESTED READINGS

Amin MB, Edge S, Greene F, et al. eds. *AJCC Cancer Staging Manual.* 8th ed. Springer International: Switzerland; 2017.

Chai CY, Cao HT, Awad S, Massarweh NN. Management of stage I squamous cell carcinoma of the anal canal. *JAMA Surg.* 2017;153(3): 209-215.

Glynne-Jones R, Sebag-Montefiore D, Meadows HM, et al. Best time to assess complete clinical response after chemoradiotherapy in squamous cell carcinoma of the anus (ACT II): a post-hoc analysis of randomised controlled phase 3 trial. *Lancet Oncol.* 2017;18(3):347-356. doi:10.1016/S1470-2045(17)30071-2.

Hojo K, Vernava AM 3rd, Sugihara K, Katumata K. Preservation of urine voiding and sexual function after rectal cancer surgery. *Dis Colon Rectum.* 1991;34(7):532-539.

NCCN Guidelines™ Version 2.2017. www.nccn.org. Accessed January 20, 2018.

Anal and Rectal Abscess

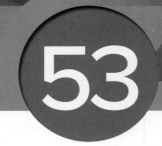

53

RICHARD E. BURNEY

Based on the previous edition chapter "Perianal Abscess" by Richard E. Burney

Presentation

A 40-year-old woman presents to your office for an urgent visit complaining of severe anal pain and tenderness that has developed over the past 2 days. She has no history of prior rectal complaints or change in bowel habit. There is no history of abdominal pain, diarrhea, or blood in her stools. On examination, she appears healthy and is afebrile. Examination of the perianal area reveals an erythematous, tender area about 1.5 cm in diameter at the posterior anal verge. It appears fluctuant. Gentle palpation is exquisitely painful precluding further rectal examination.

● DIFFERENTIAL DIAGNOSIS

In evaluating the patient with acute pain and swelling in the perianal and buttock region, one must keep in mind both the possible etiologies and the anatomy of the region, in particular the various locations or spaces where infection and abscess can arise and be manifest. There are many theories regarding the possible etiologies of perianal and perirectal infection, ranging from anal gland infection, to defecation-related anal canal trauma, to inflammatory bowel disease. The specific etiology however is not of immediate concern at the time of acute presentation when prompt diagnosis and surgical management of abscess take precedence.

The first step in the differential diagnosis of acute anal pain and swelling is to distinguish between perianal abscess, which is painful but unlikely to cause serious illness or sequelae, and perirectal or ischiorectal abscess, which can be highly morbid and life-threatening if treatment is delayed or inadequate (Figure 53-1).

Perianal abscess is limited in extent and location to the perianal tissues and intersphincteric plane, the avascular space between the internal and external sphincter muscles. Perianal abscesses are small and do not penetrate laterally through the anal sphincter into the ischiorectal fossa tissues or upward into the supralevator space. The swelling of a

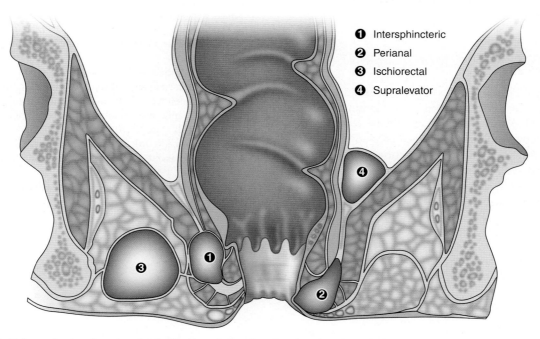

1 Intersphincteric
2 Perianal
3 Ischiorectal
4 Supralevator

FIGURE 53-1. Schematic drawing showing typical locations of perianal and perirectal abscess. Locations of abscesses can be variable and do not necessarily conform to these locations.

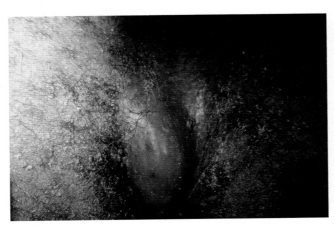

FIGURE 53-2. Perianal abscess.

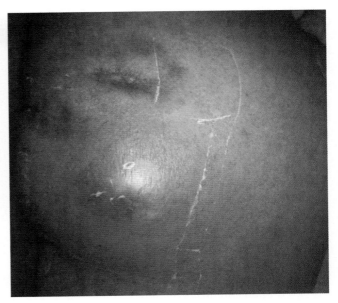

FIGURE 53-3. Appearance of ischiorectal abscess. Scar is from I&D of previous abscess.

perianal abscess is usually readily visible and easily palpable at the anal verge and does not give rise to signs of systemic infection (Figure 53-2).

Closely related to perianal abscess, and possibly its precursor, is intersphincteric abscess. An intersphincteric abscess is also small, and so named because it develops in the avascular plane between the internal and external sphincter. Unlike perianal abscess, which is usually visible under the perianal skin, it causes no outward visible signs. It causes pain and tenderness more so in the anal canal than on the surface. Tenderness is usually exquisite and located in the anal canal. The diagnosis of intersphincteric abscess can be difficult, because the signs are subtle. Intersphincteric abscess if untreated may simply evolve into a perianal abscess, which is easier to diagnose, but it could also extend upward or outward leading to a much more serious supralevator or ischiorectal abscess.

Ischiorectal abscess develops when infection, which in most theories originates in the intersphincteric space, penetrates through the external sphincter and enters the larger, fat-filled space of the ischiorectal fossa where a much larger abscess can develop (Figure 53-3). Patients with ischiorectal abscess will usually have fever, elevated white blood cell count, and may have signs of sepsis. The medial buttock will be erythematous, swollen, and tender. Because the abscess may be quite deep, more than 2 to 3 cm under the skin, obvious fluctuance is not always present. On rectal examination, one may feel a ballotable mass between the buttock and lower rectum, which is more obvious when done under anesthesia. Perirectal abscesses are easily seen on CT, but CT should not be needed to make this diagnosis in most patients.

High intersphincteric or supralevator abscesses are rare and are the most difficult to diagnose and treat. Patients will have had rectal pain, with or without fever, usually for several days or more. External examination is unrevealing. On careful rectal examination, one may be able to feel a fluctuant mass high in the anal canal at the level of the levator or anorectal ring but physical findings can be quite subtle. WBC count may be elevated. CT imaging of the pelvis, which is being done with increasing regularity in situations such as this, where one has a patient with unexplained rectal pain and signs of infection, can be very helpful in identifying the presence and exact location of these occult abscesses.

Of course, patients can also develop simple perianal carbuncles, or simple abscesses involving the perianal or buttock skin and superficial subcutaneous tissues, which have no etiologic relation to anal canal structures (Figure 53-4). Pilonidal abscess is usually located in the buttock cleft, well away from the anus. Sinus tracts arising from pilonidal cyst on occasion find their way to the perianal buttock tissues and when this happens can mimic ischiorectal abscess.

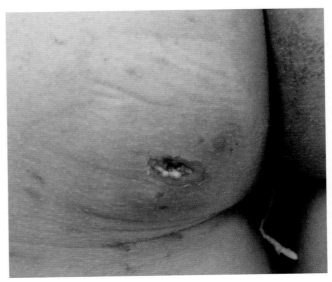

FIGURE 53-4. Carbuncle on buttock (*Staphylococcus aureus*).

Sebaceous cysts in the perianal skin can become infected and lead to abscess in the perianal region. When this happens, the patient may give a history of having had a lump there for some time that has suddenly become more tender and swollen. Finally, perianal hidradenitis suppurativa can cause anal pain and swelling. These patients rarely have disease limited to the perianal region however and almost always give a history of chronic pain, swelling, and drainage.

The differential diagnosis of patients with anal pain also includes such entities as acute hemorrhoidal inflammation, acute thrombosed hemorrhoid, acute anal fissure, anorectal inflammatory bowel disease flare, and neoplasm. None of these entities will cause fever or WBC count elevation. Patients with anorectal inflammatory bowel disease usually have other visible abnormalities and tissue distortion in the perianal area that is characteristic (Figure 53-5). Nevertheless, they may have local swelling and abscess, or ulceration that mimics abscess in its symptoms. Acute hemorrhoidal swelling and thrombosed hemorrhoids are visible and should be easily identified on external examination. By history, patients with anal fissure have anal bleeding and pain with defecation, followed by a burning or "razor blade" sensation that can last for up to an hour or more. Anal fissure can be identified most easily by simply stretching the perianal skin to expose the fissure in the anal canal. There is no swelling, and tenderness is limited to the site of the fissure itself.

Patients with fistula-in-ano will most often give a history of chronic perianal drainage or intermittent, recurrent swelling and drainage from a perianal location, usually within 3 to 4 cm of the anal verge. Acute pain and swelling may be intermittently felt but are not prominent symptoms of anal fistula. A small nubbin of granulation tissue may be present at the external fistula opening. A small proportion of patients who have undergone drainage of perianal abscess may later be found to have an associated or underlying fistula-in-ano, but in my experience, these fistulae are rarely evident at the time of surgical incision and drainage. There is no need to spend extra time looking for a possible fistula if it is not obvious at the time of initial surgical incision and drainage. If

an underlying fistula is present, it will become apparent in time. Most patients with fistula-in-ano do not initially present with an abscess; most patients with abscess do not go on to develop fistula-in-ano.

● WORKUP

The most important parts of the workup for anal pain and swelling are a complete history and a careful physical examination. The history should define the exact time course of symptoms and their specific nature. Temperature and pulse rate may give a clue as to depth and extent of abscess. Physical examination must include careful inspection and palpation of the buttock and perianal region, preferably with the patient in a knee–chest position on a sigmoidoscopy or similar table, under good lighting. In this setting, the diagnosis is frequently obvious with only simple observation and gentle palpation. Examination in lateral position in the usual exam room with poor lighting is inadequate. Lack of tenderness on rectal examination is reassuring that a high and/or deep abscess is not present.

When the diagnosis is not clear, and certainly if the patient has unexplained fever and/or elevated WBC count in conjunction with deep, unexplained rectal pain, pelvic CT is in order. Endorectal ultrasound examination might also show an abnormality but will be more uncomfortable for the patient and probably less readily available as well.

Anorectal pain, tenderness, and swelling for which there is no good explanation may require urgent or emergent examination under anesthesia. An alternative is to closely monitor the patient and reexamine for progression of signs and symptoms in 24 to 48 hours, but close observation is mandatory. Treatment is emergent not elective and should not be delayed if abscess is suspected.

● DIAGNOSIS AND TREATMENT

The treatment of perianal or intersphincteric abscess is surgical drainage. Whether the drainage procedure is done in the office, in the ED, or in the operating room is a judgment that must be made based on the size and location of the abscess, the cooperativeness and willingness of the patient, the skill and experience of the surgeon, and the resources available, such as instruments, lighting, and assistance. In general, incision and drainage in the operating room is preferred unless the abscess is quite obviously small and superficial.

When an abscess is suspected, the incision for drainage is best made over the point of maximal tenderness and swelling. Attempts to identify the presence or location of a perianal or intersphincteric abscess by exploration and aspiration with an 18-gauge needle are frequently misleading or unrewarding. While it is possible that the abscess could be small and hard to hit with a needle, more often this maneuver fails because the pus is so thick that it does not flow through the needle and cannot be aspirated. Moreover, if one does

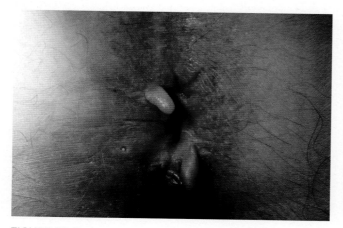

FIGURE 53-5. Anal inflammation from Crohn's disease showing inflammatory tags, edema, and ulceration.

happen to find the abscess and aspirates most of the pus from it, this will make it harder to locate after an incision is made.

In making an exploratory incision, knowledge of the perianal anatomy and how to identify the sphincters and intersphincteric plane are important. Sometimes an incision is made, and no abscess can be found. This is acceptable and preferable to missing an abscess. Close follow-up in such instances is recommended because a small abscess may have been missed.

● SURGICAL APPROACH

Perianal abscess, if superficial, small and obvious, may be drained in the office or emergency department under local anesthesia, with or without sedation. One percent lidocaine with epinephrine 1:100,000 or 1:200,000 is infiltrated into the dermis (not the subcutaneous tissue) over and around the abscess. A lanceolate or elliptical incision oriented either radially or tangentially to the anus is made over the abscess. This incision will remove a segment of overlying skin. Excision of the skin overlying the abscess helps to completely unroof it and drain it adequately (Figure 53-6). Cruciate incision is both ugly and inadequate and does not provide good drainage. A small wick of moistened plain cotton gauze is placed into the abscess cavity and removed in 48 hours. Iodoform gauze is harsh, painful, and necrosis-inducing and in my opinion should never be used. Rayon or polyester-based packing strip should be avoided as well.

If the abscess is deeper, larger, or more extensive, having expanded laterally in the intersphincteric plane and partially encircled the anal sphincter to form a horseshoe, a different approach is needed. In general, in this situation, one should avoid large or deep radial incisions, which might divide anal sphincter muscle. Tangential or circumferential incisions are preferred. In the case of horseshoe abscess, multiple small incisions are made through which a drain, such as a small Malecot catheter, rather than packing can be placed and

secured with suture. Simple packing can be placed alongside the drains and removed in 24 to 48 hours, leaving the Malecot or equivalent drains in place for a much longer period as the abscess cavity closes.

If the patient does not have an acute abscess, but rather has intermittent drainage, the surgical approach is to evaluate the patient under anesthesia, looking for a fistula-in-ano. Fine silver or lacrimal duct probes are needed. Hydrogen peroxide solution injected through a fine cannula into an external opening can be helpful in identifying an occult internal opening. If a fistula is found, treatment will depend on the depth and characteristics of the fistula. In this situation, prior measurement of the anal sphincter length by careful rectal examination prior to induction of anesthesia can be critical. If there is acute inflammation or an underlying occult abscess, or if sphincter length is unknown, the best approach is to place a seton through the fistula for drainage and allow the inflammation to subside. One should never do a fistulotomy in the face of an acute abscess and without knowing the sphincter length. Sphincter length cannot be determined under anesthesia, but rather only by examination in an awake patient. It is done by palpation of the posterior anal canal with one's finger and measuring the distance from the levator ring at one's fingertip to the anal verge. Normal sphincter length is from 2 to 5 cm. One should try to preserve at least 2 and preferably 2.5 cm of anal sphincter when doing an I&D or fistulotomy.

It is possible for a patient to have recurrent buttock abscesses as a result of unrecognized fistula-in-ano (Figure 53-7). If the abscesses are subcutaneous rather than deep (i.e., in the ischiorectal fossa), one should look for an underlying fistula (Table 53-1).

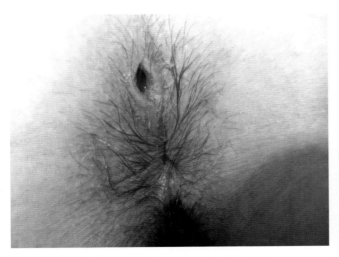

FIGURE 53-6. Appearance 2 days after incision and drainage of intersphincteric abscess demonstrating good drainage. An ellipse of skin was removed by using a lanceolate incision at time of I&D.

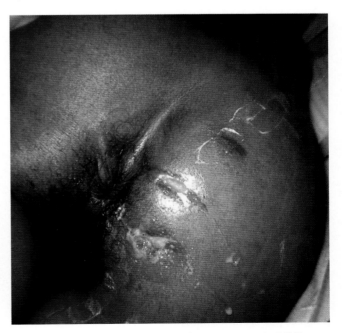

FIGURE 53-7. This patient had undergone repeated I&D procedures for buttock abscess before an underlying posterior fistula-in-ano was sought, found, and treated.

	Table 53-1 Anal and Rectal Abscess	
	Key Technical Steps	**Potential Pitfalls**
Physical examination	Prone, knee–chest position	Inadequate examination
	Proper lighting and assistance	Failure to identify subtle signs
Exam under anesthesia	Exploratory aspiration with 18-gauge needle	Failure to identify abscess with thick pus unless incision is made
Incision and drainage	Adequate anesthesia and proper positioning	Subtle abscess will be missed unless there is good exposure and muscle relaxation allowing adequate exam
	Spinal or general anesthesia, prone or lithotomy positioning is matter of surgeon preference	
	Excise an ellipse of skin over the abscess. Cruciate incision is inadequate	Incision is too small leading to inadequate drainage and/or premature closure of skin over abscess cavity
	Open and explore abscess cavity widely	Complex abscess (horseshoe) extensions may be missed
	Leave moist gauze packing for 48 h to stabilize wound opening	Once removed, packing may be difficult or impossible to replace
	Avoid fistulotomy in face of acute abscess; place seton if fistula is found	Dividing sphincter at the same time as incision and drainage leads to wide retraction of the divided sphincter muscle and can cause incontinence if too much sphincter is divided

● SPECIAL INTRAOPERATIVE CONSIDERATIONS

The position of the patient on the operating table can be a matter of personal preference. In general, my preference is to do evaluation under anesthesia in the prone position under spinal or caudal anesthesia, unless the patient has a contraindication to this, such as extreme obesity. If general anesthesia is needed in an obese patient, lithotomy position is preferred to avoid the added anesthetic risk of general anesthesia in the prone position. I position the patient prone with hips over the kidney rest, which I elevate several inches prior to flexing the table. Gel pads to support the pelvis and chest are not needed if spinal anesthesia is used unless the patient has a very obese abdomen. Pulling the buttocks apart with 3-inch adhesive tape angled about 30° toward the head improves exposure of the perianal region.

Prep solutions may obscure the skin erythema that provides a clue as to the location of the abscess. Marking the site with permanent skin marker before prepping obviates this problem. If an intersphincteric abscess is suspected, the intersphincteric plane must be identified and opened bluntly to gain access to and drain the abscess. A tangential incision parallel to the sphincter muscle helps prevent unwittingly dividing muscle unnecessarily.

If an exploratory incision is made and no pus is found, do not suture the wound closed or pack it open. Simply place a dressing over the unclosed wound. If pus is found, culture is not usually helpful in otherwise healthy individuals. Aerobic and anaerobic cultures can be obtained if you have reason so suspect resistant organisms, the patient has immune compromise, is in poor general health, or appears septic because of high fever and WBC count.

As mentioned above, avoid the use of iodoform gauze, which has no proven benefit, causes pain, and impairs wound healing. Simple saline- or plain water–moistened plain cotton gauze works quite well.

● POSTOPERATIVE MANAGEMENT

Sitz baths are traditional for comfort and to promote drainage. The initial packing can be left in place for 48 to 72 hours. If the patient has a simple perianal abscess, the packing once removed does not have to be replaced if a small ellipse of skin has been removed by the lanceolate incision, because the skin edges will not close prematurely. Antimicrobial therapy can be discontinued after a brief period unless cellulitis is present.

If the abscess is larger, more complex, and deep, it is best to use Malecot or similar catheter for drainage and to leave it in place for days or weeks. The wound can be irrigated two to three a day through the drainage tube. The tube can be downsized as the cavity closes. If the wound is superficial but extensive and/or partially circumferential, wound care consisting of shower irrigation and water-moistened plain gauze dressings changed three times a day leads to good healing (Figures 53-8 and 53-9).

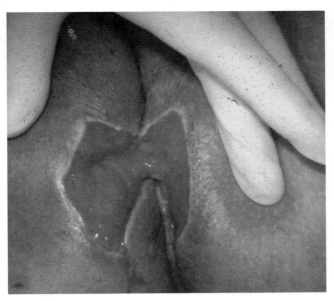

FIGURE 53-8. Appearance of large perianal wound 2 weeks after incision and drainage of superficial horseshoe abscess. Wound care consisted of plain water-moistened gauze dressings changed three times a day.

TAKE HOME POINTS

- Acute anal pain and swelling is not a trivial problem and demands urgent attention.
- Examination under anesthesia should be done if there is any question of occult or complicated abscess.
- Pelvic CT is not usually needed but is indicated if supralevator abscess is suspected. Failure to aspirate

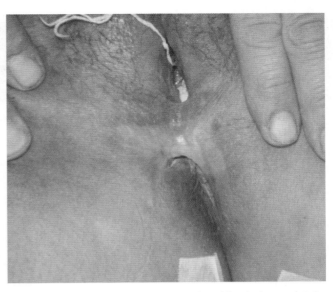

FIGURE 53-9. The wound contracted and healed completely with minimal residual scar.

pus through a needle does not mean an abscess is not present.
- Incision should be generous, with removal of overlying skin to promote adequate drainage.
- Do not attempt fistulotomy in the face of acute inflammation; place a seton if a fistula is obvious. Use plain, moist gauze packing and leave initial packing for 48 hours.
- If abscess is large and/or deep, place a Malecot or equivalent drain sutured in place.

Thrombosed Hemorrhoids

54

RICHARD E. BURNEY

Based on the previous edition chapter "Thrombosed Hemorrhoids" by Richard E. Burney

Presentation

A 49-year-old obese male presents to the emergency department with a complaint of severe anal pain for the past 24 hours. He has not had this problem before. Over the counter pain medication has not helped. He has a history of constipation and recently returned from a business trip. Past medical history includes Type 2 diabetes, hypertension, and hyperlipidemia. He reports being compliant with medications prescribed for these conditions, including an oral hypoglycemic agent, aspirin, a statin agent, and a beta-blocker.

On examination, he is afebrile. He has an exquisitely tender, swollen, edematous mass at the anal verge, with bluish discoloration, about 1.5 to 2 cm in diameter. There is no apparent cellulitis or erythema. He does not allow digital rectal examination.

● DIFFERENTIAL DIAGNOSIS

The most likely diagnosis in this man is an acutely thrombosed external hemorrhoid (Figure 54-1). Other possibilities in decreasing order of probability include: (1) prolapsed edematous internal hemorrhoid (Figure 54-2); (2) chronically prolapsed hemorrhoid (Figure 54-3); (3) perianal abscess; (4) prolapsed, strangulated internal hemorrhoid (Figure 54-4); (5) acute hemorrhoidal inflammation and edema brought on by constipation (Figure 54-5). (6) inflamed anal tag with or without associated inflammatory bowel disease; (7) infarcted hemorrhoid (Figure 54-6); (8) prolapsed anal polyp; and (9) acute anal fissure, with an edematous sentinel tag.

● WORKUP

Additional questions regarding patient's normal bowel habit, management of his chronic constipation, and medications are warranted. It is important to determine if he regularly strains when moving his bowels. The diagnosis is almost always made on the basis of physical examination. To do a good examination, the patient is best placed in prone jackknife position on a sigmoidoscopy table and examined under good light with the buttock spread apart. If a sigmoidoscopy table is not available, the patient can be placed in prone, jackknife position lying facedown with rolled blankets under the hips to elevate the buttocks. Laboratory and imaging studies are rarely helpful unless the patient has a fever or at the time of examination, an abscess seems likely. On rare occasion, examination may have to be facilitated by sedation or local

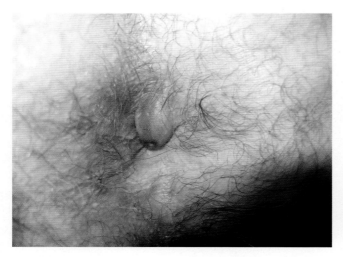

FIGURE 54-1. Thrombosed external hemorrhoid: characteristic appearance.

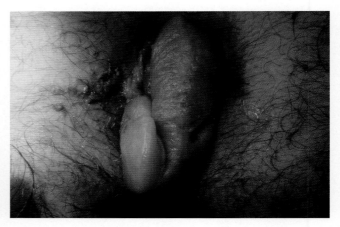

FIGURE 54-2. Chronically prolapsed mixed internal/external hemorrhoid. Bluish discoloration in places suggests underlying thromboses, but do NOT try to I&D this.

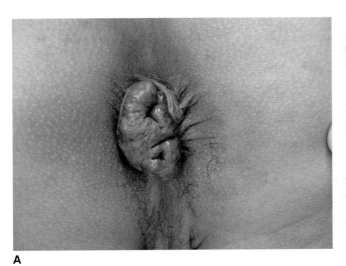

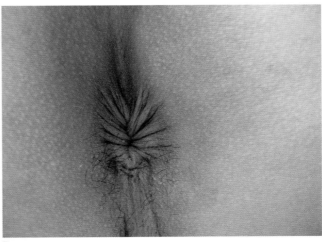

A   **B**

FIGURE 54-3. **A,B:** Chronically prolapsed left lateral internal hemorrhoid. This is NOT a thrombosed external hemorrhoid. It was manually reduced under local anesthesia, shown in **(B)**.

anesthetic injection, or evaluation under spinal or general anesthesia done in the operating room.

● DIAGNOSIS AND TREATMENT

The diagnosis in this patient, based on history and physical examination, is thrombosed external hemorrhoid. This condition, although painful, is self-limited. Although surgical treatment, consisting of incision and evacuation of clots, is something that could be done, it is not required. This is particularly true if the thrombosis is more than 48 to 72 hours old, by which time the acute inflammation and swelling are beginning to abate. With observation and attention to a proper diet, the hemorrhoidal thrombosis will reabsorb and the swelling will subside, leaving no sequelae. There is a common misconception that thrombosed hemorrhoids are

an indication that there is some kind of underlying hemorrhoidal or other disease. This is not true.

● SURGICAL APPROACH

If the acute thrombosis is <48 hours old and/or is quite large, such that one can anticipate it will take weeks for the swelling to subside, surgical treatment may be offered. The simplest and most efficacious, as well as expedient, surgical treatment is incision and evacuation of clot. This procedure can be done under local anesthesia in the office, clinic, or emergency department (Figure 54-7).

One per cent lidocaine with epinephrine is infiltrated through a very fine needle slowly into the dermis overlying the hemorrhoid. The skin will blanch as this is done. Infiltrating the subcutaneous tissue is not effective. It is not usually necessary to do a

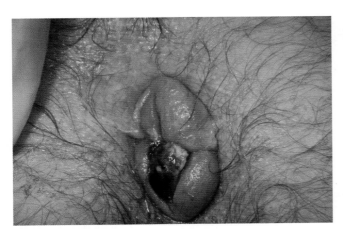

FIGURE 54-4. Prolapsed, strangulated internal hemorrhoid referred after I&D had been attempted in error. This was reduced in clinic under anal block anesthesia and eventually resolved without surgery.

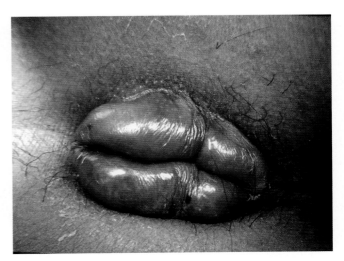

FIGURE 54-5. Acutely edematous hemorrhoids secondary to constipation and straining. Do not attempt to I&D.

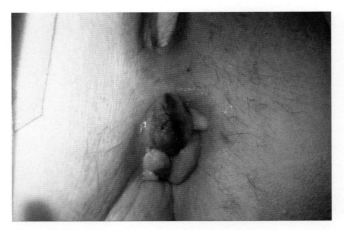

FIGURE 54-6. Infarcted mixed internal/external hemorrhoid. This was excised in the operating room.

deeper block. Allow 2 to 5 minutes for the anesthetic to take effect. An ellipse of skin is excised over the area of thrombosis, oriented to give the best exposure to the underlying thrombus. Simple, linear incision does not provide adequate exposure. Numerous small thrombi are usually present. They are intravascular, in small hemorrhoidal veins, and there are usually 3 to 6 of them. The thrombi are evacuated with a fine hemostat. The skin incision is left open. A longer-acting local anesthetic agent such as bupivacaine may be infiltrated as well. Postoperative care consists of an outer dressing to absorb any drainage, sitz baths or moist applications, and nonsteroidal pain medications. Antibiotics are not needed.

The chief potential pitfall is failure to make the correct diagnosis. Prolapsed, thrombosed, or strangulated internal hemorrhoids have been mistaken for thrombosed external hemorrhoids, leading to painful errors in management (Figure 54-4 is an example). Thrombosed external hemorrhoids are covered with dry, keratinized, normal-appearing skin, not mucosa. If this is not the case, consider another diagnosis. Other potential pitfalls are failure to have adequate lighting, assistance, and exposure, which will make the procedure more difficult, and failure to adequately anesthetize the skin overlying the thrombosed hemorrhoid or to wait long enough for the local anesthetic to be effective (at least 2 minutes); failure to make an elliptical or lanceolate incision that exposes all the thrombosed veins; and failure to carefully and completely evacuate each small thrombus (Table 54-1).

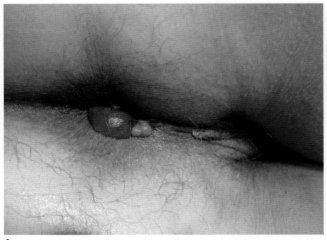

A

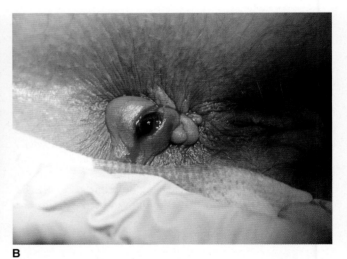

B

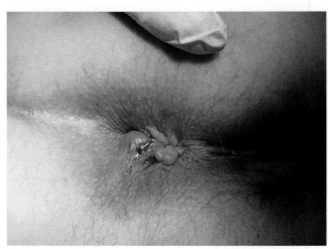

C

FIGURE 54-7. **A–C:** Incision and drainage of thrombosed external hemorrhoid. Note that ellipse of skin has been excised over the thrombosis giving good exposure. After thrombectomy, there is still residual swelling. No sutures are required.

Table 54-1	Incision and Evacuation of Hemorrhoidal Thrombi

Key Technical Steps

1. Arrange good exposure and good light. Have an assistant present.
2. If sedation is used, appropriate monitoring of blood pressure, pulse oxygen, and cardiac rhythm must be in place.
3. Infiltrate local anesthetic with epinephrine slowly and widely into the overlying dermis observing the skin as it blanches. Wait 2–5 minutes for the anesthetic agent to work.
4. Excise a generous ellipse of overlying skin to expose the thrombi.
5. Extract thrombi individually with a fine-pointed, mosquito hemostat.
6. Do not close the incision; cover with slightly moistened gauze dressing.
7. Add additional long-acting local anesthetic if desired.

Potential Pitfalls

- Incorrect diagnosis.
- Inadequate lighting, assistance, and/or exposure.
- Inadequate local anesthesia.
- Incision that does not expose all thrombi.
- Failure to extract all thrombi individually from hemorrhoidal veins.

● SPECIAL INTRAOPERATIVE CONSIDERATIONS

If you find after gaining good exposure and lighting that you are not dealing with a thrombosed external hemorrhoid, but rather with prolapsed, strangulated internal hemorrhoids (Figure 54-4) or other condition, such as abscess, the patient may need to be evaluated in the operating room under better anesthesia, such as subarachnoid block.

● POSTOPERATIVE MANAGEMENT

No special postoperative management is needed. The patient may keep a moist gauze dressing over the operative site, which usually closes within a day or two. It will, however, be painful when the local anesthetic wears off, and remain so for several days. It is a good idea to explain this to the patient. Stool softener and instructions for high-fiber diet should be given. There is no reason to subject the patient to additional examinations, such as colonoscopy. Thrombosed external hemorrhoids are rarely associated with underlying pathology of any kind, including internal hemorrhoids.

TAKE HOME POINTS

- First, be sure you have the right diagnosis. Remember that not all thrombosed hemorrhoids need surgical treatment; the majority do not.
- Treatment does not lead to rapid resolution of symptoms, especially if the thrombosis is more than 72 hours old.
- If you do decide to evacuate thrombi, have adequate positioning, light, and assistance. Infiltrate local anesthetic slowly but widely into the skin. Take an ellipse of overlying skin and extract all the thrombi individually.
- Explain to the patient that there will be continued pain and swelling for several days despite what you have done.

Breast

Palpable Breast Mass

55

JENNIFER YU AND JULIE A. MARGENTHALER

Based on the previous edition chapter "Palpable Breast Mass" by
Travis E. Grotz, Sandhya Pruthi, and James W. Jakub

Presentation

A 30-year-old female presented to the clinic for evaluation
of a new left breast mass. She discovered the mass approximately 1 month prior to presentation, and she stated that it
had not changed significantly in size since she found it. The
patient denied any change from baseline in the appearance
of her breasts. She also denied any pain, nipple discharge,
skin changes, or masses in her right breast. She had no systemic complaints and was otherwise healthy. The patient
had her menarche at age 9 and had been pregnant twice
resulting in 1 child at the age of 27. She was still menstruat-
ing, with her last menstrual cycle approximately 2 weeks
prior to presentation. She denied any history of hormone
replacement but had been using oral contraceptives for
the previous 3 years. She was on no other medications and
was a healthy young woman. Her mother was diagnosed
with cervical cancer at the age of 34 and with breast cancer at the age of 54. Bilateral breast examination revealed
normal ptotic breasts bilaterally. A firm, palpable mass measuring 2.5 cm was noted in the upper outer quadrant of
the left breast at the one-thirty position, approximately 6 cm
from the nipple–areolar border. The mass was not attached
to the overlying skin or underlying pectoralis. Examination
of the left axilla also revealed a palpable but mobile lymph
node measuring 2 cm. The right breast exam was normal
without any dominant masses, skin changes, nipple discharge, or axillary adenopathy.

● DIFFERENTIAL DIAGNOSIS

As one of the most common breast presentations, palpable
breast masses are most frequently benign in nature, but
timely evaluation and diagnosis are critical to exclude malignancy. Possible benign etiologies include fibroadenoma,
cyst, fat necrosis, or fibrocystic changes. Fibroadenomas are
solid lesions, which most often present in younger women
(age < 35) and are firm, mobile, and well-defined masses.
Though fibroadenomas are generally painless, some patients
may have discomfort given that fibroadenomas can vary in
size and may present as single or multiple nodules. Cysts are
also usually smooth, discrete masses but are fluid-filled and
may be compressible. Cysts may cause breast pain or tenderness, particularly at the beginning of the menstrual cycle,

and can also wax and wane in size. Fat necrosis of the breast
most commonly occurs due to blunt trauma, an operative
procedure, or other treatment interventions such as radiation. Since this can present as an ill-defined, palpable mass, it
is important to clearly discern the patient's medical and surgical history to determine what diagnostic measures would be
appropriate. Associated physical signs may include ecchymosis, pain, or skin tethering. Fibrocystic changes are most commonly found in premenopausal women but less commonly
present as a dominant mass. Patients may note lumpiness of
the breast or increased nodularity, which can fluctuate with
the menstrual cycle. Symptoms may be bilateral and most
frequently occur in the upper outer breast. Breast pain or discomfort, while uncommon, can also be associated with fibrocystic changes, particularly when symptoms occur just prior
to menstruation. Finally, phyllodes tumor is a unique lesion
that should be considered in this setting. These are rare, usually benign, fibroepithelial breast tumors that can be mistaken for fibroadenomas, and the majority present as smooth,
well-circumscribed, and painless masses, which can grow to
extremely large sizes. Though malignant transformation is
unusual, a high level of suspicion should be maintained when
considering the diagnostic workup and surgical resection.

Malignant lesions may present with a variety of physical findings, and while most cancers in areas with breast
screening programs are found secondary to abnormal mammograms, up to 45% of patients may have palpable tumors
either not detected by mammogram or found in the interval between mammograms. Signs suggestive of malignancy
include hard, immobile, ill-defined masses with fixation to
the chest wall, nipple retraction, asymmetry, or associated
lymphadenopathy. Skin findings such as dimpling, peau
d'orange, or erythema should also increase concern for possible inflammatory breast cancer.

Despite the low likelihood of malignancy in palpable
breast lesions, no single clinical finding is absolutely sensitive
or specific in differentiating between benign and malignant
disease. Therefore, palpable masses should always be evaluated with appropriate imaging and/or tissue biopsy confirmation as needed before giving a diagnosis.

● WORKUP

A full clinical history and physical exam should be the first
step in the evaluation of any patient with a new palpable

breast mass. Specifically, the patient should be queried on the time course of the lesion: how long it has been present, if any changes have occurred over time, and if there are any associated symptoms. Medication history should focus upon prior use of hormonal supplements or oral contraceptives, and family history must determine what types of cancer may be present in the patient's family members as well as ages at diagnosis.

Despite the recent controversy regarding the benefit of physical breast exams in breast cancer screening, it remains critical to perform a thorough exam with documentation of findings for all patients presenting with new breast symptoms. The clinical breast exam is a standard method used to systematically assess the breasts through inspection and palpation. The breasts should be examined with the patient in the sitting and supine positions, and observations should be made of any asymmetry, skin changes, or nipple findings such as inversion, retraction, or discharge. Palpation should include a bimanual examination of the entire breast area, including the axillary tail, and the regional lymph node basins (i.e., axillary, supraclavicular, infraclavicular, cervical). Timely documentation of the location, size, and nature of a palpable mass is necessary in coordinating any multidisciplinary assessment and management.

Following the clinical exam, diagnostic breast imaging is the next appropriate step in the workup of a dominant mass. When requesting imaging studies, it is important to make the distinction between diagnostic and screening imaging—given that there is a concerning finding on exam, the clinician should specify that diagnostic imaging is

needed, thereby communicating to the radiologist that additional spot compression or magnification views are needed. Diagnostic bilateral mammogram is the imaging study of choice and provides a highly sensitive and cost-efficient method of evaluation. Alternatively, in young women with clinically benign findings, it is reasonable to pursue directed ultrasound as the initial imaging study given the higher likelihood of nodular or dense breast tissue in this population of patients. Ultrasound is also frequently ordered with mammography since this provides additional information regarding the size and structure of the mass, if solid or cystic features are present, and potentially the nature of any nearby lymph nodes. Lastly, magnetic resonance imaging (MRI) is a diagnostic imaging modality, which is generally reserved for patients in whom mammography and ultrasound are not able to fully characterize the extent of disease or demonstrate discordant findings. Despite its high sensitivity, MRI is not appropriate as an initial imaging study since it has a significant false-positive rate and can lead to unnecessary biopsies.

Patients with a significant personal or family history of breast cancer should be referred to genetic testing to evaluate for the risk of a hereditary syndrome, such as BRCA1 or BRCA2. Several risk calculators are available online, and patients with elevated scores should be counseled regarding testing for familial mutations. Though uncommon in the general population, identification of a hereditary cancer syndrome may affect surgical management and subsequent therapy.

Given our patient's new palpable left breast mass on exam, she underwent bilateral diagnostic mammograms (Figure 55-1) and ultrasound (Figure 55-2)—the right breast

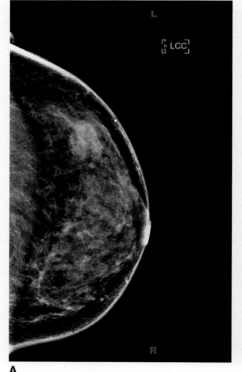
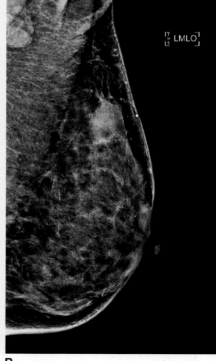

FIGURE 55-1. Diagnostic mammograms—left craniocaudal (LCC) view **(A)** and left mediolateral oblique (LMLO) view **(B)**.

A

B

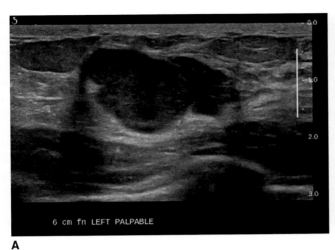
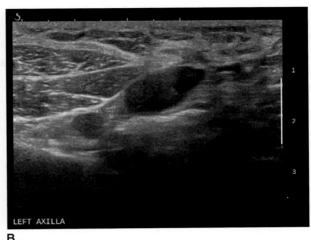

FIGURE 55-2. Ultrasound—**A:** primary left breast mass, **B:** left axillary lymph node.

was given a BI-RADS category I and the left breast was given a category V. The palpable mass corresponded with a 2.4 -cm hypoechoic lesion, located 6 cm from the nipple in the upper outer quadrant at the 12:30 position. Left axillary ultrasound also revealed a lymph node with a thickened cortex. The patient then subsequently underwent an ultrasound-guided core needle biopsy (CNB) of the left breast lesion and a fine needle aspiration (FNA) biopsy of the left axillary lymph node.

● DIAGNOSIS AND TREATMENT

Per the American Society of Breast Surgeons consensus statement, the preoperative diagnosis of breast cancer by minimally invasive methods (i.e., needle biopsy) is preferred over open surgical biopsy. This patient-centered approach is both efficient and effective, since it provides the opportunity to decide upon the need for concurrent axillary lymph node surgery while also increasing the probability of negative margins during the index procedure. Preoperative diagnosis of malignancy also assists the provider team in deciding if any further imaging is necessary or if the patient may benefit from systemic therapy prior to surgery. The surgeon, radiologist, and pathologist must be in close communication regarding concordance between clinical exam, imaging, and biopsy results, and surgical excisional biopsy may be necessary for lesions which have discordant findings. For breast lesions, CNB is generally preferred over FNA since CNB can provide the additional information of histologic architecture, marker analysis, and staining for immunohistochemistry. Placement of a clip or other markers at the time of biopsy is critical to guide future localization of the lesion, particularly if neoadjuvant therapy is planned, since treatment may cause the tumor to regress substantially and result in loss of the original target. FNA of any suspicious lymph nodes is highly useful in axillary staging and can guide surgical planning for sentinel lymph node biopsy.

Pathology from our patient's biopsy revealed grade 3 invasive ductal carcinoma with associated grade 3 ductal carcinoma in situ (DCIS). Immunohistochemistry was positive for estrogen receptor, negative for progesterone receptor, and equivocal for expression of human epidermal growth factor receptor 2 (HER2). Fluorescence in situ hybridization (FISH) testing was positive for HER2 gene amplification. The patient then underwent breast MRI (Figure 55-3) to better evaluate the full extent of disease, and results were consistent with the known malignancy. Lastly, FNA of the left axillary lymph node demonstrated adenocarcinoma, correlating with the patient's primary breast lesion.

Since no evidence of distant disease was present on clinical assessment, the patient did not undergo additional imaging. However, skeletal scintigraphy, computed tomography (CT), and fluorodeoxyglucose positron-emission tomography (FDG-PET) scanning are all modalities which can be utilized to evaluate any suspicion of metastatic involvement.

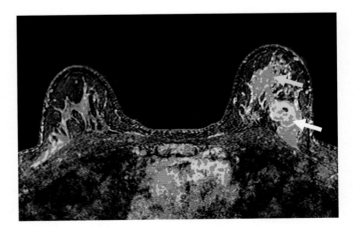

FIGURE 55-3. Breast MRI. The *white arrow* indicates the palpable mass in the left breast with MR enhancement kinetics demonstrating a washout pattern consistent with malignancy. The surrounding tissue, indicated by the *yellow arrow*, shows normal breast parenchymal enhancement.

The principles of treatment are multimodal, and surgical options include either breast conservation therapy (BCT) or mastectomy. Operative decision-making should be based upon a candid discussion of the patient's preferences and the surgeon's assessment of the patient's breast and tumor characteristics as well as the necessary follow-up care. Since BCT frequently entails radiation therapy following surgery, the surgeon should consider patient compliance with the radiation regimen and if the patient has any contraindications to radiation. For patients who are highly motivated for BCT but who are not candidates due to a large tumor-to-breast size ratio, neoadjuvant chemotherapy may be employed via hormonal therapy or systemic cytotoxic therapy, and the patient should be referred to medical oncology for evaluation. Alternatively, if the patient desires mastectomy and breast reconstruction, consultation with a plastic surgeon will provide the patient with possible options for immediate or delayed reconstruction.

● SURGICAL APPROACH

Our patient strongly desired breast conservation, and she underwent 6 cycles of neoadjuvant chemotherapy with HER2 targeted therapy with substantial tumor regression. Regarding the patient's clinical N1 status, the standard approach to posttherapy axillary staging is to perform a complete axillary dissection. However, surgical management of the axilla following neoadjuvant chemotherapy in initial node-positive patients is evolving, and recent evidence has shown that the reliability of sentinel lymph node biopsy may be comparable to axillary dissection. Given our patient's excellent response to neoadjuvant chemotherapy, she was therefore considered a candidate for sentinel lymph node biopsy for formal axillary staging in addition to partial mastectomy with needle localization.

For sentinel lymph node biopsy, a dual-agent method provides the highest rate of success in sentinel node identification. Preoperatively on the day of surgery, the patient will undergo injection of radioactive colloid into the skin or parenchyma of the breast, with or without subsequent lymphoscintigraphy. Blue dye, either dilute isosulfan blue or methylene blue, is then injected in the breast at the start of surgery. The accuracy of sentinel lymph node biopsy is comparable with a variety of injection sites (e.g., peritumoral, retroareolar, subdermal), and the breast should be massaged vigorously for 5 minutes following injection. When performed in combination with a breast-conserving procedure, sentinel lymph node biopsy is usually carried out via a separate curvilinear incision made at the edge of the axillary hairline. After carrying the incision down through the clavipectoral fascia, a blue lymphatic channel can be identified and followed to a lymph node. In addition to visual inspection for blue lymphatic channels or if no blue channels are found, the gamma probe should also be utilized to detect the area of maximal radioactivity, which can help isolate the sentinel node. Additional nodes, which have radioactivity

counts that are 10% or more of the sentinel node's count, should be excised and submitted for pathologic evaluation.

Incision for a partial mastectomy should be made in consideration of the location of the tumor in the breast and the method of localization. Tumors located in the upper half of the breast can be reached via curvilinear or transverse incisions, while those in the lower half may be best accessed through a radial incision. The incision should also be planned with awareness of the patient's possible need for later mastectomy, with avoidance of tunneling under the skin. Once the tumor specimen has been excised, it should be oriented in at least two dimensions, and particular attention must be paid to achieving hemostasis in the wound bed prior to closure.

To optimize the partial mastectomy procedure, a variety of techniques are currently utilized to assist the surgeon in tumor localization. Particularly for nonpalpable lesions, methods, such as placement of wire, biopsy clips, and radioactive tracer or seed marking and ultrasound, have shown benefit in directing the excision. With palpable masses, these techniques may still be of use in achieving clear margins on resection when used in conjunction with intraoperative palpation of the tumor. Wire or needle localization requires preoperative coordination with radiology, where a flexible wire or a needle is placed under mammographic or sonographic guidance into the lesion on the day of surgery. The patient must then be cautioned against excessive movement to avoid dislodging the wire before being taken to the operating room. Similarly, another preoperative method involves the injection of a radioactive tracer or placement of a radioactive seed into the lesion by nuclear medicine under radiologic guidance. The tracer, composed of technetium-99m–labeled particles of human serum albumin, is injected into the lesion no more than 24 hours prior to surgery, while the seed, made of titanium containing ^{125}I, can be placed up to 5 days beforehand. During the procedure, the surgeon then uses a handheld gamma probe to detect the radiation emitted by the tracer or seed, and the margins of excision are defined by where the radioactivity declines substantially.

Intraoperatively, ultrasound is a convenient and efficient tool, which can assist the surgeon in determining the boundaries of the lesion and has been shown to decrease the rate of positive margins, though this method can only be utilized for tumors which are detectable sonographically. Additional intraoperative options include frozen section or imprint cytology analysis, which both involve rapid pathologic assessment of margins and can prompt the surgeon to resect additional tissue at a compromised margin during the same procedure. Finally, cavity shave margins entail the resection of tissue from all six margins of the wound cavity immediately following excision of the main tumor. Though this technique does not provide intraoperative feedback on margin status, routine cavity shave margins have been shown to significantly decrease the rate of positive margins and of subsequent re-excision procedures. However, it may increase the length of operating time during the index procedure and does result in a larger volume of excised tissue. The ultimate impact of this on patient

Table 55-1	Partial Mastectomy with Sentinel Lymph Node Biopsy

Key Technical Steps

1. Preoperative coordination with radiology and nuclear medicine for breast lesion and axillary node localization
2. Peri- or subareolar blue dye injection and breast massage
3. Partial mastectomy incision placement with consideration of the potential need for later mastectomy
4. Intraoperative utilization of localization techniques in addition to palpation
5. Axillary sentinel lymph node identification via dual-agent method
6. Removal of all axillary nodes with gamma radiation count ≥10% of sentinel lymph node
7. Aggressive hemostasis with electrocautery
8. Inspection of specimen radiograph for biopsy clip, calcifications, and margin status

Potential Pitfalls

- Lack of identification of the sentinel node
- Inadequate hemostasis of partial mastectomy or sentinel lymph node biopsy wound cavities
- Concern for close or positive margins on specimen radiograph

outcomes remains under debate, since studies have not shown a correlation with worse cosmetic outcome due to shave margins (Table 55-1).

SPECIAL INTRAOPERATIVE CONSIDERATIONS

Several potential situations may arise which require modification of the surgical plan. For palpable lesions, localization is less challenging, but it is important to consider changes in approach when preoperative localization does not provide sufficient guidance. Wire placement is one of the most commonly utilized mechanisms due to its ease of use and relatively inexpensive implementation, but there is a substantial risk of wire movement or displacement as the patient is prepared for surgery. If this occurs before the lesion can be removed, alternative tools such as ultrasound should be employed to better define the boundaries for excision. Additionally, close examination of the specimen radiograph is warranted, particularly in cases where localization of the lesion is difficult. During the patient's preoperative needle biopsy, clip placement is highly recommended to mark the biopsy site, since, not infrequently, the area of malignancy is nearly completely removed by the biopsy itself or the patient undergoes neoadjuvant chemotherapy with complete response. The inspection of the specimen radiograph for the inclusion of the biopsy clip is critical and should be instituted as standard practice. The specimen should also always be marked in at least two dimensions, using clips, stitches, or

inking by the surgeon. Other margin assessment techniques such as frozen section, imprint cytology, or cavity shave margins may further direct the surgeon if wire localization is unsuccessful.

Another possible pitfall, which may be encountered, includes failure to identify the sentinel lymph node. While this is rare, it emphasizes the importance of using the dual-agent method to find the sentinel node. Prior ipsilateral breast or axillary procedures may result in disruption of the lymphatic system and result in failed mapping. In this situation, complete axillary dissection of level I/II lymph nodes is indicated for axillary staging.

POSTOPERATIVE MANAGEMENT

Partial mastectomy with or without sentinel lymph node biopsy is generally performed as an outpatient procedure, and the patient is seen in the clinic for postoperative evaluation 2 to 4 weeks later. In the acute postoperative setting, bleeding with hematoma formation is the most common cause for return to the operating room. This emphasizes the importance of achieving aggressive hemostasis with electrocautery prior to wound closure. Other important exam findings to note include cellulitis, seroma, or upper extremity lymphedema. Arm morbidity is less common with breast-conserving procedures compared to mastectomy and also less common with sentinel lymph node biopsy compared to axillary dissection—however, patients should be counseled regarding the still present risk of this complication.

Adjuvant therapy following primary surgical treatment is based upon multidisciplinary coordination of care. Tumor characteristics, nodal status, the patient's health state, and comorbidities play a significant role in determining the appropriate postoperative treatment plan, involving the breast surgeon, radiation oncologist, and medical oncologist. Hormonal therapy, radiation, or chemotherapy may be recommended depending upon each individual patient's tumor biology and surgical treatment.

Following partial mastectomy for invasive cancer, radiation therapy is commonly administered, either through whole breast or accelerated partial breast regimens. If systemic chemotherapy is advised, it is usually administered prior to starting radiation. A physical exam and diagnostic bilateral mammogram should be performed 6 months after the completion of all the therapy to establish a new baseline. The patient may then be followed annually with clinical exam and mammography for surveillance.

TAKE HOME POINTS

- The majority of palpable masses are benign, but there are no specific clinical findings which can differentiate between benign and malignant lesions.
- All patients presenting with palpable lesions should undergo appropriate workup, including diagnostic imaging with or without tissue biopsy (Figure 55-4).

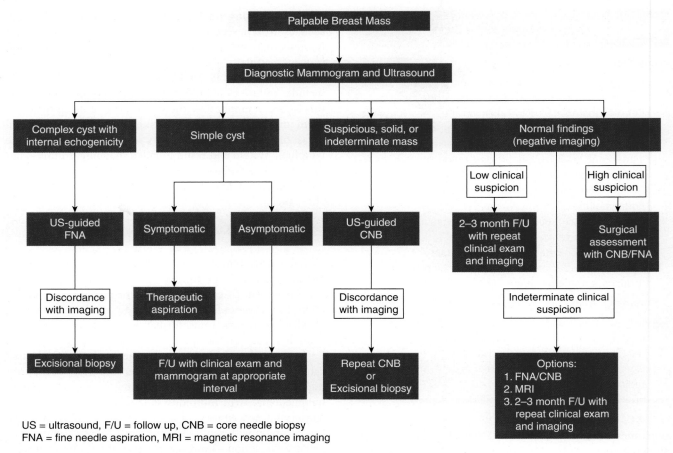

US = ultrasound, F/U = follow up, CNB = core needle biopsy
FNA = fine needle aspiration, MRI = magnetic resonance imaging

FIGURE 55-4. Palpable breast mass diagnostic algorithm.

- Minimally invasive needle biopsy is recommended as the first approach to obtaining a tissue diagnosis, followed by surgical excisional biopsy if needle biopsy results are inconclusive or discordant with imaging or clinical exam.
- Preoperative needle biopsy of both the primary tumor and any concerning lymph nodes optimizes surgical management, reduces the need for multistage procedures, and provides useful staging information for either neoadjuvant or adjuvant therapy planning. Clips should be placed in the biopsy site to assist in intraoperative identification of the lesion.
- Localization with wire placement, radioactive seed/tracer injection, or ultrasound may be helpful adjuncts in defining the boundaries of excision.
- Partial mastectomy incisions should be curvilinear or transverse in the upper half of the breast and should be curvilinear or radial in the lower half. The incision site should be cosmetically placed where it can be incorporated into a later mastectomy incision if necessary.
- The dual-agent method (blue dye, radioactive colloid) should be utilized to increase the likelihood of successful identification of the sentinel lymph node.
- Examination of the specimen radiograph provides critical confirmation of adequate excision, and the radiograph should be evaluated for inclusion of any preoperative biopsy clips and for margin status.

SUGGESTED READINGS

Dillon MF, Hill ADK, Quinn CM, O'Doherty A, McDermott EW, O'Higgins N. The accuracy of ultrasound, stereotactic, and clinical core biopsies in the diagnosis of breast cancer, with an analysis of false-negative cases. *Ann Surg.* 2005;242(5):701-707.

Goldfeder S, Davis D, Cullinan J. Breast specimen radiography: can it predict margin status of excised breast carcinoma? *Acad Radiol.* 2006;13(12):1453-1459.

McMasters KM, Tuttle TM, Carlson DJ, et al. Sentinel lymph node biopsy for breast cancer: a suitable alternative to routine axillary dissection in multi-institutional practice when optimal technique is used. *J Clin Oncol Off J Am Soc Clin Oncol.* 2000;18(13):2560-2566.

Morrow M. The evaluation of common breast problems. *Am Fam Physician.* 2000;61(8):2371-2378, 2385.

Pruthi S. Detection and evaluation of a palpable breast mass. *Mayo Clin Proc.* 2001;76(6):641-648.

Suspicious Mammographic Abnormality

56

EMILIA J. DIEGO

Based on the previous edition chapter "Suspicious Mammographic Abnormality" by Catherine E. Pesce and Lisa K. Jacobs

Presentation

A 50-year-old postmenopausal female is without breast complaints when she presents for her annual screening mammogram. Risk assessment reveals that she had menarche at 14, first pregnancy at 25, and menopause at 47. She is G2P2. She has never had a breast biopsy/procedure. Family history is significant for a paternal grandmother with postmenopausal breast cancer. She reports that she is in her usual state of health.

Physical examination reveals no palpable masses, skin changes, nipple changes, or supraclavicular, infraclavicular, or axillary adenopathy. She has a BMI of 29 and a breast cup size of C.

Screening mammogram reveals indeterminate calcifications in the lower inner quadrant of the left breast. She is recalled for diagnostic imaging, and further magnification views reveal a span of pleomorphic, clustered calcifications in the posterior aspect of the left breast (Figures 56-1 and 56-2).

● DIFFERENTIAL DIAGNOSIS

Calcifications seen on mammogram can take on different characteristics. Clustered, branching linear or pleomorphic calcifications should be viewed with suspicion. Additionally, previously present calcifications that have increased in prominence and number should further be evaluated. This is in contradistinction to calcifications that are well-rounded, solitary, diffuse and bilateral.

Patients with calcifications on mammogram have a 1.68-fold relative risk of breast cancer compared to patients without calcifications.

The differential diagnosis of calcifications seen on mammogram may be categorized according to the results of image-guided percutaneous biopsy.

Malignant pathology: these findings on percutaneous biopsy require a discussion with the patient regarding definitive oncologic, multidisciplinary management.

- Invasive ductal carcinoma
- Ductal carcinoma in situ
- Pleomorphic lobular carcinoma in situ

High-risk pathology: recommendations and management of these high-risk lesions continue to evolve with improvement in imaging and biopsy techniques. Surgical excisional biopsies are frequently performed in this setting to exclude malignancy, with the understanding that the rate of diagnosing an unexpected malignant pathology (upstaging) varies from 3% to 30% depending upon the type of lesion as well as biopsy technique, retrieval of targeted calcifications, and presence of residual calcifications on postbiopsy imaging. These pathologic findings in the absence of upstaging to carcinoma are known to confer a higher risk for future breast cancer in these patients.

- Atypical ductal hyperplasia
- Lobular neoplasia
- Papillomas, with or without atypia

Benign pathology: in the setting of radiologic–pathologic concordance, these lesions do not require surgical excision and do not appear to confer an increased risk for future breast cancer.

- Fibrocystic changes
- Sclerosing adenosis
- Fibroadenoma/fibroadenomatoid changes
- Fat necrosis
- Dermal calcifications
- Vascular calcifications

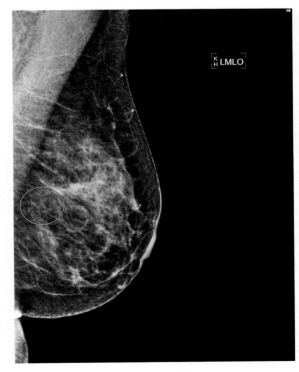

FIGURE 56-1 Left MLO view: screening mammogram.

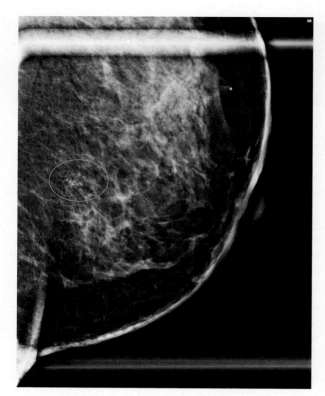

FIGURE 56-2 Left magnification ML view: diagnostic mammogram.

Other potential abnormalities that are identified on mammogram include masses, asymmetries, or architectural distortions.

● WORKUP

The workup for an asymptomatic patient with suspicious imaging includes a thorough history with particular attention paid to risk assessment, to include patient age, menstrual and obstetrical history, history of previous biopsies, and family history. Signs and symptoms to inquire include masses, skin changes, nipple inversion, or nipple discharge.

Abnormalities seen on screening mammogram should be further worked up with diagnostic imaging to characterize the findings. Magnification views help better visualize the calcifications and its morphology. Spot compression views can determine if asymmetries or architectural distortions are overlapping breast tissue, as well as better visualize mass borders.

Ultrasound and magnetic resonance imaging (MRI) can be useful adjunct screening tools in select populations of women, including those with dense breasts or with estimated lifetime risks of breast cancer exceeding 20%.

Breast imaging results are reported in a standardized fashion according to the Breast Imaging Reporting and Data System (BI-RADS) that was developed by the American College of Radiology (Table 56-1).

A percutaneous biopsy is recommended when an abnormality seen on imaging is classified as suspicious or highly

Table 56-1	Breast Imaging Reporting and Data System (BI-RADS) Classification	
BI-RADS 1	Negative	Routine follow-up recommended
BI-RADS 2	Benign findings	Routine follow-up recommended
BI-RADS 3	Probably benign findings	Likelihood of malignancy <2%. Short-term follow-up is usually recommended
BI-RADS 4	Suspicious abnormality	Likelihood of malignancy 2%–94%
BI-RADS 5	Highly suggestive of malignancy	Likelihood of malignancy >94%
BI-RADS 6	Biopsy-proven malignancy	Appropriate action should be taken

suggestive of malignancy (BI-RADS 4 or 5) (Figures 56-3 and 56-4). Current standards dictate that surgical excision should not be performed without a prior percutaneous biopsy when possible, as results will dictate the conduct of the operation.

Another important component of the workup of abnormalities seen on imaging includes radiology–pathology correlation. In addition to recommending surgical intervention for malignant or high-risk lesions, excision should also be considered for benign pathology that is found to be discordant with breast imaging.

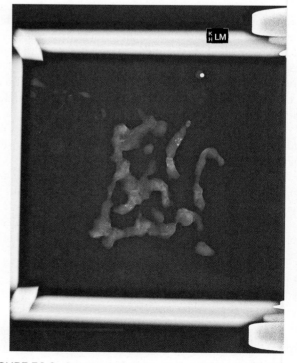

FIGURE 56-3. Specimen radiograph from stereotactic biopsy demonstrating retrieval of targeted calcifications.

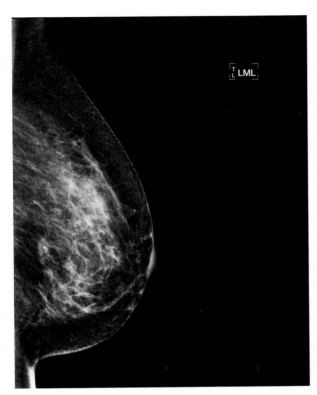

FIGURE 56-4. Postbiopsy mammogram demonstrating appropriate clip placement after the procedure.

DIAGNOSIS AND TREATMENT

For a diagnosis of breast malignancy, the standard approaches to breast surgery include a partial mastectomy or total mastectomy, with or without reconstruction. In patients who desire breast conservation but require a larger volume of tissue to be excised and have significant breast volume, an oncoplastic approach to resection may be feasible. "No tumor on ink" is considered an adequate margin for patients with invasive cancer based upon recent consensus statements included in the suggested readings. For patients with in situ carcinoma, a 2-mm margin is considered adequate with an individualized approach to patients with a single close margin, again based upon consensus statements in the suggested readings.

With appropriate patient selection, there is no difference in survival between breast conservation and total mastectomy. Patients who may not be candidates for breast conservation include those with multicentric disease, inflammatory breast cancer, pregnancy (if delivery is not feasible prior to initiation of radiation treatment), or large tumor-to-breast size ratio. Whole breast radiation is usually recommended after breast conservation. Therefore, one must be cognizant of potential contraindications to breast conservation as some patients may be ineligible for postsurgical radiation therapy, including collagen vascular diseases, genetic mutations that increase risk for secondary malignancy with radiation therapy, or history of previous breast radiation.

For this patient with a likely diagnosis of ductal carcinoma in situ, the presence of small volume disease and no contraindications to whole breast radiation make her an excellent candidate for breast conservation therapy.

Axillary staging with a sentinel lymph node biopsy would be indicated in patients with a clinically node-negative axilla and a percutaneous biopsy demonstrating invasive carcinoma. A sentinel lymph node biopsy may be considered in patients with a diagnosis of in situ carcinoma as well based upon patient/clinical or pathologic factors but is not routinely recommended.

SURGICAL APPROACH

When breast conservation will be used as the surgical approach, preoperative localization of nonpalpable lesions is essential with the marker of choice at the discretion of the surgeon/institutional practices. There are several localization tools available to date including wires, radioactive seeds, and electromagnetic reflectors. Intraoperative ultrasound localization may also be used based upon surgeon comfort with the technique. The approach to an excisional breast biopsy would be similar except that volume of tissue removed may be significantly less as the procedure is for diagnostic purposes and negative margins are not a goal of the operation.

Choice of incision is key. Very often, the oncologic outcome does not have to significantly affect cosmetic considerations. When incisions are to be done above the nipple, transverse or curvilinear incisions have excellent cosmesis. In patients with lesions that are centrally located or accessible from a periareolar approach, it is ideal to perform these incisions as it also leads to superior cosmetic outcomes. Incisions below the level of the nipple are best done in a radial fashion, because scar contracture can lead to displacement of the nipple if a transverse or curvilinear incision is used in this location.

Nonpalpable lesion excision should be confirmed with intraoperative specimen radiographs (Figures 56-5 and 56-6).

A positive surgical margin mandates re-excision except in circumstances when the anterior margin is the skin or the posterior margin is the chest wall.

When a mastectomy is necessary, an elliptical incision fashioned in a horizontal orientation has an excellent outcome and allows for patients to be fitted with a prosthesis when reconstruction is not performed. If a skin or nipple-sparing mastectomy is going to be performed, coordination with the reconstructive surgeon should be done for optimal incision placement.

The extent of surgical dissection during a mastectomy, regardless of the approach, should include the borders of the breast: clavicle superiorly, sternum medially, latissimus dorsi laterally, and inframammary crease inferiorly.

A sentinel lymph node biopsy can successfully be performed with the preprocedure injection of single or dual tracers into the breast. Our preference is to use a dilution of 1 mL methylene blue/7 mL saline into the retroareolar tissue and a 0.5-miCu dose of Tc-99 diluted to 0.3 mL solution injected intradermally in the periareolar region, after induction of general anesthesia. Modifications of this technique

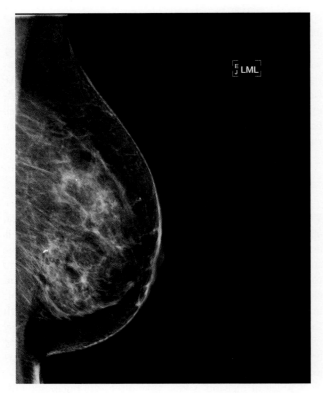

FIGURE 56-5. Presurgical mammogram demonstrating appropriate radioactive I-125 seed localization of calcifications and biopsy clip.

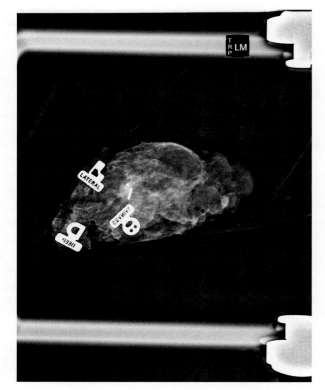

FIGURE 56-6. Radiograph showing targeted calcifications, biopsy clip, and radioactive I-125 seed centered in specimen with margin of breast tissue.

are done if the patient has undergone previous breast procedures with incisions that may affect lymphatic drainage.

In the setting of a mastectomy, the sentinel lymph node biopsy can be easily approached through the mastectomy incision. When a separate axillary incision is to be used for the axillary staging, a small incision along the lowest hair-bearing line is convenient and provides easy access to the sentinel lymph nodes. This incision can then be extended if an axillary lymph node dissection is indicated. A lymph node is excised if it is blue, radioactive with counts >10% of the highest ex vivo nodal count, or palpably suspicious (Table 56-2).

● SPECIAL INTRAOPERATIVE CONSIDERATIONS

Surgical excision of nonpalpable lesions is highly dependent upon accurate placement and retrieval of breast markers that are often radiopaque. Prominent display of the localization mammograms in the operating room is extremely helpful in the planning and conducting of the operation. Though the breast is in compression during these images, distance measurements of the skin to marker or the nipple to marker allow the surgeon to understand approximate depth of lesion in the breast.

The utmost care must be taken not to displace the wire during surgical prep as this would mandate a return of the patient to the radiology suite for a secondary wire placement.

It may also occur that the biopsy clip is displaced or lost during excision. Much as additional margins may need to be taken if the target has not been adequately excised, it is not wise to continue to blindly take margins from the breast in order to locate a displaced clip, as it may be lost in the surgical drapes, sponges, or suction canister. This can ultimately compromise the cosmesis of the breast.

The finding of biopsy site changes on final pathology confirms target retrieval, even if the biopsy clip is not found. It is therefore crucial to counsel patients preoperatively about the possibility of marker or clip displacement.

● POSTOPERATIVE MANAGEMENT

Surgical pathology should be evaluated thoroughly to ensure that the targeted lesion has been retrieved (evidence of biopsy site changes support this) and adequate margins have been obtained.

Appropriate referrals to medical oncology and radiation oncology should therefore be made based upon the need for adjuvant therapies.

This patient underwent a radioactive seed localization segmental mastectomy. Final pathology revealed 1.2-cm ductal carcinoma in situ, surgical margins >2 mm, and estrogen and progesterone positive.

She was referred to radiation oncology and medical oncology for adjuvant treatment. She will also continue breast cancer surveillance with yearly mammograms.

Table 56-2	Suspicious Mammographic Abnormality

Segmental Mastectomy

Key Technical Steps

1. Review imaging and determine localization tool (wire, seed, clip) in reference to the target.
2. Breast incision based upon location in upper or lower pole of the breast. Periareolar or inframammary incisions when lesion is accessible from these areas.
3. Consideration of surgical margins (if resecting malignancy) and intraoperative radiograph to confirm excision of target.

Potential Pitfalls

- Displacement of localization tool (wire, seed, etc.).
- Displacement of biopsy clip, particularly when no residual imaging findings are evident (e.g., small area of calcifications completely excised with core biopsy).

Total Mastectomy

Key Technical Steps

1. Total mastectomy incision placement dependent upon whether reconstruction is to be done concurrently. If so, there should be close coordination with the reconstructive surgeon.
2. Removal of tissue to anatomic borders of the breast: clavicle, sternum, latissimus dorsi, and inframammary crease. Posterior down to pectoralis fascia.
3. Single drain placement typically adequate for mastectomy without reconstruction.

Potential Pitfalls

- It is crucial to perform the mastectomy and dissect at the level of the breast capsule in order to completely remove the majority of breast tissue without compromising vascularity and viability of the skin flaps.

Axillary Staging

Key Technical Steps

1. Injection of single or dual tracer prior to surgical incision.
2. Incision in low axilla that can be extended for axillary lymph node dissection if necessary.

Potential Pitfalls

- Failure to map dye into the axilla may require axillary lymph node dissection.
- Vital structures that may be injured in the process of axillary staging include the axillary vein, long thoracic nerve, thoracodorsal nerve, and intercostobrachial nerves.
- Although rare, anaphylactic reactions can occur with the use of isosulfan blue. Isosulfan blue sometimes also causes skin tattooing.
- Methylene blue can cause skin necrosis, particularly in undiluted form.
- Blue dyes should not be used in axillary staging of pregnant patients.

TAKE HOME POINTS

- Breast cancer is the second most common cancer in women and third most common cause of cancer death.
- Participation in a screening program increases cancer detection rate and has been proven to decrease mortality from breast cancer.
- Percutaneous biopsy of imaging abnormalities determines pathology and facilitates surgical planning.
- The conduct of the operation and need to obtain adequate surgical margins will depend upon preoperative biopsy findings.
- Placement of surgical incisions should be guided by pathology and the potential to convert to mastectomy if necessary.
- Segmental mastectomy and total mastectomy, with or without reconstruction, are the options for surgical management of breast cancer.
- Axillary staging can be done through the open mastectomy wound if done concurrently.
- Axillary staging in a clinically node negative patient with invasive breast cancer should be a sentinel lymph node biopsy.
- Axillary lymph node dissection should be considered in patients when sentinel lymph node mapping fails.
- Adjuvant therapy is determined by the type of breast surgery received and breast cancer receptor status.
- Treatment and surveillance of breast cancer patients require a multidisciplinary approach and effort and should be coordinated with a medical oncologist and radiation oncologist when appropriate.
- Consideration for referral to a genetic counselor should be based upon personal and family history. The National Comprehensive Cancer Network (NCCN) guideline for "Genetic/familial high-risk assessment: breast and ovarian" is an excellent resource.

SUGGESTED READINGS

Berg WA, Yang WT. *Diagnostic Imaging: Breast*. Philadelphia, PA: Lippincott Williams & Wilkins; 2014.

Moran MS, et al. Society of Surgical Oncology-American Society for Radiation Oncology consensus guideline on margins for breast-conserving surgery with whole-breast irradiation in stages I and II invasive breast cancer. *Ann Surg Oncol*. 2014;21(3):704-716.

Morrow M, Schnitt SJ, Norton L. Current management of lesions associated with an increased risk of breast cancer. *Nat Rev Clin Oncol*. 2015;12(4):227-238.

Morrow M, et al. Society of Surgical Oncology-American Society for Radiation Oncology-American Society of Clinical Oncology Consensus Guideline on Margins for breast-conserving surgery with whole-breast irradiation in ductal carcinoma in situ. *J Clin Oncol*. 2016;34(33):4040-4046.

National Comprehensive Cancer Network. Retrieved October 1, 2016, from https://www.nccn.org/professionals/physician_gls/f_guidelines.asp.

van Roozendaal LM, et al. Sentinel lymph node biopsy can be omitted in DCIS patients treated with breast conserving therapy. *Breast Cancer Res Treat*. 2016;156(3):517-525.

Ductal Carcinoma In Situ

57

KELLY JOYCE ROSSO AND JESSICA M. BENSENHAVER

Based on the previous edition chapter "Ductal Carcinoma In Situ" by Jessica M. Bensenhaver and Tara M. Breslin

Presentation

A 56-year-old female presents with a new finding of pleomorphic microcalcifications in the upper outer quadrant of the right breast on her annual screening mammogram. She has a history of hypertension and fibroadenoma excision from the right breast 20 years ago. She has no family history of breast cancer. She smokes ½ pack of cigarettes daily and drinks one glass of wine per week. Breast exam demonstrates symmetric breasts with mild ptosis without masses, skin changes or dimpling, nipple discharge, or nipple inversion. Stereotactic core needle biopsy demonstrated high-grade ductal carcinoma in situ (DCIS), estrogen and progesterone receptor positive by immunohistochemistry.

● DIFFERENTIAL DIAGNOSIS

Calcifications on mammography can arise from multiple etiologies that include both benign and malignant disease. Morphology and distribution of the calcifications can aid in predicting the nature of the lesion, but biopsy is often necessary to establish a definitive diagnosis, especially when the calcifications are suspicious.

Typically, benign calcifications that do not require a biopsy but rather a short interval follow-up are eggshell calcifications, coarse or popcorn calcifications, calcifications arising from vasculature, large rodlike calcifications, and milk of calcium calcifications. Alternatively, amorphous, course heterogeneous, fine pleomorphic, or fine linear branching calcifications have a moderate or high suspicion for malignancy and require a biopsy, either by image-guided core or wire localized surgical excision, to establish a diagnosis.

DCIS accounts for approximately 20% of all breast cancers detected by screening mammography. The continuum of typical hyperplasia, atypical hyperplasia, and low-, intermediate-, and high-grade DCIS in the breast does not necessarily follow a predictable disease progression to microinvasive or invasive carcinoma.

● WORKUP

This patient presented with new pleomorphic microcalcifications on screening mammogram, a common presentation of DCIS. Further evaluation includes a complete history focusing on assessing the patient's individual risk for breast cancer and associated symptomatology and physical exam of *both* breasts and the axillary, supraclavicular, and cervical lymph node basins. Genetic counseling should be offered if the patient is identified as high risk for hereditary breast cancer.

Imaging evaluation consists of reviewing both previous and current bilateral breast imaging. Current diagnostic mammography should address the characteristics (calcifications, soft tissue density, mass, asymmetry) and extent (focal, multifocal, multicentric) of ipsilateral disease and rule out bilateral disease (Figures 57-1–57-3). Review of prior images is helpful for determining the stability of probably benign findings. This information is essential for guiding surgical planning.

● DIAGNOSIS

Diagnosis requires tissue biopsy. Image-guided core needle biopsy is the preferred method, typically either stereotactic or ultrasound guided. It is minimally invasive and accurate and can be performed in an ambulatory care setting under local anesthesia. Image guidance is employed for accuracy and allows placement of a marking clip in the biopsy site for future localization. It must be noted, however, that core biopsy represents just a portion of the targeted lesion, and when core biopsy reveals DCIS, there is a 10% to 20% chance of associated invasive carcinoma being present in the final surgical specimen.

● TREATMENT PRINCIPLES

The multimodal treatment for DCIS is becoming more personalized and includes a combination of surgery, radiotherapy, and hormone therapy. Unlike most cancer treatments that focus on survival, pure DCIS is associated with few deaths. In fact, any breast cancer–related mortality after a diagnosis of DCIS is related to the concomitant presence of invasive cancer or the development of ipsilateral and/or contralateral invasive breast cancer. Therefore, the focus of pure DCIS treatment is prevention of local recurrence.

Surgical options include breast conservation (BC) or simple (total) mastectomy. BC is feasible if (1) candidacy for post–partial mastectomy radiation is confirmed and (2) the size of disease is such that partial mastectomy can

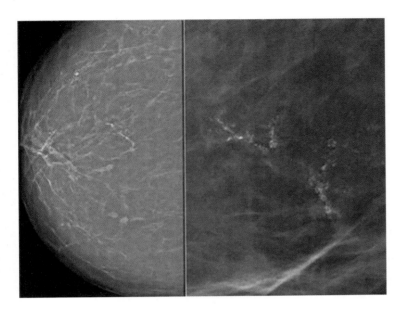

FIGURE 57-1. Mammogram images of pleomorphic microcalcifications.

be accomplished with negative margins without sacrificing cosmesis. Simple mastectomy is indicated in cases of true multicentric disease or multifocal disease for which partial mastectomy would compromise cosmesis. Patient preference can play a role in choosing mastectomy in a disease otherwise amenable to breast conservation, usually seen in highly motivated women with genetic predisposition (BRCA mutation). These patients must understand that mastectomy offers a risk reduction benefit, but no survival benefit. Patients undergoing mastectomy should also be considered for reconstruction

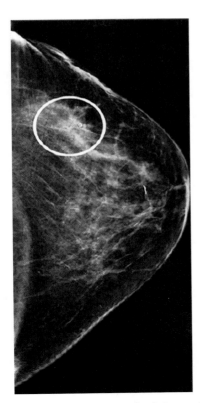

FIGURE 57-2. Mammogram image of soft tissue density.

and undergo preoperative evaluation by a plastic surgeon to access their candidacy. Lastly, in appreciation of the small but real risk of the presence of invasive carcinoma, sentinel lymph node biopsy should be strongly considered in patients who undergo mastectomy for treatment of their DCIS as the ability to perform sentinel lymph node biopsy to stage the axilla is compromised after mastectomy.

Pathologic evaluation confirms diagnosis; addresses tumor size and extent; characterizes the nuclear grade, tumor architecture, and presence or absence of comedonecrosis; evaluates for microinvasion (focus of invasion less than 0.1 cm) or occult invasive disease; establishes receptor status, and assesses surgical margins with measurements. A resection margin width for pure DCIS of 2 mL has been associated with a decreased chance of recurrence; however, clinical judgment regarding the need for re-excision is recommended when there are focally close but negative margins. DCIS is upstaged (from stage 0) by the presence of microinvasion or occult invasive disease and should be treated according to recommendation for invasive disease.

Radiotherapy is not routine after mastectomy but is routine after BC as the literature shows a 50% risk reduction in local recurrence after partial mastectomy is followed by radiotherapy—approximately half of breast cancer recurrences after treatment for DCIS occur as DCIS, and the other half are invasive cancer. However, no DCIS trial has ever demonstrated that radiation offers a survival benefit when compared with excision alone; therefore, omitting radiotherapy in some low-risk patients is an area of investigation, but to date, there are no prospective trial data or established pathologic selection criteria for identifying appropriate patients.

Hormone therapy has a role for risk reduction in patients with ER-positive and PR-positive DCIS. When used for 5 years, endocrine therapy reduces the risk of ipsilateral recurrence and contralateral disease. Therefore, noting no contraindications exist, hormonal therapy should at least be considered for ER-positive DCIS.

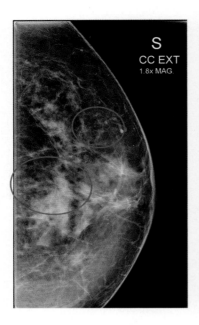
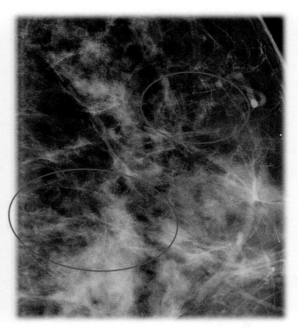

FIGURE 57-3. Multifocal, multicentric DCIS.

Studies exploring both conservative and aggressive management of DCIS are ongoing and aim to add additional evidence-based data to treatment algorithms of this heterogeneous disease.

● SURGICAL APPROACH: BREAST CONSERVATION (TABLE 57-1)

Partial mastectomy is performed with the patient in the supine position, under general anesthesia or IV sedation. Preoperative wire localization of nonpalpable lesions is performed under mammographic or ultrasound guidance the day of surgery. Postlocalization mammography is performed, allowing the surgeon to envision the depth of the lesion from the skin and from the tip of the wire (Figure 57-4). Prepping and draping include the anterior arm, breast, ipsilateral thorax, and lower neck. Orientation of the skin incision is based on the wire and lesion location, as well as the breast anatomy, with the most direct approach to the lesion in mind in order to avoid excessive tunneling. Inclusion of the skin overlying superficial lesions is recommended while appreciating that large skin excisions can affect cosmesis by causing a mastopexy-type effect. Recognizing the potential future need to incorporate the incision into a mastectomy excision, in the case of positive margins, is also considered.

After the incision is made, dissection is aimed directly down to the lesion. Gross 1-cm margins around the specimen should be the goal. Once the specimen is removed, it is oriented in space by marking sutures or ink, and a specimen radiograph is obtained to ensure intact wire and microclip and incorporation of the desired calcifications or lesion (Figure 57-5).

The lumpectomy cavity should be palpated to ensure removal of all suspicious tissue. Marking clips are placed on the borders of the specimen cavity (helpful for radiation planning). Hemostasis should be carefully ensured prior to closure.

The most common pitfall associated with partial mastectomy is inadequate margin status requiring re-excision or possibly mastectomy. Intraoperative specimen mammography helps to potentially avoid a second operation

Table 57-1	Breast Conservation

Key Technical Steps

1. Preprocedural localization of nonpalpable lesions.
2. Plan incision on lesion depth and location, with consideration of future mastectomy incision.
3. Excise the localized lesion with grossly normal 1-cm margins.
4. Orient specimen and send to mammography to ensure the wire, clip, and lesion or calcifications are in the specimen.
5. Palpate the cavity for any suspicious tissue.
6. Ensure hemostasis and close.
7. Postoperative mammogram (1 to 3 weeks postoperatively) to confirm complete excision of lesion prior to the initiation of radiation therapy.

Potential Pitfalls

- Inadequate surgical margins requiring re-excision or mastectomy.
- Inadequate hemostasis causing bleeding or hematoma.

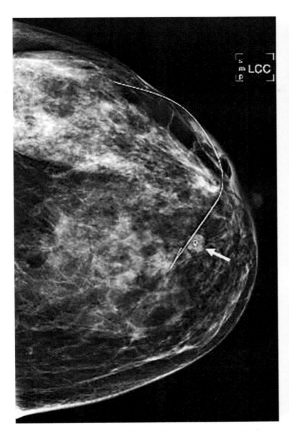
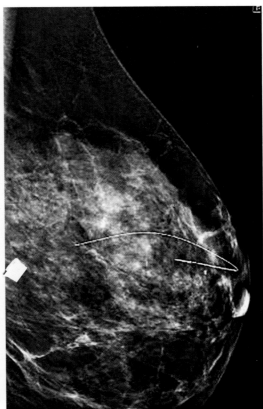

FIGURE 57-4. Wire localization with reinforced portion of wire adjacent to biopsy clip.

by providing an opportunity to identify and address margin issues at the primary operation. Re-excision to achieve negative margins is necessary; however, the resultant cosmesis may be compromised and ultimately result in the need for a mastectomy for adequate local control.

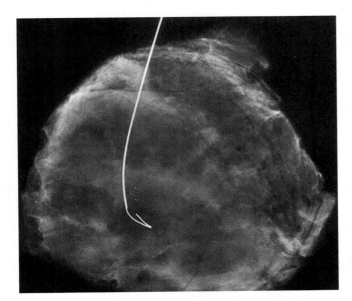

FIGURE 57-5. Intraoperative specimen radiograph (note radiographic wide margins and calcifications adjacent to reinforced portion of wire).

● SURGICAL APPROACH: MASTECTOMY (TABLE 57-2)

Mastectomy is performed under general anesthesia with the patient in the supine position. Radioisotope and/or blue dye is injected into the breast preoperatively in anticipation of sentinel lymph node biopsy. The patient is placed in the supine position with the arm abducted. Prepping and draping include the anterior arm, axilla, breast, ipsilateral thorax, and lower neck. An elliptical incision is marked including the nipple–areolar complex, the biopsy site, and the skin anterior to the tumor (Figure 57-7). Skin-sparing mastectomy is often utilized in cases with planned immediate reconstruction. The incision plan is chosen with input from the reconstructive surgeon and traditionally is adjacent to the areolar border (Figure 57-8). This smaller skin opening does somewhat limit exposure, but the rest of the procedure is performed similarly to standard mastectomy.

After incision, skin flaps are created by gently retracting the skin edges while using downward countertraction on the breast parenchyma to expose the connective tissue layer between the breast parenchyma and the subcutaneous adipose tissue of the skin. The skin flaps are developed along this connective tissue plane superiorly to the clavicle, medially to the lateral border of the sternum, inferiorly to the inframammary fold, and laterally to the anterior border of the latissimus dorsi muscle while paying close attention

Table 57-2	Mastectomy

Key Technical Steps

1. Orient elliptical incision to include nipple–areolar complex, previous biopsy site, and overlying skin.
2. Use electrocautery and gentle traction to develop the connective tissue plane superficial to the breast parenchyma in creation of the skin flaps.
3. Dissection borders are superiorly to the clavicle, medially to the lateral border of the sternum, inferiorly to the anterior rectus sheath, and laterally to the anterior border of the latissimus dorsi muscle.
4. Remove the breast from the pectoralis muscle, including the pectoralis fascia.
5. Perform sentinel lymph node biopsy utilizing the same incision.
6. Ensure hemostasis, place drain, and close.

Potential Pitfalls

- Skin flaps.
  - Overly thin flaps can lead to ischemia, necrosis, and poor wound healing.
  - Overly thick flaps may leave behind too much breast parenchyma.
- Wound closure in large resection specimens requiring undermining or grafting.

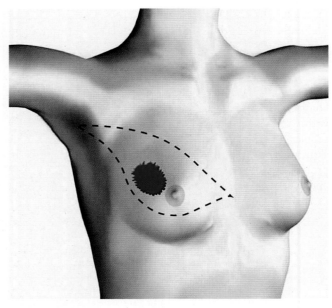

FIGURE 57-7. Mastectomy incision.

to flap thickness as overly thin flaps are at risk for necrosis and infection. Throughout dissection and removal, isolate and ligate any encountered vessels. The breast tissue is then removed off the pectoralis major muscle with the pectoralis fascia. Once completed, sentinel lymph node biopsy is performed (see details in Chapter 59: Early Stage Breast Cancer).

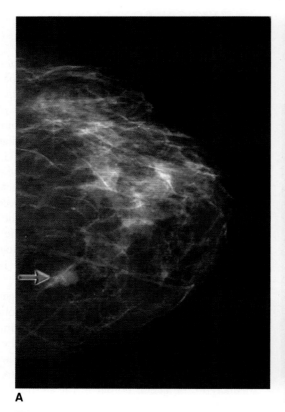

A

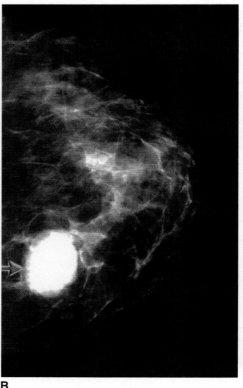

B

FIGURE 57-6. **A,B:** Pre- and postsurgery comparison mammography.

Hemostasis is ensured and drain(s) placed prior to closure. The patient is either observed overnight or discharged the same day with the drain in place. Drains are often removed once output is less than 30 to 40 mL per day.

The most common intraoperative complications of mastectomy are inadequate surgical margins and wound complications. The goal of surgical therapy is local control with complete excision of disease both grossly and microscopically. If extensive superficial disease requires a large skin resection to ensure margins, skin closure can be compromised. Undermining the subcutaneous tissues inferiorly and superiorly can better mobilize the flaps. Skin grafting is rarely necessary but also an option.

● SPECIAL INTRAOPERATIVE CONSIDERATIONS

The role of axillary surgery in DCIS is controversial. Sentinel lymph node biopsy is recommended for women undergoing mastectomy for DCIS and should be considered in women with lesions at higher risk for occult invasive disease including those with clinically palpable lesions, those with large lesions (>4 cm on imaging), or those with aggressive features including comedonecrosis. Axillary staging by SLN biopsy should be weighed against the small but significant risk of lymphedema, approximately 5% after 5 years.

Reconstruction following mastectomy is a viable option in patients undergoing mastectomy for DCIS. Options are discussed preoperatively in a multidisciplinary fashion with the plastic and reconstructive surgeon, the breast surgical oncologist, and the radiation oncologist.

Oncoplastic surgical techniques are an emerging technology offering more choices for patients with tumor characteristics that would require generous partial mastectomy to achieve negative margins. These techniques are especially beneficial as an alternative to mastectomy in women with a generous amount of breast tissue. Contralateral reduction is often necessary for symmetry.

● POSTOPERATIVE MANAGEMENT

Common complications of both partial mastectomy and simple mastectomy are infection, hematoma, seroma, chronic incisional pain, and lymphedema. Preoperative prevention practices include prophylactic antibiotics especially in high-risk patients (obese, elderly, diabetic) and cessation of anticoagulants as appropriate per medication half-life before scheduled surgery. Adequate postoperative counseling with PT/OT referral when necessary can address incisional pain and lymphedema issues. Although rare, brachial plexopathy from positioning can also occur. Two unique complications of breast conservation is the rare potential

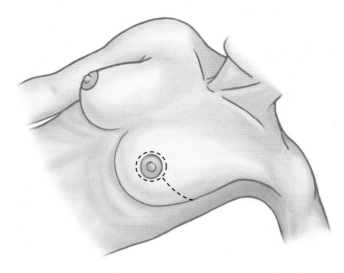

FIGURE 57-8. Skin-sparing mastectomy incision.

for pneumothorax from wire placement and Mondor's disease. Postoperative flap necrosis can occur after mastectomy, seen most often with thin flaps and in smokers. This may require debridement and chronic wound management and/or delayed closure techniques.

Partial mastectomy follow-up starts with a postsurgical mammogram 1 to 3 weeks after surgery to compare with preoperative images and confirm complete excision of calcifications (Figure 57-6). Surveillance mammography resumes 6 months after completion of radiation to evaluate treatment-associated changes and establish a new baseline. Annual bilateral screening is then re-established. Clinical breast exam is recommended every 6 months for 2 years, then annually with screening mammography. Interim self-breast exam is always encouraged.

After mastectomy, surveillance includes clinical exam (ipsilateral chest wall, contralateral breast, and bilateral nodal exam) every 6 months for 2 years, then annually. Contralateral breast screening with mammogram continues annually. Again, interim self-exam is encouraged.

Case Conclusion

The patient in this scenario opted to undergo partial mastectomy with postoperative whole breast radiation therapy. Final pathology demonstrated estrogen and progesterone receptor–positive, high-grade ductal carcinoma in situ without comedonecrosis or invasive component, with 2-mm margins, Tis (tumor in situ), stage 0. Given her ER positive DCIS, she and her treatment team elected for 5 years of endocrine therapy. She was encouraged to quit smoking and was started on a multimodal program for smoking cessation.

TAKE HOME POINTS

- Screening mammography is directly responsible for significantly increasing the preclinical identification and overall incidence of DCIS.
- Preoperative diagnostic imaging is mandatory to evaluate the extent of ipsilateral disease, to rule out contralateral disease, and to ultimately guide surgical planning.
- Diagnosis requires tissue biopsy.
- The treatment of DCIS is multidisciplinary.
- Breast conservation or mastectomy is based on the size and extent of disease, candidacy for radiation therapy, cosmesis outcome, and patient's desire for reconstruction.
- The two surgical options have equal long-term survival benefits.
- The goal of surgery is local control with clear margins.
- Sentinel lymph node biopsy is recommended in patients who are undergoing mastectomy and for those who have features considered high risk for invasive component, including clinically palpable lesions, large in size (>4 cm on imaging), or comedonecrosis.
- Adjuvant radiation therapy has been shown to decrease ipsilateral recurrence in 50% but has not been shown to increase survival.

SUGGESTED READINGS

Merrill AL, Esserman L, Morrow M. Ductal carcinoma in situ. *N Engl J Med.* 2016;374:390-392.

Morrow M, Van Zee KJ, Solin LJ, et al. Society of Surgical Oncology-American Society for Radiation Oncology-American Society of Clinical Oncology consensus guideline on margins for breast-conserving surgery with whole-breast irradiation in ductal carcinoma in situ. *J Clin Oncol.* 2016;34(33):4040-4046.

Narod SA, Iqbal J, Giannakeas V, Sopik V, Sun P. Breast cancer mortality after a diagnosis of ductal carcinoma in situ. *JAMA Oncol.* 2015;1(7)888-896.

NCCN.org. National Comprehensive Cancer Network Clinical Practice Guidelines, Breast Cancer version 1.2016.

Newman L, Bensenhaver J. *Ductal Carcinoma In Situ and Microinvasive/Borderline Breast Cancer.* New York, NY: Springer Science Media, LLC; 2015.

Lobular Carcinoma In Situ

58

LINDSAY PETERSEN AND LISA A. NEWMAN

Based on the previous edition chapter "Lobular Carcinoma In Situ" by Lisa A. Newman

Presentation

A 45-year-old African American female undergoes routine screening mammogram and is found to have scattered indeterminate microcalcifications bilaterally. One cluster in the lower left breast at the 6 o'clock position is particularly suspicious because it appears prominent and has a more branching pattern when compared to the patient's prior mammograms, which have been performed annually since age 40 years. She is referred to a surgeon for discussion of biopsy options. This patient's past medical history is noncontributory, but she does have a sister who was diagnosed with breast cancer at 40 years of age. Her clinical breast exam is negative for any skin abnormalities; there are no dominant or discrete palpable masses; there is no nipple discharge; and there is no suspicious adenopathy in either the axillary or supraclavicular nodal basins.

● DIFFERENTIAL DIAGNOSIS

Mammographically detected microcalcifications can represent benign breast findings (fibrocystic hyperplasia, vascular calcifications, cystic hyperplasia, etc.), or they can represent a breast malignancy. Patients are routinely recommended to avoid use of talc-based deodorants or topical preparations

when presenting for mammography, as these can create calcification artifact. Patients with history of prior breast surgery or radiation can also develop calcifications that are of a benign, inflammatory nature (fat necrosis). An experienced breast imaging team is necessary to distinguish the high-risk and frankly malignant patterns that require biopsy from the clearly benign patterns that can be monitored noninvasively.

● WORKUP

Additional diagnostic mammographic views (compression and magnification images) will generally be necessary for the further evaluation of microcalcifications (Figure 58-1). Calcifications that follow a linear and branching pattern, or that are associated with a spiculated density, will be considered more suspicious of a malignant etiology. Calcifications that layer out (e.g., "teacup" pattern) suggest benign cystic hyperplasia. Targeted breast ultrasound is indicated if there is any question of a coexisting mass density. Breast magnetic resonance imaging (MRI) will not be useful at this juncture because a normal MRI will not negate any mammographic indications for proceeding to biopsy. Any management decisions must be correlated with the clinical breast exam—a suspicious finding on breast exam (e.g., palpable breast mass or bloody nipple discharge) would be an indication to proceed with biopsy in order to obtain histopathologic information

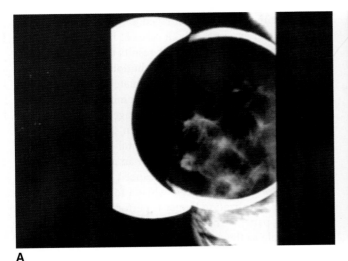
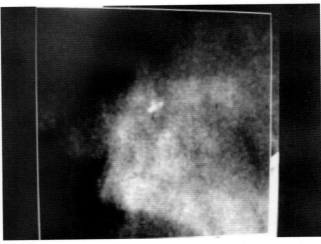

A   **B**

FIGURE 58-1. **A,B:** Patient mammogram, revealing microcalcifications in the left breast.

regarding the nature of the finding, regardless of whether or not the lesion has an imaging correlate.

This patient's additional imaging confirmed a dominant cluster of microcalcifications in the lower hemisphere of the left breast, and biopsy was recommended. Diagnostic biopsy options for nonpalpable, mammographically or sonographically detected breast abnormalities include image-guided fine needle aspiration (FNA), image-guided core needle biopsy, or wire localization surgical biopsy (Table 58-1). A diagnostic surgical biopsy is the most definitive procedure because it yields the largest pathology specimen and may result in complete extraction of the image-detected abnormality, but as a surgical volume-extracting procedure, it can result in cosmetic deformity and is less efficient compared to needle biopsy procedures. Image-guided needle biopsy procedures are generally preferred as the initial diagnostic maneuver,

Table 58-1 Breast Biopsy Options for Nonpalpable, Screen-Detected Abnormalities

Key Technical Steps

1. Image-guided percutaneous needle biopsy preferred as the most efficient maneuver.
2. Mammographically guided (stereotactic) or ultrasound-guided needle biopsy can be performed, depending on which study reveals best images of the target lesion. Core needle biopsies (14 or 16 gauge) have lower false-negative rate compared to cytologic yield from FNA biopsy.
3. Radiopaque clip must be left in place to document site-sampled breast tissue.
4. When percutaneous image-guided needle biopsy technology is unavailable, or not feasible (body habitus too large or breast too small; patient unable to tolerate percutaneous procedure), then a follow-up wire localization surgical biopsy is necessary.
5. When needle biopsy reveals high-risk pathology such as LCIS, atypical ductal hyperplasia, or atypical lobular hyperplasia, then a follow-up wire localization surgical biopsy is necessary to rule out sampling error and coexisting cancer.

Potential Pitfalls

- Images of any needle biopsy and/or surgical biopsy specimens are mandatory to confirm inclusion of the target lesion.
- If needle biopsy specimen images demonstrate failed/nondiagnostic procedure or discordant findings, then surgical biopsy is necessary.
- If surgical diagnostic wire localization specimen images demonstrate a failed procedure, then subsequent management is based upon pathology of any extracted specimen as well as postoperative imaging at a short interval.

as they are less invasive and less costly. Core needle biopsy tends to have an improved diagnostic yield compared to FNA; false-negative/sampling error rates are usually <10% for core needle biopsies (especially if vacuum assisted) but can be as high as 30% with FNA biopsy. The FNA provides a cytology sample only and therefore cannot distinguish in situ cancer from invasive cancer. Furthermore, while the spun-down cells from a cancerous FNA biopsy can be used for immunohistochemical evaluation of molecular markers (estrogen receptor, progesterone receptor, and HER2/neu), it would not be known whether these markers were expressed on the invasive or the in situ component of the cancer.

Mammography can be used to guide a percutaneous needle biopsy (the stereotactic approach), or ultrasound may be used. Patient and image factors dictate the selection of image guidance. Microcalcifications usually require mammographic, stereotactic biopsy. While upright equipment is available, most stereotactic biopsies are performed on a specially designed table and require prone positioning of the patient. The affected breast is fitted through an aperture facing the floor, and the ipsilateral arm must be raised above the head during the entire procedure. The biopsy needle is directed toward the target within the breast using stereotactic guidance, and a range of 5 to 12 core specimens are typically extracted under local anesthesia. Because of the positioning and table design prerequisites, some cases will not be amenable to the stereotactic biopsy approach: lesions that are adjacent to the pectoralis muscle, lesions that are too superficial or within the nipple, small breasts that compress to a thickness that is exceeded by the core needle trajectory, patients who cannot tolerate prone positioning for prolonged periods (half hour or longer), and patients who exceed the weight limit of the biopsy table. Solid mass lesions that are sonographically visible can be biopsied with ultrasound guidance. A radiopaque marker should be left in place at the biopsy site to document the site that was sampled. In the event that a subsequent surgical procedure is needed (and the imaged target is no longer visible on postbiopsy films), the clip would serve as the target for a wire localization resection. The core biopsy specimens should be imaged to insure adequate sampling of the target, especially in cases of microcalcifications. Specific needle biopsy pathology results that mandate a follow-up surgical resection include the following: failed procedures, where the target is not adequately sampled; benign pathologic findings that are radiographically interpreted as being discordant with the target images; and "high-risk" pathology, such as lobular carcinoma in situ (LCIS), atypical lobular hyperplasia, and atypical ductal hyperplasia. These high-risk lesions are associated with an approximately 15% to 20% frequency of coexisting cancer (ductal carcinoma in situ and/or invasive cancer) when a follow-up diagnostic surgical wire localization biopsy is performed.

In this patient, the cluster of microcalcifications was not amenable to the percutaneous needle biopsy because of small breast size, and the patient therefore underwent a wire localization surgical biopsy. It is mandatory that a specimen

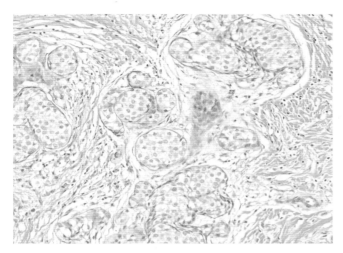

FIGURE 58-2. Biopsy slide revealing LCIS.

mammogram be obtained for this type of procedure as well, and unfortunately in this case, there were no calcifications visible in the excised breast specimen. Pathology evaluation nonetheless revealed a diagnosis of LCIS (Figure 58-2).

● DIAGNOSIS AND TREATMENT

The specimen mammography in this case documented a failed wire localization procedure. When this occurs, the surgeon can attempt to "blindly" resect or sample some breast fragments in the biopsy field, but once the wire has been extracted with the initial tissue specimen, it is extremely difficult to obtain an appropriate secondary specimen. Another option is to close the wound and await pathology results, and if these are negative for cancer, then the patient should undergo repeat mammography within the next few weeks (as chosen by the surgeon and patient in this particular case). A decision regarding any additional biopsy attempts would be made based upon the appearance of the follow-up mammogram.

In this patient, the surgical specimen revealed high-risk pathology in the form of LCIS. LCIS is identified in fewer than 5% of otherwise benign breast biopsies and is most commonly detected among women in their 40s. It may be found coincidentally with other breast pathology in up to 25% of breast surgical cases. The magnitude of the increased future breast cancer risk for LCIS is approximately 1% per year, and this risk may be higher in women with a positive family history of breast cancer in addition to the LCIS. LCIS is perceived as a microscopic pattern of breast tissue that is present diffusely and bilaterally but usually without any clinical or radiographic correlate; it therefore tends to be detected as an incidental finding in women undergoing biopsy for some other reasons. The future breast cancer risk is expressed equally in terms of laterality, and of those patients who do develop subsequent breast cancer, two-thirds will be diagnosed with ductal histopathology as opposed to invasive

lobular cancer. LCIS is therefore a marker of increased risk and not an actual precursor lesion. When LCIS is detected incidentally at the time of lumpectomy for breast cancer, the margins do not need to be free of the LCIS histology.

There are two forms of LCIS: classic and pleomorphic. Pleomorphic LCIS contains cells that are bigger with larger nuclei and have more abundant cytoplasm than classic LCIS cells. Pleomorphic LCIS can be difficult to distinguish from ductal carcinoma in situ histologically. Some clinicians advocate for more aggressive treatment with pleomorphic LCIS, including resection to negative margins and even postsurgical radiotherapy, but there is no long-term data or evidence to support this approach.

Because LCIS is a marker of risk for either breast, the management options must address the bilateral breast tissue. These management options include close surveillance/observation alone, chemoprevention with either tamoxifen (appropriate for premenopausal as well as postmenopausal women) or raloxifene (only approved for use in postmenopausal women), or bilateral prophylactic mastectomy. The surveillance options generally include annual or biannual clinical breast exam and annual mammography, and annual breast MRI may be considered as well. Chemoprevention can halve the future breast cancer risk and is usually prescribed for 5 years. Raloxifene may be used in selected postmenopausal women for longer periods if it is indicated in the control of osteoporosis. Premenopausal women must be advised to avoid pregnancy while taking tamoxifen. Both of these selective estrogen receptor modulators are associated with vasomotor symptoms (night sweats, hot flashes), thromboembolic phenomena, and uterine problems. Risk of uterine cancer is relatively greater in postmenopausal women taking tamoxifen. Patients opting for bilateral prophylactic mastectomy should meet with a plastic surgeon to assess their reconstruction options (immediate reconstruction vs. delayed, tissue expander/implant reconstruction vs. autologous tissue reconstruction). Axillary staging surgery is not necessary for LCIS patients choosing prophylactic mastectomy.

Atypical hyperplasia (ductal or lobular) represents another high-risk pathology. Future risk of breast cancer is approximately four to five times that of the general female population with benign "usual" fibrocystic hyperplasia, and most of this risk is expressed within the initial 5 to 10 years after diagnosis. In contrast to the LCIS-associated breast cancer risk, atypia is more similar to a true cancer precursor lesion—subsequent breast cancers usually occur at the site where the atypia was identified (especially in cases of atypical ductal hyperplasia).

The patient in the scenario presented in this chapter underwent follow-up mammography imaging 3 months later that was unchanged, and the patient was offered the option of continued observation at that point because of the subtle/indeterminate appearance of her microcalcifications. She opted to undergo bilateral prophylactic mastectomy with immediate reconstruction. Her final pathology revealed diffuse and bilateral LCIS (as expected) as well as extensive severe atypical ductal hyperplasia. Microcalcifications were identified in areas of atypical hyperplasia and also in areas of benign/usual hyperplasia.

● DISCUSSION POINTS/SPECIAL CONSIDERATIONS

Screening Mammography

This patient initiated annual screening mammography at age 40, despite ongoing controversy regarding whether surveillance mammography should begin prior to age 50 years. The American Cancer Society, the American College of Radiology, and the American College of Surgeons continue to advocate in favor of screening mammography beginning at age 40 or 45 years but allow for screening mammography to begin at 40 years if recommended by a patient and her doctor. Additional factors in this particular patient that support screening during the fifth decade of life include her positive family history, with breast cancer diagnosed at a young age in a second-degree relative, and her racial–ethnic identity. Lifetime incidence rates for breast cancer are lower for African American women compared to White American women, despite paradoxically higher mortality rates, and African American women have a younger age distribution. For American women younger than 45 years of age, breast cancer incidence rates are higher for African American compared to White American women.

Breast Cancer Risk Assessment

Individualized breast cancer risk is frequently estimated by use of the Gail model, a statistical tool that assesses the likelihood of a woman being diagnosed with breast cancer over the following 5 years and over her lifetime. Conventional thresholds for identifying "high-risk" women are based upon a 5-year risk estimate that exceeds 1.7% or lifetime risk estimate >20% to 25%. The Gail model calculates risk probabilities by accounting for first-degree family history of breast cancer, reproductive history (age at menarche, age at first live birth), and breast biopsy history (number of prior biopsies and whether or not any prior biopsy revealed atypical hyperplasia). The Gail model may underestimate risk in women with hereditary predisposition, since it does not account for the extended family history or the paternal family history. The Gail model is not indicated for risk assessment in

women with a personal history of breast cancer or a documented history of LCIS, as both of these features are associated with an established future, new primary breast cancer risk that approximates 1% per year.

TAKE HOME POINTS

- Annual screening mammography in women with a normal breast exam should be initiated at age 40.
- The initial, preferred biopsy approach for a mammographically detected abnormality is via image-guided percutaneous core needle biopsy.
- High-risk pathology detected on needle biopsy specimens (LCIS, atypical hyperplasia) indicates the need for follow-up diagnostic surgical wire localization biopsy. This procedure will reveal coexisting cancer in approximately 15% of cases.
- LCIS is associated with an approximately 1% risk per year of subsequent breast cancer, affecting each breast equally and diffusely. Management options include surveillance (annual clinical breast exam, annual mammography, and possible annual breast MRI), chemoprevention, and bilateral prophylactic mastectomy.
- Atypical ductal hyperplasia is associated with an approximately four- to fivefold increased relative risk of breast cancer, with most of this risk expressed within the first 5 years after diagnosis, and mainly affecting the site where the atypia was detected. Management options include surveillance (as described above) and/or chemoprevention.

SUGGESTED READINGS

King TA, Reis-Filho JS. Lobular carcinoma in situ: biology and management. In: Harris JR, Lippman ME, Morrow M, et al., eds. *Diseases of the Breast*. 5th ed. Philadelphia, PA: Lippincott Williams & Wilkins; 2014.

National Comprehensive Cancer Network. Lobular carcinoma in situ (LCIS) (Version 2.2017). https://www.nccn.org/professionals/physician_gls/pdf/breast_blocks.pdf. Accessed January 29, 2018.

Newman LA. Surgical management of high risk breast lesions. *Probl Gen Surg*. 2003;20:99-112.

Oeffinger KC, Fontham ETH, Etzioni R, et al. Breast cancer screening for women at average risk 2015 guideline update from the American Cancer Society. *JAMA*. 2015;314(15):1599-1614.

Saslow D, Boetes C, Burke W, et al. American cancer society guidelines for breast screening with MRI as an adjunct to mammography. *CA Cancer J Clin*. 2007;57:75-89.

Early Stage Breast Cancer

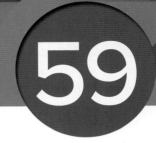

STACEY A. CARTER, KATRINA B. MITCHELL, AND HENRY KUERER

Presentation

A 39-year-old premenopausal woman with no significant past medical history palpates a firm, painless mass in the lateral aspect of her right breast. She has no history of previous breast imaging or breast biopsies. She has a family history of premenopausal breast cancer in one maternal aunt. Her physical exam is significant for a firm, irregular mass in the right breast at the 10 o'clock position, 6 centimeters from the nipple. There is no axillary, supraclavicular, or infraclavicular lymphadenopathy. The left breast and nodal basins are without significant findings.

● DIFFERENTIAL DIAGNOSIS

Breast cancer should be included in the differential diagnosis of all patients who present with a new breast mass. Careful questioning with the aid of physical exam can help guide further workup. The differential diagnoses that should be considered in this patient include the following:

- **Invasive breast cancer**: 10% of palpable breast masses are malignant. In general, early-stage breast cancer is defined as stage 0-II breast cancer (T0-2, N0-1, M0). The most common types of breast cancer are invasive ductal carcinoma and invasive lobular carcinoma. Routine mammographic screening may identify these lesions, while a portion of patients present with a palpable mass or skin and/or nipple changes. Invasive breast cancer is more common in postmenopausal women, but should remain part of the differential in younger patients as well.
- **Fibroadenoma**: The most common breast mass in young women. These lesions tend to be sharply demarcated, smooth, and mobile on exam. The lesions are often painless.
- **Phyllodes tumor**: A rare diagnosis, and may clinically resemble fibroadenomas as a discrete round or oval, firm, palpable mass. Phyllodes are usually benign, though some may demonstrate malignant potential.
- **Breast cyst**: These lesions are usually well circumscribed, smooth, and mobile, and may be associated with pain as the lesion enlarges.
- **Fibrocystic disease:** Vague thickening usually present bilaterally.

- **Fat necrosis:** May be related to prior breast trauma or a surgical procedure on the breast (augmentation or reduction mastopexy). The lesion may be hard and irregular and occasionally can mimic cancer with skin thickening and nipple retraction.
- **In situ lesions:** Ductal carcinoma in situ (DCIS) is most frequently diagnosed as calcifications on screening mammogram. Lobular carcinoma in situ (LCIS) may be mammographically occult and is more likely to be found incidentally on breast biopsy for other reasons. In situ lesions less commonly present as masses.

● WORKUP

The history initially should focus on symptomatology, such as changes of the mass with menstruation, nipple discharge, or skin changes. Patients should be assessed for risk factors for breast cancer, including a history of radiation to the chest. The history should include details of any previous breast biopsies or cosmetic procedures. A full obstetric and gynecologic history, including hormonal usage, age of menarche and menopause, age at parity, number of live births, and breast-feeding duration, is necessary in order to understand the patient's estrogen exposure over her lifetime. A complete family history (soliciting information about ovarian as well as breast cancer) and Ashkenazi Jewish heritage should be obtained.

The physical exam of the bilateral breasts and regional nodal basins should be performed in the upright and supine position. Inspection of the breasts for skin changes, asymmetry, or alterations in the nipple areolar complex is the first step in a comprehensive breast exam. The axillary, supraclavicular, and infraclavicular nodal basins should be systematically palpated. A firm mass with poorly defined margins should raise concern for a breast malignancy. Benign lesions are more likely to be well circumscribed, mobile, and soft or rubbery in texture.

The patient should undergo a bilateral diagnostic mammogram and a bilateral breast and nodal basin ultrasound. Suspicious lesions on physical exam or imaging warrant biopsy. The options include a stereotactic (mammographically guided) core needle biopsy or an ultrasound-guided core needle biopsy. A clip should be left at the biopsy site to denote the area sampled. Suspicious lymph nodes seen on ultrasound can be sampled with fine needle aspiration (FNA).

Table 59-1	Patient Workup for Invasive Early Breast Cancer

History and physical exam

Diagnostic bilateral mammogram; ultrasound as necessary

Pathology review

Determination of estrogen/progesterone (ER/PR) status and HER2 status

Genetic counseling if patient is high risk for hereditary breast cancer

Breast MRI[a] (optional)

Counseling for fertility concerns if premenopausal

Assess for distress

Labs: complete blood count, liver function studies, alkaline phosphatase

Bone scan (only if localized bone pain or elevated alkaline phosphatase)

Abdominal ± pelvic diagnostic CT scan (only if abnormal physical exam or unexplained elevated LFTs)

Chest CT scan (only if unexplained pulmonary symptoms)

[a]Breast MRI is optional, consider obtaining for patients with mammographically occult tumors.

Estrogen, progesterone, and HER2-neu status of a breast cancer should be obtained from the core needle biopsy, as it will affect adjuvant systemic therapy. If the patient is found to have metastatic disease to the axilla, she should undergo lab work (complete blood count [CBC], liver function tests [LFTs], and alkaline phosphatase) and additional imaging based on physical exam findings. All patients should have a urine pregnancy test. In selected patients, genetic counseling and referral to fertility counseling should be offered. Guidelines for the evaluation of early-stage breast cancer are outlined in Table 59-1.

Presentation Continued

The patient's mammogram shows an isodense, round mass in the right breast, upper outer quadrant measuring 1.2 cm with indistinct margins (Figure 59-1); the ultrasound shows an irregular hypoechoic mass that measures 1.2 cm with no right axillary lymphadenopathy (Figure 59-2). The patient undergoes an ultrasound-guided core needle biopsy with clip placement (Figure 59-3). The pathology shows invasive ductal carcinoma, high grade, ER/PR positive, and HER2-neu nonamplified.

● DIAGNOSIS AND TREATMENT

The patient's pathology results confirm the diagnosis of early-stage, node-negative invasive ductal carcinoma. The principles of treatment include surgery, with the possible addition of radiation and/or chemotherapy and endocrine therapy. Adjuvant therapy is guided by multiple factors beyond the scope of this chapter, and thus we will focus primarily on the surgical management of her cancer.

For early-stage breast cancer, the options for surgical management of the breast include breast-conserving surgery (BCT) with adjuvant radiation therapy versus mastectomy. If proceeding with BCT, ensure that the patient has no contraindication to radiation (previous mantle radiation or severe connective tissue disease); patients with a contraindication should be offered mastectomy with or without immediate reconstruction. Additionally, with BCT, consideration should be given to the breast size to tumor-size ratio and its impact on cosmesis, the patient's access to a radiation therapy center, and diffuse calcifications or widespread disease that would prohibit achieving a margin-negative resection.

For a small tumor, BCT followed by radiation therapy is preferred over total mastectomy. If a patient elects for or necessitates mastectomy, the options include a total mastectomy or, in appropriate candidates, a skin-sparing or nipple-sparing mastectomy with immediate reconstruction (implant based or autologous). A mastectomy may be required if a patient undergoes BCT and has persistent positive margins at a second or third attempted excision.

A patient with invasive disease and a clinically negative axilla must undergo axillary staging with sentinel lymph node biopsy (SLNB). Based on the results of the SLNB and the type of surgery performed, the patient may need no further treatment, or may undergo axillary radiation and/or axillary lymph node dissection (ALND).

Presentation Continued

The patient is counseled about her surgical options, and has no contraindication to BCT. She elects to undergo a needle-localized lumpectomy with SLNB.

● SURGICAL APPROACH

For BCT, the patient should undergo preoperative image-guided needle localization of the lesion (performed by mammogram or ultrasound guidance). Thorough review of localizing studies is necessary to estimate the trajectory of the wire and location of the mass (Figure 59-4). Though it is possible to excise a palpable lesion with or without intraoperative ultrasound guidance or without needle localization, needle localization or ^{125}I-radioactive seed localization is recommended as the safest and most conservative approach in the event the lesion is difficult to palpate in the operating room.

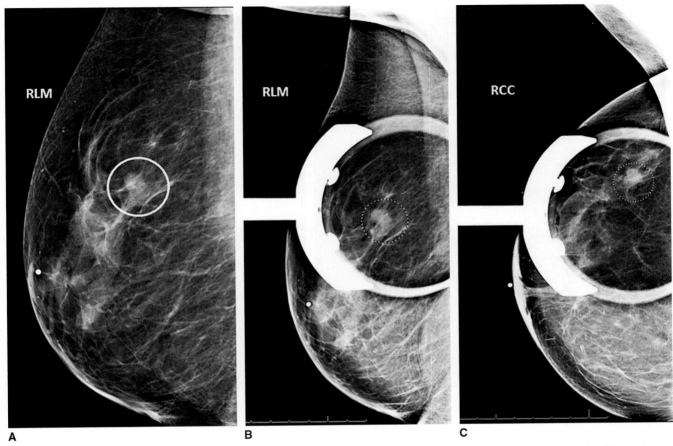

A   **B**   **C**

FIGURE 59-1. Diagnostic mammogram of the right breast, with mass lesion indicated (**A**). Spot compression views of the right breast mass (**B,C**).

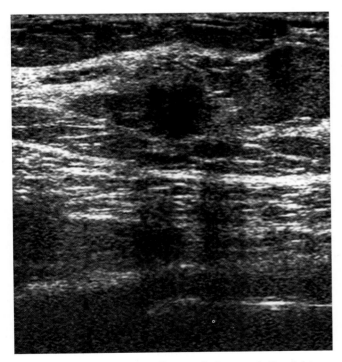

FIGURE 59-2. Ultrasound of hypoechoic mass in the right breast, upper outer quadrant.

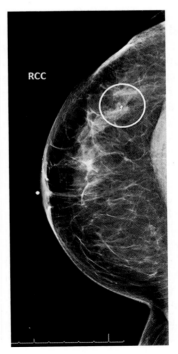

FIGURE 59-3. Postprocedure mammogram of the ultrasound-guided clip placement, confirming the clip is in the area biopsied.

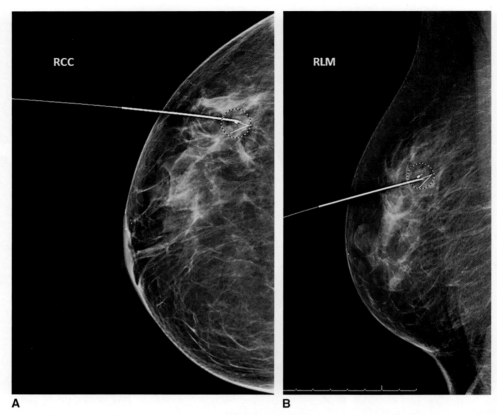

FIGURE 59-4. Mammogram after needle localization. Wire appears to be in good position near the targeted lesion and clip as seen in the craniocaudal (**A**) and medio-lateral view (**B**).

We recommended performing the SLNB with a dual tracer technique (radioactive colloid and isosulfan blue dye). Radioactive colloid may either be injected the day prior to the operation and a lymphoscintigraphy (lymphatic mapping) obtained, or it can be injected in the operating room prior to beginning the surgical procedure. Intraoperatively, we recommend injecting radioactive colloid and isosulfan blue in a peritumoral or periareolar fashion and massaging the breast for 5 minutes to optimize drainage. The gamma probe should be calibrated appropriately, and the nodal basins of the breast examined to detect a signal.

The breast incision should be placed over the lesion along Langer's lines or in a periareolar fashion to minimize cosmetic defect. Note that in order to minimize excessive undermining of the tissue, it is preferred to place the incision over the lesion rather than over the wire (which may enter the skin distant from the lesion). Once the skin is incised, superficial flaps should be raised with sharp dissection or electrocautery. Any tissue removed from the breast must be marked (usually with short superior and long lateral sutures) for pathologic inking to designate margins. Surgically, the aim is for a histologically margin-negative resection by targeting the lesion of interest and ensuring a small rim of normal tissue. A specimen radiograph should be obtained to confirm presence of the wire (or radioactive seed), clip, and targeted lesion. If any aspect of the margin appears involved, re-excision should be considered while in the operating room to avoid a second operation for positive margins. Careful hemostasis should be obtained with placement of place marker clips in the cavity. The incision is closed in layers.

The axillary dissection follows the breast excision. With the gamma probe, the area of maximal radioactive signal is located over the axilla. Using this area as a target, the axillary incision is placed below the hair-bearing area posterior to the pectoralis major. The skin is incised and the dissection carried through the clavipectoral fascia. All radioactive or blue nodes should be resected until the basin count is <10% of the node with the highest count. On average, 2 to 3 nodes are removed and either sent for permanent evaluation if BCT is performed, or for frozen section if mastectomy is performed.

A mastectomy can be performed as a simple (total) mastectomy, skin-sparing mastectomy, or nipple-sparing mastectomy. In general, superior and inferior flaps are raised to the borders of the breast tissue: the clavicle superiorly, sternum medially, latissimus dorsi laterally, and the inframammary fold inferiorly. The pectoralis fascia is excised with the breast specimen, but the muscle is left intact. Meticulous hemostasis is obtained and a drain is placed prior to closure.

● POTENTIAL PITFALLS

Potential pitfalls include poor localization of the breast lesion. For example, a wire tip may be placed beyond the targeted lesion. In most cases, the wire may fracture if manipulated, so a careful inspection of the localizing images will help determine if placement of an additional wire would be helpful. Occasionally, clips placed after biopsy may migrate and may be located away from the targeted area.

Failed localization of the sentinel lymph node with radioactive isotope and/or blue dye also may present a challenge to the surgeon. This is more common in obese patients or those who have had previous breast surgery because the lymphatic channels may be disrupted. If only one localization technique is used, the second should be added. Injecting subdermally rather than peritumoraly may help improve drainage. If all interventions fail, then the standard practice is to proceed with a full ALND; this possibility should be discussed with patients preoperatively as part of the informed consent process.

Other potential pitfalls include bleeding from one of the intercostal perforating vessels, and care should be taken to avoid these coursing medially near the sternum. If bleeding is encountered, utilize suture ligation or hemoclip placement. Allergic reaction to isosulfan dye occurs in 1% of patients and should be managed with epinephrine and steroid administration. Routine administration of prophylaxis for the isosulfan blue should be considered (steroids, H-2 blockers and diphenhydramine). Of note, isosulfan blue is teratogenic and cannot be used in pregnancy (Table 59-2).

Table 59-2	Lumpectomy with Sentinel Lymph Node Biopsy Lumpectomy
Key Technical Steps	
1.	Preoperative injection of radioactive colloid with lymphoscintigraphy for lymphatic mapping.
2.	Preoperative needle or radioactive seed localization of the breast lesion.
3.	Inject isosulfan blue dye (and radioactive colloid, if not done preoperatively) after induction and massage for 5 minutes. Use gamma probe to assess the axilla for signal.
4.	Make breast incision along Langer's lines or in a periareolar fashion. Avoid making the incision where the wire enters the skin, as this often results in excessive tunneling to resect the lesion.
5.	Dissect radial margins with the aim to preserve a small rim of normal tissue around the lesion.
6.	Orient the specimen with marking sutures for pathology.
7.	Obtain a specimen radiograph and examine for the wire (or radioactive seed), clip, and targeted lesion. Assess that there is no radiographic abnormality at the margin, if so, consider frozen section.
8.	Place marker clips in the specimen cavity to guide the radiation oncologist.
9.	Close in layers.
Sentinel Lymph Node Biopsy	
1.	Make an incision just below the hair-bearing area in the axilla over the location of the highest gamma probe signal.
2.	Continue dissection through clavipectoral fascia. Use probe to guide lymph node identification.
3.	Resect all radioactive or blue nodes until the basin count is <10% of the highest nodal count.
4.	Close the skin of axilla in layers.
Potential Pitfalls	
• Poor localization of the breast lesion	
• Failed localization using the dual-tracer technique	
• Bleeding	
• Anaphylaxis to the isosulfan blue	

● SPECIAL INTRAOPERATIVE CONSIDERATIONS

If a patient is undergoing BCT, several intraoperative issues should be considered.

If a suspicious additional mass is palpated, it should be resected and marked for margins as well. At times, the cancer may involve the anterior (skin) or posterior (muscle) margin. In this situation, a skin island (anterior) over the lesion should be resected, or a portion of the muscle (posterior) should be included en bloc with the tumor. In the case of persistently positive margins on final pathology, operation for re-excision or mastectomy is indicated.

● POSTOPERATIVE MANAGEMENT

Common potential postoperative complications include hematoma, seroma, lymphedema, infection, and more rarely wound dehiscence. Patients with large or rapidly expanding hematomas should return immediately to the operating room for evacuation and hemostasis. Small hematomas may be closely monitored for clinical change or development of infection. Seromas can be monitored, then aspirated if they become symptomatic or infected. If persistent despite repeated aspirations, drain placement may be warranted.

The risk of lymphedema after a SLNB is approximately 5% to 10%, and approximately 20% to 25% after an ALND. To reduce lymphedema risk, patients should be encouraged to perform postoperative range of motion exercises. Wound dehiscence is uncommon, but can be managed with local wound management techniques. Chest wall numbness is common after a total mastectomy and patients should be counseled that this is an expected result of surgery.

Patients with a diagnosis of breast cancer should undergo follow-up with physical exam, imaging, and possible referral to radiation and medical oncology, when appropriate. National guidelines for follow-up and surveillance for patients with breast cancer generally include a history and physical exam 1 to 4 times per year as clinically appropriate for 5 years then annually; periodic screening for changes in family history and referral to genetics as indicated; education and monitoring for lymphedema; and mammography every 12 months (after waiting at least 6 months after completion of radiation before obtaining mammogram). In the absence of signs and symptoms concerning for recurrent disease, there is no indication for laboratory or imaging studies for metastasis screening.

TAKE HOME POINTS

- A variety of benign and malignant diagnoses should be considered in a premenopausal woman with a palpable breast mass.
- Surgical options for early-stage breast cancer with a clinically negative nodal basin include lumpectomy with sentinel lymph node biopsy and postoperative radiation or total mastectomy with sentinel lymph node biopsy.
- Breast-conserving surgery should be guided by preoperative placement of a needle or other localization device and appropriate images should be reviewed prior to proceeding to the operating room.
- Any tissue removed from the breast must be marked (usually with short superior and long lateral sutures) for pathologic inking to designate margins.
- Potential intraoperative complications include allergy to blue dye (anaphylaxis), inability to localize a sentinel lymph node, and bleeding.
- Most common postoperative complications include hematoma, seroma, infection, lymphedema, wound dehiscence, and pain.

SUGGESTED READINGS

Fisher B, Anderson S, Bryant J, et al. Twenty-year follow-up of a randomized trial comparing total mastectomy, lumpectomy, and lumpectomy plus irradiation for the treatment of invasive breast cancer. *N Engl J Med.* 2002;347(16):1233-1241.

Giuliano AE, Hunt KK, Ballman KV, et al. Axillary dissection vs no axillary dissection in women with invasive breast cancer and sentinel node metastasis: a randomized clinical trial. *JAMA.* 2011; 305(6):569-575.

Kuerer HM. *Kuerer's Breast Surgical Oncology.* 1st ed. New York: McGraw Hill; 2010.

NCCN Guidelines Version 2.2016 Invasive breast cancer, 2016; Available at: https://www.nccn.org/professionals/physician_gls/ pdf/breast.pdf. Accessed May 30, 2016.

Advanced Breast Cancer

60

JUDY C. BOUGHEY AND JENNIFER RACZ

Based on the previous edition chapter "Advanced Breast Cancer" by Steven Chen and Erin Brown

Breast cancer is the second most common cause of cancer death in women in North America, second only to lung cancer. In the United States in 2013, approximately 232,300 women were diagnosed with breast cancer and 39,600 died of the disease. Approximately 5% of individuals diagnosed with breast cancer have advanced or metastatic disease at the time of their diagnosis. Locally advanced breast cancer (LABC) is a heterogeneous entity. The term includes T3, tumors >5 cm in maximum diameter; T4, tumors that directly invade the skin or chest wall, as well as inflammatory breast cancer; and N2-N3, tumors that have extensive regional lymph node involvement (matted ipsilateral lymph nodes), without evidence of distance metastatic disease at initial presentation. These tumors fall into the category of Stage IIB and III disease as per AJCC 7th edition staging. Up to 20% of patients with clinically LABC are found to be metastatic (Stage IV) after staging.

Presentation

A 42-year-old female presented with a self-detected breast mass for further investigation and discussion of treatment options. Approximately 1 month ago, she discovered an ill-defined, large mass in her right breast while bathing. She denies any symptoms related to the breast including breast pain, nipple discharge, or changes to the overlying skin. Her past medical history and family history are unremarkable. She takes no medications and is a nondrinker and nonsmoker. On physical examination, there is no evidence of supra- or infraclavicular adenopathy. There is a right breast mass measuring approximately 6 cm in size located in the upper central and upper inner quadrant. There is no evidence of overlying skin changes; however, palpation of the right axilla is remarkable for adenopathy. The nodes are firm but mobile and nontender. Examination of the left breast and axilla is unremarkable.

● DIFFERENTIAL DIAGNOSIS

A breast mass with obvious adenopathy in a premenopausal woman should be considered invasive breast cancer until proven otherwise through imaging and tissue biopsy. Both invasive ductal carcinoma and invasive lobular carcinoma

should be considered although invasive ductal carcinoma is the most common and accounts for approximately 90% of diagnoses of breast cancer. This particular subtype of cancer begins in the milk ducts of the breast. Although invasive breast cancer is the most likely diagnosis based upon clinical presentation, the differential diagnosis also includes other benign and malignant conditions. Underlying pathology of the breast that results in lymphadenopathy such as a breast abscess may be a consideration in the right clinical setting (i.e., lactation). Other malignant entities include breast lymphoma, phyllodes tumor, or metastatic disease from another primary cancer (i.e., melanoma, ovarian, medullary thyroid, pulmonary, and neuroendocrine cancer, among others). Fibroadenomas (benign breast lesions) can present as large masses; however, they are usually not associated with lymphadenopathy.

● WORKUP

A thorough history is essential in order to discern the underlying diagnosis. As invasive breast cancer is the most likely diagnosis given the clinical scenario presented, additional information that should be sought includes (a) onset and duration of symptoms, (b) relationship between the mass and the patient's menstrual cycle, and (c) presence or absence of fever and chills or systemic symptoms. Breast cancer risk stratification should also be emphasized. Important risk factors to include are age at menarche and menopause (if postmenopausal), age at first pregnancy and number of pregnancies, history of breastfeeding, previous use of oral contraceptives or hormone replacement therapy, previous breast biopsies and results, personal history of breast cancer, and family history of breast cancer and/or ovarian cancer. For premenopausal patients with breast cancer or those with a strong family history, genetic testing should be considered. Indications for genetic testing include:

- Multiple relatives with breast (especially <50 years) and/or ovarian cancer (any age)
- Age of diagnosis <35 years
- A family member diagnosed with both breast and ovarian cancer
- Breast and/or ovarian cancer in Jewish families (Ashkenazi)
- Family members with primary cancer in both breasts—especially if diagnosed <50 years

- A family member diagnosed with invasive serous ovarian cancer
- Presence of male breast cancer in the family
- Family member with an identified *BRCA*1 or *BRCA*2 mutation
- Presence of other associated cancers or conditions suggestive of an inherited cancer syndrome
- Breast cancer during pregnancy
- Triple-negative breast cancer diagnosed at age ≤60 years

Physical examination of both breasts in both the sitting and supine positions will reveal the presence of any other masses and also allow you to determine characteristics of the primary mass (i.e., size, mobility, border regularity, relationship to nipple–areolar complex, etc.). In addition to physical examination of the breast, a thorough examination of all surrounding nodal basins should be completed including axillary, infra- and supraclavicular, cervical, and submandibular. Given the presence of a palpable mass, the next step is a bilateral diagnostic mammogram in combination with ultrasound of the mass and the ipsilateral axilla. An magnetic resonance imaging (MRI) may be considered in order to assess the extent of invasive disease, which may ultimately change operative management. Image-guided (ultrasound usually or if not visible by ultrasound then stereotactic) percutaneous core needle biopsies should be obtained for histologic confirmation of the suspected diagnosis. If invasive breast cancer is identified, estrogen receptor (ER), progesterone receptor (PR), and Her2/

neu receptor status should be evaluated on the tumor from the percutaneous biopsy. The ipsilateral axilla should be evaluated with axillary ultrasound, and if sonographically abnormal lymph nodes are seen, then percutaneous ultrasound-guided biopsy (either fine needle aspiration or core needle biopsy) should be performed. In cases of clinical Stage III breast cancer, evaluation for distant metastases is recommended with use of a bone scan and computed tomography (CT) of the chest, abdomen, and pelvis (or a PET/CT scan). Metastatic workup is not indicated in Stage II breast cancer.

The patient's workup confirms the presence of a right breast mass measuring 6.5 cm in maximal dimension based on imaging studies (Figures 60-1 and 60-2). Ultrasound of the ipsilateral axilla demonstrates the presence of two large morphologically abnormal lymph nodes. No radiographic abnormalities were noted on the left breast or axilla. Core biopsy is consistent with invasive ductal carcinoma, grade III, ER negative, PR negative, and Her2 negative. FNA of the suspicious lymph nodes was positive for metastatic disease. Metastatic workup was negative for metastatic disease.

● DIAGNOSIS AND TREATMENT

Based upon the history, physical examination, and workup, invasive breast cancer involving the right breast and right axillary lymph nodes is the diagnosis. The tumor is 6.5 cm

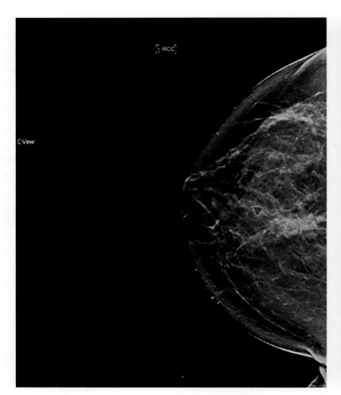 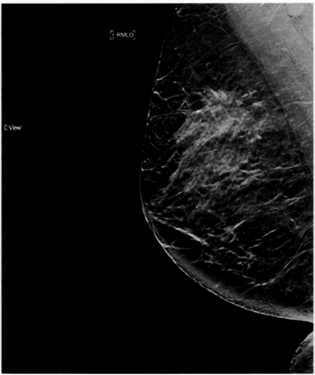

FIGURE 60-1. CC and MLO views of the right breast demonstrating a focal/regional asymmetry within the upper aspect of the right breast.

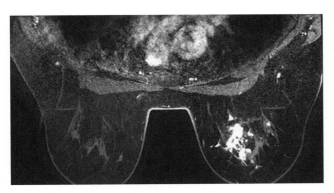

FIGURE 60-2. Bilateral breast MRI demonstrating an irregular, spiculated, and markedly enhancing mass in the upper central and upper inner right breast.

in maximum diameter (T3). There is evidence of axillary lymph node involvement in the right axilla (N1), and there is no evidence of distant metastatic disease (M0). So this is a clinical cT3N1, Stage IIIA, triple-negative breast cancer. A multidisciplinary approach is fundamental to the treatment of breast cancer, especially LABC, and several factors impact the sequence of treatment. Treatment of advanced disease should include a combination of surgery, radiation therapy, and chemotherapy. In this case of Stage IIIA, locally advanced disease, there are two options: primary surgical management followed by adjuvant chemotherapy and adjuvant radiation or neoadjuvant chemotherapy followed by surgery and adjuvant radiation. In a premenopausal patient with triple negative Stage IIIA breast cancer, neoadjuvant chemotherapy would be recommended.

Surgical management of the primary breast disease would consist of either a mastectomy or breast conservation therapy (i.e., lumpectomy, partial mastectomy, or wide local excision) and should focus on removal of all disease to negative margins. The ultimate decision between breast-conserving therapy and mastectomy should be made only after a thorough discussion between the patient and the operating surgeon has occurred. In all cases, it is essential that the surgeon inform the patient of all of the risks, benefits, and alternatives of each surgical approach. It is also imperative that the surgeon discuss the multidisciplinary treatment of breast cancer and the general sequence of care.

With a 6.5-cm tumor, the patient is not a candidate for breast conservation if surgical resection is performed first. However, with the use of neoadjuvant chemotherapy, the primary breast tumor is likely to shrink in size, and thus, the patient may be a reasonable candidate for breast conservation surgery postchemotherapy. A clip should be placed routinely in the breast lesion at the time of diagnostic percutaneous core needle biopsy; however, if one has not been placed, a clip to mark the center of the lesion should be placed before the patient starts chemotherapy. After chemotherapy, if the tumor has decreased in size, lumpectomy should be focused on resecting the residual disease, and the

total volume of the index tumor at presentation does not need to be resected. If multicentric disease is documented at presentation, then mastectomy would be recommended regardless of the response to neoadjuvant therapy.

In cases of ER-positive, PR-positive, and Her2-negative locally advanced tumors in postmenopausal women, neoadjuvant endocrine therapy rather than neoadjuvant chemotherapy may be used and similarly has been shown to decrease tumor size and increase breast conservation rates. Ultimately, the goal of neoadjuvant therapy is to reduce the disease burden in order to facilitate or enable breast conservation.

Regardless of which surgical approach of the primary breast cancer is chosen, if surgical resection is performed first, then treatment of the axillary disease will require a complete axillary lymph node dissection. If the patient receives neoadjuvant chemotherapy, then standard recommendation is axillary lymph node dissection; however, data are emerging regarding the use of sentinel lymph node surgery for patients with node-positive breast cancer treated with neoadjuvant chemotherapy with a good clinical response.

● SURGICAL APPROACH

Mastectomy

The goal of surgical resection is complete removal of all disease with adequate margins (i.e., no ink at margins in the case of invasive disease).

Key Technical Steps

1. Creation of an elliptical incision to include the nipple–areolar complex and excess breast skin. Include the skin overlying the tumor in all cases where the tumor is close to the skin.
2. Formation of superior and inferior skin flaps, using electrocautery, which extend superiorly to the clavicle, inferiorly to the inframammary fold, laterally to the anterior border of the latissimus dorsi, and medially to the lateral edge of the sternum.
3. Placement of orientation sutures on the breast.
4. Dissection of the breast off of the chest wall taking the pectoralis fascia with the breast specimen.
5. Hemostasis.
6. Placement of a drain.
7. Closure—with resection of additional skin if needed to avoid dog-ears or excess skin on the chest wall. Closure should be tight however without significant tension on the flaps.

Note: If immediate reconstruction is planned, a skin-sparing or nipple-sparing approach may be used. Nipple-sparing is not commonly used for LABC. For a skin-sparing approach, a circular incision around the edge of the areola is used and the mastectomy performed through that incision.

Potential Pitfalls

1. Formation of flaps that are too thick or too thin:
   a. Thin flaps may lead to development of flap necrosis.
   b. Thick flaps may lead to an increased risk of recurrence as breast tissue may be left behind.
2. Incomplete removal of all breast tissue, particularly the axillary tail.

Breast-Conserving Therapy

As described above, the goal of surgical resection is complete removal of all disease with adequate margins (i.e., no ink at margins in the case of invasive disease and minimum margin of 2 mm around ductal carcinoma in situ); however, with breast conservation, consideration of cosmesis is also of importance to patients. If the lesion is palpable, surgical resection is generally straightforward; however, for nonpalpable lesions, preoperative localization should be undertaken either using a wire or placing a radioactive seed or intraoperative ultrasound (if the surgeon is skilled in ultrasound). The type of preoperative localization technique is generally dependent upon surgeon preference.

Key Technical Steps

1. Incision in a location that will be incorporated in future mastectomy if required.
2. Formation of short tissue flaps circumferentially around the tumor.
3. Circumferential dissection around the tumor with the goal of negative margins.
4. Orientation of the specimen with sutures (ideally three-dimensional orientation).
5. Specimen radiograph to confirm excision of the lesion (and clip if a clip is present in the tumor).
6. Hemostasis.
7. Marking of the lumpectomy cavity with clips to facilitate radiation in the future.
8. Closure of the deep tissue defect in the breast.
9. Closure of the skin.

Potential Pitfalls

1. Incomplete resection of the tumor with inadequate or positive margins.
2. Poor cosmetic result.

Axillary Lymph Node Dissection

As mentioned above, this patient had pathologically positive nodes prior to surgery and as a result requires axillary lymph node dissection (Figure 60-3).

Key Technical Steps

1. Free draping of the arm in order to allow manipulation during the procedure.

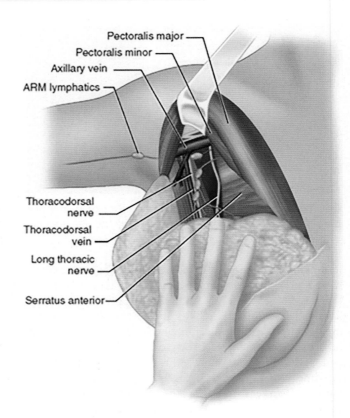

FIGURE 60-3. Axillary anatomy following axillary lymph node dissection with preserved structures including the long thoracic nerve, axillary vein, and thoracodorsal nerve.

2. Incision at the posterior edge of the pectoral fold inferior to the axillary hairline.
3. Creation of skin flaps medially, laterally, inferiorly, and superiorly.
4. Incision of clavipectoral fascia and identification of the axillary vein.
5. Identification and preservation of the thoracodorsal neurovascular bundle.
6. Identification and preservation of the long thoracic nerve.
7. En bloc removal of all level I and II lymph nodes as defined by the pectoralis minor muscle.
8. Palpation of level III nodes and Rotter's node with potential excision if suspicious.
9. Hemostasis.
10. Placement of a drain.
11. Closure of the clavipectoral fascia and skin.

Potential Pitfalls

1. Injury to the thoracodorsal or long thoracic nerves leading to weakened arm adduction and/or winged scapula.
2. Injury to the axillary vein potentially causing bleeding and hematoma and increasing the risk of upper extremity lymphedema.
3. Injury to the brachial plexus from dissection that is too high (above the axillary vein).

SPECIAL INTRAOPERATIVE CONSIDERATIONS

In patients with advanced breast cancer, the tumor may closely approximate the subcutaneous tissue or overlying skin, and as a result, a greater margin of skin may need to be excised with the specimen. Similarly, the tumor may also closely approximate or invade the deep margin (i.e., pectoralis major muscle). In this case, the involved pectoralis muscle should be excised with the specimen with a margin of normal tissue. Finally, in most cases, only level I and II lymph nodes need to be removed; however, if there are clinically palpable nodes in level III, these nodes should be excised as well.

POSTOPERATIVE MANAGEMENT

Patients who undergo breast conservation surgery and sentinel lymph node biopsy are generally managed as outpatients, whereas patients who undergo mastectomy and/or axillary lymph node dissection remain overnight in hospital to monitor the drain output. Two drains are generally left in place following a mastectomy and axillary lymph node dissection (modified radical mastectomy) in order to prevent seroma formation. Drains should be removed when draining <30 cc per day for 2 consecutive days.

Following a period of postoperative recovery (normally 4 to 6 weeks), patients should initiate adjuvant therapy. If chemotherapy was delivered prior to surgery (neoadjuvant chemotherapy), then radiation starts no later than 12 weeks after surgery and usually consists of a 6-week course of radiation to the breast or chest wall and the regional lymph nodes. For hormone receptor–positive (ER- and/or PR-positive) tumors, adjuvant endocrine therapy (tamoxifen in pre-or postmenopausal patients or an aromatase inhibitor for postmenopausal patients) is recommended for 5 to 10 years. If chemotherapy was not given in the neoadjuvant setting, then adjuvant chemotherapy should follow surgery. Radiation is then delivered after chemotherapy. The specific regimen is dependent upon the hormonal profile of the tumor and the age of the patient, and thus, a multidisciplinary approach to all cases of breast cancer cannot be emphasized enough.

After completion of treatment, patients should continue to undergo surveillance with clinical breast exams and breast imaging with mammogram (and MRI for high-risk patients). Patients who have had a mastectomy require routine imaging on the contralateral breast, but no routine breast imaging on the side of the mastectomy. Exams and imaging should begin approximately 6 months following completion of treatment.

This patient received neoadjuvant chemotherapy with Adriamycin, Cytoxan followed by Taxotere, and carboplatin. She had an excellent clinical and imaging response to neoadjuvant chemotherapy. She underwent a mastectomy and axillary dissection. The final pathology for this case demonstrated no residual viable tumor in the breast and 1 out of 18 lymph nodes positive for residual cancer. As she had positive axillary lymph nodes, she is also recommended postmastectomy radiation to the chest wall and nodal basins.

TAKE HOME POINTS

- Treatment of breast cancer requires a multidisciplinary approach as each treatment modality has the potential to impact the other modalities and patients with LABC usually require a combination of surgery, chemotherapy, and radiation therapy.
- The treatment of breast cancer continues to evolve, and as such, each patient should be considered on a case-by-case basis; tumor biology is important in decision-making.
- Tumor size and grade and nodal status are the most important prognostic factors for long-term survival from breast cancer.
- Stage I and II breast cancers have a 5-year overall survival between 90% and 100%.
- Stage III breast cancers have a 5-year overall survival between 36% and 67%.
- A patient with a Stage IV breast cancer diagnosis can expect a 5-year overall survival rate of approximately 26%.
- Monitoring for recurrence through clinical breast exams or routine imaging is essential.

SUGGESTED READINGS

Boughey JC, et al. Identification and resection of clipped node decreases the false-negative rate of sentinel lymph node surgery in patients presenting with node-positive breast cancer (T0-T4, N1-N2) who receive neoadjuvant chemotherapy: results from ACOSOG Z1071 (Alliance). *Ann Surg.* 2016;263(4):802-807.

Feig BW, Ching CD. Invasive breast disease. *The MD Anderson Surgical Oncology Handbook.* 5th ed. Lippincott Williams & Wilkins; 2012:27-84.

Gardishar WJ, et al. The NCCN Breast Cancer Clinical Practice Guidelines in Oncology Version 2.2016.

Haffty BG, et al. Patterns of local-regional management following neoadjuvant chemotherapy in breast cancer: results from ACOSOG Z1071 (Alliance). *Int J Radiat Oncol Biol Phys.* 2016; 94(3):493-502.

Inflammatory Breast Cancer

61

MIRAJ G. SHAH-KHAN AND MONICA MORROW

Based on the previous edition chapter "Inflammatory Breast Cancer" by
Walter P. Weber and Monica Morrow

Presentation

A 49-year-old woman, G2 P2, age 30 at first birth with no family history of breast cancer, presents with a 1-month history of increasing redness, heaviness, and swelling of her right breast (Figure 61-1). There was no antecedent history of trauma. Two weeks ago, she saw her primary care physician who made the diagnosis of breast infection and gave her a 10-day course of a cephalosporin. Her symptoms have not improved, and she was referred for surgical evaluation. On physical examination, there is diffuse erythema and edema of the right breast. The breast is diffusely firm compared to the left, but no discrete mass is palpable. There are no palpable supraclavicular or left axillary nodes. A firm, mobile, nontender 1-cm right axillary node is present.

● DIFFERENTIAL DIAGNOSIS

In a nonlactating woman, erythema and edema over more than one-third of the breast that does not significantly improve with antibiotic treatment is inflammatory breast cancer (IBC) until proven otherwise. Bacterial infection, including mastitis and abscess, is the most common misdiagnosis. These infections, however, are rare in nonlactating women, and treatment with antibiotics tends to be of immediate benefit. Because IBC is not a true inflammatory process, it is not associated with symptoms such as fever, localized pain, or leukocytosis.

● WORKUP

The patient undergoes bilateral mammography, which reveals only skin thickening and diffusely increased breast density on the right side (Figure 61-2). Ultrasonography demonstrates increased vascularity and minor architectural distortions in the right breast, and confirms the presence of an enlarged 1.2-cm right axillary node with abnormal architecture. A punch biopsy of the skin, ultrasound-guided core biopsy of the architectural distortion in the breast, and fine needle aspiration cytology of the right axillary node demonstrate high-grade adenocarcinoma, thereby confirming the clinical diagnosis of node-positive IBC. The estrogen

receptor (ER), progesterone receptor (PR), and HER2 are negative. Laboratory studies show that liver enzymes and lactate dehydrogenase are within normal limits. Further staging with a positron emission tomography–computed tomography (PET–CT) scan reveals no signs of distant metastases.

● DIAGNOSIS AND TREATMENT

IBC is a clinical diagnosis defined by the American Joint Committee on Cancer (AJCC) as "a diffuse erythema and edema involving approximately a third or more of the skin of the breast" and is designated cT4d. In the absence of distant metastases, staging incorporates the tumor biology, and in this case would be considered stage IIIC. Patients present with rapid enlargement of the breast, erythema, and skin edema, often with an orange-peel appearance (peau d' orange), and induration or ridging over more than one-third of the breast. The rapid evolution of breast symptoms characterizes IBC, and thus the term inflammatory breast cancer should not be used to describe a neglected locally advanced breast cancer associated with breast edema and skin ulceration. When examining a patient with IBC, the breast is warm and diffusely firm, although a discrete mass is often not palpable. In addition, physical exam often reveals palpable lymph nodes as more than 50% of IBC patients have nodal involvement at the time of diagnosis. Mammography with or

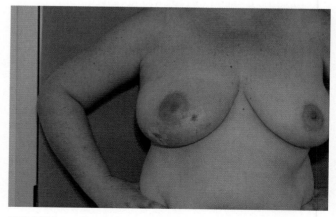

FIGURE 61-1. The findings of diffuse erythema and edema of the enlarged right breast with adenocarcinoma on biopsy are diagnostic for IBC.

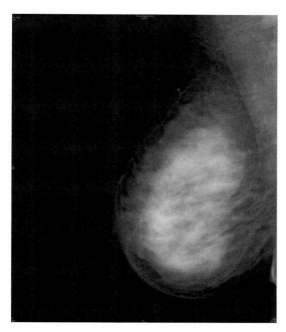

FIGURE 61-2. Mediolateral oblique view of mammogram showing inferior skin thickening and diffuse increase in density from IBC.

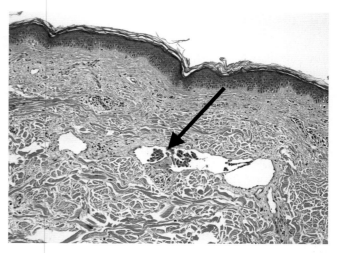

FIGURE 61-3. Photomicrograph showing tumor in the dermal lymphatic spaces (*arrow*). This finding supports the diagnosis of inflammatory cancer, but tumor in dermal lymphatic spaces without clinical inflammatory changes is not IBC.

without ultrasound is standard of care, even though imaging studies may be inconclusive. Classic mammographic features include skin thickening and increased breast density, and a discrete mass is evident in as many as 80% of cases in some reports. Ultrasonography demonstrates increased vascularity and architectural distortion in addition to mass lesions. Distant metastases are present in approximately 25% of patients at the time of diagnosis, and staging investigations should be performed on a routine basis. Laboratory tests should include a complete blood count and comprehensive metabolic profile. PET–CT is the imaging test of choice for the detection of distant metastases.

The inflammatory appearance of the breast is due to tumor emboli within the dermal lymphatics (Figure 61-3). This finding can often be demonstrated on a full-thickness skin biopsy but is not necessary to make the diagnosis of IBC when the clinical signs are present and a biopsy reveals adenocarcinoma of any subtype. Core needle biopsy of any breast mass is the preferred method of diagnosis. In the absence of a discrete mass, core biopsy of any area of architectural distortion on ultrasound is usually diagnostic. The biopsy material should be sent for hormone receptor and HER2 determination.

IBC is rare, accounting for <3% of breast cancer cases in the United States, but it is the most lethal form of primary breast cancer. Historically, mastectomy with or without radiotherapy was standard management, resulting on average 5-year overall survival rates of <5%. By the 1970s, the treatment paradigm for IBC had shifted to one involving chemotherapy followed by radiotherapy, which improved average 5-year overall survival rates to 30% or more. The use of surgery for IBC has increased again over the last two decades, but the timing of mastectomy has changed from initial cancer management to a postchemotherapy intervention, followed

by radiotherapy in all cases and hormonal therapy in hormone receptor–positive disease. The advent of multimodality therapy has significantly improved survival, with 5-year survival rates of over 40% being reported. Hence, women diagnosed with IBC should be managed in a setting where such a specialized approach can be adequately provided.

● SURGICAL APPROACH

The goals of surgery in IBC are to maintain local control and to improve survival in the absence of distant metastases. The current standard protocol for patients with IBC calls for initial treatment with neoadjuvant chemotherapy. Only patients who show complete resolution of all evidence of skin inflammation should undergo surgery. Surgery in the setting of residual inflammatory changes is associated with poor local control and survival.

The standard procedure in patients with IBC is modified radical mastectomy, which by definition includes total mastectomy with ipsilateral level I/II axillary lymph node dissection. Breast conservation is contraindicated in IBC. Skin-sparing and nipple-sparing mastectomies are contraindicated as well due to the diffuse nature of the tumor and the inability to reliably identify patients with pathologic complete response preoperatively. Moreover, sentinel lymph node biopsy is also contraindicated in patients with IBC. Even though increasing clinical experience suggests that sentinel node biopsy reliably stages the axilla after neoadjuvant therapy, the limited experience of sentinel node biopsy following neoadjuvant chemotherapy for IBC has demonstrated a false-negative rate that is unacceptably high, likely secondary to the interference of dermal lymphatics by tumor emboli. Since many of the advantages of immediate reconstruction, such as the skin-sparing approach, are lost, and because postmastectomy radiotherapy is indicated for all patients, delayed reconstruction is generally preferred.

● MASTECTOMY

The patient is placed supine, with the arm extended on a padded arm board. The arm should be prepped and draped separately to allow free rotation. The skin resection should encompass the nipple and areola, the surgical biopsy site (if present), and the excess skin of the breast. Skin flaps are then created with electrocautery or by sharp dissection with the scalpel or curved scissors. The skin flaps are raised in the plane between the subcutaneous fat and the breast tissue, and extend superiorly to the clavicle, medially to the sternal edge, laterally to the latissimus dorsi, and inferiorly to the rectus sheath. The next step is to remove the breast, which is most easily done from superior to inferior with the fascia of the pectoralis major as the deep margin of the resection. The internal mammary perforators should be ligated with clips or ties to avoid postoperative hemorrhage. The dissection is extended to the lateral aspect of the pectoralis major muscle, which is retracted, and the fascia overlying the pectoralis minor muscle is opened to allow placement of a retractor beneath the muscle. The axillary lymph node dissection is then carried out as described in detail below.

● LYMPH NODE DISSECTION

Standard axillary dissection clears levels I and II (nodes lateral to the lateral border and posterior to the pectoralis minor muscle). A full level III dissection above the pectoralis minor muscle is carried out when there is gross nodal disease as described in this case. After the breast has been taken off the chest wall as described above, the latissimus dorsi muscle is followed proximally along its anterior surface until it turns tendinous, at which time it is crossed by the axillary vein. No important structures cross this plane of dissection, making it the safest approach to the axillary vein. The anterior surface of the axillary vein is then cleared of overlying fat from lateral to medial, with care being taken not to dissect superior to the vein or to strip the vein in the vascular plane, both of which promote lymphedema. When the vein is well visualized, dissection inferior to the vein is carried out, again working from lateral to medial, dividing the fat and controlling the branches of the axillary vein entering the specimen. The thoracodorsal neurovascular bundle is usually the first deep lateral branch identified after the superficial fat and the vessels have been divided. Once the thoracodorsal bundle is identified, the pectoralis minor is retracted and the level 3 nodes are dissected from the space below the axillary vein and against the chest wall. This can be facilitated by flexion of the shoulder and elevation and adduction of the arm to provide greater access to the axillary apex. The axillary specimen is then retracted laterally; the long thoracic nerve is identified against the chest wall and dissected free from the specimen. The fat between the thoracodorsal and long thoracic nerves is then encircled with a clamp, divided, and bluntly swept inferiorly. Branches of the thoracodorsal

vessels entering the specimen are controlled with clips, and the specimen is freed from its remaining attachments to the inferior chest wall. After hemostasis is obtained, two closed suction drains are inserted, one beneath the inferior flap and one in the apex of the axilla. The deep dermis is reapproximated with absorbable sutures, and the skin is closed with a running subcuticular stitch (Table 61-1).

● SPECIAL INTRAOPERATIVE CONSIDERATIONS

Intraoperative findings that would change the operative strategy are rare after a patient has been adequately staged. If the cancer invades the pectoralis muscle, the involved muscle can be removed. There is no need for a classic radical mastectomy for limited muscle involvement, and extensive involvement is clinically evident preoperatively. If extensive axillary nodal metastases extending superiorly into the supraclavicular space are identified intraoperatively, they can be removed if they are mobile and this can be safely done. If residual disease is left behind, it should be marked with clips to assist in defining the radiotherapy fields (Table 61-2).

● POSTOPERATIVE MANAGEMENT

The patient usually requires an overnight hospital stay. The drain should be removed when the drainage is <30 mL/24 h. A single dose of antibiotic is given prior to surgery, but ongoing prophylactic antibiotics when the drains are in place are not recommended. Postoperative complications other than seroma are infrequent and include bleeding and infection. Postoperative hemorrhage can result from failure to control internal mammary perforators, axillary vein branches, or

Table 61-1	Mastectomy

Key Technical Steps

1. Plan the transverse elliptical incision to remove the nipple and areola and excess breast skin but allow tension-free closure.
2. Create the skin flaps.
3. Dissect and remove the breast with the fascia of the pectoralis major muscle.

Potential Pitfalls

- Insufficient skin removal resulting in residual disease left behind in dermal lymphatics.
- Excessive skin removal resulting in tension on the wound delaying radiotherapy.
- Failure to raise flaps to the anatomic boundaries of the breast potentially resulting in residual disease left behind in the glandular tissue.
- Bleeding from internal mammary perforators.

Table 61-2   Axillary Lymph Node Dissection

Key Technical Steps

1. Open axillary investing fascia lateral to pectoralis major and minor muscles.
2. Identify axillary vein by following the latissimus dorsi superiorly until it turns tendinous and is crossed by the vein.
3. Identify the thoracodorsal bundle and the long thoracic nerve and preserve.
4. Control vascular branches of thoracodorsal vessels entering the specimen.
5. Place suction drains.

Potential Pitfalls

- Injury to long thoracic nerve.
- Injury to thoracodorsal nerve.
- Bleeding from axillary vein or thoracodorsal branches.
- Inadequate access to axillary apex.

and occupational therapy postoperatively is recommended to improve mobility prior to radiation, as well as address any signs of early edema or axillary cording.

Case Conclusion

Following neoadjuvant therapy with dose-dense doxorubicin, cyclophosphamide, and paclitaxel with complete resolution of inflammatory skin changes, the patient underwent modified radical mastectomy and was staged ypT4dpN2a, stage IIIC. Pathology demonstrated scattered residual microscopic foci of tumor throughout the breast, with evidence of treatment effect in the remaining breast tissue. Five of fourteen nodes contained metastases, and the ER, PR, and HER2 remain negative. Adjuvant radiotherapy to the chest wall and supraclavicular, axillary, and internal mammary node fields is planned. She will be followed with clinical exam every 3 months for 2 years, then every 6 months for 3 years, and yearly thereafter, and with annual mammography.

thoracodorsal branches. Bleeding from these sites usually requires reexploration. Seroma formation can be minimized by removing drains when drainage is <30 mL/24 h rather than on some arbitrary day. If drainage is persistent at 21 days postoperatively, drain removal should be considered to avoid surgical site infection secondary to bacterial colonization of bulb or tubing. If a seroma is clinically detectable, it should be aspirated since the mastectomy flaps cannot adhere to the chest wall in the presence of seroma fluid. The chest wall is anesthetic in 100% of patients postmastectomy. This is a side effect, not a complication, and patients should be educated about this preoperatively. Skin flap necrosis is another potential complication that results from closure under tension, technical error in cutting the skin flaps, or infection. Postmastectomy infections usually present as cellulitis, and any erythema of the wound should lead to prompt antibiotic treatment to avoid flap necrosis. If flap necrosis is suspected, it should be observed until clear demarcation is present and necrotic tissue debrided at that time. With proper incision planning, major full-thickness necrosis is rare, and most necrosis is superficial and limited extent, and will heal without surgical intervention.

Axillary lymph node dissection is associated with long-term morbidity, including chronic lymphedema (5% to 25%), and shoulder dysmobility (5% to 15%). Adjuvant radiation may further increase the risk of upper extremity lymphedema, particularly in higher risk patients. Injury to the motor nerves in the axilla is rare (<1%). Injury to the long thoracic nerve results in a palsy of the serratus anterior muscle and, clinically, will create a winged scapula. Injury to the thoracodorsal nerve causes a palsy of the latissimus dorsi muscle, which may be evident during athletic activity or when trying to scratch in the midline of the back. Early referral to physical therapy

TAKE HOME POINTS

- Prompt biopsy is required for inflammatory breast changes that do not resolve with antibiotics.
- IBC is a clinical diagnosis; histologic confirmation of tumor emboli in dermal lymphatics is not mandatory.
- Multimodality treatment consists of neoadjuvant chemotherapy, surgery, radiotherapy, and hormonal therapy if indicated.
- Surgery is reserved for patients with resolution of skin erythema during neoadjuvant chemotherapy.
- Modified radical mastectomy is standard of care; breast conservation and sentinel lymph node biopsy are contraindicated.

SUGGESTED READINGS

Chia S, Swain SM, Byrd DR, et al. Locally advanced and inflammatory breast cancer. *J Clin Oncol.* 2008;26(5):786-790.

Hance KW, Anderson WF, Devesa SS, et al. Large population-based epidemiological study of IBC: trends in inflammatory breast carcinoma incidence and survival: the surveillance, epidemiology, and end results program at the National Cancer Institute. *J Natl Cancer Inst.* 2005;97(13):966-975.

Menta A, Fouad TM, Lucci A, et al. Inflammatory breast cancer: what to know about this unique, aggressive breast cancer. *Surg Clin North Am.* 2018 Aug;98(4):787-800. Epub 2018 May 24.

Merajver S, Iniesta MD, Sabel MS, et al. eds. Inflammatory breast Cancer. In: *Diseases of the Breast.* 4th ed. Philadelphia, PA: Wolters Kluwer/Lippincott; 2010:762-773.

Ueno NT, Buzdar AU, Singletary SE, et al. Combined modality treatment of inflammatory breast carcinoma: twenty years of experience at M.D Anderson Center. *Cancer Chemother Pharmacol.* 1997;40(4):321-329.

Breast Cancer During Pregnancy

ANNE E. MATTINGLY AND MARIE CATHERINE LEE

62

Based on the previous edition chapter "Breast Cancer During Pregnancy" by Jennifer E. Joh and Marie Catherine Lee

Presentation

Case 1: A 40-year-old nulliparous African American female presented to her primary care physician with a left upper outer quadrant breast mass for which 6-month follow-up ultrasound was recommended. She conceived in the interim; at the time of presentation to her obstetrician for an initial prenatal evaluation, she noted that the mass had increased in size. Her last menstrual period was approximately 6 weeks prior to presentation to the obstetrician. The palpable breast mass had increased in size over the past 6 months and had grown substantially over the past month.

Case 2: A 32-year-old G2P1 Caucasian female presented to her primary care physician in her 5th week of gestation with a palpable left breast mass and associated nipple retraction. A left breast sonogram performed at that time confirmed a 1.2-cm retroareolar breast mass. The patient was lost to follow up due to a change of insurance and presented to a new primary care physician in her 21st gestational week with complaints of a rapidly enlarging left breast mass over the prior 3 months with associated diffuse left breast pain, redness, and asymmetry compared to her normal gravid right breast. She also noted recent onset of left axillary and upper arm pain without swelling.

● DIFFERENTIAL DIAGNOSIS

The differential diagnosis of a breast mass in premenopausal women is broad and includes many benign entities such as fibroadenoma, phyllodes tumor, lipoma, fat necrosis, fibrocystic disease, galactocele, cyst, abscess, or accessory breast tissue. Many present as a palpable lump on self-exam or clinical breast exam by their primary provider, as this population does not routinely undergo breast screening. How to proceed with a diagnostic workup is often left to the surgeon. Surgical excision is recommended for phyllodes tumors and for symptomatic or enlarging fibroadenomas. Fat necrosis is usually a posttraumatic or postoperative finding. Galactoceles generally develop months after discontinuation of lactation. Breast abscesses present with skin erythema, induration, and/or fever and can be associated with lactation, smoking, diabetes, or other systemic illnesses linked with increased risk of infections. During pregnancy, accessory breast tissue may swell and present as an enlarging mass in the axillary tail of

the breast or in the axilla and may be considered for excision in the postpartum period. Breast cancer is an uncommon diagnosis in this age group, with only 0.3% of all breast cancers occurring in women between the ages of 20 and 29. However, breast cancer in the premenopausal female is more likely to be aggressive and advanced at presentation, necessitating vigilance by surgeons and primary providers for premenopausal patients who present with breast masses. Also, as women more often delay childbearing, breast cancer is now the most common malignancy diagnosed during pregnancy, occurring once in every 3,000 pregnancies.

Presentation Continued

Case 1: The patient has no prior history of breast masses or breast biopsies. She has had no prior surgery. Her father died of head and neck cancer at age 53, but she denies any additional family history of cancer, including breast or ovarian cancer. On review of systems, she denies trauma to the breast, skin changes, nipple retraction, or nipple discharge. Breast examination reveals a 4-cm mass in the upper outer quadrant. The mass is not fixed to the skin or pectoralis muscle. There is also ipsilateral palpable but movable axillary adenopathy. The contralateral breast and axilla are unremarkable. There is no cervical, supraclavicular, or infraclavicular lymphadenopathy bilaterally.

Case 2: The patient had no prior history of breast biopsy but did have incision and drainage of a right breast postpartum abscess 4 years prior with her first pregnancy. She has no family history of breast, ovarian, or any other cancers. On review of systems, she denies breast trauma but notes marked diffuse fixation and hardening of the left breast with associated skin thickening, increasing asymmetry of breast volume and contour, and worsening breast pain. Breast examination demonstrates a diffusely indurated left breast with marked retraction of the left breast and left nipple. The breast is fixed to the erythematous and thickened skin, but not to the underlying chest wall. There is also ipsilateral bulky, fixed, palpable axillary lymphadenopathy. No upper extremity lymphedema is noted. The contralateral breast is noted to be gravid and markedly larger than the affected breast but without discrete masses or skin changes. The contralateral axilla is unremarkable. There is no cervical, supraclavicular, or infraclavicular lymphadenopathy bilaterally.

● WORKUP

Diagnostic workup of a patient with a palpable breast mass includes assessment with physical exam, diagnostic breast imaging, and pathologic tissue sampling. Focused breast imaging consists of mammography and ultrasound after a thorough physical examination. Digital mammography is preferred, especially in those patients whose breast density may be increased by both lactation changes and premenopausal status. Mammography can visualize calcifications, masses, and architectural distortion and is considered safe in pregnancy, with appropriate abdominal shielding. Focused breast ultrasound, in conjunction with mammography, characterizes solid versus cystic pathology and is more sensitive than mammography in the detection of breast cancer in pregnancy.

Assessment of clinical axillary adenopathy on physical exam remains the gold standard in clinical assessment of regional disease. However, ultrasound of the axilla as an adjunct may improve sensitivity of detecting axillary metastases in high-volume centers. Regional assessment of the axilla affects recommendations for chemotherapy, surgery, and radiation therapy in patients with invasive breast cancer (Figure 62-1).

Breast magnetic resonance imaging (MRI) with gadolinium contrast is often used in evaluating the extent of disease in patients with breast cancer, especially in those with dense breast tissue and lobular histology. However, fetal effects of gadolinium-enhanced breast MRI during pregnancy are unclear. Considering the prone position and the concerns regarding fetal exposure to gadolinium, breast MRI is not considered a safe modality for diagnostic workup of a breast mass in pregnant patients.

After appropriate diagnostic imaging, pathologic tissue assessment of a breast mass is critical. The current recommended modality for pathologic diagnosis is via image-guided percutaneous biopsy with clip placement. This is most often done sonographically but can be done with mammography if the abnormality is not detected with ultrasound. If the pathology result is discordant with diagnostic imaging, surgical excision should be considered. Surgical excision in lieu of percutaneous biopsy, though feasible, is not the current standard of care for initial pathologic tissue evaluation of any patient, pregnant or not, with a palpable breast mass. Furthermore in the pregnant patient, every attempt should be made to establish the pathologic diagnosis percutaneously to avoid additional surgical procedures and anesthesia, thereby minimizing risk to the pregnant patient as well as the fetus. Regarding the axilla, any patient with sonographically abnormal axillary lymph nodes should subsequently undergo ultrasound-guided fine needle aspiration or core needle biopsy to confirm the presence of axillary metastasis pathologically.

Case Continued

Case 1: In the 9th week of gestation, the patient had bilateral mammograms and a focused breast ultrasound of the palpable mass. Left breast imaging demonstrated a 3.5 cm × 2.0 cm × 4.0 cm mass, suspicious for malignancy, in the upper outer quadrant, 5 cm from the nipple. Right breast mammogram was unremarkable. Ultrasound-guided core biopsy of the left breast mass revealed high-grade invasive ductal carcinoma that was estrogen and progesterone receptor negative and HER2/Neu negative. Ipsilateral axillary ultrasound also showed abnormal lymph nodes; fine needle aspiration diagnosed regional metastatic disease on cytology. Staging with both chest radiograph and ultrasound of the liver was negative for suspicious lesions.

Case 2: On the day she presented to her primary care physician at 21 weeks of gestation, the patient was seen by a surgeon and had a left breast core biopsy as well as a biopsy of her palpable axillary nodes. Due to the diffuse size of the mass and fixation of the breast, mammography and sonography were performed, but the images were unable to accurately size the breast mass. Left breast imaging suggested a large left breast mass at least 9 cm × 11 cm × 10 cm with associated skin thickening and calcifications involving all 4 quadrants of the breast and the nipple–areolar complex. Marked left axillary adenopathy was also noted mammographically and sonographically. Mammogram of the right breast was unremarkable (Figure 62-2). Core biopsies of the left breast and axilla confirmed high-grade invasive ductal carcinoma, estrogen and progesterone receptor negative, and Her2/Neu positive. Staging with both chest radiograph and ultrasound of the liver was negative for suspicious lesions.

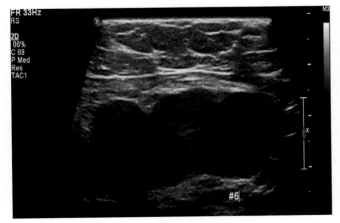

FIGURE 62-1. Axillary ultrasound demonstrates a lymph node with metastatic disease. There is complete loss of normal nodal architecture.

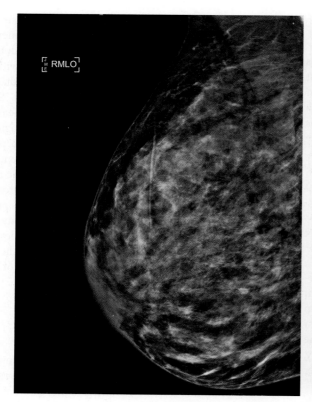
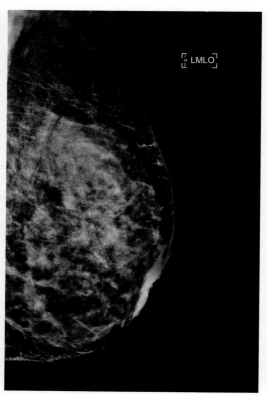

FIGURE 62-2. Bilateral digital mammography of a pregnant patient with a high-density, diffuse mass in the left breast with associated calcifications and marked skin thickening.

● DIAGNOSIS AND TREATMENT

Further evaluation and treatment of benign breast findings in pregnant patients may be deferred until the postpartum period; however, a diagnosis of breast cancer during pregnancy warrants immediate attention. Invasive breast cancer is treated in a multidisciplinary approach, which may include surgery, chemotherapy, or radiation. For the pregnant patient, the timing and order of treatment are often determined by gestational age as well as the stage of the cancer at diagnosis. Termination of the pregnancy does *not* improve outcomes and should not be recommended to patients in the context of survival from breast cancer. Patients may safely undergo both local and systemic cancer treatment while maintaining their pregnancy. Early planned delivery may be considered if felt that this can affect maternal oncologic outcomes.

Pregnant patients with an invasive breast cancer diagnosis, particularly those with biopsy-proven axillary disease, should also have staging studies performed. In the **nonpregnant** patient, either a whole body positron-emission tomography scan or a computer tomography scan of the chest and abdomen with a bone scan is considered appropriate. However, these scans should be deferred until the postpartum period in pregnant patients. Staging with a chest radiograph and an ultrasound of the liver is adequate for pregnant patients until postpartum. Any lesion noted on staging studies suspicious for distant metastatic disease warrants a percutaneous biopsy, as patients with distant metastatic disease are not considered surgical candidates and should be initially treated with systemic chemotherapy. Central to the management of breast cancer in the pregnant patient is a multidisciplinary team consisting of surgical oncology, medical oncology, radiation oncology, and maternal fetal medicine, all guiding treatment decisions.

● SURGICAL APPROACH

Patients with early-stage breast cancer that are clinically node negative at presentation should be strongly considered to proceed directly to surgery for pathologic staging. An outline of the decision-making process is illustrated in Figure 62-3.

Key Considerations in Surgical and Treatment Decision-Making

1. Gestational age at diagnosis
2. Clinical stage of disease
3. Indication and timing of systemic chemotherapy
4. Indication and timing of adjuvant radiation therapy

Gestational age at diagnosis often dictates the surgical approach. General anesthesia is considered safe in pregnancy, with no currently used anesthetic agents being shown to have teratogenic effects at standard concentrations for any gestational age. If possible, surgery should be performed in

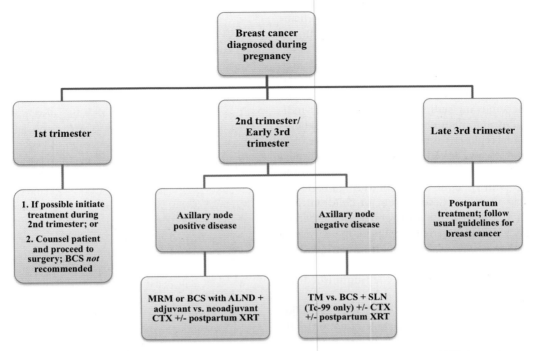

FIGURE 62-3. Surgical decision-making tree for pregnant patients diagnosed with breast cancer. BCS, breast-conserving surgery; MRM, modified radical mastectomy; ALND, axillary lymph node dissection; CTX, chemotherapy; XRT, radiation therapy; TM, total mastectomy; Tc-99, technetium-99; SLN, sentinel lymph node.

the second trimester when preterm contractions and spontaneous abortion are least likely. Nonobstetric surgical procedures at or beyond the point of fetal viability have low risk of intraoperative or immediate postoperative obstetric complications but do confer increased risk of preterm delivery. If gestational age has not yet reach fetal viability, it is sufficient to assess fetal heart tones by Doppler pre- and postoperatively. If the fetus is viable, surgery should be performed in a facility with neonatal and pediatric services and an obstetric provider readily available; electronic fetal heart rate and contraction monitoring with a trained obstetrical nurse should be done intraoperatively as well as pre- and postprocedure. Patients who present in the first trimester may proceed directly to surgery with appropriate discussion of potential risks to the fetus. Women diagnosed in the third trimester may defer surgery until postpartum and may consider early induction of labor to avoid excessive treatment delays. Surgery during later gestational age must account for the gravid uterus during patient positioning. Discussion should include maternal–fetal medicine obstetrician as to when and if to deliver early for these patients.

Surgical decision regarding breast conservation may also be directed by gestational age. Breast conservation is not recommended in the first trimester given that adjuvant radiation is absolutely contraindicated in pregnancy. Traditionally, surgical treatment for pregnant patients was limited to modified radical mastectomy; however, breast conservation may be an option for patients presenting with limited in-breast disease in the second or third trimester or if chemotherapy is indicated and initiated during pregnancy, allowing surgery and subsequent radiation to be deferred until the postpartum period. Decisions for breast-conserving surgery (BCS) require careful multidisciplinary planning due to the contraindications to radiation in pregnancy.

Clinical stage also determines surgical decisions in breast cancer patients. Mastectomy may be required in patients with multifocal disease or locally advanced breast cancer at presentation regardless of pregnancy. However, axillary surgery for breast cancer during pregnancy has evolved. Although blue dye mapping with lymphazurin or methylene blue is contraindicated in pregnancy, technetium-99 sulfur colloid for sentinel lymph node (SLN) surgery is safe and feasible in the second and third trimesters of pregnancy. Evidence estimates uterine radiation exposure for a fetus during SLN surgery to be one-fifth the daily radiation from background exposure, lending credence to the safety of SLN surgery during pregnancy. If sentinel lymph node is positive for metastasis, often this mandates axillary lymph node dissection. However, in patients with regional nodal involvement on physical exam or axillary ultrasound that is confirmed by percutaneous biopsy, axillary dissection without attempted sentinel node biopsy remains the recommended operation.

Indications for systemic chemotherapy are the same for pregnant and nonpregnant patients with breast cancer. Decision and timing for systemic chemotherapy either neoadjuvantly or in the adjuvant setting should be a multidisciplinary approach with the consulting surgeon, medical oncologist, and maternal–fetal medicine obstetrician. Systemic chemotherapy with Adriamycin and Cytoxan can be given safely during the second and third trimesters of pregnancy. Patients that are candidates for chemotherapy diagnosed in the late first trimester or second trimester could safely proceed with chemotherapy in the preoperative neoadjuvant setting. Expert consensus indicates that neoadjuvant chemotherapy in pregnant patients should be the same regimens as nonpregnant patients except that antimetabolites and trastuzumab are contraindicated in pregnancy. Evidence suggests that prenatal exposure to maternal cancer with systemic treatment during pregnancy does not lead to impaired development in children. It is important to note that patients undergoing chemotherapy during pregnancy should stop treatment prior to delivery, to avoid immunosuppression in the peripartum period. They should be followed closely by a maternal–fetal medicine obstetrician. Any chemotherapy cycles left unfinished can be completed postpartum.

Multidisciplinary treatment also often includes adjuvant radiation therapy. However, adjuvant radiation therapy is contraindicated in all trimesters of pregnancy due to the risk of teratogenesis. This impacts surgical decisions regarding breast conservation for patients diagnosed early in pregnancy as illustrated in Figure 62-3. Indications for adjuvant radiation are the same as for nonpregnant patients. Radiation, delivered postpartum, is indicated in all patients that undergo breast conservation. Also, patients may need radiation even after mastectomy if their tumor is >5 cm, margins are positive and unable to be reresected, muscle or skin are involved, or regional nodes are involved. Should a patient require adjuvant radiation, this can be completed postpartum especially for cancer diagnosed later in pregnancy.

Case Conclusion

Case 1: The patient was seen by a surgical oncologist, maternal–fetal medicine obstetrician, and a medical oncologist; because of her presentation early in the first trimester of pregnancy, she was recommended to pursue surgical resection early in pregnancy. After several discussions with the patient, her family, and a multidisciplinary team of physicians, she underwent mastectomy and axillary lymph node dissection (modified radical mastectomy) in her 14th week of pregnancy. Surgical pathology demonstrated a 4.5-cm invasive ductal carcinoma and 2 of 24 positive lymph nodes. Chemotherapy was initiated in the 20th week of pregnancy and then discontinued at week 32 for a scheduled cesarean section. The delivery was uncomplicated, and she proceeded to have adjuvant Taxol as well as chest wall radiation postpartum. BRCA mutation testing performed postpartum was negative for a deleterious mutation.

Case Conclusion Continued

Case 2: The patient was subsequently seen by maternal–fetal medicine obstetrician and medical oncologist; because of her clinically locally advanced disease, there was significant concern regarding the ability to surgically resect the disease with negative margins. Based on the patient's advanced clinical stage and gestational age at presentation, the decision to proceed with neoadjuvant chemotherapy was made. After several discussions with the patient, her family, and a multidisciplinary team of physicians, she received 4 cycles of neoadjuvant chemotherapy until her 33rd week of gestation; she was scheduled for induction at 38 weeks and the delivery was uncomplicated. Postpartum, she had a mastectomy and axillary lymph node dissection (modified radical mastectomy). Surgical pathology demonstrated innumerable foci of residual invasive ductal carcinoma involving all 4 quadrants of the breast and 10 of 37 positive lymph nodes. She proceeded to have adjuvant Taxotere, trastuzumab, and pertuzumab as well as chest wall radiation postpartum. BRCA mutation testing performed postpartum was negative for a deleterious mutation.

● POSTOPERATIVE MANAGEMENT

Both tamoxifen and Her2/neu targeted therapies (trastuzumab and pertuzumab) are contraindicated in pregnancy but can be initiated safely in the postpartum period if indicated. Postpartum, patients that have estrogen receptor–positive or progesterone receptor–positive breast cancer should be referred to medical oncology for adjuvant tamoxifen or other antihormone therapy. For patients with HER2/Neu-positive breast cancer, adjuvant treatment with trastuzumab and pertuzumab is recommended. All patients presenting with primary breast cancer before the age of 50, which includes patients with pregnancy-associated breast cancer, should be considered for genetic counseling and testing. BRCA1 and BRCA2 mutation carriers are advised to consider prophylactic bilateral oophorectomy and mastectomy due to their inherited risk of breast and ovarian carcinomas after completion of childbearing. In general, patients that are mutation carriers may consider bilateral mastectomy at the time of their definitive cancer operation, or in lieu of prophylactic surgery, they may proceed with high-risk surveillance, consisting of breast MRI and mammogram alternating every 6 months, after management of their primary breast cancer. In the case of a pregnant patient, prophylactic or reconstructive procedures should be deferred until the postpartum period to minimize fetal exposure to anesthetic agents.

Follow-up for breast cancer patients should include at a minimum a clinical breast or chest wall exam and if mastectomy was not performed, annual screening mammography as long as they are in good health. Depending on their final pathologic stage, patients with more advanced stage should also have a clinical breast exam every 3 to 6 months for the first few years after treatment.

TAKE HOME POINTS

- A multidisciplinary approach is essential to caring for the pregnant patient with breast cancer including surgical oncology, medical oncology, radiation oncology, and maternal–fetal medicine.
- Breast cancer treatment can be safely delivered during pregnancy, and termination of the pregnancy does not improve oncologic outcomes.
- Differential diagnosis is broad in pregnant patients with a breast mass, but workup to exclude breast cancer is imperative.
- Diagnostic workup initially includes bilateral mammography with abdominal shielding and focused ultrasound. Breast MRI is contraindicated in pregnancy.
- Pathologic tissue diagnosis should be done percutaneously, and clinically abnormal axillary nodes should undergo percutaneous biopsy as well.
- Evaluate node-positive patients for distant metastatic disease with a chest radiograph and ultrasound of the liver. Staging CT or nuclear scans are deferred until postpartum.
- Surgery is safest for both mother and fetus during the second trimester.
- Breast conservation is not recommended for patients presenting in the first trimester due to the need for adjuvant radiation but may be considered for appropriate patients with later gestational age at presentation.
- SLN mapping may be performed in the second or third trimester with technetium-99 only; lymphazurin and methylene blue dye are contraindicated in pregnancy.
- Systemic chemotherapy may be given during second and third trimesters in the neoadjuvant or adjuvant setting.
- Delivery should be timed to avoid delivery while immunosuppressed.

- Radiation therapy is contraindicated in all three trimesters but may be initiated in the postpartum period when indicated.
- Genetic testing should be discussed in any young woman (<50 years of age) diagnosed with breast cancer.
- All young patients with breast cancer should be followed closely posttreatment to monitor for recurrence.
- Prophylactic or elective procedures should be deferred until the postpartum period.

SUGGESTED READINGS

Ahn BY, Kim HH, Moon WK, et al. Pregnancy- and lactation-associated breast cancer: mammographic and sonographic findings. *J Ultrasound Med.* 2003;22:491-497.

Amant F, Vandenbroucke M, Verheecke M, et al. Pediatric outcome after maternal cancer diagnosed during pregnancy. *N Engl J Med.* 2015;373(19):1824-1834.

American Society of Anesthesiologists. Statement on nonobstetric surgery during pregnancy. Committee of Origin: Obstetric Anesthesia. 2009;1-2

Baldwin EA, Borowski KS, Brost BC, et al. Antepartum nonobstetric surgery at ≥23 weeks' gestation and risk for preterm delivery. *Am J Obstet Gynecol.* 2015;212:232.e1-232.e5

Berry DL, Theriault RL, Holmes FA, et al. Management of breast cancer during pregnancy using a standardized protocol. *J Clin Oncol.* 1999;17(3):855-861.

Cardonick EMD, Dougherty RMD, Grana GMD, et al. Breast cancer during pregnancy: maternal and fetal outcomes. *Cancer J.* 2010;16:76-82.

Gentilini O, Cremonesi M, Toesca A, et al. Sentinel lymph node biopsy in pregnant patients with breast cancer. *Eur J Nucl Med Mol Imaging.* 2010;37:78-83.

Kaufmann M, Von Minckwitz G, Mamounas EP, et al. Recommendations from an international consensus conference on the current status and future of neoadjuvant systemic therapy in primary breast cancer. *Ann Surg Oncol.* 2012;19:1508-1516.

Spanheimer PM, Graham MM, Sugg SL, et al. Measurement of uterine radiation exposure from lymphoscintigraphy indicates safety of sentinel lymph node biopsy during pregnancy. *Ann Surg Oncol.* 2006;16:1143-1147.

Steenvoorde P, Pauwels EKJ, Harding LK, et al. Diagnostic nuclear medicine and risk for the fetus. *Eur J Nucl Med Mol Imaging.* 1998;25:193-199.

Breast Reconstruction

63

IAN C. SANDO AND ADEYIZA O. MOMOH

Based on the previous edition chapter "Breast Reconstruction" by
Jennifer F. Waljee and Amy K. Alderman

Presentation

A 55-year-old female presents with recurrent left breast cancer. She has a history of left breast invasive ductal carcinoma, for which she underwent lumpectomy and sentinel lymph node biopsy 3 years ago. This was followed by adjuvant chemotherapy, radiation, and hormonal therapy. She detected a new lump in the upper inner quadrant of her left breast on self-breast exam approximately 3 months ago. Mammogram and ultrasound imaging revealed a 1.5 cm mass, which was percutaneously biopsied and found to be an invasive ductal carcinoma, grade 2, ER/PR positive, Her2/neu negative. She underwent staging scans, which were unremarkable. Recommendations were for mastectomy with adjuvant chemotherapy. The patient is otherwise healthy and her past surgical history includes a cesarean section, lumpectomy, breast biopsy, and sentinel lymph node biopsies. Her medications include lorazepam and loratadine. She is a nonsmoker, is married with two children, and is employed as a social worker. She currently wears a C cup size bra and desires to remain the same size. The patient is interested in pursuing contralateral prophylactic mastectomy and presents to her plastic surgery to discuss immediate bilateral breast reconstruction.

DISCUSSION

Breast reconstruction is achieved through various techniques that aim to restore the breast to an acceptable size, shape, and appearance following oncologic resection. The positive impact that breast reconstruction has on women's psychosocial functioning, mental health, and body image is well documented. The quality of breast reconstruction has improved in recent decades as surgical techniques and implant technology have evolved. Current technologies are capable of creating a breast with high aesthetic quality and limited donor site morbidity. Although most women receiving mastectomy or lumpectomy are good candidates for reconstruction, referral patterns vary geographically and there remain barriers to access based on socioeconomic status. Thus, it is important for every surgeon to introduce the idea of breast reconstruction and make the offer of a referral to a reconstructive surgeon early during preoperative consultations with the breast cancer patient. This chapter will review the current reconstructive options for breast reconstruction, including preoperative evaluation, timing of surgery, and postoperative care.

WORKUP

Breast reconstruction is achieved with use of prosthetic implants, autologous tissue, or a combination of both and can be performed either immediately at the time of cancer resection or in a delayed fashion. The type and timing of breast reconstruction is influenced by a number of oncologic and patient-specific factors, including age, family history, breast size, disease burden, need for chemotherapy and/or radiation, body mass index (BMI), medical comorbidities, and personal preferences. It is therefore vitally important for the reconstructive surgeon to be part of the multidisciplinary team caring for breast cancer patients. Consultation with a plastic surgeon should be offered at the time of initial surgical decision-making for any woman interested in breast reconstruction.

During the initial consultation, the reconstructive surgeon should elicit a woman's understanding of breast reconstruction, expectations of the reconstructive process and outcomes, concerns about reconstruction, and preferences with regard to the type and timing of reconstruction. When possible, it is helpful to provide educational material for patients to review prior to their initial consultation. Reconstruction should be discussed in the context of the overall oncologic treatment plan. Important treatment information includes the type of resection planned (lumpectomy, skin-sparing mastectomy, nipple-sparing mastectomy, etc.), anticipated laterality of mastectomy (unilateral or bilateral), need for lymph node sampling or removal, and potential plans for radiation and/or chemotherapy. Of particular importance is radiation therapy, which may result in atrophy or fat necrosis of breasts reconstructed with autologous tissue and can result in delayed healing, capsular contracture, implant exposure, and increased rates of infection in breasts reconstructed with expanders and implants. Inquiries should be made about desires for immediate or delayed reconstruction and implant-based or autologous reconstruction. In addition, aesthetic concerns need to be addressed, including the patient's ideal breast size and whether or not she would be interested in a procedure on the contralateral breast to achieve symmetry.

A thorough history should be obtained, and the surgeon should evaluate if there are any contraindications to general anesthesia or prolonged procedures. Women should be screened for conditions that may negatively impact wound healing, including diabetes, collagen vascular disease, rheumatologic disease, renal failure, and use of immunosuppressive medications. Nicotine use also leads to impaired wound healing, and patients are encouraged to refrain from smoking for at least 1 month prior to any reconstruction procedure. Women who are actively smoking at the time of reconstruction are at an increased risk of mastectomy skin flap necrosis, infection, fat necrosis, and wound dehiscence. Morbidly obese patients are also at an increased risk for surgical complications, not only at the site of the breast reconstruction but also at donor sites in cases of autologous breast reconstruction. The patient's medications should be reviewed, and any anticoagulant, immunosuppressant, or herbal medication that lead to increased bleeding, impaired wound healing, or infection should be held after consulting with the patient's primary care physician.

On physical examination, the breasts should be examined for size, symmetry, position of inframammary fold, prior incisions, degree of ptosis, quality of skin, thickness of subcutaneous tissue, position and size of nipple–areolar complex, and location of the tumor. The chest should be examined for radiation therapy-related tissue changes and for the presence of axillary or thoracotomy scars that may compromise the blood supply to potential reconstructive flap options. As a common donor site, the abdomen should be examined for the presence of scars, abdominal wall laxity, rectus diastasis, hernias, and distribution of visceral and subcutaneous adiposity.

The patient in this scenario has normal vital signs and her BMI is 32. Focused examination reveals breast volumes that approximate 300 mL bilaterally. Her breasts have moderate ptosis with good skin quality and are overall symmetric with respects to shape, nipple position, and inframammary fold height. There is a well-healed scar from her biopsy in the upper outer quadrant of the left breast. Her abdomen has a moderate amount of lipodystrophy with overall good skin quality. There are no scars, abdominal wall laxity, hernias, or rectus diastasis. The remainder of her examination is unremarkable.

● TREATMENT OPTIONS

Prosthetic Reconstruction

Breast Implant Placement Following Tissue Expansion

Currently, the staged use of tissue expanders followed by permanent implants remains the most commonly performed approach to breast reconstruction. This form of reconstruction can be performed in an immediate fashion at the time of mastectomy or in delayed fashion months to years after a mastectomy. Tissue expanders are preferred in most patients undergoing implant-based breast reconstruction due to limitations with the skin envelope following mastectomy and the

need to recruit skin in order to achieve an acceptable breast mound. Tissue expanders are textured devices often with an integrated port that allow for percutaneous injection of saline to increase the volume of the device. They come in a range of shapes and sizes depending on surgeon preference and the patient's body habitus. Placement is typically in a submuscular pocket with the possibility of complete or partial submuscular coverage (Figure 63-1). When partial submuscular coverage is performed, the superior aspect of the expander is covered with the pectoralis major muscle and the inferior and lateral aspects covered with an acellular dermal matrix (ADM) or alternative synthetic mesh material. Use of an ADM or synthetic mesh provides better control of the inframammary fold, allows for increased intraoperative expander fill (at the time of initial placement with immediate reconstruction), decreases visible rippling of the final implant, and results in easier expansion of the lower pole of the breast with increased lower pole projection and an improved aesthetic result. After a period of serial expansions, the patient returns to the operating room for a second-stage procedure, where the tissue expander is exchanged for a permanent silicone- or saline-filled implant. At this stage, a procedure such as a mastopexy, reduction, or augmentation may be performed on the contralateral breast to improve symmetry for women undergoing unilateral reconstruction. Use of tissue expander/implant reconstruction provides distinct advantages over autologous reconstruction by reducing operative and postoperative recovery length of time and eliminating an operation on a donor site. Disadvantages include implant-related complications such as capsular contracture, implant

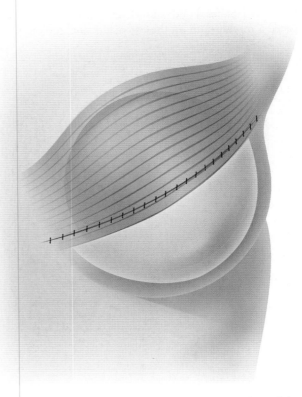

FIGURE 63-1. Illustration of subpectoral implant with partial muscle coverage.

rupture, infection, and implant malposition. Additionally, implant reconstructions tend to feel less natural to the touch, when compared to autologous tissue.

Direct to Implant Reconstruction

Although the majority of women who undergo prosthetic reconstruction require the use of tissue expanders before the insertion of permanent implants, some are candidates to have either fully filled saline or silicone implants placed at the time of a skin- or nipple-sparing mastectomy. This technique is only possible for immediate breast reconstruction. Advantages of direct to implant (DTI) reconstruction include eliminating the need for multiple clinic visits for expansions and a subsequent operation to exchange the expander for an implant. However, patients should be counseled that they may require additional revision operations to better achieve symmetry. Ideal candidates for DTI include those with either small- to medium-sized breasts with mild to moderate ptosis who are undergoing skin- or nipple-sparing mastectomies and are willing to be similar to their preoperative size or slightly smaller after reconstruction. Mastectomy flap perfusion is critical given that some degree of tension will be placed on the flaps with the use of fully filled implants. Partial muscle coverage with use of an ADM or mesh is required to accommodate and support the implant. The risks associated with single-stage implant reconstruction include infection, seroma, hematoma, skin necrosis, and capsular contracture.

At present, both saline and silicone implants are used for breast cancer reconstruction and are equally safe. In 1992, the United States Food and Drug Administration (FDA) placed a moratorium on the use of silicone implants due to the concern for increased risk of systemic illness related to the use of silicone. Multiple studies have failed to show an increased risk of systemic illness, and these regulations have been discontinued. Although silicone implants are considered safe, the FDA released a medical device safety communication in January, 2011, regarding the possible association between breast implants and the development of anaplastic large cell lymphoma (ALCL), a rare type of non-Hodgkin lymphoma that represents 0.4% to 0.5% of breast cancers. The FDA reported that women with breast implants may have a very low but increased risk of developing ALCL adjacent to the breast implant compared with women without implants. Globally, there have been approximately 80 cases of ALCL identified in women with breast implants, whereas 5 to 10 million women have received implants worldwide. Currently, additional data is required to fully evaluate the possible relationship between ALCL and breast implants. All cases of ALCL reported in women with breast implants are now tracked in the FDA MedWatch Program.

Autologous Reconstruction

Latissimus Dorsi Flap

The pedicled latissimus dorsi flap can be harvested as a muscle-only flap or as a myocutaneous flap that includes a skin paddle (Figure 63-2). The latissimus dorsi flap is most commonly used in combination with expanders/implants to reconstruct the radiated breast. Providing durable nonradiated soft tissue coverage of tissue expanders in the setting of prior radiation decreases rates of failure for reasons such as implant exposure, infection, suboptimal expansion, and poor aesthetic results. Expanding the radiated pectoralis

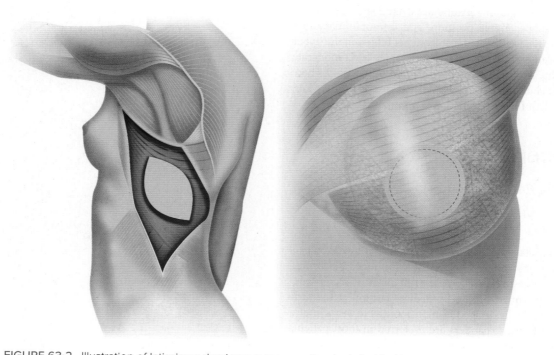

FIGURE 63-2. Illustration of latissimus dorsi myocutaneous flap for left-sided breast reconstruction.

muscle and skin is made easier with the addition of a healthy latissimus dorsi muscle (and possibly skin). This approach makes it possible to achieve a more natural-appearing breast mound even in the setting previously radiated soft tissue. Patients who have undergone prior thoracotomy are not candidates for this flap as the muscle has been divided, and patients who have previously undergone axillary node dissection should be considered for CT angiography to evaluate patency of the thoracodorsal vessels.

Deep Inferior Epigastric Perforator Flap

Similar to expander/implant reconstruction, autologous reconstruction can be performed in an immediate or delayed fashion. Complete autologous reconstruction creates a natural-appearing reconstructed breast by replacing breast tissue with tissue that is similar in softness and texture. The aesthetic results achieved are durable with high patient satisfaction that is maintained long term. Autologous reconstruction avoids the previously mentioned implant-associated complications but commits patients to a surgical donor site.

The deep inferior epigastric perforator (DIEP) flap is an abdominal-based perforator flap that has increased in popularity over the past decade. Similar to the transverse rectus abdominis (TRAM) flap, the DIEP flap uses skin and subcutaneous tissue from lower abdomen based off the deep epigastric vascular system to reconstruct the breast. However, the rectus abdominis muscle and overlying fascia are spared (Figure 63-3) by dissecting intramuscular perforating vessels from the rectus muscle prior to transferring the abdominal tissue to the chest

wall defect as a free flap. Using microsurgical techniques, the deep inferior epigastric artery and vein are anastomosed to the internal mammary recipient vessels in the chest. Compared to the pedicled TRAM flap, DIEP flaps have been shown to result in less abdominal wall morbidity such as hernias and bulges.

Complications of abdominal perforator flap reconstruction are attributed to flap perfusion when tissue viability is dependent on a few select perforators. Although total flap loss rates are low, <2% at high-volume centers, fat necrosis occurs in approximately 14% of reconstructions due to poor perfusion of segments of adipose tissue. Thus, careful intraoperative perforator selection and meticulous microsurgical technique are critical to ensure viability of the transferred tissue.

Other Flaps

Advances with microsurgical techniques and an increased understanding of soft tissue perfusion have led to the utilization of a number of other gluteal- and thigh-based perforator flaps for breast reconstruction. For example, perforator flaps based on the superior gluteal artery, inferior gluteal artery, or profunda artery systems can be used to create autologous flaps with acceptable donor site morbidity in women who may not be candidates for implant-based or abdominal wall autologous reconstruction options. Additionally, the anterior lateral thigh (ALT) flap, transverse upper gracilis (TUG) flap (Figure 63-4), and "Rubens" flap (myocutaneous flap based on the deep circumflex iliac vessels) are all other options for free tissue transfer for breast reconstruction. Although not as widely performed, these are options for women in whom the more common reconstructive options are unavailable or contraindicated.

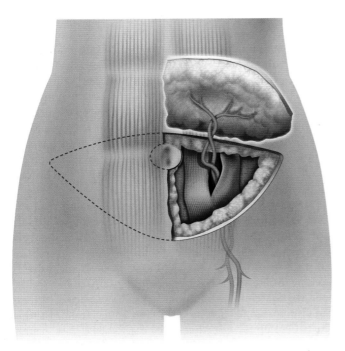

FIGURE 63-3. Deep inferior epigastric perforator (DIEP) flap. Skin and soft tissue of the abdomen are perfused by perforators of the deep inferior epigastric artery, which can be ligated, transferred to the chest, and anastomosed to the internal mammary recipient vessels.

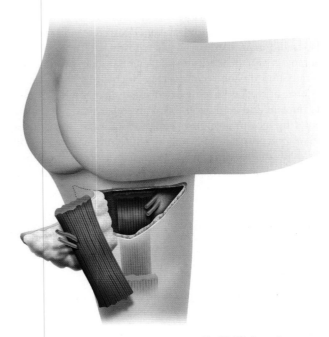

FIGURE 63-4. Transverse upper gracilis (TUG) flap. A myocutaneous flap consisting of gracilis muscle and skin and soft tissue of the medial upper thigh can be harvested based on the medial circumflex femoral vessels, transferred to the chest as a free flap, and used to reconstruct a breast.

● SURGICAL APPROACH

Timing of Reconstruction

Breast reconstruction can be performed in either an immediate or a delayed setting. Open communication with the patient and other care providers is critical to formulating a surgical plan with respect to timing. Considerations for planned adjuvant treatment are important as certain interventions, such as radiation, may have an impact on the results achieved with reconstruction. These clinical considerations are balanced with patient's choices and preferences. As most forms of breast reconstruction require multiple stages, immediate breast reconstruction initiates the first stage of reconstruction at the time of a mastectomy.

When possible, immediate reconstruction tends to be the preferred approach of a majority of women opting for postmastectomy breast reconstruction. Immediate breast reconstruction takes advantage of the skin envelope that is typically preserved with a skin- or nipple-sparing mastectomy. This reconstructive approach also provides patients with a breast mound in the immediate postoperative period, helping to ease some of the emotional and psychosocial distress experienced with loss of the breast. With specific forms of reconstruction, scars could potentially be minimized, and by combining a reconstructive procedure with the mastectomy, patients require one less surgical encounter to complete the reconstructive process.

Delayed breast reconstruction is performed weeks to months after a mastectomy. This approach to reconstruction is considered for multiple reasons, including patient choice, advanced stage of disease, significant comorbidities, and the absence of reconstructive services at an institution where the oncologic treatment in undertaken. Delayed reconstruction is also traditionally considered when postmastectomy radiation therapy is anticipated to avoid potential detrimental effects of radiation on the reconstructed breast. In recent years, a number of studies have reported some success with immediate implant and autologous breast reconstruction in patients requiring postmastectomy radiation therapy. Nonetheless, delayed reconstruction avoids specific complications associated with mastectomy such as skin flap necrosis and affords patients ample time to consider options for reconstruction.

● TECHNICAL ASPECTS

Tissue Expander/Implant Reconstruction

The patient is seen preoperatively, and markings of the breast landmarks are performed with the patient in the upright position. The chest midline and the inframammary folds are marked. Measurements of the breast base width are taken to help with expander selection. Markings for the mastectomy incision are also made and vary depending on the type of mastectomy (skin or nipple sparring) planned. The patient is placed in supine position in the operating room with arms abducted. Upon completion of the mastectomy by the oncologic surgeon, the breast pocket is prepared for tissue expander placement. The expander can be placed in either a complete or a partial submuscular pocket. Briefly, the complete submuscular coverage is achieved with use of the pectoralis major muscle (superior/medially), serratus anterior muscle (laterally), and rectus fascia (inferiorly). For the more common partial submuscular coverage, a pectoralis major muscle flap is elevated, releasing insertions for the muscle to ribs at the lower breast pole and inframammary fold. The elevated pectoralis major muscle easily covers the superior and medial half of the expander. The inferior and lateral aspects of the expander are covered with an acellular dermal matrix (ADM). The ADM is sutured to the inframammary fold and lateral chest wall at the anterior axillary line. A tissue expander is then selected based on chest wall dimensions (base width) and the patients desired breast size. One popular form of the tissue expander has a self-sealing port within the expander for access and fills. The expander and breast pockets are irrigated with an antibiotic solution (composition based on surgeon preference) prior to introducing the expander into the breast pocket. The pectoralis major muscle and ADM are draped over the expander. The muscle is then approximated to the ADM with absorbable sutures. Surgical drains are placed within the implant and mastectomy pockets. Mastectomy skin edges are then approximated with absorbable sutures in a layered fashion. The expander port is then identified with a sterile magnet, accessed with a butterfly needle, and sterile saline is introduced into the expander. The expander is filled to a volume that takes advantage of the supple skin envelope that results after the mastectomy without causing undue tension on the muscle flap and mastectomy skin flaps.

Patients are often kept in the hospital overnight and then discharged home to recover. Drains are taken out within a few weeks once their output decreases sufficiently and serial fills of the tissue expanders are performed in the outpatient clinic. The volume of each fill is limited by how much the patient can tolerate (pain) and the soft tissue response to the increased volume (blanching), with a goal to avoid vascular compromise to the skin flaps from excessive pressure on the skin. Once the desired breast volume is achieved, an overexpansion of approximately 20% of the desired volume is performed, and the implant pocket is allowed to mature for 1 to 2 months before proceeding with the next stage of reconstruction. Prior to the second procedure, information on the types of available implants related to shape, texture, and implant fill material (saline or silicone gel) is provided, and patients are able to choose with some guidance. Preoperatively, breast landmarks are marked in a similar fashion as prior. Patients are also positioned similarly, with an anticipation of sitting the patient up for a portion of the case when breast shaping is performed. Access to the expander pocket is achieved through the existing mastectomy scar, the expander is taken out, and capsulotomies are performed as needed. Release of the capsule superiorly with some dissection under the pectoralis major muscle is important to help soften the transition from the upper chest wall to the breast mound. Temporary sizers, filled with saline, are placed in the breast pocket, the capsular and skin edges are approximated temporarily, and the patient is placed in the seated position on the table. Assessments of the implant position on the chest wall, volume, and breast symmetry are performed. Adjustments to the implant volume, pocket dimensions, and skin envelope are made with the patient upright. Once appropriate changes have been made, the patient is returned to the supine position. The temporary sizers are taken out, and the breast pocket and selected implants are irrigated with an antibiotic solution prior to implant placement in the pocket. The implant capsule and skin are closed in layers with absorbable sutures. Drains are not needed for this procedure; patients are placed in a surgical brassiere and discharged home on the same day. Subsequent optional stages of reconstruction focus on nipple–areolar complex reconstruction (in the setting of a skin-sparing mastectomy).

Direct to Implant Reconstruction

The patient is seen preoperatively, and markings of the breast landmarks are performed with the patient in the upright position similar to markings for the tissue expander/implant. Positioning is also similar to the previous description for tissue expander/implant reconstruction. Once the mastectomies are complete, the specimen is weighed to get a sense of the approximate breast volume excised. The breast pocket is prepared by elevating the pectoralis major muscle and dividing its insertions at the inframammary fold, extending medially to the sternal border. Complete submuscular coverage is not an option and use of ADM is required. With plans for a full implant placement, a larger ADM than is typically used when placing an expander may be required. The ADM is first inset to the inframammary fold and lateral chest wall with absorbable sutures. A temporary sizer selected based on the breast base width and breast volume resected is then placed in the breast pocket and filled to the desired volume. With this form of reconstruction, the planned volume should be less than or equal to the preoperative breast volume due to skin perfusion concerns. With the sizer in place, the patient is sat up in bed and a process of tailor tacking of the ADM to the pectoralis major muscle is performed with interrupted sutures, with a focus on achieving the desired breast shape. Once the desired shape and symmetry has been achieved, all excess ADM is excised, and the patient is placed back in supine position. The expander is taken out and an implant selected based on the intraoperative sizing is then prepared (antibiotic irrigation of the implant and breast pocket) and introduced into the pocket under the muscle and ADM. Surgical drains are placed in the implant and mastectomy pockets. The implant pocket is closed, and the mastectomy is closed in layers with absorbable sutures.

Latissimus Dorsi Myocutaneous Flap

In addition to previously described preoperative breast skin markings, with the patient in the sitting position, the borders

of the latissimus dorsi muscle and key back landmarks including the scapula tip, posterior iliac crest, and midline are marked (Figure 63-5). The approximate pivot point of the flap adjacent to the axilla and the planned skin paddle are marked. Care is taken with the specific placement and orientation of the skin paddle on the back to ensure it reaches the mastectomy defect with ease. The mastectomy is performed in the supine position. Once complete, preparation of the breast pocket is performed. In cases of tissue expander placement in combination with the latissimus dorsi, the pectoralis major muscle is elevated in a similar fashion as described for expander/implant reconstruction. A tunnel measuring four fingerbreadths in width is created laterally for the muscle flap transfer with dissection performed in the suprafascial plane, until the lateral border of the latissimus muscle is identified. The mastectomy defect is then packed and the breast covered with an occlusive dressing. The patient is then placed in the lateral decubitus position (in the case of a unilateral flap) for the latissimus flap harvest. Incisions are made along markings for the skin paddle. Dissection is performed down to the muscle surface, beveling outward. Back skin and subcutaneous tissue are elevated off the latissimus muscle until the superior, medial, and inferior limits of the muscle are visualized. Dissection in this plain is also performed toward the axillary pivot point. The muscle is then divided inferiorly, and the submuscular flap elevation proceeds from medial to lateral taking care to avoid elevation of the serratus posterior muscle. The submuscular elevation ends at the axillary pivot point, and the vascular pedicle does not have to be identified or skeletonized. The flap is then rotated and advanced through the tunnel previously created on the lateral chest wall. A surgical drain is placed in the back donor site, which is then closed in layers with absorbable sutures. After repositioning to the supine position, all sponges in the breast pocket are taken

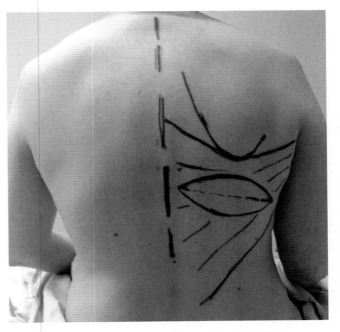

FIGURE 63-5. Preoperative markings of a right latissimus dorsi myocutaneous flap.

out, and the flap is advanced into the breast pocket. A border of the latissimus dorsi muscle is inset inferiorly at the inframammary fold with interrupted absorbable sutures. A tissue expander is selected based on considerations of preoperative measurements of the breast base width, mastectomy specimen weight, and the patient's desired breast size. The expander and breast pocket are prepared as previously described with antibiotic solution irrigation. The expander is placed deep to the pectoralis muscle (superiorly) and latissimus dorsi muscle (inferiorly). Surgical drains are placed in the mastectomy and implant pockets, and approximation of the pectoralis muscle to the latissimus muscle is performed with absorbable sutures. Approximation of the latissimus skin paddle to the mastectomy skin is performed in layers. Depending on the existing laxity of the soft tissue, some sterile saline may be introduced into the expander with care taken to avoid vascular compromise of the latissimus myocutaneous flap as a result of undue pressure. Patients are typically admitted for one or two nights prior to discharge home. Outpatient expansions and subsequent stages of reconstruction are similar to those described for the tissue expander/implant reconstruction.

Deep Inferior Epigastric Perforator Flap

Preoperative markings of the breast and chest wall landmarks are performed with the patient upright (Figure 63-6). The breast base width is measured, and markings around the areola are made in cases of a skin-sparing mastectomy. The abdominal markings are performed with the patient standing. The upper marking of the abdominal flap is made at or just above the umbilicus and extends laterally toward the anterior superior iliac spines. The breast base width is used to estimate placement of the inferior marking (midline vertical distance from superior to inferior marking). The lower marking completes the elliptical pattern of the lower abdominal flap. The patient

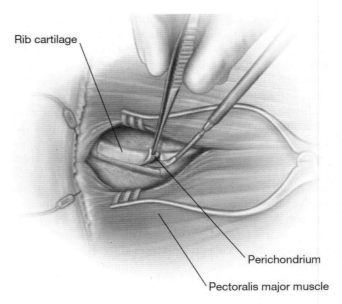

FIGURE 63-7. Harvest of rib cartilage and perichondrium to access the internal mammary vessels.

is placed in the supine position in the operating room with exposure of the breasts and abdomen. The table is turned 180 degrees from the anesthesiologist providing access for two surgical teams (oncologic and reconstructive surgeons).

With completion of the mastectomy, recipient vessels are exposed. The internal mammary vessels are the option most commonly utilized at present. The pectoralis major muscle fibers over the medial aspect of the 3rd rib are divided, exposing the underlying cartilaginous portion of the rib. The rib cartilage and perichondrium are carefully harvested to provide exposure of the internal mammary artery and vein, which are deep to the posterior perichondrium of the rib (Figure 63-7). The vessels are dissected out

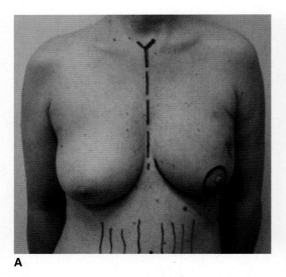
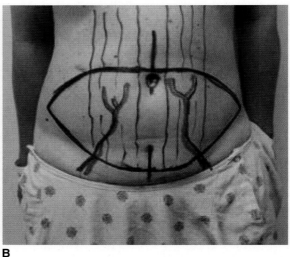

FIGURE 63-6. Preoperative marking for a deep inferior epigastric artery perforator (DIEP) flap. A: Breast markings include identifying the chest midline, measuring the breast width, and outlining the periareolar incision. B: Marking of the abdominal flap is made at or just above the umbilicus, extending laterally toward the anterior superior iliac spines and inferiorly toward the pubis at a distance equal to the breast width.

circumferentially with exposure of a length of vessels to facilitate the microvascular anastomosis.

Flap elevation begins while the mastectomies are performed. An incision is made along the superior abdominal marking with dissection down to the abdominal wall fascia. An adipocutaneous flap is elevated cephalad in the suprafascial plane to allow for advancement and closure after flap harvest. The lower abdominal incision is made and dissection performed down to the anterior abdominal wall fascia. During this portion of the dissection, the superficial inferior epigastric vessels are identified (when present), and at a minimum, the vein is dissected out to a length of 5 to 7 cm or more and clipped to provide the option of an additional outflow vessel in cases of flaps with a superficial dominant venous outflow. For bilateral breast reconstructions, the abdominal flap is split in half along the midline, incising around the umbilicus and dissecting out its stalk. Flap elevation then proceeds from lateral to medial in the suprafascial plane until the lateral row of flap perforators is identified. Elevation of the flaps from the medial border provides exposure of the medial row of perforators. Once all perforators are identified, decisions are made to select the best perforators for the flap, ideally all within one row (medial or lateral). All perforators that will not be used are clipped and divided. An incision is then made in the anterior rectus fascia adjacent to the selected row of perforators. Intramuscular dissection of the perforators down to the deep inferior epigastric pedicle is carefully performed. The superior epigastric vessels are identified and divided. The flap pedicle, deep to the rectus abdominis muscle, is dissected toward the external iliac vessels until it is of sufficient length and size for a microvascular anastomosis on the chest. At this point, the flap harvest is complete and the vessels are divided. The flap is then transferred to the chest wall where, with the aid of an operative microscope or loupes, anastomoses of the artery and vein are performed to the internal mammary artery and vein, respectively.

Flap inset and breast shaping are performed and drains are placed in the breast pocket. The flap skin paddle is approximated to the mastectomy skin with absorbable sutures placed in layers. Monitoring of perfusion is typically performed with the aid of a handheld Doppler and physical exam (color, capillary refill, temperature). The abdominal wall fascia and donor site incision are closed with drains placed prior. The OR table is reflexed to aid with closure while relieving tension on the skin closure. Postoperatively, patients are monitored for 3 to 5 days prior to discharge home. Subsequent stages of reconstruction are performed months later in a staged fashion with the goals of improving shape, breast symmetry, and nipple–areolar complex reconstruction if desired (Figure 63-8).

● POTENTIAL PITFALLS

It is vitally important to avoid violation of natural boundaries of the breast to optimize aesthetic results of any reconstruction. As such, when the inframammary fold is violated, time should be devoted to re-establishing a distinct fold with sutures. Dissection past the midline, over the sternum, can result in symmastia, and excessive lateral dissection may result in lateral displacement of implants; efforts should be made to address these problems by redefining the boundaries of the breast during the initial reconstructive procedure. Revision procedures also provide an opportunity to tackle persistent problems.

Care should be taken to account for the final location of the latissimus dorsi skin paddle on transfer and inset when the preoperative markings are made. Improper placement of the skin paddle can lead to a challenging inset with compromise to the aesthetic results. While harvesting the latissimus dorsi myocutaneous flap, muscle elevation should avoid harvest of a fat pad that is adherent to the

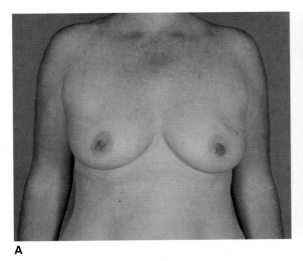
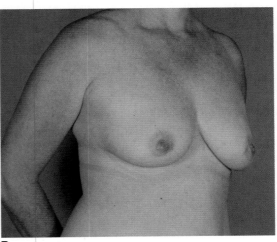

A   **B**

FIGURE 63-8. **A,B:** Preoperative photographs of a patient with a left breast cancer.

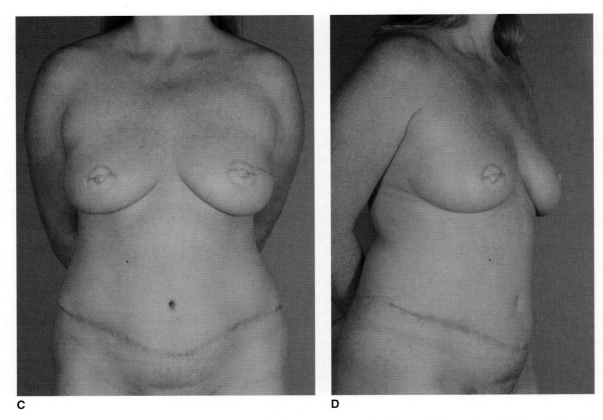

C   D

FIGURE 63-8. *(Continued)* **C,D:** Postoperative photographs of the breasts and abdominal donor site after immediate bilateral DIEP flap reconstruction with subsequent revisions including bilateral nipple reconstructions. The patient will undergo nipple tattooing for areolar pigmentation.

undersurface of the latissimus to prevent inadvertent elevation of the posterior serratus muscle.

Recipient internal mammary vessel exposure in radiated patients can be challenging. The tissue planes are often adherent, and the vessel walls are friable increasing the likelihood of vessel injury and bleeding during exposure. The friability of vessels is also a significant problem for the microvascular anastomosis or arteries in particular. Care has to be taken while placing arterial sutures to avoid intimal lacerations, which typically lead to thrombosis.

Perforator selection to provide appropriate perfusion to abdominal-based flaps should be carried out with caution to avoid intraoperative and postoperative flap compromise from arterial insufficiency or venous congestion. Prior to dividing perforators that are not likely to be used, they should be occluded temporarily with small vascular clamps with an assessment of perfusion performed by clinical exam (color and capillary refill) or with the aid of a laser indocyanine green perfusion assessment (Table 63-1).

● SPECIAL INTRAOPERATIVE CONSIDERATIONS

Close attention should be paid to mastectomy skin perfusion, particularly with implant forms of reconstruction.

In cases with compromised mastectomy skin flaps where plans were for tissue expander placement, options include placing the tissue expander without an intraoperative fill or delaying the placement for the tissue expander for a period of time. A similar approach can be employed in DTI cases, with placement of a tissue expander with limited to no intraoperative fill as opposed to a full implant.

● POSTOPERATIVE MANAGEMENT

Women undergoing immediate tissue expander placement for breast reconstruction are typically admitted overnight for pain control and routine monitoring. Hospital stays for women who undergo autologous tissue flaps usually range from 3 to 5 days. Postoperative care includes pain control, diet advancement, fluid management, early ambulation, use of incentive spirometry, and DVT mechanical and pharmacologic prophylaxis. For free flap procedures, tissue perfusion is closely monitored during the patient's hospitalization, which is particularly critical in the first 72 hours when free flaps are most likely to fail. Women are advised to refrain from strenuous exercise and activities for a period of 6 to 8 weeks following reconstruction.

Early complications following breast reconstruction include hematoma, seroma, infection, flap loss, skin necrosis,

Table 63-1	Breast Reconstruction

Tissue Expander Breast Reconstruction

Key Technical Steps

1. Precise preoperative marking of breast landmarks with patient upright
2. Selection of a tissue expander that matches the base width of the breast
3. Elevation of the pectoralis major muscle with release of its insertion to the IMF
4. Inset of ADM to the IMF and lateral chest wall
5. Insert tissue expander and approximate the pectoralis to the ADM
6. Partially fill the expander after skin closure

Potential Pitfalls

- Violation of the breast boundaries (IMF and midline over sternum)
- Overfilling of the tissue expander with compromise of perfusion to the mastectomy flap

Direct to Implant Breast Reconstruction

Key Technical Steps

1. Precise preoperative marking of breast landmarks with patient upright
2. Elevation of the pectoralis major muscle with release of its insertion to the IMF
3. Inset of ADM to the IMF and lateral chest wall
4. Place selected sizer under the pectoralis and ADM
5. Sit the patient up and shape the breast with tailoring of the ADM
6. Exchange the sizer for the selected implant

Potential Pitfalls

- Violation of the breast boundaries (IMF and midline over sternum)
- Use of an ADM size that does not account for the volume of a full implant
- Placing an implant that stretches the skin envelope with potential compromise of perfusion

Latissimus Dorsi Breast Reconstruction

Key Technical Steps

1. Precise preoperative marking of breast and back landmarks with patient upright
2. Preparation of the breast pocket and lateral chest tunnel while supine
3. Position to lateral decubitus and flap elevation
4. Selection of a tissue expander that matches the base width of the breast
5. Flap inset and tissue expander placement with the patient supine
6. Partially fill the expander after skin closure

Potential Pitfalls

- Improper placement of the flap skin paddle making for challenging inset
- Inadvertent elevation of the serratus muscle with the latissimus
- Overfilling of the tissue expander with compromise of perfusion to the mastectomy and latissimus flaps

DIEP Flap Breast Reconstruction

Key Technical Steps

1. Internal mammary vessel exposure
2. Flap elevation with perforator selection
3. Intramuscular perforator dissection and flap harvest
4. Transfer to chest wall with microsurgical anastomosis
5. Flap inset and abdominal donor site closure

Potential Pitfalls

- Injury to the recipient vessels with bleeding
- Injury to the pleura during recipient vessel exposure with resulting pneumothorax
- Improper perforator selection resulting compromise to perfusion
- Injury to selected flap perforators with potential loss of perfusion to components of the flap

and implant extrusion. Infection is a dreaded complication following tissue expander/implant reconstruction as it could lead to loss of the implant. Infections are often treated with intravenous antibiotics. Patients that fail to improve on antibiotics should undergo implant or expander removal and delayed reconstruction after the infection is cleared and the tissues have become supple. Late complications of implant-based breast reconstruction include implant rupture and capsular contracture. Current guidelines suggest that women who receive silicone implants have a baseline MRI in 3 years following placement and then every 2 years for the length of time that the implant is in place to monitor for implant rupture. Breast flap fat necrosis, mastectomy flap necrosis, infection, abdominal wall weakness and hernias, umbilical devitalization, seroma, and hematoma are potential complications that can occur after TRAM or DIEP flap breast reconstruction.

The process of breast reconstruction spans a period of months to years. Following reconstruction of the breast mound, further procedures may be required to revise the shape of the breast, create a nipple, and achieve symmetry with the contralateral breast. Such procedures may include contralateral augmentation with implants or autologous fat grafting, reduction, and mastopexy to achieve symmetry. Finally, nipple reconstruction may be performed as early as 3 to 6 months following breast mound reconstruction, in order to allow for swelling to subside and the breast mound to achieve its final shape. Multiple local flap designs can be used for nipple and areolar reconstruction and supplemented with tattooing for a more anatomic appearance.

TAKE HOME POINTS

- A majority of women undergoing mastectomy are candidates for breast reconstruction and should be referred to a reconstructive surgeon to discuss potential options.
- Breast reconstruction improves psychosocial functioning, mental health, and body image following

mastectomy and does not interfere with long-term surveillance for recurrence.
- Numerous options for reconstruction exist. The choice of reconstruction is determined based on a patient's oncologic management, body habitus, and personal preferences.
- Radiation therapy induces long-term changes in the chest wall soft tissue. Consideration should be made for delaying reconstruction and preferentially using autologous tissue reconstruction in radiated patients.
- Abdominal tissue is most commonly used for autologous breast reconstruction. Innovative perforator-based and muscle-sparing techniques can lessen donor site morbidity compared to traditional procedures.

SUGGESTED READINGS

Alderman AK, Hawley ST, Waljee J, et al. Understanding the impact of breast reconstruction on the surgical decision-making process for breast cancer. *Cancer.* 2008;112:489-494.

Breuing K, Warren S. Immediate bilateral breast reconstruction with implants and inferolateral alloderm slings. *Ann Plast Surg.* 2005;55(3):232-239.

Fisher B, Anderson S, Bryant J, et al. Twenty-year follow-up of a randomized trial comparing total mastectomy, lumpectomy, and lumpectomy plus irradiation for the treatment of invasive breast cancer. *N Engl J Med.* 2002;347(16):1233-1241

Kannchwala SK, Glatt BS, Conant EF, et al. Autologous fat grafting to the reconstructed breast: the management of acquired contour deformities. *Plast Reconstr Surg.*2009;124(2):409-418.

Kronowitz SJ, Kuerer HM, Buchholz TA. A management algorithm and practical oncoplastic surgery techniques for repairing partial mastectomy defects. *Plast Reconstr Surg.* 2008;122(6):1631-1647.

Man L, Selber JC, Serletti JM. Abdominal wall following free TRAM or DIEP flap reconstruction: a meta-analysis and critical review. *Plast Reconstr Surg.* 2009;124(3):752-764.

Maxwell GP. Iginio Tansini and the origin of the latissimus dorsi musculocutaneous flap. *Plast Reconstr Surg.* 1980;65(5):686–692.

Spear SL, Boehmler JH, Bogue DP, et al. Options in reconstructing the irradiated breast. *Plast Reconstr Surg.* 2008;122(2):379-388.

Endocrine

Palpable Thyroid Nodule

HAGGI MAZEH AND REBECCA S. SIPPEL

64

Based on the previous edition chapter "Palpable Thyroid Nodule" by Haggi Mazeh and Rebecca S. Sippel

Presentation

A 42-year-old female, without any previous medical or surgical history, presents for routine physical examination. Her vital signs are within normal limits. On neck examination, she is noted to have a palpable nodule in the front of her neck. The nodule is located two finger breadth inferior to the cricoid cartilage and 1 cm to the right of the midline. The nodule measures about 2 cm in its greatest diameter; it is firm, mobile, and nontender. When the patient swallows, the nodule moves up and down with the thyroid cartilage. There are no palpable nodules on the left side of the neck, nor is there cervical of supraclavicular lymphadenopathy. The remaining physical examination is normal.

● DIFFERENTIAL DIAGNOSIS

The description of the nodule suggests that it is located within the thyroid gland. Thyroid nodules may be of benign nature such as colloid-containing cysts, thyroid adenoma, hyperplastic nodules, or thyroiditis. Thyroid nodules may harbor malignancy including papillary, follicular, medullary, Hürthle cell, or anaplastic thyroid cancer. In rare cases, thyroid nodules may represent lymphoma, squamous cell carcinoma, or metastasis of other origin. The differential diagnosis of other neck masses is broad and is beyond the scope of this chapter.

● WORKUP

At this point, it is important to identify whether the patient has any risk factors for malignancy. The two most important risk factors for thyroid malignancy are a history of neck radiation and a family history of thyroid cancer or other endocrine tumors. Specific attention must be paid to symptoms associated with local compression or invasion such as hoarseness, cough, dysphagia, or airway compressive symptoms. Rapid growth and new onset of hoarseness raise the suspicion for malignancy.

Thyroid function testing with a thyroid-stimulating hormone (TSH) level is recommended. If the TSH is abnormal, additional testing of thyroid function is warranted. If the TSH is elevated, serum concentrations of thyroperoxidase antibody should be checked. If the TSH is suppressed, a TSH receptor antibody (TRAb) can be obtained to evaluate for Graves' disease. A thyroid scintigraphy scan can be obtained to distinguish between Graves' disease and a toxic nodule or toxic multinodular goiter. Currently, routine calcitonin testing is not recommended.

Ultrasound (US) is the imaging of choice for a newly diagnosed thyroid nodule. Ultrasound may assess nodule size, location, and other concomitant thyroid pathologies as well as the cervical lymph nodes. Ultrasonic features suspicious for malignancy include hypoechogenicity, microcalcification, irregular margins, chaotic vascular patterns, as well as extracapsular invasion and lymph node involvement. Figure 64-1 demonstrates the appearance of a malignant nodule on US.

Ultrasound-guided fine needle aspiration biopsy (FNAB) is the most important tool for evaluation of thyroid nodules. Possible FNAB results are nondiagnostic, benign, atypia or follicular lesion of undetermined significance, follicular neoplasm, suspicious for malignancy, and malignant (see Figure 64-2).

The patient's US demonstrated a 3.2-cm right thyroid lobe nodule. The nodule was hypoechoic and complex with some microcalcifications. In this patient, FNAB identified a follicular neoplasm.

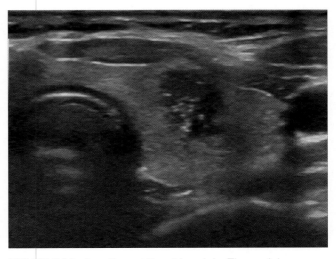

FIGURE 64-1. A malignant thyroid nodule. The nodule appears heterogeneous, cystic, hypoechoic, and irregular margins, and microcalcifications are present.

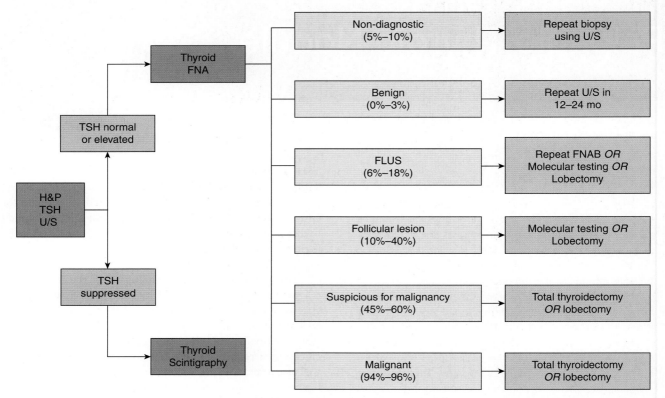

FIGURE 64-2. An algorithm for the evaluation of thyroid nodules. The six possible FNAB results are given with their associated risk of malignancy and the appropriate management. Molecular testing is considered for Bethesda categories III-IV (atypia or follicular lesion of undetermined significance or follicular neoplasm). TSH, thyroid-stimulating hormone; FNAB, fine needle aspiration biopsy.

● DIAGNOSIS AND TREATMENT

Although the prevalence of thyroid nodules on ultrasound may exceed 50%, palpable thyroid nodules can be detected in 10% of women and 2% of men. Fortunately, most nodules are of benign nature and only 5% harbor malignancy. In the last two decades, FNAB of thyroid nodules has become the "gold standard" of thyroid nodule workup. In an attempt to develop uniform terminology of FNAB reports, six categories were defined as mentioned above.

Inadequate or nondiagnostic aspirates constitute 4% to 16% of FNAB results, and FNAB should be repeated. Given the inflammation caused by the first FNAB, it is best to wait 4 to 6 weeks prior to repeating the FNAB if feasible. If the repeated aspiration is not diagnostic, surgical excision is recommended. Benign results on FNAB are the most common finding (up to 70%) and may be treated expectantly. A follow-up US should be obtained in 12 to 24 months to evaluate for interval growth. Malignant FNAB results should be treated with lobectomy or total thyroidectomy according to size and other risk factors. Follicular neoplasms (FN) are identified in 15% to 20% of all FNAB and about 10% to 40% prove to be malignant. FNAB is unable to distinguish benign from malignant FN, and in such lesions, molecular testing that takes into account the pretest probability may be

considered. In cases with positive molecular testing or cases where molecular testing is not performed, surgical removal is required. Figure 64-2 provides an algorithm for the evaluation of thyroid nodules.

● SURGICAL APPROACH

The surgical approach to a patient with a follicular neoplasm result on FNAB requires an educated decision by the patient. The appropriate surgical approach for a FN is a diagnostic lobectomy. If the final pathology reveals malignancy, then a completion thyroidectomy should be considered based on tumor features. Frozen section evaluation is usually not informative and is unnecessary unless there is a suspicion for papillary thyroid cancer. The advantages of thyroid lobectomy include avoiding possible injury to the contralateral recurrent laryngeal nerve (RLN) and parathyroid glands as well as avoiding the need for lifelong thyroid hormone replacement in the majority of patients. A major disadvantage of this approach is that it may involve the need for completion thyroidectomy if malignancy is identified on final pathology. This second procedure involves another admission and anesthetic. Patients with a history of radiation therapy to the neck, a positive family history for thyroid cancer, multinodular goiter, and those already on thyroid hormone replacement therapy may be best served with total thyroidectomy as the index procedure.

The patient in our scenario decided to undergo total thyroidectomy (Table 64-1).

The procedure is usually performed under general anesthesia. The patient is positioned in a beach chair position and the neck is extended. A horizontal neck (Kocher) incision is performed and should be located just inferior to the cricoid cartilage, ideally in a neck crease. The platysma muscle is divided, and subplatysmal flaps are elevated. The strap muscles are separated at the midline to offer access to the thyroid gland. At this point, it is preferable to begin the dissection on the side with the suspected lesion or tumor. It is important to dissect and retract the strap muscles off the thyroid gland in order to be in the correct plane. The middle thyroid vein should be divided. The upper pole of the thyroid is divided as close as possible to the thyroid gland in order to avoid injury to the superior laryngeal nerve and the upper parathyroid gland. Once the upper pole is divided, the thyroid lobe may be retracted medially and upward to assist further dissection. At this point, it is crucial to identify the RLN in the tracheoesophageal groove along its course to the cricothyroid membrane.

Parathyroid glands should be preserved with their native blood supply whenever possible. During the dissection, vessels can be divided with cautery, harmonic scalpel, clips, or ties according to surgeon preference. Once the lobe is mobilized,

the isthmus is dissected off the trachea with cautery, and the contralateral lobe is resected in a similar fashion. After hemostasis is assured, the strap muscles are reapproximated at the midline. The platysma muscle is sutured and the skin closed.

SPECIAL INTRAOPERATIVE CONSIDERATIONS

- In cases of suspected malignancy or proven malignancy, special attention must be paid to the lymph nodes in the central compartment. Lymph nodes that are grossly involved should be resected and in such cases formal central lymph node dissection should be performed.
- Failure to identify and resect a pyramidal lobe can be the source of a significant thyroid remnant with radioactive iodine treatment. The pyramidal lobe may be elongated reaching above the thyroid cartilage. Special care must be taken to correctly identify and resect it as part of the thyroid gland.
- In order to identify and preserve the parathyroid glands, it is important to understand their anatomic location, especially in relationship to the RLN. The upper parathyroid gland is located posterior and lateral to the RLN, and the lower glands are located anterior and medial to the RLN. In cases when parathyroid glands are inadvertently resected, they should be autotransplanted into the sternocleidomastoid muscle.
- Identification of the RLN during thyroidectomy is essential to avoid injury. After dividing the upper pole of the thyroid gland, it is important to avoid further dissection inferiorly prior to the nerve identification because most nerve injuries occur close to the nerve entrance to the trachea. In rare cases, the nerve is entrapped within tumor tissue, and in such cases, the nerve should be sacrificed. Nerve-monitoring devices have a role in confirming the nerve is intact, especially in complicated cases.
- The role of intraoperative frozen section is controversial. Some surgeons use it to assist in deciding on the extent of surgery for lesions with no definite malignancy on FNAB. Frozen section is most helpful in cases that have an FNAB of suspicious papillary thyroid cancer. Frozen section is rarely able to distinguish follicular adenoma from follicular carcinoma, so it is probably not useful in most cases of FN.

Table 64-1	Thyroidectomy

Key Technical Steps

1. Position the patient with the neck extended.
2. Place your incision to enable access to both the upper and lower poles.
3. Elevate subplatysmal flaps and separate the strap muscles.
4. Take the upper pole vessels first.
5. Mobilize the lobe anteriorly and medially to facilitate RLN identification.
6. Carry all dissections as close as possible to the thyroid gland.
7. Always identify the parathyroid glands and preserve their blood supply.

Potential Pitfalls

- Nerve injury usually occurs close to the nerve insertion at the cricothyroid membrane.
- Inadvertently removed or devascularized parathyroid glands should be autotransplanted and implanted in muscle tissue at the end of the case.
- Postoperative expanding neck hematoma should prompt bedside wound exploration followed by return to the operating room.

POSTOPERATIVE MANAGEMENT

Thyroid surgery may be performed in an outpatient setting or with a short admission (24 hours). Patients should be monitored for several hours after surgery to evaluate for the development of neck hematoma that may require emergent evacuation. Symptomatic hypocalcemia is not a risk after a thyroid lobectomy; however, symptomatic transient postoperative hypocalcemia occurs in 10% to 20% of patients that undergo total thyroidectomy. Postoperative hypocalcemia may be minimized with the use of oral calcium supplements. Measuring postoperative calcium and parathyroid hormone levels is typically used to identify patients who may require higher doses of calcium as well as calcitriol supplements. All patients who have the entire gland removed require thyroid hormone replacement therapy.

Follow-up varies according to the final histopathology results. Postoperative I ablation is administered for high-risk patients with differentiated thyroid carcinomas, especially those with gross residual disease, metastatic disease, or nodal involvement. In these patients, administration of levothyroxine at a suppressive dose (TSH < 0.1 mU) has been shown to improve disease-free survival. Serum thyroglobulin levels should be measured every 6 to 12 months for patients with differentiated thyroid cancer that underwent total thyroidectomy.

Case Conclusion

The patient undergoes uncomplicated total thyroidectomy as an outpatient. Postoperatively, she is treated with levothyroxine and calcium supplements, the calcium is discontinued after a week. On final pathology follicular thyroid carcinoma is identified, measuring 3.2 cm at greatest diameter with capsular invasion and extrathyroidal extension and vascular invasion. The patient is treated with radioactive iodine ablation four weeks after surgery. Five years later, the patient is noted to have elevated thyroglobulin. Workup identifies a local recurrence that is removed surgically. At 10-year follow-up, she is free of disease.

TAKE HOME POINTS

- Palpable thyroid nodules are very common in up to 10% of the population.
- Most thyroid nodules are benign.
- The single most important test for palpable thyroid nodules is FNAB with an accuracy of up to 95%.
- Thyroid nodules should be managed according to FNAB results. Accurate terminology facilitates proper treatment.
- Follicular lesions on FNAB carry a 10% to 40% malignancy and require further evaluation with molecular testing or surgical intervention.
- The appropriate surgical management for patients with a follicular neoplasm is at a minimum a thyroid lobectomy.

SUGGESTED READINGS

Cibas ES, Ali SZ. The Bethesda system for reporting thyroid cytopathology. *Thyroid*. 2017;27(11):1341-1346.

Dean DS, Gharib H. Epidemiology of thyroid nodules. *Best Pract Res Clin Endocrinol Metab*. 2008;22:901-911.

Gharib H, Papini E, Valcavi R, et al. American Association of Clinical Endocrinologists and Associazione Medici Endocrinologi medical guidelines for clinical practice for the diagnosis and management of thyroid nodules. *Endocr Pract*. 2006;12:63-102.

Haugen BR, Alexander EK, Bible KC, et al. 2015 American Thyroid Association Management Guidelines for Adult Patients with Thyroid Nodules and Differentiated Thyroid Cancer: The American Thyroid Association Guidelines Task Force on Thyroid Nodules and Differentiated Thyroid Cancer. *Thyroid*. 2016;26(1):1-133.

Papillary Thyroid Carcinoma

65

GERARD M. DOHERTY

Based on the previous edition chapter "Papillary Thyroid Carcinoma" by Gerard M. Doherty

Presentation

A 42-year-old woman in previously good health, whose only medications are oral contraceptives, presents for evaluation of a central neck mass noted on health maintenance examination. Her neck examination shows a firm mass to the right of the larynx that moves up and down with swallowing. She has no palpable lymphadenopathy. She has no family history of thyroid disease and no personal history of radiation exposure.

● DIFFERENTIAL DIAGNOSIS

A mass in the central neck that moves with swallowing is tethered to the larynx; the most common lesions are of the thyroid gland. Other possibilities include infectious or inflammatory lesions (lymphadenitis, abscess, or sarcoidosis), congenital lesions (thyroglossal duct lesions, branchial cleft cysts, cystic hygroma, or laryngocele), or neoplasms of nonthyroid origin (salivary gland, subcutaneous lipoma, sebaceous cyst, carotid body tumor, laryngeal chondroma, soft tissue sarcoma, or metastatic lymphadenopathy). The thyroid lesions can be inflammatory (lymphocytic thyroiditis most common; others

include acute thyroiditis, Riedel's thyroiditis, or suppurative thyroiditis), benign neoplastic lesions (solitary or multiple adenomas, multinodular hyperplasia), or malignant lesions (papillary, follicular, anaplastic or medullary thyroid cancer, lymphoma, or rarely metastatic lesions).

● WORKUP

Point-of-care ultrasound shows a heterogeneous, mostly hypoechoic, irregularly shaped mass in the right thyroid lobe that measures 34 mm in maximum dimension (Figure 65-1). The left lobe of the thyroid gland appears normal. Measurement of thyroid function tests show a normal TSH (thyroid-stimulating hormone) level of 1.37 mIU/L. Because of the suspicious ultrasound appearance, fine needle aspiration cytology under ultrasound guidance is performed and shows papillary thyroid carcinoma.

● DISCUSSION

Thorough initial evaluation includes ultrasound examination of the neck to clarify the physical examination findings. This can help to determine whether the lesion is thyroid in

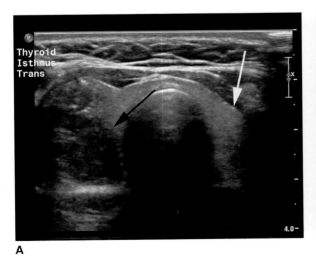

A

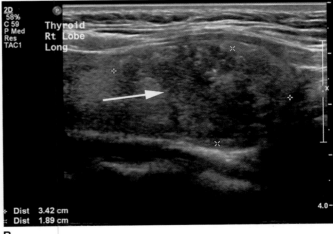

B

FIGURE 65-1. Thyroid ultrasound demonstrating the suspicious right thyroid lobe mass. **A:** Transverse view of the thyroid gland. The left lobe (*white arrow*) appears normal. The right lobe contains a hypoechoic, irregular lesion suspicious for thyroid carcinoma (*black arrow*). **B:** Sagittal view of the right thyroid lobe showing the suspicious mass (*white arrow*) in the lower portion of the right lobe.

origin and what the characteristics of the thyroid lesion are (solid vs. cystic vs. complex, smooth vs. irregular borders, solitary vs. multiple, hyper-, hypo- or isoechoic, degree of vascularity, presence or absence of microcalcification, and size). Thyroid nodules can be categorized based on these findings, and the clinical decision of whether to sample the lesion is informed by clinical management guidelines. For example, any high or intermediate suspicion nodule larger than 10 mm in diameter should be sampled, while low- or very-low-suspicion lesions should only be biopsied if larger than 15 or 20 mm, respectively.

Assessment of thyroid function is helpful, both to determine the potential need for thyroid hormone supplementation and to guide the evaluation. Patients with an elevated TSH are more likely to have malignant nodules and may require thyroid hormone supplementation even if the thyroid nodule proves to be benign. Patients with a suppressed TSH may have an overactive thyroid nodule that is extremely unlikely to be malignant. A suppressed TSH in a patient with a thyroid nodule is the only situation currently in which a nuclear thyroid scintiscan is indicated. Other than this relatively uncommon situation, scintiscan is not useful. For these hyperthyroid patients, scintiscan can help to distinguish Graves' disease with a concomitant (potentially malignant) thyroid nodule from a solitary toxic adenoma (Figure 65-2).

Fine needle aspiration cytology is the backbone of thyroid nodule assessment. This requires special expertise for interpretation but is very reliable. There are currently six standard categories for reporting of thyroid FNA results: Nondiagnostic, Benign, Follicular Lesion of Undetermined Significance, Follicular Neoplasm, Suspicious for Malignancy, and Malignant, commonly referred to as Bethesda categories 1 through 6. Nondiagnostic (1) results usually prompt repeat FNA, benign cytology (2) is followed by interval follow-up

evaluation, and suspicious (5) or definitively malignant (6) results are managed by operation. The indeterminate categories (3 and 4) have been managed by diagnostic operation, repeat needle aspiration, or follow-up monitoring depending upon the associated characteristics of the patient and the nodule.

However, the development of commercially available molecular testing of the FNA specimens has now further informed these management choices in most thyroid clinics. Molecular testing of Bethesda category 3 or 4 lesions is typically performed, and the results used to guide management to either operative intervention if results are suspicious for malignancy or ongoing follow-up if the results indicate a likely benign lesion. Though this definitely improves the management for these patients, and decreases the number of diagnostic operations performed for benign lesions, the full understanding of the implications and uses of these relatively new diagnostic tests are still in development.

● DIAGNOSIS AND TREATMENT

Preoperative cervical ultrasound to evaluate the central and lateral cervical lymph node compartments is required prior to operation for thyroid carcinoma. This is necessary in order to identify involved lymph node compartments so that a thorough initial operation can be planned. If there is lymphadenopathy on imaging in the lateral compartment, then fine needle aspiration of a lateral neck node with thyroglobulin measurement of the aspirate can determine the need for therapeutic neck dissection in that basin. Selective neck dissection based upon the levels of the involved lymph nodes should include any compartment involved (Figure 65-3).

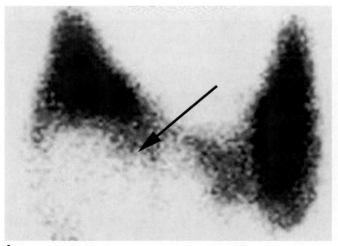

A

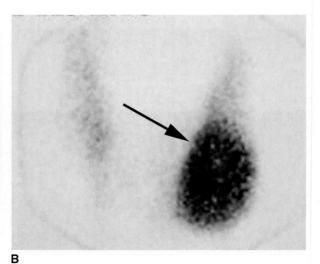

B

FIGURE 65-2. Nuclear scintiscans are only useful for, and are now reserved for, hyperthyroid patients with a thyroid nodule (low TSH). Ultrasound and cytology have replaced the routine use of scintiscan to evaluate thyroid nodules. However, hyperthyroid patients with a solitary thyroid nodule can fit one of two scenarios: Graves' disease with a thyroid nodule, that can be malignant (**Panel A**, *arrow* on the cold right lower pole nodule), or a solitary toxic adenoma with suppression of function in the remainder of the thyroid gland (**Panel B**, *arrow* on the hot left lower pole nodule).

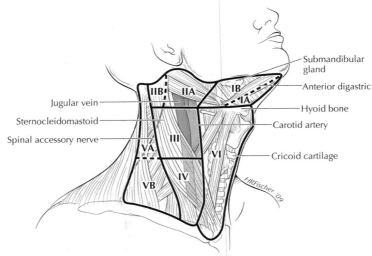

FIGURE 65-3. Lymph node compartments separated into levels and sublevels. Level VI contains the thyroid gland, and the adjacent nodes bordered superiorly by the hyoid bone, inferiorly by the innominate (brachiocephalic) artery, and laterally on each side by the carotid sheaths. The level II, III, and IV nodes are arrayed along the jugular veins on each side, bordered anteromedially by level VI and laterally by the posterior border of the sternocleidomastoid muscle. The level I node compartment includes the submental and submandibular nodes, above the hyoid bone, and anterior to the posterior edge of the submandibular gland. The level V nodes are in the posterior triangle, lateral to the lateral edge of the sternocleidomastoid muscle. (From Haugen BR, Alexander EK, Bible KC, et al. 2015 American Thyroid Association Management Guidelines for Adult Patients with Thyroid Nodules and Differentiated Thyroid Cancer: The American Thyroid Association Guidelines Task Force on Thyroid Nodules and Differentiated Thyroid Cancer. *Thyroid.* 2016;26(1):1-133, with permission.)

For those with the very best prognosis (tumor <10 mm, normal lymph nodes, age <45 years) and a normal contralateral lobe, patient with papillary thyroid carcinoma should have an initial operation that includes removal of only the ipsilateral thyroid lobe. For patients with tumors between 1 and 4 cm in size, the choice of partial or total thyroidectomy should depend upon the risks of persistent or recurrent disease and the utility of postoperative adjuvant radioiodine treatment, which can only be done after total thyroidectomy. If lymph nodes are involved by cancer based on preoperative or intraoperative assessment, they should be removed by complete compartmental dissection. This typically is also an indication for total thyroidectomy and radioiodine treatment. The utility of prophylactic level 6 lymph node dissection for those patients with apparently uninvolved lymph nodes is more controversial but may provide important prognostic information and potential therapeutic benefit for patients in higher risk categories.

Ultrasound of the neck reveals a right level 3 lymph node with suspicious features (Figure 65-4). Ultrasound-guided

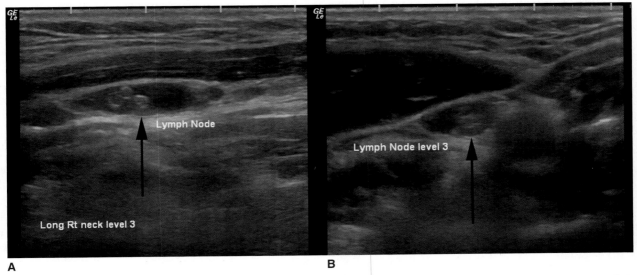

FIGURE 65-4. Ultrasound examination of the right lateral cervical lymph nodes shows an abnormal right level 3 lymph node in the longitudinal (**Panel A**) and transverse (**Panel B**) images. The *arrows* denote the abnormal lymph node.

needle aspiration of the node shows cells consistent with metastatic papillary thyroid cancer and an aspirate thyroglobulin level of 934 ng/mL. Given these findings, the patient is scheduled for a total thyroidectomy with level 6 lymph node dissection, as well as a right level 2-3-4 lymph node dissection.

● SURGICAL APPROACH

The extent of the planned operation is dictated by the locations of disease. For this patient, with a significant papillary thyroid carcinoma and an involved right lateral neck node metastasis documented, the likelihood of level 6 lymph node involvement is high, and these nodes should also be dissected. The level 6 lymph nodes can be difficult to image by ultrasound when the thyroid gland is in place.

This operation is best done under general anesthesia. Though many thyroid operations can be done using local anesthesia and sedation, the inclusion of central and lateral neck dissection makes this quite difficult. The key steps of the operation are listed in Table 65-1. Thyroidectomy can be complicated by infection, bleeding, and anesthetic reactions though these are quite unlikely. The more worrisome complications of thyroidectomy are nerve injury and hypoparathyroidism, both because they are more common and because they can cause permanent functional deficits for the patient.

The principles of the dissection are as follows:

1. Avoid dividing any structures in the tracheoesophageal groove until the recurrent laryngeal nerve is definitively identified. Small branches of the inferior thyroid artery may seem like they can clearly be safely transected, however, the distortion of tumor, retraction, or previous scar may lead the surgeon to mistakenly divide a branch of the RLN.
2. Identify the recurrent laryngeal nerve low in the neck, well below the inferior thyroid artery, at the level of the lower pole of the thyroid gland, or below. This allows dissection of the nerve at a site where it is not tethered by its attachments to the larynx or its relation to the inferior thyroid artery.
3. Keep the recurrent laryngeal nerve in view during the subsequent dissection of the thyroid gland from the larynx.
4. Minimize the use of powered dissection posterior to the thyroid gland.
5. Treat each parathyroid gland as though it were the last one.
6. Autograft any parathyroid glands that have questionable viability.

The use of nerve stimulators and laryngeal muscle action potential monitors has been investigated as a tool to try to limit or avoid nerve injuries. The data do not currently support the mandatory use of these devices; however, many experienced surgeons now routinely use a nerve monitoring system intraoperatively.

Table 65-1   Total Thyroidectomy

Key Technical Steps

1. Low collar incision within or parallel to natural skin lines.
2. Raise subplatysmal flaps.
3. Separate the strap muscles in the midline exposing the thyroid gland.
4. If using an intraoperative nerve monitoring system, expose the vagus nerve in the carotid sheath and confirm function of the monitor by stimulating the vagus nerve prior to exposure of the recurrent laryngeal nerve.
5. Separate the lateral border of the thyroid gland from the strap muscles and carotid sheath; enter the avascular plane medial to the upper pole without damaging the cricothyroid muscle fascia; isolate and divide the upper pole vessels.
6. Rotate the thyroid lobe anteriorly and identify the recurrent laryngeal nerve in the tracheoesophageal groove using the nerve monitoring system if available; dissect craniad along the nerve, separating from the thyroid, up to the cricothyroid muscle.
7. Divide the ligament of Berry anterior to the passage of the nerve into the larynx.
8. Separate the thyroid posterior surface from the trachea.
9. Identify and inspect the parathyroid glands; reimplant them if their vascularity is in question.
10. If using the nerve monitor, confirm unchanged function of the vagus nerve–recurrent laryngeal nerve–vocalis muscle system by stimulating the vagus nerve.

Potential Pitfalls

- Injury to the recurrent laryngeal or superior laryngeal nerves.
- Injury to the parathyroid glands.
- Tumor invasion into surrounding structures, such as larynx, trachea, esophagus, carotid sheath, or strap muscles.

● MANAGEMENT OF COMPLICATIONS

Nerve Injury

The main nerves adjacent to the thyroid gland that can be deliberately or inadvertently affected include the recurrent laryngeal nerve immediately adjacent to the thyroid, and the external branch of the superior laryngeal nerve (EBSLN). Damage to the RLN causes unilateral paralysis of the muscles that controls the ipsilateral vocal cord. Unilateral RLN injury changes the voice substantially in most patients and also significantly affects swallowing. Bilateral RLN injury causes paralysis of both cords and usually results in a very limited airway lumen at the cords. These patients usually have a normal-sounding speaking voice, but severe limitations on inhalation velocity because of upper airway obstruction.

RLN paresis is usually temporary and resolves over days to months. If a unilateral paresis proves to be permanent, then palliation of the cord immobility and voice changes can be achieved with vocal cord injection or laryngoplasty. These procedures stiffen and medialize the paralyzed cord, in order to allow the contralateral cord to oppose the paralyzed cord during speech. If both cords are affected, then the palliative procedures are more limited and involve creating an adequate airway for ventilation; improvements in voice quality are not likely, as there is no muscular control of the cord function.

About 10% of patients have some evidence of RLN paresis after thyroidectomy; however, this resolves in most patients. About 1% or fewer patients have permanent nerve injury when total thyroidectomy is performed by experienced surgeons.

The EBSLN courses adjacent to the superior pole vessels of the thyroid gland, before separating to penetrate the cricopharyngeus muscle fascia at it supero-posterior aspect. The nerve supplies motor innervation of the inferior constrictor muscles of the larynx. Damage to this nerve changes the ability of the larynx to control high-pressure phonation, such as high-pitched singing or yelling.

To avoid damaging this nerve, the dissection of the upper pole vessels should proceed from a space where the nerve is safely sequestered under the cricopharyngeal fascia to the superior vessels themselves, thus safely separating the nerve from the tissue to be divided.

Parathyroid Gland Injury

The parathyroid glands are small, delicate structures that share a blood supply with the thyroid gland. Their size and fragility expose them to damage during thyroidectomy. Avoidance of permanent hypoparathyroidism is far more desirable than treatment of it. This can be accomplished by preservation of the parathyroid glands on their native blood supply or autografting of parathyroid tissue to a muscular bed. If the parathyroid glands cannot be preserved on their native blood supply, then transfer of the gland to a convenient grafting site can maintain function. For normal parathyroid glands, transfer to the sternocleidomastoid muscle provides a convenient vascular bed for autograft. The parathyroid gland must be reduced to pieces that can survive on the diffusion of nutrients temporarily, while neovascular ingrowth occurs over several weeks.

The symptoms of hypoparathyroidism are those of severe hypocalcemia. Patients have numbness and tingling in the distal extremities and around the mouth or tongue in the earliest phases. For mild hypocalcemia with tingling, oral calcium supplements (calcium carbonate, 500 to 1,500 mg po, two to four times daily) are often sufficient to resolve the hypocalcemia. If supplementation beyond this level is necessary (as it is for most patients with severe hypocalcemia),

then the addition of supplemental vitamin D (calcitriol 0.25 to 1.0 mcg daily) increases the gastrointestinal absorption of calcium. Hypocalcemia not controlled by oral supplements, or accompanied by severe symptoms such as muscle cramping, is best managed by intravenous calcium administration. Intravenous calcium gluconate is the only option for intravenous calcium supplementation (calcium chloride should never be used).

Permanent hypoparathyroidism requires lifelong support with calcium supplements and vitamin D analogues. Missing doses of the supplements will usually produce symptoms, of varying severity, and which, while manageable, are often quite bothersome for patients.

Under general anesthesia, neck exploration shows a hard mass in the right lobe of the thyroid gland without evident extrathyroidal invasion. There are firm, small lymph nodes in level 6 adjacent to the thyroid gland; these are removed with the surrounding soft tissue. Both lower parathyroid glands are surrounded by abnormal lymph nodes, and so they are removed, minced into small pieces, and reimplanted into the right sternocleidomastoid muscle. The upper parathyroid glands are preserved on the native blood supply. The right level 2-3-4 lymph nodes are dissected free of the jugular vein with careful attention to preservation of the right vagus nerve (cranial nerve X), phrenic nerve, spinal accessory nerve (cranial nerve XI), and hypoglossal nerve. The ansa cervicalis nerve and omohyoid muscle are divided. At the completion of all dissection, EMG assessment of the bilateral vagus–recurrent laryngeal–vocalis muscle complex shows normal EMG signal with stimulation of the vagus nerve. There is no evidence of lymphatic leak, and no drain is placed.

● ADJUVANT THERAPY

Papillary thyroid cancer typically retains the capability of concentrating iodine. This feature can be exploited by delivering radioactive iodine in doses that will damage the cells, and cause death over a period of several weeks. Iodine is also taken up by salivary gland tissue and gastric mucosa, and is excreted mainly through the kidneys. The radioiodine is most efficiently concentrated in the thyroid tissue when the TSH is elevated, stimulating any remaining normal thyroid cells or thyroid cancer cells, to concentrate the radioiodine. The patient can be prepared with elevated TSH either by removing the thyroid gland and leaving them free of exogenous thyroid hormone, or by administering exogenous recombinant TSH. Either approach appears to be effective in the adjuvant setting. Adjuvant radioiodine is typically reserved for patients with a moderate or high risk of recurrence.

After radioiodine therapy is completed, if indicated, or immediately if exogenous TSH is administered, then the patient is treated with exogenous levothyroxine to replace their thyroid function, and to suppress their endogenous TSH. The degree of TSH suppression is determined by the risk of recurrence of the thyroid cancer. Low-risk patients can have the TSH maintained at about the lower limit of normal. Higher-risk patients may have the TSH suppressed further for several years.

The postoperative recovery is unremarkable, with mild hypocalcemia for 1 week, and normocalcemia by the 2-week follow-up. The voice is initially scratchy, but this resolves within 5 days. The final pathology shows a 35 mm papillary thyroid carcinoma with tall cell features, confined to the thyroid gland with negative margins. In level 6, 6 of 15 lymph nodes contain papillary thyroid carcinoma. In the level 2-3-4 dissection, 4 of 22 lymph nodes are involved. Because of the lymph node involvement, she subsequently receives 30 mCi of radioiodine under thyrogen stimulation. Her posttreatment radioiodine scan shows some uptake in the central neck consistent with residual thyroid tissue, and no evidence of metastases. Her thyroglobulin at that time is <0.5 ng/mL. She will have regular follow-up including physical examination, thyroglobulin measurement, and ultrasound examination of the neck.

TAKE HOME POINTS

- Assessment of a central neck mass likely to originate in the thyroid gland should include ultrasound and possibly fine needle aspiration cytology.
- Papillary thyroid carcinoma has an excellent prognosis; thorough initial treatment including operation limits the long term likelihood of recurrence and need for repeat therapy.
- Ultrasound evaluation of the lateral neck lymph nodes is important prior to operation in order to define the necessary extent of operation.
- Operation should include total thyroidectomy for most patients, and compartmental dissection of any involved lymph node basins.

- Adjuvant radioiodine and TSH suppression with levothyroxine decrease the recurrence rate of papillary thyroid cancer.
- Follow-up management and surveillance algorithms are risk based and include monitoring of serum thyroglobulin levels and cervical ultrasound examination.

SUGGESTED READINGS

Cibas ES, Ali SZ. The Bethesda System for Reporting Thyroid Cytopathology. *Thyroid.* 2009;19(11):1159-1165.

Doherty GM. Prophylactic central lymph node dissection: continued controversy. [Comment]. *Oncology.* 2010;23(7):603, 608.

Dralle H, Sekulla C, Lorenz K, Brauckhoff M, Machens A, German ISG. Intraoperative monitoring of the recurrent laryngeal nerve in thyroid surgery. *World J Surg.* 2008;32(7):1358-1366.

Haugen BR, Alexander EK, Bible KC, et al. 2015 American Thyroid Association Management Guidelines for Adult Patients with Thyroid Nodules and Differentiated Thyroid Cancer: The American Thyroid Association Guidelines Task Force on Thyroid Nodules and Differentiated Thyroid Cancer. *Thyroid.* 2016;26(1):1-133.

Hughes DT, White ML, Miller BS, Gauger PG, Burney RE, Doherty GM. Influence of prophylactic central lymph node dissection on postoperative thyroglobulin levels and radioiodine treatment in papillary thyroid cancer. *Surgery.* 2010;148(6):1100-1106; discussion 1006-1107.

Kouvaraki MA, Shapiro SE, Fornage BD, et al. Role of preoperative ultrasonography in the surgical management of patients with thyroid cancer. *Surgery.* 2003;134(6):946-954; discussion 954-945.

Kouvaraki MA, Lee JE, Shapiro SE, Sherman SI, Evans DB. Preventable reoperations for persistent and recurrent papillary thyroid carcinoma. *Surgery.* 2004;136(6):1183-1191.

Olson JA Jr, DeBenedetti MK, Baumann DS, Wells SA Jr. Parathyroid autotransplantation during thyroidectomy. Results of long-term follow-up [see comment]. *Ann Surg.* 1996;223(5):472-478; discussion 478-480.

Medullary Thyroid Cancer

66

OMEED MOAVEN AND HERBERT CHEN

Based on the previous edition chapter "Medullary Thyroid Cancer" by
Barbara Zarebczan and Herbert Chen

Presentation

A 27-year-old female presents to her primary care physician with a complaint of an enlarging neck mass. She first
noticed this mass 2 months ago and comes in concerned
because it has grown considerably larger. She denies having dyspnea, difficulty speaking, and dysphagia. She has
no known medical problems and is currently not on any
medications. She is adopted and does not know her family
history. On physical examination, her vital signs are normal.
She has a palpable, nontender neck mass, approximately
3 cm in diameter, to the left of midline just below the cricothyroid cartilage. No other masses are palpable, and the
remainder of her exam is within normal limits.

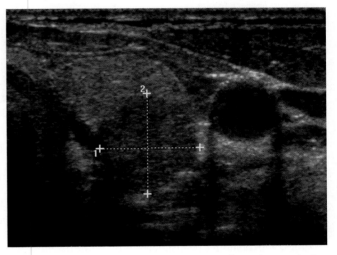

FIGURE 66-1. Ultrasound demonstrating a 3-cm, hypoechoic
left thyroid nodule.

● DIFFERENTIAL DIAGNOSIS

A nontender neck mass has a wide differential that can be
divided into three categories: neoplasms, congenital lesions,
and inflammatory masses. Neoplasms presenting as a neck
mass can be benign, such as lipomas and benign thyroid
nodules like adenomas, but in an adult, a neck mass should
be considered a malignancy until proven otherwise. Some of
the most common malignancies of the neck include thyroid
cancers, laryngeal carcinomas, and lymphomas. Congenital
masses can present at any age and include thyroglossal duct
cysts and branchial cleft cysts, which usually become apparent when they become infected. Other congenital neck lesions
include lymphangiomas, dermoid cysts, and thymic cysts.
Enlarged lymph nodes resulting from a viral or bacterial illness are the most common inflammatory masses encountered.

A comprehensive history and physical exam is an essential step to narrow the differential diagnoses. Malignancies
are more frequent in adults after their fifth decade of life
presenting as a painless, fixed and hard mass, which may be
accompanied by a clinically detectable lymph nodes, especially in medullary thyroid cancer (MTC).

● WORKUP

The patient undergoes further evaluation of her neck mass
with an ultrasound that demonstrates a 3-cm nodule in the
left lobe (Figure 66-1) and suspicious lymph nodes in the

central neck and near the left carotid artery. At this time,
a fine needle aspiration (FNA) is performed and returns as
being suspicious for MTC.

The patient undergoes laboratory testing, which demonstrates an elevated serum calcitonin of 9,091 pg/mL (normal
<5 pg/mL), an elevated carcinoembryonic antigen (CEA)
level of 320 ng/L (normal <2.5 ng/mL), and a normal calcium of 9.3 mg/dL. The patient also undergoes *RET* proto-
oncogene genetic testing, which comes back positive for a
germ-line mutation. Given this finding, the patient undergoes additional testing to evaluate for tumors associated with
multiple endocrine neoplasia (MEN)-2 syndrome. Her parathyroid hormone, plasma normetanephrine, and plasma and
urinary metanephrine levels are all normal.

Given the findings of suspicious lymph nodes on her
ultrasound as well as her highly elevated calcitonin level, the
patient undergoes a metastatic workup. Neck CT demonstrates the previously seen nodule and enlarged lymph nodes
(Figure 66-2A and B). A CT scan of her chest and abdomen
demonstrates no metastatic disease.

● DIAGNOSIS AND TREATMENT

MTC represents 3% to 10% of all thyroid cancers. Similar
to other thyroid cancers, many MTCs present as thyroid

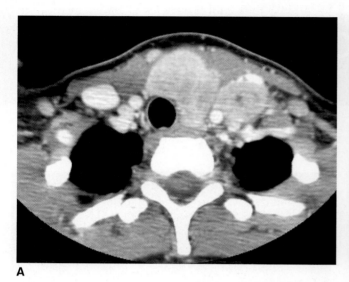

A

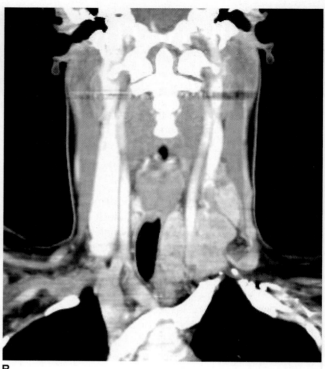

B

FIGURE 66-2. **A:** CT of the neck with a cross-sectional image demonstrating a large, left thyroid nodule and left lateral lymph nodes. **B:** Coronal views of the same CT, redemonstrating the thyroid nodule and lymph nodes surrounding the left internal jugular vein and the carotid artery.

nodules, which should be evaluated with an ultrasound and FNA biopsy (Figure 66-3).

MTCs arise from the parafollicular C cells of the thyroid, which produce calcitonin, a neuroendocrine tumor marker that is helpful in diagnosing the disease, as well as identifying recurrence. Approximately 50% of MTCs can also secrete CEA, which should also be obtained during preoperative evaluation, although it is not a good marker for early diagnosis of MTC.

The majority of MTCs occur sporadically, while about 25% of them are inherited as part of MEN2 syndromes or familial MTC (FMTC). MEN2A is the most common syndrome in which essentially all the patients develop MTC and a proportion of them may develop either or both pheochromocytoma and hyperparathyroidism. Cutaneous lichen amyloidosis and Hirschsprung are other diseases reported to be associated with MEN2A in small number of patients. FMTC is a group of hereditary MTC with germline mutations in *RET* that will not develop pheochromocytoma or hyperparathyroidism; nonetheless, many experts consider them as a variant of MEN2A. MEN2B is a more aggressive syndrome with higher rates of metastasis and is usually seen at younger ages. In addition to MTC, about half of the patients also have pheochromocytoma and marfanoid habitus, and mucosal neuromas are commonly seen.

All the patients with hereditary MTC have germ-line mutations in the *RET* proto-oncogene, while somatic mutation in *RET* is seen in 50% of sporadic MTC. *RET* mutations have been extensively studied and associated to aggressiveness and prognosis of the disease. Recent American Thyroid Association (ATA) guidelines categorize these mutations as highest risk (MEN2B with *RET* codon *M918T* mutation, ATA-HST), high risk (*RET* codon mutations *C634 and A883F*, ATA-H), and moderate risk (mutations other than the three mentioned, ATA-MOD).

The workup starts with a neck ultrasound and FNA of thyroid nodules greater than 1 centimeter (cm). The accuracy of FNA is 50% to 80% in different reports. If the FNA is suspicious or not conclusive enough, calcitonin levels should be assessed in the FNA washout fluids, and immunohistochemical (IHC) staining of the sample should be performed. Staining with calcitonin, CEA, and chromogranin and lack of thyroglobulin staining will be observed in MTC. If the patient has evidence of lymph node metastases or a calcitonin level >500 pg/mL, a metastatic workup including CT scans of the neck, chest, and three-phase contrast enhanced liver CT or liver MRI, and bone scintigraphy should be performed. PET/CT is not recommended for detection of distant metastasis in MTC.

All patients diagnosed with MTC should undergo DNA analysis to detect *RET* mutations. If a mutation is found in a presumed sporadic MTC, all the first-degree family members should undergo genetic testing as well.

Screening for hyperparathyroidism and pheochromocytoma should also be performed, as a pheochromocytoma needs to be resected prior to thyroid resection.

The mainstay of treatment for MTC remains at surgery. For patients with no evidence of lymph node and distant metastases, a total thyroidectomy and central neck (level VI)

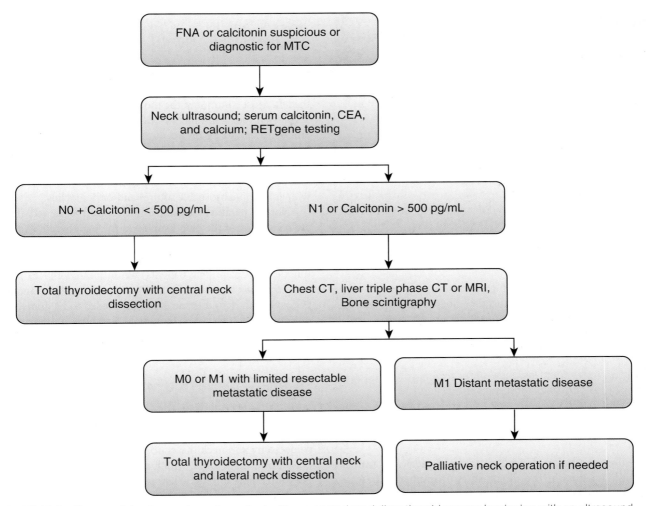

FIGURE 66-3. Chart explains the workup of a patient with suspected medullary thyroid cancer, beginning with an ultrasound and FNA, followed by measurement of calcitonin and CEA levels. Operative management is based on the extent of nodal and metastatic disease and calcitonin levels.

dissection are generally recommended. For those patients with lymph node metastases limited to the central neck compartment, a total thyroidectomy and central neck dissection are performed. Patients with suspected metastases to the lateral neck compartments should undergo a total thyroidectomy and central neck dissection, as well as a modified lateral neck (levels II, III, IV, and V) dissection. If there is involvement of ipsilateral neck with no preoperative evidence of contralateral neck involvement, the decision for contralateral neck dissection will be based on calcitonin levels. In this case, contralateral neck dissection is recommended if the calcitonin level is above 200 pg/mL.

If MTC is diagnosed after a thyroid lobectomy, completion thyroidectomy is indicated for presence of *RET* mutation, radiologic evidence of residual MTC, and postoperative elevation of serum calcitonin. If serum calcitonin is normal and there is no evidence of residual MTC, an enlarged lymph node is not an indication of a repeat surgical evaluation.

● SURGICAL APPROACH

A total thyroidectomy begins with a transverse incision made just below the cricoid cartilage, ideally in an existing neck crease (Table 66-1). In order to facilitate a modified radical neck dissection, this incision may be extended laterally or a hockey-stick incision may be made to allow for wider exposure. The total thyroidectomy should be completed in the usual manner with care taken to avoid injury to the recurrent laryngeal nerves and parathyroid glands.

Once the thyroid has been removed, attention can be turned to completing the central neck dissection. The recurrent laryngeal nerves are dissected out, and all the fatty tissue between the carotid sheaths from the hyoid bone superiorly to the brachiocephalic vessels inferiorly, including the thymus, is removed.

The lateral neck dissection is then begun by dissecting the anterior triangle, containing level II, III, and IV lymph nodes.

Table 66-1	Total Thyroidectomy with Central Neck Dissection and Modified Lateral Neck Dissection

Key Technical Steps

1. Make a transverse incision just below the cricoid cartilage and extend laterally or make a hockey-stick incision to facilitate lateral neck dissection.
2. Perform total thyroidectomy.
3. Central neck dissection is performed by dissecting out the recurrent laryngeal nerves and removing all fibroadipose tissue between the two carotid sheaths from the hyoid bone superiorly to the brachiocephalic vessels inferiorly.
4. Lymph node tissue from the anterior and posterior triangles, defined as the submandibular gland superiorly, the internal jugular vein medially, trapezius muscle laterally, and clavicle inferiorly, is removed.
5. The medial aspect of the sternocleidomastoid muscle is reapproximated to the sternothyroid muscle, followed by the platysma, and then the skin.

Potential Pitfalls

- Injury to recurrent laryngeal or superior laryngeal nerves.
- Injury to or excision of parathyroid glands.
- Injury to the brachial plexus or phrenic nerves.

The submandibular gland is retracted superiorly, and the inferior margins of the digastric and omohyoid muscles are skeletonized defining the superior aspect of dissection. The internal jugular vein is exposed, and the lateral branches are ligated or sealed, defining the medial border of dissection. The sternocleidomastoid muscle can then be retracted laterally and the tissue on its posterior surface can be dissected, with care taken to identify and preserve the spinal accessory nerve. Attention can then be turned to dissection of the posterior triangle, containing level V lymph nodes. Once the spinal accessory nerve has been identified, the posterior border of the sternocleidomastoid muscle can then be skeletonized down to the trapezius muscle, defining the lateral border of dissection. The dissection proceeds down to the clavicle, which defines the inferior border of resection. Once the fatty tissue containing the lateral neck lymph nodes has been dissected free from all adjacent structures, it can be removed en bloc.

After the lymph node tissue has been removed, if required, a drain can be placed in the lateral neck. The medial aspect of the sternocleidomastoid muscle is then reapproximated to the lateral border of the sternothyroid muscle with interrupted sutures. The platysma is reapproximated in the same manner. Finally, the skin is closed with a running subcuticular stitch.

● SPECIAL INTRAOPERATIVE CONSIDERATIONS

Due to the extent of the lymph node dissection, care should be taken to identify the thoracic duct as it enters the neck on the left. Most commonly, the thoracic duct empties into the left subclavian vein at its junction with the left internal jugular vein. Surgeons should be aware of aberrant ductal anatomy, with patients having a right thoracic duct, draining into the right subclavian vein. If the thoracic duct is inadvertently injured and a chyle leak is identified intraoperatively, it should be ligated with either nonabsorbable sutures and/or hemoclips.

Normal parathyroid glands should be all preserved. If they are resected or if the blood supply to the parathyroid glands is compromised, questionable, or cannot be preserved, the parathyroid tissue should be grafted to the sternocleidomastoid muscle. The exception is patients with MEN2A with *RET* mutations that are associated with hyperparathyroidism. In these patients, parathyroid tissue is recommended to be grafted to a muscular bed, such as brachioradialis, in which future resection would be feasible, in case hyperparathyroidism is developed.

● POSTOPERATIVE MANAGEMENT

In the immediate postoperative period, a surgeon should be aware of potential complications associated with total thyroidectomy and neck dissection. One of these complications is that of a hematoma, which could result in tracheal compression and respiratory distress. In the event of a hematoma causing tracheal compression, the incision should be opened immediately at the bedside, followed by reoperation to evaluate for the cause of bleeding.

As mentioned in the potential intraoperative pitfalls, inadvertent injury to the recurrent laryngeal does occur and if bilateral will lead to immediate respiratory distress upon extubation requiring an emergent tracheostomy. Unilateral injury of the nerve results in hoarseness and requires evaluation and treatment by an otolaryngologist.

Transient hypoparathyroidism, due to injury or removal of one or more parathyroid glands, is another complication of thyroidectomy and neck dissection, which requires short-term calcium supplementation. Rarely, this becomes permanent requiring, lifelong vitamin D and calcium supplementation.

Another complication of total thyroidectomy and neck dissection is that of a chyle leak, identified as a milky, white discharge high in triglycerides. Initially, this is managed by placing the patient on a fat-free diet, antibiotics, and application of a pressure dressing. If the chyle leak does not resolve, surgical exploration with ligation of the thoracic duct or application of a biologic sealant may be necessary.

Patients suffering from MTC will also require long-term surveillance consisting of measurements of calcitonin and CEA starting 3 months after the surgery. If the levels are not elevated, they should be rechecked every 6 months for 1 year and then annually thereafter. If the calcitonin levels is elevated but less than 150 pg/mL, an ultrasound of the neck should be performed to evaluate for recurrent local disease. Surveillance should continue every 6 months if ultrasound is negative. For calcitonin levels above 150 pg/mL, a full radiologic workup including a chest CT, triple-phase liver dedicated CT or MRI, and bone scintigraphy, in addition to a neck ultrasound should be considered.

● PROPHYLACTIC THYROIDECTOMY

Patients with a known *RET* germ-line mutation should undergo prophylactic thyroidectomy. The decision about the timing of the operation mainly depends on the risk associated with the specific mutations. Children with MEN2B and ATA-HST are at highest risk for developing aggressive MTC very early in their life. Thyroidectomy is recommended to be performed during infancy, preferably in the first few months of life. In the absence of clinically positive nodes, central neck dissection should only be performed if parathyroids are identified, which could be technically challenging at this age. Patients with ATA-H mutations should undergo surveillance from the first year of their life, and thyroidectomy is recommended at or before the age of 5 years. Serum calcitonin level dictates how soon thyroidectomy should be performed. Central node dissection should be considered for the patients with evidence of node metastasis or calcitonin levels above 40 pg/mL. Patients in the ATA-MOD category should start their annual surveillance with physical exam, ultrasound, and serum calcitonin levels at the age of 5. Thyroidectomy should be performed if serum calcitonin is elevated. Generally, it is recommended to perform prophylactic thyroidectomy in childhood or early adulthood.

Case Conclusion

The patient undergoes a successful total thyroidectomy with central and modified left lateral neck dissection. She is discharged on postoperative day 1 on thyroid hormone replacement. At 6 months, her calcitonin level is 3 pg/mL, and her CEA is 0.5 ng/mL. At her 1-year visit, her calcitonin and her CEA levels are unchanged.

TAKE HOME POINTS

- Of medullary thyroid cancers, 75% are sporadic and 25% are inherited in syndromes such as familial medullary thyroid cancer, MEN2A, and MEN2B.
- Tumors secrete calcitonin, CEA, serotonin, ACTH, and calcitonin gene-related peptide (CGRP). Calcitonin and CEA serve as diagnostic, prognostic, and guide to therapy markers.
- Tumor is of C cell origin, so radioactive iodine therapy is ineffective.
- If patients are RET mutation carriers, prophylactic total thyroidectomy is recommended based on the specific mutation and level of risk for developing MTC during childhood, with highest risk mutations requiring surgery within the first 6 months of life, high-risk mutations before age 5, and moderate risk mutations in childhood or early adulthood.
- If patients have pheochromocytoma, it is operated on first to avoid hypertensive crisis.
- Surgical treatment includes total thyroidectomy and central neck dissection; if lateral neck lymph nodes are involved, perform modified lateral neck dissection.
- Postoperative long-term surveillance includes measurement of calcitonin and CEA.

SUGGESTED READINGS

Duh Q-Y, Clark OH, Kebebew E. *Atlas of Endocrine Surgical Techniques*. Philadelphia, PA: Saunders Elsevier, 2010.

Jin LX, Moley JF. Surgery for lymph node metastases of medullary thyroid carcinoma: a review. *Cancer*. 2016;122(3):358-366.

Pinchot S, Chen H, Sippel R. Incisions and exposure of the neck for thyroidectomy and parathyroidectomy. *Oper Techniq Gen Surg*. 2008;10(2):63-76.

Roy M, Chen H, Sippel RS. Current understanding and management of medullary thyroid cancer. *Oncologist*. 2013;18(10):1093-1100.

Shaha AR. Complications of neck dissection for thyroid cancer. *Ann Surg Oncol*. 2008;15(2):397-399.

Wells SA Jr, Asa SL, Dralle H, et al. Revised American Thyroid Association guidelines for the management of medullary thyroid carcinoma. *Thyroid*. 2015;25(6):567-610.

Primary Hyperparathyroidism

67

RANDALL P. SCHERI AND JULIE ANN SOSA

Based on the previous edition chapter "Primary Hyperparathyroidism" by
Leslie S. Wu and Julie Ann Sosa

Presentation

A 29-year-old female presents to the office for evaluation of
hypercalcemia. The patient recently was treated in the emergency room for nephrolithiasis and reports a 6-month history
of fatigue, difficulty concentrating, polyuria, and polydipsia.
Her past medical history is unremarkable; she has only had
a cesarean section after a normal pregnancy and is taking
a daily multivitamin. She is adopted, and her family history is
unknown. Physical examination is unremarkable. Laboratory
values are notable for a serum calcium of 11.8 mg/dL (normal,
8.7 to 10.2), albumin 3.9 g/dL (normal, 3.5 to 4.8), phosphate 2.8 mg/dL (normal, 2.3 to 4.5), creatinine 0.8 mg/dL
(normal, 0.5 to 1.3), intact parathyroid hormone (iPTH)
180 pg/mL (normal, 14 to 72), and 25-hydroxyvitamin D
(25-OH vitamin D) 24 ng/mL (normal, 30 to 100).

● DIFFERENTIAL DIAGNOSIS

The most common cause of hypercalcemia in the outpatient
setting is primary hyperparathyroidism (HPT). Population-
based estimates reveal an overall incidence of HPT of
approximately 25 per 100,000 in the general population,
with 50,000 new cases identified annually. The incidence
of HPT is higher in Caucasian women and increases with
age. Prevalence has increased over time and is likely related
to the aging of the US population and more frequent biochemical testing. The peak incidence is in the fifth and sixth
decades of life, with a female to male ratio of 3:1. Some studies have estimated the overall prevalence of primary HPT in
the elderly at 2% to 3%, with approximately 200 cases per
100,000 population. Making the correct diagnosis requires
careful clinical evaluation coupled with biochemical testing.
After a thorough history and physical examination, laboratory measurements of serum calcium, iPTH, creatinine,
and vitamin D levels should be performed to determine if
the hypercalcemia is non–parathyroid-mediated (in which
serum iPTH levels are suppressed appropriately), or parathyroid-mediated (in which serum iPTH levels are elevated
inappropriately). Etiologies of non–parathyroid-mediated
hypercalcemia include malignancy (a parathyroid hormone-
related protein [PTHrP] level may be elevated); granulomatous disease, including sarcoidosis and tuberculosis;
hyperthyroidism; adrenal insufficiency; vitamin A or D
intoxication; thiazide diuretics; milk-alkali syndrome; and

Table 67-1	Differential Diagnosis of Hypercalcemia
Parathyroid-Mediated	**Non–Parathyroid-Mediated**
Primary HPT • Parathyroid adenoma (85%) • Parathyroid hyperplasia (15%) • Parathyroid carcinoma (<1%) Tertiary HPT Familial hypocalciuric hypercalcemia Lithium therapy	Malignancy-associated hypercalcemia • Local osteolytic hypercalcemia • Humoral hypercalcemia of malignancy (PTHrP) Granulomatous disease • Sarcoidosis, tuberculosis Endocrinopathies • Hyperthyroidism, adrenal insufficiency Drugs • Thiazides, vitamin D, calcium Immobilization

HPT, hyperparathyroidism; PTHrp, Parathyroid hormone-related protein.

prolonged immobilization leading to increased ratio of bone
resorption to bone formation. Parathyroid-mediated hypercalcemia is due to HPT, familial hypocalciuric hypercalcemia (FHH), or lithium therapy. Primary HPT generally is
caused by a benign, solitary parathyroid adenoma in 80% to
85% of patients. Approximately 5% of patients harbor two
distinct adenomas ("double adenomas"), 15% to 20% have
multigland parathyroid hyperplasia, and fewer than 1% of
patients have parathyroid carcinoma (Table 67-1).

● WORKUP

With the advent of routine serum calcium screening, the typical
presentation of primary HPT has changed from a severe, debilitating illness to an asymptomatic disease detected on routine
laboratory testing. Common manifestations of HPT include
nephrolithiasis, nephrocalcinosis, osteopenia, and osteoporosis; rarely, pancreatitis and peptic ulcer disease can occur. In
addition, there are many subtle abnormalities associated with
primary HPT, including impaired cognitive function, anxiety
and/or depression, lethargy/fatigue, myalgias and arthralgias,
constipation, polyuria, and polydipsia (Table 67-2). A medical
history should be obtained, interrogating for dietary calcium
intake, including supplements and vitamins that may cause

Table 67-2	Symptoms and Associated Conditions in Patients with Primary Hyperparathyroidism

Symptoms

Impaired cognitive function/memory
Anxiety, depression
Fatigue, depression, exhaustion
Myalgias, weakness
Arthralgias
Constipation
Polyurea, polydipsia, nocturia
Loss of appetite, nausea
Gastroesophageal reflux disease (GERD)

Associated Conditions

Fragility fracture
Nephrolithiasis
Peptic ulcer disease
Pancreatitis
Osteoporosis

hypercalcemia. If the patient is taking thiazide diuretics, they should be stopped and switched to another antihypertensive medication prior to workup for HPT.

The diagnosis of primary HPT typically is made by biochemical evidence of an elevated serum calcium concentration, usually in conjunction with an elevated or inappropriately high normal serum iPTH. Since 50% of calcium is albumin-bound, a calcium level corrected for the patient's albumin is required for diagnosis using the formula: corrected calcium = 0.8 (4.0–patient's albumin) + total calcium. Obtaining the biologically active ionized calcium concentration may be helpful in some patients with borderline hypercalcemia where the diagnosis of HPT is not clear. The clinical entity termed "normocalcemic primary HPT" recently has emerged. It appears to be an early form of primary HPT in which patients have serum calcium levels in the high-normal range associated with an elevated serum iPTH level and bone loss. When these patients are symptomatic, surgical intervention is appropriate. For asymptomatic patients, surgical intervention is recommended for those with nephrocalcinosis, impaired renal

function, osteoporosis, or worsening of bone density during observation. Approximately half of patients with primary HPT have hypophosphatemia. Because of the effect of PTH on bicarbonate excretion in the kidney, patients with primary HPT often have a hyperchloremic metabolic acidosis. To distinguish patients with FHH (who should not have surgery) from those with primary HPT, a 24-hour urinary calcium collection with fractional extraction of calcium should be performed; this measurement is low (<100 mg per specimen [normal 50 to 300 mg], fractional excretion calcium <0.01) in the setting of FHH; and normal or elevated with a fraction excretion >0.02 in primary HPT. Vitamin D insufficiency may lead to impaired urinary calcium excretion, so in patients with a deficient vitamin D level, a 24-hour urine calcium collection should be repeated after vitamin D repletion to exclude FHH. A 24-hour urine collection with biochemical stone profile should be obtained to determine if there is an increased risk of calcium-based stone formation. Renal imaging by x-ray, ultrasound, or computed tomography (CT) scan also should be obtained to evaluate for asymptomatic nephrolithiasis. Approximately 10% to 40% of primary HPT patients have elevated levels of alkaline phosphatase, which indicates some degree of increased bone turnover. Although osteitis fibrosis cystica, the classic form of parathyroid bone disease, is rarely seen today, even patients with mild disease can have biochemical or histologic evidence of bone involvement. Dual-energy x-ray absorption (DEXA) scanning of the lumbar spine, hip, and the distal 1/3 of the radius (single best metric) has become the standard method for assessing bone density to diagnose osteoporosis in the setting of primary HPT.

The etiology of HPT may be sporadic or familial. The vast majority of HPT is sporadic, of which there is a small subset of acquired disease associated with environmental exposures. Radiation exposure either through therapeutic external beam radiation or excessive environmental exposure (nuclear accident) is a risk factor for HPT; the incidence of multigland disease is similar to patients with sporadic HPT. Lithium therapy is another risk factor for HPT and occurs in approximately 15% of patients exposed to long-term lithium therapy (>10 years); multigland disease is more common than for patients with sporadic HPT. Approximately 3% to 5% of all patients will have familial HPT (Table 67-3). Patients should be evaluated for a family history suggestive of a familial syndrome, including multiple

| Table 67-3 | Hereditary Hyperparathyroidism Syndromes, Presentation of Hyperparathyroidism and Associated Features |

Disorder	Responsible Gene	HPT	Associated Tumors
MEN1	MEN1	High penetrance, multigland	Pituitary, PNET
MEN2a	RET	Low penetrance, multigland, adenoma	MTC, pheochromocytoma
HPT-JT	CDC73	Cystic tumor, parathyroid carcinoma	Jaw tumors, renal lesions
FIHPT	MEN1/CDC73	Multigland, adenoma	
FHH	CASR	Mildly hyperplastic	

MEN, multiple endocrine neoplasia; HPT-JT, hyperparathyroidism-jaw tumor syndrome; FIHPT, familial isolated primary hyperparathyroidism; FHH, familial hypocalciuric hypercalcemia; HPT, hyperparathyroidism; PNET, pancreatic neuroendocrine tumor; MTC, medullary thyroid cancer.

endocrine neoplasia type 1 (MEN1), multiple endocrine neo-plasia type 2a (MEN2a), familial isolated primary HPT, hyper-parathyroidism-jaw tumor syndrome (HPT-JT), and FHH. These patients typically present by the third or fourth decade of life. In a recent study by Starker et al., 23.5% of all patients <45 years who underwent parathyroidectomy for primary HPT referred to a tertiary medical center had a deleterious muta-tion for familial HPT. Even among patients without a suspi-cious family history, there was a 9.3% incidence of deleterious mutations. Guidelines have recommended referral for genetic counseling and testing for patients <40 years or who have pre-operative suspicion for a hereditary syndrome. The presence of a hereditary syndrome is predictive of the pattern of disease and has important implications for surgical management.

Imaging for the purpose of localization should be employed only after establishing the biochemical diagnosis of primary HPT. Imaging studies can be sorted into non-invasive and invasive techniques. Noninvasive modalities include ultrasound; sestamibi scanning, which should be combined with single photon emission computed tomog-raphy (SPECT) imaging; CT scans; and magnetic reso-nance imaging (MRI). The noninvasive localization study of choice is dependent largely on the availability and qual-ity of imaging modalities at each institution. All patients should have an ultrasound for localization (Figure 67-1) and to evaluate for concomitant thyroid pathology. Ultrasound is operator-dependent and performs best when done by an experienced ultrasonographer, with localization rates of 80% in many studies. Ultrasound is inexpensive and read-ily available but is limited by the patient's body habitus, the presence of multiple thyroid nodules, and the concomitant presence of a goiter; it is also unable to evaluate ectopic loca-tions, such as the retropharyngeal space and mediastinum. The ability of ultrasound to detect multigland disease is

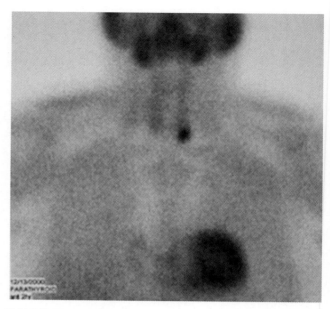

FIGURE 67-2. Sestamibi SPECT of a left inferior parathyroid adenoma.

poor. Technetium (^{99m}Tc)-sestamibi scan with SPECT, which results in a three-dimensional reconstruction, can localize an enlarged parathyroid gland in 80% of cases on average, is readily available in most hospitals and can identify ectopic parathyroid adenomas (Figure 67-2). Thyroid nodules can impact the accuracy of sestamibi scans. Thyroid disease, including thyroiditis, thyroid cancer, hürthle cell adenomas, follicular adenomas, and lymph node metastases frequently retain sestamibi and can result in false-positive studies. At the same time, early washout from pathologic parathyroid tissue may result in false-negative studies. Similar to ultra-sound, sestamibi scanning has limited success identifying multigland disease. Four-dimensional CT (4D CT), which is a high resolution multiphase contrast CT with the addi-tional "dimension" of changes in contrast perfusion over time, affords excellent localization (Figure 67-3), with a

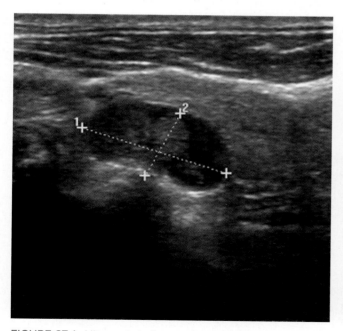

FIGURE 67-1. Ultrasound of a parathyroid adenoma with hypoechoic appearance.

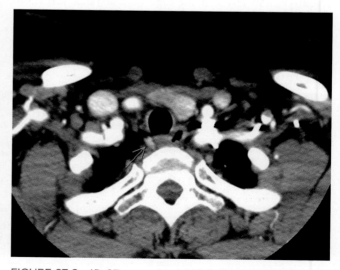

FIGURE 67-3. 4D CT scan of a right inferior parathyroid adenoma in the tracheoesophageal groove (*arrow*).

sensitivity approaching 90% for localization of pathologic parathyroid glands. 4D CT also can assess ectopic locations and identifies 45% of patients with multigland disease. The disadvantages of 4D CT are that the patient is exposed to ionizing radiation, and intravenous contrast is required, so patients with impaired renal function should not undergo 4D-CT. MRI has low sensitivity for identifying abnormal parathyroid glands, so it generally is reserved for pregnant patients with contraindications to ionizing radiation and for patients who do not localize using standard imaging modalities in remedial cases. Invasive techniques usually are reserved for reoperative cases and include angiography and venous sampling for iPTH gradients. Recently, the rapid iPTH assay has been used in the ultrasound and angiography suites, as well as the operating room. It yields real-time feedback and has become invaluable in the development of minimally invasive surgical techniques.

● DIAGNOSIS AND TREATMENT

Parathyroidectomy is the only effective long-term treatment for primary HPT. There is universal agreement that patients with clear symptoms and signs associated with primary HPT should undergo parathyroid surgery. However, controversy still exists about the management of patients with "asymptomatic" disease. In 2013, the Fourth International Workshop on HPT convened and published updated guidelines for the management of asymptomatic HPT (Table 67-4). Guidelines also were created for

Table 67-4	Surgical Indications in Patients with Primary Hyperparathyroidism

All symptomatic patients, including those with significant bone, renal, gastrointestinal, or neuromuscular symptoms typical of primary HPT

In otherwise asymptomatic patients:

- Elevation of serum calcium by ≥1 mg/dL above the normal range
- Decreased creatinine clearance (reduced to <60 mL/min)
- Significant reduction in bone density of > 2.5 standard deviations below peak bone mass at any measured site (i.e., T-score <−2.5)
- Vertebral fracture by x-ray, CT, or MRI
- 24-hour urine >400 mg per day and increased stone risk by stone risk analysis
- Presence of nephrolithiasis or nephrocalcinosis by x-ray, ultrasound, or CT
- Age <50 y
- Consistent follow-up is not possible or is undesirable because of coexisting medical conditions

CT, computed tomography; MRI, magnetic resonance imaging.

the management of patients with asymptomatic primary HPT who do not undergo surgery, including annual serum calcium and creatinine measurements, annual bone density measurements, and if renal stones are suspected, 24-hour biochemical stone profile, renal imaging by x-ray, ultrasound, or CT. In 2016, the American Association of Endocrine Surgeons published guidelines for the safe and effective operative management of primary HPT. It has been suggested that the NIH criteria for parathyroidectomy in asymptomatic patients are too limited and that all patients with primary HPT should be referred for consideration of surgical therapy.

There is no long-term effective pharmacologic treatment for primary HPT. There are several pharmacologic agents that can limit further bone loss by reducing the activation of new remodeling units in the skeleton. Estrogen replacement, bisphosphonates, and more recently, calcimimetics (cinacalcet) have been used to treat primary HPT in patients with complex comorbid medical conditions who either are unwilling or considered unfit for surgery. In addition, glucocorticoids and calcimimetics can be employed during refractory hypercalcemia of metastatic parathyroid carcinoma. For acute hypercalcemic crises (calcium typically >14 mg/dL) manifested by multiorgan dysfunction, including neurologic (mental status changes, lethargy, coma), renal (dehydration, acute kidney injury), or gastrointestinal symptoms (anorexia, nausea/vomiting, abdominal pain), patients should initially be managed with intravenous fluid hydration and pharmacologic management with calcium-lowering agents. Once the patient is adequately hydrated and calcium levels are within a more acceptable range (<13 mg/dL), parathyroidectomy should be performed prior to hospital discharge. It should be kept in mind that none of these pharmacologic therapies are definitive, and with adequate preoperative parathyroid localization, high-volume parathyroid surgeons may employ minimally invasive techniques with excellent outcomes.

Parathyroidectomy has a high rate of success (>95%), with few complications when performed by experienced parathyroid surgeons. Complications associated with parathyroidectomy include recurrent laryngeal nerve injury, persistent hypercalcemia/HPT, transient or persistent hypocalcemia, and postoperative hemorrhage. Despite this, the specific operative approach has continued to evolve through the influence of a number of synergistic factors, including improvements in preoperative localization studies and rapid intraoperative iPTH measurement. The net result has influenced patient selection, such that the majority of parathyroid explorations are very well tolerated. However, a small fraction of these explorations remain challenging and especially those with atypical gland location or previously operated fields. Therefore, any surgeon performing parathyroidectomy must be facile with standard four-gland parathyroid exploration. In fact, experienced parathyroid surgeons today achieve cure rates of around 98% with both minimally invasive and conventional techniques.

● SURGICAL APPROACH

The conventional technique for parathyroid exploration requires bilateral cervical access and four-gland exploration. This operation is usually performed under general anesthesia, although it can be performed under bilateral regional superficial cervical block with sedation. The goal is to identify all normal and abnormal parathyroid glands, thus distinguishing single-gland from multigland disease. Patients who have a single parathyroid adenoma undergo curative resection once the gland is removed. For a double adenoma, both abnormal glands should be removed, with preservation of the remaining normal glands. In the instance of four-gland hyperplasia, a subtotal parathyroidectomy (leaving a normal-sized remnant of one well-vascularized parathyroid gland in situ), or total cervical parathyroidectomy with immediate heterotopic autotransplantation of parathyroid tissue, typically into the brachioradialis muscle in the non-dominant forearm, is required (Table 67-5).

The conventional approach has been largely replaced with minimally invasive parathyroidectomy, which is dependent on high-quality preoperative imaging, usually in the form of ultrasound, sestamibi scan, or 4D CT, to identify the culprit parathyroid gland(s) in conjunction with intraoperative iPTH monitoring. A focused exploration and excision of the parathyroid gland(s) identified on preoperative imaging is performed. A decrease of intraoperative PTH from a baseline established prior to incision by over 50% and into the normal range following excision indicates sufficient removal of all hyperfunctioning parathyroid tissue. When the PTH value fails to drop by 50%, this suggests that either the hyperfunctioning gland has not been removed or the patient has additional, multigland disease. In this situation, the surgery potentially should be converted to a bilateral neck exploration with identification of the remaining parathyroid glands and removal of an adenoma or subtotal parathyroidectomy if four-gland hyperplasia is present. This technique is appropriate even for patients who have had multiple previous explorations, as long as the preoperative imaging is adequate. A bilateral neck exploration should be performed if preoperative imaging does not localize an abnormal parathyroid gland or the patient has a hereditary syndrome with suspected multigland disease. When performed by an experienced parathyroid surgeon well versed in minimally invasive techniques, this surgical procedure can be performed on an outpatient basis and can avoid the potentially increased risks associated with bilateral neck exploration and general anesthesia.

Regardless of the chosen technique of parathyroidectomy, the key steps remain constant. Parathyroidectomy can be performed under general anesthesia or under anterior superficial cervical block with mild sedation. Proper positioning of the patient on the operating table is of paramount importance. The patient should be placed in a semi-Fowler's position, with the patient's neck extended dorsally to provide optimal access to the anterior neck. The arms of the patient should lie alongside the body to allow the surgeon and assistant to stand on both sides of the neck. All appropriate pressure points should be padded for protection. A symmetric Kocher incision is made, preferentially in a natural skin crease, approximately 3 to 4 cm cranial to the suprasternal notch. Flaps are developed in the subplatysmal plane, and dissected upward to the level of the thyroid cartilage and inferiorly to the suprasternal notch. Early identification of the recurrent laryngeal nerve expedites the exploration and is invaluable in protecting the nerve. Throughout the procedure, the operative field should be kept as bloodless as possible to prevent discoloring the parathyroid glands, which may impede their identification.

In patients with a solitary enlarged parathyroid gland, the vascular stalk of the tumor should be ligated, and the tumor removed. During dissection of the parathyroid tumor, the capsule of the gland should not be opened to prevent seeding of parathyroid tissue, which can cause recurrent HPT due to parathyromatosis. In the case of double adenomas, both abnormal glands should be removed with preservation of the remaining normal glands. When four-gland hyperplasia is present, a subtotal parathyroidectomy should be performed, leaving a well-vascularized remnant of approximately 30 mg in situ, which corresponds to the dimensions of a normal gland. An alternative to subtotal parathyroidectomy is total parathyroidectomy with immediate heterotopic autotransplantation of parathyroid tissue into the brachioradialis muscle of the nondominant forearm. This alternative

---

Table 67-5   Parathyroidectomy

Key Technical Steps

1. Anesthesia: general endotracheal anesthesia or anterior cervical nerve block
2. Positioning: semi-Fowler's position with neck in extension
3. Kocher incision and development of subplatysmal flaps
4. Early identification of recurrent laryngeal nerve
5. Identification of abnormal parathyroid gland(s); careful excision without breaching parathyroid capsule
6. Intraoperative rapid iPTH monitoring if available, and meeting the Miami criteria (iPTH normalization and 50% reduction in value.)
7. Meticulous hemostasis within operative field
8. Neck incision closure
9. Overnight hospital observation or outpatient discharge to home

Potential Pitfalls

- Injury to the recurrent laryngeal nerve
- Injury to normal parathyroid glands
- Inability to localize or identify abnormal parathyroid gland
- Not meeting the Miami criteria

procedure often is combined with cryopreservation of some parathyroid tissue. In MEN1 patients, the thymus should be removed bilaterally by a transcervical approach, as supernumerary parathyroids are located in the thymus in 3% to 5% of all patients, and these patients may develop thymic carcinoid tumors.

After completion of the parathyroidectomy, the operative field is checked thoroughly to achieve meticulous hemostasis. The raphe between the strap muscles and the platysma are reapproximated with absorbable suture. The skin is closed with optimal cosmesis.

● SPECIAL INTRAOPERATIVE CONSIDERATIONS

Parathyroid carcinoma is a rare cause of primary HPT, accounting for <1% of cases. Parathyroid carcinoma should be suspected in patients who demonstrate a rapid and sustained rise in both their serum calcium and iPTH levels, which can reach very high levels. A palpable neck mass sometimes may be appreciated, whereas a parathyroid adenoma is rarely, if ever, palpable on physical examination. In addition, sestamibi scan typically demonstrates a hyperintense focus that correlates with the lesion. If parathyroid carcinoma is suspected preoperatively or is found incidentally at the time of operation, en bloc resection with the ipsilateral thyroid lobe and any tissue invaded by the tumor is performed in order to remove the entire tumor with negative margins. Although these tumors are slow-growing, they have a high propensity to recur locally, and recurrent disease is difficult to eradicate. Patients with recurrent and metastatic disease often suffer from severe, debilitating hypercalcemia, control of which may involve palliative surgical resection and the use of drugs, including bisphosphonates and calcimimetics, to lower the serum calcium level. Chemotherapy and radiation therapy rarely are effective.

If an enlarged parathyroid gland cannot be identified during neck exploration for parathyroidectomy, it is of great importance to identify the normal parathyroid glands, because a parathyroid missed at its normal location can help the surgeon predict the site of the migrated enlarged parathyroid. One must identify correctly whether a superior or inferior gland is missing. In the circumstance in which three normal parathyroid glands have been identified but a superior gland is missing, the retroesophageal space should be explored, and the carotid sheath opened from the level of the carotid bifurcation to the base of the neck. In the situation in which three normal parathyroids have been identified but an inferior gland cannot be identified, the thymus on the side of the missing gland should be exposed. The retrosternal thymus can be mobilized by gentle traction on the thyrothymic ligament, and a transcervical thymectomy can be performed. If the missing inferior gland is not contained within the mediastinal portion of the thymus, an intrathyroidal parathyroid tumor should be considered. In the circumstance in which four normal parathyroid glands have been visualized but increased levels of intact PTH exclude another cause of hypercalcemia, one must consider a hypersecreting supernumerary parathyroid gland, most commonly located within the thymus. Bilateral thymectomy is indicated.

If the abnormal parathyroid tumor cannot be identified at the time of neck exploration and the patient has persistent HPT, additional imaging techniques may be needed to localize the missing gland. These modalities include thorough neck ultrasonography with potential fine needle aspiration identification of parathyroid tissue with iPTH washout, neck and chest 4D CT or MRI studies, sestamibi scans, or selective jugular venous sampling for iPTH differential gradient measurement. The operative note and pathology report from the patient's initial exploration should be reviewed, and the patient should undergo laryngoscopy prior to remedial exploration to assure the integrity of the recurrent laryngeal nerves. Most missed glands (~40%) are located in eutopic positions. The retroesophageal space is the most frequent ectopic location of missing glands (~25%); the thyroid (~10%) and the mediastinal thymus (~13%) also are common locations for missed adenomas. Remedial parathyroidectomy is associated with increased risks of hypoparathyroidism and recurrent laryngeal nerve injury and should be performed by experienced parathyroid surgeons.

● POSTOPERATIVE MANAGEMENT

Normocalcemia generally is restored within the first 24 hours after a successful parathyroidectomy, and this may be accompanied by mild paresthesias circumorally and/or in the extremities. Symptoms may occur while the serum calcium level is within the normal range, reflecting the rapidity of change; however, this is usually transient and does not require treatment. Symptomatic hypocalcemia is more common in the elderly, in those with more severe preoperative primary HPT, or in patients with severe bone disease, often evidenced by markedly elevated preoperative blood alkaline phosphatase levels and subsequent "bone hunger." Restoration of normocalcemia can be achieved with calcitriol in combination with supplemental calcium. It is sufficient to maintain the serum calcium within the lower part of the reference range in order to control symptoms. A serum calcium should be obtained 6 months after surgery to demonstrate biochemical cure.

The rationale for parathyroidectomy is supported by evidence that in about 80% of patients, the clinical manifestations of primary HPT improve after successful parathyroidectomy. Thus, fatigue, weakness, polydipsia, polyuria, bone and joint pain, constipation, nausea, and depression regress in most patients. This is also true for associated conditions—renal stones usually stop forming, osteoporosis stabilizes or improves, pancreatitis becomes less likely, and peptic ulcer disease often resolves. In most patients, fracture risk and weakness also improve. In addition, neurocognitive impairments, confusion, spatial learning deficits, and depression have been shown to improve after successful operative intervention.

Case Conclusion

The patient had a 24-hour urinary calcium of 450 mg, and bone density was normal on DEXA. The patient was referred for genetic counseling and underwent genetic testing for MEN1, MEN2a, and HPT-JT, which were all negative for a deleterious mutation. She underwent cervical ultrasound and 4D CT scan, which revealed a normal thyroid gland and a right inferior parathyroid adenoma candidate. She underwent a minimally invasive parathyroidectomy with excision of a right inferior parathyroid adenoma. Intraoperative rapid iPTH measurement documented adequate resection, with a decline from her baseline of 220 to 35 pg/mL at 10 minutes postresection. The patient was discharged home the same day and returned 1 week later with a normal serum calcium level of 9.2 mg/dL. At 6 months postoperatively, she remained eucalcemic and did not have any further episodes of nephrolithiasis.

TAKE HOME POINTS

- In the outpatient setting, primary hyperparathyroidism is the most common reason for hypercalcemia.
- Imaging modalities to localize hyperfunctioning abnormal parathyroid glands should be undertaken only after the diagnosis of primary hyperparathyroidism has been confirmed biochemically.
- An understanding of the embryology of the parathyroid glands and the ability to distinguish between a normal and an abnormal parathyroid gland are essential for successful parathyroid surgery. A systematic approach knowing the routine and unusual locations for parathyroid glands results in successful parathyroidectomy in more than 95% of patients with primary hyperparathyroidism.
- Permanent hypoparathyroidism, injury to the recurrent laryngeal nerves, and postoperative bleeding (with possible airway compromise) are some of the more serious complications that occur after parathyroidectomy.

SUGGESTED READINGS

Adami S, Marcocci C, Gatti D. Epidemiology of primary hyperparathyroidism in Europe. *J Bone Miner Res.* 2002;17(S2):N18-N23.

Akerstrom G, Rudberg C, Grimelius L, et al. Causes of failed primary exploration and technical aspects of re-operation in primary hyperparathyroidism. *World J Surg.* 1992;16:562-568.

Bilezekian J, Brandi M, Eastell R, et al. Guidelines for the management of asymptomatic primary hyperparathyroidism: summary statement from the Fourth International Workshop. *J Clin Endocrinol Metab.* 2014;99(10):3561-3569.

Buerba R, Roman SA, Sosa JA. Thyroidectomy and parathyroidectomy in patients with high body mass index are safe overall: analysis of 26,864 patients. *Surgery.* 2011; 150(5): 950-958.

Carling T, Udelsman R. Parathyroid surgery in familial hyperparathyroid disorders. *J Intern Med.* 2005;257:27-37.

Irvin GL, Prudhomme Dl, Deriso GT, et al. A new approach to parathyroidectomy. *Ann Surg.* 1994;219:574-579.

Lo Gerfo P. Bilateral neck exploration for parathyroidectomy under local anesthesia: a viable technique for patients with coexisting thyroid disease with or without sestamibi scanning. *Surgery.* 1999;126:1011–1014.

Rodgers SE, Hunter GJ, Hamberg LM, et al. Improved preoperative planning for directed parathyroidectomy with 4-dimensional computed tomography. *Surgery.* 2006;140:932-941.

Rodgers SE, Perrier ND. Parathyroid carcinoma. *Curr Opin Oncol.* 2006;18:16-22.

Roman SA, Sosa JA, Pietrzak RH, et al. The effects of serum calcium and parathyroid hormone changes on psychological and cognitive function in patients undergoing parathyroidectomy for primary hyperparathyroidism. *Ann Surg.* 2011;253(1):131-137.

Solorzano CC, Carneiro-Pla DM, Irvin Gl. Surgeon-performed ultrasonography as the initial and only localizing study in sporadic primary hyperparathyroidism. *J Am Coll Surg.* 2006;202:18-24.

Starker LF, Akerstrom T, Long WD et al. Frequent germ-line mutations of the MEN1, CASR and HRPT2/CDC73 genes in young patients with clinically non-familial hyperparathyroidism. *Horm Cancer.* 2012;3:44-51.

Udelsman R, Aruny JE, Donovan PI, et al. Rapid parathyroid hormone analysis during venous localization. *Ann Surg.* 2003;237:714-721.

Udelsman R, Lin Z, Donovan P. The superiority of minimally invasive parathyroidectomy based on 1,650 consecutive patients with primary hyperparathyroidism. *Ann Surg.* 2011;253(3):585-591.

Wilhelm S, Wang T, Ruan D, et al. The American Association of Endocrine Surgeons Guidelines for Definitive Management of Primary Hyperparathyroidism. *JAMA Surg.* 2016 151(10): 959-968.

Persistent and Recurrent Primary Hyperparathyroidism

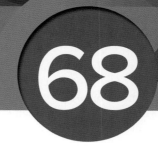

68

DAVID T. HUGHES

Based on the previous edition chapter "Persistent Hyperparathyroidism" by James T. Broome

Presentation

A 53-year-old female is referred for persistent hypercalcemia after having parathyroid surgery 3 months ago. She initially presented to her primary care physician for a routine health maintenance exam when she was noted to have an elevated serum calcium of 10.7 mg/dL (normal 8.5 to 10.2 mg/dL). Further laboratory studies demonstrated an elevated parathyroid hormone (PTH) level of 113 pg/mL (normal 12 to 75 pg/mL), a low phosphorus level of 2.6 mg/dL (normal 2.7 to 4.6 mg/dL), and normal kidney function with an estimated glomerular filtration rate of 78 mL/min (normal >59 mL/min). This was consistent with biochemical evidence of primary hyperparathyroidism.

On interview with her PCP, she did complain of several neuropsychiatric symptoms related to primary hyperparathyroidism including mood depression, memory difficulties, and fatigue. She also reported symptoms of nocturia and bone pain in the bilateral thighs. She had no history of nephrolithiasis but did have a recent DEXA bone density scan which demonstrated osteopenia in the forearm with a T-score of −1.2 (normal > −1.0). Her primary care physician diagnosed her with symptomatic primary hyperparathyroidism, and she was referred to surgery.

During her initial presurgical workup, she underwent sestamibi parathyroid scanning with planar imaging only which was nonlocalizing for a parathyroid abnormality. She did not have a cervical ultrasound prior to surgery. She underwent parathyroidectomy with planned bilateral parathyroid exploration. At the time of surgery, no definitive parathyroid abnormality was identified despite an extensive dissection and eventual left thyroid lobectomy. Intraoperative PTH (IOPTH) levels prior to exploration were 137 pg/mL and at the conclusion of surgery remain elevated at 147 pg/mL. The operating surgeon terminated the procedure suspecting persistent primary hyperparathyroidism due to failure to locate an ectopic abnormal parathyroid gland.

Postoperatively she had elevation of both serum calcium to 11.1 mg/dL and PTH level to 132 pg/mL. She was subsequently referred for persistent primary hyperparathyroidism for consideration of reoperative parathyroidectomy.

● DIFFERENTIAL DIAGNOSIS

Primary hyperparathyroidism is the most common etiology of elevated calcium levels with a prevalence of 2% to 3% in the general population. Primary hyperparathyroidism is caused by a single parathyroid adenoma in 80% to 85% of cases with the remainder of patients having multigland hyperplasia or much less commonly, double adenomas. Other causes of hypercalcemia include malignancy, hypervitaminosis D, granulomatous diseases such as sarcoidosis, iatrogenic oversupplementation of calcium, calcium sparing diuretics, and others. These other causes are typically associated with appropriately low levels of PTH.

Additional etiologies of hypercalcemia in the setting of elevated or inappropriately normal PTH levels include secondary hyperparathyroidism, tertiary hyperparathyroidism, and familial hypocalciuric hypercalcemia (FHH). FHH is caused by an inactivating mutation in the calcium-sensing receptor gene which then leads to decreased function of the receptor and subsequent hypercalcemia and hypocalciuria. FHH has an autosomal dominate inheritance pattern, and patients often have several family members with hypercalcemia, some of which may have had persistent hypercalemia after parathyroid surgery. The diagnosis of FHH can be confirmed with very–low-24-hour urine calcium levels and with mutational analysis for the calcium-sensing receptor mutation. Patients with FHH are generally not candidates for parathyroidectomy.

Confounding factors in patients with primary hyperparathyroidism include the use of medications and the presence of genetic syndromes. Treatment of bipolar disorder with long-term use of lithium has been associated with the development of primary hyperparathyroidism and is commonly associated with multigland disease. Patients taking hydrochlorothiazide may also be predisposed to the development of hypercalcemia and consideration of discontinuation of this mediation with retesting may be warranted if the diagnosis is unclear. Multiple Endocrine Neoplasia Type 1 and Type 2A are associated with primary hyperparathyroidism, and these patients commonly have multigland disease.

● WORKUP

The patient was evaluated in outpatient endocrine surgery clinic for persistent primary hyperparathyroidism. The diagnosis of primary hyperparathyroidism was confirmed with repeat labs which demonstrated an elevated serum calcium of 11.5 mg/dL, an elevated PTH of 145 pg/mL, a low 25-hydroxy vitamin D of 23 ng/mL (normal 25 to 100 ng/mL), a normal serum creatinine of 1.01 mg/dL, a GFR of >60 mL/min, and an elevated 24-hour urine calcium of 325 mg/24 hours (normal 100 to 300 mg/24 hours). The patient confirmed she was not taking cofounding medications and had no family history of hypercalcemia or primary hyperparathyroidism. Physical exam noted a well-healed lower neck incision without palpable nodules or lymphadenopathy. The patient's voice appeared normal, and flexible laryngoscopy demonstrated normal abduction and adduction of the bilateral vocal cords indicative of normal recurrent and superior laryngeal nerve function. Given her symptoms and degree of calcium elevation, reoperative parathyroidectomy was recommended.

Most cases of persistent primary hyperparathyroidism are due to the presence of enlarged parathyroid glands in the normal anatomic position. Therefore, the most common reason for persistent primary hyperparathyroidism after parathyroidectomy is the inability of the surgeon to fully visualize these areas at the time of initial surgery. Review of the operative report and the associated surgical pathology report is very beneficial in determining what locations were explored and which parathyroid glands were definitively identified. Tissue which is biopsied or excised can be confirmed to be parathyroid tissue on histology by reviewing the surgical pathology report. In some cases, removal of either diseased or normal parathyroid glands at the initial operation may mean that the persistent hyperfunctional parathyroid is the only parathyroid gland remaining. In this scenario, removal of the patient's last parathyroid may lead to permanent hypoparathyroidism. It is important to counsel the patient of this possibility and to consider reimplantation of a portion of the excised parathyroid tissue at the time of reoperative parathyroidectomy. A smaller number of patients will have an ectopic parathyroid adenoma as the cause of persistent hyperparathyroidism. Common locations of ectopic glands include inferior parathyroid glands in the thymus in the superior mediastinum, superior parathyroid glands in the paraesophageal space which have descended into the posterior mediastinum, and undescended superior or inferior parathyroid glands high in the neck or within the carotid sheath.

Review of the operative record and surgical pathology results showed that the surgeon visually identified the right superior and right inferior parathyroid glands in the normal anatomic position. The right inferior parathyroid gland was biopsied and confirmed as parathyroid tissue. The right superior parathyroid gland was not biopsied. The left superior and inferior parathyroid glands were not visually

or pathologically identified. The surgeon explored of the left central neck including the paraesophageal space, the left carotid sheath and low in the left central neck. He removed what was thought to be the left thymic horn; however, this was noted to be fibroadipose tissue on the surgical pathology report. Due to inability to identify the left parathyroid glands, there was concern for an intrathyroidal parathyroid gland and a left thyroid lobectomy was performed; however, no parathyroid tissue was noted in the thyroid on the pathology report. Despite these maneuvers, the IOPTH levels continued to be elevated at 147 pg/mL. PTH levels were drawn from both the left and right internal jugular veins and were similar: left IJ 166 pg/mL, right IJ 147 pg/mL; therefore, the residual gland could not be determined as to sidedness. The surgical pathology reported normal parathyroid tissue in the right inferior parathyroid biopsy, several biopsies from the left central neck that were fibroadipose tissue, and a left thyroid lobe with normal thyroid tissue without intrathyroidal parathyroid tissue.

Review of the operative and pathologic reports from the initial parathyroid exploration may help elucidate the location of the residual parathyroid adenoma which can help guide the next steps in workup. For this patient, the left-sided parathyroid glands were not identified; therefore, additional attention was paid to the left neck and mediastinum. The next step in workup was imaging in an attempt to localize the missing parathyroid adenoma.

● DIAGNOSIS AND TREATMENT

Image localization of the suspected missing parathyroid adenoma provides the best chance for successful reoperative parathyroidectomy for persistent primary hyperparathyroidism. Ideally, having two studies that are concordant in the location of the suspected parathyroid gland should be considered prior to proceeding with surgical reexploration. Blind reexploration for persistent primary hyperparathyroidism should be avoided as this is associated with high rates of operative failure. Available imaging studies for parathyroid localization include cervical ultrasound, parathyroid sestamibi scan with or without SPECT, 4D-CT scan, MRI, and selective venous sampling. In experienced hands, cervical ultrasound has sensitivity rates and accuracy rates of around 80% in the initial evaluation of primary hyperparathyroidism and therefore can be a useful imaging modality in persistent primary hyperparathyroidism. Areas to concentrate the ultrasound exam include the deep paraesophageal space, the lower central neck with the neck in the fully extended position, and high in the neck along the carotid arteries and internal jugular veins. Sestamibi parathyroid scans can also be useful if not previously obtained during the initial evaluation of the patient and also have sensitivity rates and accuracy rates similar to ultrasound. Sestamibi scans may be beneficial in visualizing the mediastinum and are especially helpful in localization of ectopic parathyroid glands (Figure 68-1).

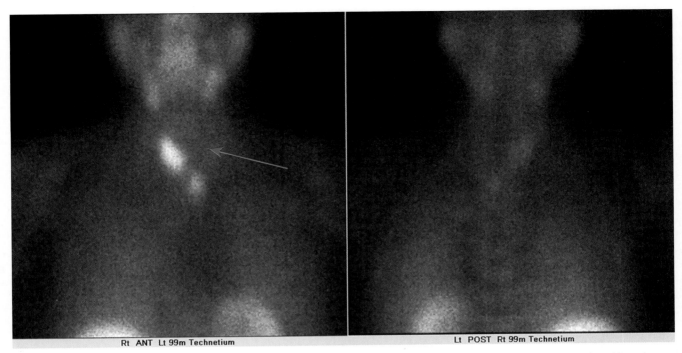

FIGURE 68-1. Sestamibi parathyroid scan demonstrating a left inferior parathyroid adenoma after previous parathyroid exploration with left thyroidectomy.

4D-CT scanning is IV contrast enhanced CT with a "4th dimension" of time. This refers to the timed arterial phases of the scan, which are obtained after IV contrast administration. Parathyroid adenomas will typically enhance on 4D-CT in the early arterial phase and have delayed washout of contrast on late arterial phase (Figure 68-2). MRI has recently been described as another useful modality for parathyroid localization for reoperative parathyroidectomy with sensitivity rates and accuracy rates of around 80%. Selective venous

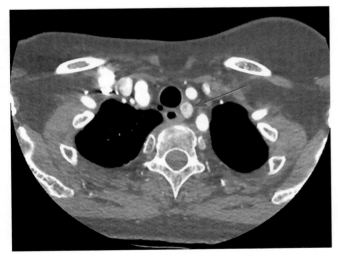

FIGURE 68-2. A 4D-CT axial imaging showing a left inferior parathryhoid adenoma (same patient as in Figure 68-1) in the left paraesophageal space, which enhances in the early arterial phase.

sampling is an invasive test that requires cannulation of the draining cervical and thoracic veins and has also been shown to be effective; however, it should typically be reserved for patients where other imaging techniques have been nonlocalizing. Ultrasound-guided FNA of the suspected lesion has been described, and if FNA aspirate washout PTH levels are very high (typically >1,000 pg/mL), this confirms the presence of parathyroid tissue in the localized nodule. Some adhesive scar can result after FNA due to periparathyroidal hemorrhage, which can make reoperation in this area more difficult.

The patient underwent cervical ultrasound by the surgeon that identified a hypoechoic nodule in the left lower neck measuring 1.1 × 1.4 cm, consistent with a possible parathyroid adenoma in the cervical thymus in the paratracheal central neck; however, this was only partially visualized in the transverse plane behind the sternal notch. A 4D-CT scan was obtained that demonstrated a 1.0 × 1.4 × 0.9 cm nodule, which enhanced with early arterial phase imaging and was suspected to be a parathyroid adenoma (Figure 68-3). Based on these imaging results, plans were made to proceed with reoperative parathyroidectomy.

● SURGICAL APPROACH

The decision to proceed with reoperative parathyroidectomy should be based on similar criteria used in recommending initial parathyroidectomy surgery; however, the increased risk of complications related to remedial surgery including an increased risk of recurrent laryngeal nerve injury and

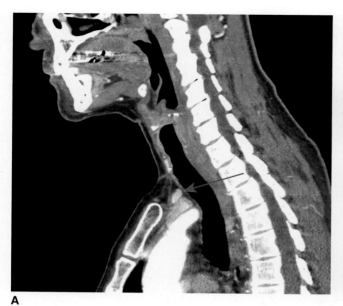

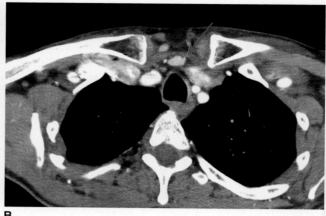

FIGURE 68-3. A 4D-CT of the patient in the case vignette demonstrating a left inferior parathyroid adenoma in the cervical thymus posterior to the sternal notch. **A:** Sagittal view. **B:** Axial view.

postoperative hypoparathyroidism should be considered. The surgeon should be sufficiently convinced of the location of the residual parathyroid adenoma prior to proceeding with exploration of a scarred operative field. Preoperative laryngoscopy should be performed prior to any reoperative thyroid or parathyroid surgery to evaluate for recurrent laryngeal nerve dysfunction from previous injury sustained at the initial operation. Intraoperative recurrent laryngeal nerve monitoring may be helpful in reoperative cases and can aid in identification of the nerves and with early detection of neuropraxia in difficult cases.

A standard anterior approach through the previous parathyroidectomy incision is commonly used and has the advantage of similarity to the traditional parathyroid surgical approach. The disadvantage of this approach is the presence of scar tissue from prior exploration which can be particularly challenging in cases where bilateral exploration is required. After making a standard Kocher incision, often through the previous incision scar, subplatysmal flaps are raised. The median raphe of the strap muscles is then divided. The strap muscles can be densely adhered to the underlying thyroid and paratracheal space making entrance into the central neck difficult. These adhesions are typically less dense lower in the central neck away from the inferior thyroid making this a good place to enter the central neck and identify the recurrent laryngeal nerve as it emanates from the mediastinum. This approach allows for access to the bilateral parathyroid glands if they reside in the normal anatomic positions as well as the cervical thymus and upper mediastinum. An approach lateral to the strap muscles and medial to the common carotid artery is an alternative approach that avoids the dense adhesion of the strap muscles to the underlying thyroid and allows access to the

paraesophageal space. Alternative incisions may be indicated for ectopic parathyroid gland locations suggested by preoperative imaging and can include a high, lateral neck incision for undescended parathyroid glands, a lateral thoracoscopic approach for parathyroid adenomas low in the mediastinum, and rarely sternotomy for mediastinal parathyroids which are inaccessible through a cervical approach.

Once the suspected abnormal parathyroid is identified and excised, frozen section can be helpful in confirmation of removal of parathyroid tissue. IOPTH monitoring is useful in confirming removal of hyperfunctional parathyroid tissue as evidenced by a drop of IOPTH level by at least 50% of the baseline value and a final value which is in the normal range (12 to 75 pg/mL). IOPTH monitoring also provides information about the functional capacity of residual normal parathyroid tissue. If IOPTH levels drop to undetectable levels (<5 pg/mL) after removal of the diseased parathyroid, reimplantation of parathyroid tissue or cryopreservation (if available) should be considered in an attempt to prevent permanent hypoparathyroidism.

In cases where preoperative imaging location is incorrect or in cases where IOPTH demonstrates persistent elevation after removal of the suspected parathyroid abnormality, a bilateral parathyroid exploration should be performed. The search for parathyroid glands should begin with exploration of the normal anatomic positions. The normal anatomic position for the inferior parathyroid gland is around the inferior pole of the thyroid gland, in the thyrothymic tract and in the cervical portion of the thymus. Most inferior parathyroid glands will be situated anterior to the course of the recurrent laryngeal nerve. Removal of the intrathoracic thymus can be accomplished via a neck incision by dissection and gentle traction of the cervical portion of the thymus to deliver the thymus from the superior mediastinum. Ectopic parathyroid adenomas in the thymus which lie at or caudal to the aortic arch may not be accessible through this maneuver; therefore, a thoroscopic approach may be required. A blind sternotomy should not be performed in the search for a missing parathyroid adenoma and should be reserved for parathyroid adenomas, which are well-localized on preoperative imaging and are not accessible transcervically or thoracoscopically.

The normal anatomic position of the superior parathyroid glands is typically within a 2 cm² area around the insertion of the inferior thyroid artery into the thyroid, near the ligament of berry and near the insertion of the recurrent laryngeal nerve into the larynx. Superior parathyroid adenomas can descend along the paraesophageal space, anterior to the fascia overlying the vertebral bodies. These parathyroids can descend posterior to the recurrent laryngeal nerve to a level below the inferior thyroid pole and occasionally down into the mediastinum and are sometimes referred to as being in a pseudoectopic position. Ectopic superior parathyroid locations include those that are intrathyroidal, those posterior to the pharynx or esophagus, and undescended parathyroid glands high in the neck near the carotid bifurcation, the hypoglossal nerve or near the submandibular salivary glands (Table 68-1).

The patient was taken to the operating room for a reoperative parathyroidectomy with intraoperative laryngeal nerve monitoring and IOPTH. The previous anterior neck collar incision was reopened. An anterior approach was used, and the median raphe of the strap muscles were opened low in the central neck. PTH levels were drawn at baseline, preexcision, and 5, 10, and 15 minutes postexcision with the criteria for biochemical cure being a drop at least 50% from the highest of the baseline or preexcision values and a final PTH level within the normal range (12 to 75 pg/mL). The left inferior parathyroid adenoma was discovered in the upper portion of the cervical thymus, posterior to the sternal notch, just left of the midline as noted on preoperative imaging. This was removed, and frozen section confirmed presence of hypercellular parathyroid tissue in a fragment of the gland, while the remainder of the parathyroid was kept on the sterile field for possible reimplantation. IOPTH levels dropped from 147 pg/mL at baseline down to 13 pg/mL at 15 minutes postexcision. The remainder of the parathyroid was not reimplanted and was sent to pathology which confirmed a 0.8-g hypercellular parathyroid with a small amount of attached thymus. The patient was discharged the same day with calcium citrate with vitamin D supplementation three times daily.

● SPECIAL INTRAOPERATIVE CONSIDERATIONS

Parathyromatosis is a rare intraoperative finding caused by previous fragmentation of a parathyroid adenoma during a previous operation. This leads to implantation of abnormal parathyroid tissue throughout the operative field. If faced

Table 68-1   Reoperative Parathyroidectomy

Key Technical Steps

1. Preoperative localization with two concordant imaging studies should convince the surgeon of the location of the suspected abnormal parathyroid prior to proceeding with reoperation
2. Preoperative assessment of laryngeal nerve function with laryngoscopy and intraoperative nerve monitoring should be considered
3. The operative approach and incision location should be dictated by location of the suspected parathyroid adenoma
4. Intraoperative PTH monitoring can confirm excision of abnormal parathyroid tissue as well as the presence of normally functioning residual parathyroid tissue
5. Drop of IOPTH to undetectable ranges after removal of abnormal parathyroid tissue should prompt consideration of reimplantation of fragments of the excised parathyroid or cryopreservation of parathyroid tissue
6. Inaccurate localization or failure of IOPTH to drop into the normal range may require extended exploration in a scarred field, and knowledge of typical locations for missed parathyroid glands is essential

Potential Pitfalls

- Ectopic parathyroid location which are not accessible through standard cervical incision parathyroidectomy approach
- Need to perform bilateral four-gland parathyroid exploration in a challenging reoperative field
- Increased risk of complications including hematoma, recurrent laryngeal nerve injury, and permanent hypoparathyroidism in reoperative parathyroidectomy

with this difficult situation, the surgeon should attempt to excise all identifiable parathyroid implants including resection of the ipsilateral strap muscles, the ipsilateral thyroid lobe, and central neck lymph nodes if required.

● POSTOPERATIVE MANAGEMENT

Postoperative management after reoperative parathyroidectomy is generally similar to that after initial parathyroidectomy. Calcium and vitamin D supplementation can be recommended for all patients or for selected patients based on IOPTH values or postoperative calcium and/or PTH levels. In patients with very low PTH values or in those who develop hypocalcemic symptoms not controlled with oral calcium supplementation, calcitriol 0.25 to 0.5 mcg once to twice daily may be beneficial. Patients should follow up in 1 to 2 weeks for evaluation of wound healing, vocal strength, hypocalcemia symptoms, and a calcium with or without PTH determination. Supplemental calcium and vitamin D can often be discontinued at this postoperative visit. Calcium and PTH levels should be monitored at 6 to 12 months postoperatively. Persistent hyperparathyroidism is defined as continued elevation of calcium and PTH within 6 months of surgery and recurrence by new onset of hypercalcemia and PTH elevation after 6 months. Persistent hyperparathyroidism rates are typically 1% to 5% with experienced surgeons, and recurrence rates are <5%.

The patient followed up in clinic in 2 weeks without complaints and stated improvements in her neuropsychiatric symptoms of primary hyperparathyroidism that were present preoperatively. She reported no hypocalcemic symptoms, and serum calcium was 9.1 mg/dL and PTH was 41 pg/mL. A calcium level 8 months after surgery was normal at 8.9 mg/dL. She was discharged from care with recommendations to have her calcium monitoring with her yearly health maintenance exams with her primary care provider.

TAKE HOME POINTS

- Patients with persistent hypercalcemia after parathyroidectomy should have confirmation of the diagnosis of primary hyperparathyroidism and queried about medication and genetic confounding factors.
- Most parathyroid adenomas causing persistent hyperparathyroidism after parathyroid exploration are found in normal anatomic positions.
- Review of prior imaging, the conduct of the initial parathyroid exploration from the operative note, and the surgical pathology report can provide clues about the potential location of the missing parathyroid adenoma.
- Two concordant imaging studies which convince the surgeon of the location of the missing parathyroid adenoma

should be considered before proceeding with reoperative parathyroidectomy.
- Reoperative parathyroidectomy has higher risks than initial surgery, and the surgeon should have appropriate experience in parathyroid surgery and remedial cervical exploration.

SUGGESTED READINGS

Kluijfhout WP, Venkatesh S, Beninato T, et al. Performance of magnetic resonance imaging in the evaluation of first-time and reoperative primary hyperparathyroidism. *Surgery.* 2016;160(3): 747-754. doi: 10.1016/j.surg.2016.05.003.

Lebastchi AH, Aruny JE, Donovan PI, et al. Real-time super selective venous sampling in remedial parathyroid surgery. *J Am Coll Surg.* 2015;220(6):994-1000. doi: 10.1016/j.jamcollsurg.2015.01.004.

Mortenson MM, Evans DB, Lee JE, et al. Parathyroid exploration in the reoperative neck: improved preoperative localization with 4D-computed tomography. *J Am Coll Surg.* 2008;206(5):888-895; discussion 895-896. doi: 10.1016/j.jamcollsurg.2007.12.044.

Okada M, Tominaga Y, Yamamoto T, Hiramitsu T, Narumi S, Watarai Y. Location frequency of missed parathyroid glands after parathyroidectomy in patients with persistent or recurrent secondary hyperparathyroidism. *World J Surg.* 2016;40(3):595-599. doi: 10.1007/s00268-015-3312-1.

Richards ML, Thompson GB, Farley DR, Grant CS. Reoperative parathyroidectomy in 228 patients during the era of minimal-access surgery and intraoperative parathyroid hormone monitoring. *Am J Surg.* 2008;196(6):937-942; discussion 942-943. doi: 10.1016/j.amjsurg.2008.07.022.

Silberfein EJ, Bao R, Lopez A, et al. Reoperative parathyroidectomy: location of missed glands based on a contemporary nomenclature system. *Arch Surg.* 2010;145(11):1065-1068. doi: 10.1001/archsurg.2010.230.

Udelsman R. Approach to the patient with persistent or recurrent primary hyperparathyroidism. *J Clin Endocrinol Metab.* 2011;96(10):2950-2958.

Incidental Adrenal Mass

69

BRIAN D. SAUNDERS AND MELISSA M. BOLTZ

Based on the previous edition chapter "Incidental Adrenal Mass" by
Brian D. Saunders and Melissa M. Boltz

Presentation

A 42-year-old woman was referred for evaluation of a
2.3-cm, left, homogeneous adrenal mass discovered when
a computed tomography (CT) scan was obtained on a visit
to the emergency room for complaints of nausea and vomiting. During her ER visit, she was noted to have a blood
pressure of 160/95. She reported a history of high blood
pressure over the past year for which she had been on
multiple antihypertensive medications. All laboratory data
were normal at that time except for low serum potassium.

● DIFFERENTIAL DIAGNOSIS

An adrenal incidentaloma is an asymptomatic adrenal
tumor found on abdominal imaging performed for another
indication. The frequency of incidentalomas is rising with
the increased use of CT scanning and other imaging modalities. Currently, between 1% and 4% of all abdominal imaging studies will reveal an incidental adrenal tumor. In adults,
incidental adrenal masses have a broad differential diagnosis
(Table 69-1). Adrenal masses may be nonfunctional or functional (hormonally active), and malignant or benign.

Although most incidentalomas are benign, a primary
adrenocortical carcinoma (ACC) is one of the most aggressive cancers, and thus, this diagnosis must be considered in
the differential diagnosis of any adrenal mass. ACC is a rare
tumor, with between 500 and 600 new cases per year in the
United States. Additionally, approximately 20% of incidentalomas are hormonally functional (albeit many with subclinical phenotypes), and although histologically benign,
failure to diagnose and treat these patients results in avoidable morbidity.

● WORKUP

The two major issues in managing a patient with an incidental adrenal mass are to evaluate for autonomous adrenal hormone production and to assess the malignant potential, both
of which are indications for operative resection. Figure 69-1
depicts a suggested algorithm for the workup of incidentalomas beginning with a complete history and physical examination with specific reference to history of prior malignancies and

signs and symptoms of adrenal hormone excess. It is especially
important to query family history of adrenal tumors producing excess catecholamines as nearly 25% of pheochromocytomas are secondary to an inherited genetic predisposition.

An adrenal protocol CT scan is ideal when assessing adrenal
masses. An adrenal protocol CT scan starts with a noncontrast
study. The noncontrast scan is followed by the rapid injection
of contrast agent, and 60 seconds later, a contrast-enhanced
CT scan is performed. Then, a delayed contrast (washout) scan
is obtained 15 minutes after the initial contrast images. The
relative percentage of contrast washout is calculated from the
Hounsfield unit values of the contrast and delayed contrast
CT scans. Benign adrenal cortical adenomas typically have
CT attenuation values of <10 Hounsfield units on noncontrast imaging or washout >60%, which indicates a lipid-rich
mass. Tumors with Hounsfield values >10 Hounsfield units are
not necessarily malignant. An abdominal MRI is an increasingly utilized and acceptable imaging modality, especially in
those patients with contrast allergies or reduced glomerular

Table 69-1	Classification of Adrenal Masses	
Functional		**Nonfunctional**
● Cortical adenoma (aldosterone/cortisol/androgen)		● Cortical adenoma
		● Cortical carcinoma
● Pheochromocytoma		● Neuroblastoma
● Cortical carcinoma (any adrenal hormone)		● Ganglioneuroma
		● Metastasis
● Congenital adrenal hyperplasia		● Cysts (true or pseudocysts)
● Nodular hyperplasia (Cushing's disease)		● Hematoma
		● Myelolipoma
		● Lipoma
		● Lymphoma
		● Granuloma
		● Amyloidosis
		● Infiltrative disease

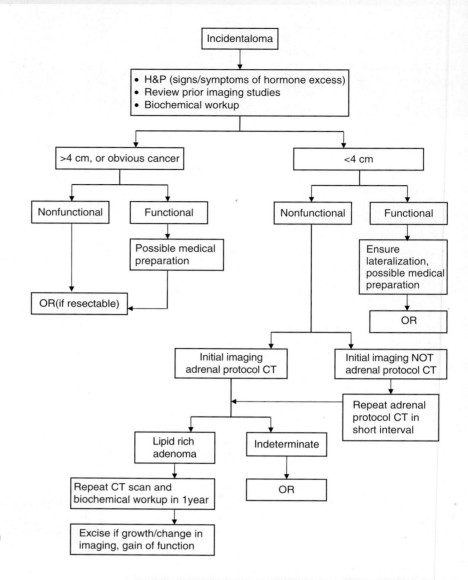

FIGURE 69-1. Algorithm for the evaluation of adrenal incidentalomas.

filtration rates. Review of imaging should account for features that would indicate malignancy, including large tumor size (>4 cm), irregular tumor margins, heterogeneity, hyperdensity, invasion into adjacent structures, lymphadenopathy, or presence of metastasis. Figure 69-2 shows a 2.3-cm left adrenal mass found on CT scan in this patient.

Regardless of radiographic appearance, all patients with an incidental adrenal mass should undergo biochemical testing to determine functional status. A comprehensive screening panel should include serum potassium, plasma aldosterone concentration, plasma renin activity, fasting AM cortisol, adrenocorticotropic hormone (ACTH), dehydroepiandrosterone sulfate (DHEAS), and plasma-fractionated metanephrines and normetanephrines. Other measures to assess increased cortisol include 24-hour urinary-free cortisol and measurements of salivary cortisol. Demonstration of hypercortisolemia should prompt suppression tests to determine the nature of the elevated endogenous cortisol (e.g., ACTH-dependent or ACTH-independent). Urinary catecholamine measurements can also be used to screen for adrenal

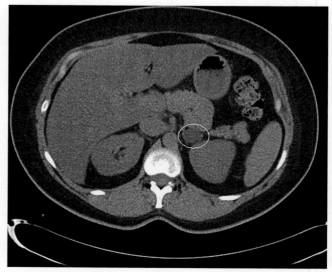

FIGURE 69-2. Axial cut of a CT scan with white circle indicating a 2.3-cm diameter left adrenal mass. Radiodensity of the mass on unenhanced images shows a Hounsfield unit of 0.

medullary hyperfunction. If the biochemical workup indicates the tumor is nonfunctional, the size of the tumor and the patient's medical condition determine further management.

● DIAGNOSIS AND TREATMENT

As stated in the case above, this patient had significant and uncontrolled hypertension, concomitant with decreased serum potassium. Further biochemical workup revealed an elevated plasma aldosterone with concurrent low plasma renin activity suggesting primary hyperaldosteronism and an aldosteronoma. Additionally, cortisol, ACTH, DHEAS, and catecholamines were normal. Therefore, adrenalectomy is indicated in this patient with a homogeneous, 2.3-cm, functional adrenal mass.

The use of laparoscopic techniques in surgery of adrenal glands has replaced the traditional open approach and is the preferred procedure for all small, benign tumors. The mortality with the laparoscopic approach is low at 0.2% 1 month after surgery. The overall morbidity rate averages 9% with a higher rate in pheochromocytoma and Cushing's syndrome. Due to the benefits associated with laparoscopic surgery, open adrenalectomy should be reserved for tumors >8 cm, as well as tumors with obvious findings consistent with malignancy on preoperative imaging.

Prior to operative intervention, medical preparation may be indicated, based on functional status of the tumor. Preoperative control of hypertension in the patient with a pheochromocytoma is necessary. Alpha-adrenergic blockade can be achieved using a nonselective agent (phenoxybenzamine) or a selective agent (doxazosin) for 10 to 14 days prior to the procedure. In addition, beta-adrenergic blockade is used after alpha-blockade to treat tachycardia and unopposed alpha-blockade. Alternatively, a calcium channel blocker may be used in lieu of both alpha and beta-blocking agents. Patients with Cushing's syndrome should receive stress dose steroids due to suppression of the hypothalamic–pituitary–adrenal (HPA) axis of the contralateral adrenal gland. For patients with severe hypercortisolism, consideration can be given to administration of an adrenolytic agent, such as ketoconazole or mitotane. In this patient with an aldosteronoma, blood pressure and hypokalemia should be controlled with a competitive aldosterone antagonist such as spironolactone or eplerenone. These agents block the mineralocorticoid receptor, promote potassium retention, and reduce extracellular fluid volume controlling blood pressure.

● SURGICAL APPROACH FOR LAPAROSCOPIC LATERAL TRANSABDOMINAL ADRENALECTOMY

In patients undergoing laparoscopic left adrenalectomy (Table 69-2), general anesthesia is induced and an orogastric tube and Foley catheter are inserted with the patient in

---

Table 69-2	Laparoscopic Left Adrenalectomy

Key Technical Steps

1. General anesthesia induced with patient in supine position.
2. Place patient in lateral decubitus position, ipsilateral side up.
3. Obtain laparoscopic access.
4. Mobilize splenic flexure of colon.
5. Divide lateral peritoneal attachments of spleen and lienophrenic ligament.
6. Reflect spleen medially and mobilize pancreatic tail.
7. Bluntly create a plane medial to adrenal gland and lateral to aorta.
8. Dissect and divide the inferior phrenic vessels and central adrenal vein.
9. Mobilize adrenal gland by dividing inferior and lateral attachments.
10. Remove adrenal gland from abdomen.
11. Inspect suprarenal fossa for hemostasis.
12. Close port sites.

Potential Pitfalls

- Inability to visualize the gland.
- Vascular injuries.
- Pancreatic injury resulting in pancreatic leak.

---

supine position. Afterward, the patient is placed in the lateral decubitus position with the ipsilateral side up. The table is flexed to widen the angle between the costal margin and iliac crest. Laparoscopic access is obtained with the camera port placed slightly superior and to the left of the umbilicus. The other two working ports are placed two fingerbreadths inferior to the subcostal margin and triangulated with the camera port.

After laparoscopic access is obtained, attention is directed toward mobilizing the splenic flexure of the colon and dividing the lateral peritoneal attachments of the spleen and lienophrenic ligament until the fundus of the stomach is in view. The spleen is then reflected medially with mobilization of the tail of the pancreas. A plane medial to the adrenal gland and lateral to the aorta is bluntly created. Then, the inferior phrenic vessels and central adrenal vein are dissected and divided. The inferior and lateral attachments of the adrenal gland are divided to mobilize the gland out of the suprarenal fossa, exposing the capsule of the superior renal pole. The adrenal gland is then placed in a specimen retrieval bag and removed from the abdomen via the camera port site. Maintaining insufflation, the suprarenal fossa is inspected for adequate hemostasis. The ports are then removed, followed by fascial closure of the camera port site, and skin closure.

Should the patient have needed a laparoscopic right adrenalectomy (Table 69-3) patient setup and positioning is the same as stated above, except the camera port is now located

Table 69-3	Laparoscopic Right Adrenalectomy

Key Technical Steps

1. General anesthesia induced with patient in supine position.
2. Place patient in lateral decubitus position, ipsilateral side up.
3. Obtain laparoscopic access.
4. Retract right lobe of liver medially.
5. Open peritoneum overlying adrenal gland inferior to superior.
6. Bluntly create a plane medial to adrenal gland and lateral to vena cava.
7. Dissect and divide the central adrenal vein (clip or linear stapler).
8. Mobilize adrenal gland by dividing inferior and lateral attachments.
9. Remove adrenal gland from abdomen.
10. Inspect suprarenal fossa for hemostasis.
11. Close port sites.

Potential Pitfalls

- Inability to visualize the gland.
- Liver injury resulting in hematomas and conversion to open procedure.
- Vascular injuries.
- Aberrant adrenal vein.

slightly superior and to the right of the umbilicus. After laparoscopic access has been obtained, the lateral attachments of the liver to the diaphragm (triangular ligament) are divided and the right lobe of the liver is retracted medially. Then, a separate medial port is placed to accommodate a laparoscopic retractor for the liver. The peritoneum overlying the medial aspect of the adrenal gland is opened inferior to superior, and a plane medial to the adrenal gland and posterolateral to the vena cava is bluntly developed. The remainder of the procedure is performed as outlined for the laparoscopic left adrenalectomy.

Sometimes, the adrenal gland is difficult to visualize due to perinephric fat, which is more common in men, obese patients, and those with small tumors. Intraoperative ultrasound may be useful in this situation to determine gland location. In addition, the gland should always be dissected with a rim of fatty tissue attached to its surface. This allows for manipulation of the gland without grasping it, which may tear the gland, causing bleeding. During laparoscopic right adrenalectomy, liver injury can easily occur during retraction causing large hematomas, which may make it impossible to proceed laparoscopically. Additionally, vena cava and other vascular injuries account for up to 7% of the complications of laparoscopic adrenalectomy, necessitating conversion to an open procedure. Consideration should also be given to the possibility of an aberrant adrenal vein, which drains into the right renal vein.

● SURGICAL APPROACH FOR LAPAROSCOPIC POSTERIOR RETROPERITONEAL ADRENALECTOMY (TABLE 69-4)

Laparoscopic posterior retroperitoneal adrenalectomy could be considered in patients with significant prior intra-abdominal operations or in patients with Cushing's disease who require bilateral adrenalectomy. The ideal patient would have a body mass index <45, and tumor size <6 cm with no more than 7 cm between Gerota's fascia and the skin on preoperative CT scan. Additionally, the 12th rib should be rostral to the level of the renal hilum.

Like the transabdominal approach, general anesthesia is induced, and an orogastric tube and Foley catheter are inserted with the patient in supine position. Afterward, the patient is placed in the prone position and the table flexed to widen the angle between the posterior ribs and iliac wing. Three ports are placed in a line about 2 fingerbreadths inferior to the costal margin, with the medial most port as close to the spine as possible just lateral to the paraspinous muscle and the lateral port as far laterally as possible. The middle port is roughly halfway between the medial and lateral ports and should be placed first.

After laparoscopic access is obtained, dissection starts superiorly sweeping the areolar tissue anterior toward the table moving medial to lateral uncovering the paraspinous muscles and peritoneum. When working medially, careful dissection is done to expose the inferior phrenic vein on the left and the inferior vena cava on the right. During the course

Table 69-4	Laparoscopic Retroperitoneal Adrenalectomy

Key Technical Steps

1. General anesthesia induced with patient in supine position.
2. Place patient in prone position.
3. Obtain laparoscopic access.
4. Sweep areolar tissue uncovering paraspinous muscles and peritoneum.
5. Expose the inferior phrenic vein or inferior vena cava medially.
6. Divide connections between adrenal gland and superior pole of kidney.
7. Ligate the adrenal vein.
8. Mobilize adrenal gland by dividing peritoneal attachments.
9. Remove adrenal gland from abdomen.
10. Inspect retroperitoneal space for hemostasis.
11. Close port sites.

Potential Pitfalls

- Inability to visualize the gland.
- Lack of traditional landmarks.
- Reduced working space.

of this dissection, adrenal arteries should also be ligated and divided. Then the superior pole of the kidney is identified and the connections between the adrenal gland the superior pole of the kidney are divided. This allows for retraction of the kidney inferiorly to facilitate identification and ligation of the adrenal vein. Once the adrenal vein is ligated, the adrenal gland can be separated from the peritoneal attachments. The adrenal gland is placed in a specimen retrieval bag and removed from the middle port. Maintaining insufflation, the retroperitoneal space is inspected for adequate hemostasis. The ports are then removed, followed by fascial closure of the middle port site, and skin closure.

The main difficulties with the retroperitoneal approach include a small working space and lack of traditional landmarks seen in the transabdominal approach. Liberal use of insufflation pressures of 15 to 30 mm Hg can increase the size of the working space. Additionally, intraoperative laparoscopic ultrasound may be used for adrenal glands that are difficult to visualize.

● SURGICAL APPROACH FOR OPEN ADRENALECTOMY

Should the patient have findings indicating the need for an open adrenalectomy, either a vertical midline incision or a subcostal incision is made. For conversion from laparoscopic to an open procedure, generally a subcostal incision is made with the patient in the lateral decubitus position. For a left adrenal mass resection via an open anterior approach, the lesser sac is entered. The splenic flexure of the colon is reflected caudad, and the spleen and tail of the pancreas are mobilized to expose the adrenal gland. The inferior phrenic vessels and central adrenal vein are dissected and divided with the remaining soft tissue attachments to complete the adrenalectomy. For adrenocortical cancers, en bloc splenectomy, distal pancreatectomy, nephrectomy, or partial diaphragmatic resection may be necessary.

An open anterior right adrenalectomy requires mobilization of the hepatic flexure of the colon and a partial Kocher maneuver to elevate the duodenum and to expose the infrahepatic vena cava. The right lobe of the liver is mobilized by dividing the triangular ligament and retracting it medially to expose the adrenal gland. The lateral and inferior margins of the adrenal gland are then mobilized. The central adrenal vein is divided and controlled with the remaining of the soft tissue attachments divided as well. Large or invasive tumors may require a thoracoabdominal incision to obtain suprahepatic vena caval control. If adrenalectomy is performed for a large adrenal cancer, en bloc resection of the right hepatic lobe, right kidney, or portion of the vena cava or diaphragm may be required.

● SPECIAL INTRAOPERATIVE CONSIDERATIONS

Unexpected finding such as unusual retroperitoneal feeding vessels and tumor invasion into surrounding structures encountered at the time of laparoscopic adrenalectomy would raise the concern of a primary adrenal cancer, and therefore, conversion to open adrenalectomy should be performed. Proceeding with the laparoscopic procedure would risk violating the tumor capsule. In addition, tumor manipulation during laparoscopic surgery causes aerosolization of cancer cells via the pneumoperitoneum and leads to seeding of the peritoneal cavity and port sites, which is known as the "chimney effect."

● POSTOPERATIVE MANAGEMENT

Postoperatively, patients who undergo laparoscopic adrenalectomy typically require less fluid replacement than those undergoing open procedures. Incentive spirometry should be used to prevent postoperative atelectasis and pneumonia. In addition, pharmacologic deep venous thrombosis prophylaxis should be started. A regular diet should be resumed as soon as possible, and the Foley catheter may be discontinued when the patient's hemodynamics, urinary output, and electrolytes are stable.

In patients with an aldosteronoma, potassium supplementation should be stopped postoperatively and antihypertensives weaned. Patients with a pheochromocytoma should be monitored in an ICU for signs of postoperative hypotension from vascular relaxation as well as hypoglycemia. Alpha-blocking medications may be discontinued immediately, beta-blockers weaned, and glycemic control initiated if necessary. Patients who underwent adrenalectomy for Cushing's syndrome should be placed on pharmacologic doses of corticosteroid replacement with a plan to wean to physiologic doses. The HPA axis should be intermittently interrogated with a cosyntropin stimulation test. In the initial postoperative period, they should also be assessed for hypotension, decreased urine output, hyponatremia, hyperkalemia, hypoglycemia, and fever.

Case Conclusion

The patient undergoes successful laparoscopic left adrenalectomy, and she is discharged on postoperative day 1. Postoperatively, her oral potassium supplement medications were discontinued immediately and antihypertensives slowly weaned over 2 months. The final pathology report showed the tumor to be a benign cortical aldosteronoma.

TAKE HOME POINTS

- Approximately 20% of adrenal incidentalomas are hormonally functional, and although histologically benign, failure to diagnose and treat these patients results in unnecessary morbidity.
- Adrenal incidentalomas, regardless of radiographic appearance, should be screened to determine their functional status.

- Laparoscopic adrenalectomy is the procedure of choice for small tumors (functional or not) without evidence of malignancy. The retroperitoneal approach should be considered when bilateral adrenalectomy is to be performed. Open adrenalectomy is indicated for masses >8 cm or obvious radiologic evidence of malignancy.
- The adrenal gland should always be dissected with a rim of fatty tissue attached to its surface so as not to tear the gland, which may cause bleeding that is difficult to control or seed tumor cells.
- Unexpected findings concerning for a primary adrenal cancer during laparoscopic adrenalectomy necessitates conversion to an open procedure.

SUGGESTED READINGS

Agcaoglu O, Sahin DA, Siperstein A, Berber E. Selection algorithm for posterior versus lateral approach in laparoscopic adrenalectomy. *Surgery.* 2012;151:731-735.

Nieman LK. Approach to the patient with an adrenal incidentaloma. *J Clin Endocrinol Metab.* 2010;95(9):4106-4113.

Shen WT, Sturgeon C, Duh QY. From incidentaloma to adrenocortical carcinoma: the surgical management of adrenal tumors. *J Surg Oncol.* 2005;89(3):186-192.

Zeiger MA, Thompson GB, Duh QY, et al. American Association of Clinical Endocrinologists and American Association of Endocrine Surgeons medical guidelines for the management of adrenal incidentalomas. *Endo Prac.* 2009;15:(suppl 1).

Adrenocortical Carcinoma

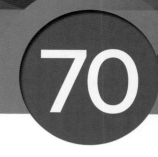

ROY LIROV AND PAUL G. GAUGER

Based on the previous edition chapter "Adrenal Cancer" by David T. Hughes and Paul G. Gauger

Presentation

The patient is a 47-year-old previously healthy female referred for management of a new right adrenal mass (Figure 70-1). Over the last 4 months, she has experienced increased appetite, weight gain, and neck fullness. She has also noticed headache, tremor, palpitations, and occasional diaphoresis. She has had no muscle weakness. She has not had diarrhea or skin changes. Her blood pressure is normal. Her BMI is 24, and she has facial plethora, moon facies, and a buffalo hump. Her abdomen is protuberant without striae or organomegaly. There is no palpable adenopathy.

● DIFFERENTIAL DIAGNOSIS

Adrenal neoplasms can develop in the cortex or medulla and may be benign or malignant. This chapter primarily concerns adrenocortical carcinoma (ACC), a malignant tumor of the adrenal cortex. The chief lesions in the differential diagnosis are adrenocortical adenoma (ACA), a benign tumor of the adrenal cortex, and pheochromocytoma, a tumor of the adrenal medulla, which may be benign or malignant. For the imaged adrenal mass, a variety of other processes must be considered as well, including: adrenal hyperplasia, granuloma, hemorrhage, cyst, ganglioneuroma, mesenchymal-lineage tumors (e.g., myelolipoma, schwannoma, etc), lymphoma, and metastasis from other primary cancers. Although ACC is a rare disease, it is essential to consider

because marked improvements in prognosis can be achieved with appropriately treated early-stage cancer, despite its reputation for aggressive behavior.

Our patient has a new right adrenal mass of moderate size with hypercortisolism and elevated DHEAS. Her history and exam are consistent with hypercortisolism, although her palpitations, headache, and diaphoresis suggest consideration of pheochromocytoma as well.

● WORKUP

Patients with ACC typically present with either an incidentally discovered adrenal mass (i.e., incidentaloma) or symptoms related to hormone excess or mass effect. Although the vast majority of adrenal incidentalomas are benign, the goal of evaluation is to rule out malignancy or hormone overproduction. All patients with adrenal incidentalomas should undergo evaluation for hypercortisolism and catecholamine production. Patients with hypertension or hypokalemia should also undergo evaluation for hyperaldosteronism. ACC may be nonfunctional or may produce any combination of steroid hormones, including intermediate metabolites. Due to the higher overall prevalence of benign lesions in general, isolated hypercortisolism, hyperaldosteronism, or catecholamine excess are most often caused by nonmalignant tumors. However, androgen production (with or without virilization) or production of multiple steroid hormones is highly suspicious for ACC. Therefore, when the likelihood of ACC is high, a complete steroid profile, including intermediate metabolites, is often obtained (Table 70-1).

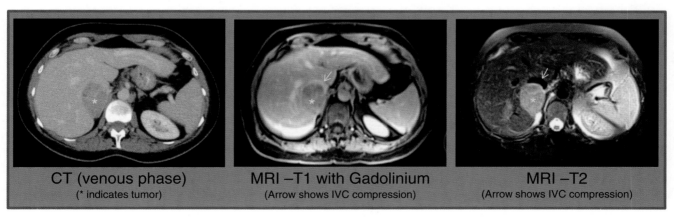

CT (venous phase)
(* indicates tumor)

MRI –T1 with Gadolinium
(Arrow shows IVC compression)

MRI –T2
(Arrow shows IVC compression)

FIGURE 70-1. CT and MRI finds for the presented patient.

Table 70-1	Comprehensive Biochemical Evaluation

Glucocorticoid excess (minimum 3 of 4 tests)

    Dexamethasone suppression (1 mg at 23:00, 8 AM cortisol level)

    24 h urine free cortisol

    Basal cortisol

    Basal ACTH

Androgen excess

    DHEA-S

    17-OH-Progesterone

    Androstenedione

    Testosterone

    17-Beta-estradiol (men and postmenopausal women)

Hyperaldosteronism (if decreased K+ or hypertensive)

    Plasma aldosterone concentration (PAC)

    Renin activity assay (RAA) (Ratio: PAC/RAA > 30 + elevated PAC => positive test)

Pheochromocytoma (either test)

    Plasma meta- and nor-metanephrines

    24 h urine catecholamines or metanephrines

Moreover, the steroid profile particular to a given tumor can have utility as biomarkers for diagnosis and surveillance.

Although many patients are referred to the surgeon with at least one form of cross-sectional imaging, patients may require additional studies to further characterize the tumor and to estimate the likelihood of malignancy. When malignancy is likely, cross-sectional imaging of the chest should always be obtained for staging purposes. Bone scintigraphy and head CT may be obtained in symptomatic patients. An adrenal-protocol CT is an important initial diagnostic study in nearly all patients with adrenal masses. It is performed with 1-mm slices in the region of the adrenal glands and in three contrast phases: noncontrast, arterial phase, and 15-minute delay. Exceedingly low enhancement on noncontrast CT (−30 Hounsfields Units, HU) is typical of myelolipoma (Figure 70-2). Small (<3 to 4 cm), homogeneous tumors with regular borders showing enhancement of <10 HU on noncontrast CT are likely to be lipid-rich ACA and may need no additional follow-up imaging. ACA may be lipid-poor in up to a third of cases however, leaving the diagnosis more elusive by this criterion alone. In such cases, the arterial and delayed-phase contrast-enhanced CT can be used to clarify the diagnosis: if the absolute percentage contrast washout (APW) exceeds 60% or relative percentage washout (RPW) exceeds 40% the lesion is more likely to be a lipid-poor ACA. More prolonged contrast retention is suspicious for ACC. Other features that are typical of ACC include larger size (usually >4 cm), heterogeneous enhancement, internal calcification, irregular margins, and decreased central enhancement suggestive of necrosis. The risk of ACC in tumors 4 to 6 cm has been reported at approximately 5%, whereas that of tumors larger than 6 cm may exceed 25%. However, size cannot be used as the sole distinguishing factor as there are numerous reports of malignant tumors <2.5 cm in diameter. MRI may also be performed as the initial diagnostic study or ordered subsequently for additional characterization. Loss of intensity within a tumor on in-and-out of phase images on chemical-shift MRI can be used to conclusively diagnose lipid-rich ACA, and high-intensity on T2 imaging is typical of pheochromocytoma. MRI can also be more accurate than CT for detection of tumor invasion or thrombus within the large neighboring veins and can have significant utility in assessing the metastatic potential of liver lesions. [18]FDG-PET is frequently used to characterize suspicious lesions identified on cross-sectional imaging

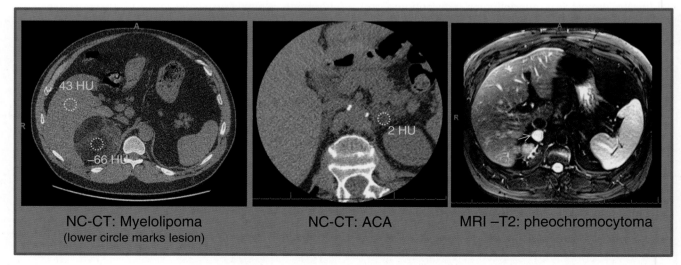

NC-CT: Myelolipoma
(lower circle marks lesion)

NC-CT: ACA

MRI −T2: pheochromocytoma

FIGURE 70-2. Imaging characteristics of commonly encountered adrenal lesions. Circles indicate measured region-of-interest. Arrow indicates right adrenal mass.

for the possibility of metastatic ACC, and as a complementary modality for assessing malignancy risk within a primary adrenal tumor itself. A threshold SUVmax ratio of adrenal to liver tissue of 1.6 has been identified as promising indicator of ACC in several studies. [18]FDG-PET can also be very helpful in suggesting the level of concern for other concordantly detected lung or liver lesions of unclear significance.

It is worth emphasizing that percutaneous adrenal biopsy should be avoided in nearly all circumstances. One possible exception is in a situation where a patient has a history of another primary tumor, other modalities have not yielded a diagnosis, and there is no alternative site amenable to biopsy. Prior to biopsy, it is imperative to biochemically exclude pheochromocytoma.

Our patient has symptoms of Cushing's syndrome but normal blood pressure. Her complete blood count and comprehensive metabolic panel are normal. Her 24–hour urine-free cortisol was elevated at 91 mcg (normal 4 to 50), and she demonstrated androgen excess, with serum DHEAS of 901 mcg/dL (normal 35 to 430). Her plasma metanephrines and normetanephrines were undetectable. An adrenal-protocol CT demonstrated a heterogeneously enhancing 5.2 × 4.3 × 5.1 cm right adrenal mass abutting segments 5 and 8 of the liver with possible IVC invasion (Figure 70-1). She underwent MRI for further characterization, which was inconclusive for invasion.

● DIAGNOSIS AND TREATMENT

Our patient has hypercortisolism, androgen excess, and a moderate-sized adrenal mass with the possibility of invasion and tumor thrombus by cross-sectional imaging; this is a constellation of findings virtually diagnostic of ACC.

Prognosis in ACC is highly dependent on stage at presentation and the delivery of optimal treatment. Lower recurrence and superior 5-year survival rates have been demonstrated in patients getting early specialized care, and therefore, experts recommend that patients with suspected ACC undergo treatment in a tertiary care facility with extensive adrenal cancer experience. The AJCC staging system for ACC introduced in 2004 has been supplanted by the ENSAT staging system (Table 70-2), which is also based on TNM criteria, but has higher predictive capability. Stages I and II are defined as a localized tumors, without invasion, metastasis,

or adenopathy, with 5 cm the size threshold for distinguishing these two stages. Stage III is defined as regionally advanced disease: a tumor of any size with either regional lymphadenopathy or evidence of infiltration or invasion, including tumor thrombus or frank tumor ingrowth into adjacent organs. Stage IV is defined by distant metastasis.

Adrenalectomy is the cornerstone of management for ACC, and preoperative optimization is essential for achieving acceptable morbidity and mortality. Patients with functional adrenal tumors may have electrolyte abnormalities, hyperglycemia, and refractory hypertension and may be predisposed to impaired wound healing and surgical site infection due to immunosuppressive effects of excessive glucocorticoid levels. Electrolyte imbalance, hyperglycemia, and hypertension should be corrected ahead of surgery. Hypertension in patients with aldosterone-secreting tumors is addressed with spironolactone, although additional agents may be necessary. Hypercortisolism should be aggressively managed; initiation of ketoconazole, mifepristone, or metyrapone may be necessary in patients not already undergoing treatment with mitotane. However, achieving optimized glucocorticoid levels should not delay surgery.

The only curative modality for patients diagnosed with ACC is an en bloc R0 resection without tumor spillage or capsular rupture. Suboptimal resection is associated with early recurrence and dismal survival. Moreover, significant controversy surrounds the efficacy of adjuvant therapies, underscoring the importance of optimal initial treatment. The agent of choice for adjuvant therapy following resection is mitotane, which is recommended for patients at higher risk of recurrence, and is currently under investigation for use as adjuvant therapy in early-stage resected ACC (ADIUVO trial, www.adiuvotrial.org). Conflicting reports have been published regarding the utility of external-beam radiation, which is also commonly used in the adjuvant setting at many centers, and frequently used as a component of multimodality palliative treatment regimens.

Patients with suspected localized ACC (stages I and II) should undergo open adrenalectomy. The question of whether a laparoscopic approach is appropriate for suspected localized ACC remains unanswered. Results following laparoscopy from even the most experienced centers include failures to achieve an R0 resection, and several earlier studies

Table 70-2 ENSAT System for Staging ACC with Published Survival

Stage	TNM	Criteria	5-year survival	Median survival (y)
Stage I	T1N0M0	Size < 5 cm	82%	24
Stage II	T2N0M0	Size > 5 cm	61%	6.1
Stage III	T3⁺NxM0 TxN1M0	Local infiltration (T3), organ invasion (T4), or node positive disease (N1)	50%	3.5
Stage IV	TxNxM1	Distant metastasis	13%	0.9

demonstrate higher local recurrence and rates of peritoneal carcinomatosis with laparoscopy. Although other studies have reported comparable oncologic outcomes with both techniques, all studies are retrospective and may not have sufficient power to support statistically robust conclusions.

Patients with locoregionally advanced ACC (stage III) are also typically offered resection, if technically feasible. Given the typically larger tumor size and involvement of other organs, achieving an R0 resection can be technically challenging but remains of paramount importance for durable recurrence-free survival. Strategies involving preoperative neoadjuvant chemoradiation for borderline resectable cases (such as those with extensive vascular involvement) are under investigation. Patients presenting with unresectable stage III or widely metastatic ACC (stage IV) are typically treated primarily with chemoradiation and locoregional ablative techniques. Symptoms of hormone excess can be debilitating for such patients. Glucocorticoid excess can be addressed with mitotane, mifepristone, ketoconazole, or metyrapone. Spironolactone, or the more selective mineralocorticoid antagonist eplerenone, can be used for management of hyperaldosteronism when it is present in the rare ACC patient. The antiandrogenic effect of spironolactone can be used to advantage in treatment of virilizing tumors, but eplerenone is preferred when an antiandrogenic effect is not desired or poorly tolerated. Uncommonly, patients with stage IV disease presenting with isolated metastasis (particularly to the lung or liver) or those with sufficient response following chemotherapy may be considered for resection and/or metastasectomy. In such situations, neoadjuvant chemoradiation may be used with short-interval (8 to 12 weeks) follow-up to determine treatment response and pace of progression. Patients with rapidly progressive disease do not generally benefit from surgical intervention, whereas short-term survival benefits and improvement in quality of life may be seen in cases with more indolent tumor behavior. Surgical debulking can also be considered for patients with medically refractory symptoms of hormone excess, although such therapy should be considered carefully in the overall context of care, and is generally avoided unless >90% of the tumor burden can be addressed. A variety of chemotherapeutic regimens for advanced ACC have been studied. The FIRM-ACT trial reported superior response and progression-free survival in patients treated with etoposide, doxorubicin, and cisplatin combined with mitotane (EDP-M) compared to an alternative regimen consisting of streptozocin and mitotane (Sz-M). EDP-M is now recommended as initial therapy for patients with advanced unresectable or stage IV ACC.

● SURGICAL APPROACH

Our approach to open adrenalectomy for ACC involves strict adherence to oncologic principles with a goal of an R0 resection. Each case is approached with the guiding principle that violation of the tumor capsule or specimen fracture is tantamount to local recurrence or carcinomatosis. The surgeon should anticipate the need for an en bloc multivisceral resection based on preoperative imaging and arrange for subspecialty intraoperative consultation in advance. Invasion of the kidney, spleen, colon, and liver can be seen. In addition, tumor thrombus may extend into the renal vein, vena cava, or right atrium. Options for management of these complex cases include venotomy and thrombectomy, partial caval resection with primary repair, and extensive caval resection with reconstruction. A thoracoabdominal approach may be necessary in cases with extensive involvement of the vena cava, and median sternotomy with cardiopulmonary bypass may be necessary in cases where tumor thrombus extends into the right atrium. Lymphatic drainage of the adrenal gland is to the ipsilateral renal hilar nodes, paracaval, and paraaortic nodes. Clinically suspicious node compartments should be resected en bloc, if technically feasible. Although there is no robust evidence to support a survival benefit, routine lymphadenectomy can provide valuable information for staging and has been advocated by many investigators.

Open adrenalectomy is typically performed with the patient supine via a midline laparotomy or bilateral subcostal incision, which typically provides better exposure. If access to the pleural cavity is necessary, a subcostal incision may be extended through the 8th or 9th intercostal space. If a thoracoabdominal approach is necessary, a partial decubitus position can facilitate exposure, with the patient's chest and upper abdomen oriented at 45° to the operating table, and the lower abdomen flat in the supine position. The thoracoabdominal incision begins 2 cm from the scapular tip and extends along the 8th intercostal space to just above the umbilicus in the midline. To approach right-sided tumors, the hepatic flexure is mobilized, and a Kocher maneuver is performed to expose the vena cava. The right lobe of the liver is retracted superiorly and the right kidney inferiorly, exposing the right adrenal gland. It is frequently necessary to widely mobilize the right lobe of the liver if the superior aspect of the gland is not palpable after the duodenum is mobilized. The right adrenal vein drains from the superomedial aspect of the gland directly into the vena cava. To approach left-sided tumors, the lesser sac is opened at the gastrocolic ligament, and the peritoneum overlying the inferior border of the pancreas is incised. Superior retraction of the pancreas and inferior retraction of the left kidney will typically reveal the left adrenal gland. The left adrenal vein drains from the inferomedial aspect of the gland into the left renal vein. On both sides, there is a superior adrenal pedicle draining to the inferior phrenic vein as well. In the course of either mobilization, the surgeon cautiously palpates to sound the depth of the underlying tumor and avoid exposing the underlying tumor capsule, which is extremely fragile. Including a margin of retroperitoneal fat and in some cases a portion of Gerota's fascia is advised in order to avoid injury to the tumor capsule. Excessive pressure on the tumor should be avoided and direct manipulation kept to an absolute minimum. A variable number of parasitized vessels may be encountered before the definitive adrenal pedicle is identified. Before ligation, the adrenal vein and vena cava should be assessed for the presence of tumor thrombus (Figures 70-3 and 70-4).

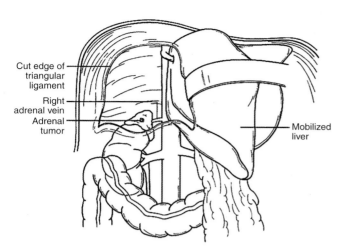

FIGURE 70-3. Right adrenalectomy. (Reprinted from Doherty GM, Skögseid B. *Surgical Endocrinology: A Clinical Syndromes Approach*. Philadelphia, PA: Lippincott Williams & Wilkins; 2001, with permission.)

● SPECIAL INTRAOPERATIVE CONSIDERATIONS

Most adrenalectomies are performed for small tumors with presumed benign disease, and for such cases, laparoscopic adrenalectomy is the gold standard. However, evidence of invasion or intraoperative suspicion for malignancy should warrant immediate conversion to open surgery and proceeding with an oncologic operation as described above (Table 70-3). In cases where malignancy is indeed likely, clinicians should be aware that cross-sectional imaging may underestimate the size and extent of the tumor by up to 40%. If the superior aspect of the left adrenal gland ascends behind the pancreatic body precluding safe exposure with simple retraction (i.e., in larger tumors), it is often necessary

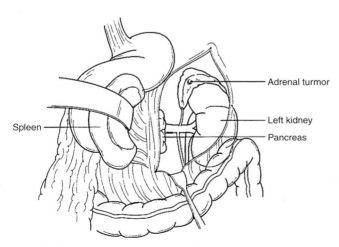

FIGURE 70-4. Left adrenalectomy. (Reprinted from Doherty GM, Skögseid B. *Surgical Endocrinology: A Clinical Syndromes Approach*. Philadelphia, PA: Lippincott Williams & Wilkins; 2001, with permission.)

Table 70-3	Open Adrenalectomy

Key Technical Steps

Ensure adequate IV access, availability of blood products, and appropriate monitoring

A bilateral subcostal incision typically provides the best exposure, although a midline laparotomy may be used in patients with a narrow costal angle, and a thoracoabdominal incision may be necessary for larger tumors with IVC invasion

Inspect and palpate to evaluate for metastasis

Right Adrenalectomy

1. Mobilize hepatic flexure and duodenum to expose vena cava
2. Retract liver superiorly and right kidney inferiorly
3. Mobilize right adrenal gland from retroperitoneal fat including a margin
4. Ligate and divide right adrenal vein (superomedial)

Left Adrenalectomy

1. Enter the lesser sac through gastrocolic omentum
2. Incise peritoneum over inferior border of pancreas
3. Retract pancreatic body superior and left kidney inferiorly
4. Mobilize left adrenal gland from retroperitoneal fat including a margin
5. Ligate and divide left adrenal vein (inferomedial)

Potential Pitfalls

- Anticipate the need for multivisceral resection and/or IVC reconstruction preoperatively
- Avoid tumor manipulation to prevent catecholamine release (PC/PGL) or capsule rupture (ACC)
- Control the right adrenal vein cautiously as it is short, easily avulsed, and drains directly into the IVC
- Additional blood supply to the adrenal may come from the inferior phrenic pedicle (often more apparent on the left side)

to mobilize the spleen and splenic flexure of the colon or perform a complete left-sided medial visceral rotation. If the left adrenal gland is located more superiorly, the gastrohepatic ligament may be opened for additional exposure. In situations where multivisceral resection is not anticipated but organ invasion is demonstrated intraoperatively, an en bloc resection should be performed if technically feasible. If the tumor is not completely resectable or if disseminated peritoneal disease is identified, it may be advisable to abort the resection and proceed with chemoradiation therapy once the patient has recovered from exploration, rather than perform a highly morbid debulking procedure without knowing the behavioral characteristics of the patient's tumor over time.

● POSTOPERATIVE MANAGEMENT

Apart from routine management following major abdominal surgery, there are a number of special postoperative considerations involved for patients undergoing adrenal surgery. Patients with hypercortisolism preoperatively will have hypothalamic–pituitary–adrenal (HPA) axis suppression and often an atrophic contralateral adrenal gland, placing them at risk of postoperative adrenal insufficiency. Symptoms include refractory hypotension, ileus, fatigue, muscle weakness, hypoglycemia, and hyperkalemia. Perioperatively glucocorticoid support should be routinely initiated prior to development of clinical signs of adrenal insufficiency. Recovery of the HPA axis may take 12 to 18 months, and a carefully monitored deescalation of glucocorticoid replacement over this timeframe is necessary. In a patient with incomplete resection, the hypercortisolism may persist, but most other patients will require significant glucocorticoid replacement.

More than half of patients with ACC will suffer recurrence despite an adequate resection. Prognostic models for recurrence have been proposed but not yet validated. The most important prognostic factors are stage at diagnosis and completeness of resection. A myriad of additional molecular prognostic markers are under investigation. Of these, Ki67 > 10% appears to have the most reliable association with decrease in disease-free survival. Patients at elevated risk for recurrence are typically treated with adjuvant mitotane, a derivative of DDT with adrenolytic and antisteroidogenic properties that has demonstrated efficacy in decreasing rates of recurrence and prolonging recurrence-free survival. Mitotane has a narrow therapeutic index with a challenging pharmacokinetic profile and poorly tolerated gastrointestinal and neurological side effects. Mitotane also induces P450-3A4, accounting for numerous drug–drug interactions, and its antisteroidogenic properties can necessitate glucocorticoid replacement during therapy (and often for some time after discontinuation). Patients are typically treated with adjuvant mitotane for at least 2 years following resection. Patients with stage III disease, close margins, or an R1 resection not amenable to reexploration are commonly offered external-beam radiation in addition to mitotane based on retrospective data suggesting significantly higher risk of local recurrence without radiation. Following complete resection of ACC, long-term surveillance is recommended for 10 years. During the first 2 years, cross-sectional imaging and a steroid panel is recommended every 3 months, but intervals may be lengthened subsequently.

Our patient underwent open right adrenalectomy with renal hilar and posterior caval lymphadenectomy. An R0 resection was achieved, and pathology demonstrated a 6 cm tumor with capsular and vascular invasion, a mitotic rate of 18/50HPFs, and Ki-67 25% (T3N0M0). Adjuvant EB-XRT and mitotane were recommended.

TAKE HOME POINTS

- A new adrenal mass requires hormonal and malignancy workup.
- When malignancy is suspected, refer to a tertiary care center with extensive experience.
- Always rule out pheochromocytoma biochemically before ordering additional studies, including imaging.
- A percutaneous biopsy of an adrenal mass is only indicated in rare circumstances, and pheochromocytoma must be ruled out first.
- An R0 resection with adherence to oncologic principles is the only curative modality for ACC, and decades-long survival can be seen with appropriate initial care.
- Avoid laparoscopy when the likelihood of ACC is high.
- Patients with glucocorticoid-producing tumors have profound HPA axis suppression and require prolonged glucocorticoid replacement.
- Mitotane has a narrow therapeutic index and requires close monitoring during therapy.
- Resected ACC patients need frequent long-term postoperative surveillance for recurrence.

SUGGESTED READINGS

Ayala-ramirez M, Jasim S, Feng L, et al. Adrenocortical carcinoma: clinical outcomes and prognosis of 330 patients at a tertiary care center. *Eur J Endocrinol.* 2013;169(6):891-899.

Berruti A, Baudin E, Gelderblom H, et al. Adrenal cancer: ESMO Clinical Practice Guidelines for diagnosis, treatment and follow-up. *Ann Oncol.* 2012;23(suppl 7):vii131-vii138.

Fassnacht M, Johanssen S, Fenske W, et al. Improved survival in patients with stage II adrenocortical carcinoma followed up prospectively by specialized centers. *J Clin Endocrinol Metab.* 2010;95(11):4925-4932.

Fassnacht M, Johanssen S, Quinkler M, et al. Limited prognostic value of the 2004 International Union Against Cancer staging classification for adrenocortical carcinoma: proposal for a revised TNM classification. *Cancer.* 2009;115(2):243-250.

Fassnacht M, Terzolo M, Allolio B, et al. Combination chemotherapy in advanced adrenocortical carcinoma. *N Engl J Med.* 2012;366(23):2189-2197.

Huynh KT, Lee DY, Lau BJ, Flaherty DC, Lee J, Goldfarb M. Impact of Laparoscopic Adrenalectomy on Overall Survival in Patients with Nonmetastatic Adrenocortical Carcinoma. *J Am Coll Surg.* 2016;223(3):485-492.

Kerkhofs TM, Verhoeven RH, Van der Zwan JM, et al. Adrenocortical carcinoma: a population-based study on incidence and survival in the Netherlands since 1993. *Eur J Cancer.* 2013;49(11):2579-2586.

Mcduffie LA, Aufforth RD. Adrenocortical carcinoma: modern management and evolving treatment strategies. *Int J Endocr Oncol.* 2016;3(2):161-174.

Miller BS, Doherty GM. Surgical management of adrenocortical tumours. *Nat Rev Endocrinol.* 2014;10(5):282-292.

Cortisol-secreting Adrenal Tumor

71

NAIRA BAREGAMIAN AND CARMEN C. SOLÓRZANO

Based on the previous edition chapter "Cortisol-secreting Adrenal Tumor" by
Hari R. Kumar and Judiann Miskulin

Presentation

A 46-year-old female presents with an enlarging left adrenal mass that was incidentally discovered on CT scan 2 years prior. She had a partial hepatectomy for a benign hemangioma. She reports headaches, anxiety, leg cramps, persistent left flank pain, unintentional weight loss, and a history of renal calculi. She lacks signs and symptoms of hypercortisolism, including weight gain, moon facies, purple stretch marks, thinning of skin, bruising, acne, fatigue, muscle weakness, and glucose intolerance. CT scan revealed a 2.6-cm left adrenal mass that has increased in size from 1.5-cm 2 years prior. Biochemical workup revealed elevated serum cortisol level after overnight dexamethasone suppression, elevated urinary free cortisol, and suppressed ACTH level.

● DIFFERENTIAL DIAGNOSIS

The most common cause of hypercortisolism is iatrogenic exogenous glucocorticoid administration to treat a variety of medical conditions. Once synthetic sources are excluded, endogenous causes of excess cortisol production include: (1) hypersecretion of adrenocorticotropic hormone (ACTH) from the pituitary (Cushing's disease), (2) adrenal-based hypercortisolism due to a single benign or malignant adrenal tumor, or bilateral adrenal hyperplasia, and (3) ectopic ACTH-producing tumors.

● WORKUP

The initial step in diagnosing hypercortisolism is to complete a biochemical workup. Screening tests to detect excess cortisol include: 24-hour urine collection for free cortisol, overnight low-dose (1 mg) oral dexamethasone suppression test, or measurement of midnight plasma and/or salivary cortisol levels. Human serum levels of cortisol demonstrate diurnal variation with peak levels occurring around 1 hour after waking (8 AM or so) and nadir at midnight. If evidence of excess cortisol is encountered, the next step is to determine if hypercortisolism is ACTH-dependent or independent. Low (<10) or undetectable serum ACTH levels suggest an adrenal source, whereas normal to high levels of ACTH suggest a pituitary or

an ectopic source. This patient's biochemical profile was consistent with an adrenal source (Elevated urine free cortisol = 109 mcg/24 hours, suppressed ACTH < 5 pg/mL).

Adrenal imaging with CT scan or MRI will help differentiate an adrenal tumor from bilateral adrenal hyperplasia. If on the scan a discrete tumor is confirmed, specific adrenal protocol CT or MRI can be used to further distinguish a benign adenoma from other adrenal neoplasms. This patient's adrenal tumor demonstrated low Hounsfield unit (HU) attenuation, suggestive of an adenoma (<10). Benign adrenal neoplasms tend to have low attenuation on unenhanced CT images due to their high lipid content. On CT scan, benign adenomas, adrenal metastases, primary adrenocortical carcinomas (ACC), and pheochromocytomas will have increasing degree of enhancement with IV contrast; however, after a 10-minute postcontrast administration period, washout of contrast in excess of 50% is seen in benign lesions. This patient's CT and MRI scans of the abdomen are shown in Figure 71-1, and resected adrenal lesion is depicted in Figure 71-2.

Biopsy of adrenal masses is typically not warranted, unless the patient has a personal history of cancer and adrenal metastases are suspected. Furthermore, a biopsy should be undertaken only if it will change management. Otherwise, once the diagnosis of a functional adrenal lesion has been made, the patient should be offered adrenalectomy.

● DIAGNOSIS AND TREATMENT

Hypercortisolism produces a wide rage of signs and symptoms known as Cushing's syndrome, including asymmetrical weight gain (truncal obesity, "buffalo hump," "moon facies"), hyperglycemia, hypertension, skin changes (striae, fragility, bruising, thinning, impaired wound healing), osteoporosis, mood lability, and sexual hormone imbalance (hirsutism, irregular menses, decreased libido, and impotence). Cortisol synthesis is regulated by the hypothalamic–pituitary–adrenal gland (HPA axis) feedback. Cortisol is essential in mediating stress response and affects the cardiovascular, metabolic, immunologic, and other systems.

This patient had subclinical autonomous glucocorticoid hypersecretion, which was characterized by unclear signs or symptoms of Cushing's syndrome, an incidentally discovered adrenal mass and two distinct alterations in the HPA axis. Interestingly, she had renal calculi, which have been observed in higher frequency in patients with hypercortisolism.

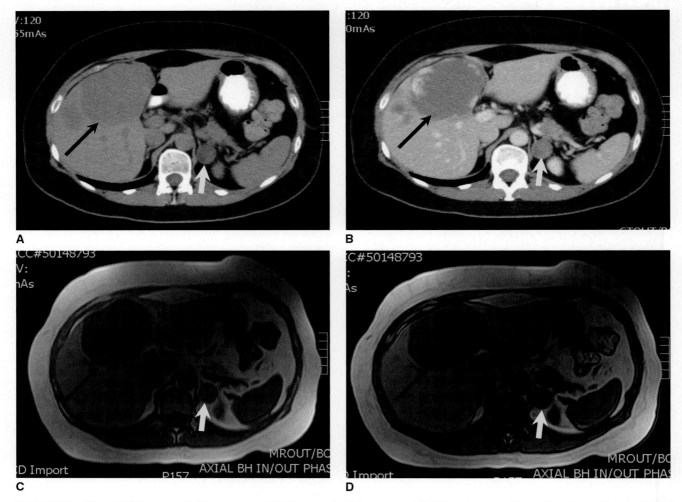

FIGURE 71-1. CT and MRI images. **A:** Noncontrasted CT image of a 2.6-cm mass left adrenal mass with very low Hounsfield units (HU) (*yellow arrow*) and nonenhanced liver hemangioma (*black arrow*). **B:** IV contrast-enhanced CT image of the same left adrenal mass (*yellow arrow*) and liver hemangioma (*black arrow*). **C:** In phase MRI image of the left adrenal mass (*yellow arrow*) and liver hemangioma (*black arrow*). **D:** Out of phase MRI image demonstrating signal dropout consistent with an adrenal adenoma (*yellow arrow*).

● SURGICAL APPROACH

Adrenal glands are retroperitoneal organs and can be approached by multiple surgical routes. Open anterior, posterior, flank, and thoracoabdominal approaches have all been well described in the past. Today, laparoscopic transabdominal adrenalectomy is the most commonly used approach.

Most patients with adrenal tumors can undergo a laparoscopic resection. Such approach is associated with shorter hospitalization, less pain and morbidity, quicker recovery, and low incidence of incisional hernias. An absolute contraindication to laparoscopic adrenalectomy is extension of the tumor into nearby structures. A relative contraindication is tumor size. From a practical standpoint, tumors >6 to 8-cm may be more difficult to mobilize and manipulate and can often result in conversion to an open procedure. In patients with suspected ACC with possible local invasion, an open approach is prudent to avoid capsule violation.

The following sections describe the more common surgical approaches to adrenalectomy: laparoscopic transabdominal, retroperitoneoscopic, robotic transabdominal, and open anterior techniques. In the case of our patient who underwent a prior liver resection, we performed a left retroperitoneoscopic adrenalectomy. Key technical steps and potential pitfalls are described in Table 71-1.

Laparoscopic Transabdominal Technique

The patient is placed on a beanbag in the lateral decubitus position. The table is flexed in order to open up the space between the costal margin and the iliac crest. The ports are placed close to the costal margin, in a line that approximates the standard open subcostal incision. A 12-mm camera port can be placed either in the middle with two 5-mm working

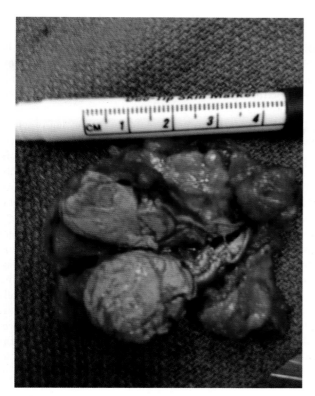

FIGURE 71-2. Typical gross appearance of an adrenocortical adenoma. The adrenal gland was bisected on the back table of the operating room to reveal the yellow cortical tumor.

Table 71-1	Adrenalectomy

Key Technical Steps

Left Adrenalectomy

1. Release lateral attachments of spleen and splenic flexure of colon to achieve medial mobilization and renal hilum exposure.
2. Dissect plane between adrenal gland and left renal vein.
3. Identify adrenal vein and inferior phrenic vein and divide close to the adrenal gland. Be aware of anatomic variations (drainage to vena cava or duplications).
4. Mobilize adrenal gland circumferentially.

Right Adrenalectomy

1. Dissect right triangular ligament of liver to the level of hepatic vein (less extensively for smaller adrenal lesions).
2. For large lesions, retract liver anteriorly and medially. If the lesion is small, cephalad liver retraction may be sufficient.
3. Dissect plane between adrenal gland and inferior vena cava.
4. Identify the right adrenal vein and divide. Be aware of anatomic variations (duplicate/triplicate venous drainage or drainage into hepatic veins).
5. Mobilize adrenal gland circumferentially.

Potential Pitfalls

- Avulsion of the right adrenal vein.
- Injury to right hepatic or caudate veins.
- Injury to renal vein.
- Injury to the renal arteries.
- Injury to the pancreas.
- Injury to the colon.
- Injury to the liver or spleen.

ports placed on either side or toward the umbilicus to avoid instrument collision during the operation.

For right-sided lesions, a fourth port is helpful to retract the liver. In order to mobilize the liver, the right triangular ligament should be taken down. The dissection begins laterally and proceeds medially until the inferior vena cava is identified. Retraction of the liver in an anterior cephalad fashion will allow for adequate exposure of the retroperitoneal space where the adrenal gland lies. Gerota's fascia can then be opened. Blunt dissection between inferior vena cava and the medial aspect of the adrenal gland will identify the right adrenal vein that is then clipped and divided. Avulsion of the adrenal vein from the cava should be avoided during this step. When a smaller caliber adrenal vein is encountered, one should look for a second adrenal vein proximally. The remaining small vessels can usually be controlled with electrocautery or ultrasonic shears. Once the adrenal gland is freed from the surrounding structures, it is placed in an endoscopic specimen bag and removed.

For left-sided lesions, the port placement is similar, though a fourth retracting port may not be necessary. The spleen and splenic flexure of the colon are taken down from their lateral attachments. Once the spleen has been mobilized medially, the plane of dissection continues posterior to the pancreatic body until the superior aspect of the adrenal is identified. The dissection should then continue at the junction of the adrenal and left renal

vein. The left adrenal vein usually empties into the left renal vein and should be ligated and divided close to the adrenal gland to avoid left renal vein injury. The phrenic vein will join the adrenal vein and may need to be ligated. The gland can then be mobilized circumferentially and removed.

Retroperitoneoscopic Technique

The patient is placed in a prone position, a 10-mm incision is made under the tip of the 12th rib, the fascia is entered sharply, and the retroperitoneum is accessed with finger dissection (Figure 71-3). A lateral 5-mm port is placed under the costal margin and aimed toward a finger placed inside the above 10-mm port site to avoid organ injury. A medial 10-mm port is then placed 3 cm caudal to the junction of

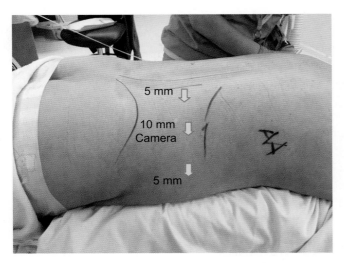

FIGURE 71-3. Port placement for a laparoscopic posterior retroperitoneoscopic right adrenalectomy (robotic or laparoscopic).

the 12th rib and the spine, near the lateral border of paraspinous muscle. A balloon port is placed in the port under the 12th rib, and insufflation is started at 20 mm Hg (up to 30). The camera is introduced into this port and Gerota's fascia dissected bluntly. The blue layer of peritoneum is seen lateral overlying the spleen or the left (or the liver on the right), while the paraspinous muscle is seen medially. Once this triangulating view is achieved, the camera is switched to the medial port looking down. The kidney is retracted caudally. The tissue above the kidney is dissected off from lateral to medial until the adrenal vein is localized. The left adrenal vein is clipped and divided. The adrenal gland is freed from the surrounding attachments. The EndoCatch bag is used via the middle port to exteriorize the adrenal gland. Desufflation and reinsufflation can be used to look for bleeding.

Robotic Transabdominal Technique

The patient positioning is similar to the laparoscopic transabdominal approach. Port placement is modified to allow for robot docking and to avoid instrument collision moving away for the costal margin. The abdomen is entered using the Optiview technique in the infraumbilical position with a 5-mm port, and insufflated to 14 to 16 mm Hg pressure. Next, a 10-mm camera port is placed under direct vision near the anterior axillary lateral to the umbilical line. Two 8-mm triangulating robotic ports are placed one lateral and one subxiphoid, with an additional 5-mm assistant port placed just below the subxiphoid robotic port for retraction. The robot is docked (Figure 71-4). The splenic flexure of the colon is taken down to expose the left kidney and its hilum. The pancreas and spleen are medialized and retracted by the assistant. Once adrenal tissue is visualized, it is pushed down toward a kidney in order to separate its most superior aspect from the pancreas. Next, the area of the kidney hilum is carefully dissected to identify and isolate the left adrenal vein. Once the adrenal vein is ligated and divided, the adrenal gland is carefully elevated off retroperitoneum. The gland is placed in the endocatch bad and exteriorized via the camera port.

Open Anterior Transabdominal Technique

The patient is supine. Either a subcostal or a midline incision can be utilized. The authors prefer a subcostal approach as it provides additional exposure, which is often needed for large tumors and en bloc resections (Figure 71-5).

On the right side, Kocherization of the duodenum and right colon/hepatic flexure mobilization will provide additional exposure. If liver or renal invasion is found, a hepatectomy and nephrectomy may also be required. If the inferior vena cava is involved, IVC resection and

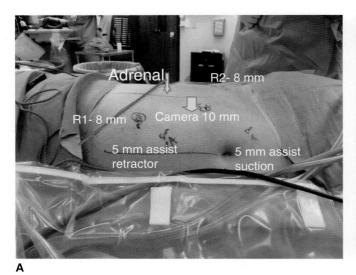

A

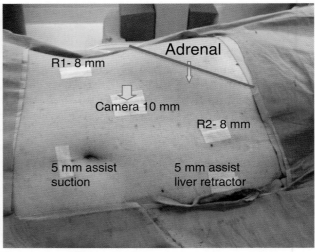

B

FIGURE 71-4. Robotic transabdominal adrenalectomy port placement. **A:** Left-sided port placement (*costal margin orange line*). **B:** Right-sided port placement.

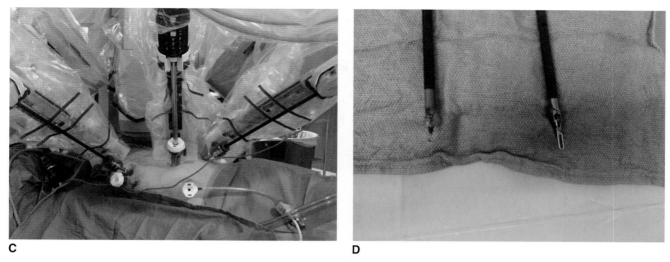

C   **D**

FIGURE 71-4. (*Continued*) **C:** Docked robotic arms in a left adrenalectomy. **D:** Robotic endo-wrist instruments, a hook and fenestrated bipolar.

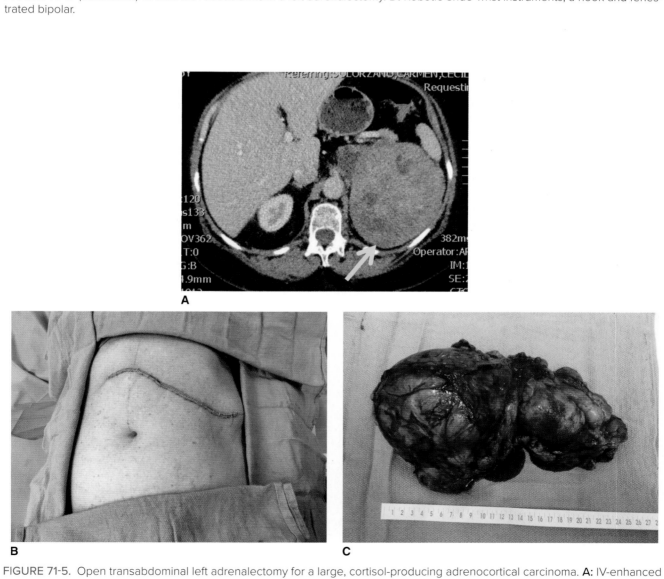

A

B   **C**

FIGURE 71-5. Open transabdominal left adrenalectomy for a large, cortisol-producing adrenocortical carcinoma. **A:** IV-enhanced CT image of a large cortisol-producing adrenocortical carcinoma (*yellow arrow*). **B:** Left subcostal incision for open radical adrenalectomy. **C:** En bloc resection of the large adrenocortical carcinoma involving the left kidney.

tumor thrombectomy with reconstruction may be needed. Description of complex multiorgan resections is beyond the scope of this chapter.

On the left side, take down of the colon splenic flexure and medial visceral rotation of the spleen and pancreas are necessary. The adrenal vein is controlled, and the tumor is removed.

● POSTOPERATIVE MANAGEMENT

Our patient tolerated a left retroperitoneoscopic adrenalectomy and was discharged the following day. Pathologic specimen measured 3.5 cm and was consistent with an adrenal adenoma (Figure 71-2). Typically, a laparoscopic approach to adrenalectomy is well-tolerated, and patients leave hospital within one or two days. Patients should be monitored for Addisonian crisis. Signs and symptoms can include nausea, dizziness, mental status changes, hypotension, hypoglycemia, and proximal muscle weakness. These symptoms occur as a result of chronic suppression of the HPA axis, leading to a state of relative hypocortisolism. The day of operation and postoperatively, patients should be supplemented with stress doses of steroids, followed by a taper regimen to oral maintenance doses. This steroid replacement (hydrocortisone or dexamethasone) regimen should be continued until the HPA axis can recover. A selective approach to steroid replacement can be used by performing a Cosyntropin test on postoperative day one, and if adequate cortisol response is detected the patient may be discharged without replacement therapy.

Biochemical recovery often lags behind clinical recovery. Discontinuation of steroid replacement therapy may take up to several months after a unilateral adrenalectomy. Typically, most of the physical and physiologic effects of hypercortisolism will improve after surgery over time, including hypertension and diabetes, and it is important to follow these patients long-term.

Case Conclusion

Our patient was placed on steroid replacement therapy, and cortisol production improved to nearly normal levels over 18 months.

TAKE HOME POINTS

- Biochemical workup for hypercortisolism in all patients with adrenal masses.
- Elevated cortisol level with suppression of ACTH production indicates an adrenal source of hypercortisolism.
- CT scan with and without contrast using adrenal protocol is our preferred approach to characterize adrenal neoplasms.
- When possible, all biochemically functional adrenal masses should be resected.
- A laparoscopic approach, whether transabdominal, retroperitoneal, or robotic, is the preferred method of adrenalectomy unless the tumor is large or involves nearby structures, which can then mandate an open approach.
- Postoperative management often includes a steroid supplementation regimen due to suppression of the HPA axis.
- Biochemical recovery and resolution of symptoms is gradual and may take up to 4 years.

SUGGESTED READINGS

Agcaoglu O, Sahin DA, Siperstein A, Berber E. Selection algorithm for posterior versus lateral approach in laparoscopic adrenalectomy. *Surgery.* 2012;151(5):731-735.

Brunt LM, Doherty GM, Norton JA, et al. Laparoscopic adrenalectomy compared to open adrenalectomy for benign adrenal neoplasms. *J Am Coll Surg.* 1996;183:1-10.

Grumbach MM, Biller BM, Braunstein GD, et al. Management of the clinically inapparent adrenal mass ("incidentaloma"). *Ann Intern Med.* 2003;138(5):424-429.

Kiernan CM, Shinall MC, Solorzano CC, et al. Influence of adrenal pathology on perioperative outcomes: a multi-institutional analysis. *Am J Surg.* 2014;208(4):619-625.

Morelli L, Tartaglia D, Bronzoni J, Mosca F, et al. Robotic assisted versus pure laparoscopic surgery of the adrenal glands: a case-control study comparing surgical techniques. *Langenbecks Arch Surg.* 2016;401:999-1066.

Ortiz DI, Findling JW, Carroll TB, et al. Cosyntropin stimulation testing on postoperative day 1 allows for selective glucocorticoid replacement therapy after adrenalectomy for hypercortisolism: Results of a novel, multidisciplinary institutional protocol. *Surgery.* 2016;159(1):259-265.

Shen WT, Sturgeon C, Duh QY. From incidentaloma to adrenocortical carcinoma: the surgical management of adrenal tumors. *J Surg Oncol.* 2005;89:186–192.

Sippel RS, Elaraj DM, Kebebew E, Lindsay S, Tyrrell JB, Duh QY. Waiting for change: symptom resolution after adrenalectomy for Cushing's syndrome. *Surgery.* 2008;144(6):1054-1060

Young WF Jr. Clinical practice. The incidentally discovered adrenal mass. *N Engl J Med.* 2007;356(6):601-610.

Zeiger MA, Thompson GB, Duh QY, et al. American Association of Clinical Endocrinologists and American Association of Endocrine Surgeons Medical Guidelines for the Management of Adrenal Incidentaloma. *Endocr Pract.* 2009;15(suppl 1):450-453.

Primary Aldosteronism

72

PRIYA H. DEDHIA AND BARBRA S. MILLER

Based on the previous edition chapter "Primary Hyperaldosteronism" by Barbra S. Miller

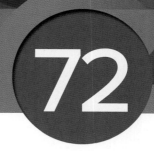

Presentation

A 45-year-old female is seen in her primary care physician's office with complaints of muscle cramps, fatigue, headaches, polyuria, polydipsia, and nocturia. She has a 10-year history of hypertension requiring four medications to achieve adequate blood pressure control. She also has long-standing hypokalemia, thought to be due to her diuretic, which is being treated with 60 mEq daily of supplemental oral potassium. She denies symptoms of chest pain, shortness of breath, or abdominal pain. She has had no episodes of flushing, tachycardia, tremors, or anxiety. Her vital signs are normal other than a blood pressure of 150/90. Her physical examination is unremarkable other than mild peripheral edema.

● DIFFERENTIAL DIAGNOSIS

Difficult-to-control hypertension should prompt investigation of secondary causes for hypertension. These include renal artery stenosis, primary aldosteronism, hyperthyroidism, intrinsic renal dysfunction, hypercortisolism, pheochromocytoma, sleep apnea, medications, and other supplements.

● WORKUP

A thorough history and physical examination should be completed, including specific questions related to symptomatology and family history of cardiac disorders, sudden death, or genetic syndromes leading to hypertension. Laboratory studies to evaluate secondary causes of hypertension include a complete metabolic profile, serum aldosterone and renin levels, and fractionated plasma metanephrines. Certain antihypertensives may confound laboratory results. Antihypertensives such as spironolactone, eplerenone, angiotensin-converting enzyme inhibitors, and diuretics affect renin–aldosterone regulation and should be discontinued for 4 to 6 weeks in advance of testing if possible. Alpha-blockers or amiloride may be substituted. Antidepressants and beta-blockers may affect plasma metanephrine levels, which should be considered when ruling out pheochromocytoma. Misdiagnosis of a pheochromocytoma and inadequate preoperative alpha blockade can lead to intraoperative complications and death.

If evidence of primary aldosteronism is identified, biochemical evaluation should be followed by radiologic evaluation of the adrenal glands. Imaging should not be obtained first without biochemical confirmation of the diagnosis, as many inconsequential "incidentalomas" are discovered on imaging studies. The adrenal glands best evaluated by adrenal protocol computed tomography (CT) may reveal normal glands, small abnormalities, thickening of the limbs of the glands, or obvious nodules. Concern for an aldosterone-producing adrenocortical carcinoma, which is extremely rare, can usually be ruled out based on size criteria and calculation of Hounsfield units (HU) of the tumor/nodule and contrast washout characteristics. Magnetic resonance images or NP-59 scans are alternative imaging modalities that may be requested.

Selective venous sampling of the bilateral adrenal veins should be obtained in most patients to biochemically investigate the unilateral or bilateral nature of excess aldosterone production (Figure 72-1). Adrenal venous sampling may not be needed in patients <35 years old with marked aldosterone excess, spontaneous hypokalemia, and unilateral adrenal adenoma because incidental adrenal nodules are rare in younger patients, but more data are needed. Venous sampling allows differentiation of unilateral from bilateral excess aldosterone production from the adrenal glands regardless of imaging findings, as CT and MRI findings tend not to correlate well with venous sampling results. Criteria suggesting unilateral excess aldosterone production are shown in Table 72-1.

● DIAGNOSIS AND TREATMENT

Primary aldosteronism is most commonly due to an aldosterone-producing adenoma or adrenal hyperplasia leading to difficult-to-control hypertension, volume excess, and hypokalemia. Primary aldosteronism is found in 5% to 13% of hypertensive patients. Hypokalemia is evident in <40% of patients with primary hyperaldosteronism. As such, the following patients should undergo testing for primary aldosteronism even if normokalemic: (1) those with severe hypertension (>150/100 resistant to three antihypertensive medications, mm Hg systolic or >100 mm Hg diastolic), (2) controlled blood pressure (<140/90) on four or more antihypertensive medications, (3) hypertension with adrenal incidentaloma, (4) hypertension with sleep apnea, and (5) hypertension with family history of early-onset hypertension or cerebrovascular

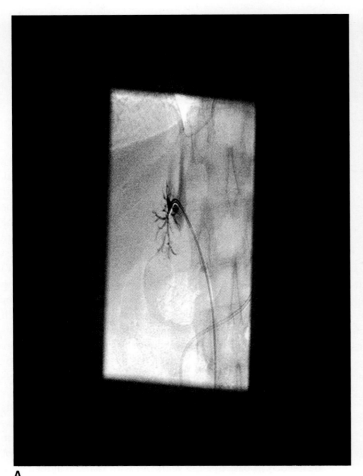
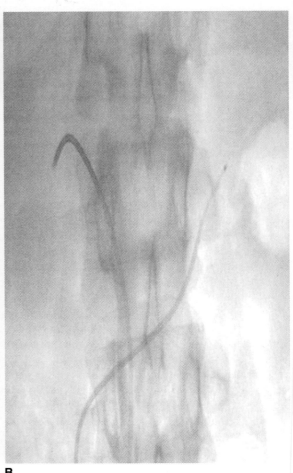

A   **B**

FIGURE 72-1. **A:** Contrast injection of right adrenal vein to confirm catheter placement prior to selective venous sampling. **B:** Catheters placed in bilateral adrenal veins.

Table 72-1	Criteria Used to Confirm Unilateral Excess Aldosterone Secretion After Bilateral Adrenal Vein Sampling	
Adrenal Vein Sampling		**Number**
Aldosterone and cortisol ratios		
Confirmation of catheter placement in adrenal vein		
Pre-cosyntropin adrenal vein C: IVC C		≥3
Lateralization		
Dominant A/C: Nondominant A/C		≥4
Supporting evidence		
Dominant A: Nondominant A		>3
Dominant A/C: IVC A/C		>1.5
Nondominant A/C: IVC A/C		<1

A, Aldosterone; C, Cortisol; A/C, aldosterone to cortisol ratio; IVC, inferior vena cava.

accident, and (6) all hypertensive first-degree relatives of someone with primary hyperaldosteronism.

Diagnosis of primary aldosteronism is suggested with identification of an elevated aldosterone level, suppressed renin level, and an aldosterone:renin ratio >20:1. Confirmatory testing should be pursued in most cases. Recognizing the inability to suppress aldosterone secretion after sodium loading or administration of captopril can be helpful in this setting. Diagnosis in patients younger than age 20 with a family history of primary aldosteronism should prompt consideration of genetic testing for familial hyperaldosteronism type 1 and testing for germ-line mutations in KCNJ5 causing familial hyperaldosteronism type 3 in very young patients.

Those patients found to have primary aldosteronism due to unilateral excess aldosterone production are usually offered surgery in an attempt to cure the disease, while those found to have bilateral production of excess aldosterone are managed medically with aldosterone receptor antagonists, as the risks of iatrogenically induced Addison's disease after bilateral adrenalectomy (despite steroid replacement) outweigh the risks of continued medical management (Figure 72-2). Selective venous sampling of the adrenal veins is imperative, especially

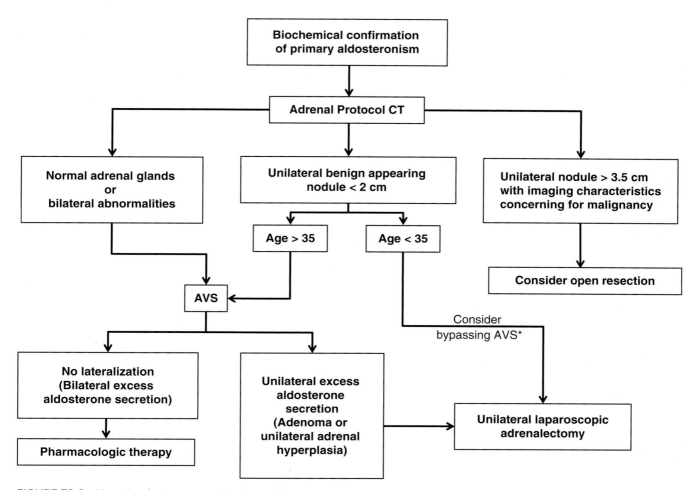

FIGURE 72-2. Algorithm for treatment of primary aldosteronism according to subtype. AVS, adrenal venous sampling. *AVS may not need to be performed in patients younger than 35 with a single benign-appearing adrenal adenoma if there is marked spontaneous hypokalemia, renin is suppressed, and aldosterone is markedly elevated.

for those with bilateral normal- or abnormal-appearing adrenal glands but also for most patients with a single adrenal nodule, as cases are described in which a nonfunctioning incidentaloma is noted on imaging studies with excess production coming from the contralateral normal-appearing adrenal gland. Adrenal venous sampling results should dictate which adrenal gland is removed rather than imaging results.

Laparoscopic resection of the affected adrenal gland has become the gold standard if malignancy is not suspected. In cases of adrenocortical carcinoma, laparoscopic resection has been associated with shorter time to local recurrence and a greater chance of margin-positive resections and is not recommended. Aldosterone-secreting adenomas seen on imaging studies are generally quite small with a median size <2 cm (Figure 72-3). Larger aldosterone-secreting adenomas are rare, and concern for an aldosterone-secreting adrenocortical malignancy (even more rare) is raised in those nodules >3 to 3.5 cm having other concerning imaging characteristics (HU, washout characteristics, in-phase/out-of-phase changes). This size criterion for concern for malignancy is smaller than the 4- to 6-cm criteria normally used for assessment of other adrenal nodules.

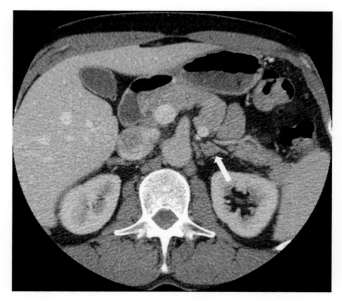

FIGURE 72-3. Typical, small, benign-appearing aldosterone-secreting adenoma in the left adrenal gland.

● SURGICAL APPROACH

The lateral transperitoneal approach to the adrenal gland is most commonly employed when performing a laparoscopic adrenalectomy. Other approaches include anterior, lateral retroperitoneal, and posterior retroperitoneoscopic. Open approaches (both anterior and posterior) may be used, but the laparoscopic approach has been shown to be associated with less pain, less morbidity, shorter hospital stay, and faster recovery.

Prior to operation, careful review of adrenal imaging should be undertaken to assess the position and course of the relevant vasculature including the adrenal veins, renal arteries, and veins. On the left side, the surgeon should note the proximity of the splenic flexure of the colon, spleen, tail of the pancreas, and the splenic artery and vein. Patients with primary aldosteronism should be prepared for surgery by correcting volume, metabolic abnormalities, and hypertension. Aldosterone receptor antagonists, such as spironolactone or eplerenone, are most useful and help correct hypertension and hypokalemia and reduce the need for other antihypertensive medications.

Left lateral transperitoneal laparoscopic adrenalectomy requires placement of the patient in the right lateral decubitus position (Table 72-2). Padding of pressure points is extremely important. The kidney rest is extended to widen the space between the pelvis and the rib cage. The left arm is extended to the right side. The peritoneal cavity is accessed in standard fashion at the junction of the lateral edge of the rectus muscle and the oblique musculature.

Once the abdomen is insufflated and examined using a 30-degree laparoscope, at least two other ports are placed in a triangulated position. Using scissors, cautery, or ultrasonic instruments, attachments of the splenic flexure of the colon and the spleen are released, and the spleen is rotated medially. The retroperitoneum is incised between the superior medial aspect of the kidney and the inferior lateral aspect of the adrenal gland. Using cautery, ultrasonic shears, and blunt dissection, the adrenal gland is mobilized from the retroperitoneal fat. At the superomedial aspect of the gland, the surgeon may encounter a branch from a phrenic vessel and should carefully ligate and divide this. Dissection at the inferior aspect should proceed cautiously to ensure no damage to the renal vessels. The adrenal vein will be found medially near a seven o'clock position draining into the renal vein. The adrenal vein should be ligated with clips and divided. The adrenal gland should be removed using an Endo-bag and inspected to ensure complete removal of the gland prior to being sent to pathology.

Right lateral transperitoneal laparoscopic adrenalectomy proceeds in a fashion similar to the left side. A fourth port is usually required to retract the right lobe of the liver using a paddle retractor after mobilizing the triangular and coronary ligaments. The right adrenal vein drains directly into the vena cava. Meticulous dissection along the vena cava is required to prevent massive bleeding.

● SPECIAL INTRAOPERATIVE CONSIDERATIONS

It may be difficult to identify the adrenal gland in obese patients with large quantities of retroperitoneal fat. The adrenal gland has a golden-rod yellow color that is darker than the surrounding fat. Laparoscopic ultrasound can be extremely helpful in these situations as well and can help identify the adrenal veins and renal vessels. On the left side, lobulations of pancreatic tissue may appear similar to adrenal tissue and be mistakenly removed although the pancreas is usually lighter in color than the adrenal gland. The splenic artery and vein are commonly visualized on the posterior surface of the pancreas. The specimen should be carefully inspected after removal to ensure the characteristic cortical and medullary tissue is identified upon incision of the gland. If at any time malignancy is suspected, convert to an open procedure. A potassium level should be checked in the preoperative area. Permissive hypokalemia to a mild degree in the operating room should be tolerated as rebound hyperkalemia may occur after resection of the adrenal gland. Communication about this between surgeon and anesthesiologist is important. If potassium supplementation is required pre- or intraoperatively, smaller than normal doses are preferred when administered.

Table 72-2	Lateral Transperitoneal Laparoscopic Adrenalectomy

Key Technical Steps

1. Position patient on beanbag in lateral decubitus position at 45-degree angle with appropriate padding over pressure points, extending bed to widen distance between rib cage and pelvis.
2. Access peritoneal cavity at lateral edge of rectus muscle and place ports in triangulated fashion.
3. Release lateral attachments of viscera from peritoneum and side wall, rolling viscera medially. A paddle retractor may be helpful, especially on the right side.
4. Dissect circumferentially around adrenal gland, ligating and dividing adrenal vein when convenient.
5. Laparoscopic ultrasound can be helpful to identify the adrenal gland in obese patients.
6. Remove specimen and inspect to confirm presence of nodule, cortical, and medullary tissue.
7. Confirm hemostasis and close port sites.

Potential Pitfalls

- Bleeding from adrenal vein, renal vein, IVC on right, splenic vessels on left.
- Removal of periadrenal fat or pancreatic tissue instead of adrenal gland.
- Laceration of liver, spleen, or perforation of other nearby viscera.

● POSTOPERATIVE MANAGEMENT

In general, patients do not require postoperative ICU management. Antihypertensive medications are held after surgery. Essential hypertension unrelated to primary aldosteronism may necessitate reinstitution of some medications. Factors including age of onset of hypertension, length of time with hypertension, and number of medications required to control the blood pressure preoperatively allow for prediction of resolution of hypertension and hypokalemia after surgery. Hypokalemia and need for potassium supplementation resolve within 24 hours, and patients may become hyperkalemic for a short time. Autodiuresis of excess volume from primary aldosteronism often occurs in the postoperative period. Most patients may be discharged on the first or second postoperative day. Aldosterone and renin levels should be checked at the postoperative visit and 2 to 3 months after surgery to ensure documented biochemical cure.

Case Conclusion

The patient is found to have an aldosterone:renin ratio of 38. CT reveals a 1.4-cm benign adenoma in the left adrenal gland. Selective venous sampling confirms unilateral excess aldosterone secretion with a dominant left A:C to nondominant right A:C ratio of 7. A left laparoscopic adrenalectomy is performed. Postoperatively, the patient's hypokalemia resolves; however, the blood pressure remains slightly elevated in the postoperative setting, and she is reinstituted on beta-blocker therapy for the perioperative period. At the postoperative visit, her blood pressure is 124/68, potassium is 4.0 mEq/L, aldosterone is 4, and renin is 1.4. Additional testing several months later remains consistent with biochemical cure.

TAKE HOME POINTS

- Secondary causes for hypertension should be sought in young patients or those with difficult to control blood pressure requiring more than three antihypertensive medications.
- Hypokalemia is not present in most patients (9% to 37%).
- Diagnosis of primary aldosteronism is by biochemical means, requiring an elevated aldosterone level and aldosterone:renin ratio >20:1. Confirmatory testing should be pursued in most cases.
- Selective venous sampling of the adrenal veins differentiates between unilateral and bilateral excess aldosterone secretion. Those with evidence of unilateral excess secretion should be offered surgery in most cases.
- Resection by a laparoscopic approach is the gold standard except in the case of malignancy.
- Resolution of hypertension is variable but predictable depending on age, severity of hypertension, and the degree to which essential hypertension contributes to the process.

SUGGESTED READINGS

Funder JW, Carey RM, Mantero F, et al. The management of primary aldosteronism: case detection, diagnosis, and treatment: an Endocrine Society Clinical Practice Guideline. *J Clin Endocrinol Metab.* 2016;101(5):1889-1916.

McKenzie TJ, Lillegard JB, Young WF Jr, et al. Aldosteronomas—state of the art. *Surg Clin North Am.* 2009;89(5):1241-1253.

Nwariaku F, Miller B, Auchus R, et al. Primary hyperaldosteronism: effect of adrenal vein sampling on surgical outcome. *Arch Surg.* 2006;141(5):497-502; discussion 502-503.

White ML, Gauger PG, Doherty GM, et al. The role of radiologic studies in the evaluation and management of primary hyperaldosteronism. *Surgery.* 2008;144(6):926-933.

Zarnegar R, Young WF Jr, Lee J, et al. The aldosteronoma resolution score: predicting complete resolution of hypertension after adrenalectomy for aldosteronoma. *Ann Surg.* 2008;247(3):511-518.

Pheochromocytoma

NATASHA HANSRAJ AND DOUGLAS J. TURNER

73

Based on the previous edition chapter "Pheochromocytoma" by Alexis D. Smith and Douglas J. Turner

Presentation

A 52-year-old male with a history of poorly controlled hypertension is referred for evaluation of a 4.5-cm left adrenal mass incidentally discovered during routine trauma computed tomography (CT) scans following a minor motor vehicle accident. Further questioning in your office reveals that he experiences episodic headaches with blurry vision, and occasional epistaxis, but denies any chest pain, palpitations, shortness of breath, or diaphoresis. He denies any history of recent weight gain or loss. He has no history of a prior cancer. He states his father died of sudden cardiac arrest in his 50s; his mother is alive and otherwise healthy. His antihypertensive regimen is currently nicardipine, lisinopril, metoprolol, and hydrochlorothiazide (HCTZ). On examination, blood pressure was 192/106 mm Hg; heart rate, 102 beats per minute; and body mass index, 29. The remainder of his examination was normal.

● DIFFERENTIAL DIAGNOSIS

Incidentally discovered adrenal masses are increasing in frequency during the current era of widespread use of thoracic and abdominal radiography. As imaging technology has evolved, adrenal incidentalomas have been reported in as high as 4% to 5% of all CT scans. In adults, an adrenal mass can represent an extensive differential diagnosis (Table 73-1). In order to determine the appropriate treatment of the mass, both biochemical testing and high-resolution imaging should be employed to differentiate between biochemically functional versus nonfunctional tumors, and malignant versus benign tumors.

● WORKUP

The patient subsequently undergoes initial evaluation of his adrenal incidentaloma with biochemical testing. Morning and 24-hour urinary cortisol levels are within normal limits. Additionally, plasma aldosterone:renin ratio is <20. Serum electrolytes are within normal limits. Subsequent 24-hour urinary fractionated metanephrines and plasma-free metanephrines return elevated at 1,800 nmol/24 hour and 2.6 nmol/L, respectively. Thus, the diagnosis of pheochromocytoma (PCC) is confirmed via biochemical testing. The patient then undergoes an adrenal–protocol CT scan for localization of the tumor that demonstrates a 4.5-cm left heterogeneous adrenal mass with a 60% contrast washout after 15 minutes.

● DIAGNOSIS AND TREATMENT

Pheochromocytomas (PCCs) are catecholamine-producing neuroendocrine tumors derived from chromaffin cells of the adrenal medulla. PCCs are rare tumors with a reported incidence of 2 to 8 per million individuals, occurring in 0.1% to 0.5% of hypertensive patients and in approximately 5% of patients with documented adrenal incidentalomas. However, the potentially lethal cardiovascular complications related to high levels of circulating catecholamines mandate biochemical testing for PCC in those found to have an adrenal incidentaloma as well as in the hypertensive population. Historically, PCC has been coined the "10% tumor" meaning that approximately 10% of cases are malignant, 10% extraadrenal, 10% bilateral, and 10% associated with hereditary tumor syndromes. However, recent literature has demonstrated that those approximations largely underestimate the incidence of hereditary PCCs and paragangliomas (PGs). Some studies have shown that up to 24% of cases are associated with familial tumor syndromes, including multiple endocrine neoplasia (MEN) types 2A and 2B, von Hippel-Lindau disease (VHL), neurofibromatosis type 1 (NF1), tuberous sclerosis, Sturge-Weber syndrome, and the familial PCC-paraganglioma (PGL) syndrome.

Table 73-1	Differential Diagnoses for Adrenal Incidentalomas	
Functioning Lesions	**Nonfunctioning Lesions**
Aldosteronoma	Cortical adenoma
Pheochromocytoma	Metastasis
Cortisol-producing adenoma (Cushing's disease)	Hemorrhage
Adrenocortical carcinoma	Cyst
Congenital adrenal hyperplasia	Infection: TB, fungal
Renin-secreting tumor	Myelolipoma
	Hemangioma

Sporadic PCC is most commonly diagnosed between the ages of 40 to 50, whereas hereditary PCC is usually diagnosed earlier, most often before 40 years of age. Twenty to thirty percent of PCC are discovered incidentally. The classic triad of symptoms associated with PCC consists of paroxysmal hypertension, palpitations, and sweating. However, the true clinical presentation of PCC varies greatly, and it is often termed a great mimicker of many other clinical conditions. Hypertension, tachycardia, pallor, headache, and anxiety usually dominate the clinical presentation. Paroxysmal signs and symptoms are a hallmark of the clinical presentation of PCC due to the episodic nature of catecholamine secretion from the tumor and are often incited by factors such as activity, stress, smoking, postural changes, anxiety, trauma, anesthesia, operative procedures, tumor manipulation, and medications.

Extra-adrenal PCC are termed paragangliomas and can be located anywhere along the sympathetic nervous system but are most commonly found at the organ of Zuckerkandl.

All patients with suspected PCC should undergo biochemical testing followed by high-resolution imaging for tumor localization and determination of the extent of disease. The preferred method of choice for biochemical assays remains a controversial topic. No current consensus exists on the best screening test and no prospective studies comparing test regimens have been published. However, current literature favors the measurement of plasma-free metanephrines and/or urinary-fractionated metanephrines for the most sensitive tests available for screening and diagnosis. However, these tests lack high specificity, and the common occurrence of false-positive results can be attributed to external stressors as well as drug and dietary interferences related to catecholamine measurements. Some common interfering substances include coffee, nicotine, labetalol, tricyclic antidepressants, and monoamine oxidase inhibitors (MAO-I). A clonidine suppression test may be utilized to confirm diagnosis in those patients with equivocal results. Fine needle aspiration (FNA) has no role in the diagnosis of PCC and should be avoided due to the risk of precipitation of a hypertensive crisis.

Once a biochemical diagnosis of PCC has been confirmed, tumor localization should be initiated in order to guide treatment planning. A CT scan of the abdomen, including pelvis (to below the level of the aortic bifurcation), is currently an appropriate initial imaging study with a >95% sensitivity for detecting adrenal PCCs. Characteristic findings include contrast uptake (40 to 50 HU) with delayed washout. Magnetic resonance imaging (MRI) is considered equally efficacious and is the procedure of choice in pregnancy and childhood with high intensity uptake on T2 imaging. A major advantage of MRI is the lack of exposure to both radiation as well as iodinated contrast, which has the potential to elicit a hypertensive crisis in patients. Since no certain histologic criteria that distinguish benign from malignant tumors exist, a critical step in the radiologic evaluation of a PCC is determination of malignancy as well as extra-adrenal extension or bilateral-

Table 73-2	Key Features on Diagnosing Pheochromocytomas

Clinical Features:

- Hypertension—paroxysmal stimulated by activity, stress, surgery, anesthesia, tumor manipulation
- Sweating
- Palpitations
- Others: tachycardia, anxiety, impending doom
- High suspicion: HTN during anesthesia, resistant HTN, <25-year old with new HTN

Laboratory Tests:

- Plasma-free metanephrines (most sensitive)
- 24-h urinary catecholamine

Imaging Tests:

- CT: increased contrast uptake with delayed washout with necrosis and calcification.
- MRI: bright lesion on T2
- MIBG—for metastasis and recurrence
- PET CT—for metastasis and recurrence

Genetic Tests:

- VHL—missense mutation—elevated normetanephrines
- NF—tumor suppressor NF 1 mutation—elevated metanephrines
- MEN 2—RET mutation—elevated metanephrines
- TMEN127
- MAX
- SDHB, SDHD—mutation in succinate dehydrogenase—elevated normetanephrines + methoxytyramine

ity. Malignancy is reported in 9% of sporadic PCC and as high as 33% in extra-adrenal PCC. PCCs that secrete only dopamine have also been noted to be at increased risk of malignancy. Therefore, functional imaging in the form of metaiodobenzylguanidine (MIBG) scanning is warranted if there exists a high probability of malignancy noted by the presence of local invasion, metastases, adrenal lesions >5 cm, extra-adrenal lesions, and contrast washout of <40% in 15 minutes on cross-sectional imaging. A review of the clinical features and of the biochemical and imaging studies is listed in Table 73-2.

● SURGICAL APPROACH

Surgical resection is the only effective treatment for PCC. Due to the high concentration of circulating catecholamines, cardiovascular lability is frequently a complicating factor during resection of these tumors. The likelihood of surgical success directly correlates to the degree of preoperative medical management. The goals of this regimen include correction of hypertension, restoration of intravascular volume, and control of dysrhythmias. The foundation of this regimen is alpha blockade, most typically phenoxybenzamine, a long-acting nonselective alpha antagonist initially dosed at 10 mg per day or twice daily with incremental increases to attain appropriate blood pressure control. A subsequent beta-blocker is added for heart rate control secondary to reflex tachycardia associated with alpha-blockade or for tachyarrhythmias. Monotherapy or initiation of therapy with a beta-blocker should be avoided due to the risk of a hypertensive crisis in the absence of β_2-adrenergic vasodilation. Calcium channel blockers may be utilized as a third agent for persistent hypertension. Some institutions prefer the use of shorter-acting selective alpha$_1$-blockers, such as doxazosin or terazosin, secondary to their avoidance of reflex tachycardia. However, no prospective head-to-head comparison trial has been done, and phenoxybenzamine remains the mainstay for alpha blockade.

In addition to adequate preoperative blood pressure control, patients should be instructed about the importance of increased fluid and salt intake prior to surgery in order to assist with repletion of intravascular volume, which is low due to the vasoconstriction accompanying their disease.

The principles of successful surgical resection of a PCC are minimization of tumor manipulation, avoidance of tumor spillage, complete extirpation of the tumor, early ligation of the adrenal vein, and close coordination with the anesthesiology team for tight control of intraoperative hemodynamics (Table 73-3). Traditionally, an open approach was utilized due to the theory of an increased risk of catecholamine surge with insufflation and tumor manipulation during laparoscopic adrenalectomy. However, over the past decade, laparoscopy has evolved as the standard of care for surgical resection of PCC especially if <6 cm and without features of malignancy.

Although multiple approaches to an adrenalectomy have been described, including open versus laparoscopic supine and lateral transabdominal as well as posterior and lateral retroperitoneal, our institution prefers the laparoscopic lateral transabdominal approach initially described by Gagner in 1992. Following induction of general anesthesia and placement of appropriate hemodynamic monitoring devices in the form of an arterial line and central line, the patient is placed in the lateral decubitus position, and the operating table is flexed at the waist to optimize the space between the lower ribs and iliac crest. A Veress needle is used to establish pneumoperitoneum. Four ports are placed between the midclavicular lines anteriorly and the midaxillary line laterally, two finger widths below the costal margin. The abdomen is inspected for hepatic or peritoneal metastases. For a right adrenalectomy, the right triangular ligament is divided, and the liver is mobilized from the diaphragm, retracting it cephalad with a fan or snake retractor; it is important to be able to visualize the inferior vena cava (IVC). It is rarely necessary to mobilize the hepatic flexure or duodenum. The adrenal gland is identified on the superomedial aspect of the kidney, and the right adrenal vein is identified at its junction with the IVC. Early identification and ligation of the adrenal

Table 73-3	Laparoscopic Adrenalectomy

Key Technical Steps

1. Pneumoperitoneum established with Veress needle
2. Three or four ports placed between midclavicular line and midaxillary line, two finger widths below the costal margin
3. Right adrenalectomy—right triangular ligament divided and mobilized cephalad. Left adrenalectomy—splenic flexure mobilized, lateral attachments of spleen and tail of pancreas mobilized medially
4. Adrenal gland identified on superomedial aspect of the kidney
5. Adrenal vein identified at its junction with either the IVC (right adrenal vein) or left renal vein (left adrenal vein)
6. Double-clip adrenal vein proximally and divide sharply
7. Continue hemostatic division of remaining arterial branches and soft tissue attachments
8. Endo-retrieval bag for removal of specimen

Potential Pitfalls

- Hypertensive crisis upon induction of anesthesia or excessive tumor manipulation
- Bleeding secondary to adrenal vein, renal vein, or IVC injury
- Hemodynamic instability following ligation of the adrenal vein

vein is paramount. It is double clipped on the IVC aspect and divided sharply with endoscopic scissors. Division of the adrenal vein may also be accomplished with a vascular stapler. The vein is often on the posterior aspect of the vena cava, and occasionally, there are accessory adrenal veins that require clipping. Hemostasis is difficult to achieve if a vein injury ensues, and retraction of the vein into the surrounding tissue may result in large volume blood loss and conversion to an open procedure. The remaining arterial branches and soft tissue attachments are then divided hemostatically. The specimen is placed in an endo-retrieval bag and brought through one of the port sites.

For a left laparoscopic adrenalectomy, patient positioning and port insertion are approached in a similar manner, although three ports often suffice on the left side. The retroperitoneum is opened by dividing the splenocolic ligament. The splenic flexure is mobilized. The lateral attachments of the spleen and the tail of the pancreas are divided for their medial mobilization. The adrenal gland is identified superior to the kidney under the mobilized pancreas and spleen. The left adrenal vein is identified when it emerges from the inferomedial aspect of the gland near to where it empties into the left renal vein. It is double clipped on the renal vein aspect and sharply divided. Any accessory adrenal veins should be handled in a similar manner.

SPECIAL INTRAOPERATIVE CONSIDERATIONS

Hemodynamic fluctuations are a common intraoperative occurrence during resection of a PCC. Open communication with the anesthesia team is a critical component of surgical success. During induction of anesthesia, insufflation with carbon dioxide, and tumor manipulation prior to ligation of the adrenal vein, the patient often experiences severe hypertension and tachyarrhythmias requiring intravenous titratable medications such as nitroprusside, nicardipine, or phentolamine (short-acting alpha blockers), with sodium nitroprusside preferred due to its rapid vasodilator effects, shorter acting and easy titration. The anesthesiologists should be notified prior to ligation of the adrenal gland is ordered to anticipate and prepare for a precipitous drop in blood pressure following abrupt cessation of the catecholamine source with large volume fluid resuscitation and vasoactive pressor support.

POSTOPERATIVE CARE

Postoperative patients require monitoring for hypotension and hypoglycemia. The average stay for patients following an uncomplicated laparoscopic adrenalectomy is approximately 2 days. Levels should be monitored every 3 months during the first year and then annually for at least 5 years. No consensus exists for extent of postoperative follow-up. Patients diagnosed with hereditary PCC should undergo yearly follow-up for their lifetime.

Case Conclusion

The patient underwent a successful laparoscopic left adrenalectomy without any postoperative pressor requirement or intensive care unit admission. He was subsequently discharged to home on postoperative day number 3. Surveillance plasma metanephrine taken 3 months following the operation was within normal limits. The patient opted for genetic testing secondary to his father's history of sudden cardiac death but returned negative for any germ-line mutations.

TAKE HOME POINTS

- Pheochromocytoma (PCC) continues to be a rare catecholamine-producing neuroendocrine tumor responsible for a surgically correctable cause of hypertension.
- The incidence of hereditary PCC has largely been underestimated with recent studies demonstrating up to a 24% association with familial tumor syndromes including MEN2a, MEN2b, NF1, and VHL syndromes.
- Plasma metanephrine levels (sensitivity of 99%) can biochemically confirm the diagnosis, and CT scans are utilized for tumor localization.
- Laparoscopic adrenalectomy has evolved as the standard of care for surgical resection of a PCC.
- Surgical resection is the treatment of choice for malignant PCC with curative intent for local disease and palliation in more advanced disease.

SUGGESTED READINGS

Amar L, Fassnacht M, Gimenez-Roqueplo AP, Januszewicz A, Prejbisz A, Timmers H, et al. Long-term postoperative follow-up in patients with apparently benign pheochromocytoma and paraganglioma. *Horm Metab Res.* 2012;44(5):385-389.

Groeben H. Preoperative α–receptor block in patients with pheochromocytoma? Against. *Chirurg.* 2012;83:551-554.

Juszczak K, Drewa T. Adrenergic crisis due to pheochromocytoma—practical aspects. A short review. *Cent European J Urol.* 2014;67(2):153-155.

Namekawa T, Utsumi T, Kawamura K, Kamiya N, Imamoto T, Takiguchi T, et al. Clinical predictors of prolonged postresection hypotension after laparoscopic adrenalectomy for pheochromocytoma. *Surgery.* 2016;159(3):763-770.

Nieman LK. Approach to the patient with an adrenal incidentaloma. *J Clin Endocrinol Metab.* 2010;95(9):4106-4113.

Nimeri AA, Brunt LM. Adrenalectomy. In: Ashley SW, Cance WG, Chen H, et al., eds. *ACS Surgery: Principles and practice.* 7th ed. Decker Intellectual Properties, 2014.

Shuch B, Ricketts CJ, Metwalli AR, Pacak K, Linehan WM. The genetic basis of pheochromocytoma and paraganglioma: implications for management. *Urology.* 2014;83(6):1225-1232.

Solorzano CC, Lew JI, Wilhelm SM, Sumner W, Huang W, Wu W, et al. Outcomes of pheochromocytoma management in the laparoscopic era. *Ann Surg Oncol.* 2007;14(10):3004-3010.

Thomas RM, Ruel E, Shantavasinkul PC, Corsino L. Endocrine hypertension: an overview on the current etiopathogenesis and management options. *World J Hypertens.* 2015;5(2):14-27.

Weiss CA, Park AE. Laparoscopic adrenalectomy technique. *Contemp Surg.* 2003;59:26-29.

Pancreatic Neuroendocrine Tumors

74

MICHAEL J. PUCCI, STACEY A. MILAN, AND CHARLES J. YEO

Based on the previous edition chapter "Pancreatic Neuroendocrine Tumors" by Stacey A. Milan and Charles J. Yeo

Presentation

Case 1: A previously healthy 40-year-old nurse presents with complaints of an 18-month history of bouts of confusion, light-headedness, diaphoresis, tremulousness, and occasional loss of consciousness. She reports a 20-lb weight gain over a similar time period. A recent episode required treatment in the emergency department, at which time her serum glucose (after an overnight fast) was 28 mg/dL (normal, 68 to 110 mg/dL). Her symptoms resolved with 10% dextrose intravenously.

Case 2: A 50-year-old female presents with a 6-month history of diarrhea. She first noted a change in her bowel habits from one or two formed stools daily to frequent loose stools of moderate volume. Over the next several months, her bowel movements became increasingly watery. She complains of mild abdominal pain, sometimes relieved with defecation, and tenesmus.

Case 3: A 54-year-old male was undergoing surveillance after treatment for prostate cancer. A CT scan identified a 2-cm mass in the head of the pancreas (Figure 74-1). He had no symptoms of abdominal pain or obstructive jaundice, no past history of pancreatitis, and no family history of pancreatic neoplasia.

● DIFFERENTIAL DIAGNOSIS

Case 1: The differential diagnosis of hypoglycemia includes reactive or postprandial hypoglycemia, surreptitious insulin or oral hypoglycemic use, noninsulinoma pancreatogenous hypoglycemia syndrome (nesidioblastosis), acute hepatic failure, and uncommon tumors such as adrenocortical carcinoma, various sarcomas, and hepatocellular carcinoma.

Case 2: The differential diagnosis of a patient who presents with voluminous diarrhea include a vasoactive intestinal peptide secreting tumor (VIPoma), laxative abuse, villous adenoma of the rectum, celiac disease, inflammatory bowel disease, infectious and parasitic causes, malabsorption from prior extensive colonic resection, gastrinoma, and carcinoid.

Case 3: Diagnoses of consideration when evaluating an incidentally discovered pancreatic mass include functional or nonfunctional pancreatic endocrine neoplasms, pancreatic adenocarcinoma, cystic pancreatic neoplasms (such as intraductal papillary mucinous neoplasm, mucinous cystadenoma, or serous cystadenoma), solid pseudopapillary tumor, pseudocyst, metastatic lymphoma, sarcoidosis, or acinar cell carcinoma.

● WORKUP

Pancreatic neuroendocrine tumors (PNETs) originate from multipotent stem cells in the pancreatic ductules and account for 1% to 2% of pancreatic neoplasms. They can be classified based on function: those associated with a functional syndrome due to ectopic secretion of a biologically active substance and those that are not associated with a functional syndrome. Functional PNETs include insulinomas, gastrinomas, VIPomas, somatostatinomas, and glucagonomas (Table 74-1). Less commonly, functional neuroendocrine pancreatic tumors may secrete adrenocorticotropic hormone, growth hormone–releasing hormone, parathyroid hormone–related protein, and calcitonin. Very rarely, neuroendocrine tumors of the pancreas may ectopically secrete luteinizing hormone, renin, IGF-2, or erythropoietin (Table 74-2). Both functional and nonfunctional endocrine tumors of the pancreas frequently secrete a number of other

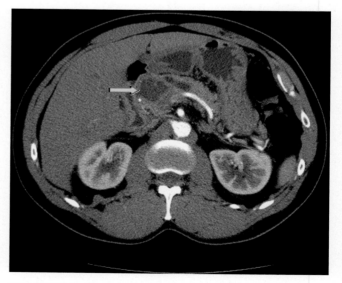

FIGURE 74-1. Asymptomatic male presenting with pancreatic head mass (*arrow*) incidentally identified on surveillance CT scan of the abdomen and pelvis following treatment for prostate cancer.

Table 74-1	Well Recognized Functional Pancreatic Neuroendocrine Tumors			
	Signs and Symptoms	**Location in Pancreas**	**Malignant**	**Incidence**
Insulinoma	Hypoglycemia Sweating Tachycardia Tremulousness Confusion Seizure	Evenly distributed head, body, tail	10%	4 per million
Gastrinoma	Gastric acid hypersecretion Peptic ulceration Diarrhea Esophagitis	Gastrinoma triangle Often extrapancreatic (duodenal) can be found anywhere in gland	50%	0.2–1 per million
VIPomas (Verner-Morrison syndrome, WDHA)	Watery diarrhea Hypokalemia Achlorhydria (or acidosis)	Distal pancreas (body and tail) Often have spread outside pancreas	Most	0.05–0.5 per million
Somatostatinomas	Gallstones diabetes (hyperglycemia) Steatorrhea	Pancreaticoduodenal groove, ampullary, periampullary	Most	1 per 40 million
Glucagonomas	Diabetes (hyperglycemia) Necrolytic migratoryerythema Stomatitis Glossitis ngular cheilitis	Body and tail of the pancreas Often large and have spread outside the pancreas	Most	1 per 20 million

WDHA, watery diarrhea, hypokalemia, achlorhydria.

substances including chromogranins (particularly chromogranin A), pancreatic polypeptide (PP), neuron-specific enolase, subunits of HCG or ghrelin, but these substances do not cause a specific hormonal syndrome.

Although there are prognostic implications to some of the functional categories (e.g., insulinomas are generally indolent), the biology of most functional pancreatic endocrine tumors (and all nonfunctioning neuroendocrine tumors) is defined by the proliferative rate of the tumor, defined by the mitotic count and measurement of Ki-67–labeling index. In 2006 and 2007, the European Neuroendocrine Tumor Society (ENETS) proposed a staging scheme accompanied by a histologic grading system. The World Health Organization (WHO) classification endorsed this scheme and divides well-differentiated pancreatic endocrine tumors into low-grade (G1) and intermediate-grade (G2) categories, while all poorly differentiated neuroendocrine tumors are consider high-grade (G3) neuroendocrine carcinomas (Table 74-3). Additionally, local invasion beyond the pancreas or metastatic spread to lymph nodes and/or distant locations mandates classification as carcinoma.

PNETs occur both sporadically and with inherited disorders, including MEN-1, von Hippel-Lindau syndrome, neurofibromatosis 1, and tuberous sclerosis (Table 74-4). In MEN-1, the majority of patients develop nonfunctional PNETs; however, gastrinoma is the most common functional PNET, followed by (in order of decreasing frequency) insulinoma, glucagonoma, VIPoma, and somatostatinoma.

Table 74-2	Secretory Products of Rare Functional Pancreatic Neuroendocrine Tumors

Adrenocorticotropic hormone (ACTH)
Growth hormone–releasing hormone
Parathyroid hormone–related protein (PTH-rp)
Calcitonin
Luteinizing hormone (LH)
Renin
Insulin-like growth factor-2 (IGF-2)
Erythropoietin

● DIAGNOSIS AND TREATMENT

Patients presenting with symptoms from a functional PNET can present a diagnostic challenge, and patients are often misdiagnosed or disregarded for years before an accurate diagnosis is made. The clinical sequelae from

Table 74-3   WHO/ENETS Classification of Pancreatic Neuroendocrine Tumors

Differentiation	Grade	Mitotic Count (per 10 hpf)	Ki-67 Index	ENETS	WHO
Well differentiated	Low grade (G1)	<2	<3%	Neuroendocrine tumor	Grade 1
	Intermediate grade (G2)	2–20	3%–20%	Neuroendocrine tumor	Grade 2
Poorly differentiated	High grade (G3)	>20	>20%	Neuroendocrine carcinoma	Grade 3

hormone hypersecretion in functional PNETs can be significant. Symptoms are often nonspecific, episodic, vary among individuals, and differ from time to time in the same individual.

Case 1: This scenario is consistent with symptoms of an insulinoma. The symptoms of hypoglycemia from an insulinoma can be divided into two categories: neuroglycopenic symptoms and neurogenic symptoms. Neuroglycopenic symptoms are due to central nervous system glucose deprivation and include behavioral changes, confusion, visual changes, fatigue, seizures, and loss of consciousness. Neurogenic symptoms are due to autonomic nervous system discharge caused by hypoglycemia and include hunger, paresthesias, sweating, anxiety, and palpitations.

Case 2: Patients with VIPomas, also known as Verner-Morrison syndrome or WDHA syndrome (watery diarrhea, hypokalemia, achlorhydria), may have diarrhea up to 20 times per day, as well as significant dehydration and muscle weakness from water and electrolyte losses.

In working up patients with suspected functional tumors, the abnormal physiology or characteristic syndrome must be recognized. Well-described clinical syndromes exist for gastrinoma (not discussed in this chapter), insulinoma, glucagonoma, VIPoma, and somatostatinoma. Hormone elevation should be detected in the serum, and commercial assays are available for measuring insulin, VIP, somatostatin, and glucagon. The next step involves tumor localization and staging in preparation for operative intervention.

The initial imaging study used by most to identify and stage a PNET is a high-quality contrast-enhanced computed tomography (CT) scan. PNETs are typically hyperdense (i.e., enhance with contrast) and spherical on the arterial

Table 74-4   Inherited Disorders Associated with Pancreatic Neuroendocrine Tumors

Syndrome	Associated Clinical Features	Chromosomal Location	Pancreatic Neuroendocrine Tumor Type
MEN1	Primary hyperparathyroidism Pituitary tumors Less commonly Adrenocortical tumors Carcinoid tumors Nonmedullary thyroid tumors	11q13	Nonfunctional Gastrinoma Insulinoma Various
von Hippel-Lindau disease (VHL)	Pheochromocytoma (often bilateral) Retinal and cerebellar hemangioblastomas Renal cell carcinoma	3p25–26	Nonfunctional Various, including cystic tumors
Neurofibromatosis 1 (von Recklinghausen's disease)	Neurofibromas Café au lait spots Pheochromocytoma	17q11.2	Somatostatinoma
Tuberous sclerosis	Cardiac rhabdomyomas Renal cysts Angiomyolipomas	9q33.34 and 16p13.3	Insulinoma

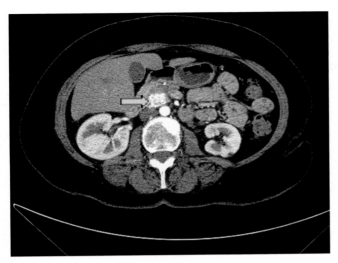

FIGURE 74-2. Hyperdense appearance of a pancreatic neuroendocrine tumor (*arrow*) on arterial phase of CT scan.

phase of imaging (Figure 74-2). CT is useful in assessing the size and location of the pancreatic tumor, peripancreatic lymph node involvement, and the presence or absence of liver metastases for staging and surgical planning. Although dependent on the size of the tumor, the sensitivity and accuracy of CT approximate 94% and 82%, respectively.

MRI is increasingly used to detect PNETs, especially small tumors. PNETs typically have high signal intensity on T2-weighted images (Figure 74-3). The sensitivity of MRI has been reported to be between 74% and 100%.

Octreotide (somatostatin) scintigraphy may also be helpful in locating pancreatic endocrine tumors, as well as in assessing for extrapancreatic metastatic disease (Figure 74-4). Neuroendocrine tumors often express large numbers of somatostatin receptors on the cell surfaces, and therefore, the tracer preferentially identifies tumors. Octreotide

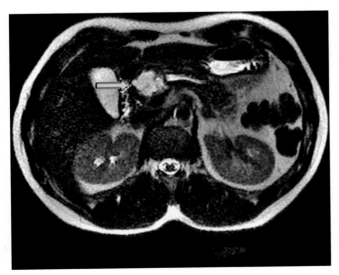

FIGURE 74-3. MRI demonstrating typical high signal intensity of pancreatic neuroendocrine tumor (*arrow*) on T2-weighted images.

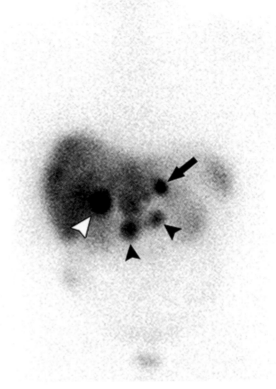

FIGURE 74-4. Octreotide scan of a patient with a VIPoma with liver metastasis (*white arrowhead*) as well as regional lymph node metastasis (*black arrowheads*). (Reprinted from Intenzo CM, et al. Scintigraphic imaging of body neuroendocrine tumors. *Radiographics.* 2007;27:1355-1369, with permission.)

scintigraphy performs well for gastrinoma, VIPoma, and glucagonoma but less frequently localizes nonfunctional tumors and insulinomas.

Endoscopic ultrasound (EUS) is also useful in localizing pancreatic endocrine neoplasms, especially in the head of the pancreas. As with all ultrasound procedures, it is operator dependent. While EUS does not accurately evaluate for liver metastasis, it has been reported, in experienced hands, to be more accurate than CT or MRI in identifying lesions <1 cm in diameter.

When all other diagnostic measures fail to localize a functional PNET, either percutaneous transhepatic portal venous sampling or arterial stimulation with hepatic venous sampling may be useful. The first technique involves placing a venous catheter percutaneously through the liver into the portal vein and sequentially sampling for hormone levels in the splenic vein, superior mesenteric vein, and portal vein, thus regionalizing the location of hormone production. Overall accuracy of this test ranges from 70% to 95%. The second technique (referred to by some as the "Imamura test") is a doubly invasive test that involves selective visceral arterial injection of calcium with concurrent hepatic venous sampling for insulin. Calcium is serially injected at low doses through an arterial catheter into the splenic, gastroduodenal, and inferior pancreaticoduodenal arteries, and samples are drawn from a hepatic vein catheter before and immediately after each injection, thereby allowing regionalization of the blood supply to the occult tumor.

Specific Case Features

Case 1: Insulinomas are the most common functional PNET. Insulinomas often present with the classic syndrome recognized as Whipple's triad: symptoms of hypoglycemia, documented serum glucose of <50 mg/dL, and relief of symptoms after administration of glucose. This can be confirmed with a monitored in-hospital fast, during which glucose and insulin levels can be checked every 4 to 6 hours, and at the time, the patient becomes symptomatic. Serum insulin levels will be elevated, and C-peptides should be checked to rule out surreptitious insulin or oral hypoglycemic use. Patients with an insulinoma will have increased insulin, proinsulin, and C-peptide levels; those with hypoglycemia secondary to surreptitious insulin use will have increased insulin levels but decreased levels of proinsulin and C-peptide. Urine tests for metformin and sulfonylurea can be performed to exclude surreptitious oral hypoglycemic use. Frequently small in size, insulinomas can be difficult to localize, although most are successfully localized with a combination of CT scan, EUS, and selective arteriography with venous sampling. In this case, a CT scan localized a 1-cm hypervascular mass in the midbody of the pancreas, with no other abnormalities.

Case 2: The classic features of a VIPoma include large-volume diarrhea (>5 L/d), severe hypokalemia with muscle weakness, and achlorhydria. Additionally, patients are often noted to be hyperglycemic. Further workup to exclude other causes of diarrhea in patient 2 includes stool samples that are negative for infectious causes of diarrhea and blood and a colonoscopy that is normal. She notes muscle weakness, and on routine labs has a potassium of 2.4 mmol/L as well as a metabolic acidosis. She has lost 25 lb in 6 months. CT scan demonstrates a large mass in the tail of the pancreas and multiple liver masses. Serum VIP was measured at 460 pg/mL (normal <50), and her serum gastrin was normal.

Case 3: Detection of nonfunctional PNETs is increasing by way of more frequent use of cross-sectional imaging. A recent study by Lahat and colleagues found that 15.6% of pancreatic "incidentalomas" are neuroendocrine in origin. However, symptomatic, nonfunctional PNETs are frequently large and at an advanced stage when first diagnosed, with as many as 60% to 85% having liver metastasis. Preoperatively, this patient was found to have elevated chromogranin A and pancreatic polypeptide levels in addition to the 2-cm mass in the head of the pancreas identified by CT.

● SURGICAL APPROACH

Surgical exploration for PNETs requires careful planning. The goals of the operation include eliminating or controlling the symptoms of hormone excess, safely resecting maximal tumor mass, and preserving maximal pancreatic parenchyma. Management strategies will vary for the different types of endocrine neoplasms, the location within the pancreas, and the presence of extrapancreatic disease. Surgical approaches include both laparoscopic and open procedures, and ranges from enucleation to pancreaticoduodenectomy, distal pancreatectomy or central pancreatectomy, with potential for debulking of metastatic disease, depending on the specific patient situation.

Case 1: Laparoscopic exploration confirmed an obvious 1-cm mass in the midbody of the pancreas. No other lesions were identified in the pancreas via visual inspection and intraoperative ultrasound, and the tumor was not intimately associated with the pancreatic duct. The tumor was successfully enucleated via the laparoscopic approach. In the postoperative period, she was noted to be euglycemic and was discharged from the hospital uneventfully. At 6-month follow-up, she remained euglycemic and had successfully lost 20 lb of excess weight.

Case 2: A discussion with the patient regarding the options of surgical debulking to control symptoms versus attempted long-term symptom control with somatostatin analog (octreotide) resulted in the patient deciding to undergo surgical debulking. Preoperatively, the patient was started on octreotide and hospitalized for correction of dehydration and metabolic abnormalities. She underwent laparotomy, distal pancreatectomy with en bloc splenectomy with careful attention to regional lymph nodes, and wedge resection of two peripheral liver metastases. A third intraparenchymal liver metastasis was treated with radiofrequency ablation to yield debulking of >95% of her disease. At 6-month follow-up, she was no longer on octreotide, her diarrhea had completely resolved, her surveillance CT scan showed no evidence of imageable disease, and her serum VIP level was 53 pg/mL.

Case 3: After counseling and education, this patient chose to undergo a pylorus-preserving pancreaticoduodenectomy, and pathology revealed a well-differentiated neuroendocrine carcinoma involving 2 of 16 resected lymph nodes. His postoperative course was complicated by a low-volume pancreatic fistula to an operatively placed drain that resolved with drain maintenance and somatostatin therapy. He was discharged from the hospital doing well, with one drain in place, on postoperative day 8. His drain was removed at his first postoperative office visit, and at 6-month follow-up, he was well. He was not advised to receive either chemotherapy or radiation therapy. His 6-month surveillance CT scan showed normal post-Whipple anatomy and no evidence of tumor.

● SPECIAL INTRAOPERATIVE CONSIDERATIONS

Approximately one-third of patients with malignant PNETs have synchronous liver metastases at the time of diagnosis.

While some of these patients remain asymptomatic and achieve long-term survival without aggressive therapy, overall 5-year survival for neuroendocrine tumors with liver metastases is <50%. In a select subset of patients where surgical resection of >90% of tumor burden can be safely achieved, surgical debulking has shown a survival advantage, with 5-year survival rates of 60% to 75%. However, the value of surgical debulking has not been rigorously tested in a prospective, randomized trial setting.

● POSTOPERATIVE MANAGEMENT

Patients following pancreatic resection are typically managed in an intensive care unit (or well-monitored bed setting) for 1 to 2 days postoperatively, with attention to multisystem organ function, fluid balance, and pain control. Close postoperative attention must be paid to common complications of pancreatic resection, including pancreatic fistula, pneumonia, myocardial infarction, venous thromboembolism, postoperative bleeding, surgical site infection, and anastomotic dehiscence. Patients undergoing extensive pancreatic resection (where a considerable portion of normal pancreatic parenchyma is sacrificed) may experience abnormal endogenous blood sugar control and ultimately require insulin therapy.

For patients with hormonally active (functioning) pancreatic endocrine tumors associated with unresectable disease, further treatment is possible to ameliorate the symptoms of hormonal excess. In patients with metastatic insulinoma, diazoxide can reduce insulin secretion and raise glucose levels. Chemotherapy regimens for insulinoma are limited but often have included streptozocin, 5-fluorouracil, and doxorubicin in combination. Continued research into developing new anticancer regimens for metastatic neuroendocrine tumors such as everolimus, sunitinib, capecitabine, and temozolomide is ongoing but has yet to become standard of care. Somatostatin can be useful in long-term management of symptoms in patients with insulinoma and VIPoma, although not all patients respond to somatostatin and others may become refractory to it. Other treatments for metastatic PNETs within the liver (not limited to insulinoma) include directed hepatic artery chemoembolization and/or radiofrequency ablation.

TAKE HOME POINTS

- Pancreatic neuroendocrine tumors may present in a variety of ways, from the five well-described clinical hormone excess syndromes to incidental discovery during imaging for an unrelated issue.
- Clinical syndromes can be difficult to recognize, and patients often elude diagnosis. Many patients experience a battery of tests over many months to years before the correct diagnosis is entertained and defined.
- Neuroendocrine tumors of the pancreas may occur sporadically or with familial syndromes such as MEN1, von Hippel-Lindau, neurofibromatosis 1, and tuberous sclerosis.
- Contrast-enhanced high-quality CT scan is the diagnostic modality of choice, but further testing may be needed to localize some tumors. EUS may be particularly helpful in identifying small tumors <1 to 2 cm in size.
- The surgical approach depends on the tumor location in the pancreas and extent of disease. In patients with liver metastases, surgical debulking to include resection of the primary lesion and either hepatic resection or ablation should be considered if ≥90% of the tumor burden can be eliminated.

SUGGESTED READINGS

Clancy TE. Surgical management of pancreatic neuroendocrine tumors. *Hematol Oncol Clin North Am.* 2016;30(1):103-18.

Imamura M. Recent standardization of treatment strategy for pancreatic neuroendocrine tumors. *World J Gastroenterol.* 2010;16(36):4519-4525.

Kennedy EP, Brody JR, Yeo CJ. *Neoplasms of the Endocrine Pancreas. Greenfield's Surgery: Scientific Principles and Practice.* 5th ed. Philadelphia, PA: Wolters Kluwer/Lippincott Williams & Wilkins; 2010:857-871.

Kulke MH, Anthony LB, Bushnell DL, et al. North American Neuroendocrine Tumor Society Treatment Guidelines: well-differentiated neuroendocrine tumors of the stomach and pancreas. *Pancreas.* 2010;39(6)735-752.

Rindi G, Kloppel G, Alhman H, et al. TNM staging of foregut (neuro)endocrine tumors: a consensus proposal including a grading system. *Virchows Arch.* 2006;449(4):395-401.

Yeo CJ, Milan SA. Neuroendocrine tumors of the pancreas. *Curr Opin Oncol.* 2012; 24(1):46-55.

Gastrinoma

75

GEOFFREY W. KRAMPITZ AND JEFFREY A. NORTON

Based on the previous edition chapter "Gastrinoma" by Geoffrey W. Krampitz and Jeffrey A. Norton

Presentation

A 22-year-old morbidly obese man with a history of peptic ulcer disease was referred to our clinic for epigastric pain. Over the past year, the pain has persisted despite a 3-month trial of omeprazole. Prior esophagogastroduodenoscopy (EGD) demonstrated a 1-cm nonhealing, solitary ulcer in the proximal duodenum with a workup that was negative for *Helicobacter pylori* infection. The patient also describes chronic loose bowel movements three to six times per day over this same time period. In clinic, the patient also divulged that he had been feeling increasingly fatigued over the last 3 years, and his mood had become progressively depressed. He also complained of persistent bone and muscle pain. He also indicated that he had a soft mobile lipoma in his right inguinal region. He had no fevers, chills, night sweats, weight loss, headaches, syncope, visual changes, galactorrhea, palpitations, shortness of breath, flushing, nausea, vomiting, hematochezia, melena, hematuria, or dysuria. His complete review of systems was otherwise negative.

His past medical history was significant for gynecomastia at the age of 16, the workup of which revealed elevated prolactin level of >280 ng/mL and a 2.1-cm pituitary macroadenoma. He underwent a surgical reduction mammoplasty, and he was started on cabergoline therapy after which his prolactin level normalized. A recent MRI showed slight reduction in tumor size, and visual field testing was normal. He also had multiple lipomas excised over the past 5 years. He was diagnosed with hypogonadotropic hypogonadism for which he was prescribed transdermal testosterone with little improvement in symptoms, morbid obesity for which he was attempting dietary changes without success, and insulin resistance not requiring medications.

Family history was significant for his mother, now aged 54, who had amenorrhea at age 35, the workup of which revealed a prolactinoma that was managed medically. Several years later, she was diagnosed with parathyroid hyperplasia for which she underwent a subtotal (3 and ½ gland) parathyroidectomy. More recently, she had progressive epigastric discomfort for which she had yet to be evaluated.

The patient's physical exam was notable for morbid obesity (BMI, 56), undisturbed visual fields, nonfocal neurologic exam, and no expressible galactorrhea; heart exam revealed a regular rate and rhythm; lungs were clear to auscultation; abdomen was protuberant but soft, nontender, and nondistended; rectal exam showed a normal prostate and no masses or blood; normal external male genitalia; a 4-cm, soft, nontender, mobile soft tissue mass in the right inguinal region; and extremities with good pulses and without clubbing or cyanosis.

● DIFFERENTIAL DIAGNOSIS

This patient has a constellation of symptoms classic for multiple endocrine neoplasia type 1 (MEN-1) and Zollinger-Ellison syndrome (ZES). The diagnosis of ZES is often delayed because it can mimic many other much more common conditions that result in peptic ulcers and/or hypergastrinemia. Ulcerogenic conditions with excessive gastric acid secretion include gastric outlet obstruction, retained gastric antrum after Billroth II reconstruction, and G-cell hyperplasia. Nonulcerogenic conditions without excessive gastric acid secretion include postvagotomy state, gastric bypass, pernicious anemia, atrophic gastritis, short gut syndrome after significant intestinal resection, renal failure, *Helicobacter pylori* infection, VIPoma, and stomach irradiation. Many of these conditions are associated with achlorhydria, in which stomach acid production is absent, resulting in hypergastrinemia, mimicking ZES. However, our patient had no obstructive symptoms, prior intra-abdominal operations, irradiation, renal failure, gastritis, or anemia. He had endoscopically proven peptic ulcers without *H. pylori* infection refractory to a standard trial of PPI therapy and in the presence of chronic diarrhea raising a suspicion of ZES.

● DISCUSSION

In 1955, Zollinger and Ellison first described a syndrome of severe peptic ulcers associated with pancreatic islet cell tumors that were refractory to conventional acid-reduction surgery. We now know that these tumors were gastrinomas causing gastrin hypersecretion and excessive gastric acid production, which in turn leads to intractable peptic ulcer disease. Gastrinoma has a yearly incidence of approximately 0.1 to 3 cases per million people, making it the second most common pancreatic neuroendocrine tumor overall. It is also the causative factor in approximately 0.1% to 1% of patients with peptic ulcer disease. In 80% of cases, ZES occurs sporadically. However, approximately 20% of patients with ZES have the familial form associated with MEN-1. MEN-1 is a syndrome first described in 1954 by Wermer caused by a mutation in a gene located on chromosome 11q13 encoding a tumor suppressor protein called menin. Patients with MEN-1 have asymmetrical parathyroid adenomas, duodenal and pancreatic neuroendocrine tumors, anterior pituitary tumors, lipomas, thyroid and adrenocortical adenomas, and bronchial and thymic carcinoid tumors. The disease occurs at a young age, and the most common causes of death in these patients is a neuroendocrine tumor of the pancreas, thymus, or bronchus. Fifty percent of patients with MEN-1 have ZES, making gastrinoma the most common functional pancreatic or duodenal neuroendocrine tumor in MEN-1. Despite increased awareness of ZES and improvements in diagnostic methodologies, the mean time from symptom onset to diagnosis is 8 years in many studies, so that improvements in detection and awareness are still needed.

● WORKUP

Any patient with peptic ulcer disease that is refractory, recurrent, atypical, requiring surgery, or in the absence *H. pylori* should undergo a workup for ZES. The presence of hyperparathyroidism, nephrolithiasis, or family history suggestive of MEN-1 should also raise suspicion for ZES. We begin our workup by obtaining a fasting serum concentration of gastrin. Hypergastrinemia occurs in almost all patients with ZES (99% sensitivity) and is defined as a serum gastrin concentration >100 pg/mL. Because PPI therapy can induce hypergastrinemia, we discontinued the patient's PPI for 1 week prior to the test and started him on a H2-receptor antagonist that we held 2 days prior to the testing. At the time of the test, the patient's gastrin level was significantly elevated at 1,210 pg/mL. Basal acid output (BAO) was also elevated at 39 mEq per hour (normal ≤ 15 mEq per hour or <5 mEq per hour in patients who have undergone previous acid-reducing operations). In addition, a gastric pH was measured at 1.7 that also indicated acid hypersecretion. Although less accurate than BAO, a gastric pH >3 essentially excludes ZES, whereas a pH ≤2 is consistent with ZES. However, many patients with ZES have gastric acid hypersecretion and minimally increased fasting serum gastrin concentrations (100 to 1,000 pg/mL). For these patients, the secretin stimulation test is the provocative test of choice to establish the diagnosis of ZES.

Twenty percent of ZES cases occur in association with MEN-1, and ZES is the presenting symptom in 40% of cases with MEN-1. Thus during the initial workup for ZES, MEN-1 must always be excluded. This was particularly relevant in our patient who exhibited other signs and symptoms consistent with MEN-1, including pituitary adenoma, lipomas, as well as fatigue, depressed mood, and musculoskeletal pain. Our initial screen was a serum calcium measurement, exploiting the high penetrance of hyperparathyroidism in MEN-1, followed by serum parathyroid hormone (PTH) concentration. In this case, our patient's serum calcium and PTH levels were elevated at 12 mg/dL and 146 pg/mL (normal < 80 pg/mL), respectively. With a biochemical diagnosis of ZES established, the next step in the workup is to treat the acid hypersecretion with proton pump inhibitors (PPI), utilizing pantoprazole at a dosage of up to 80 mg PO or IV BID.

Following the medical management of the acid hypersecretion, the next step is to localize and characterize the gastrinoma to determine resectability and the best operative approach. Approximately 80% of gastrinomas are found within the gastrinoma triangle, the apices of which are bounded by the junction of the cystic and common bile ducts superiorly, the junction of the second and third portions of the duodenum laterally, and the neck of the pancreas medially. Gastrinomas associated with MEN-1 tend to be multiple, small, and usually originate in the duodenum.

In our case, a pancreatic protocol computed tomography (CT) scan including PO and IV contrast with 5-mm cuts demonstrated a dominant 3-cm tumor in the superiomedial aspect of the head of the pancreas abutting the superior mesenteric vein (Figure 75-1). The sensitivity of CT is directly related to the size of the tumor. Tumors >3 cm are detected in 83% to 95% of cases, tumor 1 to 3 cm are detected in 30% of cases, whereas tumors <1 cm are not detectable. Another limitation of CT scanning in the setting of gastrinoma is that only 50% of liver metastases are detected.

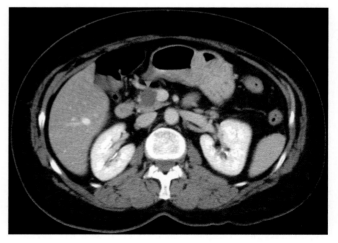

FIGURE 75-1. Computed tomography scan demonstrating 3-cm gastrinoma at the head of the pancreas and abutting the superior mesenteric vein.

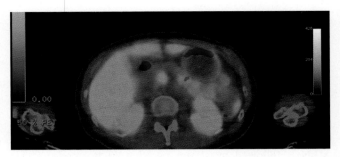

FIGURE 75-2. Gallium-68 DOTA scan that images a 3-cm hypervascular neuroendocrine tumor as seen on CT.

We then obtained a new type of somatostatin receptor scintigraphy called gallium-68 DOTA scan that revealed focal, intense tracer uptake in the region of the head of the pancreas corresponding to the 3-cm lesion seen on CT scan (Figure 75-2). In addition, it also demonstrated a 1-cm tumor in the neck of the pancreas on the anterior wall, a third tumor that was an 8-mm tumor in the inferior portion of the head of the pancreas abutting the duodenum, and no evidence of distant metastases. The additional findings seen on DOTA scan demonstrate the increased sensitivity of this modality over other modalities.

The patient's constellation of signs including pituitary adenoma, hyperparathyroidism, multiple pancreatic neuroendocrine tumors, and lipomas, as well as prolactinoma and hyperparathyroidism in his mother is strongly suggestive of MEN-1. The patient, his mother, and his two brothers underwent genetic testing for MENIN gene mutations. This testing revealed a T-278 mutation in the patient and the mother, thus establishing a genetic diagnosis of MEN-1.

● DIAGNOSIS AND TREATMENT

The first principle of treating ZES associated with MEN-1 is to control symptoms medically. Following our diagnostic workup for ZES, we reinitiated PPI therapy for our patient and titrated the dose to obtain a BAO below 15 mEq per hour, ultimately requiring 80 mg of pantoprazole orally twice per day. This dose of PPI controlled all his symptoms including abdominal pain and diarrhea.

The second principle of treating ZES associated with MEN-1 in this patient was to address the multiple parathyroid adenomas. Because ZES symptoms can be exacerbated by hypercalcemia resulting from hyperparathyroidism, the patient underwent a subtotal (3 and ½ gland) parathyroidectomy with a transcervical thyrmectomy. This allowed for decreased end-organ effect of hypergastrinemia and better medical control of ZES symptoms.

The third principle of treating ZES associated with MEN-1 is to determine if the patient is a candidate for operative intervention. Gastrinomas associated with MEN-1 have a propensity to spread to peripancreatic lymph nodes but are usually more indolent and less likely to metastasize to the liver when compared to sporadic tumors. Because hepatic involvement is the most important predictor of survival, ZES patients with MEN-1 have a more favorable long-term prognosis. Although surgery for MEN-1–associated disease is rarely curative (0% to 10%), resection may prevent liver metastases and thus affect long-term survival. Because tumor size >2 cm is predictive of progression to liver metastasis, surgery for ZES associated with MEN-1 is recommended only if there is an identifiable tumor larger than 2 cm. This is relevant to our patient because his main tumor was 3 cm in size.

● SURGICAL APPROACH

Because of tumor multifocality (both in the pancreas and the duodenum) in MEN-1 patients, there is little chance of biochemical cure. The goal of surgery is to prevent liver metastases and thus decrease tumor-related mortality. As such, we recommend operative approaches that focus on resecting tumor while preserving as much of the normal tissue as possible. In general, the operation should include resection of body and tail pancreatic tumors, enucleation of pancreatic head tumors, duodenotomy with identification and excision of duodenal tumors, and peripancreatic lymph node sampling. We do not favor routinely performing pancreaticoduodenectomy for attempted cure because long-term survival is excellent with the surgical approach described above and less morbidity. Nevertheless, pancreaticoduodenectomy may be necessary with bulky tumors in the head of the pancreas, tumors involving the ampulla, or tumor invasion into major ductal or vascular structures. Our patient had multiple pancreatic tumors, the largest of which was a bulky tumor in the head of the pancreas abutting the superior mesenteric vein. Thus, a pancreaticoduodenectomy was performed.

Operative approach includes a full abdominal exploration. The liver and peritoneal surfaces should be carefully inspected to assess for metastatic disease. Intraoperative ultrasound should be utilized to further inspect the liver for occult metastases and to aid in localization of pancreatic tumors. Standard elements of pancreaticoduodenectomy are then performed as detailed in Table 75-1.

● SPECIAL INTRAOPERATIVE CONSIDERATIONS

The first intraoperative consideration is to confirm the presence or absence of tumor metastases seen on preoperative imaging. Hepatic metastases are the primary determinant of survival in ZES patients. Thus, tumors involving the liver would require appropriate debulking via wedge resection, segmentectomy, or lobectomy depending on the extent and resectability of disease.

The second intraoperative consideration is to determine if the tumors seen on preoperative imaging indeed require a formal pancreatic resection or whether a more limited resection would be sufficient. In this case, the tumor in the head of the pancreas was of a significant size that required pancreaticoduodenectomy.

Table 75-1	**Whipple Procedure**

Key Technical Steps

1. Bilateral subcostal incisions and full abdominal exploration.
2. Mobilize the right colon and perform Kocher maneuver.
3. Open lesser sac and clear the anterior surface of the superior mesenteric vein.
4. Perform cholecystectomy, portal dissection, and ligation of gastroduodenal artery.
5. Divide proximal jejunum, duodenum, pancreas, and bile duct.
6. Dissect uncinate process from the superior mesenteric vein and artery.
7. Reconstruction with pancreaticojejunostomy, choledochojejunostomy, and gastrojejunostomy.

Potential Pitfalls

- Bleeding from the superior mesenteric or portal vein.
- Injury to the proper hepatic artery.
- Leak from pancreaticojejunostomy.

POSTOPERATIVE MANAGEMENT

The major complications of pancreaticoduodenectomy are death, anastomotic leaks, intra-abdominal abscesses, and delayed gastric emptying. With improvements in pancreatic surgery and postoperative care, the mortality for pancreaticoduodenectomy at most high-volume centers is reported as 2%. Anastomotic leaks, primarily at the pancreaticojejunostomy, occur in approximately 10% to 15% of patients and usually resolve with adequate drainage. Intra-abdominal abscesses occur in 5% to 10% of cases. Delayed gastric emptying occurs in approximately 30% of patients and usually resolves within a couple of weeks postoperatively.

Case Conclusion

The patient tolerated the procedure well and had an uncomplicated postoperative course. He tolerated a clear liquid diet on postoperative day 3 and had return of bowel function the following day. At that time, the epidural was removed and the patient's pain was well controlled on oral pain medications. On postoperative day 5, the anterior Jackson-Pratt drain was removed, and the posterior drain was removed the following day. The patient was discharged home on postoperative day 7.

The pathology showed multiple well-differentiated pancreatic neuroendocrine neoplasms, the largest measuring 3.2 cm, arising in a background of diffuse islet cell hyperplasia. The surgical margins were not involved with tumor, but there were multiple (4/12) lymph nodes with metastatic disease that gave the clinical appearance of multifocal disease. Careful pathologic examination of the duodenum did not show any tumors.

In patients with ZES who do not undergo pancreaticoduodenectomy, we routinely perform duodenotomy for detection of duodenal gastrinomas. Duodenotomy is particularly important in the detection of small duodenal tumors, allowing localization of 90% of subcentimeter tumors versus only 50% discovered on preoperative imaging. A recent prospective study of patients with sporadic ZES who underwent surgical exploration revealed a significantly higher cure rate following duodenotomy, both immediately and long term.

TAKE HOME POINTS

- ZES is a syndrome caused by gastrinoma usually located within the gastrinoma triangle and associated with symptoms of peptic ulcer disease and diarrhea.
- ZES is diagnosed by measuring fasting levels of serum gastrin, basal acid output, and secretin test.
- Due to the high association of ZES with MEN-1, hyperparathyroidism must be excluded by obtaining a serum calcium and parathyroid hormone level.
- Treatment of ZES consists of medical control of symptoms with PPIs and imaging for planning of surgical intervention.
- Noninvasive imaging studies including DOTA scan, CT, and MRI should be performed initially to evaluate for metastases and identify resectable disease. Invasive imaging modalities, such as EUS, may be performed to further evaluate primary tumors, if necessary. IOUS, palpation, and duodenotomy are used for intraoperative localization of gastrinomas.
- In patients with MEN-1, surgical resection should be pursued only if there is an identifiable tumor larger than 2 cm in contrast to resectable sporadic gastrinoma, for which all patients should undergo surgical exploration.
- In patients with liver metastases, cytoreductive surgery should be performed if more than 90% of the visible tumor can be safely removed. Figure 75-3 summarizes the workup, medical management, and surgical approach to ZES.

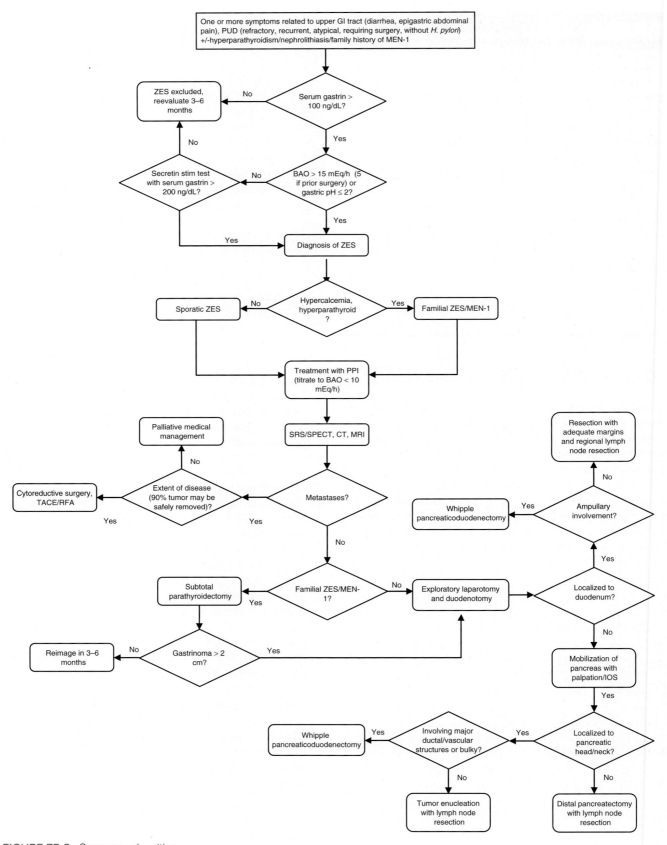

FIGURE 75-3. Summary algorithm.

SUGGESTED READINGS

Alexander HR, Fraker DL, Norton JA, et al. Prospective study of somatostatin receptor scintigraphy and its effect on operative outcome in patients with Zollinger-Ellison syndrome. *Ann Surg.* 1998;228(2):228-238.

Béhé M, Gotthardt M, Behr TM. Imaging of gastrinomas by nuclear medicine methods. *Wien Klin Wochenschr.* 2007;119(19-20): 593-596. Review.

Birkmeyer JD, Finlayson SR, Tosteson AN, et al. Effect of hospital volume on in-hospital mortality with pancreaticoduodenectomy. *Surgery* 1999;125:250-256.

Cisco RM, Norton JA. Surgery for gastrinoma. *Adv Surg.* 2007; 41:165-176.

Diener MK, Fitzmaurice C, Schwarzer G, et al. Pylorus-preserving pancreaticoduodenectomy (pp Whipple) versus pancreaticoduodenectomy (classic Whipple) for surgical treatment of periampullary and pancreatic carcinoma. *Cochrane Database Syst Rev.* 2011;5:CD006053.

Eriksson B, Oberg K, Skogseid B. Neuro-endocrine pancreatic tumors: clinical findings in a prospective study of 84 patients. *Acta Oncol.* 1989;28:373-377.

Howard TJ, Zinner MJ, Stabile BE, et al. Gastrinoma excision for cure. *Ann Surg.* 1990;211:9-14.

Imamura M, Komoto I, Ota S. Changing treatment strategy for gastrinoma in patients with Zollinger-Ellison syndrome. *World J Surg.* 2006;30(1):1-11. Review.

Li ML, Norton JA. Gastrinoma. *Curr Treat Options Oncol.* 2001; 2(4):337-346.

Meko JB, Norton JA. Management of patients with Zollinger-Ellison syndrome. *Annu Rev Med.* 1995;46:395-411.

Norton JA. Gastrinoma: advances in localization and treatments. *Surg Oncol Clin N Am.* 1998;7(4):845-861.

Norton, JA. Neuroendocrine tumors of the pancreas and duodenum. *Curr Probl Surg.* 1994;31:77-164.

Norton, JA. Surgical treatment and prognosis of gastrinoma. *Best Pract Res Clin Gastroenterol.* 2005;19:799-805.

Norton JA, Fang TD, Jensen RT. Surgery for gastrinoma and insulinoma in multiple endocrine neoplasia type 1. *J Natl Compr Canc Netw.* 2006;4(2):148-153.

Norton JA, Fraker DL, Alexander HR, et al. Surgery to cure the Zollinger-Ellison syndrome. *N Engl J Med.* 1999;341:635-644.

Norton JA, Jensen RT. Resolved and unresolved controversies in the surgical management of patients with Zollinger-Ellison syndrome. *Ann Surg.* 2004;240(5):757-773. Review.

Norton JA, Venzon DJ, Berna MJ, et al. Prospective study of surgery for primary hyperparathyroidism (HPT) in multiple endocrine neoplasia type 1. *Ann Surg.* 2008;247(3):501-510.

Norton JA, Krampitz G, Zemek A, Longacre T, Jensen RT. Better survival but changing causes of death in patients with multiple endocrine neoplasia type 1. *Ann Surg.* 2015S;262(4):632-640.

Pipeleers-Marichal M, Somers G, Willems G, et al. Gastrinomas in the duodenums of patients with multiple endocrine neoplasia type 1. *N Engl J Med.* 1990;322(11):723-727.

Pisegna JR, Norton JA, Slimak GG, et al. Effects of curative gastrinoma resection on gastric secretory function and. *Gastroenterology.* 1992;102:767-778.

Thompson NW, Vinik AI, Eckhauser FE. Micro-gastrinomas of the duodenum. *Ann Surg.* 1989;209:396-404.

Wank SA, Doppman HL, Miller DL, et al. Prospective study of the ability of computerized axial tomography to localize gastrinomas in patients with Zollinger-Ellison syndrome. *Gastroenterology.* 1987;92:905-912.

Wermer P. Endocrine adenomatosis and peptic ulcer in a large kindred: inherited multiple tumors and mosaic pleiotropism in man. *Am J Med.* 1963;35:205-212.

Wermer P. Genetic aspects of adenomatosis of endocrine glands. *Am J Med.* 1954;16(3):363-371.

Zollinger RM, Ellison EH. Primary peptic ulceration of the jejunum associated with islet cell tumors of the pancreas. *Ann Surg.* 1955;142:708-728.

Thoracic

Esophageal Cancer

76

TYLER R. GRENDA AND ANDREW C. CHANG

Based on the previous edition chapter "Esophageal Cancer" by Mark B. Orringer

Presentation

A 70-year-old man presents with a 3-month history of progressive dysphagia and a 30-lb weight loss. He has experienced heartburn symptoms for several years, worse when supine and after eating, that he has treated with over-the-counter antacids. The patient's symptoms of dysphagia have progressed to where he now has difficulty with tolerating solid foods. The patient has never had an endoscopy or formal evaluation of his symptoms. He has not experienced any abdominal pain, hematemesis, or melena. Physical examination is unremarkable.

● DIFFERENTIAL DIAGNOSIS

In an adult with new-onset dysphagia, esophageal malignancy should be the primary concern. This symptom should not be attributed to a benign etiology (e.g., gastroesophageal reflux disease [GERD]) without an evaluation for malignancy. In North America, adenocarcinoma of the esophagus has surpassed squamous cell carcinoma as the most common histologic type. Chronic GERD is a risk for development of Barrett's metaplasia and subsequent progression to dysplasia and adenocarcinoma. Barrett's esophagus is associated with a 30- to 40-fold increased risk for the development of esophageal carcinoma. The presence of high-grade dysplasia in the setting of Barrett's mucosa is a risk factor for malignant transformation. The presence of high-grade dysplasia is an indication for endoscopic or surgical intervention in appropriately selected patients. Patients with adenocarcinomas arising in Barrett's mucosa commonly present with a history of years of symptomatic GERD followed by a quiescent period as the squamous mucosa is replaced by metaplastic columnar mucosa, which is not acid sensitive. Patients may develop dysphagia related to obstruction from the subsequent development of a malignant tumor. Other causes of dysphagia in the adult patient that are included in the differential diagnosis include chronic reflux stricture, esophageal dysmotility (e.g., achalasia, diffuse esophageal spasm), reflux-induced esophageal dysmotility, benign tumor (e.g., leiomyoma), or esophageal diverticulum.

● WORKUP

Initially, the adult patient presenting with new-onset dysphagia should undergo: (1) a barium esophagogram and (2) esophagoscopy with biopsy and/or brushings for cytology to evaluate for the presence of malignancy. The esophagogram typically reveals an "applecore" constriction of the distal esophagus proximal to a sliding hiatal hernia (Figure 76-1). Laboratory studies may demonstrate anemia related to chronic GI blood loss, elevated transaminases associated with hepatic metastases, or hypoalbuminemia due to malnutrition. Once the diagnosis of esophageal carcinoma has been established, further staging should be performed to determine the recommended course of treatment. While there are few findings on physical examination specifically related to esophageal malignancy, an enlarged left supraclavicular (Virchow's) lymph node or hepatomegaly may indicate more advanced disease. If a Virchow's node is palpated, fine needle aspiration (FNA) should be performed to determine the presence of metastatic disease.

● DIAGNOSIS AND TREATMENT

Evaluation for esophageal carcinoma should include a CT scan of the chest and abdomen to determine the local extent of the tumor (e.g., local invasion or evidence of metastatic disease to mediastinal or upper abdominal lymph nodes) and to evaluate for obvious distant metastases to other organs. In addition, a PET scan should be obtained to evaluate for occult metastatic disease. Esophageal endoscopic ultrasonography (EUS) with or without FNA should be performed as well to define the depth of intramural tumor invasion (T stage) and the involvement of paraesophageal and upper abdominal lymph nodes (N stage) (Table 76-1).

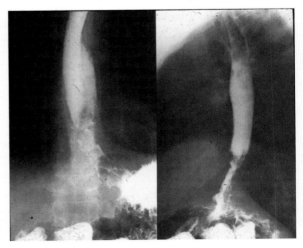

FIGURE 76-1. Barium swallow study showing a typical "applecore" constriction of adenocarcinoma proximal to a sliding hiatal hernia.

Table 76-1   TNM Staging of Esophageal Cancer

Definitions of TNM	
Primary Tumor (T)	
TX	Primary tumor cannot be assessed
T0	No evidence of primary tumor
Tis	High-grade dysplasia
T1	Tumor invades lamina propria, muscularis mucosae, or submucosa
T1a	Tumor invades lamina propria or muscularis mucosae
T1b	Tumor invades submucosa
T2	Tumor invades muscularis propria
T3	Tumor invades adventitia
T4	Tumor invades adjacent structures
T4a	Tumor invades pleura, pericardium, azygos vein, diaphragm, peritoneum
T4b	Tumor invades other adjacent structures, such as aorta, vertebral body, or trachea
Regional Lymph Nodes (N)	
NX	Regional lymph nodes cannot be assessed
N0	No regional lymph node metastasis
N1	Metastasis in one to two regional lymph nodes
N2	Metastasis in three to six regional lymph nodes
N3	Metastasis in seven or more regional lymph nodes
Distant Metastasis (M)	
M0	No distant metastasis
M1	Distant metastasis
Histologic Grade (G)	
Adenocarcinoma	
GX	Differentiation cannot be assessed
G1	Well differentiated
G2	Moderately differentiated
G3	Poorly differentiated
Squamous Cell Carcinoma	
GX	Differentiation cannot be assessed
G1	Well differentiated
G2	Moderately differentiated
G3	Poor differentiated
Squamous Cell Carcinoma L Category	
LX	Location unknown
Upper	Cervical esophagus to lower border of azygos vein
Middle	Lower border of azygos vein to lower border of inferior pulmonary vein
Lower	Lower border of inferior pulmonary vein to stomach

From the Rice TW, Kelsen DP, Blackstone EH, et al. Esophagus and esophagogastric junction. In: Amin MB, Edge SB, Greene FL, et al., eds. *AJCC Cancer Staging Manual*. 8th ed. New York, NY: Springer; 2017:185-202.

The 8th edition of the American Joint Commission on Cancer (AJCC) staging of esophageal and esophagogastric cancers has been modified from the 7th edition to include separate classifications for clinical, pathologic, and postneoadjuvant pathologic staging groups (Please see "Suggested Reading" for reference for the complete staging classification).

Endomucosal resection can be considered for patients with clinical stage IA disease. Esophagectomy alone can be discussed for select patients with early stage (IA or IB) cancers who are not candidates for neoadjuvant therapy or whose tumors demonstrate possibly aggressive histologic features such as poor differentiation, signet ring cell features or lymphovascular invasion. For those patients with stage II or more advanced-stage tumors, neoadjuvant chemoradiation therapy should be considered, typically with carboplatin, paclitaxel, and concurrent radiation therapy. For patients who are poor surgical candidates or have adenocarcinoma limited to the mucosa, evaluation for endoscopic mucosal resection can be considered. Patients with stage IV esophageal carcinoma (e.g., distant metastatic disease) are not candidates for esophagectomy and should be evaluated for definitive systemic therapy and/or supportive care.

Prior to esophagectomy, careful evaluation and preparation for surgery are imperative to successful outcome. Baseline pulmonary function tests (spirometry and diffusion capacity) should be obtained in those with a history of cigarette smoking or pulmonary disease. Evaluation for structural heart disease should be pursued as indicated by the clinical history and physical examination findings. Clinical judgment, incorporating the results of preoperative testing, functional status, and ability to tolerate an esophagectomy should guide patient selection for operation. The importance of adequate patient preparation for the operation cannot be overemphasized. Patients must abstain from cigarette smoking and use an incentive inspirometer for a minimum of 3 weeks prior to the planned operation. An exercise program that includes progressive ambulation, with a goal of walking 2 to 3 miles each day, should be instituted in the weeks leading up to surgery. Adequate preoperative hydration is key, particularly in those with radiation esophagitis, and may require insertion of temporary enteral access for administration of enteral nutritional supplements and water if swallowing is severely impaired. A gastrostomy tube should be avoided as this may complicate future esophageal conduit creation during esophagectomy.

● SURGICAL APPROACH

There are several surgical approaches to esophagectomy that have been demonstrated: open transthoracic, transhiatal, and minimally invasive approaches (e.g., VATS,

laparoscopic, robotic-assisted). Further considerations include the level of the esophageal anastomosis (thoracic or cervical) and replacement conduit (stomach, colon, or jejunum). The goals of esophagectomy are to (1) achieve a complete (R0) resection and (2) restore the ability to swallow. A transhiatal esophagectomy (THE) and cervical esophagogastric anastomosis (CEGA) offers advantages over open Ivor Lewis (right thoracotomy and intrathoracic anastomosis) esophagectomy, including (1) avoidance of a thoracotomy to reduce the morbidity of pulmonary complications and (2) CEGA to avoid mediastinitis usually associated with an intrathoracic anastomotic leak. Whether mediastinal lymph node dissection at the time of transthoracic esophagectomy translates to improved oncologic survival compared to lymph node dissection achieved with the transhiatal approach remains a point of sometimes heated debate. Minimally invasive surgery approaches may offer the advantages of accomplishing mediastinal lymphadenectomy while minimizing postoperative pain. A transhiatal resection with CEGA is the authors' preferred surgical approach to esophageal cancer.

Absolute contraindications to THE or other approaches include (1) biopsy-proven distant metastatic (stage IV) disease; (2) tracheobronchial invasion by the tumor proven at bronchoscopy; and (3) aortic invasion (documented on CT scan, MRI, EUS, or endovascular ultrasound). In addition, surgeon assessment of extensive mediastinal invasion at the time of palpation of the esophagus through the diaphragmatic hiatus could preclude safe resection of the tumor. A history of prior esophageal operation(s) or radiation therapy more than 6 to 12 months prior to the planned operation may increase the risk of encountering significant periesophageal fibrosis that also prevents safely proceeding with a transhiatal approach.

The transhiatal esophagectomy is performed in four defined phases, with key steps and potential pitfalls as outlined in Table 76-2.

1. Abdominal—(Figure 76-2) through a supraumbilical midline incision, exploration to exclude distant metastases and establish that the stomach is a satisfactory esophageal replacement; gastric mobilization, dividing and ligating the short gastric and left gastroepiploic vessels along the high greater curvature, the left gastric on the high lesser curvature, and preserving the right gastric and the right gastroepiploic vessels upon which the mobilized stomach is based; a Kocher maneuver; a pyloromyotomy; insertion of a feeding jejunostomy tube; opening the peritoneum overlying the hiatus and mobilizing the distal 5 to 10 cm of esophagus by blunt and sharp dissection

2. Cervical—(Figure 76-3A and B) through a 5- to 7-cm oblique low left neck incision along the anterior border of the sternocleidomastoid muscle, the carotid sheath is

Table 76-2	THE and CEGA

Key Technical Steps

1. Upper midline laparotomy and abdominal exploration; assess suitability of stomach as esophageal replacement.
2. Divide triangular ligament; retract liver to right with table-mounted upper hand retractor.
3. Mobilize stomach by dividing and ligating high short gastric, left gastroepiploic and left gastric vessels while preserving the right gastric and right gastroepiploic vessels.
4. Perform a generous Kocher maneuver.
5. Perform extramucosal pyloromyotomy.
6. Insert 14 French rubber jejunostomy feeding tube.
7. Open peritoneum overlying the hiatus and mobilize the distal 10 cm of esophagus under direct vision, clamping and ligating lateral attachments with long right-angle clamps and dissecting with electrocautery.
8. Through oblique left cervical incision anterior to the sternocleidomastoid muscle, mobilize and encircle cervical esophagus while *avoiding direct placement of metal retractors or instruments against the tracheoesophageal groove*.
9. Mobilize the thoracic esophagus from the posterior mediastinum with posterior, anterior, and finally lateral dissections.
10. Retract 3–4 inches of esophagus into the cervical wound, divide it with a surgical stapler, and deliver the mobilized stomach and attached esophagus out of the posterior mediastinum.
11. Through the diaphragmatic hiatus, inspect the posterior mediastinum for bleeding and assess integrity of the mediastinal pleura and the need for chest tubes (place now if needed); place gauze packs into the posterior mediastinum through the hiatus from below and the neck incision from above to encourage hemostasis.
12. Divide stomach 4–6 cm distal to the esophagogastric junction, from lesser toward greater curvature, progressively straightening the stomach by traction on the gastric tip with each application of the stapler; remove the specimen from the field and assess need for frozen section on gastric margin.
13. Oversew gastric staple suture line and transpose stomach through posterior mediastinum until 3–5 cm of gastric tip is visible in cervical wound.
14. Loosely narrow diaphragmatic hiatus and suture stomach to edge of diaphragm and left lobe of liver against the hiatus.
15. Bring jejunostomy tube through left upper quadrant of anterior abdominal wall, suture tube site to anterior abdominal wall and tube to skin, close abdomen and cover the incision with a drape to prevent contamination by oral bacteria during performance of the CEGA.
16. Perform side-to-side stapled CEGA, place Penrose drain adjacent to the anastomosis, and close cervical wound.
17. Obtain a portable chest radiograph in the operating room prior to extubation to identify and treat a previously unrecognized hemo- or pneumothorax.

Potential Pitfalls

- Abdominal phase: In the event of a hiatal hernia that displaces the greater curvature upward through the hiatus, division of the greater omentum away from the stomach may result in injury to the right gastroepiploic artery unless a conscious effort is made to pull the stomach down out of the hiatus prior to dividing any short gastric vessels to be certain this dissection is beginning high on the greater curvature; ischemic necrosis of the stomach by ligating the short gastric vessels too close to the gastric wall; splenic capsular tear due to excessive traction on the greater omentum and stomach during the gastric mobilization; inadvertent division of a "replaced left hepatic artery" due to failure to identify this structure in the gastrohepatic omentum; pyloroduodenal mucosal injury during pyloromyotomy (repaired with several 5-0 monofilament sutures and a Graham patch. This does not require conversion to a pyloroplasty.
- Cervical recurrent laryngeal nerve injury due to direct application of a metal retractor or instrument against the tracheoesophageal groove.
- Mediastinal dissection: hypotension (blood pressure monitored with a radial artery catheter) from cardiac displacement as the hand is placed into the mediastinum (the hand must consciously be kept as flat as possible parallel to the spine). A pneumothorax may occur due to entry into one or both pleural cavities during the esophageal mobilization (assessed by direct inspection through the hiatus once the esophagus has been mobilized out of the mediastinum. Placement of chest tube(s) should be performed prior to beginning preparation of gastric tube. Bleeding from injury to the aorta or azygos vein (controlled initially by packing the mediastinum, and if unsuccessful, conversion to a thoracotomy for direct clamping/suturing). Posterior membranous tracheal tear (managed by advancing the endotracheal tube down the left main bronchus and conversion to a right thoracotomy for suture repair if needed). Chylothorax (with dense periesophageal adhesions)—once esophageal mobilization is completed, perform a prophylactic "mass ligature" of thoracic duct through the hiatus with several 2-0 chromic sutures placed to the prevertebral fascia between the aorta and the azygos vein. Gastric torsion—once the tip of the stomach has been delivered into the cervical wound, be certain that the gastric staple suture line is directed toward the patient's right side and that the right gastroepiploic vascular pedicle viewed through the hiatus is toward the patient's left side.
- CEGA leaks invariably have a cause, for example, tension due to insufficient mobilization of the stomach or excessive shortening of the cervical esophagus during its division or trauma to the stomach during mobilization.

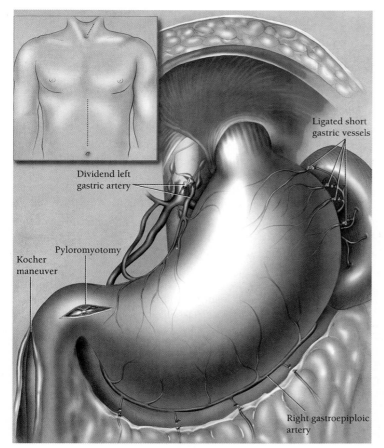

FIGURE 76-2. THE is performed through a supraumbilical midline abdominal incision and a 5- to 7-cm long oblique left cervical incision that parallels the anterior border of the left sternocleidomastoid muscle (**inset**). Gastric mobilization involves division and ligation of the high short gastric and left gastroepiploic vessels along the greater curvature and the left gastric artery and vein along the lesser curvature. The right gastric and the right gastroepiploic vessels are preserved. A pyloromyotomy, Kocher maneuver, and insertion of the feeding jejunostomy tube complete the abdominal phase of the operation. (Reprinted from Orringer MB. Transhiatal esophagectomy without thoracotomy. *Oper Tech Thorac Cardiovasc Surg.* 2005;10(1):63-83. Copyright © 2005 Elsevier, with permission.)

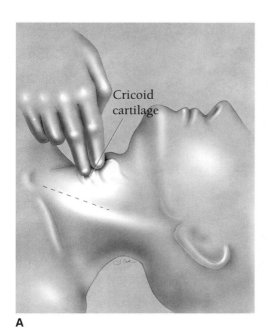

A

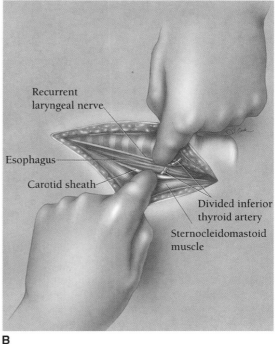

B

FIGURE 76-3. A: The cricoid cartilage is palpated and marks the level of the cricopharyngeal sphincter. The superior extent of the 5- to 7-cm incision extends no more than 2 to 3 cm superior to the cricoid cartilage. **B:** The surgeon's finger placed against the recurrent laryngeal nerve in the tracheoesophageal groove. Attention must be taken to avoid injury to the recurrent laryngeal nerve during this portion of the dissection. The cricoid cartilage is the anatomic landmark for localizing the inferior thyroid artery that occurs at the same plane but deeper in the wound. The sternocleidomastoid muscle and carotid sheath and its contents are retracted laterally, and the dissection proceeds posteriorly to the prevertebral fascia. After blunt finger dissection into the superior mediastinum, the cervical esophagus is encircled with a one-inch rubber drain carefully avoiding injury to the recurrent laryngeal nerve in the tracheoesophageal groove. (Reprinted from Orringer MB. Transhiatal esophagectomy without thoracotomy. *Oper Tech Thorac Cardiovasc Surg.* 2005;10(1):63-83. Copyright © 2005 Elsevier, with permission.)

retracted laterally and the thyroid and trachea medially; the inferior thyroid artery is divided and ligated; the dissection stays posterior to the tracheoesophageal groove and the cervical esophagus is encircled with a Penrose drain

3. Mediastinal dissection—(Figure 76-4) posterior mobilization of esophagus from the prevertebral fascia using the hand inserted through the hiatus from "below" and a "sponge-on-a-stick" from above; (Figure 76-5) anterior mobilization of the esophagus away from the pericardium and tracheobronchial tree; (Figure 76-6A and B) mobilization and division of lateral esophageal attachments; (Figure 76-7) division of cervical esophagus with surgical stapler; delivering the stomach and attached esophagus out of the abdomen; inspecting the lower mediastinum through the hiatus for bleeding or violation of the pleural requiring chest tube placement; packing the low mediastinum with a large abdominal gauze pack and the upper mediastinum with two narrow "thoracic" packs; (Figure 76-8A and B) preparing the gastric conduit by dividing the stomach with the linear surgical staple 4 to 6 cm distal to the esophagogastric junction; oversewing the gastric staple suture line; (Figure 76-9) transposing the "tubularized" stomach through the hiatus with one hand until the fundus can be palpated anterior to the spine with a finger inserted through the cervical incision; delivering 4 to 5 cm of gastric tip into cervical wound; bringing the jejunostomy tube through the abdominal wall; abdominal closure

4. CEGA—(Figure 76-10A–F) side-to-side stapled anastomosis; suture closure of the resultant esophagogastrostomy; placement of nasogastric tube into intrathoracic stomach; cervical wound drainage (1/4 inch Penrose drain) and closure

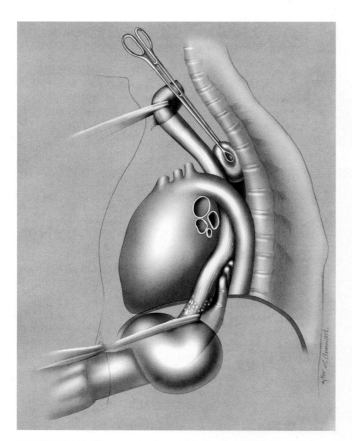

FIGURE 76-4. The cervical esophagus is retracted anteriorly and to the right as a half sponge on a stick is inserted through cervical incision posterior to the esophagus and advanced downward through the superior mediastinum along the prevertebral fascia until it meets the hand inserted through the diaphragmatic hiatus. Blood pressure is monitored during the mediastinal dissection with a radial artery catheter to prevent prolonged hypotension. (Reprinted from Orringer MB. Transhiatal esophagectomy without thoracotomy. *Oper Tech Thorac Cardiovasc Surg.* 2005;10(1):63-83. Copyright © 2005 Elsevier, with permission.)

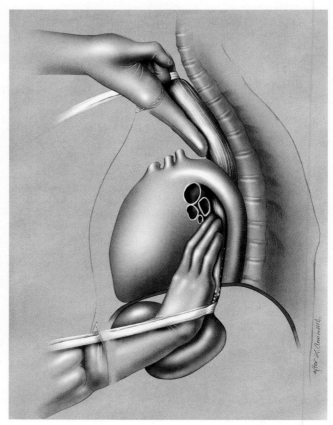

FIGURE 76-5. The anterior esophageal dissection mobilizes the esophagus away from the pericardium and the posterior membranous trachea. (Reprinted from Orringer MB. Transhiatal esophagectomy without thoracotomy. *Oper Tech Thorac Cardiovasc Surg.* 2005;10(1):63-83. Copyright © 2005 Elsevier, with permission.)

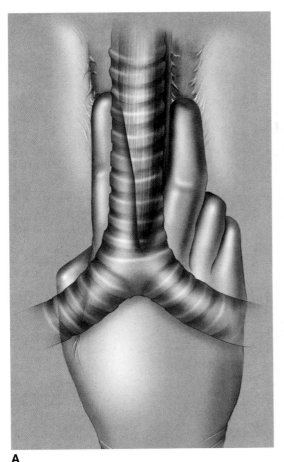

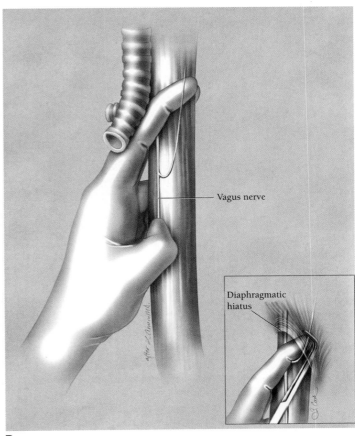

A   **B**

FIGURE 76-6. A: The surgeon's hand is inserted through the diaphragmatic hiatus along the anterior surface of the esophagus and is advanced to the level of the circumferentially mobilized cervical esophagus. **B:** The esophagus is "trapped" against the prevertebral fascia between the index and the middle fingers, and a downward raking motion of the hand avulses the small remaining upper periesophageal attachments. Small vagal branches are avulsed. Larger vagal branches below the pulmonary hila may be delivered downward closer to the diaphragmatic hiatus, visualized, clamped, and either divided with electrocautery or ligated (**inset**). (Reprinted from Orringer MB. Transhiatal esophagectomy without thoracotomy. *Oper Tech Thorac Cardiovasc Surg.* 2005;10(1):63-83. Copyright © 2005 Elsevier, with permission.)

● SPECIAL CONSIDERATIONS

Unsuspected stage IV disease discovered during the operation (e.g., an omental implant of tumor, a liver metastasis) contraindicates proceeding with an esophagectomy. The potential morbidity of an esophagectomy for palliation of dysphagia in patients with poor long-term survival is not justified. An important contraindication to THE is the surgeon's assessment of the esophagus through the hiatus suggesting significant tumor fixation or dense periesophageal fibrosis precluding safely proceeding with THE. In these situations, the surgeon should not hesitate to convert to a transthoracic approach rather than

persisting with a difficult transhiatal dissection. A right thoracotomy through the 5th intercostal space provides the best access to the mid and upper thoracic esophagus. A left posterolateral thoracotomy may be used to mobilize distal esophageal tumors. Thoracoscopic approaches may reduce pulmonary complications while allowing direct visualization of the proximal and mid-esophagus. Overly enthusiastic mediastinal lymphadenectomy should be tempered with caution when mobilizing nodal basins in proximity to the distal trachea, carina, and mainstem bronchi to avoid occult airway injury that might lead eventually to airway-enteric fistulization with its catastrophic consequences.

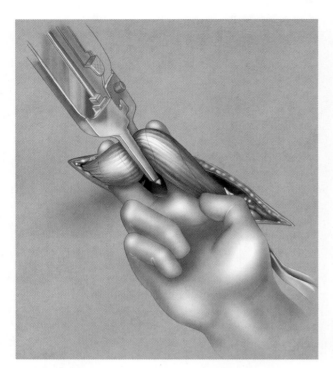

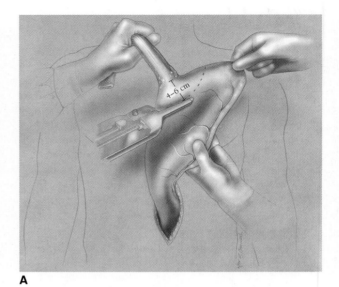

A

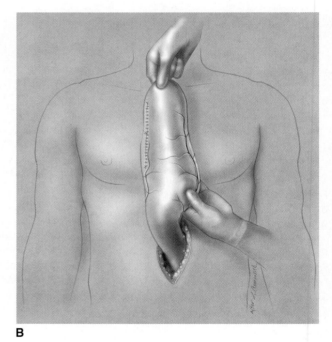

B

FIGURE 76-7. Once the entire intrathoracic esophagus has been mobilized, 3 to 4 inches are delivered into the cervical wound and the esophagus divided obliquely with a GIA surgical stapler applied from front to back with the anterior tip slightly longer than the posterior corner. (Reprinted from Orringer MB. Transhiatal esophagectomy without thoracotomy. *Oper Tech Thorac Cardiovasc Surg.* 2005;10(1):63-83. Copyright © 2005 Elsevier, with permission.)

● POSTOPERATIVE MANAGEMENT

Prior to extubation, a portable postoperative chest radiograph is obtained in the operating room to exclude an unrecognized hemo- or pneumothorax for which a chest tube is required. The routine use of epidural anesthesia is an important adjunct to consider for analgesia in this patient population. Use of the incentive inspirometer should be encouraged shortly following surgery. In addition, ambulation should begin on postoperative day one. Ice chips for throat discomfort (not to exceed 30 mL/h) are permitted the evening of surgery. The nasogastric tube is typically removed on the 3rd postoperative day. Diet is progressively advanced as tolerated, while carefully assessing for the presence of an ileus: clear liquids (day 4), full liquids (day 5), pureed diet (day 6), and soft diet (day 7). A barium swallow is routinely performed on postoperative day 7 to document the integrity of the anastomosis, adequacy of gastric emptying, and absence of obstruction at the jejunostomy tube site. Nocturnal jejunostomy tube feedings are administered if oral intake

FIGURE 76-8. A: Once the esophagus and stomach have been delivered out of the abdominal incision, the high lesser curvature of the stomach is cleared of fat and vessels at the level of the second "crow's foot." The GIA stapler is applied progressively toward the gastric fundus 4 to 6 cm distal to the esophagogastric junction, preserving as much gastric capacity and not "tubularizing" the stomach any more than necessary. **B:** After completing division of the upper stomach, the gastric staple suture line comes to rest toward the patient's right side. The gastric fundus should reach above the level of the clavicles. The staple suture line along the lesser curvature is oversewn with two running 4-0 monofilament absorbable sutures. (Reprinted from Orringer MB. Transhiatal esophagectomy without thoracotomy. *Oper Tech Thorac Cardiovasc Surg.* 2005;10(1):63-83. Copyright © 2005 Elsevier, with permission.)

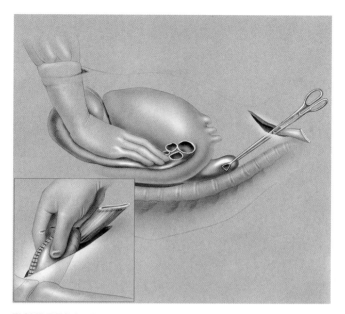

FIGURE 76-9. The gastric fundus is gently manipulated through the diaphragmatic hiatus and advanced upward into the posterior mediastinum manually until the gastric tip can be palpated with the right index finger inserted through the cervical wound. The tip of the stomach is then grasped with a Babcock forceps, but not clamped, to avoid gastric trauma. The stomach is advanced upward more by pushing it through the mediastinum from "below" rather than pulling it upward from the neck incision. Approximately 4 to 5 cm length of stomach is delivered above the level of the clavicles with the gastric staple line toward to the patient's right side (**inset**). (Reprinted from Orringer MB. Transhiatal esophagectomy without thoracotomy. *Oper Tech Thorac Cardiovasc Surg.* 2005;10(1):63-83. Copyright © 2005 Elsevier, with permission.)

is inadequate. Discharge typically is planned for the 7th postoperative day in those patients with an uncomplicated postoperative course. If the jejunostomy tube is no longer required for enteral access, it is removed 3 to 4 weeks following surgery.

If a leak of the CEGA occurs, the cervical wound is opened in its entirety at the bedside and is packed with saline moistened gauze. Enteral nutrition is delivered with jejunostomy tube feedings. Size 36, 40, and 46 French Maloney esophageal dilators are passed at the bedside within 1 week of opening the neck incision to ensure that swallowed esophageal contents pass preferentially down the esophagus and that an anastomotic stricture does not form. It is not uncommon for anastomotic leaks to close within 1 week of the esophageal dilatation. If the patient with an anastomotic leak remains febrile, has persistent purulent drainage from the neck wound, or has persistent foul odor from the wound, this heightens the concern for gastric tip necrosis. In this situation, we recommend operative exploration of the wound and flexible esophagoscopy. Reported management options also include esophageal stent placement or, more recently, use of luminal sponge vacuum therapy. Gastric tip necrosis generally requires takedown of the intrathoracic stomach through the hiatus, amputation of the devitalized stomach with a surgical stapler, and construction of an end cervical esophagostomy. Restoration of alimentary continuity is not undertaken for 6 to 12 months in order to assess for early recurrence of esophageal cancer. (In our experience, <50% of patients with esophageal cancer and gastric tip necrosis ever undergo reestablishment of alimentary continuity with a colon interposition.)

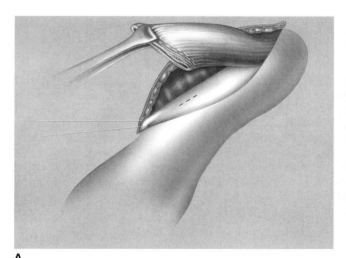
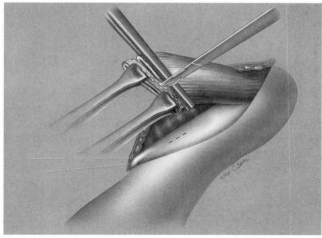

A   **B**

FIGURE 76-10. **A:** The anterior surface of the gastric fundus is elevated out of the cervical wound with a 3-0 silk traction suture that is secured to an adjacent drape. A 1.5- to 2-cm vertical gastrotomy (*dotted line*) is performed on the anterior gastric wall. **B:** The stapled tip of the divided cervical esophagus is amputated distal to an occluding DeBakey forceps that serves as a guide for the transection. The amputated tip of the esophagus is submitted to pathology as the "proximal esophageal margin."

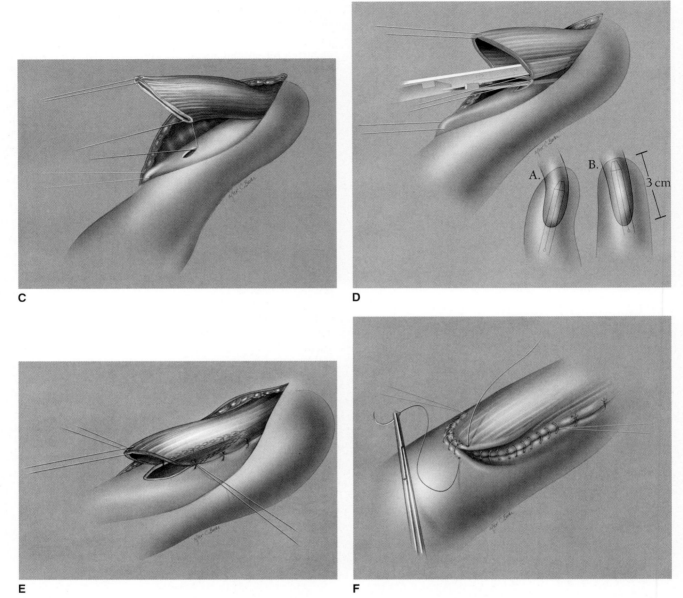

FIGURE 76-10. (*Continued*) **C:** A stay suture is placed through the anterior tip of the divided esophagus and another through the upper end of the gastrotomy and the posterior tip of the divided esophagus. These sutures align the posterior wall of the esophagus with the anterior wall of the stomach. **D:** An Endo-GIA 30-3.5 or medium/thick staple cartridge (Medtronic, Minneapolis MN) is inserted with the anvil in the stomach and the staple-bearing portion in the esophagus. **E:** After firing the Endo-GIA stapler, a 3-cm long side-to-side esophagogastric anastomosis has been constructed. The stapler is removed and a nasogastric tube inserted by the anesthesiologist and guided across the anastomosis into the stomach by the surgeon. **F:** The esophagotomy and gastrotomy are closed in two layers, an inner layer of running 4-0 monofilament absorbable suture and an outer layer of interrupted 4-0 monofilament absorbable suture. (Reprinted from Orringer MB. Transhiatal esophagectomy without thoracotomy. *Oper Tech Thorac Cardiovasc Surg.* 2005;10(1):63-83. Copyright © 2005 Elsevier, with permission)

TAKE HOME POINTS

- The properly mobilized stomach can reach to the neck for construction of a tension-free CEGA.
- Gentle, atraumatic gastric mobilization—keeping the stomach "pink in the belly and pink in the neck"—is key to preserving adequate conduit perfusion and avoiding a cervical esophagogastric anastomotic leak.
- Fingertip retraction of the thyroid and trachea medially, avoiding placement of metal retractors against the tracheoesophageal groove, minimizes the chance of recurrent laryngeal nerve injury.
- Clinical judgment and experience determine when tumor fixation or periesophageal fibrosis preclude a safe transhiatal approach. Conversion to a transthoracic approach should be considered in this setting.
- A gastric drainage procedure (pyloromyotomy) is routinely performed to avoid potential outlet obstruction, which may follow vagotomy that occurs with an esophagectomy.
- The cervical esophagus must not be divided too proximally to avoid tension on the subsequent anastomosis.
- The stomach should be divided 4 to 6 cm distal to the esophagogastric junction, preserving as much gastric volume and submucosal blood supply as possible, not "tubularizing" the stomach.
- To minimize trauma to the mobilized stomach, the conduit is positioned in the mediastinum manually; proper orientation (e.g., gastric staple line to the patient's right, right gastroepiploic pedicle to the patient's left) must be assured to avoid gastric torsion which can lead to an ischemic or obstructing conduit.
- The hiatus is closed loosely, the stomach sutured to the edge of the hiatus, and the left hepatic lobe secured back in its anatomical position to prevent herniation of the intestine through the hiatus into the chest.
- A side-to-side stapled CEGA minimizes the incidence of cervical esophagogastric anastomotic leak.

SUGGESTED READINGS

Davis J, Zhao L, Chang A, Orringer, MB. Refractory cervical esophagogastric anastomotic strictures: management and outcomes. *J Thorac Cardiovasc Surg.* 2011;141:444-448.

Iannettoni MD. White RI, Orringer MB. Catastrophic complications of the cervical esophagogastric anastomosis. *J Thorac Cardiovasc Surg.* 1995;110:1493-1501.

Orringer MB. Transhiatal esophagectomy without thoracotomy. *Oper Tech Thorac Cardiovasc Surg.* 2005;10:63-83.

Orringer MB, Marshall B, Chang AC, et al. Two thousand transhiatal esophagectomies: changing trends, lessons learned. *Ann Surg.* 2007;246:363-372.

Orringer MB, Marshall B, Iannettoni, MD. Eliminating the cervical esophagogastric anastomotic leak with a side-to-side stapled anastomosis. *J Thorac Cardiovasc Surg.* 2000;119:277-288.

Rice TW, Kelsen DP, Blackstone EH, et al. Esophagus and esophagogastric junction. In: Amin MB, Edge SB, Greene FL, et al., eds. *AJCC Cancer Staging Manual.* 8th ed. New York, NY: Springer; 2017:185-202.

Esophageal Perforation

STEPHEN W. DAVIES, ALYKHAN S. NAGJI, AND CHRISTINE L. LAU

77

Based on the previous edition chapter "Esophageal Perforation" by Alykhan S. Nagji and Christine L. Lau

Case Presentation

A 60-year-old man with a known history of alcohol abuse and binge drinking presents to the university emergency department complaining of substernal chest pain after multiple episodes of vomiting. Initial vital signs reveal sinus tachycardia along with a systolic blood pressure of 85 mm Hg. The patient is also febrile to 39.1°C. On physical examination, the patient is found to have a systolic crunching sound heard at the left sternal border (Hamman's sign) along with subcutaneous emphysema. Laboratory tests demonstrate an elevated white blood cell count of 15,000/mm³ but are otherwise normal.

● DIFFERENTIAL DIAGNOSIS

The combination of subcutaneous emphysema, vomiting, and chest pain constitute Mackler's triad, a pathognomonic sign for esophageal perforation. Potential causes of esophageal perforation include iatrogenic (most common; usually occurring at the cricopharyngeus, aortic knob, gastroesophageal junction, or other pathologic locations such as tumors or strictures), spontaneous (i.e., Boerhaave's syndrome, achalasia, malignancy, or stricture), trauma (i.e., penetrating or blunt injury, and foreign body or caustic injury), inflammation (i.e., gastroesophageal reflux, ulceration, and Crohn's disease), and infection. Cardiac, vascular, and/or other intrathoracic pathology must also be considered and ruled out.

Presentation Continued

The above patient has suffered from a spontaneous esophageal perforation attributable to Boerhaave's syndrome. This is a spontaneous, transmural esophageal perforation that may occur after an episode of forceful vomiting secondary to a rapid increase in intraluminal esophageal pressure and a concomitant negative intrathoracic pressure. It typically occurs in the left posterolateral wall of the esophagus approximately 2 to 3 cm proximal to the gastroesophageal junction. This area of the esophagus is inherently weak as the longitudinal fibers taper before passing onto the stomach wall.

● WORKUP

Clinical suspicion combined with imaging (i.e., plain radiography, contrast esophagography, and computed tomography [CT]), laboratory analysis, and in some cases direct visualization (i.e., flexible esophagoscopy) serves to confirm or refute the diagnosis of perforation. Additionally, these adjuncts assist with identifying the location and degree of perforation and resultant contamination.

The clinical presentation of esophageal perforation is highly dependent on the etiology, location, and timing of perforation. Pain is the most frequent complaint. Cervical perforations are associated with neck pain and dysphagia. Thoracic perforations are associated with pain in the mid chest and back. Distal injuries are associated with midepigastric pain and/or referred scapular pain (commonly associated with diaphragmatic irritation). Additionally, peritonitis may develop if intra-abdominal contamination occurs. Other signs and symptoms may include nausea, vomiting, hematemesis, dyspnea, and crepitus attributable to subcutaneous emphysema. Systemic signs of infection and/or inflammation (e.g., fever, tachycardia, hypotension, etc.) may be present depending upon the timing of presentation.

Radiographic studies play a significant role in establishing the diagnosis of esophageal perforation. In the case of cervical esophageal perforations, a plain film of the lateral neck may demonstrate air in the prevertebral fascial. If a thoracic or abdominal esophageal perforation is suspected, an upright abdominal along with a posteroanterior (Figure 77-1) and lateral chest radiograph should be obtained. It stands to reason that if plain films demonstrate a pleural effusion, pneumomediastinum, subcutaneous emphysema, hydrothorax, pneumothorax, or subdiaphragmatic air, the suspicion for esophageal perforation increases. However, if the plain film is normal after a suspected esophageal injury, further workup is needed.

Contrast esophagography is the study of choice for the diagnosis of esophageal perforation. Two forms of contrast are available to decipher the presence and location of a perforation. Gastrografin, being water-soluble, has traditionally been the initial contrast of choice secondary to its rapid absorption after extravasation through the perforation (Figure 77-2). In the event that no perforation is detected with a water-soluble agent, serial dilute barium esophagography should be performed. Dilute barium should be

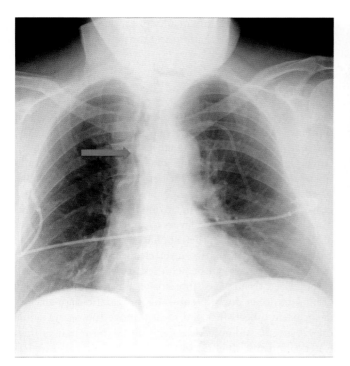

FIGURE 77-1. Chest x-ray demonstrating pneumomediastinum (*arrow*).

used exclusively in patients at high risk for aspiration or if a tracheoesophageal fistula is suspected. A negative result with suspicion of perforation requires repetition of barium contrast esophagography, and possibly a CT (Figure 77-3) and/or esophagoscopy. Flexible esophagoscopy provides direct visualization of the perforation.

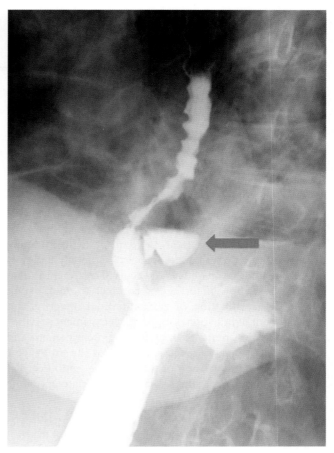

FIGURE 77-2. Esophagogram demonstrating leakage of contrast (*arrow*) into the left chest secondary to distal esophageal perforation.

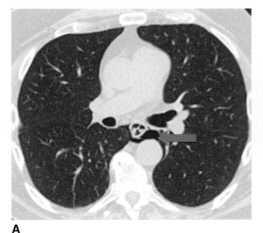 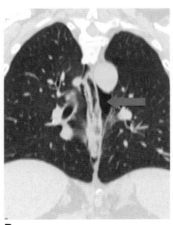 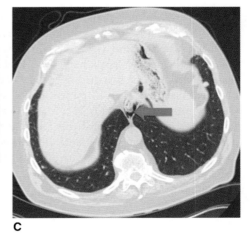

A   **B**   **C**

FIGURE 77-3. **A:** Axial computed tomography (CT) image demonstrating pneumomediastinum. **B:** Coronal CT image demonstrating pneumomediastinum. **C:** Axial CT image demonstrating air at the level of the distal esophagus and gastroesophageal junction.

Presentation Continued

Following the history and physical examination, a postero-anterior/lateral (PA/lateral) chest radiograph is obtained that demonstrates a left pleural effusion along with mediastinal air. The patient subsequently undergoes a thin barium swallow, which demonstrates extravasation into the left chest consistent with a suspected, contained, thoracic esophageal perforation (Figure 77-2).

● DIAGNOSIS AND TREATMENT

Therapy for esophageal perforation is dependent upon the age and health of the patient, the damage to surrounding tissues, and the underlying esophageal pathology and may be nonoperative or operative. The goals of treatment should include prevention of further contamination, elimination of infection, restoration of gastrointestinal integrity, and establishment of nutritional support. Management of a thoracic perforation requires the following: debridement and drainage of the pleural spaces, control of the esophageal leak, complete reexpansion of the lung, prevention of gastric reflux, nutritional support, and appropriate antibiotic treatment.

● SURGICAL APPROACH

Nonoperative Management

Nonoperative interventions (conservative therapy) involve intravenous fluid resuscitation, broad-spectrum antibiotics, drainage of fluid collections (i.e., chest tube placement for pleural effusions), cessation of oral intake, and initiation of parenteral nutrition. This approach is most successful in patients with recent, small, contained, thoracic esophageal perforation (<24 hours), minimal symptoms, and no evidence of sepsis or critical illness, malignancy, distal obstruction or stricture, or history of esophageal dysmotility. Assuming that the patient remains stable, a repeat Gastrografin swallow study is performed after seven days to evaluate leak resolution. If the leak has resolved, liquid enteral nutrition may be initiated. If the leak is still present, the above course may be repeated until the leak resolves or the patient becomes unstable, at which time surgical intervention may be needed.

Operative Approach

Surgical options include primary closure with or without buttressing repair, esophagectomy with immediate versus delayed reconstruction, esophageal exclusion and diversion, or T-tube placement and drainage. Selection of the appropriate surgical approach relies heavily on the etiology, location and timing of perforation, quality of esophageal tissue margins, degree of contamination, and the patient's overall clinical picture.

Primary Repair

The surgical treatment of choice for an otherwise normal thoracic esophageal perforation is primary repair. The perforation is to be approached using a left thoracotomy. Once exposed, the esophagus needs to be mobilized and the necrotic esophagus is debrided carefully back to viable, bleeding tissue. After proper exposure, a vertical esophageal myotomy should be performed, opening the longitudinal and circular muscle layers to appreciate the full extent of the mucosal injury. The esophageal mucosa and muscle are approximated in a two-layer closure. Reinforcement of the primary repair can be achieved using a variety of well vascularized tissues (i.e., intercostal muscle, omental onlay graft, latissimus dorsi, pleura, diaphragmatic flap, etc.). A nasogastric tube is inserted to just above the repair, while the closure is submerged under saline. The repair is than tested by insufflating air and occluding the distal esophagus. If no leak is appreciated, the nasogastric tube is then advanced into the stomach. At this time the surgeon may consider the need to obtain enteral access (i.e., gastrostomy or jejunostomy feeding tube placement) or perform additional procedures (i.e., fundoplication for significant reflux) (Table 77-1).

Table 77-1	**Primary Repair of Perforated Esophagus**

Key Technical Steps

1. Thoracotomy (dependent on location of perforation)
   a. Proximal esophageal perforation—Left neck exploration
   b. Mid-esophageal perforation—Right thoracotomy at the 4th to 6th intercostal space
   c. Distal esophagus perforation—Left thoracotomy at the 7th intercostal space
2. Harvest intercostal muscle flap—not required; decision must be made prior to thoracotomy
3. Debridement of the pleura and mediastinum
4. Mobilization of the esophagus
5. Debridement of the esophagus
6. Perform myotomy to expose entire mucosal injury
7. Two-layer closure with or without buttressing of repair
8. Enteral access

Potential Pitfalls

- Inability to perform primary repair
- Presence of a distal obstruction
- Severe undilatable reflux strictures

Presentation Continued

A left thoracotomy at the seventh interspace was used for exposure, during which an intercostal muscle flap was harvested. Care was taken to make sure the pleura and mediastinum were debrided and the distal esophagus was mobilized. The perforation was visualized and the esophagus was debrided. Subsequently, a myotomy was performed to expose the entire mucosal tear and a two-layer repair was performed. The repair was buttressed with an intercostal muscle flap. The thorax was irrigated and a chest tube was placed after which a feeding gastrostomy tube was placed for enteral access.

SPECIAL INTRAOPERATIVE CONSIDERATIONS

Resection, Diversion

When primary repair is not possible, surgical options include esophageal resection with immediate or delayed reconstruction, or exclusion and diversion. Resection should be considered when confronted with the following circumstances: megaesophagus from achalasia, carcinoma, caustic ingestion, or severe undilatable reflux strictures. The surgical approach to an esophagectomy is dictated by the surgeon's experience and underlying pathology.

In patients with a severely devitalized esophagus or when a patient is unable to tolerate definitive repair, the surgeon should consider exclusion and diversion techniques. This includes closure of the perforation, diversion, and pleural drainage, along with the creation of a cervical esophagostomy for proximal diversion. Drainage can also be achieved via the placement of a T tube distal to the esophageal perforation with the long arm directed towards the stomach and the short arm in the esophagus proximal to the site of injury. The T tube is then brought out through a separate incision.

More recently, there has been an increased use of self-expanding, covered esophageal stents as both an adjunct to some of the previously mentioned surgical interventions and as definitive management. While originally used primarily for the palliative management of spontaneous perforations secondary to malignancy, some institutions have begun to incorporate this modality, alongside of aggressive conservative therapy, for the treatment of every esophageal perforation encountered. They purport as high as 100% esophageal salvage rates without need for surgical intervention (i.e., repair or esophagectomy). Additional benefits include earlier initiation of enteral feeds, shorter hospital duration, and lower cost compared to surgical intervention. Complications encountered include stent migration, perforation/erosion, fistula formation, stent-related bleeding, and need for reintervention related to persistent leak. The most commonly reported reasons for stent failure include proximal/cervical location, gastroesophageal junction location, perforation injury >6 cm, and persistent leak. Optimal stent removal should occur approximately 4 weeks from placement as studies have shown an increased risk for stent migration, dysphagia, stent-associated bleeding, and stent fracture. Following stent removal, a repeat esophagogram is required to confirm leak resolution.

POSTOPERATIVE MANAGEMENT

Postoperative management of esophageal perforation is highly dependent upon the intervention taken. If a primary repair was attempted, a follow-up esophagogram (Figure 77-4) is needed to evaluate leak resolution. In the event that a leak is present, the chest tube placed intraoperatively should suffice for drainage. However, if not adequately drained, the surgeon should consider placement of a CT-guided pigtail. The thoracostomy tube(s) should be taken off suction, as long as the lung has completely reexpanded, and a repeat swallow study should be performed in 5 to 7 days to show that the perforation has healed.

Case Conclusion

Postoperatively, the patient did quite well. The chest tube was taken off suction, and the lung remained expanded. On postoperative day 5 the patient had an esophagogram that failed to demonstrate an esophageal leak (Figure 77-4). The patient's nasogastric tube was removed, and the patient was started on a limited diet.

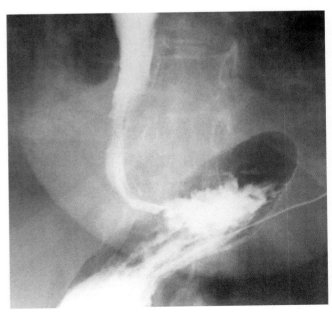

FIGURE 77-4. Esophagogram demonstrating absence of leak after primary repair of esophagus.

TAKE HOME POINTS

- Early identification of esophageal perforation is critical.
- Employment of proper imaging and direct visualization modalities is needed.
- Surgical approach is dictated by location of perforation.
- Complete intraoperative exposure of mucosal injury and two-layer closure is mandatory.
- Intraoperative recognition of circumstances that prevent primary repair.
- Postoperative imaging is performed to confirm repair of esophageal perforation.

SUGGESTED READINGS

Al Ghossaini N, Lucidarme D, Bulois P. Endoscopic treatment of iatrogenic gastrointestinal perforations: an overview. *Dig Liver Dis.* 2014;46(3):195-203.

Ben-David K, Behrns K, Hochwald S, et al. Esophageal perforation management using a multidisciplinary minimally invasive treatment algorithm. *J Am Coll Surg.* 2014;218(4):768-774.

Biancari F, D'Andrea V, Paone R, et al. Current treatment and outcome of esophageal perforations in adults: systematic review and meta-analysis of 75 studies. *World J Surg.* 2013;37(5):1051-1059.

Brinster CJ, Singhal S, Lee L, Marshall MB, Kaiser LR, Kucharczuk JC. Evolving options in the management of esophageal perforation. *Ann Thorac Surg.* 2004;77(4):1475-1483.

Bufkin BL, Miller JI Jr, Mansour KA. Esophageal perforation: emphasis on management. *Ann Thorac Surg.* 1996;61(5):1447-1451; discussion 51-52.

Dasari BV, Neely D, Kennedy A, et al. The role of esophageal stents in the management of esophageal anastomotic leaks and benign esophageal perforations. *Ann Surg.* 2014;259(5):852-860.

Derbes VJ, Mitchell RE Jr. Hermann Boerhaave's Atrocis, nec descripti prius, morbi historia, the first translation of the classic case report of rupture of the esophagus, with annotations. *Bull Med Libr Assoc.* 1955;43(2):217-240.

Foley MJ, Ghahremani GG, Rogers LF. Reappraisal of contrast media used to detect upper gastrointestinal perforations: comparison of ionic water-soluble media with barium sulfate. *Radiology.* 1982;144(2):231-237.

Freeman RK, Ascioti AJ, Dake M, Mahidhara RS. An assessment of the optimal time for removal of esophageal stents used in the treatment of an esophageal anastomotic leak or perforation. *Ann Thorac Surg.* 2015;100(2):422-428.

Freeman RK, Ascioti AJ, Giannini T, Mahidhara RJ. Analysis of unsuccessful esophageal stent placements for esophageal perforation, fistula, or anastomotic leak. *Ann Thorac Surg.* 2012; 94(3):959-964; discussion 64-65.

Freeman RK, Herrera A, Ascioti AJ, Dake M, Mahidhara RS. A propensity-matched comparison of cost and outcomes after esophageal stent placement or primary surgical repair for iatrogenic esophageal perforation. *J Thorac Cardiovasc Surg.* 2015; 149(6):1550-1555.

Han SY, McElvein RB, Aldrete JS, Tishler JM. Perforation of the esophagus: correlation of site and cause with plain film findings. *AJR Am J Roentgenol.* 1985;145(3):537-540.

Lee SH. The role of oesophageal stenting in the non-surgical management of oesophageal strictures. *Br J Radiol.* 2001;74(886): 891-900.

Lindenmann J, Matzi V, Neuboeck N, et al. Management of esophageal perforation in 120 consecutive patients: clinical impact of a structured treatment algorithm. *J Gastrointest Surg.* 2013;17(6): 1036-1043.

Menguy R. Near-total esophageal exclusion by cervical esophagostomy and tube gastrostomy in the management of massive esophageal perforation: report of a case. *Ann Surg.* 1971;173(4):613-616.

Morgan RA, Ellul JP, Denton ER, Glynos M, Mason RC, Adam A. Malignant esophageal fistulas and perforations: management with plastic-covered metallic endoprostheses. *Radiology.* 1997;204(2):527-532.

Nicholson AA, Royston CM, Wedgewood K, Milkins R, Taylor AD. Palliation of malignant oesophageal perforation and proximal oesophageal malignant dysphagia with covered metal stents. *Clin Radiol.* 1995;50(1):11-14.

Nirula R. Esophageal perforation. *Surg Clin North Am.* 2014; 94(1):35-41.

Richardson JD, Tobin GR. Closure of esophageal defects with muscle flaps. *Arch Surg.* 1994;129(5):541-547; discussion 7-8.

Sabanathan S, Eng J, Richardson J. Surgical management of intrathoracic oesophageal rupture. *Br J Surg.* 1994;81(6):863-865.

Schweigert M, Santos Sousa H, Solymosi N, et al. Spotlight on esophageal perforation: a multinational study using the Pittsburgh esophageal perforation severity scoring system. *J Thorac Cardiovasc Surg.* 2016;151(4):1002-1011.

Shaffer HA Jr, Valenzuela G, Mittal RK. Esophageal perforation. A reassessment of the criteria for choosing medical or surgical therapy. *Arch Intern Med.* 1992;152(4):757-761.

Urschel HC Jr, Razzuk MA, Wood RE, Galbraith N, Pockey M, Paulson DL. Improved management of esophageal perforation: exclusion and diversion in continuity. *Ann Surg.* 1974;179(5): 587-591.

White RK, Morris DM. Diagnosis and management of esophageal perforations. *Am Surg.* 1992;58(2):112-119.

Whyte RI, Iannettoni MD, Orringer MB. Intrathoracic esophageal perforation. The merit of primary repair. *J Thorac Cardiovasc Surg.* 1995;109(1):140-144; discussion 4-6.

Wu JT, Mattox KL, Wall MJ Jr. Esophageal perforations: new perspectives and treatment paradigms. *J Trauma.* 2007;63(5):1173-1184.

Achalasia

78

TYLER R. GRENDA AND JULES LIN

Based on the previous edition chapter "Achalasia" by Tyler Grenda and Jules Lin

Presentation

A 48-year-old male with an unremarkable past medical history presents to his primary care physician with a chief complaint of difficulty swallowing. He describes symptoms of progressive dysphagia to both solids and liquids over the past year at every meal. He regurgitates undigested food daily and has lost 20 lb over the past 9 months. He occasionally regurgitates when lying down at night and sometimes wakes up coughing. He denies any nausea, chest, or abdominal pain. His vital signs and physical examination are otherwise unremarkable.

● DIFFERENTIAL DIAGNOSIS

There are several possible etiologies for this patient's progressive dysphagia. Painless dysphagia to both solids and liquids with regurgitation of undigested food is suggestive of achalasia. However, pseudoachalasia, with obstruction secondary to a neoplasm in the distal esophagus or extraluminal compression, can present in the same manner and must be considered in the differential. Upper endoscopy is essential to evaluate for a tumor, stricture, or other esophageal or gastric pathology as the cause of his symptoms. The differential includes esophageal dysmotility, esophageal spasm, a peptic stricture, and Zenker's or epiphrenic diverticulum. Diffuse esophageal spasm results in simultaneous, frequent contractions. However, relaxation of the lower esophageal sphincter (LES) is normal, and patients complain more frequently of chest pain. Surgery is not indicated and is unlikely to resolve the patient's symptoms. Chagas' disease is clinically identical to achalasia but is caused by the parasite *Trypanosoma cruzi*, which destroys the myenteric plexus, and is common in South America.

● WORKUP

The patient undergoes a barium swallow, which reveals a dilated esophagus with a "bird's beak" narrowing at the gastroesophageal junction (Figure 78-1A). An upper endoscopy is performed, which shows no evidence of a mass or stricture. The esophagus is dilated with retained fluid and food debris. The LES is tight with mild resistance when passing the endoscope. Laboratory values are obtained and are within normal limits. He also undergoes an esophageal manometry, which reveals an aperistaltic esophageal body with an elevated integrated relaxation pressure (IRP) with incomplete relaxation of the LES in 100% of wet swallows (WS). Liquid boluses clear in 0% of swallows (Figures 78-2 and 78-3).

● DISCUSSION

Achalasia is a primary esophageal motility disorder of unknown etiology that is characterized by an aperistaltic esophagus and a LES that fails to relax in response to swallowing. Due to neural degeneration from the dorsal motor nucleus to the myenteric plexus, vagal innervation is lost. Achalasia affects approximately 1 per 100,000 people in the United States and typically presents between the ages of 20 and 50, although it may present at any age. Failure of the LES to relax results in a functional obstruction at the level of the gastroesophageal junction.

● DIAGNOSIS AND TREATMENT

Accurately characterizing the patient's symptoms are important in suggesting a diagnosis of achalasia, which is usually associated with progressive dysphagia to both solids and liquids, effortless regurgitation, and weight loss. The severity of the patient's symptoms can be assessed using the Eckardt Scoring system (Table 78-1). This patient's symptoms are consistent with achalasia with an Eckardt Score of 8.

Upper endoscopy must be performed to evaluate for pseudoachalasia caused by an esophageal carcinoma or a peptic stricture. Chest CT can also be useful to evaluate for extrinsic compression. A chest radiograph can suggest the diagnosis of achalasia with absence of a gastric air bubble or a dilated esophagus. The diagnosis is often confirmed on a barium swallow showing a dilated esophagus with an air-fluid level and narrowing of the gastroesophageal junction giving the classic "bird's beak" appearance (Figure 78-1A).

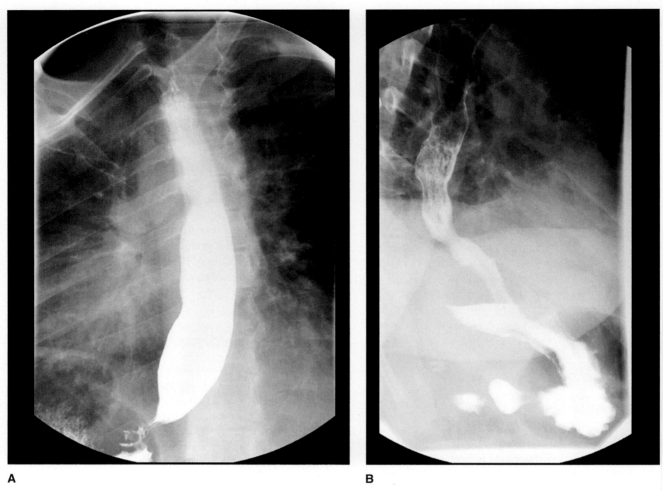

A   **B**

FIGURE 78-1.   On barium esophagram **(A)**, the distal esophagus is aperistaltic and mildly dilated. There is a bird's beak narrowing at the gastroesophageal junction with significant hold-up of contrast consistent with achalasia. Postoperative barium swallow **(B)** shows no leak and easy passage of contrast through the gastroesophageal junction.

Manometry is an important tool in the diagnosis of achalasia and shows an aperistaltic esophagus and an LES that fails to relax with swallowing (Figure 78-3). High resolution manometry is more sensitive, and an elevated median IRP > 15 mm Hg is consistent with achalasia. Achalasia has been divided into three subtypes based on findings on high-resolution manometry according to the Chicago classification system (Table 78-2). Given the findings present in this patient's workup, his symptoms are most likely secondary to type I achalasia. The manometric subtypes of achalasia differ in their responsiveness to treatment with type II being the most responsive. Type III achalasia has the highest failure rate but may respond better to esophagomyotomy than other treatments.

The primary goal of treatment is palliation of the patient's symptoms by alleviating the distal esophageal obstruction present at the LES. None of the available treatments will return the esophagus to normal, and the esophageal body remains aperistaltic. In addition, a careful balance must be achieved between alleviating the obstruction and creating gastroesophageal reflux.

Pharmacologic therapies, such as calcium channel blockers and nitrates, cause smooth muscle relaxation and decrease LES pressure. The effectiveness of these treatments is short-lived and often causes significant side effects. As a result, these should be reserved for temporizing therapy and for patients that are poor surgical candidates.

Endoscopic injection of botulinum toxin (Botox) into the LES relaxes the smooth muscle fibers. While this treatment can improve dysphagia, its effects often last <6 months and require repeat injections for continued relief of symptoms. Botox injections can also cause an inflammatory reaction, which can make a future myotomy more difficult. Therefore, Botox should be reserved for individuals that are poor candidates for endoscopy or surgery or to temporarily improve symptoms and the ability to eat until more definitive treatment.

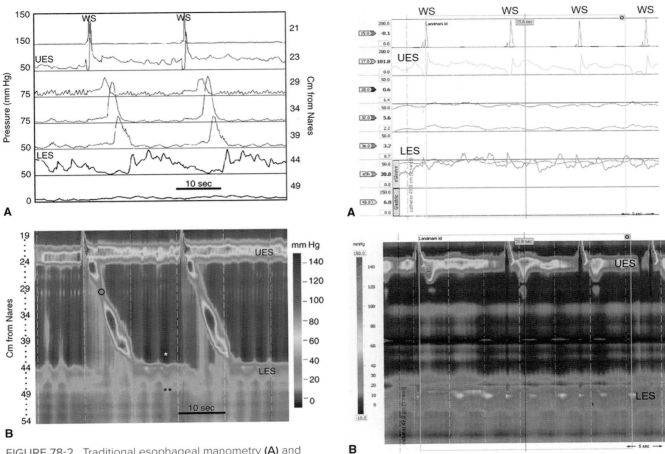

FIGURE 78-2. Traditional esophageal manometry (A) and high-resolution manometry (B) show normal peristalsis and relaxation of the lower esophageal sphincter (LES) with each wet swallow (WS). UES, upper esophageal sphincter. (From Jee SR, et al. A high-resolution view of achalasia. *J Clin Gastroenterol.* 2009;43(7):646.)

FIGURE 78-3. Esophageal manometry (A) and high-resolution manometry (B) show aperistalsis of the esophageal body on all wet swallows (WS) with no relaxation of the lower esophageal sphincter (LES). UES, upper esophageal sphincter.

Pneumatic dilation disrupts the smooth muscle fibers of the LES and is successful in relieving dysphagia in 60% to 75% of patients after a single dilation and in up to 85% after multiple dilations. The risk of perforation associated with this procedure is approximately 3% to 5%. It is typically considered to be less effective in younger patients, and 20% to 40% require repeat dilation. Pneumatic dilation should be reserved for patients that are unable to undergo myotomy.

A laparoscopic esophagomyotomy is the treatment of choice, particularly in patients younger than 40 years, and relieves symptoms in 85% to 97% initially and more than 80% at 10 years. Given this patient's degree of symptoms, findings consistent with achalasia, and limited comorbidities, a laparoscopic modified Heller myotomy with a Dor fundoplication would be the most appropriate treatment. While esophageal myotomy was performed through a

Table 78-1	Clinical Scoring System for Achalasia Symptoms (Eckardt Score)			
Score	Symptom			
	Weight Loss (kg)	Dysphagia	Retrosternal Pain	Regurgitation
0	None	None	None	None
1	<5	Occasional	Occasional	Occasional
2	5–10	Daily	Daily	Daily
3	>10	Each meal	Each meal	Each meal

Table 78-2	Chicago Classification of Achalasia Subtypes
Type	**Description**
Type I (Classic Achalasia)	Aperistalsis with incomplete LES relaxation without pressurization of the esophageal body (<30 mm Hg).
Type II (Panesophageal Pressurization)	Aperistalsis with incomplete LES relaxation. More than 20% of swallows with panesophageal pressurization (>30 mm Hg).
Type III (Spastic Achalasia)	Incomplete LES relaxation. More than 20% of swallows with spastic contractions with rapid propagation of pressurization.

LES, lower esophageal sphincter.

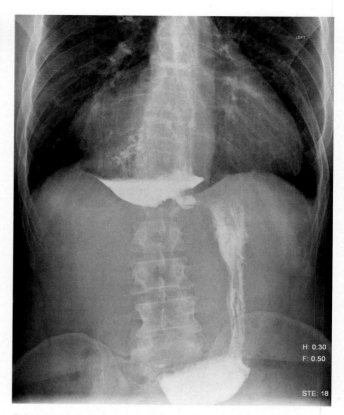

FIGURE 78-4. Barium esophagram demonstrates end-stage achalasia with a grossly dilated megaesophagus up to 12 cm with minimal flow through the gastroesophageal junction 20 years after a previous esophageal myotomy.

thoracotomy or laparotomy in the past, it is now most commonly performed laparoscopically since the angle for the myotomy is easier and allows the addition of a fundoplication to prevent reflux. Laparoscopic myotomy relieves symptoms in 90% of patients and is more effective in providing prolonged symptom relief than endoscopic therapy with a low morbidity (6.3%) and mortality (0.1%). A partial fundoplication should be performed at the time of myotomy to reduce the incidence of reflux (8.8% vs. 31.5%).

A more recent development is the peroral endoscopic myotomy (POEM). After making an endoscopic mucosotomy, a myotomy is performed through a submucosal tunnel and has had similar initial improvement in symptoms as laparoscopic myotomy. POEM may provide an alternative especially in higher risk patients; however, longer term results are needed. Recent data suggests that patients are more likely to have an increase in gastroesophageal reflux in 37.5% to 53.4% since an antireflux procedure is not performed.

Since the esophagus remains aperistaltic, patients with a megaesophagus or a sigmoid esophagus with significant tortuosity or angulation (Figure 78-4) will continue to have poor emptying despite a myotomy and should undergo an esophagectomy. In addition, patients who have had a previous myotomy should undergo transhiatal esophagectomy unless there is concern that the previous myotomy was incomplete.

● SURGICAL APPROACH

The patient is restricted to a clear liquid diet for 2 days prior to the operation. Since the dilated esophagus may contain large amounts of fluid and retained food, decompression with a nasogastric tube prior to induction of general anesthesia is critical to prevent aspiration. The patient is then placed in the supine position. A camera port is placed above the umbilicus, and pneumoperitoneum is established to 15 mm Hg. Four additional ports are placed under direct vision with

two 5-mm working ports in the epigastrium, a subxiphoid 5-mm port for the liver retractor, and a 5-mm port in the left abdomen to retract the stomach. The gastrohepatic ligament is opened, and the right crus is identified. The anterior aspect of the esophagus is bluntly dissected while the posterior planes are left intact unless there is a hiatal hernia.

The gastroesophageal fat pad is removed exposing the gastroesophageal junction. Care is taken to identify and preserve the anterior vagus nerve. The myotomy is started just above the gastroesophageal junction using the hook cautery. The longitudinal and circular muscle fibers are divided 6 cm onto the esophagus and 2 cm onto the stomach. The edges of the myotomy are bluntly separated from the mucosa for half of the esophageal circumference. The integrity of the esophageal mucosa is then tested with insufflation through the endoscope with the myotomy submerged under water. The location of the gastroesophageal junction is confirmed endoscopically to ensure that the myotomy extends at least 2 cm onto the stomach.

An anterior (Dor) or a posterior (Toupet) fundoplication is then performed after the myotomy is completed. The Dor fundoplication has the added benefit of buttressing the myotomy site and is constructed by placing two sutures on either side of the hiatus passing through the fundus, the divided esophageal muscle, and the crus (Table 78-3).

Table 78-3	Laparoscopic Heller Myotomy with a Dor Fundoplication

Key Technical Steps

1. Place a nasogastric tube prior to induction to prevent aspiration.
2. Five laparoscopic port sites.
3. Dissect the anterior aspect of the distal esophagus bluntly from the hiatus.
4. Expose the gastroesophageal junction by removing the gastroesophageal fat pad taking care to preserve the anterior vagus nerve.
5. Divide the longitudinal and the circular muscle fibers for at least 6 cm onto the esophagus and 2 cm onto the stomach.
6. Separate the edges of the myotomy from the underlying mucosa for half of the esophageal circumference.
7. Insufflate the esophagus under water to test for a leak from the myotomy site.
8. Perform an anterior (Dor) or a posterior (Toupet) fundoplication.
9. Close the laparoscopic port sites.

Potential Pitfalls

- Aspiration of retained food in the esophagus at the time of induction.
- Mucosal perforation particularly if there is scarring from previous Botox injections.
- Splenic injury due to retraction of the stomach.
- Incomplete myotomy due to failure to extend the myotomy adequately onto the stomach.

SPECIAL CONSIDERATIONS

In separating the muscle fibers from the underlying mucosa, an esophageal perforation may occur particularly if there is scarring from previous Botox treatments. The procedure should be converted to a laparotomy if the surgeon is not facile at intracorporeal suturing. The mucosal perforation should be repaired with a 4-0 absorbable suture and the overlying myotomy closed with interrupted sutures to buttress the repair. A myotomy should then be performed on the contralateral aspect of the esophagus.

POSTOPERATIVE MANAGEMENT

On postoperative day 1, an esophagram is obtained to evaluate for perforation (Figure 78-1B). If no evidence of perforation is present, a clear liquid diet is started, and the patient is discharged home. Patients are typically advanced to a mechanical soft diet, which is maintained for 3 weeks, on postoperative day 3. Mild recurrent symptoms of dysphagia, heartburn, and regurgitation may occur in up to 40% to 50% of patients. However, few of these patients will require

additional intervention other than initiation of a proton pump inhibitor or dietary modifications. Improvement in symptoms to an Eckardt score <3 is considered successful.

Case Conclusion

The patient successfully undergoes a laparoscopic Heller myotomy with a Dor fundoplication. On postoperative day 1, his esophagram shows no evidence of leak with significant improvement in esophageal emptying. He is advanced to a clear liquid diet and discharged home. At his 6-month follow-up appointment, he is tolerating a regular diet without any symptoms of dysphagia or heartburn (Table 78-1).

TAKE HOME POINTS

- Pseudoachalasia due to a carcinoma must be ruled out by upper endoscopy in a patient that presents with progressive dysphagia.
- Typical findings on esophageal manometry include an aperistaltic esophageal body with absent or incomplete relaxation of the LES.
- Botulinum toxin injection and pneumatic dilation are typically reserved for patients who are poor surgical candidates.
- Laparoscopic Heller myotomy is the standard surgical therapy for achalasia and is combined with a partial fundoplication to prevent reflux.
- Patients with megaesophagus and significant angulation or tortuosity of the esophagus should undergo a transhiatal esophagectomy.

SUGGESTED READINGS

Campos GM, Vittinghoff E, Rabl C, et al. Endoscopic and surgical treatments for achalasia: a systematic review and meta-analysis. *Ann Surg.* 2009;1:45-57.

Devaney EJ, Iannettoni MD, Orringer MB, et al. Esophagectomy for achalasia: patient selection and clinical experience. *Ann Thorac Surg.* 2001;72:854-858.

Pandolfino JE, Kwiatek MA, Nealis T, Bulsiewicz W, Post J, Kahrilas PJ. Achalasia: a new clinically relevant classification by high-resolution manometry. *Gastroenterology.* 2008;135(5):1526-1533.

Richards WO, Torquati A, Holzman MD, et al. Heller myotomy versus Heller myotomy with Dor fundoplication for achalasia: a prospective randomized double-blind clinical trial. *Ann Surg.* 2004;240(3):405-412; discussion 12-15.

Salvador R, Costantini M, Zaninotto G, et al. The preoperative manometric pattern predicts the outcome of surgical treatment for esophageal achalasia. *J Gastrointest Surg.* 2010;14(11):1635-1645.

Stefanidis D, Richardson W, Farrell TM, et al. SAGES guidelines for the surgical treatment of esophageal achalasia. *Surg Endosc.* 2012;26(2):296-311.

Swanstrom LL, Kurian A, Dunst CM, Sharata A, Bhayani N, Rieder E. Long-term outcomes of an endoscopic myotomy for achalasia: the POEM procedure. *Ann Surg.* 2012;256(4):659-667.

Williams VA, Peters JH. Achalasia of the esophagus: a surgical disease. *J Am Coll Surg.* 2009;208:151-162.

Solitary Pulmonary Nodule

79

WILLIAM Z. CHANCELLOR AND LINDA W. MARTIN

Based on the previous edition chapter "Solitary Pulmonary Nodule" by James Harris, Alicia Hulbert, and Malcolm V. Brock

Presentation

A 70-year-old man was referred to thoracic surgery clinic after a chest x-ray (CXR) performed for cough showed a 1.7-cm nodule in his right upper lobe (RUL) that was not present on previous CXR 4 years ago. Subsequent CT demonstrated a 20-mm spiculated mass without calcification (Figure 79.1). There was no mediastinal adenopathy. His medical history is significant for hypertension, and he has a 45 pack-year smoking history. He currently smokes a half-pack per day. His mother had breast cancer, but he has no family history of lung cancer. Physical examination is significant for increased AP chest diameter but is otherwise unremarkable.

● DIFFERENTIAL DIAGNOSIS

Solitary pulmonary nodules (SPNs) are well-circumscribed opacities that are <3 cm and surrounded by aerated lung. Due to the increasing volume of medical imaging, it is estimated that 150,000 SPNs are discovered incidentally every year. The majority of SPNs are benign, but the possibility of diagnosis and treating lung cancer early in its course could have life-or-death consequences for patients. Five-year survival approaches 80% for early stage lung cancer when appropriate treatment is undertaken compared to <5% survival for advanced disease. Therefore, multiple agencies have collaborated to publish guidelines that standardize the workup of pulmonary nodules to maximize early diagnosis of malignancy while avoiding unnecessary, costly, and invasive testing.

Most nodules seen incidentally on CXR or CT are benign. Benign lesions are commonly healed or nonspecific granulomas (15%), active granulomatous infections (15%), and hamartomas (15%). Other less common causes are nonspecific inflammation, abscesses, atelectasis, bronchogenic cysts, hemangiomas, and arteriovenous malformations. Imaging characteristic of benign lesions are solid appearance, heterogeneous calcification, well-circumscribed borders, symmetry, and size less that 5 mm. Malignant nodules are most often adenocarcinoma (47%), followed by squamous cell carcinoma (22%), solid metastasis (8%), undifferentiated non–small cell lung cancer (7%), and bronchioalveolar carcinoma (4%). The remaining 10% are made up of large cell carcinoma, carcinoid tumors, intrapulmonary lymphomas, adenosquamous carcinomas, adenoid cystic carcinomas, and malignant teratomas.

Imaging features, such as cavitation, irregular or spiculated borders, and size larger than 10 mm, suggest malignancy. When initally evaluating SPNs, size is the most noteworthy characteristic since only 1% of lesions <5 mm are malignant, but 80% of lesions >20 mm are cancer. Therefore, while all factors are to be considered, the driving force behind published guidelines is nodule size and growth over time.

Until recently, lung cancer was diagnosed when patients presented with symptoms such as cough, pain, or weight loss. However, lung cancer is asymptomatic until it is at an advanced stage so the 5-year survival rate has historically been very low, around 15% for all comers. Screening strategies were attempted as early as the 1960s in an effort to diagnose lung cancer at an earlier stage but they never could demonstrate an impact on lung cancer mortality. In 2011, the National Lung Screening Trial (NLST) was published, which compared annual CXR to low-dose chest CT in over 50,000 asymptomatic, at-risk patients and showed a 20% reduction in lung cancer mortality with CT scans. Based on the results of the NLST, the National Comprehensive Cancer Network (NCCN) published guidelines for lung cancer screening. Current recommendations call for annual screening with low-dose CT for adults 55 to 74 years of age who have at least a 30 pack-year smoking history and currently smoke or have quit smoking within the past 15 years, or individuals age 50 years or older with a 20 or more pack-year history of smoking with one additional risk factor (Table 79-1). Although the NCCN guidelines specify to start screening at ages 55 to

Table 79-1	NCCN Risk Factors for Lung Cancer

- Age >55 y
- Cumulative exposure to tobacco smoke
- <15 y since quitting
- Occupational exposures[a]
- Family history
- History of pulmonary fibrosis
- History of chronic obstruction pulmonary disease

USPSTF recommends annual screening for adults aged 55–80 y who have a 30 pack-year smoking history and currently smoke or have quit smoking with the past 15 y.

[a]Includes exposure to indoor cooking fumes, radon, asbestos, arsenic, chromium, and coal tar.

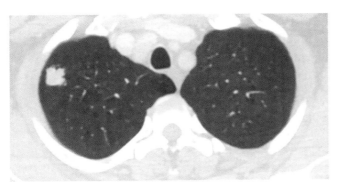

FIGURE 79-1. CT scan confirming a 1.7-cm lesion in the patient's RUL.

74 years old, there is no limit on how long patients should be screened. The current agreed upon recommendation is that screening should continue until patients are no longer candidates for definitive treatment (Figure 79-1).

● WORKUP

In the course of your initial encounter for an SPN, you should perform a complete history and physical examination with an emphasis on smoking history, occupational exposures, and personal and family history of cancer. At minimum, a chest CT, complete metabolic panel, and complete blood count should be obtained to help determine the cause

of the nodule, evaluate operative suitability, and assess for paraneoplastic syndrome or metastatic disease. All previous imaging should be reviewed to determine progression and doubling time. Volumetric assessment over time can enhance sensitivity for detecting malignant versus benign nodules. In a spherical lesion, a 30% increase in diameter represents a doubling in volume. Infectious or inflammatory lesions typically double in volume within 20 days, and nodules that take more than 400 days to double in volume are rarely malignant.

It is important to discuss imaging findings and risks of malignancy candidly with patients and to ascertain their desire for curative treatment before continuing with further workup. It is also important to determine a patient's ability to endure definitive treatment before subjecting them to further invasive and inconvenient testing. It is appropriate to assess functional status and obtain pulmonary function testing early in the process to guide decision-making. If patients with a suspicious lesion are healthy enough to undergo surgery, the need for further workup is determined by their clinical probability of having lung cancer. Although studies have shown that expert opinion is accurate for this purpose, there are validated models and online tools that can assist in quantifying a patient's lung cancer risk. Commonly used risk calculators include the Mayo Clinic Model, Brock University Nodule Malignancy Risk Calculator, and the VA SNAP Cooperative Study Group Model. Interestingly, the only factors common to all three are age and nodule size, but the Mayo and Brock University models both include spiculation and upper lobe location (Table 79-2). Each model has been validated individually but

Table 79-2	Mayo Clinic, Brock University, and VA Cooperative Study Group Models for Calculating Preoperative Probability of Lung Cancer	
Mayo Clinic	**Brock University**	**VA Cooperative Study Group**
• Age • Current or former smoker • History of extrathoracic cancer • Nodule diameter • Spiculation • Upper lobe location	• Age • Sex • Family history • Emphysema • Nodule diameter • Nodule type (ground glass, part solid, or solid) • Upper lobe location • Spiculation • Nodule count	• Age • History of smoking • Time since quitting smoking • Nodule diameter
Probability of malignancy = $100 \times e^{(X)}/(1 + e^{(X)})$ $X = (0.0391 \times \text{Age}) + (0.7917 \times \text{smoker}) + (1.3388 \times \text{cancer}) + (0.1274 \times \text{nodule diameter}) + (1.0407 \times \text{spiculation}) + (0.7838 \times \text{upper lobe}) - 6.8272$	Probability of malignancy = $100 \times (e^{(\text{Log odds})}/(1 + e^{(\text{Log odds})}))$ Log odds = $(0.0287 \times (\text{Age} - 62))$ + Sex + Family History Lung Ca + Emphysema $- (5.3854 \times ((\text{Nodule size}/10)^{-0.5} - 1.58113883))$ + Nodule type + Nodule Upper Lung $- (0.0824 \times (\text{Nodule count} - 4))$ + Spiculation $- 6.7892$	Probability of malignancy $= e^x/(1 + e^x)$ $X = -8.404 + (2.061 \times \text{smoke}) + (0.779 \times \text{age}/10) + (0.112 \times \text{diameter}) - (0.567 \times \text{years quit}/10)$

| Table 79-3 | Recommended Follow-up Based on Imaging Characteristics and Nodule Size Based on ACCP Guidelines (2013) |

Composition	Size	Risks		Recommendation
Solid	<4 mm	No RF for cancer		No further imaging
		>/=1 RF for cancer		LDCT in 12 mo
	4–6 mm	LDCT in 6–12 mo then 18–24 if no change		
	6–8 mm	LDCT in 3–6, then 9–12, then 24 mo if no change		
	>8 mm	Very low risk (<5%)		LDCT in 3–6 mo, then 18–24 mo if no change
		Low/moderate risk (5%–65%)		FDG-PET scan
		High risk (>65%)		Surgical biopsy
Part-solid	≤8 mm	LDCT in 3, 12, and 24 mo then annual LDCT for 1–3 y		
	>8 mm	Repeat CT in 3 mo then PET and biopsy if nodule persists		
Nonsolid (ground glass)	≤5 mm	No further evaluation		
	>5 mm	Annual Surveillance with LDCT for at least 3 y		

should be used with caution since they can be affected by the prevalence of cancer in your patient population.

In general, low-risk patients with solid lesions <8 mm can be followed with serial imaging and do not require further testing. Although guidelines vary (Tables 79-3–79-5), when lesions are larger than 8 mm and patients have a moderately high pretest probability of malignancy, a PET scan should be obtained to further characterize the lesion. Decision analysis modeling has shown that PET-CT at this juncture in the workup of incidentally discovered nodules decreases the number of invasive tests due to the increased sensitivity and specificity of PET-CT over CT alone. Tissue diagnosis is recommended if the lesion is PET avid, thus concerning for malignancy. Otherwise, patients can be relegated to routine surveillance imaging. It is recommended that patients with solid lesions >8 mm with high pretest probability of malignancy should forgo PET scan and have surgical biopsy. However, in our practice, it is unusual for patients to undergo resection without first undergoing a staging PET scan.

| Table 79-4 | Recommended Follow-up of Incidentally Discovered Pulmonary Nodules Based on Patient Risk Profile and Nodule Size Based on Fleischner Guidelines (2017) |

Solid	<6 mm	Low risk	No routine follow-up
		High risk	Optional LDCT in 12 mo
	6–8 mm	Low risk	LDCT at 6–12 mo, consider LDCT at 18–24 mo
		High risk	LDCT at 6–12 mo, then LDCT at 18–24 mo
	>8 mm	Low risk	Consider CT at 3 mo, PET/CT, or tissue sampling
		High risk	Consider CT at 3 mo, PET/CT, or tissue sampling
Part-solid	<6 mm		No routine follow-up
	≥6 mm		CT at 6–12 mo to confirm persistence, then CT every 2 y until 5 y
Nonsolid (ground glass)	<6 mm		No routine follow-up
	≥6 mm		CT at 3–6 mo to confirm persistence. If unchanged and solid component remains <6 mm, annual CT for 5 y.

Table 79-5	Recommended Follow-up of Screening Detected Nodules Based on Imaging Characteristics and Nodule Size Based on NCCN Lung Cancer Screening Guidelines (2017)		
Solid	≤5 mm	LDCT in 12 mo	
	6–7 mm	LDCT in 6 mo	
	8–14 mm	LDCT in 3 or consider PET-CT	
	>15 mm	Low suspicion of lung cancer	LDCT in 3–6 mo
		High suspicion of lung cancer	Biopsy or Surgical excision
Part-solid	≤5 mm	Annual LDCT until no longer candidate for definitive treatment	
	≥6 mm with solid component ≤5 mm	LDCT in 6 mo	
	≥6 mm with solid component 6–7 mm	LDCT in 3 mo or consider PET-CT	
	Solid component ≥8 mm	Chest CT with or without contrast and/or PET-CT	
Nonsolid (ground glass)	≤19	Annual LDCT until no longer candidate for definitive treatment	
	>20	LDCT in 6 mo	

Presentation Continued

According to the Mayo Clinic Solitary Pulmonary Nodule Malignancy Risk Model, our patient's pretest probability of having lung cancer is 75% based on his age, smoking history, nodule size of 20 mm, spiculation, and RUL location. PET scan demonstrates a solitary lesion in his RUL with a maximum standard uptake value (SUV) of 11.26 (Figure 79-2). At this point, a transbronchial or transthoracic biopsy would either demonstrate lung cancer or be discordant with his clinical risks and imaging features. Therefore, after a discussion including the risk and benefits of nonsurgical versus surgical biopsy, he elects to proceed with video-assisted thoracoscopic surgery (VATS) wedge resection.

● DIAGNOSIS AND TREATMENT

Incidentally discovered nodules that are likely to be cancer and nodules that exhibit malignant growth since previous imaging should have tissue diagnosis. Nonsurgical biopsy techniques include transthoracic CT-guided needle biopsy, standard bronchoscopic biopsy with fluoroscopy or ultrasound guidance, and electromagnetic navigational bronchoscopic biopsy. Bronchoscopic biopsy is limited to larger, more central lesions, while transthoracic biopsy has excellent sensi-

tivity, specificity, and positive predictive value for peripheral lesions, even when they are smaller than 2 cm. Nonsurgical biopsy techniques are recommended when there is discordance between the clinical risk of lung cancer and imaging characteristics or when the pretest probability of malignancy is moderate. Possible outcomes of a nonsurgical biopsy are malignancy, benign specific, benign nonspecific, or indeterminate. A specific, benign diagnosis, such as hamartoma or granuloma, can avert the need for surgery but suspicion should remain when the results are nonspecific, atypical, or show "normal lung"—indicating the lesion wasn't sampled.

As was mentioned previously, surgical biopsy is recommended for patients with lesions >8 mm who have high pretest probability of malignancy. Likewise, surgical biopsy is recommended when functional imaging is concerning for malignancy, nonsurgical biopsy is suspicious for malignancy, or when a fully informed patient prefers a definitive diagnostic approach. Patients who are high risk often have staging PET-CT prior to their operation. NCCN guidelines no longer recommend invasive staging procedures for all patients in light of evidence that it may not be beneficial when lesions are smaller than 3 cm or peripheral, and there is no evidence of nodal disease on PET-CT. If these criteria are not met, however, complete staging with invasive mediastinal lymph node sampling is indicated for biopsy-proven lung cancer as it can help determine the need for induction therapy prior to resection. Mediastinoscopy has been the gold standard for lymph node sampling but

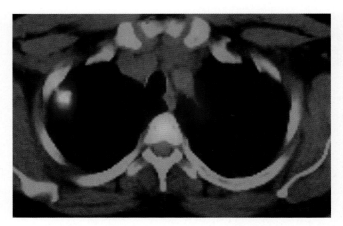

FIGURE 79-2. PET-CT showing 11.26 SUV FDG uptake of the previously seen RUL lesion.

is being replaced by endobronchial ultrasound guided transbronchial fine needle aspiration (EBUS-TFNA). Mediastinoscopy is now used mainly with EBUS samples are inadequate (Figure 79-2).

SURGICAL APPROACH

Surgical biopsy can be accomplished via open thoracotomy or VATS wedge resection. VATS biopsy offers the potential for lower morbidity and shorter hospitalization than open surgery. For VATS procedures, patients are intubated a double lumen endotracheal tube to allow ventilation of the nonoperative side only. Flexible bronchoscopy is routinely performed to ensure appropriate tube position and rule out concurrent endobronchial disease. Patients are placed in lateral decubitus position and prepped widely from the axilla to the costal margin and from the midclavicular line to the tip of the scapula transversely. A camera port is placed through a 1.5-cm incision in the eighth intercostal space at the anterior axillary line. CO_2 insufflation is used to facilitate lung collapse then secondary ports can then be placed to triangulate the lesion under direct visualization. For upper lobe lesions, working ports are centered over the superior pulmonary vein and at the sixth intercostal space near the scapula. At this point, our institution utilizes intercostal nerve block with liposomal bupivacaine intraoperatively, which is part of a larger nonnarcotic-focused pain management strategy and enhanced recovery pathway.

Peripheral nodules can often be seen and digitally palpated through the port site after lung collapse. However, advanced localization techniques may be required for central lesions or peripheral nodules that are small or otherwise difficult to identify. Once identified, nodules are resected with serial firings of an endoscopic stapler. The specimen is then removed from the thorax though a wound protector and sent to pathology for frozen section.

In this case, the pathology came back as adenocarcinoma with negative margins. A benefit of surgical biopsy is that, based on preliminary pathology results, you can proceed with staging and definitive resection during the same procedure. At this point, we performed lymph node sampling of levels 2R, 4R, 7, 8R, and 9R. All sampled nodes were negative for malignancy, which suggests early-stage NSCLC so definitive resection could be achieved with completion right lobectomy. At the end of the case, a chest tube was placed posteriorly through the camera port and the lung was reinflated carefully under direct visualization to avoid RML torsion (see Table 79-6).

SPECIAL INTRAOPERATIVE CONSIDERATIONS

Peripheral lung lesions are often easily visualized and palpated even through small thoracoscopic incisions. However, the smaller lesions that are often found incidentally or with screening can be difficult to locate intraoperatively. These lesions can be identified using hook wires, methylene blue dye, or fiduciary markers like metal coils placed using CT guidance or navigational bronchoscopy. The coils can then be localized by palpation or with fluoroscopy. Complications after localization procedures are uncommon and often clinically insignificant but include marker dislodgement, pneumothorax, hemorrhage, and air embolus. An option for localization that is gaining popularity is CT-guided transthoracic injection of a radiotracer that can be localized intraoperatively using a gamma probe. Stiles et al found this method to be effective and accurate with minimal morbidity in their early studies. While there is still a risk of pneumothorax with transthoracic injection, radiotracer localization does not require fluoroscopy and eliminates the risk of dislodgement of fiducials.

POSTOPERATIVE CARE

Following definitive resection with right upper lobectomy, our patient was sent to the floor with one chest tube in place. The most common complication after VATS lung resection is persistent air leak and the most worrisome is hemorrhage (<1%), both of which will be obvious with a properly placed chest tube. As a general rule, chest tubes are removed when there is no air leak, blood, or chyle regardless of the volume of serious drainage. It should also be noted that even small thoracotomy incisions are quite painful so the need for pain control adjuncts should be anticipated. Enhanced recovery pathways are new in thoracic surgery but are showing great potential to improve pain control and time to recovery. With adequate pain and can often be discharged in 1 to 2 days rather than 4 to 7, even after lobectomy. This patient went home a few hours after chest tube removal on postoperative day 2.

Table 79-6   Solitary Pulmonary Nodule

Key Technical Steps

1. Place patient in lateral decubitus position with reverse Trendelenburg allowing chest wall to be parallel to the floor and intercostal spaces to be maximized.
2. Intubation with double lumen endotracheal tube to allow for single lung ventilation.
3. Flexible bronchoscopy to confirm correct placement of double lumen endotracheal tube.
4. Placement of camera port through eighth intercostal space at the anterior axillary line and secondary ports through the fourth intercostal space at the midclavicular line and the sixth intercostal space near the scapula to triangulate the lesion.
5. 5–10 mmHg of CO_2 insufflation to facilitate lung collapse and allow a larger working space.
6. Identify target lesion and control proximally with lung grasper; minimize manipulation of lung to avoid causing hematoma and obscuring the nodule.
7. Resection of nodule with endoscopic stapler.
8. Removal of specimen using endoscopic retrieval bag or through wound protector. Do not pull directly through an unprotected port.
9. Send for frozen section if there is any concern about margins and if nature of the lesion will change your operative plan (i.e., conversion to lobectomy).
10. Assessment of staple line for pneumostasis and hemostasis.
11. Chest tube placement through camera port and closure of remain ports in layers.

Potential Pitfalls

- Damage to intercostal neurovascular bundle or intravascular injection of local anesthesia.
- Damage to lung/abdominal/mediastinal structures during port placement, especially if adhesions are present.
- Improper endotracheal tube placement leading to hypoxemia or poor lung isolation.
- Inability to locate nodule or remove with a clean margin.
- Failure to remove sample using retrieval bag or wound protector may lead to port site recurrence.

Case Conclusion

Final pathology showed a 1.9-cm adenocarcinoma with negative margins and 13 nodes from 6 different nodal stations that were negative for malignancy. Because he had completely resected stage 1A NSCLC, he will not require adjuvant chemotherapy or radiation therapy. According to NCCN guidelines, he should continue to have chest CT every 6 months for 2 to 3 years then annual low-dose, noncontrast CT until he is no longer a candidate for definitive treatment. Continued smoking cessation is also critical and should be reinforced at every visit.

TAKE HOME POINTS

- Greater than 90% of solitary pulmonary nodules <2 cm are benign.
- NCCN guidelines for lung cancer screening call for annual screening with low-dose CT for adults 55 to 74 years of age who have at least a 30-pack-year smoking history and currently smoke or have quit within the past 15 years or individuals age 50 years or older with a 20 or more pack-year history of smoking with one additional risk factor.
- The National Lung Screening Trial showed that annual screening with low-dose chest CT reduces mortality due to lung cancer by 20%.
- Five-year survival after complete resection of screening-detected lung cancer is >80%.
- Individuals with a solid nodule >8 mm with low to moderate risk of lung cancer should be referred for functional imaging with a PET scan.
- Individuals with a solid nodule >8 mm with high risk of lung cancer and those with PET avid lesions should be referred for surgical biopsy.
- One advantage of surgical biopsy is the potential to diagnose, stage, and definitively resect lung cancer during a single operation. This is reserved for good-risk surgical candidates.

SUGGESTED READINGS

Ettinger D, Wood D, Aisner D, et al. Non–Small Cell Lung Cancer, Version 5.2017, NCCN Clinical Practice Guidelines in Oncology. *J Natl Compr Canc Netw.* 2017;15:504-535.

Gao SJ, Kim AW, Puchalski JT, et al. Indications for invasive mediastinal staging in patients with early non-small cell lung cancer staged with PET-CT. *Lung Cancer.* 2017;109:36-41.

Gould M, Ananth L, Barnett P; for the Veterans Affairs SNAP Cooperative Study Group. A clinical model to estimate the pretest probability of lung cancer in patients with solitary pulmonary nodules. *Chest.* 2007;131(2):383–388.

Gould M, Donington J, Lynch WR, et al. Evaluation of individuals with pulmonary nodules/when is it lung cancer? Diagnosis and management of lung cancer, 3rd ed: American College of Chest Physicians Evidence-Based Clinical Practice Guidelines. *Chest.* 2013;143(5 suppl):e93S-e120S.

Gould M, Fletcher J, Iannettoni M, et al. Evaluation of patients with pulmonary nodules: when is it lung cancer? ACCP evidence-based clinical practice guidelines (2nd Edition). *Chest.* 2007;132(3 suppl):108S-130S.

MacMahon H, Austin J, Gamsu G, et al. Guidelines for management of small pulmonary nodules detected on CT scans: a statement from the Fleischner Society. *Radiology.* 2005;237:395-400.

McWilliams A, Tammemagi M, Mayo J, et al. Probability of cancer in pulmonary nodules detected on first screening CT. *N Engl J Med.* 2013;369:910-919.

Ost D, Fein AM, Feinsilver SH. The solitary pulmonary nodule. *N Engl J Med.* 2003;348:2535-2542.

Stiles BM, Altes TA, Jones DR, et al. Clinical experience with radiotracer-guided thoracoscopic biopsy of small, indeterminate lung nodules. *Ann Thorac Surg.* 2006;82:1191–1197.

Swensen S, Silverstein M, Ilstrup D, Schleck C, Edell E. The probability of malignancy in solitary pulmonary nodules. Application to small radiologically indeterminate nodules. *Arch Intern Med.* 1997;157(8):849-855.

Spontaneous Pneumothorax

HUBERT YIU-WEI LUU AND PIERRE R. THEODORE

Based on the previous edition chapter "Spontaneous Pneumothorax" by Pierre Theodore

Presentation

A 65-year-old man with a history of chronic obstructive pulmonary disease (COPD), hypertension, and a 50 pack-year history of smoking presents with acute onset shortness of breath. He regularly has dyspnea on exertion but suddenly became short of breath at rest 1 hour ago. He has new right-sided chest pain, which he describes as knife-like and worse on inspiration. He has no history of pneumothorax, acute coronary syndrome, or stroke. He denies recent chest trauma. He smokes one pack of cigarettes per day. On physical examination, he is tachycardic, hypertensive, tachypneic, and his oxygen saturation is 85% on room air. He has decreased breath sounds on the right side, decreased chest expansion on the right, and hyperresonance to percussion on the right. His trachea is midline.

● DIFFERENTIAL DIAGNOSIS

The two main groups of spontaneous pneumothorax are primary or secondary spontaneous pneumothorax. Primary pneumothorax usually occurs in a young person without underlying lung disease, as a result of rupture of an apical subpleural bleb. Classically, these patients are tall, young men who are light to moderate smokers and are often physically active.

This patient likely experienced a secondary spontaneous pneumothorax due to underlying lung disease. Other causes of secondary spontaneous pneumothorax include airway diseases, such as cystic fibrosis or asthma; significant lung infections, such as *Pneumocystis jiroveci* (*P. carinii*) pneumonia or tuberculosis; and other intrapulmonary diseases such as lung tumors, inflammatory lung disease, and connective tissue diseases of the lung. Pneumothoraces may also be due to trauma or iatrogenic causes such as subclavian line placement, percutaneous lung biopsy, chest tube clamping, or barotrauma such as deep-sea diving or mechanical ventilation.

In the elderly patient presenting with chest pain or shortness of breath, myocardial infarction, pulmonary embolism, aortic dissection, and pneumonia must be ruled out. The workup must include a physical examination with EKG, cardiac enzymes, chest x-ray, bedside chest ultrasound, and a CT scan of the chest as directed by the findings.

In young women, two additional causes of pneumothorax are lymphangioleiomyomatosis (LAM) and catamenial pneumothorax. LAM, also known as pneumothorax of pregnancy, is hormonally driven smooth muscle proliferation along lymphatic channels, which obstructs bronchioles and leads to air trapping, bullae formation, and pneumothorax. Catamenial pneumothorax occurs in young women due to ectopic migration of endometrial tissue to the thorax, forming cysts that can rupture during menses. The recurrence rate of catamenial pneumothorax is high and often requires surgical management for definitive treatment.

A leading differential diagnosis should always be tension pneumothorax, which may result in a mediastinal shift and decreased venous return leading to circulatory collapse, should always be on the differential diagnosis. Any evidence of tracheal deviation on examination requires immediate needle decompression without waiting for a chest x-ray. An audible escape of air under pressure from the thorax confirms the diagnosis. The requisite chest tube placement can thus be subsequently performed on a less emergent basis. Patients with a hemodynamically significant spontaneous pneumothorax who require intubation and ventilation should first have a small chest tube placed to prevent conversion to tension pneumothorax when positive pressure ventilation is initiated.

● WORKUP

The patient in this case should first have supplemental oxygen administered and a peripheral intravenous catheter placed. An EKG and upright chest x-ray are performed that reveal the presence of sinus tachycardia without evidence of acute ischemia and a visible partial collapse of the right lung and pneumothorax without evidence of deviation of the mediastinum, respectively. His oxygen saturations improved with the administration of supplemental oxygen through nasal cannula. An urgent CT scan of his chest reveals a right-sided pneumothorax, emphysematous changes throughout both lungs, and no evidence of malignancy (Figure 80-2).

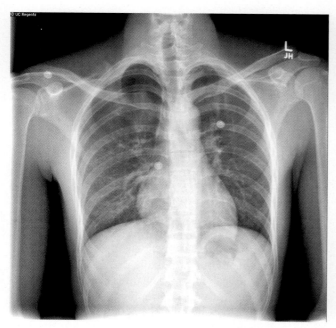

FIGURE 80-1. Chest x-ray of right-sided spontaneous pneumothorax.

● RADIOGRAPHIC FINDINGS

A pneumothorax can be most easily observed on an upright chest x-ray (Figure 80-1). An apex-to-cupola distance of <3 cm is considered a small pneumothorax. The key findings are the absence of lung markings peripheral to the visceral pleural edge and the increased radiolucency of the thoracic space compared to the lung parenchyma. One possible error

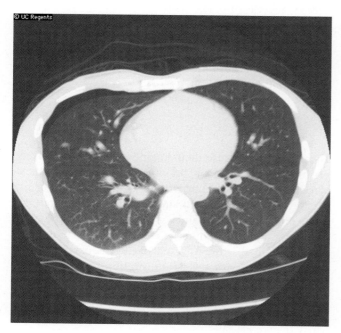

FIGURE 80-2. CT chest through the midlung showing pneumothorax.

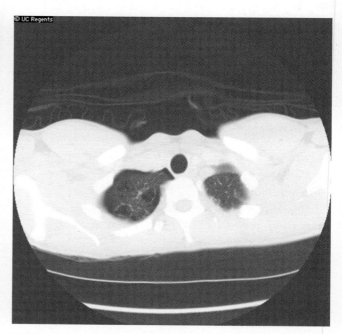

FIGURE 80-3. CT chest through the lung apex showing bullae.

in chest x-ray interpretation is to confuse a skin fold for a pneumothorax. Skin folded against the x-ray cassette appears almost as a vertical line that does not follow the contour of the rib cage. A skin fold has a different radiographic density than a pneumothorax, and vascular markings may be seen lateral to the skin fold.

In the patient with preexisting lung disease, a CT scan of the chest can help differentiate between large bullae, cystic lesions, and pneumothoraces, which may all appear similar on routine chest x-ray (Figure 80-3). The CT scan can also guide operative management by providing information about underlying lung disease. A CT scan of the chest may be omitted for younger patients with their first presentation of primary spontaneous pneumothorax. However, a CT scan may be highly useful for older patients with chronic lung disease in order to describe the severity and extent of the pathology for surgical planning.

Lung ultrasonography may also be useful in trauma or critically ill patients. Although it is not yet well established for routine use in primary spontaneous pneumothorax, recent studies in trauma patients demonstrate high sensitivity (98%) and positive predictive value (100%) but moderate negative predictive value (82%).

● MANAGEMENT AND TREATMENT

According to the 2001 management guidelines by the American College of Chest Physicians, the main goals of management are to treat the pneumothorax and to reduce the risk of recurrence by achieving visceral and parietal pleural symphysis by pleurodesis or pleurectomy. The risk of recurrence after a first episode of primary spontaneous pneumothorax is approximately 32%. These patients do not necessarily need surgical treatment or pleurodesis aimed at reducing recurrence *unless* they have bilateral pneumothoraces or are exposed to significant changes in transpulmonary pressure (e.g., pilots or divers). Any anticipated lack of access to advanced health care or long periods of travel distant from adequate health services should also prompt definitive surgical treatment. The recurrence rate after spontaneous pneumothorax associated with underlying lung disease is approximately 43%, but these patients carry a higher risk of morbidity and mortality due to their baseline respiratory compromise.

Operative management or pleurodesis is typically indicated at first presentation. For all patients, the risk of further recurrence increases with each episode. After the second pneumothorax, the recurrence risk is as high as 75% and exceeds 80% after the third pneumothorax. As such, most clinicians recommend intervention following a second episode of pneumothorax.

Clinically stable patients with small primary pneumothoraces can be observed; if the pneumothorax is radiographically stable over 6 hours and there is no progression of symptoms, they may be sent home with follow-up in 1 to 2 days. Most patients with large primary pneumothoraces will be treated with tube thoracostomy or a small "pigtail catheter" inserted into the fifth intercostal space and placed to suction for 24 to 48 hours. Early conversion to water seal drainage is sufficient for the vast majority of pneumothoraces. With radiographic resolution of the pneumothorax and no evidence of ongoing air leak, the catheter or tube may be removed, and the patient may be discharged with follow-up in 1 to 2 days. Generally, a 16 to 24 French chest tube is sufficient, although patients with a large air leak or receiving mechanical ventilation may require larger or multiple chest tubes.

If an air leak persists for more than 3 days, the patient should be evaluated for persistent or recurrent pneumothorax. The patient should be considered for surgical intervention: video-assisted mechanical or talc pleurodesis, blebectomy, or a pleural tenting procedure. Another treatment option for persistent air leak is to perform a blood patch of 50 mL of the patient's own blood instilled through the chest tube under sterile conditions and flushed with saline. The tube is clamped for 30 minutes and then returned to water seal. This procedure should not be performed if the lung is incompletely reexpanded or if the patient has evidence of infection in the pleural space. The patient should be monitored for conversion to tension pneumothorax during the procedure, as this has been reported.

Patients with pneumothoraces in the setting of severe underlying lung disease should receive prompt evaluation, supplemental oxygen, and small chest tube placed urgently. For loculated or complicated pneumothorax, placement of the chest tube under CT scan guidance may be required. The standard approach to surgical management of pneumothorax is video-assisted thoracoscopic surgery (VATS). In addition to shorter hospital stays, less pain, and disability in comparison to open thoracotomy, studies demonstrate similarly low recurrence rates of 5% after VATS. Patients who are poor surgical candidates or refuse surgery may be managed with tube thoracostomy and receive bedside pleurodesis through their chest tube.

A novel approach is the use of endobronchial valve technology to specifically obstruct the segmental orifice leading to the site of the classic air leak, though this has not been sufficiently evaluated.

Chemical pleurodesis can be performed by direct instillation of talc or doxycycline into the pleural space. Talc pleurodesis is particularly effective and has rarely been associated with acute lung injury. However, recent studies associating talc pleurodesis chronic lung injury have shifted favor to intrapleural doxycycline to promote pleurodesis.

● SURGICAL APPROACH FOR BULLECTOMY AND PLEURODESIS USING VATS

The operation for bleb/bulla resection is similar to a standard wedge resection of the lung using VATS (Table 80-1). The patient is intubated with a double-lumen endotracheal tube,

Table 80-1	Video-Assisted Thoracoscopic Bleb/Bullae Resection and Pleurodesis

Key Technical Steps

1. Prepare the patient with general anesthesia and a double-lumen endotracheal tube.
2. Commence the operation with a thorough bronchoscopy of the tracheobronchial tree.
3. For the resection, position the patient in the lateral decubitus position with single lung ventilation.
4. Place the VATS camera port at the 5th intercostal space in the anterior axillary line.
5. Depending on the location of the pathology, additional ports may be placed in the 4th intercostal space or the 7th intercostal space.
6. Similar to a wedge resection, grasp the affected tissue and apply the endoscopic stapler across the base of the bullae/bleb. Use a reinforced, linear GIA staple load.
7. After resection, abrade the parietal pleura through the VATS ports. This can be accomplished by using the electrocautery scratch pad, the electrocautery, or the argon beam coagulator.
8. Chemical pleurodesis can be accomplished by evenly distributing 1–5 mg of aerosolized sterile talc or 500 mg of powder doxycycline in 50 mL sterile saline to the pleural space.
9. Upon completion of the procedure, remove the ports and insert a single chest tube into the inferior VATS port.

which permits single-lung ventilation. Epidural catheters are not generally necessary, and the patient is placed in the lateral decubitus position. The operation commences with a thorough bronchoscopy of the tracheobronchial tree, looking for neoplasm, infectious processes, or aberrant anatomy. In order to access the lung apex, a camera port is placed at the 5th intercostal space in the anterior axillary line. Additional instrument ports may be placed in the 4th intercostal space or the 7th intercostal space depending on the location of the pathology. Apical bullae are resected using reinforced, linear GIA staple loads.

The second part of the operation is to create the conditions for pleural symphysis through mechanical or chemical means. The parietal pleura including the diaphragmatic surface can be gently abraded using the electrocautery scratch pad introduced through at VATS incision. Alternate means of mechanical abrasion of the pleura include electrocautery or the argon beam coagulator. Chemical pleurodesis is an important adjunct to mechanical pleurodesis and can be performed with 1 to 5 mg of aerosolized sterile talc or 500 mg of powder doxycycline in 50 mL sterile saline evenly distributed to the pleural space.

Pleurectomy is an option for recurrent pneumothorax particularly in younger patients and can be performed through the VATS ports. After making a small incision in the pleura, a ring forcep may be used to grasp the pleural edge, followed by a gentle stripping motion moving along the curvature of the thoracic wall.

Finally, the conventional 24 or 28 French straight chest tube should be placed aiming superoposteriorly. Alternatively, the usage of 19 French flexible silastic drains instead of the conventional plastic thoracostomy tube has increased due to acceptable results and outcomes. However, choosing the right patient for this type of tube is critical due to their higher likelihood of occluding in the presence of coagulum or pus.

● INTRAOPERATIVE COMPLICATIONS

The main intraoperative complication is a large air leak after resection of the tissue. Prior to closure, the lung should be reinflated and examined for persistent air leak. Reinforcing the lung tissue with additional stapling, fibrin glue, or both may be necessary. Approved pulmonary sealants may reduce the risk of air leak. Bleeding and infections in the pleural space represent important potential complications. However, the most common concern is a persistent air leak following resection of diseased tissue.

Intraoperative management issues also include the approach to the "trapped lung." A lung incapable of expanding to reach the parietal pleural surface creates a judgment challenge for the clinician. If trapped by infection, decortication can be performed in a thoracoscopic or, more frequently, an open procedure. Patients with trapped lung as a result of carcinoma often can be only managed with a pleural tent.

● POSTOPERATIVE MANAGEMENT

Postoperatively, the chest tube can be placed to water seal upon radiographic resolution of the pneumothorax and can be removed as early as postoperative day 3 should there be no air leak.

If the patient has a persistent air leak after postoperative day 4, then the chest tube should be connected to an outpatient suctionless device, such as a Heimlich valve. If the patient can tolerate this device for 24 hours inpatient without reexpansion of the pneumothorax or clinical deterioration, then they may be discharged home with the suctionless device and strict return precautions for any worsening of symptoms. Two weeks postoperatively, the patient should follow-up in clinic. If they remain asymptomatic on the outpatient suctionless device, the chest tube may be removed even if a small pneumothorax persists. Clamping the chest tube is not necessary prior to removal. To demonstrate stability of the pneumothorax, the patient should have a chest x-ray in 4 hours, or earlier if the clinical condition worsens.

● COMPLICATIONS

Patients should be monitored for arrhythmias, air leaks, chest tube malfunction, reexpansion pulmonary edema, or conversion to tension pneumothorax. Additionally, the presence of an air leak can progressively lead to empyema, although this is not common. The risk of empyema increases with the amount of time the chest tube remains in place and can develop in as little as 2 weeks. Antibiotics have not been shown to reduce empyema risk when given longer than 24 hours after surgery.

Fibrin deposition on an incompletely expanded lung can begin as soon as 7 days after lung collapse, creating a fibrous rind that may require decortication. Patients with infections of the pleural space are at risk of developing a trapped lung. These patients should be considered for VATS or open thoracotomy and surgical decortication. Particular attention to pain management is important as respiratory compromise, such as atelectasis or pneumonia, is common in patients with poor pain control and hypoventilation.

TAKE HOME POINTS

- A first presentation of a spontaneous pneumothorax should be managed based on size and clinical presentation with either observation or tube thoracostomy.
- All patients with pneumothorax due to significant underlying lung disease should be admitted and most should have operative management to reduce their recurrence risk.
- VATS is now the standard operative approach for bullectomy and pleurodesis.
- For nonoperative and postoperative patients, place chest tubes to water seal as soon as possible.
- Clinically stable patients with persistent air leaks postoperatively can be discharged home with an outpatient suctionless device and seen back in clinic in 2 weeks.

● ACKNOWLEDGMENTS

Our thanks to Dr. Brett Elicker, UCSF, for the radiographic images.

SUGGESTED READINGS

Baumann MH, Strange C, Heffner JE, et al. Management of spontaneous pneumothorax: an American College of Chest Physicians Delphi Consensus Statement. *Chest.* 2001;119: 590-602.

Casali C, Stefani A, Ligabue G, et al. Role of blebs and bullae detected by high-resolution computed tomography and recurrent spontaneous pneumothorax. *Ann Thorac Surg.* 2013;95(1):249-255.

Cerfolio RJ, Minnich DJ, Bryant AS. The removal of chest tubes despite an air leak or a pneumothorax. *Ann Thorac Surg.* 2009;87(6):1690-1694; discussion 1694-1696.

Jiang L, Jiang G, Zhu Y, et al. Risk factors predisposing to prolonged air leak after video-assisted thoracoscopic surgery for spontaneous pneumothorax. *Ann Thorac Surg.* 2014;97(3):1008-1013.

Tschopp JM, Bintcliffe O, Astoul P, et al. ERS task force statement: diagnosis and treatment of primary spontaneous pneumothorax. *Eur Respir J.* 2015;46:321-335.

Vascular

Pulsatile Abdominal Mass

ANNA Z. FASHANDI AND GILBERT R. UPCHURCH JR.

81

Based on the previous edition chapter "Pulsatile Abdominal Mass" by Paul D. Dimusto and Gilbert R. Upchurch Jr.

Case Presentation

A 75-year-old man with a history of hypertension, hyperlipidemia, and a 40-pack-year history of smoking presents for routine physical examination. His vital signs are normal. On abdominal examination, a pulsatile mass is noted in the epigastric region. In addition, he has a well-healed right lower quadrant scar from a prior open appendectomy. He denies any symptoms of abdominal pain, back pain, or claudication. He is having normal bowel movements and denies melena. He has palpable femoral, popliteal, dorsalis pedis, and posterior tibial pulses bilaterally. The patient is retired, but active, and able to work in his yard and climb a flight of stairs without shortness of breath.

● DIFFERENTIAL DIAGNOSIS

A pulsatile abdominal mass typically represents aneurysm disease of the arteries of the abdomen, most commonly of the aorta. Less common causes of pulsatile abdominal masses include various abdominal tumors, pancreatic pseudocysts, and hepatomegaly from heart failure.

● WORKUP

The patient undergoes further evaluation of his pulsatile abdominal mass with a CT scan of the abdomen and pelvis with intravenous contrast, which reveals a 5.8-cm abdominal aortic aneurysm (AAA) that begins 2 cm below the renal arteries (Figure 81-1). The iliac arteries are not aneurysmal, with a diameter of 1 cm bilaterally. Femoral and popliteal aneurysm scan by duplex ultrasound does not reveal any evidence of aneurysm. Serum laboratory studies reveal a hemoglobin of 14 g/dL, a normal platelet count, and creatinine of 0.9 mg/dL.

● DIAGNOSIS AND TREATMENT

AAA is defined as an aortic diameter of >50% larger than normal, with the normal abdominal aorta being 2 to 2.5 cm. Thus, a diameter of 3 cm is typically defined as an aortic aneurysm. Men are affected approximately four times as often as women. Additional risk factors for AAA formation

include smoking, hypertension, chronic obstructive pulmonary disease, atherosclerosis, dyslipidemia, advanced age, and a family history of AAA. AAAs are often discovered incidentally on imaging for workup of another disease, with only 30% to 40% of patients having abnormal physical exam findings or symptoms.

Aortic diameter is used to determine the risk of rupture and the indications for repair. One-year rupture rate rises quickly with increasing diameter: 0.5% to 5%/year for 4 to 5 cm, 3% to 15%/year for 5 to 6 cm, 10% to 20%/year for 6 to 7 cm, and as high as 50%/year once the aneurysm is 8 cm in size. Other factors that increase the likelihood of AAA rupture at a given diameter are chronic obstructive pulmonary disease, female gender, rapid expansion rate on serial imaging, hypertension, and smoking. Most recommend that the average patient with AAA < 5.5 cm in diameter be followed, unless rapid expansion is noted.

Aortic aneurysms extend into the common iliac arteries in 20% to 25% of patients. Patients with an AAA have an approximately 14% risk of also having femoral or popliteal aneurysms. In contrast, AAA may be present in up to 85% of patients with known femoral aneurysms or 62% of those with popliteal aneurysms. Therefore, all patients with these lower extremity aneurysms should be screened for AAA. Males who are hypertensive should also likely undergo a duplex for screening for femoral and popliteal artery aneurysms.

Repair is indicated in this patient with a 5.8-cm AAA. Because of its minimally invasive nature and early benefit in terms of perioperative mortality, endovascular aneurysm

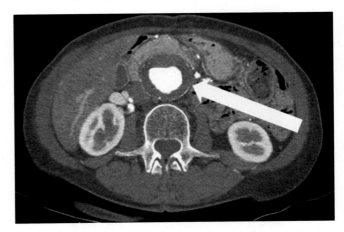

FIGURE 81-1. Axial cut of a CT scan documenting an infrarenal AAA.

repair (EVAR) has become the preferred method of AAA repair for patients who meet the appropriate anatomic criteria. It should be noted, however, that meta-analyses of studies comparing open and endovascular AAA repair show a loss of the early mortality benefit of EVAR once a patient has survived 2 years after surgery. Additionally, the rate of secondary intervention in EVAR patients is considerably higher than in open surgery patients.

In order for a patient to be considered a candidate for EVAR, their aneurysm neck (the area between the lowest renal artery and top of the aneurysm) must be at least 10 to 15 mm in length and have a diameter of <32 mm. Fenestrated endografts are now available for pararenal aortic aneurysms that meet strict anatomic criteria. The proximal neck should also have an angulation of <60° in order to decrease the risk of device migration and endoleak. Additionally, the iliac arteries must be of appropriate diameter (6 to 8 mm) and without significant tortuosity to allow for delivery of the endograft device. This patient meets criteria for EVAR, and this approach would therefore be recommended.

● SURGICAL APPROACH FOR ENDOVASCULAR ANEURYSM REPAIR

In order to choose an appropriately sized endograft and plan the operation, the patient first needs a 3D reconstruction of his CT scan (Figure 81-2). The diameter of the graft should be oversized by approximately 10% to 20% based on the diameter of the proximal landing zone. Standard endograft

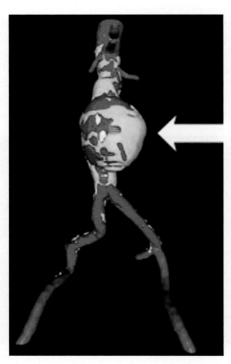

FIGURE 81-2. 3D reconstruction of the patient's CT scan demonstrating an infrarenal AAA.

configurations are bifurcated, terminating in the common iliac arteries bilaterally. This type of graft can be used if the common iliac arteries are not aneurysmal. If anatomically required to get an appropriate seal distally, an internal iliac artery (IIA) can be coiled or occluded and the graft extended past the orifice of the IIA, as it is generally acceptable to exclude one IIA. If, however, both common iliac arteries are aneurysmal, most would agree that an external to IIA bypass be performed on one side in order to avoid debilitating pelvic pain, erectile dysfunction, and potential spinal cord or mesenteric ischemia. New endografts are available that allow for preservation of IIA flow, but similar to the fenestrated aortic endografts, certain anatomic criteria are required for these IIA preservation grafts.

EVAR is typically performed under general anesthesia for patients who are not of prohibitive risk. However, it can also be performed under regional or local anesthesia with sedation, if necessary. The patient is supine on the angiography table with an arterial line and good peripheral intravenous access (Table 81-1). The locations of the distal lower extremity pulses are marked. The patient is prepped from the nipples to the toes and draped so that both groins are exposed. Bilateral cut downs exposing the common femoral arteries (CFAs) are performed. The patient is systemically heparinized, and wires are placed into the thoracic aorta via the CFAs. Bilateral iliofemoral sheaths are introduced, and a marking catheter is placed in the aorta at the level of the renal arteries. An aortogram is performed to define the location of the

Table 81-1	EVAR

Key Technical Steps

1. Choose appropriate endograft based on 3D reconstruction of CT scan
2. Expose the common femoral arteries bilaterally or place closure devices
3. Insert sheaths and catheters; perform abdominal and pelvic aortogram
4. Administer heparin
5. Insert main body of endograft just below renal arteries
6. Obtain wire access of contralateral side gate of endograft
7. Place contralateral iliac limb
8. Balloon angioplasty sealing zones and joints
9. Perform completion angiogram and assess for presence of endoleaks
10. Administer protamine to reverse heparin
11. Close arteriotomies and groin wounds or deploy closure devices, check distal pulses

Potential Pitfalls

- Endoleak
- Vascular injury
- Distal embolism

Table 81-2   Types of Endoleaks

- Type Ia—Failure of seal at proximal aortic neck
- Type Ib—Failure of seal at one of the distal iliac landing sites
- Type II—Continued flow into aneurysm sac via a branch artery, typically a lumbar artery or the inferior mesenteric artery
- Type III—Leak at junction of the main body of the graft and iliac limb
- Type IV—Pressure in the aneurysm sac due to leak from small holes in graft material
- Type V—Seroma or hygroma

renal arteries and internal iliac arteries, as well as to verify the aortic lengths obtained by CTA. The main body of the endograft is inserted over a stiff wire and deployed just below the renal arteries. Once the contralateral gate is opened, it is cannulated, and a stiff wire is introduced. The contralateral limb is then introduced over the wire, docked into the main body, and deployed. Balloon angioplasty is then performed at the upper and lower fixation sites, as well as at the graft joints, to smooth out any folds in the endograft. Completion angiography is performed to document the absence of endoleaks (Table 81-2) and confirm exclusion of the AAA and patency of all graft components (Figure 81-3). Once the wires and sheaths are removed, arteriotomies are closed, flow is confirmed distal to the arterial closures, and protamine is administered to reverse the heparin. The groin wounds are closed in multiple layers. Recent studies have documented the use of closure devices for the femoral arteries instead of open femoral artery exposure. Data have suggested that patients are discharged to home earlier with this approach and have fewer groin complications. Distal extremity pulses are checked before leaving the endovascular suite.

The most common potential pitfall during EVAR is the documentation of endoleak on completion angiography. Endoleaks typically seen at this time are type II endoleaks but also include type I and type III endoleaks, both of which are normally addressed at the time of the original surgery as they represent a direct communication between systemic circulation and the aneurysm sac. A type I leak at either the proximal or distal landing zones of the endograft is treated with either balloon angioplasty or graft extension. Recent studies have also suggested that staple devices may be effective at sealing type I endoleaks. A type III leak at the junction of graft components is typically addressed with placement of a new stent–graft component across the defect with subsequent balloon angioplasty.

The rate of vascular injury during EVAR is low (~0% to 3%), as is the rate of distal embolism now that lower profile graft introducer systems are in regular use. Vascular injury during the procedure is often related to small caliber iliac vessels, which are more commonly seen in female patients.

● POSTOPERATIVE MANAGEMENT AFTER EVAR

Patients whose endovascular procedures are without complication can typically be cared for on the acute care floor, rather than in an intensive care unit (ICU). Their diets are quickly advanced following appropriate recovery from anesthesia, with patients typically discharged home on postoperative day 1 or 2.

A common complication following EVAR is the development of an endoleak, documented during postoperative surveillance. Current recommendations are for an abdominal and pelvic CT scan with intravenous contrast at 1 and 12 months following EVAR, and then, annually thereafter if no endoleaks have been noted. There are five types of endoleaks (Table 81-2). As stated previously, type I and type III endoleaks are typically identified on completion angiogram at the time of the initial EVAR and should be immediately repaired, as the aneurysm is still subjected to arterial pressure. Type IV endoleaks typically resolve without intervention and are most often the result of small holes where the stent was sewn onto the graft material. Type V endoleaks result from porosity in the graft material leading to a seroma in the aneurysm sac. These were more common with early endograft materials and are rare when using the endografts currently on the market. Occasionally, an older endograft will need to be "re-lined" with a second endograft to resolve a type V endoleak. Type II endoleaks, while not always visualized on completion angiogram, are often detected on postoperative surveillance CTAs in the delayed phase. Type II endoleaks may seal spontaneously in up to 50% of cases, but they require intervention,

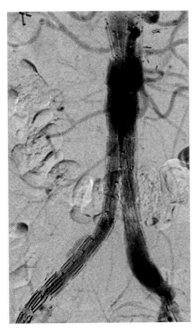

FIGURE 81-3. Completion angiogram following EVAR.

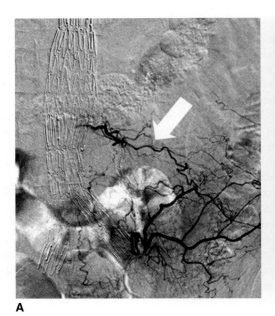
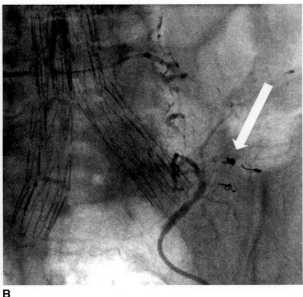

A   **B**

FIGURE 81-4. **A:** Selective angiogram demonstrating a lumbar artery causing a type II endoleak (*arrow*). **B:** Angiogram following placement of embolic coils in the offending lumbar artery (*arrow*) demonstrating no flow in the vessel.

most often with an endovascular approach, if they are associated with an increasing aneurysm sac size (Figure 81-4). Those that are associated with no change in sac size or a decreasing sac size can be followed with imaging.

● SURGICAL APPROACH FOR OPEN ANEURYSM REPAIR

Should the patient not be anatomically eligible for EVAR, open AAA repair is indicated (Table 81-3). In this operation, the abdomen is widely prepped and draped after marking the distal extremity pulses. Typically, a midline incision is made; however, a transverse or retroperitoneal incision may also be used. A retroperitoneal approach is particularly well suited for a patient with an aneurysm that involves the renal or visceral arteries, or a patient with a "hostile" abdomen from multiple prior abdominal operations. Multiple randomized trials have not shown a convincing difference in the incidence of postoperative complications between transperitoneal and retroperitoneal approaches.

The small bowel is reflected to the right, the transverse colon superiorly, and a self-retaining retractor is placed. After the duodenum is dissected off the aorta, proximal exposure of the aorta below the renal arteries and distal exposure of the common iliac arteries is obtained. The left renal vein may be divided, if necessary, to provide appropriate exposure of the aorta. Brisk diuresis is established with mannitol and furosemide. Following heparin administration for a goal-activated clotting time (ACT) > 250, the iliac arteries are clamped distally, then the aorta proximally. The aneurysm sac is opened longitudinally opposite the inferior mesenteric artery (IMA) and aortic thrombus is removed. All lumbar arteries are oversewn. A prosthetic tube or bifurcated graft is used to replace

the aneurysmal aorta, depending on the extent of aneurysmal disease in the iliac arteries. The graft is sewn in place proximally first, then distally, with monofilament suture. The IMA may be ligated if there is good back bleeding suggesting

Table 81-3	Open AAA Repair

Key Technical Steps

1. Midline abdominal incision
2. Reflect small bowel to right, transverse colon superiorly, insert self-retaining retractor
3. Dissect duodenum off of the aorta, and define proximal clamp site
4. Dissect distal aorta and proximal iliac arteries, taking care to avoid sympathetic nerves
5. Choose appropriate graft size, administer heparin, furosemide, and mannitol
6. Clamp iliac arteries followed by proximal aorta
7. Open aneurysm sac opposite IMA, remove thrombus, and oversew back bleeding lumbar arteries
8. Sew in graft starting proximally, then distally, with monofilament suture
9. Reestablish blood flow through graft, administer protamine, obtain hemostasis
10. Close aneurysm sac and retroperitoneum over graft
11. Close abdomen, check distal pulses

Potential Pitfalls

- Embolus to lower extremities
- Significant aortoiliac occlusive disease (AIOD)
- Aberrant venous anatomy
- Ischemia–reperfusion injury to lower extremities

adequate mesenteric collateral circulation; an IMA with poor back bleeding should be reimplanted onto the aortic graft at the end of the case (selective IMA implantation) in order to avoid left colonic ischemia. Selective IMA implantation may also be necessary if one of the internal iliac arteries must be ligated. Blood flow is then reestablished to the legs in a staged fashion. Once the graft is in place and the patient is hemodynamically stable, heparin is reversed. The aneurysm sac and the retroperitoneum are closed over the graft to prevent subsequent aortoenteric fistula. The abdomen is closed in the standard fashion, and the distal extremity pulses are checked prior to leaving the operating room.

One common pitfall of open AAA repair is lower extremity embolism resulting from dislodgement of atheromatous plaque or mural thrombus from the aortic wall upon placement of vascular clamps or from concurrent aortoiliac occlusive disease (AIOD). Distal pulses should always be documented before and after an aortic operation to detect this problem. Placing vascular clamps on the iliac arteries before the proximal aortic clamp may help to decrease the incidence of embolism, although there is no strong evidence to support this. If an embolus causes significant hemodynamic compromise to the leg and foot, indicated by absent pulses and a cool or discolored extremity, embolectomy should be performed before leaving the operating room. If an embolus lodges in a small vessel, such as to a single toe, no further operative intervention is typically performed and antiplatelet therapy is indicated.

Review of CT scanning prior to open AAA repair is critical to assess for aberrant venous anatomy. Retroaortic left renal vein or circumferential left renal cuffs are common anomalies and can be associated with voluminous bleeding if injured inadvertently. It is also important to recognize a left-sided inferior vena cava as division of a left renal vein crossing the aorta may really be the left-sided IVC, and ligation of this important vein is not suggested.

Ischemia–reperfusion injury may also occur following open AAA repair, as a result of the ischemic insult to the legs during the operation. Clinically, ischemia–reperfusion injury is typically heralded by hypotension, acute renal failure, and an increasing serum creatinine phosphokinase (CK) level. Minimizing ischemic time and restoring blood flow to the lower extremities in a staged fashion can help to reduce the incidence of this injury. Treatment is supportive with administration of intravenous fluids, maintenance of adequate urine output, and initiation of renal replacement therapy, if necessary.

● SPECIAL INTRAOPERATIVE CONSIDERATIONS FOR OPEN AAA REPAIR

Several unexpected findings may be encountered at the time of open AAA repair. The discovery of a previously unknown colon cancer or other intra-abdominal malignancy is not uncommon. In this scenario, the most immediately life-threatening condition is treated first. Generally, it is ill advised to perform a contaminated procedure and aortic repair simultaneously, given the risk of prosthetic graft infection. Typically, the AAA should be repaired first followed by recovery and subsequent operation for resection of the malignancy 6 to 12 weeks later, unless a near-obstructing colon cancer is discovered. If the malignancy is discovered on preoperative imaging and the patient is a candidate for EVAR, endovascular repair should be undertaken first followed by resection of the malignancy. Recovery from EVAR is typically much faster than from open repair and avoids the difficulties encountered in a repeat open abdominal operation.

● POSTOPERATIVE MANAGEMENT AFTER OPEN AAA REPAIR

Patients are typically cared for in the ICU for at least 1 to 2 days following open AAA repair, depending on their clinical status and comorbidities. Patients' volume status and renal function should be closely monitored and managed in the postoperative period. Ischemia of the left colon can occur following AAA repair, regardless of the need for IMA reimplantation and is more common following ruptured AAA repair. Bloody bowel movements, abdominal pain out of proportion to exam, or unexplained elevated leukocyte count or a drop in the platelet count should prompt urgent evaluation of the colon by sigmoidoscopy. Resection is indicated if transmural necrosis of ischemic bowel is found.

Open AAA repair is durable with limited graft complications (5% to 10%) at 10 years. The most common graft complications include pseudoaneurysm at anastomotic sites and limb thrombosis. Graft infection occurs in <1% of open AAA repairs. Secondary aortic rupture is extremely rare, unlike in EVAR. Approximately 20% of patients who undergo open AAA repair will develop a ventral hernia. Patients should be counseled about this complication and examined for development of a hernia at each of their postoperative visits.

Case Conclusion

The patient described in our scenario undergoes successful EVAR and is discharged from the hospital on postoperative day 2. Surveillance CT scan at 1 month demonstrates a type II endoleak. The endoleak is still present at 6 months, and there is now an enlarging aneurysm sac. The patient is returned to the endovascular suite where the offending vessel is successfully embolized via a transfemoral approach with selective coiling of an IIA branch supplying the aneurysm (Figure 81-4). Repeat CT 1 month later shows no evidence of an endoleak and a shrinking aneurysm sac.

TAKE HOME POINTS

- Abnormal physical examination findings are only present in 30% to 40% of patients with AAAs.
- AAA should be repaired when the diameter is larger than 5.5 cm, the aneurysm is rapidly expanding or ruptured, or if the patient has unexplained or new back or abdominal pain.
- Endovascular repair has become the standard of care in patient who have suitable arterial anatomy.
- Patients need surveillance CT scans at 1 and 12 months following EVAR, then annually thereafter to check for endoleaks.
- Incisional hernia, colon ischemia, and aortoenteric fistula are some of the more serious complications that occur after open aneurysm repair.

SUGGESTED READINGS

Chaikof EL, Brewster DC, Dalman RL, et al. The care of patients with an abdominal aortic aneurysm: the Society for Vascular Surgery practice guidelines. *J Vasc Surg.* 2009;50(4 suppl):S2-S49.

Dangas G, O'Connor D, Firwana B, et al. Open versus endovascular stent graft repair of abdominal aortic aneurysms: a meta-analysis of randomized trials. *JACC Cardiovasc Interv.* 2012;5(10):1071-1080.

Eliason JL, Upchurch GR Jr. Endovascular abdominal aortic aneurysm repair. *Circulation.* 2008;117(13):1738-1744.

Erbel R, Aboyans V, Boileau C, et al. 2014 ESC guidelines on the diagnosis and treatment of aortic diseases: document covering acute and chronic aortic diseases of the thoracic and abdominal aorta of the adult. The Task Force for the Diagnosis and Treatment of Aortic Diseases of the European Society of Cardiology (ESC). *Eur Heart J.* 2014;35(41):2873-2926.

EVAR Trial Participants. Endovascular aneurysm repair versus open repair in patients with abdominal aortic aneurysm (EVAR trial 1): randomised controlled trial. *Lancet.* 2005;365(9478):2179-2186.

Lederle FA, Freischlag JA, Kyriakides TC, et al. Outcomes following endovascular vs open repair of abdominal aortic aneurysm: a randomized trial. *JAMA.* 2009;302(14):1535-1542.

Lederle FA, Freischlag JA, Kyriakides TC, et al. Long-term comparison of endovascular and open repair of abdominal aortic aneurysm. *N Engl J Med.* 2012;367(21):1988-1997.

Ruptured Abdominal Aortic Aneurysm

82

LILY E. JOHNSTON AND GILBERT R. UPCHURCH JR.

Based on the previous edition chapter "Ruptured Abdominal Aortic Aneurysm" by Adriana Laser, Guillermo A. Escobar, and Gilbert R. Upchurch Jr.

Case Presentation

A 71-year-old male smoker presents to the emergency department complaining of a sharp, continuous pain in his left back and groin starting earlier in the evening. His vital signs are significant for tachycardia and decreased mental status, but he is normotensive and oxygenating appropriately. He reports no associated trauma. He has a history of coronary artery disease and hyperlipidemia. He is taking aspirin and an HMG-CoA reductase inhibitor (statin) daily. He smokes approximately one pack of cigarettes per day and has done so for 40 years. On physical examination, the patient is neurologically intact but lethargic. He is tachycardic, and this is confirmed on EKG to be sinus with no other significant abnormalities; no appreciable murmur on auscultation. His abdomen is obese with diffuse voluntary guarding, but no rebound or focal tenderness. A pulsatile midabdominal mass is noted, and no hernias are identifiable. He has palpable femoral pulses but decreased popliteal and dorsalis pedis pulses with livedo reticularis of bilateral lower extremities.

● PRESENTATION AND DIFFERENTIAL DIAGNOSIS

The incidence of ruptured abdominal aortic aneurysm (rAAA) in the United States is 1 to 3/100,000. Mortality after rAAA repair remains high despite advances in screening, medical therapy, operative technique, and postoperative management and ranges typically from approximately 20% to 50% in larger series. The mean age for a patient with rAAA is 70.6 years in males and 77.3 years in females.

Presentation and therefore differential diagnosis of an rAAA is varied. If the AAA ruptures intraperitoneally, presentation is usually acute with hemodynamic instability. Cardiovascular collapse often ensues. An AAA can also rupture retroperitoneally, and the patient can present with relative hemodynamic stability. Retroperitoneal rupture is most often posterior and can at least temporarily be contained via clotting, plugging by the aneurysm's mural thrombus being ejected, and tamponade by the retroperitoneal periaortic and perivertebral tissues. One study of 226 patients found that rAAA bleed into the retroperitoneum 85% of the time, the peritoneum 7%, the inferior vena cavae (IVC) 6%, and enterically in 2% of cases.

Some studies report that up to three-quarters of patients are asymptomatic before rupture. Presentation, either with or without preceding symptoms, including 45% of patients with hypotension, 72% with back and abdominal pain, and 83% with a pulsatile abdominal mass. Less than 50% of patients present with the classic triad of hypotension, abdominal pain, and pulsatile abdominal mass. However, symptomatic but intact aneurysms are considered high risk for imminent rupture and should be repaired urgently; patients should be counseled that outcomes are not as good as elective repair but considerably better than those following repair of a ruptured aneurysm. Symptoms of rAAA can include those resulting from hematoma on adjacent structures or signs of hypovolemic shock, such as diaphoresis, emesis, syncope, pallor, flank ecchymosis, and vital sign abnormalities. Contained or sealed rupture can even exist chronically before being discovered. Chronic ruptures can present with chronic lower back pain, lower extremity neuropathy, or can be asymptomatic. Another complication of chronic rAAAs are IVC fistulae. These can occur in as many as 2% to 6% of patients with rAAA, can present as lower extremity swelling, congestive heart failure, or a left varicocele. Atypical presentations of rAAA can include pain radiating to the groin, thigh ecchymosis or acute femoral neuropathy, partial upper GI obstruction (third part of the duodenum), lower extremity ischemia from emboli from mural thrombi or aortic thrombosis, visceral thromboembolism, aortoenteric fistula, and gross hematuria. Trauma can also be a cause of acute rupture of a previously stable AAA. The differential diagnosis of rAAA can be seen in Table 82-1.

Largely because many AAA patients are asymptomatic, it is believed that 33% to 50% of patients with rAAA die before arriving at the hospital. In-hospital mortality can reach 40% including patients who die before repair or in the perioperative period. This brings the overall mortality of patients with rAAA to a reported range of 50% to 94% and essentially 100% for *untreated* true rAAA.

One major predisposing risk factor for rupture of an existing AAA is female sex, with a three- to fourfold higher risk when compared with males. Current smoking also predisposes to rupture, with a 2.7-fold increased odds of rupture; current smoking is an independent predictor and associated with higher risk than previously smoking. Aortic morphology, such as an eccentric or saccular shape leading to increased wall stress, less tortuosity, greater cross-sectional diameter asymmetry, and increased aortic compliance, also

Table 82-1	Differential Diagnosis for rAAA

System	Differential Diagnosis
Gastrointestinal	Initial GI bleed, pancreatitis, cholecystitis, perforated ulcer or viscus, appendicitis, diverticulitis, acute strangulated hernia
Genitourinary	Ureteral obstruction, nephrolithiasis or renal colic, pyelonephritis
Vascular	Aortic rupture or dissection, symptomatic AAA, ruptured visceral or iliac artery aneurysm, myocardial infarction, mesenteric ischemia
Musculoskeletal	Lumbar radiculopathy, vertebral fracture, paravertebral muscle spasm
Other	Lymphoma

predispose to rupture. Other factors that have been associated with an increased probability of rupturing an existing AAA include (Table 82-2) large size at initial diagnosis, rapid progression in size with an expansion rate >1 cm/year, chronic obstructive pulmonary disease (COPD), and/or a lower forced expiratory volume in one second (FEV-1),

Table 82-2	Risk Factors for Rupture

Risk Factors for Rupture	
Female Gender	
Smoking	
COPD	Low FEV_1
Hypertension	Uncontrolled
Aortic diameter	
AAA expansion rate	>1 cm/y
Aortic morphology	Saccular
	Less tortuosity
	Greater cross-section diameter asymmetry
Peak wall	Increased stress
	Increased tension
Decreased wall strength	Decreased stiffness, increased thickness
Increase in intraluminal thrombus	Thickness
	Volume
	Extension

hypertension, pain upon manual palpation of aneurysm, a mycotic AAA, family history of aneurysm, and uninsured status. It was also noted that more ruptures occur in winter, likely due to lower atmospheric pressure. Diabetes has been found to be associated with a greater risk of rupture of a small AAA, although it is negatively associated with the development of AAAs.

Once AAA is diagnosed, size becomes one of the most important determinants for planning surgical repair. The VA cooperative Natural History of Large Abdominal Aortic Aneurysms Study determined the incidence of rupture in patients with large AAA > 5.5 cm. One-year incidence of rupture by initial aortic diameter was 9.4% for 5.5 to 5.9 cm, 20% for 6.5 to 6.9 cm, and 29.5% for ≥7.0 cm AAA. The annual rupture risk of observed small aneurysms (4 to 5.5 cm) was 0.6% per ADAM (Aneurysm Detection and Management) screening program and 3.2% per UKSAT (UK Small Aneurysm Trial). Other studies have also reported that one-third to one-half of all AAAs eventually rupture. Although the above factors describe who is at risk of rupturing an AAA, most are too prevalent and nonspecific to be used to identify patients for management or treatment. Risk of aneurysm rupture relates to hemodynamic stresses placed on a degenerative aortic wall and the capacity of the tissue to resist tensile stress. Berguer et al. numerically analyzed wall thickness, herniation of soft plaque through elastic coats of aneurysm, and local stress concentrators due to rigid calcium plaques using finite element analysis to determine that hemodynamic stresses are better than periodic diameter changes at predicting rupture. Although it is more time consuming, volume analysis is more sensitive than change in diameter alone in predicting rupture; however, diameter remains the predominantly used determinant of rupture risk clinically.

On a molecular level, the cause of AAA rupture involves many other complex processes. Choke et al. discovered increased angiogenesis at the rupture site and HIF-1-alpha up-regulation with relative hypoxia at the aneurysm rupture edge. Other changes seen within the ruptured aortic wall are decreased elastin; changes in the extracellular matrix (ECM), such as increased collagen turnover; and an imbalance of matrix metalloproteinases and their inhibitors. Thrombosis-associated enzymes (tissue plasminogen activator), lipids (lysophosphatidic acid), and inflammatory mediators (C-reactive protein) may also be associated with AAA expansion and rupture.

● WORKUP

If available, an unstable patient without a diagnosis can undergo ultrasound examination in the emergency room, especially when there is unclear etiology of hemodynamic instability. Contrast-enhanced computed tomography angiography (CTA) should be performed in all stable patients where rAAA is suspected to both confirm the presence of an

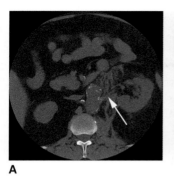 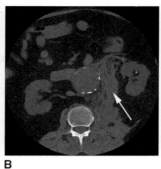 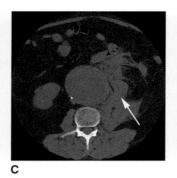 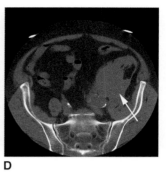

A   **B**   **C**   **D**

FIGURE 82-1. Axial noncontrast CT image of a 60-year-old male with a rAAA preoperatively. **A:** Aneurysm is shown with left renal artery (*arrow*) and stranding. **B:** Further high attenuation stranding and retroperitoneal blood. **C:** Retroperitoneal blood contained. **D:** Extravasation of blood from the aorta.

AAA and determine operative planning and suitability for endovascular aneurysm repair (EVAR). This also allows for evaluation of the iliac arteries and any venous anomalies, should open repair be undertaken. If ultrasound or CTA is unavailable, and the unstable patient has a history of an AAA or a current pulsatile abdominal mass, he should be taken to the endovascular hybrid suite directly for immediate endovascular or surgical repair based on angiography, recognizing that aortography often underestimates the true size of an AAA because laminated clot obscures the outer limit of the wall. If the receiving facility is unable to perform surgical repair, then immediate transfer should be undertaken.

The patient was deemed stable for transport to CT. Figure 82-1 shows a rAAA with an indistinct border on the left side and a likely site of rupture. There is left perinephric stranding and a fluid collection with increased attenuation in the retroperitoneum. The patient is believed to have suitable anatomy for EVAR.

● DIAGNOSIS AND TREATMENT

Arrival to the endovascular suite or operating room (OR) should occur immediately. Fluids should be minimized, allowing for permissive hypotension, as blood pressure needs only to maintain cerebral and end-organ perfusion. Resuscitation beyond this can increase bleeding, and crystalloid dilutes the coagulation factors. Patient should have blood products type and crossed, labs drawn for a blood count and creatinine, placement of two large-bore peripheral intravenous catheters and an arterial blood pressure monitoring line, bladder catheter placement, and antibiotics given. A dedicated vascular OR team should be involved from beginning to end of the case. The patient should be prepped and draped from chest to toes, and the surgical team should be ready to make an incision before anesthesia is induced since sudden hypotension can occur due to reversal of the tamponade, vasodilatation from the anesthetic agents, abdominal wall muscle relaxation, and decompression by the incision.

Traditionally, open rAAA repair has been the only option with its attendant high mortality (44%) and morbidity (56%). EVAR is now becoming the preferred option for repair of rAAA at facilities where it is available on an emergency basis. Although only 8.8% of rAAA were repaired endovascular in 2003 (vs. 43% for unruptured AAA), a recent meta-analysis illustrated that 34% to 100% of patients presenting with rAAA met criteria for EVAR via CT. A 2010 study found that implementing an algorithm favoring endovascular repair over open repair for rAAA significantly improved mortality. A significant mortality advantage, a reduction by 25%, was also found in another study of EVAR-suitable patients undergoing EVAR as compared with open repair, though follow-up was a short 6 months.

● SURGICAL APPROACH

For open repair, a transperitoneal approach via midline incision is most commonly undertaken. The primary goal is to first control the inflow and limit hemorrhage, so rapid supraceliac aortic control can be undertaken by manual (or sponge-stick) aortic compression at the level of the diaphragm. This is complimented by dividing the gastrohepatic ligament and left crus of the diaphragm, then bluntly dissecting through the crus and around the aorta to place a clamp. Then, the third and fourth portion of the duodenum is rotated to the right to expose the perirenal aorta for assessment of infrarenal clamping. Heparin is often omitted if the patient is actively bleeding, but lasix and mannitol are frequently given for renal protection after the cross-clamp is placed. Distal control of the aorta is obtained by dissecting the iliac arteries free and clamping them. Then, the aneurysm can then be opened and any lumbar and inferior mesenteric arteries that are bleeding into the sac are ligated. If at all possible, a tube graft is selected to serve as the repair conduit as this configuration requires the least length of anastomosis (when compared to a bifurcated graft). The graft is anastomosed proximally with 3-0 monofilament suture. After checking this anastomosis, the distal anastomosis is created in an end-to-end configuration as well. Iliac clamps should be removed after informing the anesthesiologists and done one at a time to decrease hypotension from sudden perfusion to the lower extremities. The aneurysm sac is closed over the graft to decrease the risk of graft-enteric fistulae later on. Typically, the retroperitoneal hematoma is not decompressed. Distal pulses are checked before abdominal closure. There should be a low threshold for considering the patient at risk for abdominal compartment syndrome (ACS), and the abdomen may need to be left open.

EVAR can be performed under local, regional, or general anesthesia, depending on patient comfort, hemodynamic status, respiratory status, and level of consciousness. The patient should be placed supine on the table, preferably in a hybrid OR. Prep should be from chest to toes. Bilateral femoral artery cut downs are done before giving systemic heparin. Bilateral iliofemoral sheaths are placed, and wires are placed into the thoracic aorta along with a marking catheter. An angiogram of the aorta is performed using either iodinated contrast dye or carbon dioxide (to minimize injury to the kidneys) in order to identify the anatomy and location of the renal arteries. At this time, a decision is made regarding whether to use an aortouniiliac (tube) or a modular, bifurcated endograft. Once this is done, the endograft body is inserted over a stiff guidewire and deployed below the renal arteries. Assuming a bifurcated graft is chosen, the contralateral gate is opened, cannulated, and a contralateral limb is docked into the endograft and deployed. Balloon angioplasty is performed at the proximal and distal fixation sites, as well as in the gate area. Completion angiogram is performed to confirm there are no leaks and ensure exclusion of the ruptured aneurysm. All wires and sheaths are removed, and the femoral arteriotomies are closed. Flow is confirmed distal to the arteriotomy closures by hand-held Doppler. Protamine is given to reverse the heparin if used. Groin incisions are closed in multiple layers, and lastly pulses are checked prior to leaving the endovascular suite. These steps are highlighted in Table 82-3. Conversion to open repair may be necessary due to continuing blood loss, difficult access, graft migration, and other anatomic challenges.

The patient in this scenario underwent endovascular repair under general anesthesia. The postprocedure angiogram was undertaken with CO_2 angiography, and no endoleaks were detected (Figure 82-2). He was then transported to ICU in stable condition for recovery.

● SPECIAL INTRAOPERATIVE CONSIDERATIONS

If the patient is bleeding and hypotensive, rather than depend on open control of the aorta, an endovascularly placed aortic occlusion balloon catheter (inserted either transfemoral or transbrachial) can be utilized as an alternative for rapid proximal aortic control. It can be placed using local anesthesia alone, so it can be used to minimize the acute drop in blood pressure during general anesthesia. It can be used in

Table 82-3	EVAR for rAAA

Key Technical Steps

1. Expose bilateral common femoral arteries (or insert percutaneous closure devices)
2. Introduce wires and sheaths
3. Perform aortogram
4. Systemic heparin
5. Main body of endograft inserted and deployed just below renal arteries
6. Contralateral limb inserted and deployed
7. Balloon angioplasty
8. Completion angiogram
9. Administer protamine
10. Close arteriotomies, check pulses, and close wounds

Potential Pitfalls

- Endoleak (type I or III)
- Embolism
- Dissection or rupture of iliac, femoral arteries
- Abdominal compartment syndrome
- Ischemic colitis

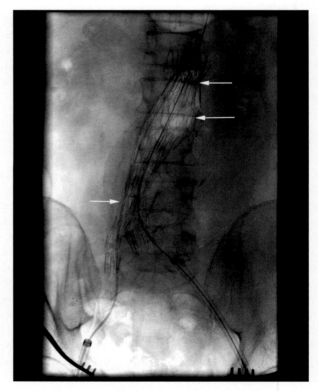

FIGURE 82-2. Intraoperative angiography with CO_2 at completion of endograft placement for rAAA. Endograft successfully excluding aneurysm with no leaks (*arrows*).

conjunction with a stent for endovascular repair but can also be used alone as an adjunct for hemorrhage control prior to an open repair. Some institutions find that balloon occlusion is necessary in up to one-third of rAAAs treated, and in one study was associated with a significant reduction in intraoperative mortality compared to aortic cross-clamping in unstable patients with rAAA. Care must be taken to minimize renal, mesenteric, and spinal ischemic time during all occlusions of the proximal aorta. Other scenarios that may be encountered intraoperatively are an infection, which preceded the rupture, an aortoenteric fistula, or an aortic-IVC fistula. These are rare occurrences, and in the acute setting, may be treated as other rAAA, although higher morbidity and mortality are expected.

Endoleaks occur after elective and ruptured endovascular AAA repairs and are the primary indication for reintervention. Type I, II, or III are seen in up to one-half of patients by 1 year after AAA repair, compared to approximately 25% in electively repaired AAA. As endoleaks appear to be more common following rAAA repair, frequent and long-term follow-up is mandatory.

● POSTOPERATIVE MANAGEMENT

Morbidity after rAAA repair has been documented at 61%, including respiratory failure, tracheostomy, renal failure, sepsis, myocardial infarction, congestive heart failure, and bleeding. Less commonly seen postoperative complications are stroke, ischemic colitis, lower extremity ischemia, and paraplegia. Late vascular complications are also higher after rAAA, 17% as compared with 8% after elective AAA repair. As well, there is a high rate (20%) of secondary operations: 50% get laparotomy and 50% undergo other procedure. Complications, notably the prevalent respiratory and renal failure, are seen more frequently in open as compared with endovascular rAAA repair.

Ischemia of the sigmoid colon is one of the most serious complications following rAAA repair, as compared with elective AAA repair (presumably from ligation or covering of the inferior mesenteric artery during the repair). Ischemic colitis may present as hypotension, thrombocytopenia, bloody diarrhea, or metabolic acidosis. Sigmoidoscopy is performed at the bedside to evaluate for transmural ischemia. Mild cases may be treated with antibiotics and supportive care alone; however, severe cases may require resection. Bowel ischemia is described as occurring in 42% of patients after open rAAA repair and 22% after endovascular rAAA repair.

Another complication, ACS, can result if the abdomen is closed under excessive tension or due to massive resuscitation in the setting of EVAR or open repair for rAAA. ACS is defined as bladder pressure >20 mm Hg with associated new-onset organ dysfunction (e.g., oliguric renal failure, increased peak ventilator pressures). ACS may occur in the setting of an rAAA as a result of an expanding retroperitoneal hematoma, but it is not clearly defined if risk is greater from endovascular or open repair. Presumably, the risk of ACS after rAAA would be higher following EVAR as compared with open repair

due to unligated aortic branch vessels causing an enlarging hematoma. However, a recent study found that rAAA treated with open repair had significantly higher postoperative intra-abdominal pressures than those undergoing EVAR. The state of shock associated with AAA-free rupture and the insult of an open repair also contribute to tissue edema via microvascular permeability alterations. Since increased abdominal pressure leads to bowel ischemia and respiratory, cardiac, and renal dysfunction, immediate intervention is required. This consists of intra-abdominal pressure monitoring, early recognition, and abdominal decompression at the bedside if the patient is unstable. In a recent study of rAAA, factors associated with increased risk of developing ACS included need for occlusion balloon, greater transfusion requirement, higher partial activated thromboplastin time, and higher use of aortouni-iliac grafts. These patients, and those with massive bowel edema or a large retroperitoneal hematoma, should be considered intraoperatively for temporary abdominal closure with vacuum-assisted closure (VAC) or mesh if undergoing open repair.

Mortality rates after rAAA open repair have been shown to be 35% to 65% (95% if present in extremis) and are not decreasing like the mortality rates of unruptured AAA. In contrast, elective AAA repair mortality is 1% to 3%. Consecutive patient series have found rAAA mortality to be associated with age >80 years, history of hypertension, angina, or MI, APACHE II score, low hematocrit, preoperative cardiac arrest or loss of consciousness, pre- or intraoperative hypotension, estimated blood loss ≥6 L or resuscitation with ≥12 L, and postoperative renal or respiratory failure. Traditionally, the majority of postoperative mortality is attributed to other cardiovascular disease, such as coronary artery disease.

However, EVAR has become the new gold standard for rAAA. Veith et al. took patients with rAAA and, utilizing hypotensive hemostasis, performed arteriography. EVAR was undertaken if anatomy was deemed suitable. Supraceliac balloon occlusion was used if circulatory collapse ensued (10 of 29 patients required it). Operative mortality was only 13%. More recently, mortality was shown to be 33% for rAAA patients undergoing EVAR versus 41% for open repair. The advantage for EVAR remained significant for patients >70 years old (36% vs. 47%, $p < 0.001$). One-year data from the IMPROVE trial, a multicenter pragmatic trial that randomized over 600 patients with rAAA to endovascular-first or open repair, demonstrate equivalent 1-year all-cause mortality as well as rates of reintervention, but a significantly shorter length of stay in the EVAR-first arm.

Elevated operative risk for patients undergoing open repair of rAAA as compared with EVAR has been attributed to aspects of the procedure. General anesthesia induction and sudden decompression of the aorta may both lead to hypotension. Increased hypothermia and blood loss leading to coagulopathy are also often involved. Cost-effectiveness analyses for rAAA repair suggest that EVAR may not be more cost-effective than open repair, though this is contrary to the early IMPROVE trial results; this remains an active area of investigation and should prompt broad discussions of resource utilization as technology evolves.

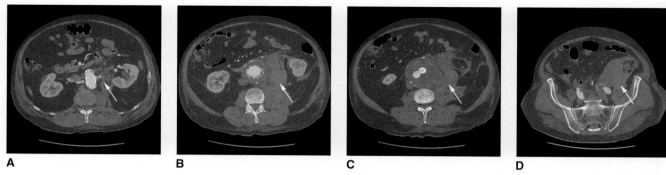

FIGURE 82-3. Axial CT image with contrast enhancement of a 60-year-old male with a rAAA post-EVAR. **A:** Aneurysm is shown with endograft in place, stranding (*arrow*). **B:** Aneurysm sac around endograft with residual blood in the retroperitoneum (*arrow*). **C:** Retroperitoneal blood (*arrow*) with possible site of rupture. **D:** Residual blood in the pelvis (*arrow*).

Case Conclusion

The patient recovered uneventfully from his surgery except for mild renal dysfunction. He developed azotemia but did not require dialysis. He underwent CT imaging on postoperative day 2, which showed no endoleaks (Figure 82-3). He had no neurologic sequelae, was eating a regular diet, had no signs of infection, and had adequate blood pressure control. He was able to be discharged home on postoperative day 5 with smoking cessation information and a follow-up visit in 1 month with CT.

TAKE HOME POINTS

- Rupture risk increases with age, female sex, and increased aortic diameter.
- Presentation is varied. However, patients uncommonly present with the classic triad of hypotension, abdominal pain, and pulsatile abdominal mass.
- CT imaging for stable patients; ultrasound or operating room for unstable patients.
- Endovascular aortic occlusion can be used to provide hemorrhage control prior to either open or endovascular repair.
- Abdominal compartment syndrome and bowel ischemia are severe complications following rAAA repair.
- Endovascular repair shows morbidity and mortality advantage over open repair for rAAA.

SUGGESTED READINGS

Burgers LT, Vahl AC, Severens JL, et al. Cost-effectiveness of elective endovascular aneurysm repair versus open surgical repair of abdominal aortic aneurysms. *Eur J Vasc Endovasc Surg.* 2016;52(1):29-40. http://doi.org/10.1016/j.ejvs.2016.03.001

Cho J-S, Gloviczki P, Martelli E, et al. Long-term survival and late complications after repair of ruptured abdominal aortic aneurysms. *J Vasc Surg.* 1998;27(5):813-820. http://doi.org/10.1016/S0741-5214(98)70260-5

De Martino RR, Nolan BW, Goodney PP, et al. Outcomes of symptomatic abdominal aortic aneurysm repair. *J Vasc Surg.* 2010;52(1):5.e1-12.e1. http://doi.org/10.1016/j.jvs.2010.01.095

Dua A, Kuy S, Lee CJ, et al. Epidemiology of aortic aneurysm repair in the United States from 2000 to 2010. *J Vasc Surg.* 2014;59(6):1512-1517. http://doi.org/10.1016/j.jvs.2014.01.007

Giles KA, Hamdan AD, Pomposelli FB, Wyers MC, Dahlberg SE, Schermerhorn ML. Population-based outcomes following endovascular and open repair of ruptured abdominal aortic aneurysms. *J Endovasc Ther.* 2009;16(5):554-564. http://doi.org/10.1583/09-2743.1

Harris LM, Faggioli GL, Fiedler R, Curl GR, Ricotta JJ. Ruptured abdominal aortic aneurysms: factors affecting mortality rates. *J Vasc Surg.* 1991;14(6):812-820. http://doi.org/10.1067/mva.1991.33494

Investigators IT, Hassan TB, Hinchliffe R, et al. Endovascular strategy or open repair for ruptured abdominal aortic aneurysm: one-year outcomes from the IMPROVE randomized trial. *Eur Heart J.* 2015;36(31):2061-2069. http://doi.org/10.1093/eurheartj/ehv125

Mehta M, Byrne J, Darling RC III, et al. Endovascular repair of ruptured infrarenal abdominal aortic aneurysm is associated with lower 30-day mortality and better 5-year survival rates than open surgical repair. *J Vasc Surg.* 2013;57(2):368-375. http://doi.org/10.1016/j.jvs.2012.09.003

Mehta M, Darling RC III, Roddy SP, et al. Factors associated with abdominal compartment syndrome complicating endovascular repair of ruptured abdominal aortic aneurysms. *J Vasc Surg.* 2005;42(6):1047-1051. http://doi.org/10.1016/j.jvs.2005.08.033

Quanstrum KH, Upchurch GR Jr. Mesenteric ischemia following abdominal aortic aneurysm repair. In: Upchurch GR Jr, Criado E, eds. *Aortic Aneurysms: Pathogenesis and Treatment. Contemporary Cardiology.* New York, NY: Humana Press, 2009:325-336.

Raux M, Marzelle J, Kobeiter H, et al. Endovascular balloon occlusion is associated with reduced intraoperative mortality of unstable patients with ruptured abdominal aortic aneurysm but fails to improve other outcomes. *J Vasc Surg.* 2015;61(2):304-308. http://doi.org/10.1016/j.jvs.2014.07.098

Veith FJ, Ohki T, Lipsitz EC, Suggs WD, Cynamon J. Treatment of ruptured abdominal aneurysms with stent grafts: a new gold standard? *Semin Vasc Surg.* 2003;16(2):171-175. http://doi.org/10.1016/S0895-7967(03)00003-6

Visser JJ, van Sambeek MRHM, Hamza TH, Hunink MGM, Bosch JL. Ruptured abdominal aortic aneurysms: endovascular repair versus open surgery—systematic review. *Radiology.* 2007;245(1):122-129. http://doi.org/10.1148/radiol.2451061204

Wakefield TW, Whitehouse WM, Wu SC, et al. Abdominal aortic aneurysm rupture: statistical analysis of factors affecting outcome of surgical treatment. *Surgery.* 1982;91(5):586-596.

Lifestyle-Limiting Claudication

RYAN M. SVOBODA AND PHILIP P. GOODNEY

83

Based on the previous edition chapter "Lifestyle-Limiting Claudication" by Edouard Aboian and Philip P. Goodney

Presentation

A 54-year-old male construction worker presents to the vascular surgery clinic with 6 months of cramp-like right calf pain with ambulation. The pain consistently occurs after walking about 50 yards and is remitted with rest. Despite the pain, he is able to perform the duties of his job and carry out normal activities of daily living. He has a history of hypertension for which he is on hydrochlorothiazide and has been smoking one pack of cigarettes per day since age 18.

● DIFFERENTIAL DIAGNOSIS

A wide variety of disease processes can manifest clinically as lower extremity pain. Atherosclerotic *intermittent claudication*, the most likely diagnosis in this patient, occurs when reduced arterial perfusion leads to inadequate blood supply to meet the increased metabolic demands of the lower extremity musculature during exertion. It typically manifests as a burning or cramping sensation that occurs with a given level of exertion and is remitted by rest. It can occur in either the calves or the thighs/buttocks, depending on the location of the atherosclerotic plaques. *Critical limb ischemia* (CLI), a more severe manifestation of peripheral arterial occlusive disease (PAOD), occurs when arterial perfusion is severely diminished to the point that blood supply is inadequate even at rest. CLI typically manifests as severe foot pain at rest or ischemic ulceration and is a marker of limb threat.

Nonatherosclerotic causes of claudication include *popliteal artery entrapment syndrome, adventitial cystic disease of the popliteal artery, iliac artery endofibrosis, and chronic exertional compartment syndrome.* These pathologies can all present similarly to claudication caused by atherosclerosis and should be suspected in younger patients who do not exhibit the classic risk factors for PAOD, such as smoking, hypertension, and hyperlipidemia. *Thromboangiitis obliterans (Buerger's disease)* is another nonatherosclerotic etiology of diminished perfusion, caused by vasculitis of the small- and medium-sized vessels of the hands and feet. Thromboangiitis obliterans can present with severe, unremitting lower extremity pain but is commonly associated with digital necrosis. This diagnosis most commonly occurs in young men in the third through fifth decades of life with a history of heavy tobacco use.

Finally, nonarterial etiologies of lower extremity pain should be considered. *Venous insufficiency* can lead to aching lower extremity pain but is often associated with edema and is relieved by elevation. Other signs of venous valvular incompetency, such as varicosities and lipodermatosclerosis (brawny skin discoloration), may be present. *Diabetic neuropathy* often leads to a burning sensation or paresthesias of the forefoot. Unlike ischemic rest pain, neuropathic pain tends to be constant and is not relieved by placing the extremity in a dependent position. *Neurogenic claudication*, caused by compression of the lumbosacral nerve roots in patients with lumbar spinal stenosis, also presents as burning and cramping with ambulation. Unlike vascular claudication, it typically extends from the buttocks to the feet and is relieved by sitting or bending over while walking, the so-called "shopping cart sign."

● WORKUP

Patients with suspected intermittent claudication should undergo a full history and physical examination. The history should specifically focus on atherosclerotic risk factors: smoking history, hypertension, hyperlipidemia, diabetes, as well as their family history of cardiovascular disease. Certain comorbidities, in addition to making PAOD more likely, can also provide clues to the most likely level of disease. For example, smokers have a predisposition toward atherosclerosis of the aortoiliac segment, and diabetics are more likely to have tibial disease. Exacerbating and remitting factors should be elicited in an attempt to rule out competing diagnoses such as neurogenic claudication. Physical examination should include a full pulse exam of both lower extremities, including femoral, popliteal, and pedal pulses. The finding of diminished arterial pulses can not only help diagnose an arterial pathology, but it can also help localize the level of the disease. Asymmetry should be noted. The distal extremities should be inspected closely for signs of hypoperfusion, such as hairlessness, pallor, and poikilothermia. Signs of more severe arterial insufficiency such as dependent rubor (redness that disappears with elevation of the foot) and ulceration should also be noted. Attention should be paid to signs of alternative diagnoses, such as the edema and lipodermatosclerosis associated with venous insufficiency.

In addition to a comprehensive history and physical examination, additional diagnostic tests are valuable in confirming the diagnosis and planning treatment. Ankle–brachial indices (ABIs) should be obtained in all patients in whom PAOD is suspected (Figure 83-1). An ABI of <1.0 is considered abnormal and is indicative of reduced perfusion. Patients with lifestyle-limiting intermittent claudication typically have an ABI in the 0.50 to 0.80 range, while patients with an ABI of <0.5 often present with symptoms of CLI and have multilevel disease. Segmental pressures, or at the very least, waveforms, can help pinpoint the levels of disease. In patients in who atypical causes of claudication, such as endofibrosis or chronic exertional compartment syndrome, are suspected, exercise (treadmill) ABIs can be helpful. In diabetic patients, ABIs can be falsely elevated due to medial calcinosis of the tibial vessels; Doppler waveforms and toe photoplethysmography ("toe pressure") are useful in delineating the severity of disease in these patients.

Presentation Continued

Physical exam revealed palpable femoral pulses bilaterally and absent popliteal and pedal pulses on the right. The right foot was slightly cool, with noted pallor and hair loss. There was no evidence of dependent rubor or tissue loss. Sensation and motor function was normal in both feet. Noninvasive vascular laboratories were ordered and on the right, the ABI was diminished at 0.68. On the left, ABI was slightly diminished at 0.90. At this point, the most likely diagnosis is lifestyle-limiting intermittent claudication.

● DIAGNOSIS AND TREATMENT

The diagnosis of intermittent claudication should be made based upon clinical history, physical examination, and noninvasive vascular laboratory studies (typically ABI). Once claudication is diagnosed, treatment options should be discussed. For all patients with claudication, optimal medical therapy with aspirin and a statin should be prescribed. For patients with cardiovascular disease, even those with normal lipid profiles, statins have been shown to carry a benefit in terms of improved survival and slower progression of disease. This is likely due to the pleiotropic effects of statin medications on matrix metalloproteinases. Additionally, cilostazol, a phosphodiesterase-3 inhibitor, is approved for the treatment of intermittent claudication. It is associated with modest improvements in claudication-free walking distance of up to 50% in some patients, although it typically takes several weeks before improvement is noted. Common side effects include headaches, flushing, and diarrhea, although these typically resolve with continued use of the drug. The typical dose of cilostazol is 100 mg twice daily, and this can be reduced if patients suffer side effects such as edema. Of note, the FDA has issued a black box warning against the use of cilostazol in patients with congestive heart failure, in whom the medication has been shown to increase all-cause mortality. Another medication, pentoxifylline, is also FDA approved for the treatment of claudication, but multiple postmarket studies have called into question its effectiveness; it is not currently recommended for use in patients with claudication. Beyond medical therapy, intense,

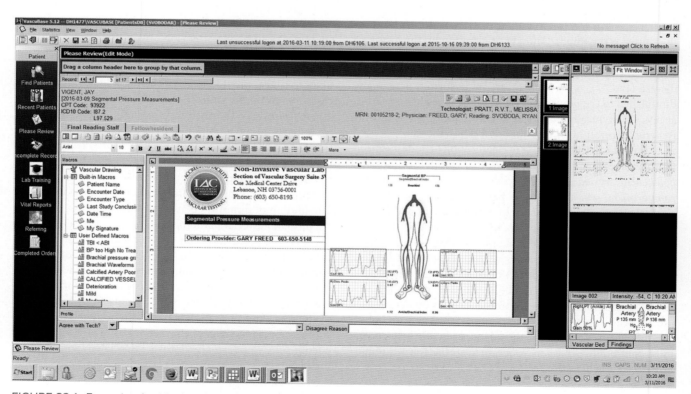

FIGURE 83-1. Example of ankle–brachial index (ABI) vascular laboratory report.

structured exercise therapy has been shown to improve maximum walking distance, presumably through increasing collateral circulation.

In addition to direct medical treatment of claudication, it is important that these patients be screened and treated for concomitant coronary and cerebrovascular arterial disease. Although only roughly 10% of patients with intermittent claudication ever progress to the state of limb-threat, approximately 20% to 25% of these patients will experience death within 5 years of a diagnosis of claudication. This is because the development of peripheral atherosclerosis is an overall marker of cardiovascular health; these patients are at risk for disease in other arterial beds.

In patients with lifestyle-limiting claudication and in those whose medical therapy and structured exercise therapy do not sufficiently relieve symptoms, intervention is indicated. Prior to (or as part of) revascularization, arterial imaging is necessary for case planning. Options for arterial imaging include digital subtraction angiography (DSA), computed tomographic angiography (CTA), and magnetic resonance angiography (MRA). CTA and MRA are noninvasive but are prone to artifact and may not be sufficient for planning infrapopliteal interventions. Angiography is invasive but has the added advantage of being both diagnostic and therapeutic. If a lesion is amenable to endovascular therapy, intervention can be performed at the time of the initial arteriogram. If disease of the aortoiliac segment is suspected based on an absent femoral pulse, a CTA or MRA of the abdomen and pelvis with lower extremity runoff is of utility to ensure access vessel patency prior to any attempts at angiography.

Presentation Continued

The patient was continued on his daily aspirin and statin. Cilostazol therapy was also initiated. The importance of claudication as a marker of cardiovascular risk was emphasized, and he was given a referral for local tobacco cessation services. Three months later, he returns to clinic and states that despite adhering to his medications and successfully quitting smoking, his claudication has worsened and now occurs after walking 50 yards. Additionally, the pain is now interfering with his ability to reliably do his job. He wishes to discuss the options for intervention. Given that there is minimal concern for iliac occlusion based on clinical history and physical exam, he is scheduled for angiography in order to image his right lower extremity arterial vasculature and possibly intervene.

● APPROACHES FOR REVASCULARIZATION

Endovascular Therapy

Endovascular treatment of lower extremity atherosclerotic lesions in patients with lifestyle-limiting claudication is typically performed through retrograde femoral access of the contralateral extremity in patients with suspected infrainguinal disease. In patients with diminished femoral pulses, a CTA should be performed preoperatively to rule out significant iliac disease.

Additionally, prior to invasive angiography, all prior noninvasive studies and arterial imaging should be reviewed in detail. Prior interventions can significantly impact the available interventions and approaches; preoperative planning in these instances is particularly important. For example, prior placement of "kissing" common iliac stents with advancement of the aortic bifurcation can be prohibitive of a retrograde femoral approach from the contralateral groin when targeting infrainguinal disease and may necessitate an antegrade puncture of the ipsilateral common femoral artery.

After all preoperative imaging has been reviewed, the lower abdomen, bilateral groins, and affected extremity are prepped and draped in sterile fashion. In our practice, intravenous antibiotics are reserved for therapeutic endovascular procedures and are given after the culprit lesion is crossed, unless the patient has indwelling intravascular stents or a previous bypass. Retrograde, or antegrade, common femoral arterial access is then obtained with a micropuncture needle and sheath. In our practice, all access is performed under ultrasound and fluoroscopic guidance. Care is taken to puncture the common femoral artery overlying the medial two-thirds of the femoral head in order to ensure an adequate platform for compression following sheath removal. Typically, 4 or 5 French sheath access is sufficient for diagnostic procedures, and thus, it is our practice to always begin with this smaller size of sheath, upsizing only after the initial arteriogram is performed and the decision to attempt intervention is made. After aortic aortography and selective lower extremity imaging, the arterial anatomy is studied closely to determine if the lesion is amenable to percutaneous intervention based on Trans-Atlantic Society Consensus (TASC) II classification (Figure 83-1, Table 83-1). In general, TASC A and B lesions are easily amenable to percutaneous intervention. TASC C and D lesions represent more difficult technical challenges, and while endovascular therapy is not necessarily contraindicated, open surgery should be considered after considering important patient-related factors such as patient preference, comorbidities, and conduit availability.

If a lesion is deemed to be amenable to endovascular therapy, a long sheath—typically 6 French for most interventions—is placed over the aortic bifurcation into the contralateral, target extremity after heparinization. The lesion is carefully crossed under fluoroscopic guidance and then treated. Intervention typically consists of angioplasty +/− stent placement. Atherectomy may be a helpful adjunct prior to stent placement in patients with very dense, calcific plaque. Following successful treatment, heparinization is reversed with protamine. The sheath can be removed primarily with application of direct pressure to the puncture site for a minimum of 15 minutes, or an arterial closure device can be used (Figure 83-2).

Table 83-1	Trans-Atlantic Society Consensus (TASC) II Criteria for Infrainguinal Lesions	

TASC II Classification	Lesion Characteristics	Typical Treatment of Choice*
TASC A	• Single stenosis ≤10 cm OR • Single occlusion ≤5 cm	Endovascular
TASC B	• Multiple stenoses or occlusions, each ≤5 cm OR • Single stenosis 10–15 cm or occlusion 5–15 cm (of the SFA or suprageniculate popliteal artery) OR • Heavily calcified occlusion ≤5 cm OR • Single infrageniculate stenosis or occlusion	Endovascular
TASC C	• Multiple stenosis or occlusions >15 cm total OR • Recurrent stenosis or occlusions that have undergone ≥2 prior endovascular interventions	Open, endovascular if not a good surgical candidate or if local expertise exists
TASC D	• Chronic total occlusion of the superficial femoral artery ≥20 cm, with extension into the popliteal artery OR • Chronic total occlusion of the popliteal artery and proximal tibial vessels	Open

TASC, Trans-Atlantic Inter-Society Consensus.

* Actual treatment of choice should be tailored to individual patient based on hospital, surgeon, and patient factors.

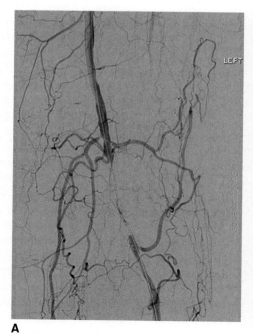 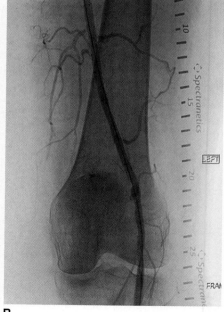

FIGURE 83-2. Approximately 5 cm occlusion of distal SFA prior to (A) and after (B) bare metal stent deployment.

A

B

Open Surgical Revascularization

If a lesion is deemed to be most appropriate for open surgical revascularization, additional preoperative planning is required. Patients with unstable coronary artery disease, active decompensated heart failure, uncontrolled arrhythmias, or severe valvular disease, they require preoperative cardiac evaluation and likely have a cardiac risk prohibitive to elective bypass for claudication. Additionally, vein mapping should be performed to assess for adequate ipsilateral great saphenous vein conduit. Vein is considered to be suitable for bypass if it is 3 mm or greater in diameter. It is our practice to have the vascular laboratory measure and mark the course of suitable vein to ensure adequate length for a tension-free bypass. If no suitable vein is found in the ipsilateral lower extremity, we typically vein map the upper extremities, although use of upper extremity vein should be avoided in patients with chronic kidney disease, as it should be preserved for potential dialysis access. In our practice, we avoid use of contralateral lower extremity GSV, as PAOD is often bilateral and there is a significant chance of requiring a contralateral procedure in the future. If no suitable veins are available, consideration is given to alternative conduit choices, such as prosthetic material.

After preoperative planning is complete, the lower abdomen and extremity of interest are prepped and draped in sterile fashion. It is our practice to routinely prep the contralateral groin in case endovascular access is required. The inflow and outflow target vessels are then dissected prior to assessing the conduit, to ensure that adequate targets for bypass exist. The common femoral artery is the most common inflow artery utilized for infrainguinal bypass. To expose the common femoral artery, a vertical incision is made over the pulse in the groin and extended one-third above and two-thirds below the inguinal ligament. The femoral sheath is exposed and opened, and the artery and its branches are carefully dissected out and controlled with silastic vessel loops. In our experience, the most common distal target utilized for bypass in patients with claudication is the infrageniculate popliteal artery, although the precise target is chosen based upon preoperative angiographic imaging. To expose the infrageniculate popliteal artery, a longitudinal incision is made 1 cm posterior to the posterior border of the tibia. Care must be taken to avoid injury to the great saphenous vein at this site. The fascia of the superficial posterior compartment is opened, and the gastrocnemius muscle is retracted posteriorly. The anterior attachments of the soleus are dissected carefully off of the tibia, and the popliteal artery is identified medial to the popliteal vein and tibial nerve. Vena communicantes often must be divided in order to gain access to the artery. Once proximal and distal target vessels are assessed and deemed appropriate for clamping and anastomosis, the conduit must be harvested (if a venous conduit is being utilized).

After the target vessels are exposed and the conduit is harvested, decisions must be made in terms of orientation and tunneling of the bypass. Although reversed, nonreversed, and in situ great saphenous vein bypasses all have certain advantages and disadvantages, there appears to be no major differences in outcomes in the existing literature. If nonreversed vein is used, intraoperative valve lysis must be performed. It is our practice to do this under direct vision using an angioscope and remote valvulotome. After establishment of a tunnel, the patient is heparinized, and the distal anastomosis is the anastomoses performed after careful tunneling to avoid kinking or twisting of the graft. After completion of both anastomoses, it is our routine practice to perform intraoperative duplex ultrasonography to evaluate technical adequacy of the bypass graft as well as the outflow (Table 83-2).

● SPECIAL INTRAOPERATIVE CONSIDERATIONS

In patients undergoing infrainguinal bypass who are found to have significant common femoral artery calcification, endarterectomy is performed with bovine pericardial patch angioplasty, and the bypass graft is sutured to the patch. This increases flow through the origin of the graft. Additionally, endarterectomy of a diseased profunda origin ensures an adequate source of collateral flow should the bypass graft experience acute thrombosis.

Table 83-2	Lower Extremity Endovascular Intervention

Key Technical Steps

1. Carefully review all preoperative imaging and prior vascular procedures
2. Perform *ultrasound-guided* access of contralateral common femoral artery with a micropuncture kit
3. Perform aortography, lower extremity angiography
4. Heparinize patient, place appropriately sized long access sheath (e.g., 55 cm) over the aortic bifurcation into target extremity over a stiff wire (e.g., Amplatz)
5. Carefully cross the lesion of interest using appropriate wire/catheter combination
6. Pretreat lesion with adjunctive therapy (e.g., atherectomy) if necessary
7. Perform balloon angioplasty or stent placement
8. Perform completion arteriogram
9. Reverse heparin with protamine; remove access sheath or deploy closure device
10. Hold manual pressure until hemostasis is deemed satisfactory

Potential Pitfalls

- Improper placement of arterial puncture resulting in inability to properly compress and increased likelihood of retroperitoneal hematoma or arterial pseudoaneurysm
- Contralateral iliac artery occlusion not appreciate preoperatively
- Iatrogenic arterial dissection from balloon angioplasty

● POSTOPERATIVE MANAGEMENT

Aspirin 81 mg is prescribed for all patients undergoing lower extremity arterial intervention. If a patient is not on aspirin preoperatively, we make sure that it is administered in the preoperative holding area prior to the procedure. Additionally, based on findings of better patency of arterial interventions on patients receiving statin therapy, likely due to the pleiotropic effects, we routinely prescribe statin agents for all patients undergoing lower extremity endovascular or open surgical intervention. Although there is little data examining the precise effects of clopidogrel in patients undergoing lower extremity endovascular intervention, we routinely prescribe 1 month of clopidogrel therapy for patients undergoing infrainguinal stent placement. Additionally, there are some data suggesting that twice-daily cilostazol may prevent restenosis of lower extremity stents. Anticoagulation is not routinely prescribed for patients undergoing lower extremity arterial intervention. However, if a patient undergoing open surgical bypass is deemed to have a "disadvantaged" bypass graft due to poor conduit or poor outflow, we will typically institute indefinite anticoagulation, starting several hours after the surgical procedure. In our practice, routine surveillance of intravascular stents and lower extremity bypass grafts is performed 1 month after the procedure and yearly henceforth to monitor for restenosis. However, the precise frequency of surveillance imaging should be determined based on individual patient characteristics.

Case Conclusion

The patient underwent right lower angiography revealing a 5-cm superficial femoral artery occlusion with distal reconstitution in the region of Hunter's canal. The lesion was successfully crossed and treated with bare metal stent placement. Postoperatively, he was maintained on aspirin, a statin medication, and 1 month of clopidogrel therapy. He returned to clinic 1 month after the procedure with complete resolution of his claudication symptoms and normalization of his right ABI to 1.01.

TAKE HOME POINTS

- Nonatherosclerotic causes of claudication should be ruled out in younger patients and in the absence of atherosclerotic risk factors.
- Progression to limb-threatening ischemia is relatively uncommon in patients with intermittent claudication, but risk of a major cardiovascular event such as myocardial infarction or stroke within 5 years is high.
- Prior to undergoing invasive treatment of claudication, risk factor medication, optimal medical therapy, and structured exercise therapy should be employed.
- Most lower extremity atherosclerotic lesions are amenable to either endovascular or open surgical intervention; careful preoperative planning is essential, and therapy should be tailored based upon individual patient-related factors.

SUGGESTED READINGS

Apigian AK, Landry GJ. Basic data underlying decision making in nonatherosclerotic causes of intermittent claudication. *Ann Vasc Surg.* 2015;29(1):138-153.

Chowdhury MM, McLain AD, Twine CP. Angioplasty versus bare metal stenting for superficial femoral artery lesions. *Cochrane Database Syst Rev.* 2014;(6):CD006767.

Norgren L, Hiatt WR, Dormandy JA, Nehler MR, Harris KA, Fowkes FG. TASC II Working Group: inter-society consensus for the management of peripheral arterial disease. *J Vasc Surg.* 2007;45S:S5-S67.

Ravin RA, Faries PL. Chapter 114: infrainguinal disease: endovascular treatment. In: Cronenwett JL, Johnston KW, eds. *Rutherford's Vascular Surgery.* 8th ed. Philadelphia, PA: Elsevier; 2014.

Selvin E, Erlinger TP. Prevalence of and risk factors for peripheral arterial disease in the United States: results from the National Health and Nutrition Examination Survey, 1999-2000. *Circulation.* 2004;110(6):738-743.

Varcoe RL, Taylor CF, Annett P, Jacobsen EE, McMullin G. The conundrum of claudication. *ANZ J Surg.* 2006;76(10):916-927.

Warner CJ, Greaves SW, Larson RJ, et al. Cilostazol is associated with improved outcomes after peripheral endovascular interventions. *J Vasc Surg.* 2014;59(6):1607-1614.

Tissue Loss from Arterial Insufficiency

84

RORI E. MORROW AND WILLIAM P. ROBINSON III

Based on the previous edition chapter "Tissue Loss Due to Arterial Insufficiency" by William P. Robinson III

Presentation

A 74-year-old white male with a history of hypertension, diabetes mellitus (DM), tobacco abuse, coronary artery disease, atrial fibrillation, and end-stage renal disease on hemodialysis presents to the emergency department with a 3-week history of spontaneous ulceration of the left great toe and increasing rest pain in the left foot (Figure 84-1). Vital signs are normal. On physical examination, there is dry gangrene at the base of the left great toe with mild surrounding cellulitis. The patient has dry and hairless skin of the bilateral lower extremities with dependent rubor and elevation pallor of the left foot. Bilateral femoral and popliteal pulses are palpable. Pedal pulses are absent to palpation, but there is an audible Doppler signal at the left dorsalis pedis. The patient has intact strength and sensation of the lower extremities. He walks independently and performs his own activities of daily living.

● DIFFERENTIAL DIAGNOSIS

Tissue loss due to arterial insufficiency most often affects the foot due to the predilection of atherosclerotic occlusive disease to occur in the lower extremity vessels. The prevalence of peripheral arterial disease (PAD) is 3% to 10% overall and 15% to 20% in those over age 70. Of those aged >50 with PAD, 1% to 3% will have critical limb ischemia (CLI) in the form of rest pain or tissue loss. The incidence of CLI ranges from 220 to 1,000 new cases per year in a European or an American population of 1 million people. The risk factors for infrainguinal occlusive disease include those for the development of atherosclerosis in general: age, male gender, hypertension, DM, smoking, dyslipidemia, family history, and homocysteinemia. Trauma secondary to diabetic neuropathy and venous hypertension can also lead to lower extremity ulceration or coexist with arterial insufficiency. People with diabetes are four times as likely to develop CLI, while smokers are three times as likely. The rate of amputation is 10 times higher in patients with diabetes than without diabetes.

Tissue loss secondary to arterial insufficiency typically occurs on the distal aspect of the extremity, such as the digits, and is often associated with underlying ischemic rest pain of the affected extremity. It represents the most advanced form of ischemia as perfusion is not adequate to maintain tissue integrity. Ischemic ulcerations usually begin as small, dry ulcers of the toes or heel area and progress to frank gangrene of the forefoot or heel with greater degrees of arterial insufficiency (Figure 84-2). Such progressive disease, affecting multiple levels of the peripheral vasculature, is more frequently encountered in the elderly. Patients with diabetes or renal failure are more susceptible to the development of ischemic pedal ulcers. Disease progression can be very rapid, as up to 50% of patients with CLI are asymptomatic 6 months before onset of pain or ulceration.

Foot ulcers are classified based on their extent and depth as well as the presence or absence of infection. Evaluation of the limb with tissue loss should include assessment of the wound severity, any degree of ischemia, and the presence of foot infection. These factors are captured in the Society for Vascular Surgery WIfI (Wound, Ischemia, foot Infection) Classification System, which helps in staging the degree of limb threat and assessing the risk of amputation and wound healing time. As diabetes increases in prevalence throughout the world, the importance of a multidisciplinary team approach to diabetic foot ulcers and the limb is essential to aid in wound healing and limb salvage. Multidisciplinary team care and aggressive wound care including revascularization in those with both diabetes and PAD show promise in reducing wound healing time and ultimately amputation rates compared to historical results.

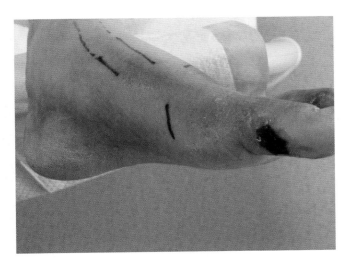

FIGURE 84-1. Left foot with dry gangrene of great toe, dependent rubor, and erythema on dorsum of foot.

497

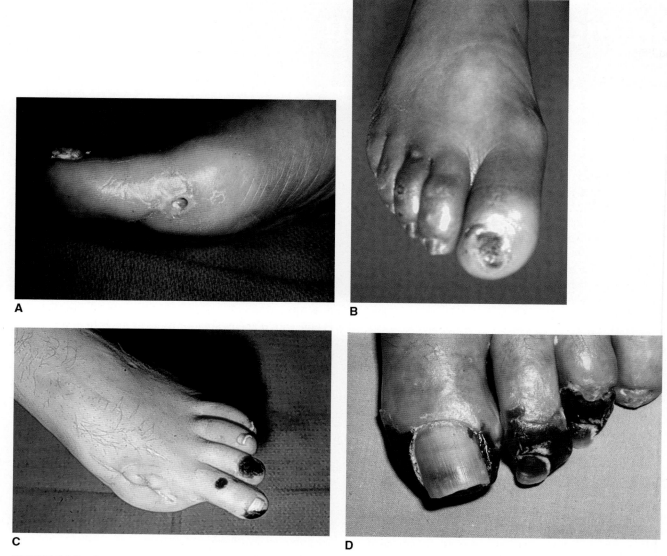

FIGURE 84-2. Progressive stages of tissue loss from small ischemic ulcerations (**A,B**) to gangrene (**C,D**).

CLI is associated with an extremely high risk of limb loss and mortality as it is a marker of advanced comorbidities and cardiovascular disease—including a 25% risk of death and 25% risk of major amputation within 1 year of diagnosis. Rutherford's stage V (minor tissue loss) and VI (major tissue loss) arterial insufficiency are associated with a 50% amputation-free survival at 1 year. The 5-year survival rate for patients with CLI is approximately 50% to 60%.

Because of the extremely high risk of limb loss, tissue loss from arterial insufficiency must be expeditiously and accurately diagnosed. Clinical experience indicates that in some patients, minor ulcerations may heal with improved cardiac hemodynamics and optimal local wound care even without revascularization, with wound closure rates in approximately half of patients. Successful closure often depends on the severity of ankle–brachial index (ABI) and the initial wound size. Major tissue necrosis inevitably progresses to limb loss without revascularization.

● WORKUP

A careful physical examination can diagnose the extent of tissue loss and the presence of arterial insufficiency. A lack of a pedal pulse indicates abnormal arterial perfusion and, in the presence of ulceration or gangrene, warrants further investigation. An ABI is an essential part of the detailed vascular examination. An ABI of <1.0 is considered abnormal and <0.4 is generally considered consistent with the potential for tissue loss. Further workup can be conducted using noninvasive arterial testing, most often in a vascular laboratory. Segmental pressures measured at the level of the upper thigh, lower thigh, calf, ankle, and metatarsal level can diagnose the anatomic level of occlusive disease. If vessels prove noncompressible with cuff pressures of 225 mm Hg, related to severe calcification of vessels in the setting of diabetes and end-stage renal disease, then the ABI and segmental pressures are not reliable indicators of perfusion. Pulse volume recordings, which measure the volume of blood delivered to each segment of the lower extremity, are then utilized to assess perfusion. In addition, toe blood pressures remain a reliable indicator of distal perfusion. According to the TASC II guidelines, toe–brachial index <0.3 or absolute toe pressure of <30 mm Hg is indicative of severe ischemia and strongly predictive of inability to heal a lower extremity wound, although a single "cutoff" value cannot be advocated for all patients and the perfusion needed to achieve healing increases with increasingly severe tissue loss. Extensive tissue loss frequently requires the restoration of palpable pulses in the foot for healing.

Presentation Continued

The patient is started on broad-spectrum intravenous antibiotics. Ankle–brachial indices and segmental pressures are nondiagnostic due to noncompressible vessels. Pulse volume recordings are consistent with severe ischemia and indicate disease at the tibial and pedal levels (Figure 84-3). The patient has an absolute toe pressure of 0 mm Hg.

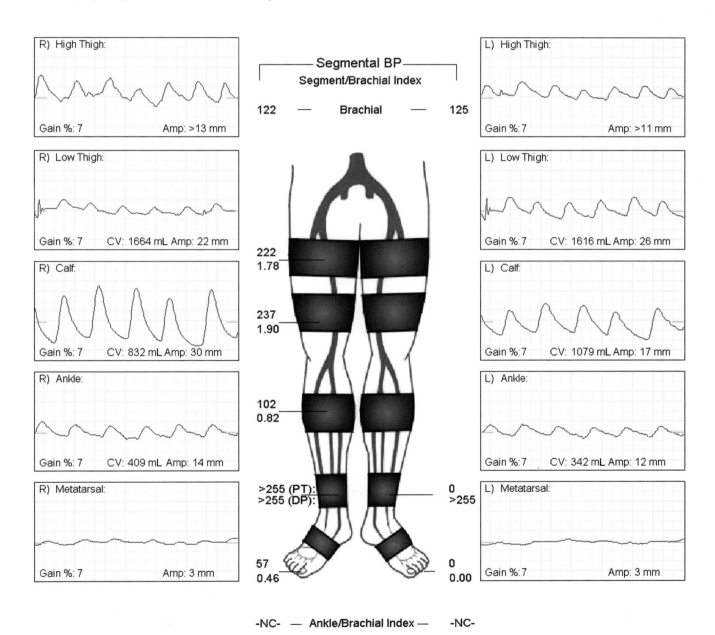

FIGURE 84-3. Arterial noninvasive testing including measurement of segmental pressures and toe pressure and pulse volume recordings.

● DIAGNOSIS AND TREATMENT

The diagnosis of tissue loss secondary to arterial insufficiency is based upon history, physical examination, and noninvasive arterial testing. The objective of arterial imaging is to plan revascularization and is usually indicated only if physiologic testing has indicated significant ischemia, and the decision has been made to pursue revascularization. Imaging options include digital subtraction angiography, magnetic resonance angiography (MRA), and computed tomographic angiography (CTA). Although MRA and CTA are noninvasive, they are subject to artifact and may not provide the anatomic detail necessary to adequately plan infrainguinal bypass or endovascular intervention. Digital subtraction angiography provides optimal vessel detail, especially in calcified tibial vessels, and remains the gold standard for evaluation of occlusive disease and distal targets. In addition, percutaneous endovascular therapy can often be performed at the time of diagnostic angiography if the patient and anatomy is deemed suitable.

Revascularization options for lower extremity occlusive disease include percutaneous endovascular therapy, open surgical therapy, and combinations of the two modalities, known as a "hybrid approach." The optimal treatment is dependent primarily upon the extent and location of occlusive disease and on the patient's operative risk. Regardless of means of therapy, the overarching theme of revascularization is to provide in-line or straight-line flow from adequate inflow vessels to the outflow vessels supplying the area of tissue loss to optimize the local environment for wound healing.

Not all options apply to all patients. Expected outcomes vary based on patient anatomy, vein quality (for conduit), and comorbidities. General health and life expectancy of the patient should be considered. Choosing the best option includes balancing surgical risk considering the short-term benefit of endovascular therapy versus the durability of bypass. Primary amputation may be appropriate in select patients.

Autogenous vein grafts to the above-knee and below-knee popliteal artery have primary patency rates of >80% at 1 year and >70% at 5 years. Tibial or pedal targets have primary patency rates >60% and assisted patency rates of about 70% at 3 to 5 years. Both popliteal and infrapopliteal bypass with autogenous vein is associated with limb salvage rates of 80% at 5 years. Wound complications occur in 10% to 20% of patients. Endovascular therapy is increasingly utilized and is thought to be advantageous because of its less invasive nature and lower morbidity and is often preferred in high-risk patients. However, the durability of endovascular intervention has not been well studied, and current evidence demonstrates that it is inferior to that of lower extremity bypass. It must also be realized that stents at preferred inflow or outflow anastomotic sites or distal embolization to the outflow may indeed limit surgical options. The cost of endovascular therapy is relevant to the patient and the health care system, especially when these therapies fail and prolong tissue loss and delay ultimate interventions.

Thirty-day mortality rates for endovascular intervention (2% to 8%) and surgical bypass (2% to 6%) are similar, while somewhat higher for primary amputation (6% to 12%). In deciding between endovascular therapy and infrainguinal bypass, algorithms have proposed that a life expectancy of at least 2 years and a good-quality GSV or alternative vein favor bypass. In addition, factors such as major tissue loss, multilevel TASC C/D anatomic lesions, and <5% surgical risk would also favor open surgical bypass.

The choice of endovascular or open revascularization is also largely dependent on the anatomic extent of disease. The Trans-Atlantic Inter-society Consensus Document on the management of Peripheral Arterial Disease (TASC) classifications attempt to categorize lesions according to a preference for endovascular therapy (TASC A and B) or open bypass (TASC C and D). Type A lesions include a single stenosis ≤10 cm in length or single occlusion ≤5 cm in length. Type D lesions include those that are chronic total occlusions (CTO) of common femoral or superficial femoral arteries >20 cm, involving the popliteal artery or CTO of popliteal artery and proximal trifurcation vessels. Type B and C lesions are of intermediate severity.

Level I data comparing infrainguinal bypass and endovascular therapy are limited. The BASIL trial (British Angioplasty vs. Surgery in Ischaemic Legs) randomized patients with CLI to an endovascular revascularization first or bypass-first strategy. Amputation-free survival at 5 years was not different between the two strategies. Among patients who lived >2 years, overall survival was significantly improved in patients who underwent bypass and there was a trend toward improved amputation-free survival in patients who underwent bypass. A significant number of patients required bypass after failed initial angioplasty, and this group fared more poorly than patients who underwent initial bypass therapy. Current trials are ongoing to define optimal clinical practices and include the Best Endovascular versus Best Surgical Therapy in patients with Critical Limb Ischemia (BEST CLI) trial.

In summary, percutaneous endoluminal therapy is best utilized for those with less extensive lesions and high surgical risk. The technical success and the durability of endovascular therapy are best for iliac and superficial femoral artery lesions. Extensive popliteal and tibial disease can be treated via endovascular means, but their durability is quite limited. In addition, long-segment stenoses and occlusions are less favorable for endovascular therapy than more limited lesions.

Extensive occlusive disease at multiple levels of the circulation is generally required to develop tissue loss secondary to arterial insufficiency. Therefore, open surgical therapy in the form of endarterectomy and surgical bypass is often required. Surgical revascularization provides durable patency and limb salvage.

NOVEL THERAPIES

Stem cell therapies have been utilized in clinical trials and remain in development. Safety and efficacy appear promising. The utilization of bone marrow mesenchymal cells is one of many future directions that target the local tissue hypoxia and angiogenesis mechanisms via paracrine signaling to build collaterals and improve wound healing at a cellular level.

SURGICAL APPROACH

Percutaneous Endovascular Therapy

Endovascular treatment of iliac disease is generally performed through ipsilateral retrograde femoral access. Infrainguinal lesions are generally treated via a sheath placed "up and over" the aortic bifurcation from the contralateral femoral artery. In general, the principle of endovascular therapy is to cross the diseased segment with a wire and then successively dilate the stenosis or the occlusion with balloon catheters and/or stents over the wire. Keys to success include stable placement of a sheath, which allows controlled wire and catheter manipulation in traversing lesions and accommodates the passage of balloon catheters and stents of adequate caliber for restoring flow. Potential complications of endovascular therapy include atherothromboembolism to distal arteries, access site hematoma and pseudoaneurysm, and contrast-induced nephropathy. Alternative endovascular approaches include arterial access through antegrade common femoral and pedal accesses to traverse difficult occlusive lesions through either intraluminal or subintimal planes. Atherectomy devices can aid in luminal gain. Drug-coated balloon angioplasty shows promise in reducing neointimal hyperplasia.

Infrainguinal Bypass

The principle of successful bypass is to perform the shortest bypass possible to reestablish in-line flow to the foot. The importance of "inflow," "outflow," and "conduit" are repeatedly emphasized by vascular surgeons. First, flow must be unobstructed to the level of the proximal anastomosis. Second, a site distal to significant disease must be chosen for the distal anastomosis. In general, the target vessel should be the least diseased artery that is the dominant angiosome supply to the foot. Finally, the conduit for the bypass must be adequate to support pulsatile flow. For bypass to below the level of the knee, optimal conduit is paramount and is described as a single-segment of nondiseased autogenous ipsilateral greater saphenous vein with a diameter of at least 3.5 mm. Prosthetic conduit is preferred for aortoiliac reconstruction and acceptable for femoral to above-knee popliteal bypass when autogenous conduit is not available.

Infrainguinal surgical bypass can be performed under general, spinal, or occasionally regional anesthesia. It is our practice to work from proximal to distal, first exploring the inflow artery and exposing the venous conduit. We then explore the site proposed as a suitable target vessel for the distal anastomosis, which was identified on high-quality preoperative imaging or intraoperative angiogram through proximal artery access. Vein of sufficient length is then harvested and prepared for use by gentle dilation and testing for leaks with heparinized saline solution. The proximal anastomosis is performed prior to the distal anastomosis. This allows for confirmation of adequate inflow before the bypass is performed and allows the graft to be tunneled and tailored to the appropriate length under arterial pressure. Prior to vessel occlusion for the proximal anastomosis, the patient is systemically anticoagulated with weight-based 100 units/kg of intravenous heparin and additional heparin is given as necessary. Blunt tunneling with placement of umbilical tapes through the tunnels is completed before heparin is administered to prevent bleeding. Atraumatic vascular clamps are placed proximally and distally, and the donor artery is incised. The vein is then spatulated and a beveled proximal anastomosis carried out. Typically, a 5-0 polypropylene suture is used for the femoral anastomosis and a 6-0 used at the popliteal level. If a nonreversed orientation is used to improve size match, the vein valves are then lysed with a valvulotome under arterial pressure. The vein is carefully brought through the tunnel under pressure and pulsatile flow confirmed with brief release of the clamp. The graft is then tailored to appropriate length, and the distal anastomosis is then completed after occluding the target vessel, often utilizing a sterile tourniquet for tibial vessels to minimize dissection and prevent clamp injuries. 7-0 Prolene suture is generally used at the tibial or pedal level. If there is extensive calcification, proximal control can be achieved using occlusion balloons placed intraluminally. Flow through the graft and the outflow artery is assessed following completion of the bypass with a continuous wave Doppler and pulse examination. If there is inadequate augmentation, completion angiogram is performed by directly cannulating the proximal graft. This allows for immediate repair of any technical defects that are identified. Intraoperative duplex ultrasonography is an additional sensitive screen for hemodynamically significant abnormalities within the graft.

Pitfalls of infrainguinal bypass that lead to early graft failure include attempted anastomosis to highly calcified vessels and use of inadequate conduit. Technical defects not corrected at time of operation guarantee early graft failure. In addition, adequate hemostasis and meticulous attention to wound closure are necessary to prevent hematoma and wound dehiscence, which incur significant morbidity and can precipitate graft failure. Key steps of infrainguinal bypass with ipsilateral saphenous vein are outlined in Table 84-1.

Table 84-1	Infrainguinal Bypass Graft with Nonreversed Greater Saphenous Vein

Key Technical Steps

1. Expose inflow artery for proximal anastomosis and evaluate suitability for proximal anastomosis.
2. Expose target artery for distal anastomosis and evaluate suitability for distal anastomosis.
3. Expose saphenous vein of adequate length through skip incisions or endovein harvest. Ligate side braches with fine silk and divide. Ligate and divide vein distally and at sapheno-femoral junction.
4. Prepare vein for bypass with gentle distension of heparinized saline and repair any leaks. Excise proximal valves under direct vision. The vein is the case!
5. Create bypass graft tunnel between donor and target arteries with blunt clamp or tunneling device. Place umbilical tape through tunnel.
6. Systemically heparinize.
7. Perform proximal anastomosis:
   - Clamp donor artery distally and then proximally.
   - Make arteriotomy.
   - Fashion proximal vein to match arteriotomy.
   - Perform anastomosis with running polypropylene suture.
8. Lyse valves in vein under arterial distension using valvulotome. Confirm pulsatile flow.
9. Bring graft through tunnel under arterial pressure. Avoid kinks. Confirm pulsatile flow.
10. Perform distal anastomosis:
    - Occlude target artery (clamps or pneumatic tourniquet).
    - Make arteriotomy.
    - Trim vein under distention and fashion to match arteriotomy.
    - Perform anastomosis with running polypropylene suture.
11. Confirm flow through graft and outflow arteries with pulse exam and continuous wave Doppler.
12. Perform completion angiography and/or duplex ultrasonography.

Potential Pitfalls

- Poor preoperative planning: donor and target arteries unsuitable for anastomosis.
- Use of conduit of inadequate quality or caliber.
- Poor hemostasis and wound closure.

Special Intraoperative Considerations

Adequate preoperative planning based on high-quality angiography generally avoids unanticipated intraoperative findings. Occasionally, the necessity of improving the inflow to support an infrainguinal graft is determined intraoperatively, either by direct visual assessment of inflow at the desired donor site, angiography, or by comparison of a transduced pressure tracing from the donor site with that of a systemic pressure tracing. Aortoiliac angioplasty and stenting is increasingly becoming the preliminary or combined procedure performed to attain sufficient inflow prior to construction of a more distal bypass graft. At times, the ipsilateral greater saphenous vein will be found to be inadequate on exploration despite appearing adequate on preoperative mapping. Alternative autogenous conduit, such as contralateral saphenous vein and arm vein, must then be available and utilized for below-knee bypass. Especially in young females, vasospasm of distal vessels can also affect graft failure and thrombosis. Intraoperative use of papaverine or nitroglycerin can relax the smooth muscle and relieve the spasm.

Postoperative Management

The most common major complications of infrainguinal bypass surgery are cardiac in nature. These are best prevented with perioperative optimization including appropriate use of beta-blockade, statin therapy, and careful attention to volume status. Wound infection, dehiscence, and skin flap necrosis can best be avoided by gentle tissue handling and avoidance of skin flaps during vein harvesting. Leg elevation in the early postoperative period minimizes leg swelling and healing complications. Aggressive mobilization and rehabilitation maximizes return to function. All patients are maintained indefinitely on aspirin or clopidogrel following surgical bypass. When a graft is at increased risk of failure, as in cases in which there is compromised outflow or only marginal conduit available, the antithrombotic agent may be supplemented with an anticoagulant such as heparin and then warfarin or new oral anticoagulant agent. Serial duplex ultrasound scanning is necessary to identify hemodynamically significant stenoses within the vein graft that threaten graft patency. Duplex

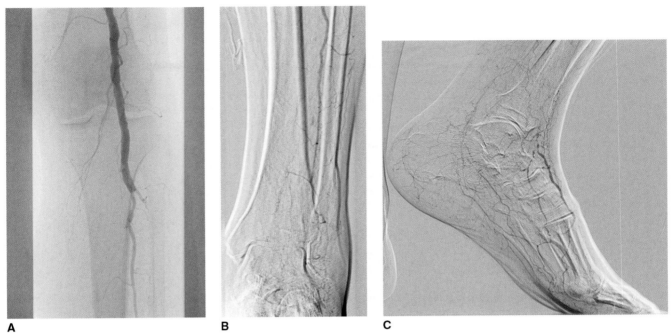

A   **B**   **C**

FIGURE 84-4. Lower extremity angiogram showing preservation of below-knee popliteal artery with posterior tibial and anterior tibial artery occlusion and single vessel runoff via the peroneal artery (**A**), occlusion of the peroneal artery in the distal calf (**B,C**), and reconstitution of the dorsalis pedis artery in the foot (**C**).

ultrasonography is generally done at 1, 6, and 12 months with yearly scans thereafter.

Debridement is avoided or deferred until after revascularization is complete unless foot sepsis is evident. Small,

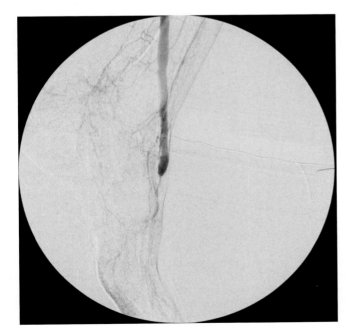

FIGURE 84-5. Intraoperative completion angiogram demonstrating excellent result of below-knee popliteal to dorsalis pedis vein bypass graft.

uninfected ulcerations of the toe or foot often can be safely managed conservatively. Larger, gangrenous lesions of the toe, forefoot, or heel usually require debridement of all necrotic tissue before and after revascularization. If the ischemia is particularly severe or infection is present, a toe or transmetatarsal amputation may be necessary in order to achieve a margin of healthy tissue. Pressure offloading for up to a month is often necessary to facilitate healing. Local wound care must be diligent and frequent.

Case Conclusion

The patient underwent left lower extremity angiography via a right common femoral artery approach. There were no significant stenoses in the iliac, femoral, and popliteal vessels. There was severe tibial disease with single vessel run-off via a peroneal artery that was occluded in the distal leg (Figure 84-4A and B). A dorsalis pedis artery reconstituted in the foot with patent vessels in the pedal arch (Figure 84-4C). He underwent below-knee popliteal to dorsalis pedis bypass with ipsilateral reversed greater saphenous vein. Intraoperative angiogram revealed no technical defects (Figure 84-5). Bypass resulted in a palpable pulse in the dorsalis pedis artery distal to the graft and greatly improved perfusion of the foot. He was discharged on postoperative day 3 on aspirin. The wound healed with gentle serial debridement completed as an outpatient.

TAKE HOME POINTS

- The diagnosis of tissue loss due to arterial insufficiency is made based on patient symptomatology, physical examination, and noninvasive tests, such as segmental pressure measurements and pulse volume recordings.
- Patients with tissue loss secondary to arterial insufficiency are at high risk for limb loss and death.
- Tissue loss secondary to arterial insufficiency represents the most advanced form of CLI and mandates revascularization for limb salvage.
- Percutaneous endovascular therapy is often applied as first-line therapy in appropriate patients with limited extent of anatomic disease and/or prohibitive operative risk.
- In patients with extensive, multilevel atherosclerotic occlusions and tissue loss, open surgical revascularization remains the gold standard for restoring durable perfusion to the threatened limb.
- Infrainguinal bypass surgery performed with autogenous vein conduit offers durable patency and excellent limb salvage.
- Debridement of nonviable tissue should be delayed until perfusion is restored to the limb unless uncontrolled infection is present. Many patients will require one or more adjunctive operative procedures for salvage of their foot.

SUGGESTED READINGS

Conte MS. Critical appraisal of surgical revascularization for critical limb ischemia. *J Vasc Surg.* 2013;57(2, suppl S):S8-S13.

Conte MS, Belkin M, Upchurch GR, et al. Impact of increasing comorbidity on infrainguinal reconstruction: a 20-year perspective. *Ann Surg.* 2001;233(3):445-452.

Criqui MH, Fronek A, Barrett-Connor E, et al. The prevalence of peripheral arterial disease in a defined population. *Circulation.* 1985;71(3):510-515.

Halperin JL. Evaluation of patients with peripheral vascular disease. *Thromb Res.* 2002;106(6):V303-V311.

Hingorani A, LaMuraglia GM, Henke P, et al. The management of diabetic foot: a clinical practice guideline by the Society for Vascular Surgery in collaboration with the American Podiatric Medical Association and the Society for Vascular Medicine. *J Vasc Surg.* 2016;63(suppl S):S3-S21.

Hirsch AT, Haskal ZJ, Hertzer NR, et al. ACC/AHA 2005 guidelines for the management of patients with peripheral arterial disease (lower extremity, renal, mesenteric, and abdominal aortic): executive summary. *J Am Coll Cardiol.* 2006;47(6):1239-1312.

Lu D, Chen B, Liang Z, et al. Comparison of bone marrow mesenchymal stem cells with bone marrow-derived mononuclear cells for treatment of diabetic critical limb ischemia and foot ulcer: a double-blind, randomized, controlled trial. *Diabetes Res Clin Pract.* 2011;92(1):26-36.

Mathioudakis N, Hicks CW, Canner JK, et al. The Society for Vascular Surgery Wound, Ischemia, and foot Infection (WIfI) classification system predicts wound healing but not major amputation in patients with diabetic foot ulcers treated in a multidisciplinary setting. *J Vasc Surg.* 2017;65(6):1698-1705.

Mills JL Sr, Conte MS, Armstrong DG, et al. The Society for Vascular Surgery Lower Extremity Threatened Limb Classification System: risk stratification based on wound, ischemia, and foot infection (WIfI). *J Vasc Surg.* 59(1):220-234.e1-2.

Norgren L, Hiatt WR, Dormandy JA, et al. Inter-Society Consensus for the Management of Peripheral Arterial Disease (TASC II). *Eur J Vasc Endovasc Surg.* 2007;33(1 suppl S):S1-S75.

Schaper NC, Andros G, Apelqvist J, et al. Diagnosis and treatment of peripheral arterial disease in diabetic patients with a foot ulcer. A progress report of the International Working Group on the Diabetic Foot. *Diabetes Metab Res Rev.* 2012;28:218-224.

Selvin E, Erlinger TP. Prevalence of and risk factors for peripheral arterial disease in the United States: results from the National Health and Nutrition Examination Survey, 1999–2000. *Circulation.* 2004;110(6):738-743.

Taylor LM Jr, Edwards JM, Porter JM. Present status of reversed vein bypass grafting: five-year results of a modern series. *J Vasc Surg.* 1990;11(2):193-205; discussion 205-206.

Wengerter KR, Veith FJ, Gupta SK, et al. Prospective randomized multicenter comparison of in situ and reversed vein infrapopliteal bypasses. *J Vasc Surg.* 1991;13(2):189-197; discussion 97-99.

Wolfe JH, Wyatt MG. Critical and subcritical ischemia. *Eur J Vasc Endovasc Surg.* 1997;13(6):578-582.

Acute Limb Ischemia

JONATHAN R. THOMPSON AND PETER K. HENKE

Based on the previous edition chapter "Acute Limb Ischemia" by Peter K. Henke and John W. Rectenwald

Presentation

A 68-year-old active man presents to the emergency room (ER) with a 4-hour history of left limb pain and numbness. He had fallen out of bed and noticed worsening limb symptoms ever since. He notes no prior leg problems and no history of claudication, walking at least 2 miles daily without stopping. His past history is significant for a myocardial infarction 7 years ago and subsequent CABG. Past medical history includes tobacco use and hypertension, but no diabetes or stroke. Medications include an aspirin, a calcium channel blocker, and a statin agent. He describes feeling as though his heart is beating fast, but denies chest pain. He was able to ambulate with assistance to the car and ER, but now has a difficult time moving his foot due to pain and neurologic impairment.

● DIFFERENTIAL DIAGNOSIS

At this point, lower limb etiologies include direct trauma and possible fracture, deep vein thrombosis (DVT), spinal cord compression, and arterial ischemia (embolism, thrombosis, dissection) are all possible.

● EVALUATION

Physical Examination

On physical examination, his cardiac rhythm is irregularly, irregular with a rate of 130, BP = 130/90, and RR = 20. His abdomen is soft and nontender. Pulse exam is +2/4 bilateral radial, left femoral, and right pedal pulses, left femoral +2/4 but 0/4 for left popliteal and pedal pulses. He has no dopplerable signals in this left popliteal, dorsalis pedis, and posterior tibial arteries. The left common femoral artery has a water hammer sound on auscultation. He has a normal neurologic exam on the right. On the left, his foot is cool, discolored with a blue hue, and demonstrates delayed capillary refill. He has diminished sensation below the knee on the left and decreased foot dorsiflexion. No external trauma is noted, and no swelling is noted in either limb (Figure 85-1).

Presentation

Acute limb ischemia (ALI) is a common vascular emergency that all physicians should be able to recognize and treat in a timely fashion (Figure 85-2). Delays in diagnosis and lack of anticoagulation are causes of limb loss in ALI. At this point, the history and pulmonary embolism give a clear picture of ALI. In this case, lack of external trauma, swelling, and DVT makes fracture less likely. Nerve root compression is possible but would usually be associated with a distinctly different neurologic exam usually involving a whole-leg motor deficit. The most significant finding suggesting ALI is that he has a total pulse deficit below the femoral artery on the symptomatic side but a normal exam on the nonaffected side. This patient has several of the "6" "P's" of ALI, namely paresthesia, pulselessness, poikilothermia, and paralysis. The specific cause for ALI is broad (Table 85-1), and this will alter the treatment strategy. According to the Society for Vascular Surgery (SVS) limb ischemia grading system, he has a level IIb ischemia and requires rapid revascularization to save his leg. The grading system is listed in Table 85-2.

Laboratory/EKG

As comorbid diseases and conditions account for much of the mortality of ALI, it is important to evaluate for common problems that may compromise the patient acutely. These are primarily cardiac and renal diseases, including a potential for hyperkalemia, anemia, and acute myocardial infarction after ischemia reperfusion injury. Standard blood assessment includes CBC, electrolytes, BUN, creatinine, troponin, and CPK. A hypercoagulable panel can also be considered but is not necessary. A baseline CXR is optional.

Other Imaging and Noninvasive Tests

These should not delay definitive treatment, the urgency of which is dictated by the history and physical examination findings. If immediately available, duplex ultrasonography can image the arterial flow and demonstrate the location and extent of the occlusive embolus. An echocardiogram, if rapidly available, may also be useful for confirming the

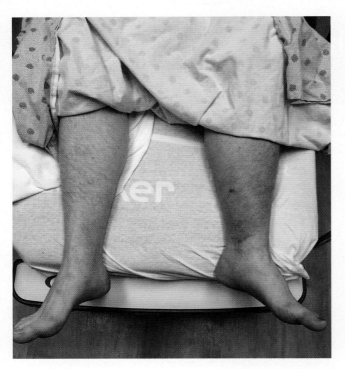

FIGURE 85-1. A patient presenting with grade IIA ischemia of left lower extremity. Notice discoloration of the left leg and toes compared to the normal right leg.

presence of cardiac thrombus and overall function but is not necessary preoperatively and should not delay revascularization. An ankle–brachial index can be done as well, but in most cases of true ALI is zero. With new-generation high-speed multidetector CT scanners, CT angiography can further aid in distinguishing the type of ALI. One should order a CT angiography with caution as this can have a detrimental effect on renal function and further delay definitive treatment.

● THERAPY

Medical

Hydration with normal saline is standard practice. Urine output should be monitored, with a goal of at least 1 mL/kg/h. An oral aspirin should be administered and a heparin bolus given, approximately 80 U/kg, followed by 18 U/kg/h continuous infusion for a goal aPTT 2 to 2.5× baseline or to a Xa level of 0.3 to 0.7 units/mL. Most institutions have a protocol for heparin infusions. It is common for patients with ALI to have multiple acute medical problems that must be treated appropriately, and saving life before limb is paramount. First and foremost is evaluation and stabilization of cardiac issues and ensuring adequate renal clearance.

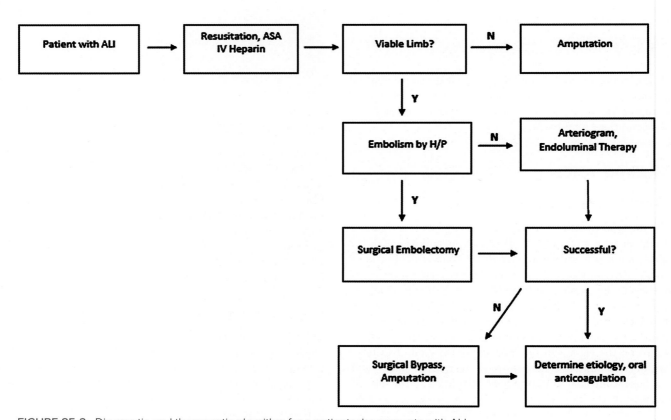

FIGURE 85-2. Diagnostic and therapeutic algorithm for a patient who presents with ALI.

Table 85-1	Etiologies of Acute Limb Ischemia

1. Embolism
   a. Cardiac
      i. Atrial and ventricular
      ii. Paradoxical (clot from venous system migrating to arteries)
      iii. Endocarditis
      iv. Cardiac tumor
   b. Noncardiac
      i. Atheroembolism (clot from native arteries)
      ii. Aortic mural thrombus
2. Thrombosis
   a. Atherosclerotic obstruction
   b. Hypercoagulable state
   c. Vasospasm
3. Aortic or arterial dissection

Reprinted from Earnshaw JJ. *Acute Ischemia: Evaluation and Decision Making.* In: Cronenwett JL, Johnston KW, eds. *Rutherford's Vascular Surgery.* 8th ed. Philadelphia, PA: Saunders; 2014: Ch 161, 2518-2527.

Interventional

The most likely etiology of ALI in this case is a cardiac embolism, and the lower extremity is the most common site of origin in general. Arteriography with thrombolysis is an option, but given the patient's classic history for an arterial thromboembolism (an antecedent cardiac event, lack of history of claudication, and normal vascular exam on his contralateral asymptomatic leg), this step may delay reperfusion achieved more readily with surgery. For cases where the etiology is not clear or points toward a nonembolic etiology (e.g., graft thrombosis or occluded aneurysm), proceeding to the arteriogram suite is best.

Procedural Basics

A longitudinal incision in the groin (or in the medial upper thigh, or below the knee, depending on the clinical circumstances) is made, and the femoral artery is exposed to include the common, deep, and superficial femoral artery. These are controlled with vessel loops. After ensuring the patient's ACT is >250, the loops are secured and the artery opened transversely if not significantly diseased. After adequate pulsatile arterial inflow is established by embolectomy, attention is turned to the distal embolectomy. The use of the embolectomy catheter relies on the catheter traversing a thrombus, and pulling it out with gentle inflation of the balloon in a continuous motion. The typical sizes are 4F and 5F for larger arteries, such as femoral and iliacs, and smaller with 2F and 3F size for distal arteries. After ensuring adequate back bleeding and having passed the catheter at least twice without retrieving thrombus, the arteriotomy is flushed with heparinized saline and closed with nonabsorbable monofilament suture in an interrupted fashion. Blood flow is reestablished to the distal limb, and Doppler signals are checked.

When the etiology of ALI is not clear by history and physical examination, arteriography with thrombolysis or catheter-assisted extraction is the best option (Figures 85-3 and 85-4). Versatile equipment in well-outfitted endovascular, hybrid rooms includes over-the-wire embolectomy catheters, suction embolectomy catheters, and high-resolution C-arm fluoroscopy that allows concurrent endovascular and open techniques. This scenario is generally the standard of care at properly equipped hospitals. Proper case selection is essential, as failed lysis or frivolous persistence at endoluminal approaches confers a significantly increased risk of limb loss and death. Thrombolytic agents may cause a systemic fibrinolytic state and potentially release thrombus

Table 85-2	Clinical Categories of Acute Limb Ischemia

Category	Description/Prognosis	Findings: Sensory Loss	Muscle Weakness	Doppler Signals: Arterial	Venous
I. Viable	Not immediately threatened	None	None	Audible	Audible
II. Threatened					
a. Marginally	Salvageable if promptly treated	Minimal (toes) or none	None	Inaudible	Audible
b. Immediately	Salvageable with immediate revascularization	More than toes, associated with rest pain	Mild, moderate	Inaudible	Audible
III. Irreversible	Major tissue loss or permanent nerve damage inevitables	Profound, anesthetic	Profound, paralysis (rigor)	Inaudible	Inaudible

Reprinted from Rutherford RB, Baker JD, Ernst C, et al. Recommended standards for reports dealing with lower ischemia: revised version. *J Vasc Surg.* 1997;26(3):517-538. Copyright © 1997 Society for Vascular Surgery and International Society for Cardiovascular Surgery, North American Chapter, with permission.

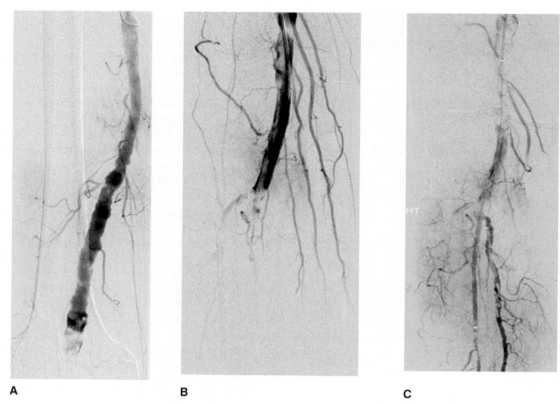

A   **B**   **C**

FIGURE 85-3. A: Appearance of a patient with underlying mild peripheral arterial disease who presented with severe right lower ischemia. **B:** Later DSA arteriogram after 5 mg of tPA intra-arterially. **C:** Shows wire traversal and approximately 8 hours after thrombolytic started with opening of tibial vessels. This patient went on to have full resolution, with the underlying etiology thought to be a hypercoagulable state.

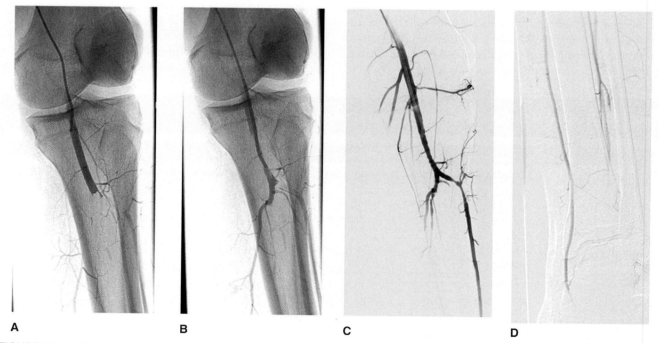

A   **B**   **C**   **D**

FIGURE 85-4. This patient with modest bilateral PAD presented with ALI and underwent percutaneous suction catheter embolectomy for ALI. **A:** The arteriogram shows a complete thrombotic obstruction at the distal popliteal artery. **B,C:** A 5 French guide catheter is advanced into the thrombus with aspiration, followed by pulsed infusion of thrombolytic agent. Repeat arteriogram shows opening of the tibial–peroneal trunk and tibial vessels. **D:** Completion arteriogram with tibial vessels showing arterial patency and no evidence of distal thromboemboli.

from the atrium or ventricle and may cause a stroke or other complications. Thus, an echocardiogram should be obtained prior to beginning thrombolysis if the suspected source of the embolus is intracardiac. A head CT should be performed if there is concern for intracranial pathology (mental status changes, recent trauma/fall, history of cancer, new headaches, or headaches without a complete workup).

It is important to continue therapeutic heparin throughout the case, as well as maintain adequate hydration. Determining a postoperative CPK and urine myoglobin may aid with resuscitation. Consideration of a four-compartment fasciotomy to treat postreperfusion compartment syndrome should be given to any patient with ALI >6-hour duration, as the morbidity is low. With good wound care, these can often be closed by delayed primary closure.

Routine follow-up with history and physical examination, but no specific imaging protocol, is needed for the affected and contralateral limb if palpable pulses returned. Standard cardiovascular risk factor modification therapies should be pursued.

Presentation

Laboratory evaluation reveals a normal hematocrit (HCT) of 38, and a normal BUN/Cr, and potassium. An EKG shows atrial fibrillation with no obvious ST elevation or depression. Baseline CPK is elevated at 1,000. The patient also denies any chest pain, and a rapid troponin I level is within normal limits. Thus, it is unlikely he has suffered a recurrent major myocardial infarction. His urine output is >30 mL/h. If his blood pressure tolerates it, an intravenous (IV) beta-blocker or calcium channel blocker is reasonable with his tachycardia.

The embolic location is likely below the femoral artery as his femoral pulse is normal (if not prominent), and no pulses or signals are present distally. The patient needs revascularization within 1 to 2 hours, as it is likely he has had approximately 4 hours of total ischemia, or he may suffer permanent muscle and nerve damage, rendering a nonsalvageable limb. As this patient has critical late ischemia, surgical embolectomy is the most appropriate means to rapidly restore limb blood flow, as compared with thrombolysis, which may take several hours before adequate reperfusion.

After cardiac rate control and heparinization, he is taken to the operating room and both lower extremities are prepped and draped to allow potential inflow site, as well as vein for conduit, should these be necessary. An open left thromboembolectomy via a femoral approach under local anesthesia with IV sedation is performed. Pedal signals are present at close. The patient undergoes four-compartment fasciotomy (Table 85-3).

Table 85-3 Open Femoral Thromboembolectomy

Key Technical Steps

1. Systemic heparinization (PTT 2–2.5× baseline or Xa 0.3–0.7 units/mL) immediately when ALI diagnosed.
2. Book patient for hybrid operative suite if available.
3. The abdomen, both groins and both legs (circumferentially) are prepped into the operative field.
4. Vertical skin incision below the inguinal ligament over the femoral pulse. If no pulse is present, the vertical incision is made vertically just medial to the midpoint of the inguinal ligament.
5. Lymphatic channels should be ligated with silk ties, and arterial circumflex branches should be preserved.
6. The common femoral, superficial femoral, and profunda femoris arteries should be controlled circumferentially with elastic vessel loops.
7. The patient should be systemically heparinized further to an ACT of >250.
8. Vessel loops are secured and a transverse arteriotomy is made over the femoral bifurcation.
9. A 4F or 5F Fogarty embolectomy is passed proximally until it returns clean twice. This is repeated distally, down the superficial femoral and profunda femoris arteries.
10. Once inflow and outflow has been reestablished, the arteriotomy is closed with several interrupted 5-0 monofilament permanent sutures (such as Prolene).
11. The groin is closed in layers, femoral sheath, Scarpa's, deep dermal, and subcuticular using absorbable suture.
12. Strong consideration should be given to four compartment fasciotomies on the operative side, particularly in a patient with no evidence of chronic peripheral arterial disease.

● DISCUSSION

Several important issues with ALI should be kept in mind; first, major errors occur with lack of timely diagnosis, anticoagulation, documentation of the exam pre- and postoperatively, and focusing too much on the limb salvage at the expense of the life (Table 85-4). Second, the same principles hold if the patient presents with upper extremity ALI. The operative approach is usually the medial distal brachial artery in the upper arm, or at the confluence of the radial and ulnar in the forearm. Third, recurrent on table or early recurrent ALI suggests an incomplete thrombectomy, or a persistent nidus of thromboembolism. For this, it is important to proceed with an on-table angiogram to visualize the inflow anatomy. Similarly, if no signals are present after reestablishing blood flow to the limb (after full embolectomy), an arteriogram is best for imaging the outflow. An intraoperative thrombolytic agent can be given (e.g., 10 mg tPA) intra-arterially, and/ or vasodilator, nitroglycerin (50 to 100 µg), may be helpful. Fourth, never force the embolectomy catheter in the artery,

Table 85-4   Acute Limb Ischemia Pitfalls

- Choosing the wrong diagnosis and attempting an embolectomy in a patient with peripheral arterial disease in whom a catheter cannot be passed subsequently limits thrombolytic agent administration.
- Be aware of reperfusion in patients with anuria, as fatal hyperkalemia may result. Communication with the anesthesiologist is critical.
- Use fluoroscopy over the wire technique to traverse areas where stenosis may be present.
- Thrombolectomize and embolectomize inflow first, flow followed by distal embolectomy.
- Do not forget fasciotomies after reperfusion.

as dissection of the artery is a major problem that often requires endoluminal techniques or an open bypass to repair. Lastly, ALI in the setting of trauma is particularly challenging because of the disrupted operative field with limited, if any, soft tissue graft coverage, the frequent inability to give heparin, and the common need to perform a bypass rather than simple embolectomy. In these cases, proceeding as expeditiously without heparin or local small doses is reasonable.

Case Conclusion

Postoperatively, the patient was maintained on heparin and then systematically anticoagulated with a vitamin K antagonist for 3 months. He was also discharged on a beta-blocker for heart rate control with early follow-up with his local cardiologists. Reassessment can be done at that time in relation to source control; that is, if he is in sinus rhythm and his ECHO shows no thrombus, it is reasonable to stop the anticoagulation at this time. His fasciotomy sites were closed by delayed primary closure on his initial inpatient admission, and his mild foot drop has since resolved.

TAKE HOME POINTS

- Early recognition of ALI is critical.
- Determine the site of occlusion based on examination and ease of anatomical exposure.
- Do not limit your therapy options; consider contrast imaging intraoperatively if available.
- Start with the small catheter first, followed by a larger embolectomy catheter and do not force the catheter if encountering persistent obstruction.
- Any of the embolectomy procedures can be done under local anesthesia to minimize cardiovascular stress.
- Do not hesitate to proceed to a distal arterial exposure if thrombosis is extensive.
- Always pass a thrombectomy catheter proximally—regardless of inflow. A lesion proximally may be the source of thromboemboli.

SUGGESTED READINGS

Earnshaw JJ. Acute ischemia: evaluation and decision making and medical treatment. In: Johnston W, Cronenwett JL, eds. *Rutherford's Vascular Surgery*. 8th ed. Philadelphia, PA: Elsevier; 2014: 2518-2527.

Eliason JL, Wainess RM, Proctor MP, et al. A national and single institutional experience in the contemporary treatment of acute lower extremity ischemia. *Ann Surg*. 2003;238:382-390.

Henke PK. Contemporary management of acute limb ischemia: factors associated with amputation and in-hospital mortality. *Semin Vasc Surg*. 2009;22(1):34-40.

Ouriel K, Veith FJ, Sarahara AA. A comparison of recombinant urokinase with vascular surgery as initial treatment for acute arterial occlusion of the legs. *N Engl J Med*. 1998;338:1105-1111.

Palfreyman SJ, Booth A, Michaels JA. A systematic review of intra-arterial thrombolytic therapy for lower limb ischemia. *Eur J Vasc Endovasc Surg*. 2000;19:143-157.

Panetta T, Thompson JE, Talkington CM, et al. Arterial embolectomy: a 34-year experience with 400 cases. *Surg Clin North Am*. 1986;66:339-352.

Rutherford RB, Baker JD, Ernst C, et al. Recommended standards for reports dealing with lower ischemia: revised version. *J Vasc Surg*. 1997;26:517-538.

Asymptomatic Carotid Artery Stenosis

86

CARLIN WILLIAMS AND GILBERT R. UPCHURCH JR.

Based on the previous edition chapter "Asymptomatic Carotid Stenosis" by Paul D. Dimusto, John Rectenwald, and Gilbert R. Upchurch Jr.

Presentation

A 70-year-old man arrives to clinic having been referred by his family physician who auscultated a left-sided cervical bruit on routine physical examination. His past medical history includes hyperlipidemia and hypertension managed medically with atorvastatin and carvedilol. He takes a baby aspirin daily. The patient has a 50-pack-year smoking history and continues at a rate of 1 pack/day. He has never had difficulty with speech, sensory or motor deficits, or transient monocular blindness. He denies any other symptoms of transient ischemic attack or stroke. On physical examination, there is a left carotid bruit, and bilateral upper extremity pulses are equal. There are no neurologic deficits.

● DIFFERENTIAL DIAGNOSIS

Given this patient's age, comorbidities and concomitant tobacco use, asymptomatic internal carotid artery stenosis is the most likely diagnosis. Other pathologies that can cause a neck bruit include a carotid aneurysm, dissection, carotid body tumor, or vertebral artery flow reversal secondary to "subclavian steal." In addition, referred bruits from heart valve abnormalities can often be heard in the neck.

● WORKUP

Duplex ultrasonography is the initial test of choice for presumed carotid artery stenosis. It carries a sensitivity of 90% and a specificity of 94% for its ability to detect a stenosis ≥70% stenosis. Gray scale imaging of the carotid arteries can provide anatomic information about plaque morphology and the location of the stenosis but have limited reproducible accuracy to estimate an artery's percentage of stenosis. This is extrapolated from Doppler flow velocity measurements. The peak systolic velocity (PSV) and end-diastolic velocity (EDV) values in the ICA and the internal carotid to common carotid artery peak systolic velocity ratio (ICA/CCA ratio) are all used to measure the severity of stenosis in the internal

carotid artery (Table 86-1). These values can then be translated to a percent stenosis range with charts that are based on data from studies correlating flow velocities with visible stenoses on angiographic imaging. Although differences in measurement methods between ultrasound and angiography can result in significant discrepancies, a commonly used chart with velocities are found in Table 86-1. The degree of stenosis can be estimated based on duplex velocity values.

Computed tomography angiogram (CTA) is useful in further defining the extent of the lesion and degree of stenosis (Figure 86-1). While the gold standard for measuring the degree of carotid stenosis is angiography, it is rarely used now given the reliable results from noninvasive duplex ultrasound scanning and CTA. Many surgeons will make operative decisions based on ultrasound alone. However, angiography does have a roll in carotid stenting.

● DIAGNOSIS AND TREATMENT

The patient's carotid duplex results reveal a high-grade left internal carotid artery stenosis and no significant disease on the right side. The combination of history, physical examination, and duplex ultrasound findings make the diagnosis of high-grade asymptomatic internal carotid artery stenosis in this case (Figure 86-2). A left carotid endarterectomy (CEA) is recommended. Smoking cessation is recommended, and the patient is continued on his statin, beta-blocker, and aspirin.

The patient is told he has a risk of 3% for combined ipsilateral stroke and death and a risk of 5% to 10% for cranial nerve injury. The patient signs consent for a left CEA with patch angioplasty. An EKG and cardiopulmonary function are normal. He is able to walk up two flights of stairs without dyspnea. No further cardiac testing is indicated given his young (<70 years) age, normal EKG, and good functional capacity.

● DISCUSSION

The current recommendations for performing CEA or carotid artery stenting (CAS) in asymptomatic carotid stenosis are derived from studies that compared the risk

| Table 86-1 | Ultrasound Criteria for Determining Carotid Stenosis |

Stenosis (%)		Duplex Velocity Criteria				Plaque and Lumen
NASCET	ECST	PSVic	EDVic	PSVic/PSVic	PSVic/EDVcc	
Normal	Normal	<125	<40	<2	<8	Absent
<50	<70	<125	<40	<4	<8	Present
50–59	70–76	125–230	40–100	2–4	8–10	Narrowing
60–69	77–82	125–230	40–100	2–4	11–14	Narrowing
70–79	83–89	230–400	100–125	5–5	15–20	Narrowing
80–89	90–94	230–400	>125	>4.0	21–30	Narrowing
90–99	95–99	>400*	>125*	>4.0	>30	Narrowing

Note: This table incorporates the guidelines of the Society of Radiologists in Ultrasound published in 2003 and the Joint Recommendations for Reporting Carotid Ultrasound Investigation in the United Kingdom published in 2009 as used in this chapter. The ECST percent stenosis column has been added for ease of use for those who want to grade lesions in terms of stroke risk (ECST stenosis is linearly related to stroke risk, but NASCET stenosis is not).

* In cases of trickle flow, these velocities might not be detectable (see text).

cc, Common carotid artery; EDVic, end-diastolic velocity in internal carotid artery; ECST, European Carotid Surgery Trial; ic, internal carotid artery; NASCET, North American Symptomatic Carotid Endarterectomy Trial; PSVic, peak systolic velocity in internal carotid artery.

of stroke with either adherence to medical management alone or medical management with the addition of CEA or CAS.

The Asymptomatic Carotid Atherosclerosis Study (ACAS) compared the risk of transient ischemic attack (TIA) and stroke between those treated with medical therapy alone or to medical therapy plus CEA. One thousand six hundred and sixty-two asymptomatic patients with a carotid stenosis ≥60% by angiography (correlating to ~75% on ultrasound) were randomized to aspirin and risk factor management alone or aspirin and risk factor management plus CEA. The 5-year aggregate risk of ipsilateral TIA and perioperative stroke or

death was 5.1% in the patients undergoing CEA versus 11.0% in patients receiving only medical therapy. The aggregate risk reduction for CEA was 53%.

The Asymptomatic Carotid Surgery Trial (ACST) was a European study that randomized 3,120 patients with a >60% internal carotid artery stenosis by ultrasound to medical therapy and immediate CEA versus medical therapy and deferred CEA, performed after symptomatic conversion. The medical therapy in this study targeted known atherosclerotic risk factors but was not standardized throughout the study period. Antiplatelet, antihypertensives, and lipid-lowering therapy were used more commonly in the study's later years.

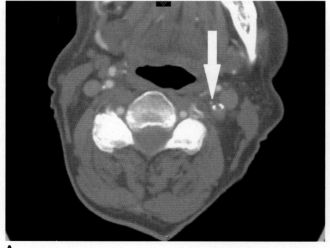

A

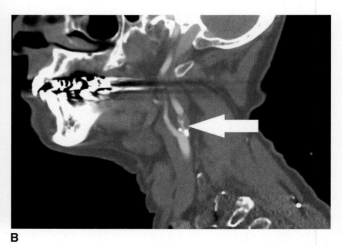

B

FIGURE 86-1. CT angiogram demonstrating high-grade left carotid artery stenosis in **(A)** axial cross section (*arrow*) and **(B)** sagittal cross section (*arrow*).

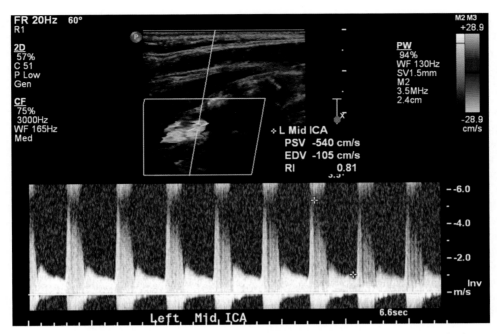

FIGURE 86-2. Preoperative duplex ultrasonography demonstrating high-grade left carotid stenosis with elevated peak systolic velocity and high EDV in left internal carotid artery.

After 5 years, the combined perioperative event and overall stroke risk for the immediate CEA group was 6.9% compared to 10.9% for deferred CEA group. The perioperative risk of stroke or death within 30 days was 3.0% among patients who underwent CEA.

The Stenting versus Endarterectomy for Treatment of Carotid-Artery Stenosis (CREST) trial randomized 2,502 patients with symptomatic or asymptomatic carotid stenosis to undergo CAS or CEA. The primary end points were perioperative stroke, MI, or death as well as any ipsilateral stroke within 4 years of randomization. Results of this study revealed a higher perioperative stroke rate for CAS (4.1% vs. 2.3%, $P = 0.01$) and a higher perioperative MI rate for CEA (2.3% vs. 1.1%, $P = 0.03$). For both CAS and CEA, ipsilateral stroke rates and contralateral stroke rates were similar after the periprocedural period (30 days).

These trials form much of the foundation on which medical and surgical management of asymptomatic carotid artery stenosis stands today. There are today, however, distinct differences in medical management worth taking into account. ACAS and ACST were studies that compared the stroke risk of CEA and medical management to that of medical management alone in an era where medical management in carotid stenosis was not standardized. The CREST trial compared the stroke risk in CEA to that of CAS and was devoid of a medical arm of therapy. The medical nuances in these studies are limiting in that, current best medical therapy could potentially be proven superior to any intervention for asymptomatic carotid disease. These studies, while cited in management guidelines for extracranial carotid disease, are controversial in that the medical management of asymptomatic carotid disease and

its associated stroke risk differ today than when these studies were published. Current medical management consists of hypertension control, diabetes mellitus treatment, lipid-lowering medications, antiplatelet therapy, and smoking cessation.

The CREST-2 trial is a randomized controlled trial that at the time of this publication, is actively comparing a standardized modern intense medical therapy, CEA and CAS in patients with asymptomatic carotid stenosis. It is currently tasked with providing evidence that will answer questions regarding current treatment algorithms in asymptomatic carotid disease. As of now, current SVS guidelines recommend intense medical therapy and CEA as the first-line treatment for asymptomatic patients with stenosis of 60% to 99% by carotid ultrasound with the caveat that the surgeon's perioperative risk of stroke and death must be <3% to ensure benefit to the patient.

● SURGICAL APPROACH

CEA is performed under local or general anesthesia depending on the surgeon's preference. Intraluminal carotid shunting can either be routinely or selectively employed. If an awake CEA is performed, the literature supports there being no significant difference in the 30-day periprocedural incidence of stroke, myocardial infarction, or death when compared to a CEA done under general anesthesia. When performed awake and under local anesthesia, clinical neurologic status can be monitored by asking a patient to perform physical and verbal tasks such as squeezing a ball and engaging in conversation. Deterioration in neurologic status during carotid clamp time warrants shunt insertion. Most carotid endarterectomies, however, are performed under general anesthesia, with the majority of the evidence supporting the use of intraoperative EEG monitoring or carotid stump pressure measurements to predict the need for enhanced cerebral perfusion and thus shunting.

If the decision is made to perform the CEA under general anesthesia, the patient is induced and endotracheally intubated. If a high carotid lesion is seen on preoperative imaging and mandibular subluxation is a consideration, nasotracheal intubation can be performed. If laryngoscopy has not been performed for a patient who has had a previous contralateral CEA, it should be performed prior to induction. The patient is positioned supine or in a beach chair position, and the patient's head is turned away from the lesion. A radial arterial line is placed, usually on the contralateral arm for accessibility. A shoulder roll is helpful in providing neck extension. Appropriate neurologic monitoring is introduced. Sterile preparation and draping is performed so that the sternal notch, chin, earlobe, and clavicle are all visible. After time-out and prepping/draping, an incision is made slightly anterior to the sternocleidomastoid muscle. The incision is deepened to the platysma muscle, which is divided. The sternocleidomastoid is retracted laterally, and entrance into the carotid sheath is obtained revealing internal jugular vein. Ansa cervicalis fibers are usually encountered prior to entering the carotid sheath and are sacrificed if necessary. Electrocautery is usually avoided as thermal spread can injure nearby cranial nerves. The facial vein tributary to the internal jugular vein is identified anteriorly and is usually ligated and divided. The facial vein is generally superficial to and at the same level as the carotid artery bifurcation. Carotid artery dissection is performed with care to avoid iatrogenic

embolization. The vagus and hypoglossal nerves are identified and preserved. The CCA and the external carotid artery (ECA) are encircled with vessel loops with care not to incorporate the vagus nerve posterior in the carotid sheath. The patient is systemically heparinized (100 units/kg), and the ICA is encircled distal to the plaque. After therapeutic heparinization, a test clamp of the ECA and ICA is performed. If the patient remains neurologically intact, the CCA is clamped during awake CEAs. A longitudinal arteriotomy is made in the CCA extending into the ICA until the distal end of the plaque is reached. The endarterectomy is begun in the CCA, includes an eversion endarterectomy of the ECA, and ends in the distal ICA as a gradual transition from endarterectomized artery to normal artery occurs. Debris is removed from the endarterectomized vessel with forceps and heparinized saline or dextran solution. Tacking sutures can be placed in the proximal and distal end points at areas that do not have a gradual, feathered taper. A 6-0 nonabsorbable monofilament suture and a patch are used to repair the arteriotomy. Prior to completing the patch, the ECA and ICA are back bled and the CCA is forward bled. Heparinized saline may be used to flush the repair of any remaining air or debris, and the patch is completed. The clamp on the ECA is released first to test the patch for leaks. The CCA is then released to flush any remaining debris into the ECA. The ICA is released last after a few heartbeats. This order is to prevent cerebral embolic events. An intraoperative duplex scan should show normal velocities (Figure 86-3) and no evidence of residual debris or stenosis. The incision is closed with the platysma layer as the strength layer. A closed-suction drain can be placed in the subplatysma space. If the patient is neurologically intact when awakened, he/she is transferred to the postanesthesia care unit. The patient is placed in an

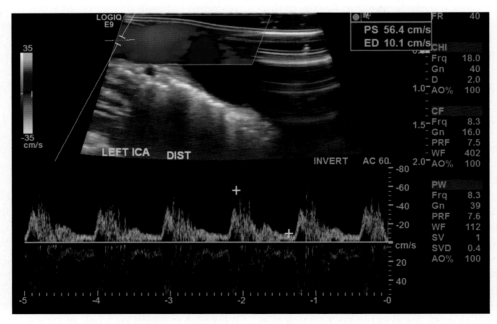

FIGURE 86-3. Intraoperative duplex scan following CEA demonstrating no residual debris or stenosis in the left internal carotid artery.

Table 86-2	Asymptomatic Carotid Artery Stenosis

Key Technical Steps

1. Establish arterial line blood pressure monitoring and neurologic monitoring, position the patient
2. Incise the skin and platysma, retract the sternocleidomastoid laterally, identify the internal jugular vein and ligate the facial vein
3. Expose the CCA, ECA, and ICA with sharp dissection and minimal manipulation, identifying and preserving the vagus and hypoglossal nerves
4. Administer heparin, clamp the ICA, CCA, and ECA, respectively, and insert shunt if needed. *Note: if performing stump pressure measurements, clamp the CCA and ECA and transduce ICA pressures by sticking the CCA above the clamp; ICA pressure will transmit across stenosis*
5. Make arteriotomy starting on CCA and extending to ICA; perform the endarterectomy
6. Flush with heparinized saline, assess the end points of endarterectomy, place tacking sutures if needed
7. Sew in patch, back bleed ICA and ECA, forward bleed CCA prior to completion of patch angioplasty
8. Unclamp ECA, CCA, and ICA, respectively
9. Assure hemostasis; perform completion study
10. Place closed suction drain in subplatysma space; close incision in layers
11. Check neurologic status prior to leaving the OR

Potential Pitfalls

- Cranial nerve injury
- Perioperative stroke
- Perioperative myocardial infarction

intermediate care setting and monitored for any neurologic changes or blood pressure lability. Systolic blood pressures are kept between 100 and 140 mm Hg. The drain is removed the following postoperative day, and the patient is usually discharged on postoperative day 1 (Table 86-2).

● SPECIAL INTRAOPERATIVE CONSIDERATIONS

It is important to identify and protect the cranial nerves encountered during the operation to avoid even temporary paralysis. The vagus and hypoglossal nerves are the most commonly encountered, but the glossopharyngeal nerve can also be injured, especially in exposures higher in the neck. Care should be taken to ensure accurate carotid clamp placement on the artery, without including the vagus nerve.

It is crucially important to see the distal end of the plaque to create a smooth, feathered end to the endarterectomy.

Interrupted sutures with knots tied extraluminally can assist in tacking down the intima distally that may be at risk for dissecting. If preoperative imaging shows a high lesion where adequate visualization of the distal end point may be difficult, subluxation of the mandible and nasotracheal intubation can be performed before starting the operation to allow for enhanced exposure. If high disease is unexpectedly encountered intraoperatively, the digastric muscle can be divided, the hypoglossal nerve mobilized, the styloglossus and stylopharyngeus muscles can be divided, and finally the styloid process can be fractured to provide adequate exposure.

● POSTOPERATIVE MANAGEMENT

Patients are usually monitored in an intermediate care setting with arterial line blood pressure monitoring overnight as intraoperative manipulation of the carotid bulb and changes in the flow dynamics can cause blood pressure lability. Blood pressure parameters are generally kept between 100 and 140 mm Hg systolic. Antiplatelet therapy with aspirin is employed as it was preoperatively. Clopidogrel is neither added or continued unless used to treat non–carotid-related disease processes. Neurologic function should also be monitored, as a change could represent a postoperative stroke related to an embolus from thrombus formation at the operative site or propagation of a dissection plane created by an inadequately tapered end point. Any new neurologic deficit within 24 hours of CEA is considered technical in etiology, and the patient should be promptly returned to the operating room for exploration and repair. Most patients, however, are discharged home on postoperative day 1 after restarting their home medications. Blood pressure, glucose, and lipid control, as well as continued smoking cessation, are the goals of postoperative medical management.

The patient can be seen in 2 weeks for an incision check and then in 3 months for a repeat carotid duplex to check for restenosis, as well as to surveil any contralateral stenosis if present. Up to 85% of patients with a moderate contralateral stenosis will progress to severe stenosis and require intervention. Therefore, yearly carotid duplex monitoring is recommended.

TAKE HOME POINTS

- Duplex ultrasound scan is the best initial diagnostic test for assessing carotid stenosis.
- Patients with high-grade asymptomatic carotid stenosis (80% to 99% by ultrasound) should be considered for CEA along with modern intense medical therapy to reduce their risk of stroke.
- CEA can be performed under local anesthesia with awake neurologic monitoring, under general anesthesia with EEG or stump pressure monitoring, or with routine shunt use.

- Fastidious management of the proximal and distal end points is crucial to the technical success of the CEA and clinical outcome of the patient.
- Blood pressure control, glucose control, antiplatelet, and statin therapy, as well as smoking cessation are the major tenets of postoperative success after CEA.

SUGGESTED READINGS

Brott TG, Hobson RW, Howard G, et al. Stenting versus endarterectomy for treatment of carotid-artery stenosis. *N Engl J Med.* 2010; 363(1):11-23.

CREST-2. http://www.crest2trial.org

Nicolaides AN, Griffin M, Labropoulos N. Duplex scanning and spectral analysis of carotid bifurcation atherosclerotic disease. In: Stanley JC, Veith F, Wakefield TW, eds. *Current Therapy in Vascular and Endovascular Surgery.* 5th ed. Philadelphia, PA: Elsevier Saunders; 2014:22-25.

Endarterectomy for asymptomatic carotid artery stenosis. Executive Committee for the Asymptomatic Carotid Atherosclerosis Study. *JAMA.* 1995;273(18):1421-1428.

Halliday A, et al. 10-year stroke prevention after successful carotid endarterectomy for asymptomatic stenosis (ACST-1): a multicentre randomised trial. *Lancet.* 2010;376(9746):1074-1084.

Jahromi AS, Cinà CS, Liu Y, Clase CM. Sensitivity and specificity of color duplex ultrasound measurement in the estimation of internal carotid artery stenosis: a systematic review and meta-analysis. *J Vasc Surg.* 2005;41(6):962-972.

Symptomatic Carotid Artery Stenosis

87

MARTYN KNOWLES AND CARLOS H. TIMARAN

Based on the previous edition chapter "Symptomatic Carotid Stenosis" by Sarah M. Weakley and Peter H. Lin

Presentation

A 57-year-old female presented to the Emergency Department after an episode of left-sided weakness, confusion, and aphasia. The patient has a history of coronary artery disease, hypertension, hyperlipidemia, and smoking. On evaluation, the patient is still slightly weak in the left upper and lower extremities, with aphasia. Her initial workup included a computerized tomography (CT) without contrast of the brain. She was admitted to the neurology service, and a carotid duplex ultrasonography (DUS) was performed among other studies. The duplex shows a <50% internal carotid stenosis on the left. On the right, there was a stenosis with a peak systolic velocity (PSV) of 294 cm/sec, with an end diastolic velocity (EDV) of 103 cm/sec. The DUS showed a complex heterogeneous plaque (Figures 87-1 and 87-2).

● DIFFERENTIAL DIAGNOSIS

The differential diagnosis for a patient with similar symptoms includes cardiac arrhythmias (atrial fibrillation being the most common), cardiac embolization, carotid dissection,

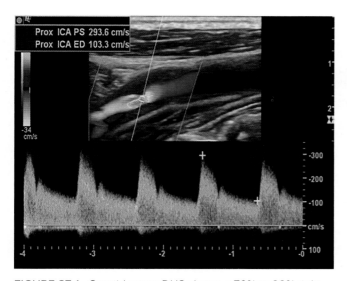

FIGURE 87-1. Carotid artery DUS shows a 70% to 99% right ICA stenosis with a complex heterogeneous plaque involving the distal CCA and proximal ICA. (Courtesy of Patrick Washko BSRT, RDMS, RVT, FSVU.)

extracranial carotid aneurysm, vasculitis, carotid trauma, vertebrobasilar disease, vasculitis, seizure disorder, and migraine headaches.

Carotid disease is broken down into asymptomatic and symptomatic. Symptomatic carotid artery disease is most classically associated with a transient ischemic attack (TIA), cerebrovascular accident (CVA), or amaurosis fugax. A TIA is a neurologic event that exhibits stroke-like symptoms, such as arm or leg weakness or numbness, aphasia, or facial droop, for <24 hours. These events are considered a herald of a more serious event that may progress to a CVA. Once the symptoms progress past 24 hours, the TIA has become a full CVA. The full severity of a stroke can take weeks to manifest as the penumbra evolves. Symptoms correspond with a focal deficit that can be related to a carotid lesion. These symptoms typically involve the anterior or middle cerebral artery circulations. Motor symptoms can include hemiparesis contralateral to the affected hemisphere. Sensory deficits can also occur in a similar fashion, such as numbness or paresthesia. Aphasia, dysphagia, or dysarthria can also occur. Amaurosis fugax is the temporary monocular blindness from cholesterol embolization to the retinal artery via the ophthalmic artery. Other symptoms, such as syncope, vertigo, dizziness, seizures, bowel or bladder incontinence, or migraines, are not normally related to carotid disease, and other causes must be pursued.

● WORKUP

Carotid DUS is the preferred diagnostic tool for the evaluation of carotid disease. The benefits of DUS include the ease to easily follow patients with progressive disease and excellent sensitivity for the diagnosis of occlusive carotid disease. Furthermore, DUS allows the avoidance of radiation, rapid availability, and ease of evaluation. Often, DUS is a standalone test for the decision for carotid intervention in patients with carotid disease. A complete examination includes evaluation of the common, external, and internal carotid arteries as well as the vertebral arteries and often the subclavian arteries. The PSV, EDV, and the ratio of the common carotid artery to internal carotid artery (CCA/ICA) is used to determine the severity of stenosis (Table 87-1). Although labs differ in their ranges, patients are typically classified into normal, 1% to 49%, 50% to

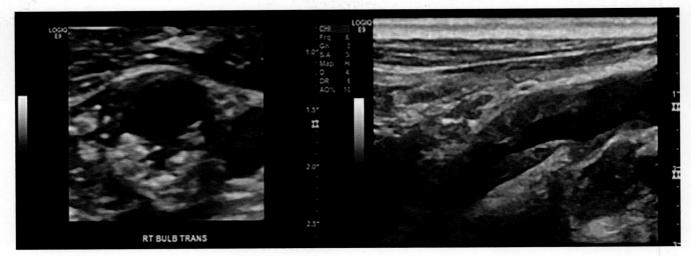

FIGURE 87-2. Complex heterogeneous plaque with appearance of a ruptured plaque. (Courtesy of Patrick Washko BSRT, RDMS, RVT, FSVU.)

69%, 70% to 99%, or occluded. Additionally, the DUS can provide important information regarding the plaque morphology. DUS allows for the identification of high-risk lesions that are worrisome in symptomatic patients, such as echolucent plaques. The degree of stenosis corresponds with the risk of stroke and can easily be identified on DUS. Concerning findings such as ruptured or heterogeneous plaques can increase the risk of neurologic symptoms. Magnetic resonance angiography (MRA) and computerized tomographic angiography (CTA) are becoming more popular for diagnosis in carotid disease and continue to have improvements in technology. These imaging modalities can provide important information regarding anatomic issues and verify the degree of stenosis, as well as provide information related to intracerebral collateral circulation. They can, however, overestimate the amount of stenosis, and often correlation to the DUS is required. Angiography

remains the gold standard for diagnosis; however, the procedure itself carries approximately 1% risk of neurologic complications.

● DIAGNOSIS AND TREATMENT

Patients with symptomatic lesions are at the highest risk of ipsilateral CVA, and the degree of stenosis corresponds with the risk. As seen in the North American Symptomatic Carotid Endarterectomy Trial (NASCET) study, the degree of stenosis correlates with CVA risk. A stenosis <50% was extremely unlikely to cause neurologic manifestations. In the NASCET study, symptomatic patients were assigned to medical therapy or endarterectomy with symptomatic disease and a stenosis >50%. In patients with >50% stenosis, those treated with medical therapy with aspirin were more likely

Table 87-1	Carotid Artery Stenosis Duplex Criteria			
Degree of Stenosis (%)	**ICA PSV (cm/sec)**	**ICA EDV (cm/sec)**	**ICA/CCA Ratio (%)**	**Carotid Plaquse**
Carotid artery duplex criteria				
Normal	<125	<40	<2.0	None
<50%	<125	<40	<2.0	<50%
50–69%	125–230	40–100	2.0–4.0	>50%
70–99%	>230	>100	>4.0	>70%
Occlusion	Undetectable	Undetectable	Not applicable	100%

From Knowles M, Timaran CH. Cerebrovascular disease. In: *Greenfield's Surgery: Scientific Principles and Practice*. 6th ed. Philadelphia, PA: Wolters Kluwer; 2017:1622-1637.

ICA, internal carotid artery; PSV, peak systolic velocity; EDV, end-diastolic velocity; CCA, common carotid artery.

to progress to ipsilateral stroke than those that underwent carotid endarterectomy (CEA). In patients with a 70% to 99% stenosis range, the benefit of surgery was even stronger. After 2 years, there was a significant reduction in ipsilateral stroke in those who underwent a CEA; among patients with 50% to 69% stenosis, the stroke and death rates were 22.2% in medical patients vs. 16.7% in surgical patients, whereas in those with 70% to 99% stenosis the rates were 26% in medical patients and 9% in surgical patients. The European Carotid Surgery Trial (ECST) showed similar findings for severe stenosis; however, no benefit was found to surgery over medical management with the more moderate stenosis. Medical therapy has advanced since the NASCET trial with the introduction of improved antiplatelet medications such as clopidogrel and HMG Co-A reductase inhibitors. In the NASCET trial, aspirin was the only agent used and is not currently the standard of care. Most neurologists recommend aspirin and clopidogrel in symptomatic patients for prevention of stroke until surgical intervention is performed. Statins lower stroke risk by 30% by plaque stabilization and are important for the overall reduction of stroke.

The timing of intervention after CVA continues to be debated. Traditionally, surgeons waited at least 6 weeks prior to intervention. However, the chance of recurrent stroke increases with waiting. Unfortunately, the consequences of surgery too soon can lead to hemorrhagic conversion of an ischemic lesion. In patients who have returned to baseline from their symptoms, the current thought is to undergo surgery between 2 days and 2 weeks after the event. If the patient does not return to normal or has a dense lesion on imaging, it is best to wait a few weeks. Crescendo TIA or evolving stroke are different entities entirely, and urgent revascularization is warranted to prevent a major stroke.

There are two options for the repair of symptomatic carotid stenosis, carotid artery stenting (CAS), and CEA. CAS was initially considered as a substitute of CEA in high-risk patients from anatomic or medical reasons, as well as elderly patients. Trials comparing CAS versus CEA in high-risk patients such as the Stenting and Angioplasty with Protection in Patients at High Risk for Endarterectomy (SAPPHIRE) trial revealed CAS was associated with a lower risk of major events at 1 year, with a greater advantage in asymptomatic patients. The Carotid Revascularization Endarterectomy versus Stenting Trial (CREST) examined CAS versus CEA in standard-risk patients with both symptomatic and asymptomatic carotid disease. Overall, there was no difference between CAS and CEA in the primary end point of the study because of a higher rate of myocardial infarction with CEA and a higher rate of periprocedural CVA with CAS. Despite the similar rate of complications overall, stroke-related complications portended a worse long-term survival. CREST and similar trials in Europe confirmed that elderly symptomatic patients, particularly those older than 70 years, have a higher risk of stroke and death after CAS and improved outcomes after CEA, which is currently the preferred

treatment option for these patients. With the mixed data with these trials, CREST 2 is underway to further ascertain the role of CAS in the management of patients with asymptomatic carotid stenosis.

There are some subpopulations that do better than others with a CEA. Despite increasing age being a reason early in the experience to perform a CAS, age ≥68 was associated with a significantly higher risk of stroke and death. Additionally, symptomatic patients undergoing CAS appear to have a higher risk of stroke or death if performed within 7 days after the symptomatic event. At this time, there are insufficient data to support CAS for asymptomatic and symptomatic patients outside high-risk criteria for CEA associated with anatomical factors (stoma, previous neck radiation, contralateral vocal cord paralysis, or high lesion) or severe medical comorbidities (coronary or pulmonary disease). Conversely, patients with significant anatomical factors that put them at risk for CAS should undergo CEA, such as thrombus, unstable plaque, circumferential calcification, and difficult aortic arch configurations.

● SURGICAL APPROACH

Anesthesia options for CEA include local, regional, or general. Depending on the choice of anesthetic, there is a choice of cerebral monitoring. For local or regional, the patient can be continually assessed clinically for changes after clamping. In patients under general anesthesia, electroencephalogram (EEG), transcranial Doppler (TCD), stump pressure measurement, or somatosensory-evoked potentials (SSEPs) can be performed based on the surgeon's preferences or capabilities.

Correct patient positioning is critical for a successful endarterectomy, especially for a high lesion (Table 87-2). The patient's neck is slightly hyperextended and turned away, with a roll under the shoulder. A longitudinal incision is made along the anterior border of the sternocleidomastoid muscle (SCM). The use of ultrasound intraoperatively can help guide the surgeon to perform a limited incision over the bifurcation. The platysma is divided. By retracting the SCM laterally, the internal jugular vein (IJV) is identified close to the carotid sheath. The facial vein, a branch off the IJV, is an important landmark for identification of the bifurcation and is divided. Inferior and medial to the IJV is the common carotid artery (CCA), which is carefully exposed. Care must be taken to avoid injuring the vagus nerve that is typically posterior to the artery. After the CCA is dissected out, the external carotid artery (ECA) and superior thyroid arteries are controlled. Often, dissection at the carotid bifurcation can cause reactive bradycardia, which can be improved with administration of 1% lidocaine directly into the bifurcation adventitia. Care must be taken in dissecting out the internal carotid artery (ICA) to avoid excessive manipulation to prevent embolization and avoid injury of the hypoglossal nerve. For high lesions, division of the posterior belly of the

Table 87-2 Carotid Endarterectomy with Shunting

Key Technical Steps

1. The patient's neck is slightly hyperextended and turned away, with a roll under the shoulder to open the neck.
2. A longitudinal incision is made along the anterior border of the SCM.
3. The use of ultrasound intraoperatively can help guide the surgeon to perform a limited incision over the bifurcation.
4. The platysma is divided.
5. By retracting the SCM laterally, the IJV is identified in the carotid sheath.
6. The facial vein is an important landmark for identification of the bifurcation and is divided.
7. Care must be taken to avoid injuring the vagus nerve that is typically posterior to the artery but can travel anteriorly in some cases.
8. The CCA is carefully dissected and controlled with a vessel loop.
9. The ECA and superior thyroid arteries are identified and controlled.
10. The ICA is then carefully dissected out well above the most cranial plaque and controlled with a vessel loop.
11. The hypoglossal nerve is carefully avoided. This is especially prudent if the lesion is high and requires division of the posterior belly of the digastric muscle.
12. The patient is systemically heparinized, and clamps are placed on the ICA, CCA, ECA, and superior thyroid arteries.
13. An arteriotomy is made from the CCA onto the ICA anteriorly.
14. A shunt is placed into the ICA and CCA and secured with Rommel tourniquets. A Doppler is used to interrogate the shunt to ensure blood is flowing.
15. An endarterectomy is performed removing plaque.
16. Loose debris is removed, and a distal end point is carefully accomplished. Intimal flaps are secured with tacking sutures.
17. The repair is closed with a patch angioplasty using most likely Bovine pericardium.
18. Prior to completion of the patch repair, the shunt is removed.
19. Backbleeding is performed from all vessels sequentially to remove air or debris that could serve as embolic sources.
20. Arterial flow is returned to the ECA, followed by the ICA.
21. Duplex ultrasonography is performed intraoperatively to ensure the quality of the repair.

Potential Pitfalls

- Aggressive dissection at the bulb can cause bradycardia. Injection of 1% lidocaine into the bulb adventitia can relieve the bradycardia.
- Tacking sutures should be used on the distal end point if while checking with pressurized heparinized saline, if it appears to lift.
- Avoid injury to the vagus nerve when getting control of the CCA and the hypoglossal nerve when getting ICA control.

digastric, or preoperative nasotracheal intubation and mandibular subluxation with temporary fixation, can assist in exposure of the distal ICA.

Once all vessels are controlled, intravenous heparin is administered prior to clamping. The ICA is clamped first to avoid embolization after ensuring the clamp site is above palpable plaque. The ECA and CCA are then clamped. A longitudinal arteriotomy is created from the CCA into the ICA anteriorly. A shunt can be placed from the ICA to the CCA to maintain antegrade flow. An endarterectomy is then performed to remove the plaque. The plaque extending into the ECA is most easily dealt with by way of an eversion technique. The entire endarterectomized surface must be examined to remove flaps or debris. This is of most importance at the distal aspect in the ICA. If needed, tacking with 7-0 Prolene sutures can be used to keep down a concerning end point to avoid a flap once flow resumes.

At this point, the arteriotomy is closed. Primary repair is not recommended due to improved short- and long-term outcomes with patch closure. The patch is either synthetic material, such as Dacron or polytetrafluoroethylene, or biologic material, such as bovine pericardium or autogenous vein. Prior to closure, the shunt is removed, and careful sequential flushing of each of the vessels is performed to remove air and debris. Additionally, after patch closure, flow is restored to the ECA for a few seconds prior to removal of the ICA clamp to allow flushing through the ECA to ensure any remaining debris or thrombus does not proceed into the cerebral circulation. The heparin is typically reversed with protamine sulfate. Once hemostasis is accomplished, closure is performed by approximating the sternocleidomastoid back, closing the platysma and skin. A full neurologic exam is performed prior to extubation or exit from the operating room if performed under local anesthesia (Figure 87-3).

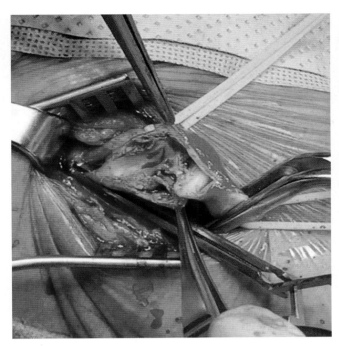

FIGURE 87-3. Intraoperative picture showing a severe stenosis and irregular complex plaque.

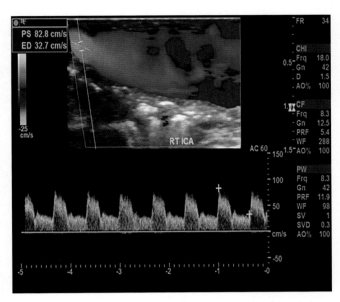

FIGURE 87-4. Intraoperative DUS showing a good result from endarterectomy with patch repair with excellent ICA waveform and no evidence of remaining stenosis or flap. (Courtesy of Patrick Washko BSRT, RDMS, RVT, FSVU.)

● POST-OPERATIVE MANAGEMENT

The patient is evaluated with a limited neurologic exam prior to extubation. Subsequently, the patient undergoes a full neurologic evaluation once in recovery. The patient is typically maintained on aspirin throughout the perioperative period. Blood pressure parameters must be carefully followed over the first 24 hours given dissection of the carotid bifurcation. Furthermore, hypotension could cause vessel thrombosis, and hypertension could cause reperfusion injury or bleeding. Frequent neurologic checks allow rapid identification of patient changes as the patient has a chance of CVA after surgery.

Case Conclusion

The patient underwent a right carotid endarterectomy 5 days after her initial symptoms. The endarterectomy was performed under general anesthesia with a shunt. She awoke without any new neurologic deficits. She was discharged to home with no residual motor deficits. Speech therapy continued to work with the patient regarding her improving aphasia (Figure 87-4).

SUGGESTED READINGS

Barnett HJ, Taylor DW, Eliasziw M, et al. Benefit of carotid endarterectomy in patients with symptomatic moderate or severe stenosis. North American Symptomatic Carotid Endarterectomy Trial Collaborators. *N Engl J Med.* 1998;339:1415-1425.

Brott TG, Hobson RW II, Howard G, et al. Stenting versus endarterectomy for treatment of carotid-artery stenosis. *N Engl J Med.* 2010;363:11-23.

Endarterectomy for asymptomatic carotid artery stenosis. Executive Committee for the Asymptomatic Carotid Atherosclerosis Study. *JAMA.* 1995;273:1421-1428.

Gurm HS, Yadav JS, Fayad P, et al. Long-term results of carotid stenting versus endarterectomy in high-risk patients. *N Engl J Med.* 2008;358:1572-1579.

Mas JL, Chatellier G, Beyssen B, et al. Endarterectomy versus stenting in patients with symptomatic severe carotid stenosis. *N Engl J Med.* 2006;355:1660-1671.

Knowles M, Timaran DE, Timaran CH. Cerebrovascular disease. In: Mulholland MW, Lillemoe KD, Doherty GM, Maier RV, Simeone DM, Upchurch GR, eds. *Greenfield's Surgery: Scientific Principles & Practice*, 6th ed. Lippincott Williams & Wilkins: Philadelphia, PA. 2015:1622-1637.

Rerkasem K, Rothwell PM. Systematic review of operative risks of carotid endarterectomy for recently symptomatic stenosis in relation to timing of surgery. *Stroke.* 2009;e564-e725

Warlow CP. Symptomatic patients: the European Carotid Surgery Trial (ECST). *J Mal Vasc.* 1993;18:198-201.

Diabetic Foot Infection

88

PATRIC LIANG, DOUGLAS JONES, JEFFREY KALISH, AND ALLEN HAMDAN

Based on the previous edition chapter "Diabetic Foot Infection" by Jeffrey Kalish and Allen Hamdan

Presentation

A 65-year-old man with a history of hypertension, hyperlipidemia, and non–insulin-dependent diabetes mellitus presents with a 3-day history of pain in his left foot. He reports that his blood sugars, while normally very well controlled, have been very difficult to manage over the past day. His vital signs are normal. On physical examination, he has palpable femoral and popliteal pulses bilaterally. His right dorsalis pedis and posterior tibial arteries are palpable, but on the left foot, the dorsalis pedis and the posterior tibial arteries have no palpable pulses, and Doppler signals are monophasic. He has redness around the left second toe, with a small 5-mm ulcer on the dorsal surface of the toe.

● DIFFERENTIAL DIAGNOSIS

The lifetime risk of acquiring foot lesions (ulcers/gangrene) in diabetic patients has been estimated at 15% to 25%, with an annual incidence of approximately 1.0% to 4.1%. The clinical presentation of peripheral arterial disease (PAD) is represented by a wide range of symptoms, including intermittent claudication, rest pain, and ulcers with or without gangrene. Diabetic patients may exhibit these typical symptoms, but more often they present with a wound that fails to heal or with pain at the site of a callus, pressure point, or other bony prominence. It is imperative to identify the presence of neuropathic ulcers, which arise at points of increased pressure and weight bearing leading to progressive bony destruction and joint deformity known as Charcot foot.

● WORKUP

The pathologic components leading to diabetic foot complications frequently occur in combination as an etiologic triad; ischemia, neuropathy, and infection. Thorough clinical examination of foot ulcers is necessary to evaluate the depth and extent of involvement, anatomic location, etiology, and presence of ischemia or infection. Diabetic patients typically suffer from tibial level arterial occlusive disease with relative sparing of the foot arteries. Ischemia results from both

atherosclerotic macrovascular disease and microcirculatory dysfunction. Diabetic neuropathy has multiple manifestations in the foot because it encompasses damaged sensory, motor, and autonomic fibers. Because of a blunted neuro-inflammatory response and poor blood supply, diabetic patients lack a crucial component of the body's natural first-line defense against pathogens and thus are more susceptible to an ensuing foot infection.

The typical inflammatory signs of infection may be absent or diminished (e.g., erythema, rubor, cellulitis, or tenderness), and the systemic manifestations of infection (e.g., fever, tachycardia, or elevated white blood cell count) may be absent as well. Unexplained hyperglycemia should prompt an aggressive search for a source of infection because the elevated glucose may be the only sign of impending problems. Careful palpation of the foot for areas of tenderness or fluctuance is important in order to detect undrained abscesses in deeper tissue planes. All ulcers must be carefully inspected and probed, and superficial eschar unroofed, to look for potential deep space abscesses. Osteomyelitis occurs after the spread of superficial infection of the soft tissue to the adjacent bone or marrow. Although numerous expensive radiologic techniques are available to diagnose osteomyelitis (e.g., MRI, bone scan, tagged white blood cell scan), a simple sterile metallic probe will usually suffice; if this sterile probe reaches bone, then osteomyelitis can be diagnosed with a sensitivity of 66%, a specificity of 85%, and a positive predictive value of 89%. Plain radiographs of the foot should be obtained in every patient with suspected foot infection. X-rays can reveal the presence of a foreign body, gas, osteolysis or joint effusion, as well as delineate anatomy for surgical planning.

A complete vascular exam is essential in any patient reporting symptoms consistent with claudication or rest pain and in any patient with extremity ulcers or gangrene. All nonpalpable pedal pulses should be confirmed with handheld Doppler probe. A normal Doppler signal is triphasic in the lower extremity, due to a high resistance arterial bed. In those cases where the vascular status is unclear, noninvasive vascular laboratory studies (ankle–brachial indices/pulse volume recordings [ABI/PVR]) are particularly useful. Patients with severe ischemia usually have ABI of <0.4, but many diabetic patients have noncompressible tibial vessels due to medial calcinosis, resulting in artificially elevated ABIs. In these situations, PVRs can be helpful as an indirect measurement of arterial flow within segmental levels of the leg. Toe pressures and transcutaneous oximetry (TcPO$_2$) can also be helpful in diabetic patients to evaluate for healing potential. Toe pressures <30 mm Hg are not compatible with healing.

Arterial duplex ultrasound combines gray scale ultrasound to visualize plaque morphology and color Doppler to measure velocity of blood flow and estimate degree of stenosis. Lower extremity computed tomography angiography (CTA) and magnetic resonance angiography (MRA) are additional modalities used to visualize lower extremity vasculature, but concerns for contrast-induced nephropathy with CTA and nephrogenic systemic fibrosis with MRA remain. Furthermore, these modalities are of limited value in the evaluation of tibial and peroneal arteries. Intra-arterial digital subtraction arteriography (DSA) is the most accurate method to evaluate the lower extremity arterial circulation, particularly the infrapopliteal segments. A carefully performed arteriogram must show the appropriate inflow source and outflow target artery, and it must incorporate the complete infrapopliteal circulation, including foot vessels. Additionally, angiography uses less contrast compared to CTA and allows ability for therapeutic intervention.

● DIAGNOSIS AND TREATMENT

In the absence of deep infection or necrosis, minor infections or ulcers may be managed conservatively with local wound care and/or antibiotics. Topical dressings, typically saline-impregnated gauze, should be aimed at maintaining a moist environment. The ulcer should be protected from excessive pressure by placement of an accommodative pad around the lesion to distribute pressure to surrounding tissues. Patients with limb-threatening infections require immediate

hospitalization, immobilization, and intravenous antibiotics. Wound swabs are unreliable and should not be performed. However, bone cultures and deep tissue cultures can be helpful if deep debridement or amputation is performed. Empiric broad-spectrum antibiotic therapy (dictated by institutional preferences, local resistance patterns, availability, and cost) is often needed to cover the polymicrobial infections seen in diabetic patients. However, not every diabetic patient who is admitted with a foot ulcer requires broad-spectrum intravenous antibiotics. Patients with minimal signs of local, superficial infection may be managed with oral antibiotics. Although various trials have tried to compare various antibiotic regimens, they fail to focus on an inherent weakness of simply using antibiotics alone, that is, the reported "failure rates" in these trials of 11% to 12% for moderate infections and 19% to 30% for severe infections. Furthermore, the presence of PAD predicts a higher failure rate for healing any diabetic foot lesion after 1 year (31% failure vs. 16% failure). Mild infections usually require only 7 to 10 days of antibiotic therapy, whereas moderate and severe infections may require 2 to 3 weeks of treatment. Traditional therapy for osteomyelitis was accepted as 4 to 6 weeks of intravenous antibiotics, but studies have documented a >30% recurrence rate using this modality alone.

Presentation Continued

The patient is admitted to the hospital and placed on an insulin drip. The ulcer and surrounding cellulitis worsen (Figure 88-1), and he does not respond to the intravenous broad-spectrum antibiotics. An arteriogram shows patency of vessels to the level of the below-knee popliteal but long-segment occlusions in his anterior and posterior tibial vessels with a large reconstituted dorsalis pedis artery (Figure 88-2).

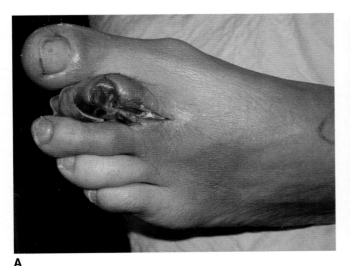

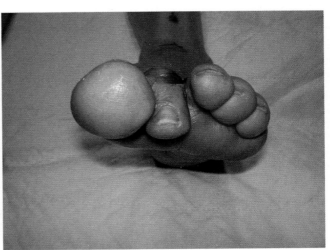

A   **B**

FIGURE 88-1. **A,B:** Left second toe ulcer and surrounding cellulitis.

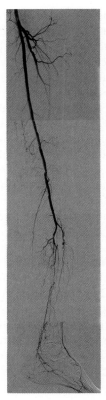

FIGURE 88-2. Composite arteriogram of left lower extremity revealing tibial artery occlusions with reconstitution of dorsalis pedis artery in foot.

● SURGICAL APPROACH

Debridement/Drainage Procedures

Presentation Continued

The patient undergoes an open second toe amputation, continues intravenous antibiotics, and has resolution of the surrounding cellulitis. Vein mapping shows adequate ipsilateral greater saphenous vein for a planned below-knee popliteal to dorsalis pedis artery bypass.

Patients with abscess formation or necrotizing fasciitis must undergo prompt incision, drainage, and debridement including partial open toe, ray, or forefoot amputation. In the setting of severe systemic infection, guillotine below- or above-knee amputation may be necessary. Tendon sheaths should be probed as proximally as possible and excised if infected. Despite fears to the contrary, long and extensive drainage incisions will heal when infection is controlled and foot circulation is adequate. It is imperative to make any necessary incision initially but at the same time to consider the implications of those incisions on the potential completion amputation. Wounds should be packed open with saline-moistened gauze, and dressings should be changed two to

three times a day. Wounds should be examined daily, and additional bedside or operative debridement should be repeated as needed. Adequate dependent drainage is crucial, and limited incisions with drains (closed suction or penrose) should be avoided.

Patients with salvageable ischemic foot lesions and concomitant active infection need the infection controlled prior to vascular surgical intervention. In addition to instituting broad-spectrum antibiotics, options include open debridement and drainage or partial foot amputation. A short delay (usually <5 days) before revascularization in order to control active infection is justified; however, longer waits in order to "sterilize wounds" is inappropriate and may result in further necrosis and a lost opportunity to save the foot. On the contrary, patients with dry eschar or gangrene and no active signs of infection can undergo revascularization first before considering debridement or amputation.

Lower Extremity Bypass

When considering revascularization, the most important difference in lower extremity atherosclerosis in the patient with diabetes is the anatomic location or distribution of the arterial lesions. While patients with diabetes who abuse cigarettes may manifest iliac or femoral occlusive disease, diabetic patients typically have significant occlusive disease in the infrapopliteal arteries, while arteries of the foot are spared. This "tibial artery disease" requires a different approach to arterial reconstruction and presents special challenges for the surgeon (Table 88-1).

Table 88-1	Lower Extremity Bypass

Key Technical Steps

1. Identify greater saphenous vein and harvest with full-length leg incision.
2. Obtain control of proximal and distal anastomotic sites.
3. Create tunnels for bypass (subcutaneous or subfascial).
4. Dilate vein with heparinized saline, check for any holes requiring repair.
5. Heparinize patient systemically.
6. Perform proximal anastomosis, tunnel vein, and confirm pulsatile flow.
7. Perform distal anastomosis.
8. Confirm unobstructed Doppler signal in distal artery and at anastomosis.
9. Reverse heparin with protamine.
10. Close incisions and confirm pulses or signals in foot prior to leaving OR.

Potential Pitfalls

- Inadequate caliber or length of vein conduit.
- Inadequate hemostatic control of target vessels.
- Need to combine an open/endovascular hybrid approach to revascularization.

Each operation must be individualized, based on the patient's available venous conduit and arterial anatomy. In 10% of cases, a foot artery, usually the dorsalis pedis artery, is the only suitable outflow vessel; in an additional 15% of patients, the dorsalis pedis artery will appear to be the best target vessel in comparison to other patent but diseased tibial vessels. Although pedal bypass represents one of the most "extreme" types of distal arterial reconstruction, it is almost always possible, particularly when the surgeon is flexible in terms of venous conduit and location of proximal anastomosis. Primary patency, secondary patency, and limb salvage rates approach 57%, 63%, and 78% at 5 years and 38%, 42%, and 58% at 10 years.

Endovascular Therapy

Although surgical reconstruction has traditionally been the gold standard for diabetic foot revascularization, endovascular intervention has become a viable alternative. With the potential pitfalls accompanying traditional surgical approaches to limb salvage, as well as the overall poor health and life expectancy of patients with PAD, less invasive endovascular therapy is an attractive option. Balloon angioplasty and stenting are well suited to focal, short-segment iliac stenoses or occlusions, which exist in 10% to 20% of diabetic patients. With regard to outflow procedures, the morbidity of open surgery can be quite significant, and not simply limited to local wound complications or myocardial infarctions. Readmissions to the hospital, reoperations, slow time to healing, and time spent in rehabilitation must be factored into the risk–benefit analysis. In fact, the ideal outcome (patent graft, healed wound, no additional operations in a fully ambulatory patient who can sustain independent living) may only be obtainable up to 20% of the time. Although patency rates of bypass grafts have been shown to be equivalent in diabetics and nondiabetic patients, endovascular interventions may be associated with worse patency rates in diabetics due to their higher prevalence of limb-threatening ischemia as the presenting symptom.

The bypass versus angioplasty in severe ischemia of the leg (BASIL) trial compared outcomes between open bypass versus angioplasty as the initial choice for revascularization. This prospective randomized trial enrolled 452 patients over a 5-year period. Perioperative (30-day) morbidity was higher with bypass; all-cause mortality trended higher with bypass for the first 6 months but then trended lower for the next 6 months; amputation-free survival was similar in both groups. Two-year post hoc analysis revealed that surgery was associated with a reduced risk of future amputation and/or death. The trialists concluded that although the strategies are roughly equivalent at medium-term follow-up with regard to mortality and amputation-free survival, angioplasty should be used first for patients with significant comorbidities and with a life expectancy of <1 to 2 years. Moreover, longer-term results favor surgery over angioplasty if there is a "good" vein and a medically fit patient. Other reviews have shown that after 2 years, tibial angioplasty requires repeat endovascular intervention in up to one-third of patients, and another 15% of patients go on to have a surgical bypass. However, as technology continues to develop, the effectiveness of endovascular intervention will likely improve. The Best Endovascular versus Surgical Therapy in patients with Critical Limb Ischemia (BEST-CLI) is a prospective, multicenter, randomized trial that is in its enrollment stages, which will help determine whether current endovascular therapy or surgical bypass results in better outcomes in patients who are candidates for either intervention.

Amputation

The last alternative, though not necessarily the worst, is amputation. Closed minor amputations (toes or transmetatarsal) are practical following infection control and revascularization and typically leave the patient with a functional foot for walking (Figure 88-3). In situations involving extensive tissue loss precluding a functional foot, when there are nonhealing wounds in the setting of patent grafts, and for control of sepsis, amputation below the knee is necessary. Thirty-day mortality from above knee amputation and below knee amputation is 16% and 6%, respectively. Survival after amputation is worse in patients with diabetes and end-stage renal disease. Surgeons should strive to preserve the knee joint because of its functional significance for rehabilitation. Above-knee amputations are reserved for debilitated patients with severe tissue loss or with no capacity to ambulate. Because of modern advances in prostheses coupled with aggressive approaches to rehabilitation, amputation should be viewed as an acceptable modality to treat diabetic foot complications and not as a treatment failure.

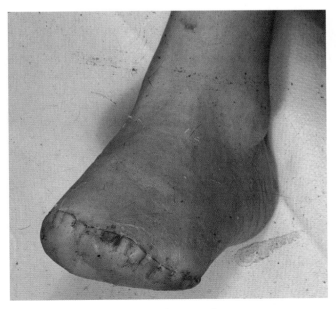

FIGURE 88-3. Transmetatarsal amputation.

● SPECIAL INTRAOPERATIVE CONSIDERATIONS

Several unexpected findings may be encountered during a lower extremity revascularization procedure. If an artery is found to be too heavily calcified or does not have an adequate lumen, then the surgeon must reevaluate the preoperative arteriogram to find a more suitable target. If the venous conduit is not of suitable quality or length to perform the planned bypass, then the surgeon must consider splicing the greater saphenous vein with alternative venous conduits or using an alternative conduit altogether (such as contralateral greater saphenous vein, ipsilateral or contralateral lesser saphenous vein, basilic or cephalic arm veins, or even a composite sequential bypass with prosthetic and vein). Vein conduits should always be preferred over prosthetic grafts for infrapopliteal bypasses given the poor patency rates of infrapopliteal prosthetic grafts. Vein diameter of >3 mm is considered adequate for bypass conduit. Another current option involves hybrid procedures to achieve revascularization; this involves the combination of a shorter bypass with either an inflow or outflow endovascular procedure (such as a superficial femoral artery angioplasty/stent coupled with a popliteal to distal bypass, or a prosthetic femoral to popliteal bypass coupled with a tibial angioplasty/stent). Vascular surgeons have many tools and technologies available, and these should all be used in the efforts to achieve limb salvage.

● POSTOPERATIVE MANAGEMENT

Patients should be observed in a monitored setting overnight following lower extremity bypass, and neurovascular checks should be performed every 1 to 2 hours. Endovascular procedures can usually be performed in the outpatient setting. Arterial lines and foley catheters can usually be discontinued after 1 to 2 days once blood pressures have stabilized, and urine output has been adequate. Patients should get out of bed to chair by postoperative day 1 and typically can ambulate on postoperative day 2. Physical therapy consults should be involved early in order to facilitate a patient's transition home or to rehabilitation. Because these vascular surgery patients typically have significant comorbidities, practitioners must be vigilant for postoperative complications such as myocardial infarction, pneumonia, wound infection, hematoma, etc.

Surveillance studies should typically be done on both lower extremity bypass grafts and endovascular interventions in order to monitor for recurrent stenoses or impending failure. Exact algorithms are debatable, but the basic premise relies on surveillance duplex ultrasounds in regular intervals (such as every 3 months for 1 year, then every 6 months for 1 year, then yearly) in order to identify grafts that are at risk for failure. This allows for certain patients to undergo arteriograms to identify and treat potential areas of intimal hyperplasia or new atherosclerotic lesions.

Case Conclusion

The patient undergoes a successful bypass and is discharged to rehabilitation on postoperative day 5. His wound improves with local wound care, and his wound eventually granulates and heals secondarily. Surveillance duplex shows a patent bypass graft with no areas of elevated velocities.

TAKE HOME POINTS

- Ischemia, neuropathy, and infection often occur in combination, leading to diabetic foot complications.
- The typical inflammatory signs and systemic manifestations of infection may be absent or diminished in diabetic patients, and unexplained hyperglycemia may be the only indicator of a foot infection.
- Patients with salvageable ischemic foot lesions and concomitant active infection need the infection controlled for a short period (usually no more than 5 days) prior to vascular surgical intervention.
- Source control requires prompt incision and drainage with minor toe or forefoot amputation as necessary. In cases of severe, uncontrolled infection, guillotine below- or above-knee amputation may be the only effective means of source control.
- Each lower extremity bypass operation must be individualized, based on the patient's available venous conduit and arterial anatomy, with diabetic patients typically manifesting tibioperoneal disease with sparing of foot arteries.
- Although surgical reconstruction has been the current gold standard for diabetic foot revascularization, endovascular intervention has become a viable alternative.

SUGGESTED READINGS

Adam DJ, Beard JD, Cleveland T, et al. BASIL trial participants. Bypass versus angioplasty in severe ischaemia of the leg (BASIL): multicentre, randomised controlled trial. *Lancet.* 2005;366(9501):1925-1934.

Gibbons GW, Eliopoulos GM. Infection of the diabetic foot. In: Kozak GP, Campbell DR, Frykberg RG, et al., eds. *Management of Diabetic Foot Problems.* 2nd ed. Philadelphia, PA: WB Saunders; 1995:121-129.

Mills JL, Armstrong DG, Andros G. Strategies to prevent and heal diabetic foot ulcers: building a partnership for amputation prevention. *J Vasc Surg.* 2010;52(3 suppl):1S-103S.

Pomposelli FB, Kansal N, Hamdan AD, et al. A decade of experience with dorsalis pedis artery bypass: analysis of outcome in more than 1000 cases. *J Vasc Surg.* 2003;37:307-315.

Acute Mesenteric Ischemia

89

JOSEPH M. WHITE, DAVID R. WHITTAKER, AND JAMES H. BLACK III

Based on the previous edition chapter "Acute Mesenteric Ischemia" by Babak J. Orandi and James H. Black III

Presentation

A 71-year-old woman with a remote but significant smoking history presented to the emergency department (ED) with 24 hours of abdominal pain, nausea, vomiting, and diarrhea. She was discharged from the hospital 1 week prior after an elective coronary artery bypass graft, which was significant only for an episode of new-onset atrial fibrillation, which resolved after administration of an amiodarone bolus. In the ED, her vitals were as follows: "T= 38.1°C, HR 101, BP 148/67, RR 16, and 98% saturation" 98% saturation on 2 L of oxygen via nasal cannula. On physical examination, she was clearly uncomfortable. She had a number of well-healed incisions on her abdomen, including a right subcostal incision from an open cholecystectomy, a left lower quadrant incision from an open appendectomy, a Pfannenstiel incision from two prior cesarean sections, and a lower midline incision from a total abdominal hysterectomy. Her abdomen was obese, distended, and without focal point tenderness. Rectal exam revealed no gross blood, but the stool sample was guaiac positive.

DIFFERENTIAL DIAGNOSIS

Acute abdominal pain can pose a diagnostic challenge to clinicians as the presenting symptoms for a variety of etiologies are often nonspecific and overlapping. The differential diagnosis includes acute pancreatitis, abdominal aortic aneurysm, aortic dissection, myocardial infarction, acute diverticulitis, small bowel obstruction, peptic ulcer disease with perforation, and gastroenteritis. Though not applicable to this patient given her past surgical history, the differential also includes acute cholecystitis and appendicitis.

WORKUP

The patient underwent CT angiography (CTA) for further evaluation of her abdominal pain, which revealed an abrupt cutoff in the superior mesenteric artery (SMA) approximately 4 cm distal to the vessel's takeoff from the aorta. The small bowel was dilated, there was evidence of bowel wall thickening, and there was trace free fluid in the pelvis.

Laboratory testing was significant for a serum lactate level of 2.8 mmol/L (elevated), a leukocytosis of 16,200 cells/mL, a serum bicarbonate level of 19 mEq/L, an INR of 1.1, a partial thromboplastic time (PTT) of 22 seconds, and a prothrombin time (PT) of 13 seconds.

CTA has become the most important diagnostic test for acute mesenteric ischemia (AMI). While angiography has been the historic gold standard and has the benefit of allowing for simultaneous endovascular revascularization options, CTA has the advantages of being more readily available and rapid. CTA has demonstrated 93% sensitivity and 96% specificity for the diagnosis of AMI in a large systematic review and meta-analysis. Additionally, CTA also permits simultaneous evaluation of the bowel and the vasculature, as well as allowing for a more thorough evaluation of the abdominal cavity which may rule out other etiologies, as the diagnosis is often in question prior to performing the CTA. Of particular interest for acute vascular etiologies, CTA is extremely helpful in identifying the presumed level of occlusion, which will have direct implications on treatment approaches.

A number of laboratory abnormalities are variably present in AMI. Unfortunately, no specific, rapidly available serum marker exists for AMI in the way that cardiac enzymes are available for myocardial ischemia. Worse yet, most of the markers that do rise in AMI only do so after transmural bowel infarction has already occurred. AMI-associated leukocytosis, lactic acidosis, and serum amylasemia are often seen later in the course of the disease process.

DIAGNOSIS AND TREATMENT

AMI is a relatively uncommon diagnosis, accounting for <1 in every 10,000 admissions; however, maintaining a high index of suspicion is critical given the high mortality associated with this disease process and a significant delay in diagnosis and treatment can result in a fatal outcome. The mortality rate is 50% when the diagnosis is achieved with 24 hours of clinical presentation, and it climbs to over 70% if the diagnosis is established after that time frame. The missed diagnosis of AMI is a frequent cause of medical malpractice litigation. AMI is typically the clinical manifestation of one of four processes: embolism, thrombosis, nonocclusive mesenteric ischemia (NOMI), or mesenteric venous thrombosis (MVT).

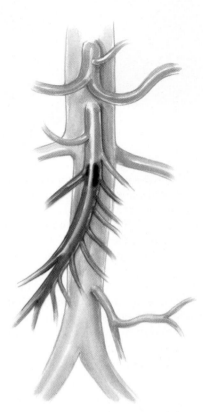

FIGURE 89-1. Acute embolus to the SMA usually lodges in the region of the first branches of the SMA, with the length of small bowel ischemia less affected, usually only portions of the distal jejunum, ileum, and colon. (From Cameron JL, Sandone C. *Atlas of Gastrointestinal Surgery.* Vol. 2, 2nd ed. 2011, used with permission from PMPH-USA, Ltd., Raleigh, North Carolina.)

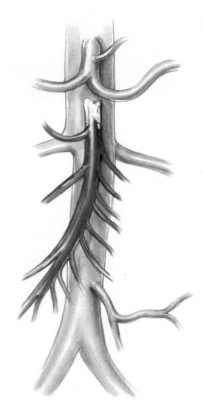

FIGURE 89-2. Acute thrombotic occlusion of the SMA usually occurs secondary to a proximal atherosclerotic plaque, yielding extensive ischemia of the entire small bowel and large bowel. (From Cameron JL, Sandone C. *Atlas of Gastrointestinal Surgery.* Vol. 2, 2nd ed. 2011, used with permission from PMPH-USA, Ltd., Raleigh, North Carolina.)

An embolic event, usually to the SMA, is the most common cause of AMI, accounting for approximately half of all cases (Figure 89-1). Risk factors include atrial fibrillation, congestive heart failure, a history of prior embolic events, and recent myocardial infarction. Emboli tend to lodge in the SMA distal to the takeoff of the middle colic artery, which results in ischemia of the distal jejunum through the ascending colon, with sparing of the proximal jejunum and transverse colon.

Arterial thrombosis accounts for 20% of AMI cases. Many of these patients have extensive atherosclerotic disease in the mesenteric vasculature. A thorough history will often reveal abdominal pain after meals (postprandial abdominal pain), weight loss, and food avoidance. Compared with SMA embolism, which tend to occur slightly more distal, SMA thrombosis typically occurs at the origin of the vessel, which creates ischemia from the mid-duodenum to the splenic flexure (Figure 89-2).

NOMI results from a relative low-flow state and vasoconstriction, creating an imbalance between mesenteric oxygen supply and demand. NOMI accounts for 20% of all presentations of AMI. These patients typically have a greater burden of atherosclerotic disease and are critically ill.

These contributing factors predispose the patient to the development of impaired intestinal perfusion in the absence of occlusion of the celiac, superior mesenteric, and inferior mesenteric arteries. CTA usually demonstrates narrowing of multiple branches of the SMA, alternating dilation and narrowing of the mesenteric vessel, spasm of the SMA mesenteric arcades, and impaired filling of intramural vessels. CTA often will show a flattened inferior vena cava, consistent with the low-flow etiology of NOMI.

MVT is the least common cause of AMI and accounts for approximately 10% of all causes. This ischemia is secondary to impaired venous outflow resulting in venous congestion and engorgement. MVT is typically caused by primary or idiopathic thrombosis with 90% of cases related to thrombophilia, traumatic injury, or local inflammatory process (i.e., acute pancreatitis, acute diverticulitis, inflammatory bowel disease, or infections within the biliary system). Significant ascites is often appreciated on imaging.

In general, the cornerstones of treatment for AMI include fluid resuscitation, correction of electrolyte abnormalities, intravenous antibiotics, initiation of therapeutic anticoagulation, immediate revascularization, and resection of irreversibly necrotic bowel. Patients with NOMI and MVT typically only require surgical intervention for clinical deterioration as a result of bowel necrosis. NOMI patients may benefit from endovascular stenting of the splanchnic vessels and intra-arterial papaverine infusion to promote vasodilation. MVT patients require immediate anticoagulation.

For the patient in our particular scenario, the recent history of atrial fibrillation, cardiac disease, leukocytosis, low-grade fever, tachycardia, lactic acidemia, and pain out of proportion to physical exam, an emergent exploratory laparotomy was indicated.

● SURGICAL APPROACH

Historically, open surgical exploration and revascularization with either catheter embolectomy or retrograde SMA bypass (Table 89-1) was the sole treatment for AMI, and while it remains the gold standard, a number of authors are advocating endovascular approaches to the treatment of AMI as the collective experience with catheter-based interventions grows. Given how infrequently this disease process presents, there are no prospective, randomized studies to direct the optimal approach. The minimally invasive nature of endovascular surgery may be beneficial to patients who are often already critically ill; however, the strongest argument against this approach is that it does not permit the surgeon to assess bowel viability and perform bowel resections when indicated. If an endovascular approach is to be pursued, patient selection must be stringent, and intensive perioperative monitoring for the development of peritonitis or clinical deterioration is mandatory. More often than not, even with successful endovascular revascularization, a laparotomy is still required to assess the bowel. Arthurs et al. reported an 87% technical success rate regarding endovascular management of AMI over a 9-year experience. Successful endovascular therapy resulted in a significant mortality reduction of 36% compared to traditional (open revascularization) therapy of 50%. Additionally, 31% of patients treated with endovascular therapy avoided laparotomy. This report also revealed a significant decrease in the median length of bowel requiring resection, and lower rates of acute renal failure and pulmonary failure (Figures 89-3–89-8).

Table 89-1	SMA Revascularization (Figures 89-3 to 89-8)

Key Technical Steps

1. Liberal midline incision and full abdominal exploration
2. Exposure of SMA by cephalad retraction of the transverse mesocolon, rightward retraction of the small bowel, and division of the ligament of Treitz
3. Obtain proximal and distal control of the SMA and administer systemic heparin
4. Perform an embolectomy via transverse arteriotomy and passage of a Fogarty catheter
5. If inflow is reestablished, close the SMA utilizing a patch angioplasty if vessel narrowing is anticipated
6. If inflow fails to be reestablished, the etiology is likely SMA thrombosis and a retrograde SMA bypass should be performed
7. Create the distal anastomosis on the SMA first, ideally with saphenous vein graft
8. Proximal anastomosis can be performed either on the infrarenal aorta or the iliac vessels
9. Assess bowel viability after 30 minutes using visual inspection, Doppler probe, and/or fluorescein

Potential Pitfalls

- Failure to efficiently recognize the diagnosis
- Not adhering to "damage control" principles
- Resecting too much bowel at the index operation
- Metabolic disturbances once the affected bowel has been revascularized

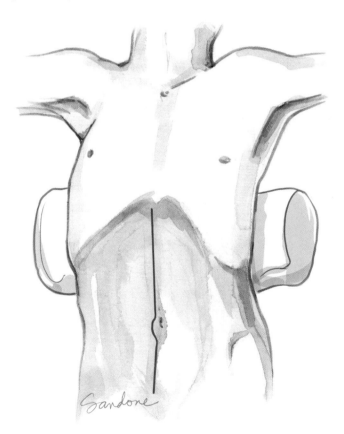

FIGURE 89-3. A long midline incision is best used to evaluate the viscera and provide ample exposure to identify suitable targets for revascularization. The towel rolls lifts the costal margin upward and facilitates exposure of the supraceliac aorta, which is usually spared from significant plaque burden and thus may provide suitable inflow for SMA revascularization. (From Cameron JL, Sandone C. *Atlas of Gastrointestinal Surgery.* Vol. 2, 2nd ed. 2011, used with permission from PMPH-USA, Ltd., Raleigh, North Carolina.)

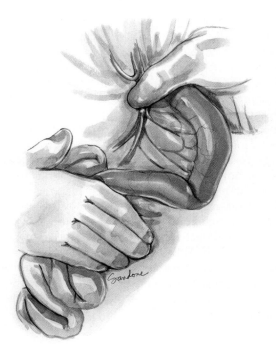

FIGURE 89-4. Palpation of the root of the mesentery is the first step to determine the status of the mesenteric circulation. In thrombotic occlusion from proximal plaque, the pulse will be absent and a revascularization will be necessary. In acute embolus, a pulse will be palpable via transmission through fresh clot. (From Cameron JL, Sandone C. *Atlas of Gastrointestinal Surgery*. Vol. 2, 2nd ed. 2011, used with permission from PMPH-USA, Ltd., Raleigh, North Carolina.)

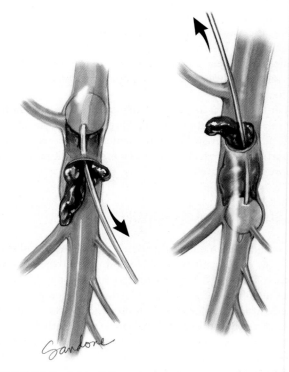

FIGURE 89-6. A 4 to 5 French embolectomy catheter is used to clear the clot and restore inflow from the SMA. Distally, careful passes of a 3 to 4 French embolectomy catheter is used for clot extraction. (From Cameron JL, Sandone C. *Atlas of Gastrointestinal Surgery*. Vol. 2, 2nd ed. 2011, used with permission from PMPH-USA, Ltd., Raleigh, North Carolina.)

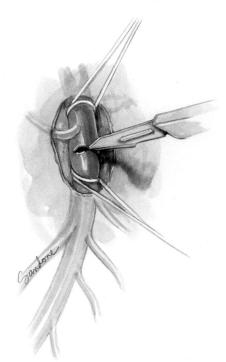

FIGURE 89-5. A transverse arteriotomy on the mid-SMA in the region of the middle colic can be used to extract the clot. (From Cameron JL, Sandone C. *Atlas of Gastrointestinal Surgery*. Vol. 2, 2nd ed. 2011, used with permission from PMPH-USA, Ltd., Raleigh, North Carolina.)

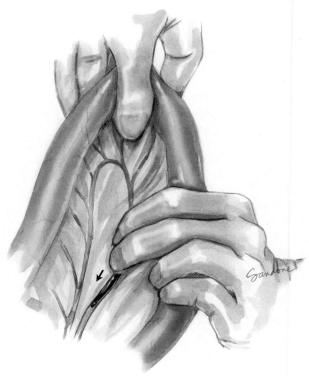

FIGURE 89-7. Distant clot in the mesenteric arcade can be milked back to the arteriotomy to extract the clot burden. (From Cameron JL, Sandone C. *Atlas of Gastrointestinal Surgery*. Vol. 2, 2nd ed. 2011, used with permission from PMPH-USA, Ltd., Raleigh, North Carolina.)

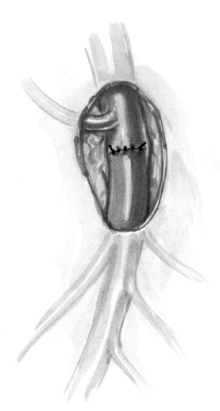

FIGURE 89-8. Interrupted, nonabsorbable, monofilament closure of the arteriotomy is preferred to avoid narrowing the closed SMA. (From Cameron JL, Sandone C. *Atlas of Gastrointestinal Surgery.* Vol. 2, 2nd ed. 2011, used with permission from PMPH-USA, Ltd., Raleigh, North Carolina.)

A large retrospective review incorporating the Nationwide Inpatient Sample (NIS) database evaluated endovascular and traditional open therapy for AMI. Patient mortality was significantly associated with open repair with a rate of 39% compared to endovascular management which revealed a reduction in mortality rate to 25%. Both bowel resection and use of total parenteral nutrition significantly favored endovascular therapy. An alternative, hybrid approach (retrograde open mesenteric stenting) combines traditional open exploration with retrograde stenting of the SMA. This technique incorporates open surgical exploration and the ability to inspect the bowel with subsequent isolation of the SMA followed by retrograde recanalization and stenting of the occluded proximal SMA. Although limited to small case series, the reported results demonstrate technical feasibility.

Regarding traditional open therapy, the patient is taken to the operating room for a general anesthetic. If feasible, the operative theater should have endovascular/fluoroscopic capabilities (i.e., hybrid operating room) allowing endovascular diagnostic and therapeutic options. The abdomen is opened via a large midline laparotomy incision. The bowel is initially inspected for viability, and segments of frankly necrotic or perforated bowel are efficiently resected. In order to achieve access to the infra-pancreatic portion of the SMA, the transverse colon is retracted cranially, and the small bowel is gathered into the right side of the abdomen. The SMA is exposed at the base of the transverse mesocolon through a transverse incision across the base of the mesentery. The middle colonic artery can act as a guide by following this structure to the SMA proper. Additionally, complete mobilization of the duodenum by dividing the ligament of Treitz facilitates greater exposure. The patient is therapeutically anticoagulated. Once proximal and distal SMA control has been achieved, either a transverse arteriotomy for embolectomy or longitudinal arteriotomy for bypass can be performed. In cases of arterial embolism, catheter embolectomy is completed antegrade and retrograde until appropriate flow is reestablished with the return of brisk bleeding. The transverse arteriotomy is closed primarily. In cases of arterial thrombosis, a right common iliac artery bypass to the SMA using greater saphenous vein is constructed with the incorporation of a gentle C-loop to avoid kinking and to reestablish visceral perfusion. Considerations regarding a planned second-look operation are completed.

It is important to consider damage control techniques and implement these strategies when faced with a clinically ill patient following visceral reperfusion. Optimizing operating room efficiency, utilization of temporary abdominal closures, and continued meticulous perioperative monitoring and resuscitation with subsequent correction of associated metabolic disturbances are key to minimizing complications.

● SPECIAL INTRAOPERATIVE CONSIDERATIONS

Many surgeons advocate a mandatory "second-look" operation within 24 to 36 hours with minimal bowel resection at the time of the initial surgery. While no data support or refute this approach, supporters suggest that it minimizes the amount of bowel resected as this waiting period after revascularization renders salvageable bowel that at first glance might have been removed. In addition, avoiding bowel resection and leaving the patient with a temporary abdominal closure facilitates a more rapid return to the ICU for continued resuscitation and stabilization, as many of these patients are critically ill at the time of their initial operation. Other authors have reported the use of a selective second-look strategy.

● POSTOPERATIVE MANAGEMENT

Patients should be continued on systemic heparin therapy in the immediate postoperative period. All patients will require anticoagulation and/or antiplatelet therapy. Because these patients tend to have systemic vascular disease, they require aggressive risk factor modification as much as possible.

Case Conclusion

The patient underwent an exploratory laparotomy, which revealed extensively threatened bowel from the jejunum through the ascending colon. An embolectomy was performed, which reestablished blood flow after the removal of a large embolus. The patient's abdomen was left open with a wound vacuum system providing a temporary abdominal closure. She returned to the Surgical Intensive Care Unit for aggressive resuscitation. Approximately 36 hours later, she returned to the operating room for a planned second-look procedure. Much of the previously threatened bowel demonstrated significant improvement, though she still required resection of the distal ileum. At that time, her abdomen was definitively closed. She was discharged to a rehabilitation facility on postoperative day seven, with warfarin anticoagulation, aspirin, a statin, and monthly vitamin B_{12} injections to compensate for the distal ileum resection.

TAKE HOME POINTS

- AMI is a relatively rare disease, but its high mortality rate mandates a low threshold for action.
- CTA is the diagnostic study of choice.
- The four most common causes of AMI are embolic, thrombotic, nonocclusive mesenteric ischemia, and mesenteric venous thrombosis.
- Patients should receive IV heparin, fluid resuscitation, and broad-spectrum antibiotics as soon as possible.
- Open revascularization with bowel resection is the gold standard treatment for AMI. A second-look operation may minimize the amount of bowel requiring resection.

- Endovascular revascularization has been used successfully in a number of cases, though careful patient selection and close patient monitoring is necessary when implementing this therapeutic technique.

SUGGESTED READINGS

Arthurs ZM, Titus J, Bannazadeh M, et al. A comparison of endovascular revascularization with traditional therapy for the treatment of acute mesenteric ischemia. *J Vasc Surg.* 2011;53:698-705.

Beaulieu RJ, Arnaoutakis KD, Abularrage CJ, Efron DT, Schneider E, Black JH. Comparison of open and endovascular treatment of acute mesenteric ischemia. *J Vasc Surg.* 2014;59(1):159-164.

Brandt LJ, Boley SJ. AGA technical review on intestinal ischemia. American Gastrointestinal Association. *Gastroenterology.* 2000;118:954-968.

Clair DG, Beach JM. Mesenteric ischemia. *N Engl J Med.* 2016;374(10):959-968.

Horton KM, Fishman EK. Multidetector CT angiography in the diagnosis of mesenteric ischemia. *Radiol Clin North Am.* 2007;3(9):677-685.

Meng X, Liu L, Jiang H. Indications and procedures for second-look surgery in acute mesenteric ischemia. *Surg Today.* 2010;40:700-705.

Resch TA, Acosta S, Sonesson B. Endovascular techniques in acute arterial mesenteric ischemia. *Semin Vasc Surg.* 2010;23:29-35.

Sise MJ. Mesenteric ischemia: the whole spectrum. *Scand J Surg.* 2010;99:106-110.

Wyers MC. Acute mesenteric ischemia: diagnostic approach and surgical treatment. *Semin Vasc Surg.* 2010;23:9-20.

Wyers MC, Powell RJ, Nolan BW, Cronenwett JL. Retrograde mesenteric stenting during laparotomy for the management of acute thromboembolic occlusion of the superior mesenteric artery: autopsy findings in 213 patients. *Ann Surg.* 2005;241:516-522.

Chronic Mesenteric Ischemia

90

ANNE LAUX AND MATTHEW J. SIDEMAN

Based on the previous edition chapter "Chronic Mesenteric Ischemia" by Maureen K. Sheehan, Matthew J. Sideman, and Kevin E. Taubman

Presentation

A 67-year-old woman is referred as she has a 10-month history of postprandial abdominal pain, which has led to a fear of food and a 30 lb weight loss. Her past medical history is significant for hypertension, hyperlipidemia, and a 60-pack-year smoking history. She has had multiple tests including an EGD, colonoscopy, barium swallow, CT scan, abdominal ultrasound, and a HIDA scan. She underwent a laparoscopic cholecystectomy 4 months ago for biliary dyskinesia without improvement in her symptoms.

● DIFFERENTIAL DIAGNOSIS

The diagnosis of chronic mesenteric ischemia (CMI) is usually made late in the course of the disease. Most patients have had multiple tests before the diagnosis is considered. Peptic ulcer disease, biliary disease, enteritis, colitis, and gastrointestinal (GI) tumors should all be ruled out before settling on a diagnosis of CMI. However, in the patient with classic symptoms and significant risk factors, a high index of suspicion for CMI should be maintained and explored. The most common etiology is atherosclerosis, which accounts for >90% of cases. Less frequent causes are arcuate ligament syndrome, fibromuscular dysplasia, aneurysm, and radiation-induced vasculitis.

● PRESENTATION

Patients with CMI tend to have the same risk factors as other individuals with atherosclerosis including hypertension, dyslipidemia, and smoking. The classic CMI symptom is postprandial abdominal pain, which typically occurs 15 to 45 minutes after food intake with severity frequently linearly related to the size of the meal. The pain is most often dull and located in the mid-epigastrium but may have some radiation. Due to the postprandial pain, many patients will develop fear of food and avoidance of food to avoid pain. As a result, significant weight loss tends to be a prevalent symptom as well. Because symptoms are often nonspecific, patients will

frequently have undergone extensive work up and perhaps treatment for their abdominal pain prior to presentation to a vascular surgeon.

Physical examination of patients with CMI tends not to be significantly telling. Patients in general will be thin secondary to their ongoing weight loss. They may have other sequelae of peripheral vascular disease, such as carotid bruits or diminished lower extremity pulses. Patients may have an abdominal bruit present, but that is neither sensitive nor specific.

● DISCUSSION

CMI is a relatively rare disease. Estimates show mesenteric atherosclerosis to affect only 17% of patients over 65 years of age, with many of the affected patients having asymptomatic disease. Open intervention was first described in 1958 followed by percutaneous intervention in 1980. Since the introduction of endovascular treatment, there has been debate regarding the best treatment for CMI. Open bypass has longer durability but carries significant morbidity and mortality. On the other hand, endovascular treatment has significantly less morbidity and mortality but also increased restenosis rates. Therefore, treatment choice needs to be individualized to the patient.

● WORKUP

Duplex ultrasonography is an excellent screening modality for mesenteric occlusive disease. As noted previously, patients tend to have an ongoing history of weight loss and tend to be thin if not near cachectic so that imaging the celiac artery and superior mesenteric artery (SMA) with the ultrasound probe is not as difficult as usual; however, there remain the challenges of intra-abdominal gas and respiratory variation. Moneta et al. have reported that a PSV of 275 cm/sec or greater in the SMA detects a 70% or greater stenosis with sensitivity of 92% and specificity of 96%, while a PSV of 200 cm/sec or greater in the celiac artery detects a 70% or greater stenosis with a sensitivity of 87% and specificity of 80%. In a separate study, Zwolak et al. found that an EDV of 45 cm/sec in the SMA

533

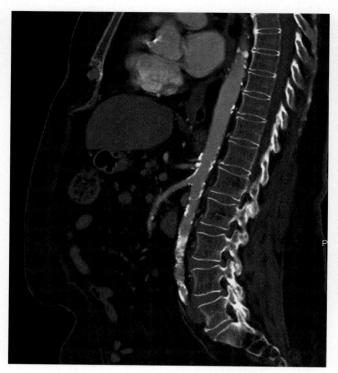

FIGURE 90-1. Aortic atherosclerotic disease with mesenteric "spillover."

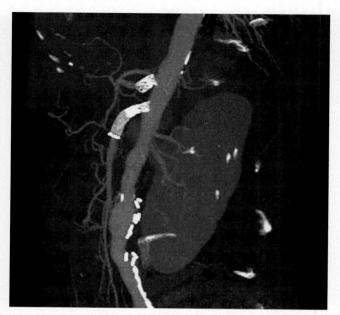

FIGURE 90-2. Celiac and SMA stenting.

correlated with a >50% stenosis, while the same was true of an EDV of 55 cm/sec in the celiac artery. However, each vascular laboratory needs to determine their own criteria for diagnosis of mesenteric artery stenosis with validation.

Angiography is the gold standard diagnostic test and allows for definitive planning. Complete angiography requires both anteroposterior and lateral aortic views and may require selective injections of the celiac, superior mesenteric, and inferior mesenteric arteries. Atherosclerotic disease in the celiac artery and SMA tends to be orificial and may result from "spillover" disease from the aorta (Figure 90-1). Presence of well-developed collaterals supports the diagnosis of mesenteric ischemia. Generally, occlusion or significant stenosis of at least two of the vessels needs to be present for the patient to have symptoms; however, if the patient lacks adequate collateral pathways, symptoms may be present with disease of only one vessel.

Presentation Continued

CT angiogram of the patient showed atherosclerotic disease of the abdominal aorta with involvement of the visceral vessels. Lateral abdominal aortogram showed significant stenosis of the celiac and SMA. Endovascular stents were placed in the orifices of the celiac and SMA with resolution of abdominal pain, and the patient was able to regain her weight (Figure 90-2).

● ENDOVASCULAR REPAIR OF CMI

CMI can be treated endovascularly with angioplasty, or more commonly, stenting of the diseased vessels. This can be done for stenosis and occlusions, assuming that the occlusions can be crossed with a wire. Endovascular treatment is attractive because it is minimally invasive, can be performed at the same time as the diagnostic angiogram, and it can be done without general anesthesia. Benefits include the potential to reduce morbidity, mortality, length of hospital stays, and costs. Limitations of endovascular repair include questionable long-term durability. Restenosis within mesenteric stents is common (Figure 90-3).

Technical considerations for endovascular repair include access site and stent choice (Table 90-1). Femoral access can be used, but access of the mesenteric vessels can be difficult

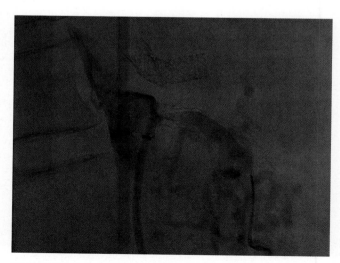

FIGURE 90-3. In-stent stenosis of an SMA stent.

Table 90-1	Endovascular Treatment of CMI

Key Technical Steps

1. Choose appropriate access site
2. Insert sheaths and catheters
3. Perform AP and lateral abdominal aortogram
4. Administer heparin
5. Obtain wire access of mesenteric vessel
6. Place long guiding catheter or long sheath into target vessel
7. Chose appropriate type and sized stent (consider IVUS to assist selection)
8. Treat addition mesenteric vessel as above if indicated
9. Perform completion angiogram
10. Surrender wire access and remove sheaths
11. Consider use of closure devices
12. Check distal pulses and monitor postoperatively

Potential Pitfalls

- Access site complications
- Inability to access target vessel
- Distal embolization

from this approach due to the angle of origin from the aorta of the celiac and SMA. A reverse curve angiographic catheter is used to access the orifice of the vessel that can be difficult given the disease. Once the vessel is accessed, a stiff wire and either a guide or long sheath should be advanced into the vessel to maintain access for the intervention. An easier approach is from the brachial artery that yields a more direct access angle to the mesenteric vessels; however, sheath size needed for intervention must be taken into consideration in relation to the size of the brachial artery. If stenting is planned, a 6 French sheath will likely be required which may be too large for a small brachial artery in an elderly female making brachial artery thrombosis postintervention an unacceptable risk or necessitating a brachial cutdown for sheath removal.

Once the diagnostic angiogram is completed, the decision made to intervene, and access to the target vessel accomplished, the distal vessel is assessed with angiogram and the appropriate-sized stent chosen. Intravascular ultrasound (IVUS) can be an extremely useful adjunct in choosing the appropriate-sized stent. Orificial lesions that are heavily diseased and or calcified are best treated with balloon expandable stents given their superior radial force. If the disease extends beyond the bend in the SMA, consideration should be given to self-expanding stents to accommodate the tortuosity and motion of the artery. After successful deployment of the stent(s), a completion angiogram is performed and access surrendered. Closure devices for the access site are used at the discretion of the physician.

Success of the intervention is ultimately determined by symptomatic improvement in the patient. Function of the stents can be followed with duplex surveillance or by CT angiograms. Both modalities have their benefits and limitations.

Duplex is inexpensive and noninvasive, but it is highly operator dependent and visualization of the stents can be problematic. CT is more reliable for imaging but is expensive and carries the risks of repeated radiation and contrast exposure.

Outcomes of endovascular treatment have shown good initial results, but poorer long-term patencies compared to open repair. Up to 30% of endovascular repairs will require secondary interventions for recurrent symptoms due to failing or failed stents. Despite these results, Medicare utilization studies have shown that mesenteric angioplasty/stenting has surpassed open surgical repair as the treatment of choice.

● SURGICAL REPAIR OF CMI

There are multiple options for surgical treatment of CMI (Table 90-2). Since the disease is most often caused by "spillover" atherosclerosis of the aorta into the origins of the celiac and SMA, one surgical treatment is endarterectomy. To perform this operation (Table 90-3), a left-sided medial visceral rotation and retroperitoneal dissection are done to expose the abdominal aorta from the hiatus to the iliac bifurcation. The supraceliac aorta, infrarenal aorta, celiac, SMA, and left renal arteries are controlled with vessel loops. The patient is systemically heparinized and the vessels clamped. A "trap door" incision is made in the aorta by making transverse arteriotomies proximal to the celiac and distal to the SMA and then connecting them longitudinally on the left lateral side of the aorta. The anterior wall of the aorta with the visceral vessels is then reflected anteriorly, and the atherosclerotic plaque is removed from this segment as well as the celiac and SMA. The newly endarterectomized portion of the aorta is then closed primarily with running monofilament suture and flow reestablished to the bowel.

The other surgical option for treatment of CMI is bypass. There are multiple options and configurations for bypass of the mesenteric arteries (Table 90-2). One option is an antegrade bypass with the inflow arising from the supraceliac aorta. The bypass can either be to one vessel or be a bifurcated graft to the celiac and SMA. If only one vessel is to be revascularized, the most important vessel to bypass is the SMA as it supplies the majority of the blood flow to the gut and has collaterals to the celiac and inferior mesenteric distributions. For this operation (Table 90-3), a laparotomy is performed, and the supraceliac aorta is exposed through the lesser sac. The crura

Table 90-2	Surgical Options for Treatment of CMI

1. Aortomesenteric endarterectomy
2. Antegrade aortomesenteric bypass
   a. Conduit—autogenous or prosthetic
   b. Target—single or multiple vessels
3. Retrograde bypass
   a. Inflow—infrarenal aorta or iliac artery
   b. Conduit—autogenous or prosthetic
   c. Target—single or multiple vessels

Table 90-3	Surgical Treatment of CMI

Key Technical Steps

1. Midline abdominal incision
2. Expose inflow vessel
   a. Left medial visceral rotation for aortomesenteric endarterectomy
   b. Through the lesser sac for antegrade bypass
   c. Infrarenal aorta or iliac artery for retrograde bypass
3. Expose target (outflow) vessel
   a. Through lesser sac for celiac
   b. Root of mesentery for SMA
4. Confirm decision on number of vessels to revascularize
5. Choose appropriate bypass conduit including type and size
6. Systemically heparinize patient
7. Clamp inflow vessel, perform arteriotomy, and complete proximal anastomosis with running monofilament suture
   a. Alternatively, clamp aorta and mesenteric vessels; perform trapdoor incision and endarterectomized flap
8. Clamp target vessel, perform arteriotomy, and complete distal anastomosis with running monofilament suture
   a. Close trapdoor incision with running monofilament suture
9. Reestablish blood flow through graft
10. Assess mesenteric pulses and viability of the bowel
11. Obtain hemostasis, consider reversal of heparin
12. Close abdomen and transfer to ICU for postoperative care

Potential Pitfalls

- Kinking of bypass graft
- Ischemia–reperfusion injury to bowel
- Significant aortoiliac occlusive disease (AIOD)
- Distal embolic events

of the diaphragm are dissected to gain full exposure of the aorta in this location. The distal targets are exposed and controlled. The celiac can be exposed through the lesser sac on the anterior surface of the aorta. The SMA needs to be exposed in the root of the mesentery. A tunnel is then created behind the pancreas connecting the exposed SMA in the root of the mesentery with the exposed supraceliac aorta. After completing the dissection, the patient is systemically heparinized, and the vessels are controlled. A side-biting aortic clamp can be used to partially occlude the supraceliac aorta and either a bifurcated graft or a solitary graft sewn with running monofilament suture. Autogenous venous grafts can be used instead of prosthetic if desired. The distal anastomoses are then completed in a standard fashion with running monofilament suture as well.

Another bypass option is a retrograde bypass to the mesenteric arteries (Table 90-2). In a retrograde bypass, the inflow is taken from either the infrarenal abdominal aorta or an iliac artery. Again, the bypass can be to a solitary mesenteric vessel or it can be bifurcated to two vessels. The operation is begun with a laparotomy and exposure of the inflow vessel with proximal and distal control (Table 90-3). The target vessel(s) are then exposed as described above. The patient is systemically heparinized and then the proximal and distal anastomoses are completed with running monofilament suture. Prosthetic graft material is generally used, but autogenous grafts can be used as well. If vein is used for the bypass, it is preferable to make the length of the bypass as short as possible to prevent kinking of the graft. Care must be taken to measure the length and angle to prevent this complication after the retractors have been removed and the bowel returned to its normal location. Again, if only one vessel is to be revascularized, the SMA is the most important vessel to bypass. A prosthetic graft has a theoretic advantage in this scenario. An externally reinforced PTFE graft can be used in a gentle reverse "C" configuration from the infrarenal aorta (or iliac) to the SMA. The gentle curve allows the graft to lie within the bowel without kinking.

The choice of treatment, endovascular versus open, should be based on lesion anatomy, the nutritional status, and the life expectancy of the patient. Complete occlusion with the inability to cross the target lesion, long segment stenosis, and choice of access vessel affects the technical success rates of endovascular treatment. Assessing the nutritional status of the patient is critical in these malnourished patients, and some propose that endovascular revascularization be performed as a bridge to open repair in suitable patients with a >5-year life expectancy. A meta-analysis by Cai et al. demonstrates that the 30-day mortality and 3-year cumulative survival rate is similar between endovascular therapy and open surgical treatment groups. As one might expect, the endovascular therapy group has a significantly lower rate of inhospital complications that comes with the trade off of a greater recurrence rate within 3 years of revascularization.

Regardless of the surgical approach to mesenteric revascularization, all patients need to be carefully monitored postoperatively for signs of visceral ischemia. Large volume resuscitation may be necessary, especially if patients have sustained prolong bowel ischemia times. Lactate levels, urine output, and volume status all need to be closely monitored. The ICU setting is typically best suited for the initial postoperative care.

Case Conclusion

Approximately 1 year after stenting of the celiac and SMA, the patient experienced recurrent symptoms of postprandial abdominal pain, fear of food, and weight loss. She continued to smoke heavily. CTA showed near occlusion of both stents (Figures 90-4 and 90-5). Conversion to surgical bypass was recommended. She underwent antegrade aortoceliac and aorto-SMA bypass without sequelae. She recovered well and had complete resolution of her symptoms. Postoperative CT scan showed good function of her bypass grafts (Figure 90-6).

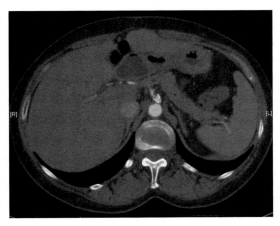

FIGURE 90-4. Stenosis of celiac stent.

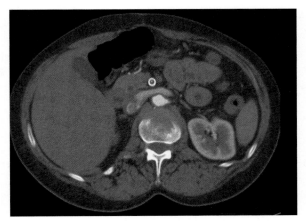

FIGURE 90-5. In-stent stenosis of SMA stent.

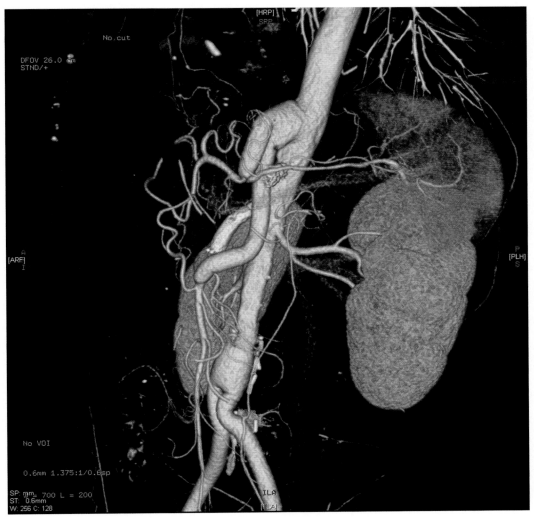

FIGURE 90-6. Reconstructed CTA of an antegrade aortoceliac and aortomesenteric bypass.

TAKE HOME POINTS

- Chronic mesenteric ischemia (CMI) is a rare disease.
- The triad of postprandial pain, fear of food, and weight loss must be present to entertain the diagnosis.
- Atherosclerotic disease with "spillover" into the visceral vessel orifices is the main cause.
- Lateral aortogram is the gold standard test.
- Open surgical treatments include endarterectomy, antegrade bypass, and retrograde bypass.
- The superior mesenteric artery is the most crucial artery to revascularize.
- Endovascular treatment caries lower morbidity but also has lower long-term patency rates.

SUGGESTED READINGS

Cai W, Li X, Shu C, et al. Comparison of clinical outcomes of endovascular versus open revascularization for chronic mesenteric ischemia: a meta-analysis. *Ann Vasc Surg.* 2015;29(5):934-940.

Ernst CB. Bypass procedures for chronic mesenteric ischemia. In: Ernst CB, Stanley JC, eds. *Current Therapy in Vascular Surgery.* 4th ed. Mosby: Philadelphia, PA. 2001:682-685.

Moneta GL, Yeager RA, Dalman R, Antonovic R, Hall LD, Porter JM. Duplex ultrasound criteria for diagnosis of splanchnic artery stenosis or occlusion. *J Vasc Surg.* 1991;14(4):511-518.

Oderich GS. Current concepts in the management of chronic mesenteric ischemia. *Curr Treat Options Cardiovasc Med.* 2010;12(2):117-130.

Oderich GS, Malgor RD, Ricotta JJ II. Open and endovascular revascularization for chronic mesenteric ischemia: tabular review of the literature. *Ann Vasc Surg.* 2009;23(5):700-712.

Pecoraro F, Rancic Z, Lachat M, et al. Chronic mesenteric ischemia: critical review and guidelines for management. *Ann Vasc Surg.* 2013;27(1):113-122.

Schermerhorn ML, Giles KA, Hamdan AD, Wyers MC, Pomposelli FB. Mesenteric revascularization: management and outcomes in the United States, 1988-2006. *J Vasc Surg.* 2009;50(2):341-348.

Zwolak RM, Fillinger MF, Walsh DB, et al. Mesenteric and celiac duplex scanning: a validation study. *J Vasc Surg.* 1998;27(6): 1078-1087.

Deep Venous Thrombosis

91

JUSTIN B. HURIE

Based on the previous edition chapter "Deep Venous Thrombosis"
by Justin Hurie and Thomas W. Wakefield

Presentation

A 35-year-old man presents to the emergency department with a few days of left leg swelling and pain. The patient first noticed the swelling 3 days ago after returning on a long car trip from Florida. The patient describes his pain as an ache in his left leg, and he has no prior episodes. The patient is otherwise healthy except that he smokes a half a pack of cigarettes a day. The patient takes no medications and has no family history of clotting and/or hypercoagulable conditions. The patient's physical examination is essentially normal other than extensive asymmetric left leg swelling that does not involve the foot. The patient's neurovascular examination is unremarkable, although pulses are only dopplerable and not palpable due to swelling.

● DIFFERENTIAL DIAGNOSIS

In this scenario, the most likely diagnosis is deep venous thrombosis (DVT), which also carries the highest risk associated with a delay in diagnosis, given its association with pulmonary embolism. In an extreme form, phlegmasia cerulea dolens involves extensive DVT causing massive lower extremity swelling and leg threat (see Figure 91-1). The patient is relatively young without a history of trauma or use of anticoagulation, which if positive could indicate a hematoma as an underlying etiology. Another cause of leg swelling is lymphedema, which tends to include swelling on the dorsum of the foot. Although it may arise spontaneously, lymphedema may also be iatrogenic, after surgery or radiation therapy. Other possible causes of leg swelling include congestive heart failure or nephrotic syndrome, but these generally involve bilateral leg swelling.

● WORKUP

Venous thromboembolism (VTE) is a common diagnosis encompassing deep vein thrombosis and pulmonary embolism, with a yearly incidence >900,000 in some estimates. The most widely utilized test to diagnose DVT is duplex ultrasound imaging with a sensitivity and specificity >95%. First, an ultrasound is performed using gray scale to image the external iliac, femoral, and popliteal veins. The veins below the knee are able to be imaged, although with less reliability. Under direct vision, compression is applied, which causes normal veins to collapse completely indicating patency (see Figure 91-2). When veins fail to collapse, either partially or completely, this indicates intraluminal material, usually either acute thrombus or chronic scar tissue (see Figure 91-3). There are rough guidelines to distinguish acute from chronic clot, but none are definitive or absolute (see Table 91-1). Acute clot generally appears echolucent, and the vein that contains the clot may appear enlarged on ultrasound. As DVT becomes chronic, its ultrasound appearance changes and

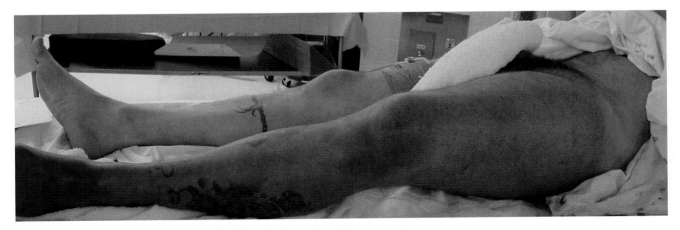

FIGURE 91-1. Photograph of a patient with phlegmasia cerulea dolens.

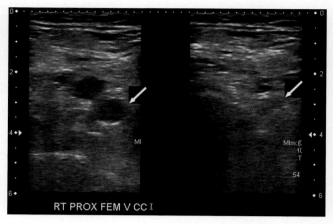

FIGURE 91-2. Ultrasound demonstrating complete collapse with compression indicating a patent femoral vein.

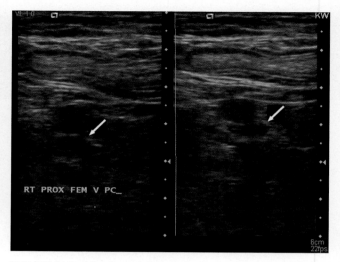

FIGURE 91-3. Ultrasound demonstrating only partial collapse with compression indicating intraluminal thrombus.

becomes echodense and heterogeneous, and the vein shrinks in size. Subacute thrombus generally represents a noncompressible vein with a combination of features of both acute and chronic clot.

The second component of duplex evaluation involves using color flow Doppler. Color flow may give additional information regarding partial versus complete occlusion. In addition, color flow may give indirect evidence of occlusions not directly visualized. Lack of respiratory variation indicates an obstruction cephalad to the vessel that is being imaged. Flow augmentation is used to evaluate patency of caudad vessels.

● DIAGNOSIS AND TREATMENT

The leading diagnosis is DVT, and the main modality of treatment is anticoagulation. According to the CHEST guidelines, dabigatran, rivaroxaban, apixaban, and edoxaban are now the first-line treatment for patients with DVT and no evidence of cancer. For patients with DVT and cancer, low molecular weight heparin (LMWH) is recommended as the first line of treatment. Patients with a new diagnosed VTE should be treated for a minimum of 3 months of anticoagulation. In patients with an unprovoked DVT, the duration of treatment depends on the patient's underlying coagulability and risk of bleeding and may benefit from longer treatment. More details regarding duration of treatment are found in the CHEST guidelines (see Suggested Readings).

Newer treatment modalities include the use of thrombolysis with the goal of reduction of clot burden. The goal of thrombolysis is to decrease the chance of developing one of the long-term sequelae of DVT, chronic venous insufficiency. Chronic venous insufficiency is due to long-standing venous hypertension, due to valvular incompetence, obstruction, or both. Postthrombotic syndrome (PTS) occurs in up to 30% to 40% of patients 5 years after developing a DVT, with an even higher incidence in those with iliofemoral DVT and

those with ipsilateral recurrent DVT. Risk factors for chronic venous insufficiency include multiple DVTs, advanced age, cancer, recent surgery, immobilization or trauma, pregnancy, hormone replacement therapy, obesity, and gender. The preliminary results of the ATTRACT trial have shown no decrease in the primary outcome of overall incidence of PTS with the use of catheter-directed thrombolysis. There may be up to a 25% decrease in moderate to severe PTS with catheter-directed thrombolysis in a subset analysis of patients with iliofemoral disease.

In younger patients without a clear etiology, it is important to look for anatomic risk factors, such as May-Thurner syndrome, defined as compression of the left iliac vein by the overlying right iliac artery, which forms an area of narrowing predisposing to thrombosis. Treatment of the May-Thurner syndrome includes venoplasty and stenting and, if thrombosis, thrombolysis, venoplasty, and stenting (see Figure 91-4).

● SURGICAL APPROACH

The primary determinant of the level of intervention is guided by the degree of symptoms. Systemic anticoagulation is the primary treatment for DVT. In patients who are unable

Table 91-1	Acute Versus Chronic DVT	
Acute	**Chronic**
Loss of compressibility	Loss of compressibility
Echolucency	Increased echogenicity
Lack of collateral vessels	Presence of collateral vessels
Venous distension	Shrunken fibrous cord
Surrounding inflammation	No inflammation

Left Iliac Vein Compression and Stent Repair

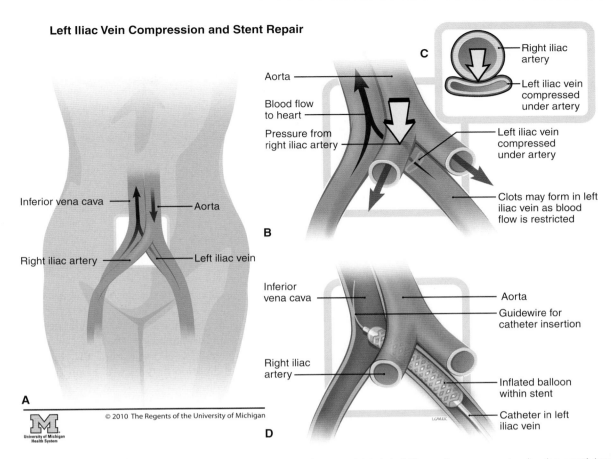

FIGURE 91-4. **A-D:** Depiction and treatment of May-Thurner syndrome, which is left iliac vein compression by the overlying right iliac artery.

to be anticoagulated, DVT is an indication for placement of an inferior vena cava filter. In patients with severe symptoms of leg swelling and extensive DVT, more aggressive intervention is indicated. In the most severe form, patients with phlegmasia cerulea dolens require venous decompression in order to decrease the chance of venous gangrene and the associated 20% to 50% amputation rate. One modality involves catheter-directed thrombolysis, which more quickly restores patency compared to anticoagulation alone. In patients who fail to respond to thrombolysis, open venous thrombectomy remains a good option. There are a variety of adjunctive measures that may be required in order to correct any underlying anatomic abnormality.

The patient should be placed on full anticoagulation involving heparin including a bolus (80 U/kg) or LMWH (1 mg/kg). Thrombolysis involves prepping the bilateral lower extremities circumferentially. The venous system may be accessed in the femoral, popliteal, or posterior tibial veins. Once a guidewire is passed across the lesion and position confirmed within the proximal vein, an infusion catheter may be placed with an infusion of TPA run overnight. Along with pharmacologic thrombolysis, today, mechanical catheters are also used. These catheters use various physical principles to help obliterate thrombus, and when used in combination, they may decrease both the amount of thrombolytic medication needed and also the time thrombolysis is required (pharmacomechanical thrombolysis).

If these methods fail to reestablish outflow, open surgery may be indicated. The femoral vein is exposed through a groin incision. Cephalad and caudad control is obtained with vessel loops, and a venotomy is made through the vein itself or a side branch. Five or six French venous thrombectomy catheters may be carefully passed in order to remove thrombus and reestablish venous flow. In patients with a chronic DVT, the femoral vein often contains webs (scar tissue) that requires removal. Once adequate flow is established, the venotomy may be closed primarily with a polypropylene suture or with a patch of vein or polyester. A completion duplex is performed in order to evaluate for technical problems. In some patients, an additional venogram may be needed in order to confirm adequate clearance of clot.

Given the required use of postoperative anticoagulation, there is a significant risk of bleeding. This requires careful postoperative observation and adequate drainage. Another

Table 91-2	Thrombectomy/Thrombolysis

Key Technical Steps

1. Prep widely including the full extent of the involved leg.
2. Use mechanical thrombolysis catheters.
3. May require overnight thrombolysis and serial fibrinogen levels.
4. Adjunctive stenting may be necessary, especially in cases of May-Thurner syndrome.
5. Intraoperative duplex and drain placement if open surgery is required.
6. Compression/elevation/sequential compression devices in order to assure adequate inflow.

Potential Pitfalls

- Adequate length of infusion catheter to cross the lesion.
- Bleeding due to technical reason, anticoagulation, HIT, or DIC.
- Importance of a technically perfect result.

HIT, heparin-induced thrombocytopenia; DIC, disseminated intravascular coagulation.

potential pitfall involves the unforgiving nature of venous interventions and a low-flow state. This requires the use of intraoperative duplex in order to evaluate for technical errors that may be easily remedied at the time of the initial procedure but may be catastrophic at a later point (Table 91-2).

● SPECIAL INTRAOPERATIVE CONSIDERATIONS

As with most vascular cases, potential difficult situations will usually involve bleeding or the lack thereof. In terms of postoperative bleeding, one potential source is technical or another is generalized oozing due to ongoing anticoagulation. Additional causes of bleeding include the development of heparin-induced thrombocytopenia (HIT) or disseminated intravascular coagulation (DIC). HIT usually manifests 3 to 10 days after administration of heparin, although the time can be reduced with prior exposure. DIC can complicate thrombolysis and requires the serial measurement of fibrinogen levels. Finally, lack of flow can be just as detrimental predisposing the patient to vein and stent thrombosis. Outflow into pelvic veins can usually be treated using a combination of stenting and venoplasty. A more troubling problem can be lack of adequate inflow. Adjunctive measures can include additional stent placement across the inguinal ligament or creation of an arteriovenous fistula in order to augment inflow (see Figure 91-4).

Case Conclusion

Compression stockings have been shown not to be effective in reducing the incidence of PTS and are no longer recommended outside of the role of symptomatic improvement. In the case presented, the patient underwent thrombolysis and stenting for May-Thurner syndrome. The patient had resolution of his symptoms and improvement in his leg swelling. Postoperatively, the patient was treated with anticoagulation for 3 months and continues to wear compression stockings for comfort.

TAKE HOME POINTS

- VTE is common with an incidence of more than 900,000 cases per year.
- Duplex evaluation is the cornerstone for diagnosis of DVT.
- Evaluate for phlegmasia given the high rate of associated gangrene and amputation.
- Anticoagulation is a cornerstone for the treatment of DVT, and duration of therapy depends on etiology and risk of bleeding.
- Consider thrombolysis for significant symptoms or limb threat in order to reduce thrombus burden for patients with extensive iliofemoral deep vein thrombosis.
- Excessive bleeding may be due to technical problems but may also occur with HIT or DIC.
- May-Thurner syndrome is a common etiology of left lower extremity swelling in patients without other risk factors for disease.
- Chronic venous insufficiency is a challenging problem with a range of symptoms from pain and swelling to non-healing ulcers.

SUGGESTED READINGS

Cronenwett JL, Johnston W. *Rutherford's Vascular Surgery*. 8th ed. Philadelphia, PA: Saunders; 2014.

Gloviczki P. *Handbook of Venous Disorders. Guidelines of the American Venous Forum*. 3rd ed. Oxford, UK: Oxford University Press; 2009.

Kahn SR, Shapiro S, Wells PS, et al. Compression stockings to prevent post-thrombotic syndrome: a randomized placebo-controlled trial. *Lancet*. 2014;383(9920):880-888.

Kearon C, Akl EA, Ornelas J, et al. Antithrombotic therapy for VTE disease: CHEST guideline and expert panel report (10th ed). *Chest*. 2016;149(2):315-352.

Pellerito J, Polak JF. *Introduction to Vascular Ultrasonography*. 6th ed. Philadelphia, PA: Saunders; 2012.

Wakefield TW. Venous thrombosis. In: Bope ET, Kellerman RD, Rakel RD eds. *Conn's Current Therapy*. Philadelphia, PA: Elsevier, 2011.

Wakefield TW, Caprini J, Comerota AJ. Thromboembolic disease. *Curr Probl Surg*. 2008;45(12):833-900.

Need for Hemodialysis Access

92

ALEXIS D. JACOB AND THOMAS S. HUBER

Based on the previous edition chapter "Need for Hemodialysis Access" by Alexis D. Jacob and Thomas S. Huber

Presentation

A 71-year-old female with a history of hypertension, congestive heart failure, and chronic kidney disease secondary to Goodpasture's disease presents to the emergency room with shortness of breath and bilateral lower extremity swelling. Her past medical history is otherwise significant for breast cancer treated with a left modified radical mastectomy and axillary node dissection. She states that she has not been compliant with her medical regimen and has not seen either her primary care physician or nephrologist for the past few months. She is hemodynamically stable but requires 2 L of oxygen by nasal cannula to maintain an oxygen saturation of >90%. Her physical examination is notable for bibasilar rales and pitting edema in both lower extremities. Her laboratory studies are remarkable for a blood urea nitrogen of 102 mg/dL, a serum creatinine 6.8 mg/dL, and a serum potassium of 6.1 mmol/L. An electrocardiogram demonstrates a normal sinus rhythm with slightly peaked T waves, and chest radiograph demonstrates findings consistent with fluid overload and congestive heart failure.

● DIAGNOSIS AND RECOMMENDATION

The patient appears to be in acute renal failure with the diagnosis based upon her generalized fluid overload, elevated blood urea nitrogen, and elevated potassium. She requires acute hemodialysis and needs dialysis access.

● DISCUSSION

The National Kidney Foundation Kidney Disease Outcome Quality Initiative (KDOQI) and the Fistula First Breakthrough Initiative (FFBI) have helped define the care of patients with chronic kidney disease (CKD) and end-stage renal disease (ESRD), emphasizing the role of autogenous hemodialysis access. These guidelines suggest that patients with stage 4 CKD (GFR < 30 mL per minute) should be referred to an access surgeon for a permanent access well in advance of their anticipated dialysis start date. The guidelines recommend that autogenous arteriovenous access (AVF) should be constructed 6 months prior to initiation while prosthetic access (AVG) should be constructed 3 to 6 weeks prior to initiation with the ultimate goal that patients start dialysis with a permanent access. The longer lead time for AVF allows for access maturation and any necessary remedial procedures to facilitate maturation. Additionally, patients with advanced CKD should be educated about the various options for renal replacement therapy (i.e., hemodialysis, peritoneal dialysis, transplantation) and engaged to preserve the veins on their nondominant arm for future access options. Despite the national initiatives, the majority of patients in our country initiate dialysis with a catheter according to the United States Renal Data System. Although these dialysis catheters facilitate life-sustaining treatment, they are associated with a variety of complications including thrombosis, infection, and central vein stenosis/occlusion. The associated catheter patency rates are limited (i.e., primary patency rates 2 to 3 months), and the limited flow rates can lead to ineffective dialysis. Long-term catheter use is associated with increased mortality when compared to AVFs or AVGs, and the percentage of patients dialyzing through tunneled catheters is used as a quality metric for dialysis units. Noncuffed catheters are frequently placed in the urgent or emergent setting to facilitate the initiation of dialysis. However, their use should be restricted to the inpatient setting because of the concern for dislodgement. Cuffed, tunneled catheters are more resistant to infection and can be used for time periods ranging from weeks to months. Both the noncuffed and cuffed catheters should be inserted through the internal jugular vein opposite the side of the proposed permanent access, typically the right internal jugular vein. Notably, insertion of a dialysis catheter into the subclavian vein is associated with a significant risk of stenosis/occlusion that can preclude an ipsilateral permanent access.

Presentation Continued

A noncuffed hemodialysis catheter is placed in the interventional radiology suite, and the patient is admitted to the nephrology service for initiation of dialysis. The noncuffed catheter is replaced with a cuffed tunneled catheter after several dialysis sessions.

● DIAGNOSIS AND RECOMMENDATIONS

A permanent hemodialysis access should be constructed after the patient is "stabilized" on hemodialysis and her volume and electrolyte abnormalities are corrected.

● DISCUSSION

As noted above, the KDOQI and the FFBI have emphasized the use of AVFs and have set ambitious national targets (AVF prevalence: KDOQI—65%, FFBI—68%; tunneled dialysis catheters (>90 days): FFBI—<10%). This strong emphasis is based upon the impression that AVFs are associated with improved patency, fewer complications, lower mortality, and lower costs relative to both cuffed tunneled catheters and AVGs. However, there are several disadvantages with AVFs that partially offset these purported advantages including the obligatory maturation period that can last several months (frequently mandating the use of a cuffed tunneled catheter as a "bridge") and the frequent need for remedial procedures to facilitate maturation. Although most providers would concede that a "mature" AVF is the optimal access choice, the ultimate goal should be a functional, durable permanent access rather than specifically an AVF. Notably, there has been an evolution across the country from the concept of "fistula first" to "catheter last" and more recently to a "functional permanent access."

There are patients who are better suited with an AVG rather than an AVF and a small subset of patients with advanced comorbidities that are best suited with a tunneled catheter. Maintaining effective hemodialysis access is a difficult problem that really requires a lifelong plan and committed providers, best reflected by the current access mantra that the goals should be the "right access for the right patient at the right time."

The evaluation of patients presenting for permanent hemodialysis access includes a focused history and physical examination in combination with noninvasive imaging. Indeed, the noninvasive imaging has been the cornerstone of our preoperative evaluation. Special attention should be directed at documenting the access history including procedures, revisions, and associated complications. Physical examination should include a detailed pulse examination with an Allen's test to determine the forearm vessel responsible for the dominant arterial supply to the hand. The noninvasive testing in the diagnostic vascular laboratory includes examination of both the arterial and venous circulation. Although the preoperative arterial imaging is not as well accepted, we would contend that it is equally important given the prevalence of upper extremity and forearm occlusive disease in the dialysis population. The arterial studies include blood pressure measurements of the brachial, radial, ulnar, and digital arteries along with the corresponding Doppler waveforms of all but the digital vessels (Figure 92-1). Additionally, the Allen's test is

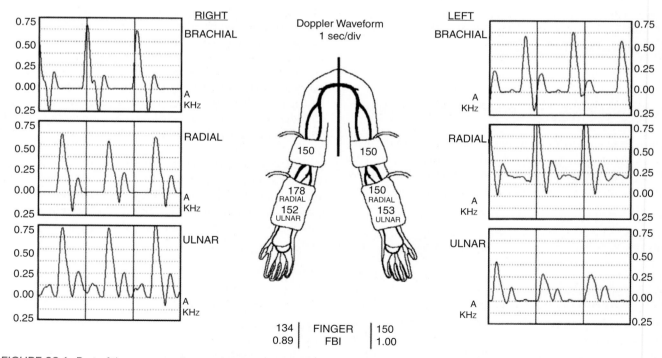

FIGURE 92-1. Part of the preoperative noninvasive arterial imaging studies are shown. The brachial, radial, and ulnar arterial pressures (mm Hg) are shown on the diagram of the upper extremities while the finger pressures are shown in the center of the figure at the bottom. The corresponding Doppler waveforms (sec/div) are shown for the brachial, radial, and ulnar arteries. The FBI denotes the finger/brachial index and is the ratio of the finger pressure to the ipsilateral brachial artery pressure. Note the symmetric brachial artery pressures and the corresponding normal appearing triphasic Doppler waveforms.

repeated and the diameters of both the radial and brachial arteries are measured at the wrist and antecubital fossa, respectively. Venous imaging includes the interrogation of the cephalic and basilic veins from the wrist to the axilla complete with diameter measurements similar to the preoperative vein survey obtained prior to infrainguinal arterial revascularization (Figure 92-2). Admittedly, the interrogation of the central veins is somewhat limited by the bony thorax cavity.

An operative plan is then generated based upon the results of the history/physical and noninvasive imaging with a relatively strong emphasis on autogenous access as emphasized by the guidelines. Our objective has been to select the combination of the artery and vein that would most likely result in a successful AVF. We have not felt constrained by the usual conventions of using the nondominant > dominant extremity and the forearm > arm, although we have followed these standard approaches when the choices are equivocal. The criteria for an adequate artery and vein include an adequate diameter, no hemodynamically significant arterial inflow stenoses, no venous outflow stenoses, and a peripheral vein segment of suitable length and diameter (Table 92-1). Our preferences in descending order include the radiocephalic, radiobasilic, brachiocephalic, and brachiobasilic autogenous accesses prior to use of prosthetic material (Table 92-2). Notably, these preferences are consistent with

the current KDOQI guidelines. Contrast arteriography and venography can be used to confirm the preliminary access choice although these are usually reserved for select patients with suspected arterial inflow or venous outflow lesions, respectively. Our overall approach has evolved along with the national trends with the ultimate goal of establishing a functional permanent access, and we readily concede that some patients are better suited with an

Table 92-1 Criteria to Determine Suitability of Artery and Vein for Autogenous Access

Vein

Diameter ≥ 3 mm without evidence of significant stenosis. Suitable segment from wrist to antecubital fossa (forearm access) or antecubital fossa to axilla (upper arm access). Absence of significant central vein stenosis in the ipsilateral extremity.

Artery

Diameter ≥2 mm.
Absence of hemodynamically significant inflow stenosis.[a]
Nondominant radial artery for wrist access.

[a]≥15-mm Hg pressure gradient between the brachial arteries for proposed arm accesses or between the ipsilateral brachial and radial arteries for proposed forearm accesses.

Cephalic Mapping

Location	Right Diameter	Thrombus	Depth	Left Diameter	Thrombus	Depth
Cephalic at UA	2.9	None		3.4	None	
Cephalic at Mid UA	3.7	None		3.1	None	
Cephalic at AF	4.1	None		3.4	None	
Median Cubital	3	None		2.7	None	
Cephalic at Mid LA	1.1	None		2	None	
Cephalic at Wrist	1.3	None		2	None	

Basilic Mapping

Location	Right Diameter	Thrombus	Depth	Left Diameter	Thrombus	Depth
Basilic at UA	5.4	None		4.1	None	
Basilic at Mid UA	5	None		4.3	None	
Basilic at AF	2.4	None		1.6	None	
Median Cubital	3	None		2.7	None	
Basilic at Mid LA	2.7	None		2.6	None	

Incidental Observations

The right brachial artery measures 3.3mm. The right radial artery measures 2mm. The left brachial artery measures 3.4mm. The left radial artery measures 2.1mm.

FIGURE 92-2. Part of the preoperative noninvasive venous imaging studies are shown. The diameters (mm) of both the basilic and cephalic veins in the forearm and upper arm are shown. Note that the cephalic basilic vein segments in both upper arms are likely suitable for autogenous access using our diameter criteria. The diameters of the brachial and radial arteries at the antecubital fossa and wrist, respectively, are shown under the Incidental Observations.

Table 92-2	Hierarchy for Permanent Hemodialysis Accesses Configurations

Autogenous radial–cephalic
Autogenous radial–basilic
Autogenous brachial–cephalic
Autogenous brachial–basilic
Forearm prosthetic
Upper arm prosthetic

AVG and even a tunneled catheter. The role of AVGs in our practice is similar to that outlined by a thoughtful review discussing the role of AVGs in the KDOI and FFBI era (Table 92-3).

Presentation Continued

The patient undergoes further evaluation including non-invasive imaging in the vascular laboratory. Of note, she is right hand dominant but refused to have any type of access in her left arm because of her prior left modified radical mastectomy and axillary node dissection. She is found to have suitable cephalic and basilic veins in both upper arms for a possible AVF on her noninvasive imaging based upon our size criteria outlined above. Her brachial artery measures 3.3 mm at the antecubital fossa on the right and 3.2 mm on the left. She has no evidence of arterial inflow stenosis based upon her Doppler waveforms and pressure measurements. Additionally, she has no evidence of venous outflow stenosis on either side.

• DIAGNOSIS AND RECOMMENDATION

The patient could potentially have a brachial–cephalic or brachial–basilic autogenous access on either size, but has a relative contraindication on her left side because of her prior mastectomy and axillary node dissection. A right brachial–cephalic autogenous access should be constructed.

• SURGICAL APPROACH

The patient undergoes routine preoperative evaluation with optimization of her underlying medical problems and consultation with the anesthesiologists (Figure 92-3 and Table 92-4). The procedure is performed on a nondialysis day under regional anesthesia using a short acting agent to allow assessment of the hand motor and sensory function in the early postoperative period. The cephalic vein in the upper arm is interrogated with ultrasound prior to the skin preparation, and the course of the vein is marked on the skin. We have found the intraoperative ultrasound to be a valuable adjunct to the preoperative vein assessment and can frequently identify veins that are suitable for autogenous access, having been deemed non suitable by the initial imaging, likely due to the vasodilatory effects of the anesthetic agents. An incision is made across the antecubital crease and incorporating the previously marked cephalic vein. Care should be exercised during the skin incision since the cephalic and median antecubital veins are very superficial. The cephalic vein is dissected free for approximately 3 cm by creating superior and inferior skin flaps. The cephalic vein, and its continuation as the median antecubital vein, bifurcates or trifurcates in the

Table 92-3	Factors Influencing the Choice of Autogenous or Prosthetic Arteriovenous Hemodialysis Access in the KDOQI and FFBI Era		
Clinical Scenarios Favoring Autogenous Success	**Clinical Scenarios Favoring Prosthetic Access**	**Factors That Adversely Influence Autogenous Access Maturation**
Young patient age	Imminent need for or currently on hemodialysis	Diabetes mellitus (radial and ulnar-based accesses)
Favorable vascular anatomy (artery >2.0 mm: vein >3.0 mm)	Short life expectancy	Arterial diameter <2.0 mm
Chronic skin diseases	Morbid obesity	Calcified radial artery
History of multiple previous access infections	Unfavorable vascular anatomy	Vein diameter <3.0 mm
Immunosuppression/HIV		Congestive heart failure
Hypercoagulability		Advanced patient age
Multiple prior prosthetic access failures		Female gender

HIV, human immunodeficiency virus.

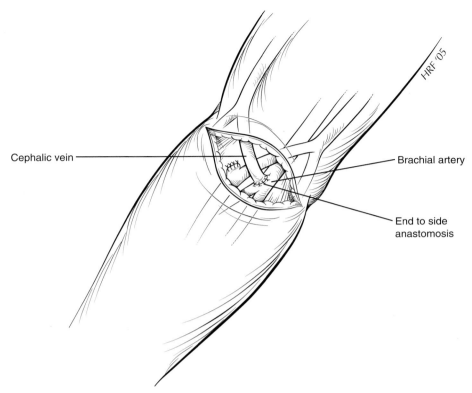

FIGURE 92-3. Brachial–cephalic AVF. (Reprinted from Englesbe MJ, Campbell DA. Upper extremity arteriovenous hemodialysis access. In: Zelenock GB, Huber TS, Lumsden A, Messina LM, Moneta GL, eds. *Mastery of Vascular and Endovascular Surgery.* Philadelphia, PA: Lippincott Williams & Wilkins, 2006; with permission.)

Table 92-4	Need for Hemodialysis Access

Key Technical Steps

1. Intraoperative ultrasound to mark course of cephalic vein
2. Antecubital incision through crease
3. Dissection of cephalic and median antecubital vein
4. Mobilization of cephalic vein with ligation of proximal branch
5. Dissection of brachial artery
6. Distension of the outflow vein and spatulation of orifice
7. Vascular control of brachial artery and arteriotomy
8. Tension-free anastomosis
9. Confirmation of adequate access thrill and arterial Doppler signal at wrist

Potential Pitfalls

- Injury to cephalic or median antecubital vein with skin incision
- Excess tension on the outflow cephalic vein
- Kinking or compressing the outflow vein with skin closure
- Absence of a thrill in access

antecubital fossa. It can be helpful to preserve the proximal aspects of these branches to help create a generous hood for the anastomosis. These large, deep branches should be suture ligated since they tend to retract into to muscle and soft tissue. The brachial artery is exposed by incising the overlying bicipital aponeurosis, and approximately 2 to 3 cm of the artery is dissected free. The vein is distended with saline using an olive-tipped catheter, spatulated, and all defects are repaired. Patients are administered 5,000 units of heparin intravenously, and the brachial artery is occluded proximally and distally with the appropriate-sized vascular clamps (e.g., Cooley microvascular or Gregory bulldogs). A 0.75- to 1-cm incision is created in the artery using a no. 11 blade scalpel blade and arteriotomy scissors. The anastomosis is performed using a 6-0 monofilament vascular suture and standard surgical technique. Upon completion, the fistula and the arterial signals at the wrist are interrogated with the continuous wave Doppler. A thrill should be detected in the proximal aspect of the fistula. The absence of a thrill or a pulsatile Doppler signal in the AVF merits further investigation. A diminished or monophasic Doppler signal at the wrist suggests that the hand may be ischemic. It is impossible to determine at this point whether this is due to reversible vasospasm or frank hand ischemia. All patients with suspected hand ischemia merit very close observation throughout the immediate postoperative period with aggressive remedial treatment as necessary. The wound edges are reapproximated with an interrupted 3-0 braided, absorbable suture, and the skin is closed with a subcuticular stitch (e.g., 4-0 monofilament, absorbable) to complete the procedure.

The proximal radial artery can be used as an alternative arterial inflow source for upper arm cephalic- or basilic-based autogenous access procedures. The potential advantages of using the proximal radial artery include a lower access flow rate that may result in less venous hypertension and potentially a lower incidence of access-related hand ischemia. The proximal radial artery can be exposed by dissecting further distal on the brachial artery than outlined above. The median antecubital vein and its deep branches should be preserved and can be used for the anastomosis.

Case Conclusion

The patient undergoes a right brachial–cephalic AVF and is discharged home from the recovery room after the anesthetic agent wears off and her hand function is found to be intact. Follow-up to the vascular surgery clinic is arranged in 2 weeks.

● DISCUSSION

The radial–cephalic and brachial–cephalic AVFs are usually performed as an outpatient, but we typically admit patients undergoing single-stage brachial–basilic AVFs overnight for observation and pain control. The inpatients are placed on a telemetry bed with continuous pulse oximetry and their serum electrolytes are checked. Patients are monitored throughout the postoperative period for the development of the usual complications inherent to all surgical procedures (e.g., hematoma, wound infection) along with those more specific to the access procedure. The latter including upper extremity edema from venous hypertension and access-related ischemia or "steal." Some type of mild edema is relatively common after all access procedures due to the surgical trauma although this usually resolves early in the postoperative period. Persistent edema suggests a venous outflow stenosis, commonly from a central vein stenosis or occlusion. This merits further evaluation with catheter-based contrast study. Moderate or severe hand ischemic occurs in approximately 10% of the brachial artery-based procedures. The diagnosis of access-related hand ischemia is a clinical one that can be corroborated with noninvasive testing for equivocal cases. Preoperative predictors include advanced age, female gender, the presence of peripheral vascular occlusive disease, large conduits, and a prior episode of hand ischemia. Treatment options include access ligation, distal revascularization and interval ligation (DRIL), proximalization of the anastomosis, correction of any arterial inflow stenosis, and limiting the flow through the access (e.g., "banding").

Patients are seen in the outpatient clinic 2 weeks after their operative procedure and at monthly intervals thereafter until their accesses are usable for dialysis. The KDOQI recommendations ("rule of 6's"—6 mm in diameter, 6 mm depth below the skin, 600 mL per minute) are used to determine when the access is suitable for cannulation. We have found duplex ultrasound to be a particularly helpful adjunct to physical examination to "clear" the AVF for initial use or cannulation. Accesses that fail to dilate and those without a thrill are investigated with a catheter-based fistulagram to identify potential problems. Open surgical or endovascular procedures (e.g., balloon angioplasty, vein patch angioplasty) are performed as necessary based upon the fistulagram. When the accesses are ultimately deemed suitable for cannulation, the patients are provided with a diagram of their specific access configuration and instructions for cannulation while a similar facsimile is sent to their dialysis unit. The cuffed, tunneled catheter is removed when the AVF can be cannulated consistently.

TAKE HOME POINTS

- Patients with stage 4 and 5 chronic kidney disease should be referred to an access surgeon well in advance of their anticipated hemodialysis initiation date.
- Cuffed tunneled catheters should be inserted into the internal jugular vein contralateral to the site of the planned permanent access.
- A mature autogenous arteriovenous hemodialysis access is likely the best access option for most patients, but the primary goal should be a functional permanent access.
- Preoperative arterial and venous noninvasive imaging can help identify the optimal artery and vein combination for a permanent access.
- Patients should be followed in the surgical clinic until the access is suitable for cannulation and monitored closely for access-related hand ischemia and ipsilateral edema.
- The construction and maintenance of hemodialysis access is a challenging problem that requires a lifetime plan and committed providers.

SUGGESTED READINGS

Beathard GA, Lok CE, Glickman MH, et al. Definitions and endpoints for interventional studies for arteriovenous dialyses accesses. *Clin J Am Soc Nephrol.* 2018;13(3):501-512.

Cull DL. Role of prosthetic hemodialysis access following introduction of the dialysis outcome quality and Fistula First Breakthrough Initiatives. *Semin Vasc Surg.* 2011;24:89-95.

Feezor RJ, Huber TS. Autogenous hemodialysis access, in Fischer JE (ed.). *Mastery of Surgery*, 7th ed. Wolters Kluwer; 2018.

Fistula First Catheter Last. Available at: https://www.esrdncc.org/en/fistula-first-catheter-last.

Huber TS, Ozaki CK, Flynn TC, et al. Prospective validation of an algorithm to maximize native arteriovenous fistulae for chronic hemodialysis access. *J Vasc Surg.* 2002;36:452-459.

Lok CE, Allon M, Moist L, et al. Risk equation determining unsuccessful cannulation events and failure to maturation in arteriovenous fistulas (REDUCE FTM I). *J Am Soc Nephrol.* 2006;17: 3204-3212.

National Kidney Foundation. K/DOQI Clinical Practice Guidelines for Vascular Access, 2006 Updates. *Am J Kidney Dis.* 2001;37: S137-S181.

Scali ST, Huber TS. Treatment strategies for access-related hand ischemia. *Semin Vasc Surg.* 2011;24:128-136.

United States Renal Data System Annual Report. 2017. Available at: https://www.usrds.org/adr.aspx.

Woo K, Ulloa J, Allon M, et al. Establishing patient specific criteria for selecting the optimal upper extremity vascular access procedure. *J Vasc Surg.* 2017;65:1089-1103.

SECTION 10

Pediatric

Emesis in an Infant

93

CHASEN J. GREIG AND ROBERT A. COWLES

Based on the previous edition chapter "Emesis in an Infant"
by Erica R. Gross and Robert A. Cowles

Presentation

A 4-week-old male infant is brought to the emergency room by his parents for persistent emesis. The mother reports that the baby began spitting up several days ago and that over the past day it has become more frequent and noticeably more forceful. It now occurs following nearly every feeding and is described as faint yellow in color, much like his formula, without blood or bile. The baby is still having wet diapers but not as frequently, and he is quieter than usual. The infant has no significant medical history, was delivered full-term without complications, and is otherwise healthy and developing normally. Vital signs are remarkable for tachycardia. On physical examination, the baby is sleeping but easily aroused. The anterior fontanelle is depressed. His abdomen is soft, nondistended, and nontender. No masses are palpable, but gastric peristaltic waves are visible on inspection of the abdomen. No inguinal hernias are detected. A complete blood count and chemistry panel are ordered, and the results are given in Table 93-1. The patient is admitted for treatment of dehydration and electrolyte imbalance.

● DIFFERENTIAL DIAGNOSIS

In an infant presenting with emesis, determination of the presence or absence of bile in the vomitus is critical. Bilious emesis is concerning for malrotation with volvulus, a true surgical emergency that must be ruled out. In the presentation above, however, the infant presents with nonbilious emesis, leading to the following differential diagnoses: formula intolerance, gastroesophageal reflux, pyloric stenosis, pylorospasm, antral or duodenal web, gastric volvulus, and gastroparesis. Recurrent emesis can also be associated with metabolic disorders, inborn errors of metabolism, or elevated intracranial pressure due to brain tumors; however, emesis is rarely the isolated symptom in these systemic or neurologic disorders. Thus, based on the history, examination, and simple laboratory test results provided, pyloric stenosis is the most likely diagnosis. Pyloric stenosis can often be identified with a fair degree of certainty by clinical history that the infant is hungry after emesis, that

the emesis is forceful and nonbilious, and that the baby is otherwise well. As emesis persists over days, lethargy may develop secondary to hypovolemia.

● WORKUP

The clinical history and the physical exam alone are sufficient to make a diagnosis of pyloric stenosis in the majority of infants with the condition. To optimize the examination of an infant with suspected pyloric stenosis, the examiner should do their best to make the infant calm, warm, and in the proper position. The infant should be supine with legs flexed to relax the abdominal musculature. Palpation of the liver edge should then be possible, and slowly moving toward the umbilicus in the midline should reveal the palpable pylorus, classically referred to as the "olive."

Despite best efforts, however, a palpable mass is not always present, and with the improvement in ultrasound technology, there has been a decline in reliance on physical exam findings in diagnosis of pyloric stenosis. Not only is ultrasound extremely sensitive and specific, but it is quick, available, inexpensive, noninvasive, and does not expose the child to radiation. A pylorus is considered hypertrophied if the thickness is ≥3 mm and if the pyloric channel length is ≥15 mm (Figure 93-1). In addition to these static measurements, the radiologist can often assess whether fluid is able to pass from the stomach into the duodenum.

In the uncommon situation that the diagnosis is not clear after physical exam and ultrasound, an upper gastrointestinal series can show a distended stomach that cannot empty due to pyloric obstruction ("shoulder sign") and a narrowed pyloric channel ("string sign") (Figure 93-2). Along with ultrasound, initial workup includes evaluation of serum electrolytes, as a vast majority of patients with pyloric stenosis will have imbalances ranging from mild to severe.

● DISCUSSION

Infantile hypertrophic pyloric stenosis is the most common cause of gastric outlet obstruction in infancy with a reported incidence ranging between 2 and 5/1,000 live births in the Western world. This disorder has a male

Table 93-1   Laboratory Values

Complete Blood Count		Chemistry Panel	
WBC	8.3	Sodium	136
Hemoglobin	13.7	Potassium	3.3
Hematocrit	38.6	Chloride	95
Platelets	301	Bicarbonate	33
		BUN	7
		Creatinine	0.4
		Glucose	93

predominance between 2:1 and 5:1 and occurs more frequently in Caucasians. Etiology has been well investigated, but no definitive causative factors have been identified, although both genetic and environmental factors seem to have a role.

● DIAGNOSIS AND TREATMENT

The ultrasound of this patient showed that the pyloric muscle is 5 mm thick with a channel length of 20 mm, thus confirming the diagnosis of pyloric stenosis. Although surgery is the gold standard for treatment of pyloric stenosis, it is not a surgical emergency, and correction of electrolyte abnormalities and hypovolemia is the priority in initial management of these infants. As is classically described, this

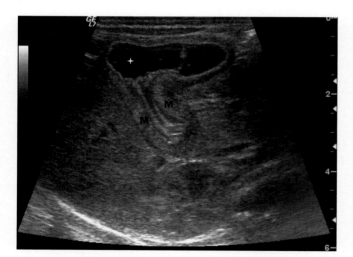

FIGURE 93-1. Abdominal ultrasound of hypertrophied pylorus. The patient has taken Pedialyte® by mouth, and the stomach appears the density of water (*white asterisk*). Mucosa is radiopaque and is seen outlining the pyloric channel (*black asterisk*). The hypertrophied pyloric muscle (*M*) measures 5 mm in thickness and 20 mm in length.

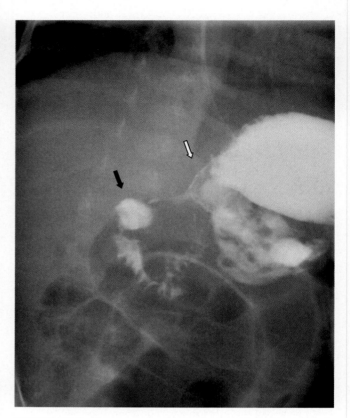

FIGURE 93-2. Fluoroscopy after oral contrast. A string sign is seen between the antrum (*white arrow*) and the duodenal bulb (*black arrow*) indicating pyloric stenosis.

child has a hypokalemic, hypochloremic metabolic alkalosis. Prolonged emesis can lead to significant dehydration and a worsening of the alkalosis and hypokalemia through an aldosterone-mediated loss of H^+ and K^+ in the kidneys, referred to as paradoxical aciduria and typically a late finding. Despite frequently being present, it is important to remember that these derangements depend upon duration of symptoms, and the absence of electrolyte abnormalities in patients with pyloric stenosis has been described. Normal electrolytes do not rule out the diagnosis, and they should not be used to assess which infants with pyloric stenosis are dehydrated or not.

It is safest to assume that all infants with pyloric stenosis are fluid depleted. Approach to resuscitation and correction of electrolyte abnormalities can differ slightly but is centered around aggressive volume repletion and careful correction of electrolyte abnormalities. All infants diagnosed with pyloric stenosis should receive a 20 mL/kg bolus of normal saline (NS). Closely monitor urine output and administer additional fluid boluses until adequate urine output is achieved (1.5 to 2 mL/kg/h). Intravenous (IV) fluids, D5 ½ NS, should also be started at 1.5 times maintenance rate. Potassium supplementation can be given in initial IV fluids or after adequate urine output is reestablished in an attempt to prevent rebound hyperkalemia. Either approach should be done in combination with careful monitoring of serum potassium.

Emesis should cease once the infant is taking nothing by mouth, and therefore, a nasogastric tube (NGT) is generally not necessary.

SURGICAL APPROACH TO OPEN PYLOROMYOTOMY

After the electrolyte imbalances have been corrected, the surgeon must relieve the gastric outlet obstruction. Medical treatment with atropine and endoscopic dilatation has been described, but these therapies have not met the standard set by surgical pyloromyotomy. The gold standard approach has been the Fredet-Ramstedt pyloromyotomy. Classically, the procedure was performed through a transverse right upper quadrant incision, although a supraumbilical curvilinear incision is currently the preferred approach and is described here (Table 93-2).

The infant is placed in a supine position on the operating table, an NGT is placed, and general anesthesia is induced. After the infant is relaxed, the pylorus should be palpable in the epigastric region. An incision is made over this area in the right upper quadrant or above the umbilicus and is carried down through the muscle and fascia. The omentum is retracted downward to retract the transverse colon and reveal the stomach. Then, the antrum and the pylorus are identified and brought through the incision. Holding the duodenum with the left index finger supporting the pylorus, the serosa is incised approximately 2 mm proximal to the pyloric vein extending onto the gastric antrum (Figure 93-3). A blunt instrument is then used to divide the remaining circular muscle fibers without injuring, or violating, the underlying mucosa. When separation is complete, bulging of the mucosa is often seen, and the two sides of the pyloric muscle can be moved independently. The anesthesiologist can then fill the stomach with air to assess for perforation. The pylorus

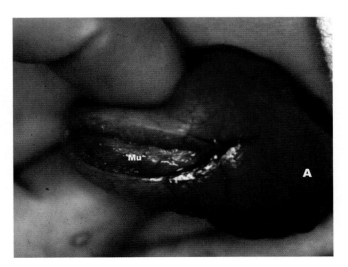

FIGURE 93-3. Externalization of pylorus during open pyloromyotomy. The duodenum is being held, and the pyloromyotomy has been extended onto the gastric antrum. Mucosa (*Mu*) is seen ballooning through the completed incision.

is then placed back into the abdomen, and the fascia and the skin are closed.

If the pyloric incision is not deep enough or long enough, the child may show signs of persistent pyloric obstruction and require reoperation. Incomplete myotomy commonly occurs proximally, close to the gastric antrum. If the incision is too deep, through the mucosa, leakage of gastric or duodenal contents will occur. This most commonly occurs at the distal aspect of the incision, on the duodenal bulb. If this is identified intraoperatively, the mucosa should be closed with interrupted sutures and covered by the omentum. In the case of perforation, the NGT can be left for 24 hours after repair to ensure gastric decompression.

SURGICAL APPROACH TO LAPAROSCOPIC PYLOROMYOTOMY

The first laparoscopic pyloromyotomy was described by Alain in 1991. Studies have shown that the laparoscopic approach is safe and effective and few differences compared to open pyloromyotomy with the exception of improved cosmetic outcome in laparoscopy. Newer techniques for pyloromyotomy have been described, including endoscopic and single-incision laparoscopic pyloromyotomy, but experience and long-term outcomes are limited. Standard three-port laparoscopic pyloromyotomy is described here (Table 93-3).

General anesthesia is induced, and the infant is placed transversely on the operating table. The monitor is placed at the baby's head, across from the operating surgeon, who stands at the infant's feet. An incision is made through the umbilicus or inferior to it. The Veress needle is then placed into the peritoneal cavity through this incision. A 4-mm

Table 93-2	Surgical Approach to Open Pyloromyotomy

Key Technical Steps

1. Palpate the limits of the pyloric muscle. Identify the pyloric vein. Start the pyloromyotomy superficially, taking care to avoid the duodenum.
2. Extend the incision onto the antrum of the stomach.
3. Bluntly separate the deep muscle fibers.
4. Look for a bulge of the mucosa after completely separating muscle fibers.
5. Test for duodenal perforation with insufflation via an NG tube.

Potential Pitfalls

- Incomplete myotomy.
- Perforating the duodenal mucosa.

Table 93-3	Surgical Approach to Laparoscopic Pyloromyotomy

Key Technical Steps

1. Using an umbilical port, select the location of two working port sites in the epigastrium (left and right); these often do not require trocars.
2. Identify the limits of the pylorus, and map incision by scoring serosa with electrocautery.
3. Bluntly separate muscle fibers.
4. Ensure that muscle fibers are freely mobile and underlying mucosa is visualized.
5. Test for duodenal perforation with insufflation via an NG tube.

Potential Pitfalls

- Incomplete myotomy.
- Perforating the duodenal mucosa.
- Allowing herniation of the omentum through trocar sites during closure.

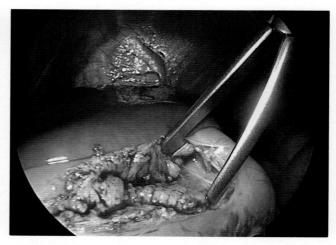

FIGURE 93-5. Spreading of the muscle fibers to complete the myotomy. Mucosa can be seen deep to the muscle layers between tips of the instrument.

trocar is inserted after inflation, and a 4-mm, 30° scope is inserted. The abdomen is insufflated to 8 to 10 mm Hg. Two stab incisions are made in the right and left epigastrium under direct visualization, and 3-mm instruments are placed directly via the skin incisions without trocars. The proximal duodenum is grasped with the left hand, and more recently electrocautery is used in place of an arthrotomy knife to incise the serosa of the pylorus (Figure 93-4). The same landmarks are used for the pyloric incision. A laparoscopic pyloric spreader is used to spread the deep muscular layers (Figure 93-5). Again, the stomach should be insufflated with the duodenum occluded to evaluate for mucosal perforation. The carbon dioxide is then evacuated from the abdominal

cavity, and the umbilical fascia and the skin are closed. The epigastric incisions may be closed with Steri-Strips or Dermabond.

● SPECIAL INTRAOPERATIVE CONSIDERATIONS

While diagnostic error is unusual, a normal pylorus can be an unexpected intraoperative finding. This error in diagnosis is likely due to pylorospasm, a condition expected to resolve with bowel rest. When this occurs, patency of the stomach, pylorus, and proximal duodenum should be confirmed. This can be achieved by passage of an orogastric tube across the pylorus or by performing an intraoperative fluoroscopic gastric emptying study. In addition, other etiologies of upper gastrointestinal obstruction, discussed above, should also be ruled out.

● POSTOPERATIVE MANAGEMENT

Pain control with oral acetaminophen is typically sufficient. While the optimal approach to postoperative feeds following pyloromyotomy may not be clear, there is good evidence to support early reinstitution of feeds, whether in the form of a protocol or ad libitum. The following is an example of a postoperative feeding protocol. Intake begins 4 to 6 hours postoperatively with small volumes of Pedialyte® and is increased at every feed as tolerated, typically by 10 to 15 mL. Once the infant is able to tolerate an adequate volume of Pedialyte® (usually 60 to 90 mL), he or she can be transitioned to breast milk or formula. It is common for an infant to vomit after surgery. If the infant vomits a feeding, allow 3 hours and reattempt the same volume. Continue maintenance IV fluids until the infant is tolerating oral feedings well. Most patients

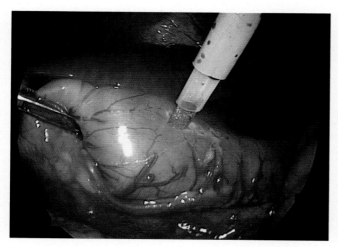

FIGURE 93-4. Serosal incision over the pylorus during laparoscopic pyloromyotomy, extending from the antrum proximally to the duodenum distally.

are discharged 24 to 48 hours after surgery. Very few patients have long-term complications, such as gastric dysmotility. Any infant with persistent emesis 1 week after surgery should be evaluated for an incomplete myotomy or for severe gastroesophageal reflux.

Case Conclusion

The baby is adequately rehydrated, and electrolytes normalize over the first 36 hours. On hospital day 2, a laparoscopic pyloromyotomy is performed. Oral feeding with Pedialyte® is started 4 hours postoperatively and administered in increasing volumes every 3 hours. The baby has one episode of emesis, but does well, and is discharged home on the first postoperative day. At a 4-week follow-up appointment, the child is gaining weight appropriately according to growth curves.

TAKE HOME POINTS

- In any newborn, differentiate bilious from nonbilious vomiting. Bilious emesis is intestinal obstruction secondary to volvulus, a true surgical emergency, unless proven otherwise.
- The morbidity associated with pyloric stenosis comes from the dehydration and electrolyte disturbances rather than the gastric outlet obstruction alone. The classic disturbance is a hypokalemic, hypochloremic metabolic alkalosis with paradoxical aciduria, although actual presentation is variable. These abnormalities require IV fluid resuscitation and careful monitoring of electrolyte correction prior to surgery.
- Postoperative vomiting is usually self-limited and does not indicate surgical failure unless it becomes persistent with failure to gain weight.
- Incomplete myotomy most often occurs proximally (gastric antrum). Perforation most often occurs distally (duodenal bulb).

SUGGESTED READINGS

Adibe OO, et al. Protocol versus ad libitum feeds after laparoscopic pyloromyotomy: a prospective randomized trial. *J Pediatr Surg.* 2014;49:129-132; discussion 132. doi: 10.1016/j.jpedsurg.2013.09.044.

Iqbal CW, Rivard DC, Mortellaro VE, Sharp SW, St Peter SD. Evaluation of ultrasonographic parameters in the diagnosis of pyloric stenosis relative to patient age and size. *J Pediatr Surg.* 2012;47:1542-1547. doi: 10.1016/j.jpedsurg.2012.03.068.

Jobson M, Hall NJ. Contemporary management of pyloric stenosis. *Semin Pediatr Surg.* 2016;25:219-224. doi: 10.1053/j.sempedsurg.2016.05.004.

Schwartz MZ. Hypertrophic Pyloric Stenosis. In *Pediatric Surgery*, 7th ed. Coran AG (ed). Elsevier, Philadelphia, PA; 2012, pp1021-2028.

Siddiqui S, Heidel RE, Angel CA, Kennedy AP Jr. Pyloromyotomy: randomized control trial of laparoscopic vs open technique. *J Pediatr Surg.* 2012;47:93-98. doi: 10.1016/j.jpedsurg.2011.10.026.

Touloukian RJ, Higgins E. The spectrum of serum electrolytes in hypertrophic pyloric stenosis. *J Pediatr Surg.* 1983;18:394-397. http://dx.doi.org/10.1016/S0022-3468(83)80188-2

Malrotation and Midgut Volvulus

94

RICHARD J. HENDRICKSON AND BARTHOLOMEW J. KANE

Based on the previous edition chapter "Malrotation and Midgut Volvulus" by Adam S. Brinkman and Dennis P. Lund

Presentation

A 5-day-old male infant is brought to the emergency department with bilious emesis. The child was born via an uncomplicated spontaneous vaginal delivery following a full-term pregnancy and had been discharged home on day of life 2 after tolerating feeds. At home, the infant had intermittent fussiness and feeding intolerance with emesis. On day of life 5, the symptoms progressed to bilious emesis and inconsolability. The child has no other medical history, and there is no associated family history of bowel dysfunction. In the emergency department, the mother shows you the child's blanket that is stained with green emesis. The infant is inconsolable. He is afebrile with a heart rate of 152 bpm and a blood pressure of 82/48 mm Hg. Abdominal examination revealed mild abdominal distention and tenderness to palpation. The child's diaper is dry.

● DIFFERENTIAL DIAGNOSIS

Malrotation is the result of an error in development wherein the midgut fails to complete normal conformational changes. The primary developmental steps of normal midgut rotation and fixation begins in the 5th week of development when the midgut elongates, protrudes into the umbilical coelom, and makes a ¼ (90°) counterclockwise rotation. Between the 10th and 11th weeks, the proximal limb returns to the abdominal cavity, making two 90° counterclockwise turns for a total of 270° in counterclockwise rotation. Fixation of the bowel continues from the 11th week until after birth, including the formation of a broad base of the small bowel mesentery and the ligament of Treitz is formed, thereby tethering the duodenojejunal junction (DJJ) in the left upper quadrant. The anatomic abnormalities resulting from malrotation are determined by the stage at which the development happened and occur within a spectrum, ranging between normal rotation and relatively severe reverse rotation. The normally rotated midgut is shown in Figure 94-1A. As the result of malrotation, the DJJ is either located in the right hemiabdomen or at an abnormally low (caudal) position in the left hemiabdomen, and the cecum is typically not located in the right lower quadrant. Atypical malrotation, shown in Figure 94-1B, represents a less

severe form wherein the DJJ is located caudal to the gastric outlet but remains to the left of the vertebral pedicles. In typical malrotation, shown in Figure 94-1C, the DJJ is located to the right of the vertebral pedicles. The cecum is commonly displaced out of the right lower quadrant in both atypical and typical malrotation. Malrotation also results in the formation of Ladd's bands—fibrous peritoneal tissue spanning between the malpositioned cecum and the right abdominal wall that can cause duodenal obstruction. Also seen in Figure 94-1B and C are the fibrous Ladd's bands. In nonrotation, shown in Figure 94-1D, the DJJ is located in right hemiabdomen and colon is commonly located in the left hemiabdomen but can be located anywhere within the abdomen. Reverse rotation, seen in Figure 94-1E is the result of an abnormal 90° clockwise rotation of the midgut, resulting in the ascending colon located in the right hemiabdomen and the transverse colon located posterior to both the duodenum and the superior mesenteric artery (SMA). In addition, the small bowel mesentery in patients with malrotation has a narrow stalk, predisposing the 3rd and 4th portion of the duodenum, the jejunum, the ileum, and the ascending colon to twist on its self or volvulized.

The differential diagnosis list for bilious emesis is age dependent. Infants and toddlers with malrotation commonly present in a classic manner with bilious emesis. The most frequent cause of emesis in an infant is gastroesophageal reflux due to physiologically normally incomplete development of the lower esophageal sphincter. Pyloric stenosis can be confused with malrotation as it is characterized by nonbilious, projectile emesis and occurs with a high prevalence (1:400–1:1,600). True bilious emesis is associated with obstruction or dysfunction of the bowel distal to the ampulla of Vater and includes duodenal atresia/web/stenosis, annular pancreas, jejunal atresia, necrotizing enterocolitis, incarcerated hernia, meconium ileus, and duplication cyst. Pathological processes located in the distal bowel are typically associated with abdominal distention and include imperforate anus, colonic atresia, meconium plug, Hirschsprung's disease, and small left colon syndrome. The estimated prevalence of malrotation in live births ranges broadly between 1:200 and 1:6,000. Malrotation of some form has been found in 0.5% to 1% of subject who underwent an autopsy. Associated congenital gastrointestinal tract anomalies occur in 15% to 20% of infants with malrotation, including intestinal atresia, duodenal web, paraduodenal hernia, Meckel's diverticulum,

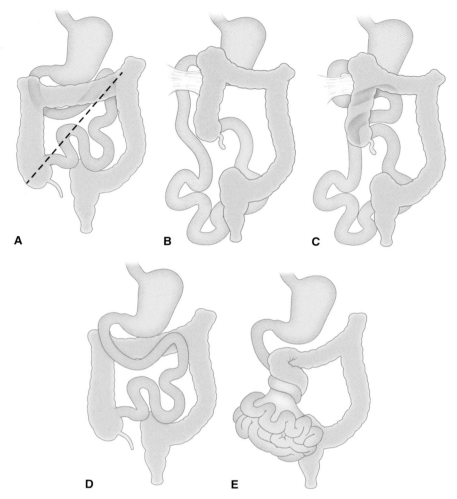

FIGURE 94-1. Intestinal malrotation occurs with a spectrum, with variability in the relative positioning of the stomach, duodenum, small bowl, and colon, including normal rotation **(A)**; nonrotation of the duodenum, small bowel, and colon **(B)**; nonrotation of the colon **(C)**; midgut volvulus due to narrow small bowel mesenteric root **(D)**; and Ladd's fibrous bands between the right lateral abdominal wall and the ascending and right colon overlying and compressing the duodenum **(E)**. This variability in the resulting anatomy can be linked to the variability in the presenting symptoms and timing for presentation. (Reprinted by permission from Springer: Lampl B, Levin TL, Berdon WE, et al. Malrotation and midgut volvulus: a historical review and current controversies in diagnosis and management. *Pediatr Radiol.* 2009;39(4):359-366. Copyright © 2009 Springer-Verlag.)

ileal stenosis, rectal duplication, and Hirschsprung's disease. Individuals with Down's syndrome are 45 times more likely than the general population to have intestinal malrotation (Tables 94-1 and 94-2).

● WORKUP

All patients with suspected malrotation must undergo a focused history and physical exam as well as laboratory value assessment, followed by the prompt performance of an appropriate imaging study. The workup of a patient with suspected malrotation is somewhat age dependent. Malrotation is most commonly diagnosed in the neonatal period, 30% within the first 3 days of life, 50% within the first week, 75% to 80% within the first month, and approximately 90% of symptomatic cases occur before 1 year of life. The classic presentation of infants and pre–school-aged children with malrotation and possible

volvulus is bilious emesis. Because of the significant potential for morbidity and mortality, infants and toddlers with bilious emesis should have an expedited workup under the directed guidance of the consulting surgeon. Only after malrotation and volvulus have been ruled-out in the child, should other causes of the bilious emesis be actively considered.

Determining the timing, quality, and frequency of GI tract–related symptoms is at the forefront in making the correct diagnosis. Ladd's bands cause extrinsic duodenal obstruction, leading to recurrent and episodic feeding intolerance, dehydration, and bilious emesis. Without volvulus, malrotation does not always produce abdominal pain. The extent of the symptoms related to volvulus are dependent on the duration and degree of mesenteric twisting. Initially, mesenteric twisting can lead to obstruction of the enteric lumen and lymphatic system, resulting in abdominal pain, recurrent emesis, dehydration, ascites formation, and abdominal distention. Further twisting leads to venous outflow obstruction,

Table 94-1	Differential Diagnosis for Neonate with Bilious Emesis

Malrotation with midgut volvulus
Gastroesophageal reflux disease
Pyloric stenosis
Duodenal atresia
Duodenal stenosis
Duodenal web
Annular pancreas
Jejunal atresia
Necrotizing enterocolitis
Incarcerated hernia
Duplication cyst
Meconium ileus
Meconium plug
Small left colon syndrome
Colonic atresia
Imperforate anus
Hirschsprung's disease
Congenital adhesions

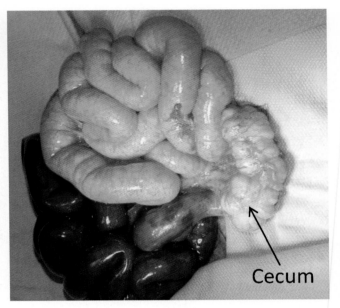

FIGURE 94-2. Appearance of bowel in a 21-month-old boy with malrotation and midgut volvulus resulting in small bowel necrosis.

resulting in compromised mucosal perfusion, bacterial translocation, mucosal sloughing, and bloody bowel movements. With prolonged or severe volvulus, arterial inflow obstruction leads to bowel hypoperfusion, ischemia, transmural necrosis, bowel perforation, peritonitis, and gram-negative sepsis. Bowel ischemia and necrosis as the result of volvulus in a 21-month-old boy is shown in Figure 94-2.

In contrast to infants, the symptoms in school-aged children and adults with malrotation can be vague, intermittent, and subtle including nonspecific abdominal pain, nausea, weight loss, as well as bilious and nonbilious emesis. As a result, it can be much more difficult to diagnose older patients with malrotation. These vague symptoms can be falsely attributed to a psychiatric disorder or to a less specific bowel dysfunction diagnoses such as irritable bowel, cyclical vomiting, and abdominal migraine. This can lead to delay in diagnosis and treatment. A high index of suspicion for malrotation is needed in older patient with vague and chronic abdominal symptoms.

Table 94-2	Congenital Anomalies Associated with Malrotation

Duodenal atresia
Duodenal web
Jejunal atresia
Paraduodenal hernia
Meckel's diverticulum
Ileal stenosis
Rectal stenosis
Hirschsprung's disease
Trisomy 21 (Down's syndrome)
Congenital diaphragmatic hernia
Gastroschisis
Omphalocele
Heterotaxy

Just as is the case with the presenting symptoms, there is a spectrum of physical exam findings in patients with malrotation, ranging from a benign, scaphoid abdomen to an acute abdomen with profound distention, diffuse peritonitis, and abdominal wall erythema. Acute abdomen is less commonly encountered in infants with malrotation. In an infant, abdominal pain is manifest through fussiness and inconsolability. Lethargy in an infant with malrotation is a sign of physiologic decompensation and a harbinger of ongoing bowel hypoperfusion and shock physiology. In school-aged children and adult patients who are capable of verbal communication, the physical exam findings can be subtle, including episodic abdominal distention and epigastric tenderness. For patients with suspected malrotation, complete blood count, basic metabolic panel, and specimen for type and cross should be obtained while the patient is being stabilized and fluid resuscitated. In infants with dehydration due to emesis, the basic metabolic panel may reveal elevated BUN and creatinine, as well as decrease chloride. If volvulus is present, the laboratory values may demonstrate signs of metabolic acidosis with diminished CO_2 and elevated lactate. Laboratory values consistent with metabolic acidosis may not be present if the volvulus has entirely occluded the mesenteric vein.

The most effective way to radiographically evaluate for malrotation and volvulus in an infant or toddler is a prompt upper gastrointestinal (UGI) study performed with barium or water-soluble contrast. The UGI study is used to demonstrate the position of the DJJ in both the frontal and lateral projections. The radiologist must take care to observe and record the first passage of contrast through the entire duodenum. It can be very helpful for the consulting surgeon to be present while the UGI is being performed. As is shown

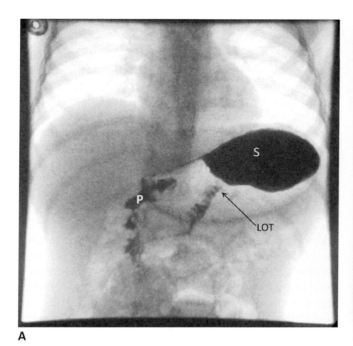

A

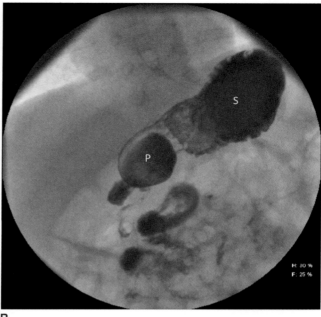

B

FIGURE 94-3. A contrast studies of the upper gastrointestinal tract including the stomach, duodenum, and proximal small bowl. A normal UGI with normally positioned duodenojejunal junction defined by the ligament of Treitz is shown in **(A)**. An abnormal UGI with a low lying duodenojejunal junction is demonstrated in **(B)**.

in Figure 94-3A, the normal position of the DJJ on the frontal view of an upper GI study is to the left of the left-sided vertebral pedicles at the level of the duodenal bulb in the craniocaudal axis. As seen in Figure 94-3B, in patients with malrotation, the DJJ will be abnormally positioned caudal to the duodenal bulb and/or to the right of the left vertebral pedicle. The Ladd's bands produce findings of a dilated, contrast-filled proximal duodenum with z-shaped course of distal duodenum and proximal jejunum. Findings on an UGI consistent with volvulus include a "corkscrew"-shaped course of the distal duodenum in the midabdomen, duodenal luminal narrowing with partial or complete obstruction, or a proximally dilated bowel that tapers to a "bird's beak." In some cases of complete volvulus, none of these patterns are seen because the contrast does not enter the bowel loops.

The most common finding on an abdominal x-ray in a child with malrotation is "normal bowel gas pattern." A normal abdominal x-ray does not preclude further workup for malrotation. A double bubble can be seen on an abdominal x-ray due to duodenal obstruction. A gasless abdomen on abdominal x-ray in conjunction with abdominal distention and tenderness is concerning for midgut volvulus. Adults and school-aged children who are being worked up for malrotation are likely to undergo an abdominal CT scan than any other imaging study. An abdominal CT can effectively diagnose malrotation with demonstration of malpositioned viscera and mesenteric vasculature, as well as volvulus. Finding on abdominal ultrasound (US) of a superior mesenteric vein (SMV) to the left of the SMA or the SMV anterior to the SMA is suggestive of malrotation with a 2% to 3% false-negative rate.

● DIAGNOSIS AND TREATMENT

The decision to operate on a patient with malrotation is dependent upon the age and symptoms. A patient with tachycardia, hypotension, acidosis, and peritonitis with a compelling history for malrotation needs no imaging workup and should be taken immediately to the operating room for Ladd's procedure. Stable patients with symptoms and imaging studies consistent with malrotation are clearly best served by undergoing surgical intervention. In patients with compelling symptoms, but an equivocal imaging study, it is prudent to proceed to the operating room for exploration to directly visualize the anatomy and treat the condition. Laparoscopy is helpful in such cases. Because volvulus rates are reported as high as 70% in infants and toddlers with malrotation, asymptomatic patients with malrotation in this age group are best served by undergoing Ladd's procedure.

The clinical manifestations of malrotation in school-aged children and adults can be chronic, vague, intermittent, and subtle including episodic abdominal pain, distention, nausea, and vomiting. Some patients with malrotation live their entire lives without discernible symptoms. Making the decision to operate in an asymptomatic school-aged child or adult can be challenging. The diagnosis of malrotation in asymptomatic patients is typically made incidentally through imaging studies obtained during the workup of another disease process or vague abdominal symptoms. Some patients thought to be asymptomatic actually have intermittent symptoms that were not previously brought to attention or recognized. Because of this, it is critical to ask focused questions regarding symptoms to distinguish mildly symptomatic patients from asymptomatic patients.

There remains controversy regarding the need for surgery in school-aged children and adults with asymptomatic malrotation. Researchers have attempted to determine the age range in asymptomatic individuals with malrotation where the risks of Ladd's procedure outweigh the benefits. The rates of Ladd's procedure in the general population decrease with age—15 per million in 1-year-olds, 10 per million in 2-year-olds, and approximately 3.5 per million in ages 3 to 17. It is known that adults undergoing Ladd's procedure have lower rate (15% to 20%) of acute volvulus or ischemia. Major complications and reoperation occur at a higher rate in adults than in children (50% vs. 7% and 40% vs. 0%, respectively). Based upon Markov's decision analysis with input from administrative databases, performing Ladd's procedure in an asymptomatic patient with malrotation provides a benefit when the patient is younger than 20 years old.

There are currently no reliable diagnostic studies that accurately predict the risk for volvulus in asymptomatic patients with malrotation. Several studies have demonstrated that asymptomatic patients with atypical malrotation have a lower risk of volvulus relative to those with typical malrotation (2% vs. 16%). Atypical malrotation, shown in Figure 94-1B, is identified on UGI when the DJJ found to be located below the level of the gastric outlet but to the left of the left-sided spinal pedicles. The risk for post-Ladd's procedure complications is elevated in patients with atypical malrotation (22% vs. 13%). Though these data suggest that there may be a role for observation in patients with atypical malrotation, further study is needed. As there is no accurate way to predict the risk for volvulus in older asymptomatic patients with malrotation, in order to make a decision regarding operative intervention, it is critical to have a thorough discussion that includes the patient, their family, and any involved consulting services such as gastroenterology or cardiology.

● SURGICAL APPROACH

In infants and toddlers with suspected malrotation, access to the abdominal cavity for Ladd's procedure is achieved through a generous horizontal supraumbilical incision that extends from the right upper quadrant to cross the midline. In school-aged children and adults, assess to the abdomen for Ladd's procedure can be obtained through a generous upper midline incision. The presence of ascites is a sign of volvulus with lymphatic and possible vascular obstruction. Foul-smelling ascites or pneumoperitoneum are signs of bowel ischemia and necrosis. Upon initial inspection, it can be difficult to sort out the gastrointestinal anatomy. Herniating the small bowel from the abdomen can aid in clarifying the anatomy. As is shown in Figure 94-4A, the first step of Ladd's procedure is to reduce the small bowel volvulus by rotating the volvulized small bowel between 1 and 3 complete 360° rotations, most commonly in a

counterclockwise direction. Following reduction of the volvulus, the bowel is inspected for signs of ischemic injury, necrosis, or perforation. Clearly necrotic bowel should be resected at that time. Bowel with any question regarding viability should remain and be inspected at the end of the case. The second step of the procedure is to take down Ladd's bands, the fibrous adhesive bands spanning between the ascending or right colon and the right abdominal side wall. As illustrated in Figure 94-4B, these bands are taken down completely with either electrocautery or sharply with scissors. Following lysis of Ladd's band, the duodenum can be visualized and is often found to have a redundant, accordion-like configuration. The root of the small bowel mesentery is then assessed. If it is narrow, it can be broadened by opening the peritoneum that makes up the anterior surface to mesenteric leaflet. Incising the mesenteric peritoneum results in increased distance between the duodenum and the cecum as well as an increased distance between the branches of the SMA. An incidental appendectomy is then performed to prevent a future diagnostic dilemma. The bowel on a broad-based mesentery can then be placed in the nonrotated configuration with the duodenum and small bowel located in the right hemiabdomen and the colon located in the left (Figure 94-4C and D).

The laparoscopic Ladd's procedure has been shown to be safe, effective, and associated with shorter hospital stays. With the laparoscopic approach, a primary port is placed in the umbilical region and two additional ports or stab incisions are then placed symmetrically lateral to the rectus abdominis muscles and at approximately the same level as the umbilical port in the craniocaudal axis. The same basic steps are performed in both the laparoscopic and the open approaches; with the exception that it can be easier to divide the Ladd's bands *before* reducing the volvulus in a counterclockwise direction. The approach should be converted to open if anatomy cannot be fully clarified, volvulus cannot be reduced, or if bowel is compromised, friable, necrotic, or perforated.

● SPECIAL INTRAOPERATIVE CONSIDERATION

The classic pitfalls that can be encountered in either the laparoscopic or open approach to the Ladd's procedures are outlined in Table 94-3. The first pitfall can be interpreting the often-confusing gastrointestinal anatomy encountered when entering the abdomen of a patient with malrotation and volvulus. In the open approach, the anatomy can be clarified by eviscerating the bowel entirely out to the abdomen. If a surgeon has limited experience with malrotation, they should have a low threshold to consult with an experienced pediatric or general surgeon. The second potential pitfall is inadequate lysis of Ladd's bands that can result in persistent duodenal obstruction and increases the potential need for a second operation. A third pitfall is to attempt to eliminate the accordion-like redundancy of the duodenum. The duodenal redundancy typically remains following lysis

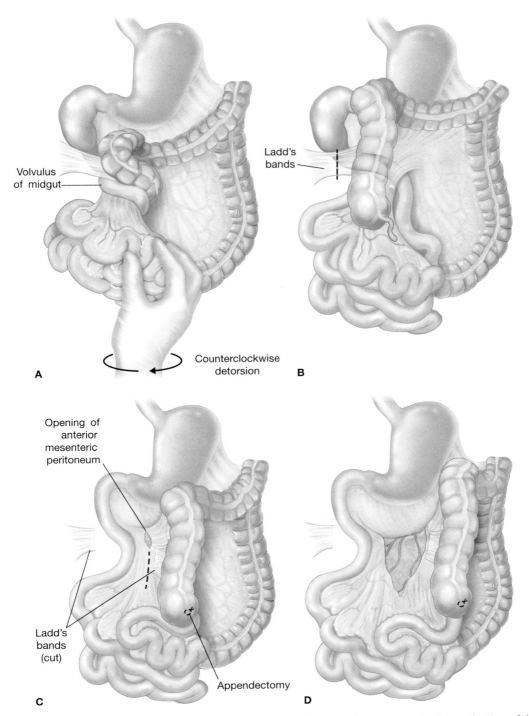

FIGURE 94-4. The primary operative maneuvers performed during Ladd's procedure, demonstrating reduction of the volvulized bowel **(A)**, lysis of the Ladd's bands **(B)**, broadening of the mesentery **(C)**, performance of appendectomy and placement of the bowel into the nonrotated configuration **(D)**.

of Ladd's bands. Attempts to eliminate it are typically unsuccessful and result in duodenal edema, leading to delay in return of bowel function. It is, therefore, not recommended that the operating surgeon persist in attempts to eliminate this redundancy.

While opening the mesenteric peritoneum in order to broaden the narrowed small bowel mesentery, great care

must be taken to avoid damaging the underlying vessels as this can result in loss of blood supply to the bowel, leading to ischemia and necrosis. This peritoneal opening is most easily accomplished in an area where there is protective mesenteric fat overlying the SMA and vein within the narrowed mesenteric root. A fine right angle should be used to elevate the peritoneum, thereby allowing the peritoneum to be divided

Table 94-3   Ladd's Procedure

Key Technical Steps

1. Access to the abdomen through a generous supraumbilical horizontal incision biased to the right in infants and toddlers, upper midline incision in school-aged children and adults.
2. Manual reduce volvulized bowel, typically with 1–3 counterclockwise rotations.
3. Take down Ladd's bands between the right colon and the right abdominal side wall.
4. Perform appendectomy.
5. Broaden small bowel mesentery by opening peritoneum overlying the anterior leaflet of the mesentery with care to prevent damage to underlying vessels.
6. Place bowel in nonrotated configuration with the colon on the left hemiabdomen and small bowel on the right.
7. Resection of clearly compromised bowel with either creation of ostomies or primary anastomosis.

Potential Pitfalls

- Incomplete reduction of volvulus.
- Inadequate lysis of Ladd's bands results in persistent duodenal obstruction.
- Attempts to eliminate redundancy of duodenum resulting in increased duodenal edema.
- Injury to the superior mesenteric artery during broadening of small bowel mesentery resulting in ischemia and necrosis of bowel.
- Fixation of bowel to the abdominal wall can result in an internal hernia.
- Persisting with laparoscopic approach in a case where significant progress has not been made after 30–40 min unnecessarily prolongs procedure.

without damaging the underlying tissue and vessels. No attempts should be made to surgically fix the colon or small bowel to the abdominal side wall as rates of recurrent volvulus after a traditional Ladd's procedure without fixation are low, ranging from 0% to 2.4%. A pitfall that is specific to the minimally invasive approach is the tendency to persist with laparoscopic approach even when no significant progress is being made. To prevent this, the operating surgeon should mark the start time of the case. If little progress has been made after 30 to 40 minutes, the approach should be converted to open.

● POSTOPERATIVE MANAGEMENT

For patients without suspected bowel compromise, postoperative management is largely supportive. The patients are maintained with intravenous fluids, pain medication,

and possibly gastric decompression with a nasogastric tube pending the operative findings. The timing for return of bowel function depends upon the severity of the preoperative obstruction and the overall health of the patient. If there were no intraoperative sign of bowel compromise, enteral feeds typically can be started by postoperative days 2 to 3. Patients with midgut volvulus requiring bowel resection can be critically ill, necessitating admission to the pediatric intensive care unit (PICU) and a longer hospital stay. Critically ill patients such as this require calorie and protein support with total parenteral nutrition (TPN). Pediatric patients with two ostomies may benefit from refeeding of the enteric contents from the proximal ostomy into the distal ostomy.

If there was a question regarding bowel during the initial Ladd's procedure, a reexploration is performed between 24 and 48 hours after the initial laparotomy. During this second laparotomy, the bowel is assessed and any bowel that is found to be compromised or is suspected of compromise is resected. If a postoperative patient decompensates in the PICU with progressive hypotension, tachycardia, and acidosis, or necrotic ostomies, they should be promptly taken back to the operating room for reexploration.

TAKE HOME POINTS

- Bilious emesis in infants and toddlers is malrotation with volvulus until proven otherwise. The prompt performance of a contrast upper GI study is imperative to preserving bowel mass.
- Infants and toddlers with bilious emesis, peritonitis, and hypotension do not need to undergo an upper GI study and should be taken to OR emergently.
- The symptoms of malrotation are variable because the extent the anatomic abnormality is variable, from mild nonrotated colon to a complete nonrotated duodenum, small bowel, and colon with volvulus.
- Making the diagnosis of malrotation in school-aged children and adults requires a high index of suspicion as symptoms can be subtle, vague, intermittent, and vary from patient-to-patient.
- When determining the utility of operative intervention in an asymptomatic patient, it is critical to have an inclusive discussion with the patient, their family, and appropriate consultants.
- For surgeons with limited experience managing malrotation, the open approach is highly suggested as is early herniation of the bowel out of the abdomen and intraoperative consultation with an experienced surgeon.
- Though the laparoscopic approach to Ladd's procedure is safe and effective, the operating surgeon should have low threshold to convert to an open approach if progress has not been made over a span of 30 to 40 minutes.
- Midgut volvulus with compromised bowel viability may require bowel resection, second look laparotomy, open abdomen, admission to PICU, and support with TPN.

SUGGESTED READINGS

Andrassy RJ, Mahour GH. Malrotation of the midgut in infants and children. *Arch Surg.* 1981;116(2):158-160.

Bax NM, van der Zee DC. Laparoscopic treatment of intestinal malrotation in children. *Surg Endosc.* 1998;12:1314-1316.

Dassinger MS, Smith SD. Malrotation. In: Holcomb GW, Murphy JP, Ostlie DJ, eds. *Ashcraft's Pediatric Surgery.* 6th ed. Philadelphia, PA: Elsevier Saunders; 2014:430-438.

Dassinger MS, Smith SD. Disorders of intestinal rotation and fixation. In: Coran AG, et al., eds. *Pediatric Surgery.* 7th ed. Philadelphia, PA: Elsevier Saunders; 2012:1111-1125.

Ford EG, Senac MO, Srikanth MS, Weitzman JJ. Malrotation of the intestine in children. *Ann Surg.* 1992;215(2):172-178.

Fraser JD, Aguayo P, Sharp S, Ostlie D, St. Peter S. The role of laparoscopy in the management of malrotation. *J Surg Res.* 2009;156(1):80-82.

Kapfer SA, Rappold JF. Intestinal malrotation—not just the pediatric surgeon's problem. *J Am Coll Surg.* 2004;199(4):628-635.

McVay MR, Kokaska ER, Jackson RJ, Smith SD. The changing spectrum of intestinal malrotation: diagnosis and management. *Am J Surg.* 2007;194(6):712-718.

Lampl B, Levin TL, Berdon WE, Cowels RA. Malrotation and midgut volvulus: a historical review and current controversies in diagnosis and management. *Pediatr Radiol.* 2009;39:359-366.

Snyder WH, Chaffin L. Embryology and pathology of the intestinal tract: presentation of 40 cases of malrotation. *Ann Surg.* 1954;140(3):368-379.

Strouse PJ. Malrotation. *Semin Roentgenol.* 2008;43(1):7-14.

Neuroblastoma

95

IHAB HALAWEISH AND ERIKA A. NEWMAN

Based on the previous edition chapter "Neuroblastoma" by Erika Newman and Ihab Halaweish

Presentation

A 19-month old baby is brought to her pediatrician with irritability and poor feeding. Abdominal examination reveals a large right-sided abdominal mass. An abdominal ultrasound reveals a large retroperitoneal mass crossing the midline. Urine catecholamines are elevated.

● DIFFERENTIAL DIAGNOSIS

The differential diagnosis of neuroblastoma (NB) is broad and varies according to the location of the mass. Suprarenal and retroperitoneal masses include NB, Wilms' tumor, undifferentiated soft tissue sarcoma, and lymphoma. Metastatic disease in the bone marrow must be distinguished from lymphoma, osteosarcoma, Ewing's sarcoma, and primitive neuroectodermal tumors. NB is the most common cancer in infants and the most common extracranial solid tumor in all children, accounting for 8% to 10% of childhood malignancies. Further cross-sectional imaging to characterize the anatomic nature of the mass is warranted.

● WORKUP

NB is an embryonal cancer of the peripheral sympathetic nervous system with signs and symptoms reflecting the tumor site and extent of disease. Over 50% of cases occur in children <2 years, and 90% of cases are diagnosed by 8 years of age. The majority of NB arises in the retroperitoneum (75%) with 50% in the adrenal gland and 25% in the abdominal and pelvic paravertebral ganglia. The remaining cases are found in the paravertebral ganglia in either cervical or thoracic locations.

In addition to a complete abdominal and pelvic examination, including an evaluation for hypertension, the workup of NB involves a series of radiographic and chemical studies. A plain radiograph of the affected area may reveal stippled calcification within the tumor, common with NB. In children, ultrasound is typically the first imaging modality for solid masses and may reveal a lobulated mass of mixed echogenicity. Computed tomography (CT) with intravenous contrast can provide valuable information regarding the resectability of the mass as detailed by its relationship with surrounding structures and blood vessels, as well as presence of metastases. An intravenous urogram can be obtained during the same study. Large thoracic and abdominal tumors that encase any major blood vessels, encroach the spinal canal, or cross the midline are generally unresectable at diagnosis. Magnetic resonance imaging (MRI) will determine whether spinal extradural tumor extension has occurred. A ^{131}I-metaiodobenzylguanidine (MIBG) nuclear medicine scan is the preferred study for evaluating bone and bone marrow for metastasis. ^{131}I-MIBG is an analogue of norepinephrine and is specifically taken up and stored in the tumor. If imaging confirms a mass suspicious for NB, biopsy or resection of the primary mass and bilateral iliac crest bone marrow aspiration and biopsy are required for staging.

NB is characterized by secretion of catecholamine products, such as vanillylmandelic acid (VMA) and homovanillic acid (HVA), which can be elevated in up to 95% of patients. Urinary levels of VMA and HVA can be used as markers of tumor progression, relapse, and prognosis. Other nonspecific markers include neuron-specific enolase, ferritin, and serum lactate dehydrogenase (LDH).

Presentation Continued

CT scan reveals a right inferior retroperitoneal mass measuring 5.5 cm, with infiltration into the right psoas muscle (Figure 95-1) and extension into the right neural foramina of the L4-L5 disc space without frank intradural extension of the mass (Figure 95-2). Diagnostic MIBG reveals diffuse long bone metastasis and bone marrow infiltration. An open transabdominal biopsy of the mass shows neuroblastoma with unfavorable histology and poor differentiation. Cytogenetics revealed amplification of the *MYCN* oncogene. Bone marrow biopsy is positive for metastatic disease.

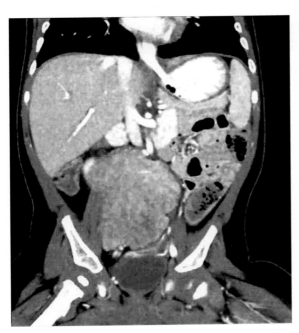

FIGURE 95-1. CT shows a right inferior retroperitoneal mass measuring 5.5 cm, with infiltration into the right psoas muscle.

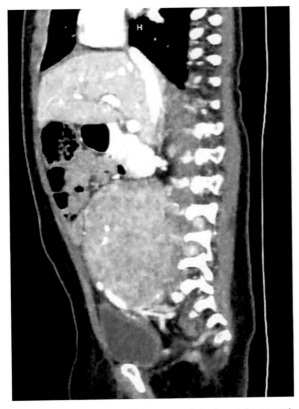

FIGURE 95-2. Extension of the tumor into the right neural foramina of the L4-L5 disc space is demonstrated on CT.

● DIAGNOSIS AND TREATMENT

Patient stratification is important in guiding therapeutic options, and results of the diagnostic workup are used to assign stage. The International Neuroblastoma Staging System (INSS), which takes into account the resectability of the tumor and the lymph nodal status, was previously the most widely accepted staging system. This was supplemented by the Children's Oncology Group (COG) stratification system based on INSS stage, age, *MYCN* status, and Shimada histology that classifies patients into low risk, intermediate risk, and high risk. Because the INSS is a postsurgical staging system, the International Neuroblastoma Risk Group (INRG) classification system was developed to establish a consensus approach for pretreatment risk stratification. The INRG staging system (Cohn et al., 2009) (Table 95-1) is based on a pretreatment risk stratification using image-defined risk factors (IDRFs), rather than resectability (Monclair et al. 2009) (Table 95-2).

There are several karyotypic abnormalities including chromosomal deletions, translocations, and gene amplifications that have been shown to affect prognosis. Aneuploidy of tumor DNA carries a favorable prognosis, whereas amplification of the *MYCN* oncogene (>10 copies) adversely correlates with prognosis independent of clinical stage in up to 30% of patients. Gain of 17q and deletion of the short arm of chromosome 1 (1p deletion) are also associated with poor prognosis.

Treatment modalities used in the management of NB are surgery, chemotherapy, and radiation therapy. Treatment approaches are based upon the previously described risk stratification scheme, which has decreased therapy-related toxicities and improved outcomes. For most patients with

Table 95-1	International Neuroblastoma Risk Group Staging System
Stage	**Definition**
L1	Localized tumor contained within one body compartment without IDRF, including intraspinal tumors not meeting IDRF definition
L2	Local–regional tumor with one or more IDRF, ipsilateral contiguous body compartments
M	Distant metastases excluding MS disease (see below), contralateral contiguous body compartments
MS	L1 or L2 primary, <18 months of age with metastases confined to skin, liver, and/or bone marrow (<10% of nucleated cells) and negative MIBG for bone/bone marrow

IDRF, image-defined risk factor; MIBG, metaiodobenzylguanidine.

Table 95-2   Image-Defined Risk Factors

Anatomic Region	Image-Defined Risk Factors
Multiple body compartments	Ipsilateral tumor extension into two body compartments, includes neck and chest, chest and abdomen, abdomen and pelvis
Neck	Tumor compressing trachea or encasing carotid or vertebral artery or internal jugular vein, tumor extending to the skull base
Cervicothoracic area	Tumor compressing trachea or encasing brachial plexus, carotid or vertebral artery or subclavian vessels
Chest	Tumor compressing trachea or principal bronchi or encasing aorta or major branches, tumor infiltrating costovertebral junction between levels T9 and T12
Thoracoabdominal	Tumor encasing aorta or vena cava
Abdomen/pelvis	Tumor infiltrating porta hepatis; hepatoduodenal ligament or renal pedicles; tumor encasing superior mesenteric artery at mesenteric root; origin of celiac axis, aorta, inferior vena cava, or iliac vessels; tumor crossing sciatic notch
Intraspinal	Tumor extension in any location that invades more than one-third of the spinal canal in the axial plane; the perimedullary leptomeningeal spaces are not visible, or there is abnormal signal intensity of the spinal cord
Adjacent organ infiltration	Infiltration of the pericardium, diaphragm, kidney, liver, duodenopancreatic block, or mesentery

localized disease (L1), complete resection of the tumor may be sufficient. Achieving complete macroscopic clearance is not essential as minor residual disease is usually acceptable with cure rates of >90% without further therapy. Chemotherapy is indicated in the event of relapse or in the presence of *MYCN* amplification with unfavorable histology.

Upfront resection of L2 tumors has been associated with an increased rate of surgical complications without significant improvement in survival. Tumor resection should be delayed until after four cycles of induction chemotherapy with agents, such as cyclophosphamide, vincristine, dacarbazine, doxorubicin, cisplatin, and teniposide, to improve resectability and minimize complications. Initial surgery for L2 tumors is usually limited to a biopsy of the tumor, bone marrow biopsy for staging, or placement of vascular access.

Up to 40% to 50% of patients have metastatic disease at diagnosis. In older patients, NB has a pattern of metastatic disease to the bone marrow, lymph nodes, and bone. In such cases, diagnosis of NB is usually confirmed by bone marrow biopsy and elevation of catecholamines in the urine. As with L2 tumors, surgery of the primary and metastatic disease is delayed until after four cycles of induction chemotherapy.

In patients with stage MS disease, only supportive therapy is recommended because of the overall good prognosis and high incidence of spontaneous regression. Complications are usually secondary to complications of the disease. Limited chemotherapy, low-dose radiotherapy, or minimal resection may be required in the face of large tumors or life-threatening

hepatomegaly, mechanical obstruction, or respiratory compromise. For those infants with life-threatening symptoms of hepatomegaly, placement of a temporary abdominal wall silastic pouch can reduce the intra-abdominal pressure until initiation of chemotherapy.

Presentation Continued

In this scenario, given the *MYCN* status and locoregional disease with extension into the spinal canal, the disease is staged as L2 and high risk. The patient is started on four cycles of chemotherapy with carboplatin and etoposide. Repeat imaging shows reduction of tumor size with continued extension into the right L4-L5 neural foramina.

● SURGICAL APPROACH

The goal of surgical resection, either upfront or after induction chemotherapy, is complete tumor resection without harm to contiguous structures or disability. Epidural anesthesia is often considered and provides excellent pain control in the postoperative period. For abdominal tumors, a full inspection of the liver with biopsy of any suspicious lesions and a sampling of lymph nodes are warranted for adequate staging and treatment planning. A minimum of six to nine nodes should be obtained from the paraaortic

Table 95-3	Neuroblastoma Resection

Key Technical Steps

1. The operation is approached as a "vascular" operation where identification and skeletonization of the major intra-abdominal vessels is crucial. The tumor can generally be separated from the vessel via a subadventitial plane dissection.
2. Careful handling of the tumor during dissection is important to avoid tumor spill and hemorrhage.
3. For retroperitoneal and pelvic tumors, dissection commences distal to the inferior edge of the tumor, along the common or external iliac artery, and proceeds proximally along the aorta, identifying the major arterial branches and left renal vein.
4. Excessive torque on the renal artery when clearing the tumor can lead to intimal injury of the artery and vessel spasm or thrombosis, leading to renal ischemia.
5. The tumor can typically be removed en bloc off of the mesenteric and renal vessels; however, piecemeal resection with splitting of the tumor may be necessary to avoid injury to the liver, bowel, spleen, and kidneys.
6. Routine retroperitoneal lymph node dissection is usually not performed; it is important, however, to excise suspicious paraaortic and perirenal lymph nodes for staging purposes.

Potential Pitfalls

- It is essential to make all attempts to preserve the kidney in cases of suprarenal NB or renal vascular encasement.
- Postoperative renal failure can significantly delay initiation of chemotherapy. Additionally, patients with postoperative renal failure are not candidates for myeloablative chemotherapy with autologous bone marrow transplant, a critical adjuvant therapy impacting survival outcomes.

region (hiatus to the bifurcation). The same principles apply to tumors in the cervical and thoracic regions, though sampling of contralateral nodes is not required. During thoracotomy for thoracic tumors or laparotomy for abdominal/pelvic masses arising from the sympathetic ganglia, it may be impossible to avoid leaving small amounts of gross or microscopic residual disease along the nerve roots at the foramina. The areas are marked with titanium clips for postoperative monitoring. A small amount of residual disease with negative lymph nodes could still result in a good prognosis.

For tumors with vascular encasement encountered intraoperatively, the tumor rarely invades into the tunica media of major blood vessels. The key principle is to identify major blood vessels early before they enter the tumor and then proceed with a careful and meticulous dissection performed outside the subadventitial plane.

The use of minimally invasive surgical techniques for resection of NB has become a viable alternative to open surgery, especially with adrenal NB. Data from several case series show that thoracoscopic and laparoscopic techniques are safe with equivalent long-term oncologic outcomes in carefully selected patients. Tumor size >6 cm and vascular invasion are relative contraindications to minimally invasive techniques. Laparoscopic biopsy of NB is an attractive alternative for advanced tumors (Table 95-3).

Presentation Continued

The patient underwent exploratory laparotomy with finding of tumor involving the right psoas paraspinal muscles, right iliac vein, inferior vena cava, and right iliac artery. The tumor, along with paraaortic lymph nodes, was resected with gross negative margins except for tumor extension into the neural foramina at L4.

● SPECIAL INTRAOPERATIVE CONSIDERATIONS

NB can often extend into the spinal canal (dumbbell tumors). Cord compression can occur in children who are at low risk and is an oncologic emergency requiring rapid intervention. Extraction of tumor from this location is controversial and can be associated with significant complications. Retrospective analyses show similar neurologic outcomes for patients treated with chemotherapy versus laminectomy. Current management in the presence of an intraspinal component of NB is chemotherapy to avoid the need for laminotomy or laminectomy at the time of resection of the primary tumor. Neurosurgery interventions should be reserved for patients with rapid neurologic deterioration or worsening symptoms while receiving chemotherapy.

The aggressiveness with which to pursue gross total resection, especially in the setting of bulky or extensive intra-abdominal involvement, remains intensely debated. Some research suggests that accepting incomplete resection to avoid serious complications may not impact local control rate and outcome in high-risk patients who are treated with intensive multimodality therapy. Future clinical trials are ongoing.

Presentation Continued

It was elected not to remove the tumor in the laminar space due to the morbidity risk. Pathology revealed viable tumor with extension to the margins as well as angiolymphatic invasion and positive adjacent lymph nodes.

● POSTOPERATIVE MANAGEMENT

Postoperative care follows the same principles as any major laparotomy or thoracotomy. Pain management is through epidural infusion or intravenous opiate infusion. Arterial and central venous pressures are typically monitored for 24 to 48 hours. Intake and output are monitored closely. Postoperative ileus usually lasts 3 to 4 days postoperatively. Drainage tubes can be checked for amylase/lipase or creatinine if there is a concern for pancreatic or urinary leak. Chemotherapy can be initiated 7 to 10 days postoperatively if patient is sufficiently recovered without fever, wound complications, or signs of infection.

Case Conclusion

The patient undergoes four additional cycles of chemotherapy and completed all adjuvant therapy based on current COG recommendations. Since completion of therapy, the patient has been doing well. At 1-year follow-up, MRI of the abdomen and pelvis continues to show no evidence of disease recurrence, and MIBG reveals no active metastatic bone lesions.

TAKE HOME POINTS

- NB is the most common tumor in infants and the most common extracranial solid neoplasm in all children.
- Most NB arises in the abdomen, with the adrenal gland being the most common primary site. Half of the patients will present with metastatic disease.
- NB is a clinically heterogeneous tumor with a natural history that ranges from regression and complete

resolution to progression with metastasis and eventual death.

- The outcomes for patients with low- and intermediate-risk NB has improved, largely through the recognition of the significant therapy-related complications and a subsequent reduction in therapy intensity, although the survival for high-risk disease remains poor.
- NB is staged using a pretreatment risk stratification based on image-defined risk factors.
- Unless the tumor is localized, initial therapy for NB is induction chemotherapy with myeloablative therapy after surgery based on risk stratification.
- In the absence of complications, stage MS patients usually receive supportive care because of the high rate of regression.
- Complete surgical excision is the goal of operative therapy though effort should be made to preserve adjacent organs and organ function.

SUGGESTED READINGS

Baker DL, Schmidt ML, Cohn SL, et al. Outcome after reduced chemotherapy for intermediate-risk neuroblastoma. *N Engl J Med.* 2010;363(14):1313-1323.

Brisse HJ, McCarville MB, Granata C, et al. Guidelines for imaging and staging of neuroblastic tumors: consensus report from the International Neuroblastoma Risk Group Project. *Radiology.* 2011;261(1):243-257.

Cohn SL, Pearson ADJ, London WB, et al. The International Neuroblastoma Risk Group (INRG) classification system: an INRG task force report. *J Clin Oncol.* 2009;27(2):289-297.

Davidoff A. Neuroblastoma. In: Holcomb G, Murphy J, Ostlie D, eds. *Ashcraft's Pediatric Surgery.* 6th ed. Philadelphia, PA: Elsevier; 2014:883-905.

Irtan S, Brisse HJ, Minard-Colin V, et al. Image-defined risk factor assessment of neurogenic tumors after neoadjuvant chemotherapy is useful for predicting intra-operative risk factors and the completeness of resection. *Pediatr Blood Cancer.* 2015;62(9): 1543-1549.

Monclair T, Brodeur GM, Ambros PF, et al. The International Neuroblastoma Risk Group (INRG) staging system: an INRG task force report. *J Clin Oncol.* 2009;27(2):298-303.

Nuchtern JG, London WB, Barnewolt CE, et al. A prospective study of expectant observation as primary therapy for neuroblastoma in young infants: a Children's Oncology Group study. *Ann Surg.* 2012;256(4):573-580.

Schmidt ML, Lukens JN, Seeger RC, et al. Biologic factors determine prognosis in infants with stage IV neuroblastoma: a prospective Children's Cancer Group study. *J Clin Oncol.* 2000;18(6): 1260-1268.

Simon T, Haberle B, Hero B, et al. Role of surgery in the treatment of patients with stage 4 neuroblastoma age 18 months or older at diagnosis. *J Clin Oncol.* 2013;31(6):752-758.

Strother DR, London WB, Schmidt ML, et al. Outcome after surgery alone or with restricted use of chemotherapy for patients with low-risk neuroblastoma: results of Children's Oncology Group study P9641. *J Clin Oncol.* 2012;30(15):1842-1848.

Palpable Abdominal Mass in a Toddler

96

SCOTT S. SHORT AND DOUGLAS C. BARNHART

Based on the previous edition chapter "Palpable Abdominal Mass in a Toddler" by Douglas C. Barnhart

Presentation

A 15-month-old boy who was born prematurely at 28 weeks' gestation is growing and developing normally. He has no other medical problems or long-term sequelae of prematurity. While giving him a bath, his mother notes a large mass that seems to be left sided. He is examined by his pediatrician who confirms the presence of large abdominal mass that is not tender. His vital signs including blood pressure are normal. Routine laboratories including a CBC and urinalysis are normal.

● DIFFERENTIAL DIAGNOSIS

The sudden recognition of a large abdominal mass in an infant or a young child is not an uncommon occurrence and is the typical presentation for most intra-abdominal malignancies in this age group. These masses are often very large at presentation and are typically nontender and apparently asymptomatic. The most common malignancies of early childhood, which present with large abdominal masses, are Wilms' tumor (nephroblastoma), neuroblastoma, and hepatoblastoma. Less common primary pediatric renal tumors include congenital mesoblastic nephroma (infants <6 months), clear cell sarcoma, rhabdoid tumor, and renal carcinoma. Rhabdomyosarcoma may also present with a large abdominal mass, although this is more typically located in the pelvis as it often arises from the genitourinary tract. Less common abdominal malignancies in a young child are germ cell tumors and lymphoma.

It is important to recognize that not all palpable abdominal lesions in the young child are malignancies. Massive hydronephrosis can present with a large unilateral abdominal mass. However, it would be common for these to be detected on prenatal ultrasound. Autosomal dominant polycystic kidney disease can present with bilaterally enlarged kidneys that may be palpable on physical examination. Large omental cysts, duplication cysts of the gastrointestinal tract, lymphatic malformations, and ovarian cysts may also present with abdominal fullness and possibly a palpable mass.

● WORKUP

Given the lifelong risk of malignancy associated with radiation exposure in children, CT scans should be used judiciously. Abdominal ultrasound is the preferred initial study in a child presenting with a palpable abdominal mass. Most of the benign diagnoses can be made with the use of ultrasound alone. Patients with hydronephrosis, polycystic kidney disease, and ovarian cysts are not likely to require a CT scan for diagnosis and management. Children with solid or mixed (solid and cystic) lesions on ultrasound should undergo a CT scan with oral and intravenous contrast to characterize the organ of origin and anatomic extent of the mass. In some cases, it can be difficult to discern if a large tumor is arising from the liver (hepatoblastoma), adrenal gland (neuroblastoma), or kidney (Wilms' tumor).

Presentation Continued

This patient underwent a contrast CT scan that demonstrated a 7-cm mass arising from the left kidney. The CT scan demonstrated a "claw sign" in which the remaining renal parenchyma encircles the mass (Figure 96-1). This suggests a primary renal tumor even if the mass abuts and displaces the liver, and the adrenal gland is not visualized. As Wilms' tumor can occur bilaterally (5% of all children with Wilms' tumors), it is important to assure that the contralateral kidney is normal. The CT scan often demonstrates compression of the inferior vena cava (IVC) by the mass. Wilms' tumor is prone to develop tumor thrombi, which can extend into the vena cava and even the right atrium. A Doppler ultrasound is typically obtained to evaluate the renal vein and the IVC. The lungs and liver are the most common sites of distant metastases. A chest CT is therefore obtained as part of the preoperative staging evaluation. The child's ultrasound demonstrated no signs of tumor thrombus in the IVC, and there were no distant metastases.

● DIAGNOSIS AND TREATMENT

Based on the age at presentation and appearance on CT scan, this toddler is presumed to have a Wilms' tumor and should be managed accordingly. The treatment of Wilms' tumor is multimodal and has been defined initially through the National Wilms' Tumor Study and subsequently through Children's Oncology Group trials in North America. Similar organizations in Europe (International Society of Paediatric

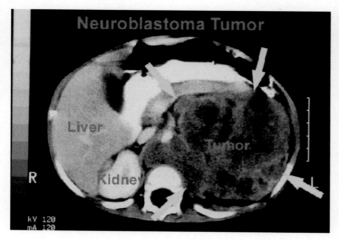

FIGURE 96-1. The child's CT scan demonstrates a large solitary mass involving the left kidney. The renal parenchyma is displaced by the tumor. This "claw sign" is seen more clearly on the coronal images. The right kidney is normal. There was no evidence of hepatic or pulmonary metastases.

Table 96-1	Wilms' Tumor Staging

Stage	Description
I	Tumor limited to the kidney and resected without disruption of the capsule or the biopsy.
II	Tumor extends beyond the kidney but is resected completely without spillage of tumor. Tumor may extend into renal sinus or beyond renal capsule but is contained within a pseudocapsule. All margins and lymph nodes are free of tumor.
III	Residual nonhematogenous tumor confined to the abdomen. Occurs in several ways: preoperative rupture, peritoneal implants, intraoperative spill, biopsy (preoperative or intraoperative), residual tumor left due to involvement of adjacent structures, resection margin positive on final pathology, lymph nodes involved.
IV	Hematogenous metastases (most commonly to the lung or liver).
V	Bilateral renal tumors.

Oncology [SIOP]) and the United Kingdom have conducted clinical trials as well. Essentially, all children are treated with surgical resection and chemotherapy. Radiation therapy is used to treat pulmonary metastases and selectively to enhance intra-abdominal local control. There are fundamental differences between the North American and European approaches to Wilms' tumor. The American approach favors upfront resection to provide immediate local control and accurate staging. This strategy may potentially diminish the required chemotherapy. The European strategy treats with chemotherapy presumptively without biopsy or initial resection in many cases. This strategy simplifies resection as there is often a dramatic response to chemotherapy. This may decrease the rate of intraoperative tumor rupture but confound accurate staging as lymph node status prior to treatment is unknown. The remainder of this discussion will focus on the American approach.

All children with Wilms' tumor should be treated in a center with a multidisciplinary team. Survival in children with Wilms' tumor is principally determined by the stage at presentation and the presence or absence of diffuse anaplasia (Table 96-1). More recent studies suggest that loss of genetic material at 1p and 16q may also be associated with poorer outcomes. Children with favorable histology (lack of anaplasia) and lower stages (I to II) have excellent outcomes with standard two-drug chemotherapy (vincristine and dactinomycin). Typical therapy for children with higher stages of favorable histology Wilms' tumors adds a third drug such as doxorubicin. More complicated regimens using multiple other combinations are also used in stages III and IV. Children with favorable histology even stage IV do well having overall survival of near 90%. Anaplasia is associated with resistance to chemotherapy. These children do more poorly with overall survival in stage IV patients approximately 50%. Due to the markedly

decreased survival associated with this histology, adjunctive chemotherapy regimens for these patients remain an active area of research.

Abdominal radiation therapy is used to improve local control in patients with local stage III disease. Whole-lung radiation is standard therapy for children with pulmonary metastases, but current research is directed to see whether this can be eliminated in those who have complete response to a more intensive chemotherapy regimen.

Management of children with bilateral Wilms' tumors (stage V) requires preservation of renal function, while not jeopardizing oncologic cure. Decisions regarding biopsy and resection in these complicated children must be done as part of multidisciplinary approach and are beyond the scope of this discussion. In brief, the contemporary approach begins with neoadjuvant therapy without biopsy. The timing and operative approach for subsequent nephron-sparing resections are based on the response to chemotherapy.

Decisions regarding local control are made independently of the presence of distant metastases. The three principal goals of laparotomy for Wilms' tumor are to (1) obtain accurate diagnosis and staging, (2) resect the primary tumor without causing local upstaging (i.e., tumor spillage), and (3) avoid resection of adjacent organs. Many Wilms' tumors present as very large masses, and size per se should not be considered a contraindication to upfront resection. Contraindications to initial resection include extensive venous tumor thrombus, invasion of adjacent organs, pulmonary compromise due to extensive pulmonary metastasis, or if nephrectomy would result in unnecessary morbidity or tumor spill. Tumor thrombus in Wilms' tumor can be extensive with involvement of the retrohepatic IVC and the right atrium. In such cases, operative biopsy and pre-resection chemotherapy are recommended as they typically reduce the thrombus facilitating resection. Tumor thrombus in the renal vein and infrahepatic vena cava can typically be extracted after obtaining vascular control of the IVC. The extent of tumor thrombus can be accurately characterized preoperatively using CT scan and ultrasound. In contrast, extension to adjacent organs can often not be determined preoperatively. With the exception of the adrenal gland, other involved organs should not be resected as a part of the initial operation. Rather in such cases, an operative biopsy should be performed, and nephrectomy deferred until chemotherapy is given.

● SURGICAL APPROACH

Given the large size and fragility of Wilms' tumors, generous exposure is required to avoid tumor rupture during resection. The importance of this cannot be overstated as tumor rupture will necessitate abdominal radiation even if the child was stage I or II preoperatively. Additionally, the large size of the mass frequently distorts relationships with adjacent visceral vessels making exposure essential for protection of the mesenteric and the contralateral renal vessels. The ureter must be resected with an adequate margin to assure that it is free of tumor. Finally, proper staging must include aortocaval lymph node sampling and inspection of the peritoneal surfaces.

In order to accomplish these goals, a generous transverse laparotomy is typically performed (Table 96-2). For large right-sided tumors, a thoracoabdominal exposure may facilitate vascular control and mobilization of the tumor. A retroperitoneal, flank approach is not appropriate due to the large size of these tumors and the clinical significance of an intraoperative rupture. Laparoscopic resection is not appropriate for upfront resection but is being explored using the European approach of delayed resection after preoperative chemotherapy.

Upon entry into the peritoneal cavity, inspection and palpation are performed for staging, and all findings are documented. Any bloody fluid in the peritoneum is recorded and collected. The peritoneum is inspected for tumor implants. Either of these findings would suggest preoperative tumor rupture. The liver is inspected and palpated, although most lesions would be identified on preoperative imaging. In the past, the contralateral kidney was exposed, inspected, and palpated on both the anterior and the posterior surfaces. This maneuver placed this typically normal and soon-to-be solitary kidney at risk of injury. Given the accuracy of current CT scans, this is not necessary and should be avoided. If there is no obvious invasion of adjacent organs on this initial examination, it is appropriate to begin mobilization for nephrectomy. In the case of obvious invasion of other organs, a wedge biopsy should be performed. A generous biopsy should be obtained as core needle biopsies may fail to detect

Table 96-2	Palpable Abdominal Mass in a Toddler

Key Technical Steps

1. Generous transverse supraumbilical laparotomy or thoracoabdominal approach.
2. Inspection of the peritoneum for evidence of rupture, peritoneal implants, or other metastases.
3. Mobilize the colon and duodenum to expose tumor and involved kidney.
4. Mobilize tumor and kidney without disruption of capsule.
5. Control renal artery and vein. Palpate vein to evaluate for tumor thrombus. Divide artery followed by vein.
6. Mobilize the ureter into pelvis to allow resection en bloc.
7. Aortocaval lymph node sampling.

Potential Pitfalls

- Unnecessary biopsy of mass.
- Disruption of tumor capsule resulting in spillage of tumor.
- Resection of adjacent organs (except adrenal gland) (invasion should prompt biopsy and chemotherapy prior to resection).
- Misidentification and subsequent division of mesenteric or contralateral renal vessels.
- Failure to perform aortocaval lymph node sampling.

anaplasia. Any type of biopsy is considered to cause rupture of the tumor and results in upstaging of the tumor (stage III). Therefore, a tumor that can be resected should not be biopsied simply to confirm the diagnosis prior to resection.

After resection is decided upon, the peritoneal reflection of the ipsilateral portion of the colon is divided to allow the colon to be mobilized medially. The duodenum is similarly mobilized to allow exposure of the renal hilum, IVC, and aorta. If the aorta can be exposed initially, the renal artery should be isolated and divided after mobilization and retraction of the renal vein. This is followed by ligation of the vein. In most cases, however, the tumor is sufficiently large that the IVC and the aorta will be obscured. In these cases, initial mobilization of the tumor will be required to allow access to the aorta and the IVC.

The tumor is mobilized typically in a gradual circumferential fashion. It is common for there to be neovascularity from the retroperitoneum. Vessel-sealing devices are helpful in this mobilization. Careful attention must be paid to avoid traction on the mass as the tumor capsule is easily disrupted resulting in spillage of tumor. If the ipsilateral adrenal gland is adherent to the tumor, it should be resected along with the nephrectomy specimen. No attempt to separate the adrenal gland should be made if this may increase the risk of tumor rupture. As the nephrectomy specimen is circumferentially mobilized, the ureter will become apparent. The ureter should be dissected distally to allow resection en bloc with the nephrectomy specimen. The ureter is divided as distally as possible, but it is unnecessary to resect a cuff of bladder. Mobilization of the tumor allows it to be rolled medially to provide posterior exposure of the renal artery. Duplicated renal arteries are common and should be sought. Dissection of the renal vein allows it to be retracted to provide anterior exposure of the renal artery was well. With left-sided tumors, the gonadal vein may be divided to facilitate this exposure.

Ideally, the artery is ligated prior to division of the renal vein to avoid engorgement of the tumor. There can be marked distortion of the mesenteric and the contralateral renal vessels with large Wilms' tumors, so it is essential to achieve adequate exposure of the aorta to verify the anatomy prior to ligation of the purported renal artery. The renal vein should be palpated for tumor thrombus prior to ligation. If there is tumor thrombus present, proximal and distal control of the IVC must be obtained so that renal vein/IVC junction can be opened for a tumor thrombectomy. Typically, the tumor thrombus is not densely adherent and can be withdrawn through the venotomy with forceps. Division of the renal vessels and ureter provides access to any remaining retroperitoneal attachments that can be divided with electrocautery to complete the nephrectomy.

The nephrectomy specimen should be sent intact to pathology. As an important part of the pathologic staging of Wilms' tumor is a systematic microscopic examination of inked margins, bivalving the specimen in the operating room is contraindicated.

After removal of the nephrectomy specimen, the aorta and IVC are clearly visible allowing aortocaval lymph node sampling. As 40% of stage III tumors are due to lymph node involvement only, this node sampling is essential to correct staging. All visible aortocaval lymph nodes are removed, but it is not necessary to perform a formal lymph node dissection that may be associated with increased morbidity. Mesenteric lymph node sampling is likely to be of little value unless enlarged or pathologic in appearance. Hemostasis is verified and lymphatic leaks sought prior to closure of the laparotomy.

Consideration should be given to placing a subcutaneous venous access port at the time of nephrectomy. This should be decided in discussion with the pediatric medical oncologist as some children with stage I tumors may be successfully managed with only a peripherally inserted central catheter. Further, data from the ARENO532 study demonstrated that chemotherapy may be safely eliminated in children under age 2 with stage I tumors <550 g in 85% of cases. Future studies are likely to evaluate elimination of chemotherapy in children up to age 4 with tumors <1,000 g. All others can typically be treated with a single-lumen central venous access device.

POSTOPERATIVE CARE

Children may be admitted to the acute care floor or intensive care dependent upon local practice with particular attention to assuring adequate analgesia and fluid resuscitation. Many children will benefit from epidural analgesia if it is available. It is essential to assure adequate intravascular volume to provide perfusion to the now solitary kidney, and urine output should be carefully monitored typically with a Foley catheter. Most children's postoperative ileus is relatively brief (2 to 4 days), and nasogastric decompression is not routinely required. Small bowel: small bowel intussusception can occur in the immediate postoperative period in children who underwent resection of retroperitoneal tumors. This should be sought if the child seems to have a prolonged postoperative ileus or an immediate postoperative bowel obstruction.

Chemotherapy is typically initiated prior to discharge home from the operation (usually by postoperative day 5). After completion of chemotherapy and possible radiation therapy, surveillance is performed using chest and abdominal CT scans. Local recurrences in the renal bed are managed with resection and radiation in addition to chemotherapy.

Case Conclusion

The boy undergoes a laparotomy and is found to have an intact tumor capsule without evidence of metastatic disease. A tumor nephrectomy is performed without spillage. There was no involvement of the renal vein. Final pathology showed stage I favorable histology Wilms' tumor. He was treated with a standard course of vincristine and dactinomycin and is currently in remission.

TAKE HOME POINTS

- Wilms' tumor is the most common renal tumor in children. Renal masses in children are managed presumptively as Wilms' tumor.
- Outcomes are dependent on the stage and the presence or absence of diffuse anaplasia.
- Decisions about local control via nephrectomy are independent of hematogenous metastases.
- Preoperative or intraoperative biopsy should be avoided to not upstage tumor and mandate abdominal radiation.
- Primary resection of the tumor should be performed avoiding disruption of the tumor capsule or resection of adjacent organs.
- Aortocaval lymph node sampling is essential for accurate staging.
- Adjunctive chemotherapy is routine, while radiotherapy is used to supplement local control in stage III tumors and for pulmonary metastases.

SUGGESTED READINGS

Davidoff AM. Wilms' tumor. *Curr Opin Pediatr.* 2009;21(3):357-364.
Ehrlich PF. Wilm's tumor: progress and considerations for the surgeon. *Surg Oncol.* 2007;16(3):157-171.
Melkan AD. An approach to renal masses in pediatrics. *Pediatrics.* 2015;135(1):242-258.

Hepatoblastoma

TERRY LYNN BUCHMILLER

97

Based on the previous edition chapter "Hepatoblastoma" by Terry L. Buchmiller

Presentation

A 2-year-old previously healthy girl presents to her pediatrician with a right upper abdominal fullness discovered yesterday by her mother during bathing. She has seemed a bit more tired than usual after playing and has been eating less at mealtimes for a week. She has had no fevers, no recent travel, and no other family members are ill. On physical examination, she is listless, though well hydrated and afebrile. She has no scleral icterus and no adenopathy. Her lungs are clear to auscultation. A firm, nonmobile mass is palpated in the right upper quadrant (RUQ) just under the costal margin. It is not tender but moves with respiration. Her abdomen is otherwise soft and nondistended, and she has no peritoneal signs.

● DIFFERENTIAL DIAGNOSIS

The differential diagnosis of an RUQ abdominal mass in a pediatric patient is broad and includes hydronephrosis, nephroblastoma (Wilms' tumor), liver masses and tumors, choledochal cysts, intestinal duplication cysts, and retroperitoneal tumors. Liver masses include hemangiomas, focal nodular hyperplasia, and liver tumors, both benign and malignant. The most common malignant tumor in young children is hepatoblastoma. Hepatocellular carcinoma is more commonly seen in those over 5 years of age. Liver sarcomas, rhabdoid tumors, immature teratomas, and choriocarcinomas are more uncommon.

● WORKUP

Evaluation of a potential abdominal mass in children may include plain films to detect calcifications, displacement of the stomach or the intestine, and assessment of the bowel gas pattern. As these findings will likely be nonspecific, further imaging includes an abdominal ultrasound to narrow the differential diagnosis and ascertain organ involvement as well as characteristics of the mass. An abdominal CT with intravenous and oral contrast can further define vascular involvement and assess lymphadenopathy. MRI may ultimately be an important adjunct in hepatic lesions in determining tumor relationship to biliary anatomy and the hepatic vasculature. A chest x-ray or a CT should be obtained

to rule out metastatic disease. Laboratory evaluation should include a CBC, electrolytes, serum transaminases, α-fetal protein (AFP), β-HCG, and a urinalysis. Serum AFP is produced in the fetal liver and yolk sac and gradually declines to adult levels after age 6 months. Elevated AFP occurs in 90% of patients presenting with hepatoblastoma and can be used as an adjunct to assess response to treatment and disease recurrence.

Presentation Continued

CBC and electrolytes were normal. Her ultrasound showed normal kidneys without hydronephrosis and a solid mass measuring 4 × 4.5 cm confined to the right hepatic lobe with mildly increased vascular flow. An abdominal CT with contrast confirmed this solitary hepatic mass and showed no vascular impingement or invasion. There was no obvious adenopathy. The following day, the β-HCG returned at 1 (normal, <6 mIU/mL), while the AFP was significantly elevated at >50,000 (normal, 1 to 15 ng/mL).

● DIAGNOSIS AND TREATMENT

Based on the workup demonstrating a large solid hepatic mass in a toddler with a markedly elevated AFP, the single leading diagnosis is hepatoblastoma. Hepatoblastoma is the most common malignant hepatic tumor in children <3 years of age, and complete surgical resection offers the best chance for cure. However, approximately 20% of children with hepatoblastoma have metastatic disease at presentation. Histologically, hepatoblastomas are classified as either epithelial or mixed epithelial/mesenchymal lesions. Epithelial tumors are further classified as pure fetal, embryonal, macrotrabecular, or small cell undifferentiated lesions. Tumors with pure fetal histology carry a more favorable prognosis. A chest CT should be obtained to exclude pulmonary metastases. Evaluation by both a pediatric surgeon and a pediatric oncologist is warranted, and assessment for inclusion in clinical trials is encouraged.

Imaging is scrutinized to assess for primary tumor resection. If there is metastatic disease and/or obvious unresectability, then the tumor should be biopsied and neoadjuvant chemotherapy initiated. The PRETEXT system, based on Couinaud's segments and other anatomic factors, has now been internationally adopted as a way to assess upfront tumor resectability and assign patients to risk groups. If the tumor is unresectable at presentation, restaging after chemotherapy will reassess for subsequent resection. In select cases of bilobar disease in the absence of metastasis, primary liver transplantation may be considered.

Presentation Continued

The chest CT was negative, and all abdominal imaging suggested the solitary tumor being contained in the right hepatic lobe. Therefore, the patient is a candidate for a formal right hepatic lobectomy.

● SURGICAL APPROACH

Although preoperative imaging may suggest respectability, only surgical exploration is confirmatory. Nonanatomic liver resections are typically avoided because of a higher rate of incomplete resection and local relapse.

Operative steps include careful preparation with the placement of several large bore intravenous lines (preferably in the upper extremity), an arterial line, and a urinary catheter as blood loss should be anticipated. An epidural catheter for postoperative pain management should be considered. Blood products including packed RBCs, FFP, and platelets should be available. Positioning should allow the surgeon access to the neck, chest, abdomen, and groins.

A right subcostal incision is used to evaluate the tumor location and extent. The abdomen is explored for any regional or metastatic disease not detected on preoperative imaging studies. Suspicious extrahepatic lesions should be biopsied and sent for frozen section prior to proceeding with hepatic resection. If the lesion is deemed resectable, an appropriate anatomic hepatic lobectomy or trisectionectomy is undertaken.

The liver is completely mobilized by dividing the triangular ligament and attachments to the bare area, allowing anterior displacement of the liver and access to the retrohepatic vena cava. Attachments to the right adrenal and small branches to the IVC are divided. The IVC is mobilized and the resection plane assessed for vascular invasion. The hepatic veins are palpated to assure clearance from tumor. Intraoperative ultrasound may be useful in completing the vascular assessment.

The porta hepatis is dissected, and the appropriate branches of the hepatic artery, portal vein, and bile duct are isolated. Assuring resectability after complete vascular assessment, the respective portal structures are now ligated. After vascular ligation, a demarcation line is evident, and the parenchyma is then divided. Anatomic liver resection is undertaken proceeding from the portal structures, up the retrohepatic cava, toward the hepatic veins. Many different techniques and instruments for parenchymal division exist

subject to surgeon experience and preference. Small vascular branches and bile ductules within the liver substance are ligated as encountered. The hepatic veins should be approached by dissection within the liver substance. Once the hepatic vein(s) are ligated, the final parenchymal attachments are divided completing specimen resection.

The raw surface of the remaining liver is closely scrutinized, and small bile leaks or vessels are ligated. Omentum may be placed over this raw surface in older children. Drains are left.

The major morbidity and mortality with hepatic tumor resection are from intraoperative hemorrhage. Potential pitfalls include inaccurate assessment of vascular invasion leading to hemorrhage and tumor recurrence. Variations in vascular anatomy are common as the right hepatic artery arises from the superior mesenteric artery and the left hepatic artery from the left gastric artery in 15% each, respectively (Table 97-1).

● SPECIAL INTRAOPERATIVE CONSIDERATIONS

Should tumor be suspected at the resection margin, intraoperative frozen section should be performed as complete resection is the goal. Explicit knowledge of hepatic segmental anatomy will assist in resection options.

Presentation Continued

The patient's right hepatic lobectomy was performed with a 150 mL blood loss and no transfusion requirement. Gross tumor resection was achieved, and no suspicious extrahepatic lesions were encountered. She was extubated at the termination of the operation and taken to the ICU for management.

● POSTOPERATIVE MANAGEMENT

Most children readily adapt to major hepatic resection with compensatory hypertrophy of the remaining liver mass. Postoperative hepatic insufficiency may manifest by hypoglycemia, hypoalbuminemia, and hypoprothrombinemia and requires meticulous surveillance. Neonates remain a susceptible population. Intravenous fluids should contain 10% dextrose, and supplemental albumin and vitamin K are provided as needed the first week. Close attention to vital signs, urine output, and hemoglobin levels assures no occult postoperative bleeding. Oral feeding may be resumed when the ileus resolves, typically within 2 to 3 days. When the patient is tolerating a regular diet, the abdominal drain can be removed when it is low volume and free from bile. If needed, chemotherapy is usually initiated after several weeks to allow for hepatic regeneration and recovery.

Table 97-1   Hepatic Lobectomy

Key Technical Steps

1. Right subcostal incision and full exploration.
2. Mobilize the liver anteriorly by dividing all attachments to the diaphragm and the abdominal wall.
3. The IVC is mobilized and, in addition to the hepatic veins, palpated to assure clearance from tumor. Intraoperative ultrasound may be a useful adjunct.
4. Perform portal dissection and ligation of the appropriate branches of the hepatic artery, portal vein, and bile duct.
5. The parenchyma is divided following the line of vascular demarcation. Small vascular branches and bile ductules within the liver substance are ligated.
6. The hepatic veins are dissected within the liver substance. Once the appropriate branch is ligated, the final parenchymal attachments are divided completing specimen resection.
7. Small bile leaks and/or vessels on the remaining raw surface are ligated. Omental placement over the raw surface is optional.
8. Drains are left, and the abdomen is closed.

Potential Pitfalls

- The major morbidity and mortality from pediatric liver resection is from intraoperative hemorrhage. Thorough preoperative evaluation and planning minimizes risk.
- Be aware of common anatomic variations of a replaced right or left hepatic artery.
- Inaccurate assessment of vascular invasion may lead to hemorrhage and tumor recurrence.
- Unexpected invasion of the remaining hepatic vein is the most common cause of positive resection margins, severe hemorrhage, and postoperative liver failure from the Budd-Chiari syndrome. Intraoperative US is a useful adjunct if assessment is uncertain.
- The course of the hepatic veins is extremely short as they originate close to the liver surface. Divide the veins within the parenchyma if tumor margins allow. Supradiaphragmatic IVC control is encouraged should the ability to control the hepatic veins be challenging.

Case Conclusion

Her recovery was uneventful, and she maintained normal serum glucose levels. She was transferred to the floor, and her ileus resolved on postoperative day (POD) 3. Her nasogastric tube was removed, and her diet advanced. Her drain output was <30 mL of serous fluid and was removed on POD 6. She was discharged home on oral narcotics. Her final pathology returned as pure fetal-type hepatoblastoma with clear tumor margins. She is being closely observed without chemotherapy and monitored for tumor recurrence with serum AFP and imaging. A >85% cure rate is anticipated.

TAKE HOME POINTS

- More than 70% of all pediatric liver tumors are malignant, accounting for 1% of all pediatric malignancies. Hepatoblastoma is the third most common abdominal malignancy following neuroblastoma and Wilms' tumor.
- Hepatoblastoma presents between ages 6 months to 3 years and can be associated with the Beckwith-Wiedemann syndrome, familial adenomatous polyposis, hemihypertrophy, and a low birth weight. Serum AFP is elevated in 90%. Children with associated conditions should be considered for tumor screening with serum AFP and US to increase the likelihood of earlier detection.
- The PRETEXT system is used to determine upfront tumor resectability and to risk stratify patients accordingly. Approximately 20% of patients have metastatic disease at presentation with the lung, brain, and/ or bone marrow involvement. Only one-third to one-half of children diagnosed with hepatoblastoma have tumors amenable to primary resection.
- Diagnostic imaging with US, CT, and MRI is used to assess resection. Chest CT is most commonly used to rule out pulmonary metastasis.
- Complete surgical resection remains the ultimate goal as the only effective cure.
- Several chemotherapeutic regimens exist that are based on cisplatin. Although most patients receive postoperative chemotherapy, it may be avoided in those with completely resected tumors with pure fetal histology. Radiation therapy has a very limited role.
- Preoperative chemotherapy may shrink bulky tumors rendering them amenable to complete resection.
- The best survival rate approaches 95% in those with stage I disease (complete resection) with pure fetal histology. Overall survival rates are 75%.
- Children with unresectable tumors in the absence of metastasis may be strongly considered for liver transplantation. Transplantation is ultimately utilized in 6% of patients with hepatoblastoma and may be combined with neoadjuvant chemotherapy.

SUGGESTED READINGS

Essentials of pediatric surgery. In: Marc I. Rowe, James A. O'Neill Jr., Jay L. Grosfeld, Eric W. Fonkalsrud, Arnold G. Coran. eds. *Liver Tumors.* St. Louis, MO: Mosby-Year Book; 1995:278-290.

Kremer N, Walther AE, Tiao GM. Management of hepatoblastoma: an update. *Curr Opin Pediatr.* 2014;26(3):362-369.

Meyers RL, Tiao G, de Ville de Goyet J, Superina R, Aronson DC. Hepatoblastoma state of the art: pre-treatment extent of disease, surgical resection guidelines and the role of liver transplantation. *Curr Opin Pediatr.* 2014;26(1):29-36.

Roebuck DJ, Aronson D, Clapuyt P, et al.; International Childhood Liver Tumor Strategy Group. 2005 PRETEXT: a revised staging system for primary malignant liver tumours of childhood developed by the SIOPEL group. *Pediatr Radiol.* 2007;37(2):123-132.

Intussusception

98

KEVIN N. JOHNSON AND JAMES D. GEIGER

Based on the previous edition chapter "Intussusception" by
Sabina Siddiqui and James D. Geiger

Presentation

A 26-month-old previously healthy female is brought to
the emergency department for a 24-hour history of intermittent abdominal pain and a bloody bowel movement.
The patient is slightly lethargic and has an episode of
nonbilious emesis in the emergency room. The patient's
abdomen is soft on examination with a palpable mass in
the right upper quadrant.

● DIFFERENTIAL DIAGNOSIS

Differential diagnosis for this patient includes intussusception, Meckel's diverticulum, perforated appendicitis, incarcerated hernia, gastroenteritis, and abdominal
trauma.

● WORKUP

Laboratory studies are nonspecific for patients with intussusception but can show evidence of dehydration or infection
depending on the length of illness. Laboratory studies may
be completely normal, however.

Abdominal x-ray may be normal in intussusception, but
it may show evidence of obstruction with air–fluid levels,
absent distal bowel gas, or evidence of a soft tissue mass in
the right lower quadrant (Dance's sign). X-ray may also show
evidence of free air, which changes the management strategy
of intussusception, as outlined below. Air that outlines the
cecum argues against ileocolic intussusception.

An abdominal ultrasound may show evidence of intussusception with a "target sign" (Figure 98-1). Dilated proximal loops may also be seen. Leadpoints are not reliably seen
or excluded with any imaging modality. Despite the fact that
85% of occurrences of intussusception are idiopathic, in

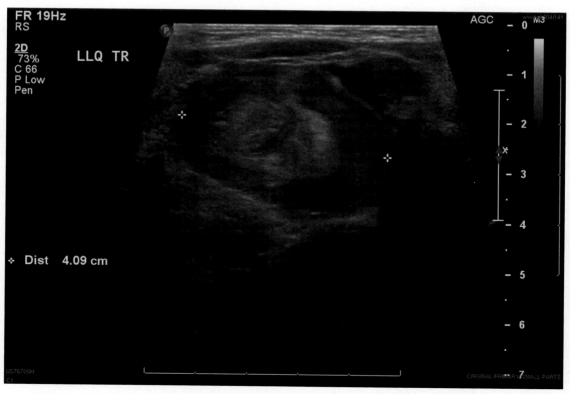

FIGURE 98-1. Abdominal ultrasound illustrates a "target sign" with hypoechoic rim (edematous bowel wall) surrounding hyperechoic central area (intussusceptum and mesenteric fat).

Table 98-1	Imaging for Intussusception

Abdominal X-ray

Normal

Air–fluid levels

Soft tissue mass in RUQ (Dance's sign)

Ultrasound

Target sign (transverse view)

"Pseudokidney" (oblique view)

Air-Contrast Enema

Intussuscipiens seen within the colon

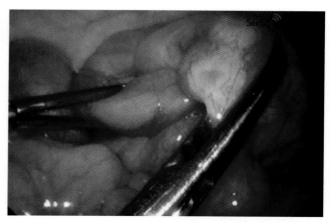

FIGURE 98-2. Gentle traction being applied for reduction of the intussusception.

patients with multiple recurrences, or presentation outside of the standard ages for the presence of intussusception (3 months to 3 years), consideration should be taken to surgical exploration for a leadpoint. Of note, asymptomatic patients with small bowel intussusception found incidentally on cross-sectional imaging can be observed as they are almost always transient in nature.

In patients with evidence of ileocolic intussusception and no free air or peritonitis on initial workup, an air-contrast enema can be both diagnostic and therapeutic.

Air-contrast enema allows visualization of the intussusceptum within the colon and allows for reduction in over 90% of cases (Table 98-1).

Presentation Continued

Following fluid resuscitation and laboratory studies, the patient has an abdominal x-ray performed, which show fluid. Ultrasound is performed, and a "target sign" is seen in the right upper quadrant, consistent with ileocolic intussusception.

● DIAGNOSIS AND TREATMENT

Intussusception is a clinical phenomenon in which one segment of the bowel (intussusceptum) telescopes into another segment of bowel (intussuscipiens, Figure 98-2). This causes obstruction of the bowel at that point and also leads to venous and lymphatic congestion within that segment that leads to mucosal ischemia, and the resultant "currant jelly" stools. Rarely, the ischemia will progress and become full thickness, leading to perforation of the bowel.

Treatment of intussusception depends on the initial resuscitation. Most patients will have some degree of dehydration, and fluid resuscitation is appropriate. In patients with evidence of bowel obstruction, nasogastric tube placement for decompression may be indicated. If there is evidence of free air on abdominal x-ray, or peritonitis on physical exam, the patient should proceed directly to the operating room for

exploration following resuscitation and antibiotic administration. All other patients can proceed to radiology for air-contrast enema. Air-contrast enema involves placement of a rectal tube for insufflation of air up to 120 mm Hg while under fluoroscopy (see Figure 98-3). This procedure allows for visualization of the intussusceptum and reduction in around 90% of cases. Reduction is confirmed by the passage of air into the small bowel seen on fluoroscopy and the resolution of clinical symptoms. Air-contrast enema can be repeated up to three times prior to proceeding to surgery, although this is up to the surgeon's discretion, with success rates of around 50% for subsequent attempts in published series. Patients are admitted to the hospital or kept for observation for several hours after reduction as recurrence of the intussusception occurs in 5% to 10% usually within 2 weeks, whether the reduction is performed by air-contrast enema or surgery.

Presentation Continued

The patient is taken for air-contrast enema. The intussusception is reduced, and air is seen entering the small bowel. The patient is admitted to the floor for observation. Subsequently, you are called to the patient's bedside as they have recurrent abdominal pain. Repeated air-contrast enema is unsuccessful, and the patient is taken to surgery for operative reduction.

● SURGICAL APPROACH

Surgical intervention for intussusception is reserved for patients with evidence of perforation or nonviable bowel, including free air and peritonitis; patients with intussusception not reducible by radiographic methods; or patients with multiple recurrences. Intussusception can be addressed either by a laparoscopic or an open approach.

The laparoscopic approach to intussusception includes a port placed at the umbilicus, a port in the right upper quadrant, and a port in the left lower quadrant. After inspecting

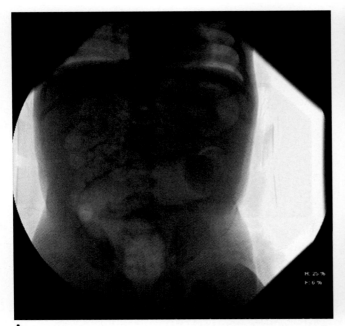
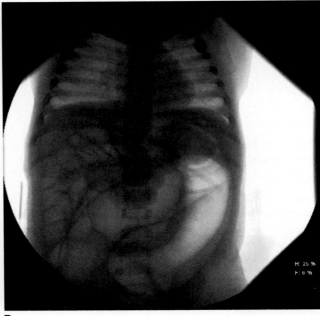

A   **B**

FIGURE 98-3. Air-contrast enema demonstrates a long ileocolic intussusception with intussusceptum encountered in sigmoid colon **(A)** and reduced now to the splenic flexure **(B)**.

the bowel, the intussusception is reduced by placing one blunt grasper into the folds of the intussuscipiens and applying gentle pressure to the terminal ileum (see Figure 98-2). The tension must be held constant for a few minutes before it starts to reduce. Gentle squeezing of the bowel proximal to intussusception can also be done. Combined hydrostatic reduction with grasping may be beneficial. Appendectomy can be performed, but this has not been shown to affect outcomes or rates of recurrence and is not commonly performed. Following reduction of the intussusception, the bowel is inspected for viability and any evidence of a leadpoint. Lymphoid thickening of the terminal ileum is common and should not be mistaken for a mass requiring resection.

For the open approach, a transverse laparotomy is performed in the right upper quadrant. The intussusception is deliver through the wound, and pressure is held against the tip of the intussuscipiens in the colon. Generally, the bowel is not directly grasped and pulled to try and reduce the intussusception as the bowel will be markedly edematous and friable and may lead to deserosalization or perforation (Table 98-2).

● SPECIAL INTRAOPERATIVE CONSIDERATIONS

If the intussusception is not able to be reduced with gentle traction, the bowel should be resected as further manipulation can lead to perforation and subsequent systemic illness. Nonviable bowel or a leadpoint should also be resected. A minilaparotomy can be performed to externalize the bowel to be resected.

While most cases of intussusception are idiopathic (85%), leadpoints for intussusception do occur and can

include Meckel's diverticulum, intestinal polyp, enteric duplication cyst, hemangioma, or lymphadenopathy related to lymphoma (most commonly Burkitt's lymphoma). These lead points should be resected if found.

Table 98-2	Reduction of Intussusception

Key Technical Steps

Laparoscopic Approach

1. Ports at umbilicus, right upper quadrant, left lower quadrant.
2. Reduction of intussusception by unfolding the intussuscipiens and holding gentle counter traction on the intussusceptum.
3. If unable to reduce the intussusception, perform an ileocolic resection.
4. Examine bowel for leadpoint, viability.

Open Approach

1. Right upper quadrant transverse incision.
2. Delivery of intussusception into the wound.
3. Milk out intussusceptum with gentle distal pressure.
4. If unable to reduce the intussusception perform an ileocolic resection.
5. Examine bowel for leadpoint, viability.

Potential Pitfalls

- Pulling on the bowel causing deserosalization or perforation.
- Mistaking bowel with lymphoid hyperplasia or edema as nonviable.

● POSTOPERATIVE MANAGEMENT

Following reduction of the intussusception, patients should either be admitted to the hospital or kept under observation for several hours to evaluate for evidence of recurrence, which occurs in 5% to 10% of patients. Return of clinical symptoms or intolerance to oral feeds should prompt further evaluation for recurrence. Generally, patients are given approximately 6 hours following reduction before a trial of oral feeds is given. Patients who are discharged following this trial should be given instructions to return if symptoms recur.

For patients who undergo surgery with resection, feeds are started after evidence of return of bowel function usually flatus. For patients who had evidence of obstruction, enteral decompression with nasogastric tube may be indicated even after surgery. Patients with perforation should be given a broad-spectrum antibiotic and will likely require a longer recovery as postoperative ileus is common.

Case Conclusion

The patient is taken to the operating room, and the intussusception is reduced laparoscopically. A Meckel's diverticulum is found to be the leadpoint of the intussusception. The diverticulum is exteriorized through an extension in the umbilical port site and is resected. The patient has return of bowel the following day and is discharged home on postoperative day 3.

TAKE HOME POINTS

- Classic presentation is intermittent abdominal pain, emesis, and "currant jelly" stools.
- Air-contrast enema is both diagnostic and therapeutic.
- Patients with free air or peritonitis should forego air-contrast enema and be taken to surgery.
- Failure to reduce the intussusception or recurrence of the intussusception is also indications for surgery, although air-contrast enemas can be repeated.
- For operative reduction "milk," the intussuscipiens back instead of pulling the bowel out to avoid injury.

SUGGESTED READINGS

Apelt N, Featherstone N, Guiliani S. Laparoscopic treatment of intussusception in children: a systematic review. *J Pediatr Surg.* 2013;48(8):1789-1793.

Jen HC, Shew SB. The impact of hospital type and experience on the operative utilization in pediatric intussusception: a nationwide study. *J Pediatr Surg.* 2009;44(1):241-246.

McAteer JP, Kwon S, LaRiviere CA, et al. Pediatric specialist care is associated with a lower risk of bowel resection in children with intussusception: a population-based analysis. *J Am Coll Surg.* 2013;217(2):226-232.

Rubenstein JC, Liu L, Caty MG, Christison-Lagay ER. Pathologic leadpoint is uncommon in ileo-colic intussusception regardless of age. *J Pediatr Surg.* 2015;50:1665-1667.

Sandler AD, Ein SH, Connolly B, et al. Unsuccessful air-enema reduction of intussusception: is a second attempt worthwhile? *Pediatr Surg Int.* 1999;15(3-4):214-216.

Necrotizing Enterocolitis

99

PATRICK MELMER AND SARA K. RASMUSSEN

Based on the previous edition chapter "Necrotizing Enterocolitis" by Richard Herman and Daniel H. Teitelbaum

Presentation

The patient is a former 26-week premature infant who is now 14 days old in the neonatal intensive care unit. The infant weighs 1,000 g and presents with abdominal distention, feeding intolerance, and a bloody stool. On physical examination, the child has a distended abdomen, with moderate erythema over the lower abdomen and scrotum. Additionally, the abdominal wall is edematous with a tense, brawny appearance to it. The flank is dusky on the right side. Laboratory studies are significant for a white blood cell count of 55,000, a hematocrit of 33%, platelets of 60,000, and a significant metabolic acidosis with a bicarbonate of 14 and serum sodium of 130. An abdominal radiograph demonstrates pneumatosis intestinalis, a fixed loop of bowel, and portal venous gas is evident.

● DIFFERENTIAL DIAGNOSIS

Necrotizing enterocolitis (NEC) should be suspected in the premature infant who presents with acute abdominal distention. It is among the leading causes of morbidity and mortality seen in the neonatal intensive care unit and should be considered a surgical emergency. The incidence of NEC ranges from approximately 3% to 12% in neonates weighing between 500 and 1,500 g, with lower weight infants having a higher risk of developing NEC. Mortality ranges from approximately 16% to 42% and is inversely proportional to weight.

The presentation of NEC may consist of nonspecific signs, and a broad differential diagnosis must be considered. Infectious enterocolitis, anatomic and functional congenital anomalies leading to abdominal distension (e.g., Hirschsprung's disease, intussusception, ileal meconium plug or atresia, malrotation with volvulus, etc.), and ileus secondary to sepsis may all present with findings similar to NEC. An additional entity, spontaneous intestinal perforation (sometimes called SIP), also must be considered. SIP needs to be distinguished from NEC given its similar and sometimes overlapping presentation. It tends to present with a bluish hue discoloration of the abdomen and pneumoperitoneum with an absence of pneumatosis intestinalis. The risk of SIP is increased in infants who received indomethacin or ibuprofen treatment to prompt closure of a patent ductus arteriosus (PDA). As such, there is not necessarily a correlation to timing of feeding advancement, discussed below.

There does exist a small number of characteristic physical examination and radiographic findings. Classic NEC findings are abdominal wall erythema and crepitus on physical examination, and pneumatosis intestinalis on radiograph. Additionally, abdominal radiographs in NEC may demonstrate "fixed" loops of bowel and portal venous gas (discussed below). These signs are more diagnostic of NEC.

● WORKUP

A thorough history and physical examination should begin the clinical investigation. The initiation of enteral feeds in premature infants and the rate at which they are advanced is correlated with the development of NEC. As such, details in the history that raise suspicion for NEC include a history of prematurity, recent advancement of enteral formula feeds, and the development of feeding intolerance. Maternal factors, such as drug abuse and placental insufficiency, have been implicated in the development of NEC, and sometimes SIP, as well. On physical examination, significant findings include abdominal distention and tenderness, erythematous discoloration of the abdominal wall and scrotum, and crepitus (Figure 99-1).

Following this, laboratory and radiographic investigations may take place. A complete blood count, a coagulation panel, a metabolic panel, blood gas, inflammatory markers, and cultures for the workup of sepsis are indicated. While laboratory values are commonly nonspecific in NEC, abnormalities such as metabolic acidosis, elevated C-reactive protein, thrombocytopenia, and an elevated or depressed white blood cell count should raise suspicion. Imaging should always begin with abdominal radiographs both in the supine and decubitus positions in order to assess for the presence of pneumoperitoneum.

Pathognomonic findings on imaging are pneumatosis intestinalis (gas within the wall of the bowel) and portal venous gas (indicating air has been absorbed into the mesenteric circulation). Early signs of NEC include dilated loops of bowel or a paucity of gas within the bowel lumen suggestive of an ileus. Another potentially alarming sign is

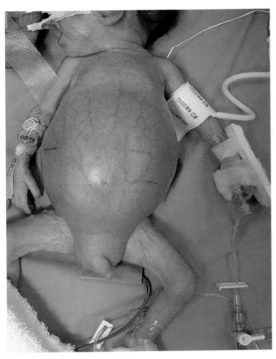

FIGURE 99-1. Physical examination findings including distention and abdominal wall erythema. (Photo courtesy of David Notrica, MD, Phoenix Children's Hospital. Used by permission.)

the "sentinel loops" of bowel that do not change across serial radiographs, suggesting bowel necrosis. Pneumoperitoneum indicates perforation secondary to bowel necrosis. Two important considerations should be noted: first, if malrotation with volvulus is high on the differential, then it is prudent to consider an upper gastrointestinal series to rule out such a diagnosis. The second consideration is that contrast enemas are contraindicated when working up suspected NEC given the increased risk of colonic perforation (Figure 99-2).

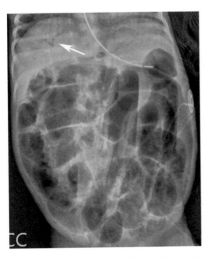

FIGURE 99-2. Necrotizing enterocolitis in a 2-week-old male. Left lateral decubitus abdominal x-ray showing widespread pneumatosis, diffuse bowel distension, and portal venous gas (*arrow*). (With permission from Iyer R, Chapman T. *Pediatric Imaging: The Essentials*. Philadelphia, PA: Wolters Kluwer Health, 2015.)

● DIAGNOSIS AND TREATMENT

The mechanism by which NEC occurs and causes intestinal mucosal damage and eventual tissue necrosis and perforation is incompletely understood. It is thought to be a result of a combined picture of infection and ischemia to the bowel that occurs when an unstable infant has a low-flow state in their splanchnic circulation. Though a sizeable percentage of patients, as high as 40% in some series, will progress to surgical intervention, medical management is the first line of treatment in infants who do not have an indication for surgical intervention (perforation or uncontrolled sepsis from an abdominal source). Findings suggestive of an early NEC process, such as mild or absent physical exam signs, absent pneumatosis intestinalis, or an indolent history, would also point to starting with medical therapy and close clinical observation. A conservative approach includes abdominal decompression, bowel rest, broad-spectrum antibiotic coverage, and parenteral feeding along with serial abdominal exams and radiographs. Bell's criteria can be used to stratify the severity of NEC in patients, which assists in planning for optimal management.

Even with an initial nonsurgical approach, the serious nature of NEC and high associated morbidity and mortality often mandates surgical therapy. Grave findings on initial presentation or decompensation following a period of clinical observation will require operative intervention. The optimal surgical management of NEC has been controversial over time and is addressed in the next section.

In the present scenario, the child has a history of prematurity and progressive intolerance to formula feeds while being cared for in the neonatal intensive care unit. Characteristic abdominal distension with typical skin changes is present. Laboratory studies suggest sepsis and profound metabolic acidosis. Classic pneumatosis intestinalis is evident from abdominal imaging. Together, the single leading diagnosis in this 14-day-old, formerly 26-week premature male is NEC. Two hours after abdominal decompression and bowel rest is initiated, abdominal distension worsens. A repeat abdominal radiograph in the left lateral decubitus position is positive for pneumoperitoneum.

● SURGICAL APPROACH

After electing to intervene, the first major decision is whether to pursue laparotomy with resection of affected intestine or primary peritoneal drainage. For infants weighing 1,500 g or greater, the former is the preferred approach. In infants weighing <1,500 g, the advantage of each option is less clear. In 1977, Ein et al. first described five infants for whom peritoneal drainage alone was sufficient for the treatment of NEC. This approach was utilized for many years with the argument that it reasonably allowed decompression of the abdomen, drainage of infected fluid, and stabilization of the patient while possibly sparing the risks of laparotomy and general anesthesia.

However, two recent, prospective, multicenter, randomized controlled trials demonstrated conflicting data on this issue. In 2006, Moss et al. found no statistical advantage for primary peritoneal drainage versus laparotomy with bowel resection in terms of survival, dependence on parenteral feeds, or length of hospitalization for infants who weighed <1,500 g. A concurrent study by Rees et al. published a short time after found that primary peritoneal drainage was instead associated with increased mortality and argued that it was not a safe alternative to early laparotomy. Still another series reported by Blakely et al. found that neurodevelopmental impairment may be increased in infants who undergo drainage versus those who are openly resected. While there is no incontrovertible data pointing to an optimal approach in children with NEC, clinical evidence seems to suggest some advantage to intervention with laparotomy. Local protocols and surgeon expertise along with clinical correlation should guide the ultimate decision-making. It is important to remember that even if upfront exploration is required, long-term management may involve surgical exploration as post-NEC strictures can develop, which cause mechanical bowel obstructions.

Preoperative resuscitation is paramount once operative intervention is elected. Fluid shifts and third spacing are typical for these infants, and their fluid requirements may be considerable. Once a laparotomy is undertaken, key technical aspects involve proper positioning, draping, and entrance into the abdomen via a transverse midline incision focus on the preservation of as much intestine as possible. All grossly necrotic areas should be removed, and any bowel thought to be viable should be preserved. For viable intestine, the creation of an ostomy without primary reanastomosis is the usual approach. Additionally, the liver in a premature infant often extends well below the costal margin, and care must be taken to avoid injury to the organ. A bleeding liver can be arduous to control and requires blood transfusion. Glisson's capsule is fragile and thin and requires little tension to tear.

Various techniques have been utilized including end stomas, double barrels, and loop enterostomies with mucous fistulas depending on the specific sections of affected intestine. A potential pitfall of this operation is seen when small bowel is more affected than large bowel. In general, ileal and jejunal resections fare worse than colonic resection. The ileum has the greatest ability to adapt and increase absorption postoperatively, and it has been debated as to whether or not the preservation of the ileocecal valve improves outcomes. Regardless, the primary goal is to remove the necrotic bowel that is the source of sepsis and preserving much bowel as possible. A return to the OR for "second-look" procedures if necessary is common for reevaluation of areas with questionable viability.

For patients undergoing primary peritoneal drainage, penrose drains are placed in the abdominal cavity and allowed to drain over the course of several days. Volume and character of the drain output is monitored and correlated clinically. If a conversion to "rescue" laparotomy is not required in the setting of clinical improvement, the drain may be slowly backed out and removed (Table 99-1).

Table 99-1	Necrotizing Enterocolitis

Key Technical Steps

1. Transverse midline incision and entrance into the abdomen
2. Thorough examination of the entire intestine and resection of necrotic areas
3. Resection of necrotic bowel with careful preservation of any potentially viable sections of bowel
4. Creation of ostomy(ies)
5. Second-look operations

Potential Pitfalls

- Involvement and resection of a large portion of the small bowel
- Involvement and resection of the ileocecal valve
- Injury to the liver capsule precipitating dangerous bleeding

● SPECIAL INTRAOPERATIVE CONSIDERATIONS

In the surgical treatment of NEC, one nonroutine intraoperative finding in particular may drastically change management. Should the special case of pannecrosis of the intestine or so-called NEC totalis be encountered, a frank discussion of the goals of care must be entertained. Infants with this disease process have very little viable bowel beyond the ligament of treitz. This carries a risk of extreme morbidity and mortality. Outcomes not resulting in death are few and will necessarily require prolonged hospitalization, long-term parenteral feeding, and probable bowel transplant if survival is to occur at all. In these patients, excellent comfort care measures may be a reasonable option.

● POSTOPERATIVE MANAGEMENT

The two most common complications that can arise following surgery for NEC are strictures and short bowel syndrome. Scarring in and around inflamed or ischemic tissue can cause strictures to develop postoperatively. Should clinical suspicion be raised by abdominal distention, bilious vomiting, or other suggestive signs following the restarting of feeds, a contrast study should be performed and the need for surgical resection evaluated. NEC is the leading cause of short bowel syndrome, which occurs when there is not enough bowel for absorption of nutrients required for proper growth. This minimum length of viable and functioning bowel is traditionally believed to be 40 cm and again highlights the important of preserving as much bowel as possible intraoperatively. Infants with short bowel syndrome are dependent on parenteral nutrition and therefore subject to its risks such as sepsis and hepatobiliary complications including cholestasis and liver failure. Long-term surveillance following survival of NEC also includes monitoring for neurodevelopmental delay, a significant cause of morbidity in this population.

Case Conclusion

The child is taken to the operating room for an exploratory laparotomy. A single area of necrotic ascending colon is noted with otherwise viable intestine throughout. Resection of this portion of bowel is followed by creation of a stoma with mucous fistula. The infant is maintained postoperatively with bowel rest, antibiotics, and TPN until the slow restarting of enteral feeds on postoperative day 14. Output from the proximal ostomy is "refed" through the mucous fistula for several weeks as the child grows and is ultimately able to be discharged from the neonatal intensive care unit. Two months out from the operation, a contrast enema does not demonstrate any strictures and so continuity of the gastrointestinal tract is reestablished. Recovery is uneventful, and the child is followed for proper growth and attainment of milestones.

TAKE HOME POINTS

- NEC should be suspected in the premature infant who presents with acute abdominal distention.
- Abdominal radiographs help assess for pneumatosis intestinalis or pneumoperitoneum.
- Careful consideration should be given for medical versus surgical management.
- Careful consideration should be given for exploratory laparotomy with bowel resection versus primary peritoneal drainage.
- Preserve as much bowel as possible.
- Maintain a high degree of clinical suspicion for complications such as strictures following surgery for NEC.

SUGGESTED READINGS

Blakely ML, Tyson JE, Lally KP, et al. Laparotomy versus peritoneal drainage for necrotizing enterocolitis or isolated intestinal perforation in extremely low birth weight infants: outcomes through 18 months adjusted age. *Pediatrics.* 2006;117(4):E680-E687.

Ein SH, Marshall DG, Girvan D. Peritoneal drainage under local anesthesia for perforations from necrotizing enterocolitis. *J Pediatr Surg.* 1977;12(6):963-967.

Fitzgibbons SC, Ching Y, Yu D, et al. Mortality of necrotizing enterocolitis expressed by birth weight categories. *J Pediatr Surg.* 2009;44(6):1072-1076.

Moss RL, Dimmitt RA, Barnhart DC, et al. Laparotomy versus peritoneal drainage for necrotizing enterocolitis and perforation. *N Engl J Med.* 2006;354:2225-2234.

Rees CM, Eaton S, Kiely EM, Wade AM, McHugh K, Pierro A. Peritoneal drainage or laparotomy for neonatal bowel perforation? A randomized controlled trial. *Ann Surg.* 2008;248:44-51.

Wilmore D. Factors correlating with a successful outcome following extensive intestinal resection in newborn infants. *J Pediatr.* 1972;80(1):88-95.

100

Rectal Bleeding in a Young Child

IAN C. GLENN, GAVIN A. FALK, AND OLIVER S. SOLDES

Based on the previous edition chapter "Rectal Bleeding in a Young Child" by Gavin A. Falk and Oliver S. Soldes

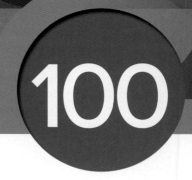

Presentation

An 18-month-old boy with an unremarkable past medical history presents to the emergency department (ED) with a 3-day history of episodic bright red bleeding per rectum. On examination, the child is quiet, tachycardiac, and normotensive. His abdomen is soft, nontender, and nondistended, without palpable masses. He does not seem to be in pain, but appears pale and lethargic. He has not had any episodes of hematemesis. His distressed mother confirms that there is no family history of clotting disorders, inflammatory bowel disease, or polyposis syndromes. A nasogastric (NG) tube was placed and the aspirate is clear.

● DIFFERENTIAL DIAGNOSIS

The causes of lower gastrointestinal (GI) bleeding in neonates (<30 days of age), infants (30 days to 1 year), children (1 to 12 years), and adolescents (13–adult) are diverse and vary by age. Most causes in otherwise healthy children are self-limited. A child (1 to 12 years) who presents with bleeding per rectum has a differential diagnosis that includes anal fissures, Meckel's diverticulum (MD), inflammatory bowel disease, intestinal polyps, and intestinal duplications. Uncommon causes of rectal bleeding include arteriovenous malformation, varices due to portal hypertension and liver disease, and upper GI bleeding from peptic disease. In a young child (<4 to 5 years), MD is the most common cause of clinically significant lower GI bleeding. Occasionally, the degree of hemorrhage is impressive and may require transfusion.

● WORKUP

After a full physical examination and comprehensive history taking, the patient undergoes further evaluation in the ED with basic laboratory tests including a complete blood count, coagulation studies, and type and screen. His serum hemoglobin is reported as 11 g/dL, with a normal platelet count and BMP. His PT/INR and aPTT are within normal limits. The patient undergoes a technetium (Tc)-99m pertechnetate scan ("Meckel's scan"), the diagnostic modality of choice to investigate for an MD with heterotopic gastric mucosa.

● DISCUSSION

Complications associated with MD are most readily understood in the context of the embryologic origin of these diverticula. MD is the most frequently encountered diverticulum of the small intestine (Figure 100-1). It is a true diverticulum containing all of the layers of the normal small intestinal wall. During the embryologic development of the midgut, the omphalomesenteric (vitelline) duct connects the yolk sac to the intestinal tract and usually obliterates by the 7th week of life. Arrest of the obliteration of the duct may lead to a number of omphalomesenteric anomalies, the most common of which is MD. The blood supply of the MD is derived from the paired vitelline arteries. The left vitelline artery involutes and the right artery (which also gives rise to the superior mesenteric artery) may persist and travel to the tip of the diverticulum. Incomplete involution of the duct and vitelline artery remnants, with failure to separate from the abdominal wall, may produce connections to the base of the umbilicus. These may give rise to draining ileoumbilical vitelline duct fistulas, vitelline duct cysts, blind-ending umbilical sinuses, and fibrous umbilicodiverticular bands, depending on the extent of involution

The "rule of 2s" is often quoted as an aide-mémoire to the features of MD: The incidence is 2% of the general population; it is located within 2 feet of the ileocecal valve, is

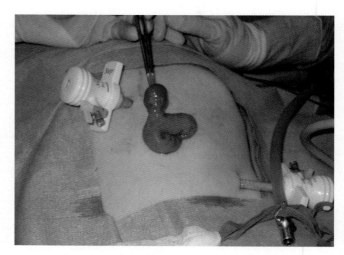

FIGURE 100-1. The Meckel's diverticulum is delivered via the umbilicus when laparoscopically assisted extracorporeal diverticulectomy is performed.

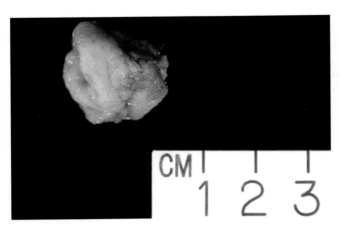

FIGURE 100-2. Meckel's diverticulum with heterotopic gastric mucosa. There is ulceration of the ileal mucosa adjacent to the heterotopic gastric mucosa.

2 inches in length, is usually symptomatic by 2 years of age, is two times as common in boys, and can contain two types of heterotopic mucosa. The heterotopic mucosa is most commonly gastric (80%), pancreatic (5%), or both. The gastric mucosa is metabolically active and secretes hydrochloric acid. The pathogenesis of hemorrhage is thought to be ulceration of the normal ileum adjacent to the gastric mucosa (Figure 100-2).

Although MD is the most common cause of significant rectal bleeding in young children, intestinal obstruction is actually the most frequent presenting symptom of MD (30% obstructive vs. 27% hemorrhagic presentation). Fibrous umbilicodiverticular bands to the abdominal wall produce a point of fixation around which the midgut volvulus may occur. Mesodiverticular bands arising from vitelline artery remnants extending from the tip of the diverticulum to the mesentery may give rise to internal hernias. Heterotopic mucosa within the diverticula can act as a lead point for intussusception.

Inflammation related to the heterotopic mucosa may produce Meckel's diverticulitis, which may be confused with acute appendicitis and may rarely lead to perforation with peritonitis and abscess formation. Enteroliths within the diverticula and incarceration of an MD within an inguinal hernia (Littre's hernia) may also rarely occur.

● DIAGNOSIS AND TREATMENT

Given the varied presentation of patients with MD, several different diagnostic modalities may be used in an attempt to arrive at the diagnosis. The correct diagnosis of MD is made more often in children presenting with bleeding versus other symptoms.

Tc-99m nuclear scan is the most accurate way to detect the heterotopic gastric mucosa frequently found in MD. The usefulness of the Tc-99m Meckel's scan derives from the finding that approximately 95% of diverticula excised for bleeding contain gastric mucosa. The patient is injected intravenously with Tc-99m pertechnetate and a nuclear scan is performed. This isotope is selectively taken up by gastric mucosa and, if present, produces a positive scan (Figure 100-3A and B). Scintigraphy has a sensitivity of 85%, specificity of 95%, and accuracy of 90% in children. Pentagastrin stimulation, H2

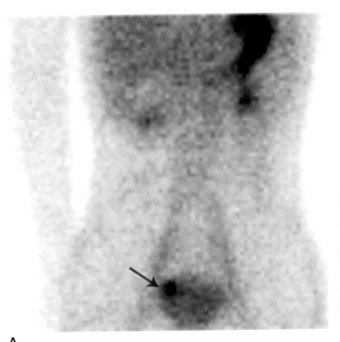

A

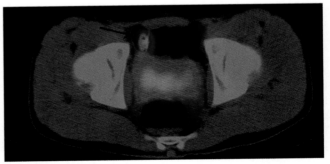

B

FIGURE 100-3. **A,B:** Meckel's scan demonstrating heterotopic gastric mucosa. Heterotopic gastric mucosa within an MD with uptake of radiotracer. There is also uptake in the mucosa of the stomach and the bladder. (Courtesy of Sankaran Shrikanthan, MD.)

histamine blockers, and glucagon may enhance the accuracy of the scan. Angiography is infrequently used due to its invasive nature and because it is useful only if there is brisk active bleeding. Tagged red blood cell scans are less sensitive and specific than Meckel's scans and are seldom used.

MANAGEMENT OF THE SYMPTOMATIC MD

The bleeding related to an MD is often episodic and surgery can usually be briefly delayed until the patient is stabilized and diagnostic evaluation can be performed. Adequate intravenous access and volume resuscitation are the first step in management. Infrequently, a blood transfusion may be required. An NG tube should be inserted early in the evaluation to help rule out an upper GI source and confirm lower GI bleeding. A Meckel's scan should be obtained and, if positive, the patient should proceed to operation without delay. A child with an unexplained source of lower GI bleeding may require exploratory operative intervention (preferably diagnostic laparoscopy) even if the nuclear scan is negative due to a significant false-negative rate of Meckel's scan.

MANAGEMENT OF AN INCIDENTALLY DISCOVERED MD

It is not definitely clear from the medical literature how a surgeon should proceed when he/she finds an MD incidentally. The vast majority of incidentally discovered Meckel's diverticula will remain asymptomatic, especially if it has been asymptomatic into adulthood. The lifetime complication rate from Meckel's diverticula is estimated to be 4% to 6%, with obstruction and hemorrhage occurring most frequently. It is recommended by some that Meckel's diverticula be palpated for the presence of ectopic tissue, and the MD be resected if tissue thickening or a mass is felt. However, ectopic tissue is likely to be discovered by palpation in only two-thirds of cases where it is actually present. Furthermore, from an oncologic perspective, an MD has a 70-fold higher lifetime rate of developing malignancy (most frequently carcinoid tumor) than the rest of the ileum. Resection of incidental MD offers a high probability of curative resection for a group of diseases unlikely to be diagnosed preoperatively. These arguments are further bolstered when operating on younger children, where it can be argued that an incidentally found MD should be removed given the child's greater lifetime risk of developing complications. Operative morbidity and mortality for resection of an MD are lower when the MD is incidentally identified. Asymptomatic incidentally discovered MD without a mass should generally only be resected under optimal conditions, in the absence of peritonitis and shock, because of the limited benefits and the small risk of suture line leak and peritonitis.

SURGICAL APPROACH

Surgical resection is the treatment of choice for symptomatic MD, and the approach is dependent on the patient's presentation and clinical condition (Table 100-1). Preoperative intravenous antibiotics are administered. The operation for bleeding or intussuscepted MD can be performed either as a laparoscopic, laparoscopic-assisted with extracorporeal resection, or open procedure. In slender children, the

Table 100-1 Meckel's Diverticulum

Key Technical Steps

1. Laparoscopic, laparoscopically assisted extracorporeal or open technique.
2. With laparoscopically assisted extracorporeal technique, the diverticulum is easily delivered via a minimal umbilical incision in slender children.
3. Remove the appendix in open procedures with a right lower quadrant incision.
4. If there is a mesenteric vessel to the tip of the diverticulum, it should be ligated prior to resection.
5. For a bleeding diverticulum, it is safest to begin with incision and wedge resection with direct inspection of the mucosa. Include adjacent ulcerated ileum in the resection.
6. For nonbleeding long diverticula with a moderate or a narrow base width (HDR > 2.0), stapler excision may be used. Avoid transverse stapler excision in short, wide MD.
7. Transverse resection and Heineke-Mikulicz type closure of the ileum is preferred to avoid narrowing the lumen.
8. Segmental resection and primary anastomosis is appropriate for short, wide diverticula, extensive ulceration and ulceration on the mesenteric ileal wall, or bulky heterotrophic mucosa that extends to the base of the diverticulum.
9. Standard anastomotic/closure technique for small bowel is utilized. In small diameter bowel, a single-layer hand-sewn technique may be advantageous to minimize luminal narrowing.

Potential Pitfalls

- Failure to control hemorrhage from areas of ulceration and residual ectopic mucosa with stapler excision without direct examination of the ileal mucosa.
- Narrowing the lumen of the ileum.
- Leak at suture or staple lines.
- Perforation of the diverticulum or ileum with primary umbilical ports when a connection to the base of the umbilicus is suspected (volvulus, patent ducts).
- Unnecessarily large incisions.

diverticulum is readily externalized by minimally enlarging the umbilical trocar incision, allowing palpation, examination, and excision of the diverticulum by conventional technique while conferring the benefits of a small abdominal incision. An initial minimally invasive approach is usually possible and preferred in children and is associated with a shorter hospital stay and decreased cost.

Regardless of approach, the first step is to inspect and assess the diverticulum. There is often a large mesenteric vessel, which extends to the tip of the diverticulum and should be ligated. Resection of the MD can then be achieved either by diverticulectomy or segmental bowel resection with primary anastomosis by stapled or hand-sewn techniques. Open resection is generally performed via a transverse right lower quadrant incision. An incidental appendectomy is generally performed when this incision is used, to eliminate the diagnosis of appendicitis in the evaluation of abdominal pain later in life.

When the patient presents with acute hemorrhage, it is safest to perform a wedge resection of the diverticulum and adjacent area of ileal ulceration. The ileal mucosa should be visually inspected to identify and control the sight(s) of bleeding. The closure is generally performed transversely by hand-sewn technique in young children. However, longer narrow diverticula may be stapled if the base of the diverticulum is narrow and the bowel lumen is large enough to avoid narrowing. A segmental ileal resection is indicated if there is evidence of intestinal ischemia, extensive inflammation, irreducible intussusception, the base of the diverticulum is very wide, or there is palpable ectopic tissue near the diverticular opening. Ileal mucosa with significant ulceration and bleeding opposite the diverticulum (on the mesenteric side) usually requires segmental resection. In cases where diagnostic testing has failed to make a definitive diagnosis, an exploratory laparoscopy is a safe way to proceed to localize the lesion.

Pitfalls associated with resection of a bleeding MD include failure to control hemorrhage from areas of adjacent ulceration if the diverticulum is excised with a stapler without opening the ileum and inspection of the mucosa. Simple transverse resection (stapled diverticulectomy) is not recommended for short MD, with a height-to-diameter ratio (HDR) <2.0 due to the risk of ectopic mucosa at the base being left behind. Simple wedge excision (diverticulectomy) with longitudinal closure of a wide-based diverticulum may create a stenosis. Leaks from suture or staple lines may occur and offset the limited benefits of excision of asymptomatic MD especially in acutely ill, elderly patients, who are unlikely to develop complications of the MD late in life. Caution should be observed in placement of the primary laparoscopic trocar in cases where attachment to the umbilical abdominal wall is suspected (volvulus, draining ileoumbilical vitelline duct fistulas, vitelline duct cyst, or sinuses). A nonumbilical site for the primary trocar may be selected in these cases.

● POSTOPERATIVE MANAGEMENT

Postoperative care following Meckel's diverticulectomy or segmental resections consists of conventional care for small bowel surgery with supportive care consisting primarily of intravenous fluids, 1 or 2 doses of postoperative antibiotics, a brief period of nothing by mouth (NPO), and sometimes NG suction (in the case of segmental bowel resection) until any ileus resolved. If a simple wedge resection or diverticulectomy is performed with laparoscopic or laparoscopically assisted extracorporeal technique, an NG tube is usually not needed and clear liquids may be initiated the following day.

Case Conclusion

The patient undergoes successful laparoscopic-assisted Meckel's diverticulectomy with wedge resection. At follow-up in the outpatient clinic 3 weeks later, the child was well, with no further bleeding, and a benign abdominal examination. Pathologic analysis of the surgical specimen confirms a gastric mucosa containing MD with ulceration. Further follow-up is unnecessary.

TAKE HOME POINTS

- MD is the most common cause of clinically significant rectal bleeding in young children (<4 to 5 years of age). Bleeding may be impressive and require transfusion.
- With the exception of tachycardia, hypotension, and pallor, the physical exam in patients with MD is often normal. The NG aspirate is usually clear.
- MD often presents with episodic painless rectal bleeding, but obstructive symptoms are more common (with volvulus, internal hernia, or intussusception). An acute abdomen (diverticulitis and perforation), or umbilical fistulas/cysts/sinuses may occur.
- A positive Meckel's nuclear scan is diagnostic in the child with significant lower GI bleeding and is the test of choice.
- Wedge resection of the diverticulum and adjacent ulceration with direct inspection of the ileal mucosa is safest in MD presenting with hemorrhage. A laparoscopically assisted extracorporeal approach is usually possible in the slender child.
- Segmental resection may be necessary to control hemorrhage from extensive ulceration, ulceration opposite the diverticulum, for ischemia, or when narrowing of the ileal lumen will result from diverticulectomy.

SUGGESTED READINGS

Brown RL, Azizkhan RG. Gastrointestinal bleeding in infants and children: Meckel's diverticulum and intestinal duplications. *Semin Pediatr Surg.* 1999;4:202-209.

Dassinger MS. Meckel's diverticulum. In: Mattei P, ed. *Fundamentals of Pediatric Surgery*. 1st ed. New York, NY: Springer; 2011.

Ruscher KA, Fisher JN, Hughes CD, et al. National trends in the surgical management of meckel's diverticulum. *J Pediatr Surg*. 2011;46:893-896.

St. Vil D, Brandt ML, Panis S, et al. Meckel's diverticulum in children: a 20-year review. *J Pediatr Surg*. 1991;11:1289-1292.

Thirunavukarasu P, Sathaiah M, Sukumar S, et al. Meckel's diverticulum—a high-risk region for malignancy in the ileum: insights from a population-based epidemiological study and implications in surgical management. *Ann Surg*. 2011;253(2): 223-230.

Vane DM, West KW, Grosfeld JL. Vitelline duct anomalies: experience with 217 childhood cases. *Arch Surg*. 1987;122: 542-547.

Varcoe RL, Wong SW, Taylor CF, Newstead GL. Diverticulectomy is inadequate treatment for short meckel's diverticulum with heterotopic mucosa. *ANZ J Surg*. 2004;74:869-872.

Omphalocele

SARA SCARLET, EMILY M. FONTENOT, AND SEAN E. McLEAN

101

Based on the previous edition chapter "Omphalocele" by
Emily M. Fontenot and Sean E. McLean

Presentation

A 34-year-old prima gravida woman is referred to your
office by her obstetrician after an abdominal wall defect
was noted on her first trimester ultrasound. The ultrasound demonstrated herniation of small bowel and liver
through the defect. She presents for counseling concerning the child's delivery and options for surgical repair. A
repeat fetal ultrasound is performed which demonstrates
an omphalocele, but no other fetal anomalies. Karyotyping
is consistent with the normal male karyotype (46, XY).

Frequent ultrasounds are continued throughout the
gestational period. The remainder of the pregnancy is
unremarkable. She gives birth to a 34-week estimated gestational age (EGA) male infant via normal spontaneous vaginal delivery. APGAR scores are 8 and 9 at 1 and 5 minutes,
respectively. The child's lower extremities and abdomen
are placed into a sterile abdominal bag, and he is transferred to the neonatal intensive care unit for resuscitation.

● DIFFERENTIAL DIAGNOSIS

Omphalocele and gastroschisis are the most common
abdominal wall defects in neonates. *Omphalocele* is characterized by a defect in the midline anterior abdominal wall
fascia and skin that is >4 cm in diameter. In omphalocele,
the rectus muscles are present and normal, but insert widely
on the costal margins and do not meet centrally at the
xiphoid process. The resultant defect allows for herniation
of the midgut and other abdominal viscera. The herniated
organs are contained within a membranous sac that consists
of peritoneum on the inside, Wharton's jelly, and amnion
externally. The umbilical cord inserts on the apex of the sac.
Omphaloceles are classified by size. A *small omphalocele* has
a fascial defect <5 cm and will usually contain only bowel. A
giant omphalocele often contains bowel, stomach, and liver
and has a defect 5 cm or greater. *Ruptured omphalocele* is a
presentation of omphalocele in which the sac has ruptured
in utero or during birth. Within utero rupture and exposure
to amniotic fluid, there is associated inflammation of the
intestines.

Gastroschisis is a full thickness abdominal wall defect
that occurs to the right of a normally inserted umbilical
cord. In this case, herniated bowel and abdominal viscera

are not covered by a membrane, and the viscera are exposed
to amniotic fluid during gestation. An *umbilical hernia* is an
abdominal wall defect caused by a persistent umbilical ring
and is covered by skin. *Pentalogy of Cantrell* is a rare congenital abnormality characterized by omphalocele, anterior
diaphragmatic hernia, malformation or absence of the pericardium, a sternal cleft, and cardiac anomalies. *Ectopia cordis
thoracis* is characterized by partial or complete failure of midline fusion of the sternum. This results in protrusion of the
heart from the chest through a split sternum. In *ectopia cordis
thoracis*, the heart is not covered by a membrane. In contrast,
in Pentalogy of Cantrell, the heart is covered by a membrane.
Prune belly syndrome is a constellation of anomalies including deficient or absent abdominal wall muscles, bilateral
cryptorchidism, and a dilated and dysmorphic urinary tract.

● WORKUP

On physical examination, the newborn has a fascial defect
6 cm in diameter. The herniated viscera—small bowel and
liver—are covered by a translucent sac with the umbilical
cord inserted at its apex (Figure 101-1). Chest x-ray, echocardiogram, renal ultrasound, and skeletal radiography are performed. Aside from the omphalocele, no other anomalies are
noted. Routine laboratory tests are within normal limits, and
no hypoglycemia is observed.

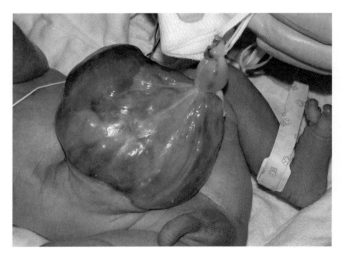

FIGURE 101-1. Giant omphalocele with small bowel and a
large portion of the liver herniated through the defect.

● DISCUSSION

Omphalocele occurs due to a failed midline fusion of the lateral embryonic abdominal folds and unsuccessful return of the midgut into the abdominal cavity at approximately 5 weeks gestation. The incidence of omphalocele is 1 in 5,000 live births. Omphalocele occurs more commonly in males, infants born to multiparous women, multiple births, infants born to African American women, families with a history of omphalocele, and with extremes of maternal age (<20 years and ≥35 years). Omphalocele can present as a part of a syndrome, as with Beckwith-Wiedemann syndrome, OEIS (omphalocele, cloacal exstrophy, imperforate anus, and spinal anomalies) complex, Gershoni-Baruch syndrome, and Donnai-Barrow syndrome. Chromosomal abnormalities are also associated with omphalocele (trisomy 13, 14, 15, 18, or 21). Of patients with an omphalocele, 50% to 70% will have at least one associated anomaly. Cardiac defects are the most frequent associated anomaly, occurring in 30% to 50%. Of these, ventricular septal defect, atrial septal defect, and patent ductus arteriosus are most commonly observed. Aside from cardiac defects, musculoskeletal, gastrointestinal, and genitourinary defects are common. Chromosomal abnormalities occur in 30%. For children with omphalocele and a chromosomal abnormality, trisomies 13, 18, and 21 are most common, collectively occurring in 87%. Omphalocele has been observed in cases of Turner's syndrome and triploidy. Beckwith-Wiedemann Syndrome is associated with an umbilical defect (umbilical hernia or omphalocele), macroglossia, hyperinsulinemia, and organomegaly. Additionally, Beckwith-Wiedemann syndromes carry an increased risk of pediatric malignancies (Wilms' tumor, hepatoblastoma, and neuroblastoma). Lower midline syndrome is characterized by exstrophy of the bladder or cloaca, vesicointestinal fissure, colonic atresia, imperforate anus, sacral vertebral defects, and lipomeningocele or meningomyelocele.

Omphaloceles that are large in size are associated with worse outcomes. Compared to children with small omphaloceles, those with giant omphaloceles are more likely to have an associated congenital abnormality (37% to 67%) and have higher mortality rates.

● MANAGEMENT

Most cases of omphalocele are diagnosed via prenatal ultrasound. Omphalocele can be detected by ultrasound after 10 to 14 weeks gestation. The sensitivity of antenatal ultrasound for detecting an omphalocele is approximately 75%. After the diagnosis is established, further prenatal testing is performed to assess for the presence of other congenital abnormalities and genetic alterations that may lead to intrauterine fetal demise or death postnatally. Elevated maternal serum and amniotic fluid alpha fetoprotein can be found with omphalocele and other abdominal wall defects. A fetal karyotype should be performed. Given the high likelihood of congenital cardiac disease, fetal echocardiography is recommended. Serial prenatal ultrasounds and close prenatal surveillance must be performed because a fetus with omphalocele is at increased risk for fetal growth retardation, polyhydramnios, and intrauterine death.

After the diagnosis of omphalocele is confirmed, prenatal counseling should be provided by a multidisciplinary team that includes a pediatric surgeon to provide the parents with an overview of the postnatal and surgical management of the future newborn patient. Delivery for omphalocele should occur in a tertiary care center with advanced neonatal and pediatric surgical support. To the extent that it is possible, mode and timing of delivery is determined by the obstetrical team. There is no benefit to delivery prior to 37 weeks gestation. During delivery, there is a risk of dystocia, sac rupture, and injury to abdominal viscera; therefore, special care and preparation must be taken. Cesarean section should be performed if a giant omphalocele is present. Vaginal delivery is appropriate for children with a small omphalocele.

Initial postnatal care and management should focus upon stabilization of the newborn. For babies born outside of tertiary care institutions, transport after initial stabilization is necessary. After birth, care must be taken to prevent injury to the sac and its contents. Rupture of the sac increases the risk of infection, intestinal injury, and hepatic trauma. If the sac is compromised, the option for delayed closure is lost. After birth, infants must be evaluated immediately for pulmonary or cardiac anomalies by routine birth assessment. Some infants may require supplemental oxygen or intubation and ventilator support. Patients with a giant omphalocele are at risk for pulmonary insufficiency secondary to pulmonary hypoplasia. Such patients may require prolonged ventilation, advanced modes of ventilator support, or extracorporeal membrane oxygenation.

After delivery and upon confirmation of cardiovascular and pulmonary stability, intravenous (IV) access is established. Peripheral IV catheters are sufficient for immediate postnatal resuscitation. However, many infants with omphalocele will require parenteral nutrition, and obtaining central venous access early is preferable. Umbilical vessels should not be used for central access because the course of the umbilical vessels is abnormal in omphalocele. Furthermore, the vessels are ligated at the time of surgical repair.

Patients with omphalocele can be hypovolemic at birth—the risk of hypovolemia is increased in cases of ruptured omphalocele. With established IV access, patients are immediately placed on D10/0.25 normal saline at a rate of 140 to 150 mL/kg/d. With the demonstration of adequate hydration, the fluid rate can be reduced to a maintenance rate of 80 to 100 mL/kg/d. If the omphalocele sac remains intact, fluid loss is not excessive. However, a ruptured sac can lead to continued high fluid loss. In these cases, patients should be maintained at the higher fluid rate (140 to 150 mL/kg/d), and fluid boluses (20 mL/kg of 0.45 normal saline) should be administered when clinically indicated.

There are two critical aspects of management of babies with omphalocele. First, there is a significant risk for hypothermia. The patient's temperature must be closely monitored, temperature in the resuscitation room should be elevated, the newborn should be placed in an isolette with a warmer, and the omphalocele should be covered with plastic wrap to maintain body heat. Second, frequent glucose monitoring is essential. Due to the association of omphalocele with Beckwith-Wiedemann syndrome, glucose monitoring should be performed until Beckwith-Wiedemann syndrome can be ruled out.

Further management includes the placement of a Repogle and urinary catheter for gastric and bladder decompression. Antibiotics and vitamin K are administered. A physical examination and appropriate imaging are necessary to assess for other anomalies. After the initial resuscitation, all infants with omphalocele receive an echocardiogram to evaluate for cardiac abnormalities.

Once the child is deemed stable from a cardiorespiratory standpoint, the membranous sac is evaluated for areas of disruption. The diameter of the fascial defect is measured. The omphalocele sac should be covered for protection, to prevent insensible fluid losses, and to minimize heat loss. Wet dressings can accelerate hypothermia; thus, a nonadherent dressing should be placed around the sac. A second layer with dry mildly compressive gauze should be wrapped around the omphalocele. A third layer of plastic wrap may also be applied. If the child requires transfer to a tertiary care center, the lower extremities and abdomen should be placed into a sterile bowel bag.

As long as omphalocele remains intact, closure is not urgent and should be delayed until the neonate has been stabilized and other anomalies are been ruled out. If the membrane has been violated, the viscera should be placed in a spring-loaded silastic silo. The silo can be placed in the operating room or in a sterile setting in the neonatal intensive care unit with the support of an operating room team.

● SURGICAL APPROACH

Emergent repair of omphalocele is not indicated, rather, the defect should be repaired under planned and controlled circumstances. Prior to repair, patients should be stable from a cardiopulmonary standpoint. Patients with Beckwith-Wiedemann syndrome require aggressive management of hypoglycemia. Children should undergo karyotype analysis—given that the presence of Trisomy 13 or 18 has the potential to change goals of care (Table 101-1).

The goals of surgery for correction of omphalocele are to reduce the viscera into the abdominal cavity and to close the skin and fascia. Up to half of omphalocele defects can be closed primarily. Children with omphalocele will have reduced intraabdominal domain. Forced placement of the viscera into the abdomen places the patient at risk for abdominal compartment syndrome. The amount of viscera that requires reduction in relation to the size of the abdomen, referred to as visceroabdominal disproportion, is a key factor in determining the timing and type of surgical closure. Other

Table 101-1	Omphalocele

Key Technical Steps

1. Sharp dissection of the membranous sac from the fascial and skin edges
2. Reduction of the herniated viscera
3. Evaluation for increased intra-abdominal pressure
4. Primary closure of the fascia in a tension-free manner
5. Primary closure of the skin

Potential Pitfalls

- Increase in intra-abdominal pressure resulting in respiratory compromise or abdominal compartment syndrome
- Injury to the liver capsule and resulting hemorrhage
- Disruption of portal, mesenteric, or central venous vessels

equally important factors are the size of the fascial defect and the overall physiologic state of the patient.

For an omphalocele <5 cm, a primary closure is the best option for treatment. Closure involves removal of the sac at the level of the skin. If there is residual sac covering the liver, this can be left in place to avoid injury to the liver capsule. The umbilical vessels and urachus are suture ligated. Skin flaps are raised to expose the fascia. Some surgeons will manually stretch the muscles and fascia to increase abdominal domain. As the viscera are reduced, the anesthesiologist must be kept abreast, as it is essential to monitor for signs of abdominal compartment syndrome. Early signs of abdominal compartment syndrome include increased peak inspiratory pressures. Oliguria or anuria is also possible. With respiratory or hemodynamic compromise, temporizing measures must be taken prior to closure of the abdomen. The neonatal liver must be handled carefully during reduction to avoid torsion of the hepatic veins, disruption of portal vein inflow, or hemorrhage due to injury to the liver capsule. The bowel is inspected for anomalies. However, adhesiolysis or dissection is not performed for the purpose of inspection. The midgut should be reduced first, followed by the liver. Once the viscera are reduced and there is no signs of abdominal compartment syndrome are observed, the fascia is closed in the midline. If midline closure is not possible, transverse closure is acceptable. Simple or mattress stitches are placed through the abdominal wall (except the skin) with absorbable suture. The skin is closed with a running absorbable suture. An umbilicoplasty is performed if there is sufficient skin.

Primary closure may not be an option in the setting of increased intraabdominal pressure or a wide fascial gap. If primary closure is not possible, several options exist. Skin closure with incomplete fascial closure can be completed. In this case, incomplete fascial closure is completed at the edges of the defect to the extent that is possible. Skin flaps are raised, and the skin is closed over the remaining defect. If a small ventral hernia remains it can be repaired at a later date. Another temporizing method is to bridge the fascia with nonabsorbable (Gore-tex, Marlex), absorbable (Vicryl, Dexon), or biologic mesh (Alloderm, Surgisis). Skin flaps are mobilized to cover the mesh. Nonabsorbable mesh is a temporary option. The mesh is removed and fascia closed after the child has grown, and closure is possible. The potential complications of using nonabsorbable mesh are infection, seroma, and fistula. Absorbable graft material (Vicryl, Dexon) provides favorable short-term results, but the repair will weaken over time leaving a ventral hernia. Such hernias should be repaired when the child has grown sufficiently to allow for a fascial closure. Biologic mesh will incorporate into the fascia and stimulate fibroblast ingrowth. There are no large series that demonstrate the efficacy and complication rates associated with biologic mesh repair.

A ruptured omphalocele requires urgent coverage of the viscera, usually with a silastic silo or a biologic mesh. If a biologic mesh is used, topical therapy is applied to its exterior to facilitate granulation.

A single operative repair may not be feasible, as with small omphalocele that cannot be closed primarily, a large omphalocele with a high volume of herniated viscera, or a wide fascial defect. In such cases, staged closure is required. Different methods of staged closure exist. The key principle of staged closure is to provide temporary coverage while the viscera are gradually reduced into the abdomen. Temporary coverage can be achieved using a silastic silo sewn to the edges of the fascia or a spring-loaded silo suspended from an isolette. Gradual pressure is applied by placing ties or sutures along the silo that push the viscera into the abdomen over time. Another methods involves sewing sheets of Gore-tex or silastic to opposite ends of the fascia. The closure is gradually tightened by cutting out a portion of each sheet in the center and closing it with a new suture line. This is done every 2 to 3 days until the fascial edges are close enough to perform a primary closure.

For patients with a giant omphalocele or those that are too unstable for surgery, the "paint and wait" technique with or without compression of the sac is recommended. The hernia sac is coated with an antimicrobial agent that allows the sac to toughen into an eschar and contract the sac. As the child grows, the sac becomes smaller, and the viscera slowly return to the abdomen. Currently, silver sulfadiazine (Silvadene) is the topical treatment of choice due to its broad spectrum antimicrobial activity, decreased toxicity compared to other potential agents, and ease of daily application. Daily application of silver sulfadiazine facilitates granulation tissue formation and subsequent epithelialization of the sac. Complete epithelialization of the sac generally occurs within 3 months. Some pediatric surgeons have begun to use betadine rather than silver sulfadiazine, crediting ease of application and quicker eschar formation; however, recent studies have demonstrated superior results with silver sulfadiazine. Mercurochrome and silver nitrite are no longer used because they create metabolic and electrolyte derangements. With the "paint and wait" technique, a large ventral hernia develops that can later be repaired primarily with or without component separation or with placement of a biocompatible mesh. Compression is accomplished via wrapping an

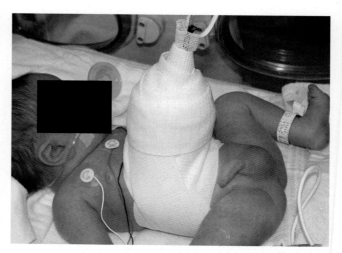

FIGURE 101-2. Elastic compression bandages are wrapped around the omphalocele and the back of the infant to gradually reduce the herniated viscera.

elastic bandage around the sac. The bandage should assume the conformation of a cone and is carried around the back of the infant to create compressive forces toward center of the abdominal cavity. The addition of an elastic bandage for compression may speed the process of reduction of the viscera and increase the likelihood of a delayed primary fascial repair. The "paint and wait" technique usually necessitates a delay of 6 to 12 months before definitive closure.

● POSTOPERATIVE MANAGEMENT

The use of systemic antibiotics is at the discretion of the surgeon and is based on intraoperative findings. IV fluid at an initial rate of 150 mL/kg/h should be started and titrated for goal urine output of at least 1 mL/kg/h. Parental nutrition administered via a central venous catheter should continue until bowel function returns. Prolonged postopertative ileus often occurs. If bowel function fails to return by 3 weeks after surgery, a contrast bowel study should be ordered to rule out other gastrointestinal pathology.

Case Conclusion

In this case, primary closure of the defect was impossible. As the patient had no other congenital anomalies, we chose to perform a staged repair using the "paint and wait" technique. Parenteral nutrition was initiated at birth.

Over the next several weeks, silver sulfadiazine was applied daily. An external compression bandage was utilized. Enteral feeds were slowly titrated to goal, and parenteral nutrition was discontinued. By 2 months of age, the sac was completely epithelialized, and visceroabdominal disproportion was considerably decreased. At 8 months of age, the infant was taken to the operating room for primary closure. The child's postoperative course was uncomplicated (Figure 101-2).

● COMPLICATIONS

Complications can occur after omphalocele repair. Most often, these occur early on are attributed to an increase in abdominal pressure after reduction of the herniated viscera into an abdomen. Left unaddressed, abdominal compartment syndrome and associated respiratory compromise can result. Infants can develop indirect inguinal hernias following omphalocele repair, as increases in intraabdominal pressure may lead to dilation of the internal inguinal rings. Unless there is evidence of incarceration or strangulation of the bowel, there is no need for immediate repair. In fact, inguinal hernias may act as a "pop off" valve to reduce intra-abdominal pressure. Thus, inguinal hernia repair is delayed until comorbid conditions resolve. An increased incidence of gastroesophageal reflux may also occur due to the increased intraabdominal pressure.

As with any abdominal operation, postoperative adhesions can develop. Intraabdominal infections or infections within the abdominal wall can lead to wound separation, dehiscence, or sepsis. The presence of a prosthesis increases the risk of infection. Complications associated with prolonged parental nutrition include central venous catheter infection and hepatic dysfunction. Due to abnormal fixation and rotation of the intestine, a child with omphalocele has malrotation. However, corrective repair does not take place at the time of the abdominal wall defect repair. Therefore, complications related to malrotation and midgut volvulus are occasionally observed following repair.

● OUTCOMES

The overall mortality in live birth with omphalocele is 13% to 25%. Patients with giant omphalocele more commonly have associated anomalies, higher mortality rates, and possibly higher rates of neurocognitive delays. Additionally, unfavorable outcomes are associated with exteriorization of the liver. Oftentimes, the presence of associated congenital anomalies influence outcomes. Irrespective of omphalocele size, infants with an isolated omphalocele have a 75% to 95% likelihood of survival. In children with giant omphalocele, prognosis and outcome are closely related to associated anomalies and pulmonary complications, such as pulmonary hypoplasia.

TAKE HOME POINTS

- Fifty to Seventy percent of infants with omphalocele have an additional congenital anomaly. Cardiac defects occur in 30% to 50% of cases. Congenital anomalies are more common with giant omphalocele.
- Early strict glucose monitoring is required until Beckwith-Wiedemann Syndrome is ruled out.
- When the membrane covering the viscera is intact, repair can be delayed until other pathology is ruled out.
- The goal of repair is primary closure with no increase in intraabdominal pressure. If this is not possible, mesh closure of the defect or staged closure may be required.
- In the unstable infant, or for infants with giant omphalocele, the "paint and wait" technique is preferred.
- Morbidity and mortality are often due to concurrent anomalies, rather than the omphalocele itself.

SUGGESTED READINGS

Baird R, Gholoum S, Laberge J, Puligandia P. Management of a giant omphalocele with an external skin closure system. *J Pediatr Surg.* 2010;45(7):E17-E20.

Bauman B, Stephens D, Gershone H, et al. Management of giant omphaloceles: a systematic review of methods of staged surgical vs. nonoperative delayed closure. *J Pediatr Surg.* 2016;51:1725-1730.

Frolov P, Alali J, Klein M. Clinical risk factors for gastroschisis and omphalocele in humans: a review of the literature. *Pediatr Surg Int.* 2010;26(12):1135-1148.

Heider A, Strauss R, Kuller J. Omphalocele: clinical outcomes in cases with normal karyotypes. *Am J Obstet Gynecol.* 2004;190(1):135-141.

Isalm S. Clinical care outcomes in abdominal wall defects. *Curr Opin Pediatr.* 2008;20(3):305-310.

Kumar H, Jester A, Ladd A. Impact of omphalocele size of associated conditions. *J Pediatr Surg.* 2008;43(12):2216-2219.

Ledbetter D. Gastroschisis and omphalocele. *Surg Clin North Am.* 2006;86(2):249-260, vii.

Mac Bird T, Robbins J, Druschel C, Cleves M, Yang S, Hobbs C; National Birth Defects Prevention Study. Demographic and environmental risk factors for gastroschisis and omphalocele in the National Birth Defects Prevention Study. *J Pediatr Surg.* 2009;44(8):1546-1551.

Mann S, Blinman T, Douglas Wilson R. Prenatal and postnatal management of omphalocele. *Prenat Diagn.* 2008;28:626-632.

Marshall J, Salemi JL, Tanner JP, et al. Prevalence, correlates, and outcomes of omphalocele in the United States, 1995-2005. *Obstet Gynecol.* 2015;126(2):284-293.

Marvin S, Owen A. Contemporary surgical management strategies for congenital abdominal wall defects. *Semin Pediatr Surg.* 2008;17(4):225-235.

Whitehouse J, Gourlay D, Masonbrink A, et al. Conservative management of giant omphalocele with topical povidone-iodine and its effects on thyroid function. *J Pediatr Surg.* 2010;45(6):1192-1197.

Gastroschisis

KEVIN N. JOHNSON AND JAMES D. GEIGER

Based on the previous edition chapter "Gastroschisis"
by Samir K. Gadepalli and James D. Geiger

Presentation

A child is born via spontaneous vaginal delivery to a 17-year-old mother with abdominal contents open to the air. Prenatal ultrasound had shown polyhydramnios and thickened, echogenic loops of bowel outside of the abdomen. On examination, the child weighs 2.5 kg, is on room air, and is in no acute distress. Bowel is seen protruding from a fascial defect measuring approximately 2 cm in size just to the right of the umbilicus without a membranous covering.

DIFFERENTIAL DIAGNOSIS

Congenital abdominal wall defects are classified as either gastroschisis or omphalocele. Gastroschisis occur to the right of midline, do not have a protective covering, and rarely have organs other than bowel outside of the abdomen (see Figure 102-1). Gastroschisis is also associated with atresias of the bowel, although these cannot be reliably diagnosed at the time of birth. Omphalocele is a midline defect that does have a membrane covering the bowel, and commonly has liver in the defect as well. Additionally, omphalocele may be associated with upper midline defects, including diaphragm, pericardium, cardiac, and sternal defects, known as the pentalogy of Cantrell. Bladder exstrophy may also occur

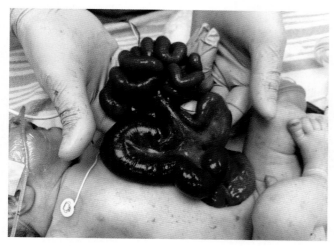

FIGURE 102-1. Gastroschisis.

in omphalocele. Omphalocele is also associated with several genetic disorders, including trisomies 13, 18, and 21, and Beckwith-Wiedemann syndrome.

WORKUP

Children with gastroschisis are more likely to be born to young mothers (<20 years of age), mothers who smoke or use drugs or alcohol during pregnancy, and those who are born with low birth weight for gestational age. Prenatal factors that can be found with gastroschisis include elevated alpha-fetoprotein (77% to 100%) and polyhydramnios. Along with the presence of the bowel outside of the abdomen, echogenic bowel loops can often be seen on fetal ultrasound late in pregnancy, and about half of patients with gastroschisis will have intrauterine growth restriction. Familial cases of gastroschisis are exceedingly rare. Neonates with gastroschisis can be born via vaginal delivery without increased risk of bowel injury when compared to cesarean section.

Little workup is performed initially for patients with gastroschisis. No membrane is present over the bowel in gastroschisis, although care must be taken not to mistake a ruptured omphalocele for gastroschisis, as this requires a much different workup. There are few congenital anomalies associated with gastroschisis outside of intestinal atresias, most commonly jejunoileal atresias. While initial examination of the bowel prior to reduction and closure of the abdomen can reveal areas of the bowel, which appear to be atretic, this evaluation is not reliable, and the bowel should be reduced regardless. Persistent feeding intolerance can prompt contrast studies to evaluate for the presence of intestinal atresias in the future (Table 102-1).

DIAGNOSIS AND TREATMENT

For children who are born with gastroschisis, the main principles are to resuscitate the child as they are often dehydrated at birth and to provide coverage of the exposed bowel. The bowel is examined for any evidence of twisting of the mesentery (which has a narrow base), which must be promptly reduced to avoid bowel compromise. Tension must also be avoided on the mesentery by turning the baby or supporting the bowel with towels to keep it up on the abdomen before it

Table 102-1	Differences Between Gastroschisis and Omphalocele	
	Gastroschisis	**Omphalocele**
Location of defect	Right of midline	Midline
Presence of sac	No	Yes
Contents	Small bowel only	Bowel, liver (usually)
Associated anomalies	Intestinal atresias	Heart, bladder Genetic (trisomy, Beckwith-Wiedemann)

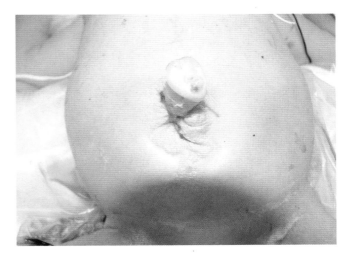

FIGURE 102-2. Primary closure of gastroschisis.

is placed into a silo. Failure to recognize a mesenteric twist or tension can lead to catastrophic bowel injury. The lower half of the child will often be placed in a bag to minimize fluid losses until a more definitive solution can be performed. Enteral decompression with a nasogastric or orogastric tube is performed, and a Foley catheter is placed to monitor resuscitation.

Initial resuscitation involves placement of an intravenous line and the administration of IV fluids containing sodium (usually ¼ to ½ NS) at around 150 mL/kg/d or 1.5 times maintenance. Urine output and electrolytes should be closely followed to guide resuscitation. Central access for administration of parenteral nutrition is needed in almost all cases. Endotracheal intubation is not an absolute but is needed in the majority of cases

Presentation Continued

Following placement of an orogastric tube, Foley catheter, and a peripheral IV, the patient is intubated for attempted reduction of the small bowel. As the bowel is reduced, peak airway pressures begin to rise and the patient's oxygen requirements begin to increase. The decision is made to place the bowel in a silo and transport the patient to the NICU for further care.

● SURGICAL APPROACH

Following initial resuscitation of the child including gastric decompression, options for closure are considered. Attempted reduction of the bowel into the abdomen is often performed in the neonatal recovery room, while monitoring overall hemodynamics and peak airway pressures in intubated patients to monitor for signs of abdominal compartment syndromes. Decompression of dilated bowel loops can be accomplished when the bowel is not thickened by "milking" succus proximal into the stomach and meconium distally out the anus. Often 100 to 500 mL of volume can be

evacuated increasing the likelihood of primary reduction. In patients in who the bowel can be completely reduced, the umbilical stalk can be used to cover the residual defect, and an occlusive dressing placed over the top to be left in place for 7 days (see Figure 102-2). To facilitate primary reduction or silo placement, it is necessary to enlarge a small fascial defect. This can be done either in the midline superiorly or transversely to the right of the defect.

In patients in who there is a significant rise in intra-abdominal pressure with reduction of the bowel, or when the bowel cannot be completely reduced without significant tension on the wound, a silo should be placed (Figure 102-3). It is important the defect is open enough to avoid a funnel effect. Antibiotic prophylaxis is not routinely used while the silo is in place. Once the silo is in place, gradual reduction of the bowel into the abdomen can be performed using umbilical tape tied around the silo. Once the bowel has been nearly completely reduced, the patient is brought to the operating room for formal closure. Undermining of the skin is often needed to maximize the amount of fascia that can be closed.

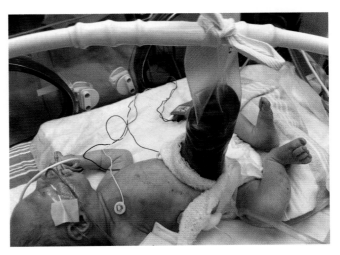

FIGURE 102-3. Silo placement.

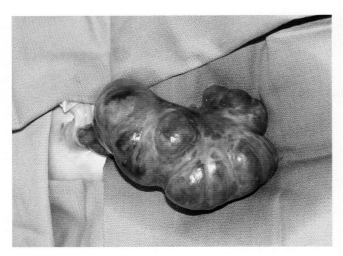

FIGURE 102-4. Matted bowel with gastroschisis.

Table 102-2	Gastroschisis Closure

Key Technical Steps

1. Decompress the bowel
2. Reduce the bowel while monitoring peak airway pressures and tidal volumes
3. Undermine the skin if needed
4. Determination if a patch is needed for closure, for either a staged or primary closure
5. Closure fascia and skin
6. Creation of an umbilicus

Potential Pitfalls

- Bowel injury
- Abdominal compartment syndrome

The silo spring can lead to a large abdominal wall defect that has to be closed in a stage manner or with mesh.

Common pitfalls of closure for gastroschisis include inadvertent bowel injury, which is common given the inflamed and matted nature of the bowel (Figure 102-4). Minimizing manipulation of thickened bowel aids in minimizing this risk. Additionally, mesenteric ischemia can be avoided by paying careful attention to the orientation and tension on the mesentary. Also, careful monitoring of peak airway pressures and tidal volumes intraoperatively will aid in the decision is made whether the fascial defect can be closed primarily or if a synthetic patch (vicryl or polytetrafluoroethylene) should be used for closure in order to not create an abdominal compartment syndrome with the closure (Table 102-2).

Presentation Continued

Following several days of cinching, the bowel is nearly completely reduced and the patient is taken to the operating room for formal closure. After undermining the fascia, the bowel is reduced and peak airway pressures and tidal volumes remain adequate. The fascia is closed primarily, and the patient is returned to the NICU.

● SPECIAL INTRAOPERATIVE CONSIDERATIONS

If a suspected atresia is seen during closure of a gastroschisis, the temptation may be to either create an ostomy or attempt primary repair of the atretic area. However, this should only be considered when the bowel is not thickend and matted. In most cases, the thickened and matted nature of the bowel in gastroschisis due to it being outside of the abdomen in utero and since birth makes it difficult to create an ostomy. Additionally, visual inspection of the bowel has been shown to not be a reliable indication that an atresia is present, and

attempting to operate on the bowel, either to create ostomies or anastomose, the atretic segment is not recommended due to the friable nature of the bowel. Once the bowel has been reduced, waiting at least 4 weeks is traditionally done prior to operating for an atresia if it is confirmed on contrast study; although if the patient is developing cholestatic liver disease as the results of parenteral nutrition, surgery can be performed earlier.

Management of bowel perforations in patients with gastroschisis is particularly challenging. As the bowel is inflamed and matted in most cases, primary repair is not an option and also makes ostomy creation challenging. Additionally, if the bowel is present within a silo, catheters can be placed into the bowel perforation to try and control the output, in addition to keeping the perforation near the top of the silo if possible to minimize spillage.

● POSTOPERATIVE MANAGEMENT

Feeding intolerance is common following closure of gastroschisis. Patients commonly have some element of gastroparesis, intestinal dysmotility, and gastroesophageal reflux. In patients with prolonged feeding intolerance, the possibility of an atresia should be addressed by performing a contrast study. Standard measures to improve feeding include keeping the head of the bed elevated, administration of H_2 blockers or PPI, placement of a postpyloric feeding tube, and occasionally the use of a promotility agent such as erythromycin or metoclopramide.

Life-threatening complications for patients with gastroschisis include the development of necrotizing enterocolitis (NEC) and line sepsis. Patients with gastroschisis are more likely to develop NEC, and treatment of NEC in these patients does not differ from standard patients. In patients who become ill, but do not have evidence of NEC, the presence of line sepsis is the most common cause among this population.

Wound breakdown is another common occurrence following gastroschisis closure. Peri-incisional erythema is common following closure, so careful monitoring of the wound is needed to identify surgical site infections. Wound breakdown can often be managed conservatively with wet-to-dry wound packing in many cases.

Case Conclusion

Two weeks postoperatively, the patient develops bloody movements and has evidence of pneumatosis on an abdominal film consistent with NEC. Feeds are held, and the patient is placed on antibiotics for 10 days. Following the course of antibiotics, the patient is restarted on feeds and is discharged several days later after reaching goal feeds.

TAKE HOME POINTS

- Fundamentals of initial care include coverage of the bowel to limit heat and fluid loss and aggressive resuscitation.
- Intestinal atresias occur in about 10% of patients with gastroschisis.
- Monitor peak airway pressures and tidal volumes while reducing the abdominal contents for closure to avoid abdominal compartment syndrome.
- Feeding intolerance is very common postoperatively, with several measures that can be taken to improve tolerance.
- Closely monitor for NEC and line sepsis during the postoperative period.

SUGGESTED READINGS

Almman R, Sousa J, Walker MW, et al. The epidemiology, prevalence and hospital outcomes of infants with gastroschisis. *J Perinatol.* 2016;36(10):901-905.

Kong JY, Yeo KT, Abdel-Latif ME, et al. Outcomes of infants with abdominal wall defects over 18 years. *J Pediatr Surg.* 2016;51(10):1644-1649.

Safavi A, Skarsgard ED. Advances in the surgical treatment of gastroschisis. *Surg Technol Int.* 2015;26:37-41.

Skarsgard ED. Management of gastroschisis. *Curr Opin Pediatr.* 2016;28(3):363-369.

Stoll C, Alembik Y, Dott B, Roth MP. Risk factors in congenital abdominal wall defects (omphalocele and gastroschisis): a study in a series of 265,858 consecutive births. *Ann Genet.* 2001; 44(4):201-208.

Tracheoesophageal Fistula

STEVEN W. BRUCH

103

Based on the previous edition chapter "Tracheoesophageal Fistula" by Steven W. Bruch

Presentation

A newborn baby boy, born to a healthy 28-year-old female at 37 weeks' estimated gestational age with APGAR scores of 8 and 9, had difficulties with his first feed. He coughed and sputtered after the feeding appearing to choke and then almost immediately spit up all of the feeding. There was no bile in the emesis. A nasogastric tube was passed but met resistance. A chest x-ray revealed the tube curled up at the thoracic inlet, a slightly distended stomach, but otherwise a normal abdominal gas pattern.

● DIFFERENTIAL DIAGNOSIS

Failure to tolerate feeds and an x-ray showing a nasogastric tube coiled in a proximal esophageal pouch with air in the bowel is typical in a baby born with esophageal atresia (EA) and a distal tracheoesophageal fistula (TEF). There are five variations of EA with or without TEF as seen in Figure 103-1, with the most common being EA with a distal TEF. An iatrogenic esophageal perforation can mimic an EA with difficult passage of a nasogastric tube. These perforations are almost always in the proximal esophagus, just proximal to the cricopharyngeus muscle, and heal on their own with intravenous antibiotics, nothing per mouth, and placement of a tube past the perforation into the stomach to help drain the saliva.

● WORKUP

Preoperative workup attempts to answer three questions: Are there associated anomalies? What side of the chest is the arch of the aorta located? And what is the exact anatomy of the trachea, esophagus, and their connections?

Anomalies associated with EA and TEF include chromosomal anomalies and a sequence of anomalies referred to as the VACTERL sequence that includes vertebral, anorectal, cardiac, tracheal, esophageal, renal, and limb anomalies. A karyotype will look for chromosomal anomalies the most frequent being trisomies 13 and 18, which are lethal, and trisomy 21, Down's syndrome. The VACTERL anomalies are evaluated with physical exam looking for the anorectal anomalies, usually imperforate anus, plain x-rays for the vertebral and limb anomalies, an abdominal ultrasound for renal anomalies and to look for tethering of the spinal cord, and an echocardiogram for cardiac abnormalities.

The echocardiogram is also used to locate the aortic arch. If the arch is located on the right side, it makes it difficult to complete the esophageal anastomosis over the arch making a left thoracotomy optimal for a tension-free esophageal anastomosis.

The anatomy of the trachea and esophagus can be defined in a number of ways. The initial plain x-ray determines if a distal TEF is present. If there is a gasless abdomen as seen in Figure 103-2, there is no distal TEF, whereas if there is gas in the bowel, a connection between the trachea and the distal esophagus is present. A proximal fistula can be evaluated with a "pouchogram," rigid bronchoscopy, or both. A pouchogram, depicted in Figure 103-3, involves placing a small amount of barium in the proximal esophageal pouch to evaluate its size and to look for a connection between the pouch and the membranous portion of the trachea. A small pouch implies that fluid swallowed by the fetus exited the pouch via a proximal fistula, therefore not providing the pressure required to distend the proximal esophageal pouch. Rigid bronchoscopy will allow visualization of the distal fistula, which is usually seen at the carina as shown in Figure 103-4. A close look should be undertaken for a proximal fistula, which is rare and quite a bit more subtle than the distal fistulas. An H-type fistula is often suspected later and is diagnosed with an esophagram as seen in Figure 103-5 and/or with rigid bronchoscopy.

● DIAGNOSIS AND TREATMENT

With the diagnosis made and the workup completed, the newborn is taken to the operating room for repair of the EA and TEF. In children with EA without a distal TEF, a gastrostomy tube placement with evaluation of the gap length between the two ends of the esophagus is the first step in treatment. If the gap length is ≥3 vertebral bodies, repair is delayed. With time, the gap length may shorten allowing primary repair, or remain "long" leading to creative techniques

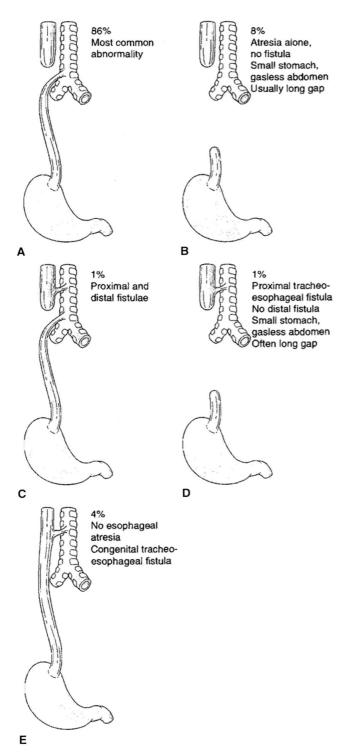

A 86%
Most common abnormality

B 8%
Atresia alone, no fistula
Small stomach, gasless abdomen
Usually long gap

C 1%
Proximal and distal fistulae

D 1%
Proximal tracheo-esophageal fistula
No distal fistula
Small stomach, gasless abdomen
Often long gap

E 4%
No esophageal atresia
Congenital tracheo-esophageal fistula

FIGURE 103-1. The five varieties of EA with and without TEFs with their rates of occurrence. **A:** EA with a distal TEF. **B:** Pure EA. **C:** EA with a proximal and a distal TEF. **D:** EA with a proximal TEF. **E:** H-type TEF.

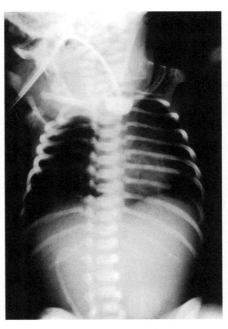

FIGURE 103-2. The gasless abdomen of pure EA. The proximal pouch is outlined with contrast.

● SURGICAL APPROACH

A right posterolateral thoracotomy is used unless a right-sided aortic arch is identified on echocardiography, when a left posterolateral thoracotomy provides optimal exposure. A muscle-sparing technique minimizes rib cage and spinal abnormalities later in life. The chest is entered through the fourth interspace using a retropleural approach. This allows for more easy retraction of the lung during the case and prevents intrapleural soilage in case of an anastomotic leak postoperatively. The azygos vein is identified and divided exposing the connection between the trachea and the distal esophagus. The esophagus will distend with each breath helping identify its location. The fistula is divided close to the tracheal wall. The proximal pouch is then identified by asking the anesthesiologist to push on the nasogastric tube located in the pouch. It will be found at the thoracic inlet. A suture, used to provide traction, is placed through the esophageal pouch and the nasogastric tube. The proximal pouch is dissected circumferentially as proximal as possible keeping in mind the possibility of a proximal fistula located between the pouch and the membranous portion of the trachea. The dissection should avoid opening the membranous tracheal wall by staying on the thick muscular wall of the esophageal pouch. Cautery should be minimized to avoid injury to the recurrent laryngeal nerves. At this point, an assessment of the length of the gap between the two ends of the esophagus should be made. If the two ends can be brought together, an anastomosis is performed. If extra length is required, the distal esophagus may be mobilized. Although the blood supply to the distal esophagus, which is segmental from the

to bring the esophageal ends together, or to the creation of an esophageal spit fistula in the left side of the neck and an eventual esophageal replacement with either a gastric or colon conduit.

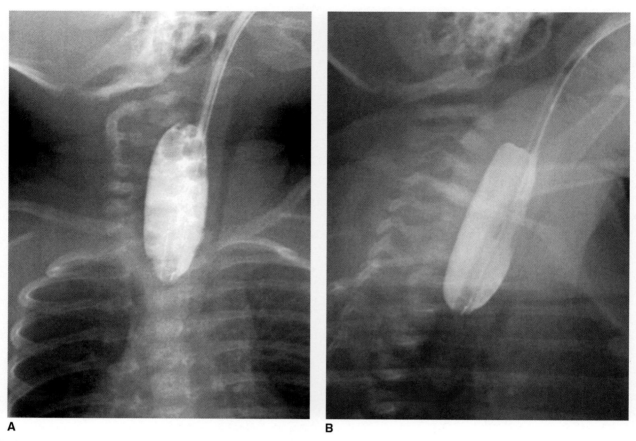

A   **B**

FIGURE 103-3. AP (**A**) and lateral (**B**) views of a pouchogram revealing no connection between the upper esophageal pouch and the trachea.

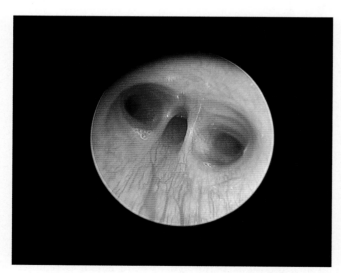

FIGURE 103-4. Bronchoscopic view of the distal TEF emanating from the carina between the right and the left mainstem bronchi.

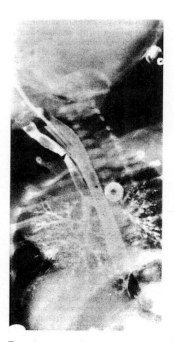

FIGURE 103-5. Esophogram demonstrating an H-type TEF denoted by the *arrow*. Contrast placed in the esophagus entered the tracheobronchial tree via the H-type fistula.

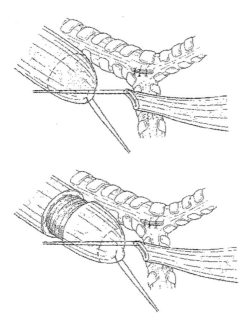

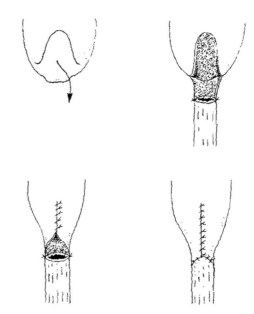

FIGURE 103-6. Use of a circular esophageal myotomy on the upper pouch to gain length and close the esophagus primarily.

FIGURE 103-7. Use of an anterior muscle flap of the upper pouch to gain length and close the esophagus primarily. (Reprinted from Gough MH. Esophageal atresia—use of an anterior flap in the difficult anastomosis. *J Pediatr Surg.* 1980;15(3):310-311. Copyright © 1980 Elsevier, with permission.)

descending aorta, is more tenuous than that of the proximal esophagus, which arises from the thyrocervical trunk, the distal esophagus may safely be mobilized if length is required but only after complete mobilization of the proximal esophagus. Other techniques to gain length include circular myotomies of the proximal pouch and tubularization of the proximal pouch as seen in Figures 103-6 and 103-7. When adequate length is obtained, an eight-stitch anastomosis is performed with absorbable suture material. The five back row sutures are placed, and a nasogastric tube is placed through the anastomosis and into the stomach. Then, the remaining three anterior sutures are placed to complete the anastomosis as shown in Figure 103-8. A chest tube is placed, and the thoracotomy incision is closed. Recently, thoracoscopic techniques have been developed to complete the repair in a minimally invasive fashion.

● SPECIAL INTRAOPERATIVE CONSIDERATIONS

Babies born with pure EA without a connection between the trachea and the distal esophagus present unique problems. The gap between the two ends of the atretic esophagus is often too long to bridge in the neonatal period. The first operative step in a pure EA is the placement of a gastrostomy tube to gain access to the stomach for enteral feeds. The stomach in these babies is very small making the placement technically challenging. When the gastrostomy tube is placed, an estimate of the gap length can be

obtained by placing a tube in the upper pouch and a neonatal endoscope in the distal esophagus via the gastrostomy site and looking at the gap distance with fluoroscopy. If the gap is within two vertebral bodies, a primary repair may be attempted. Most of the time, this gap will be too long to close, and the baby will be nursed with a Replogle tube in the proximal pouch, the head of the bed elevated 45°, while using the G-tube for feedings. Evaluation of the gap length should then be carried out every 4 to 6 weeks. Most agree that if the gap is not close enough to attempt repair by 3 months of age, then it is time to think about an esophageal replacement. This would include creating a spit fistula in the left neck in preparation for a gastric transposition or a colon conduit. The spit fistula allows sham feeds in these babies while they await their replacement operation. An option to consider prior to going to replacement of the esophagus is the "Foker" technique. This technique uses tension on the esophageal ends over time to lengthen the proximal and distal esophageal remnants. Multiple sutures with pledgets are placed on the proximal and distal esophageal ends. These sutures are then brought out the back of the baby (the lower pouch sutures out the upper back and the upper pouch sutures out the lower back) where they are placed on traction and shortened a small incremental amount each day until the ends are close enough to allow primary anastomosis as shown in Figure 103-9. A second option to avoid the spit fistula is to attempt a primary closure by fully mobilizing both the upper and lower esophageal segments, opening the crura, consider proximal and distal myotomies, and

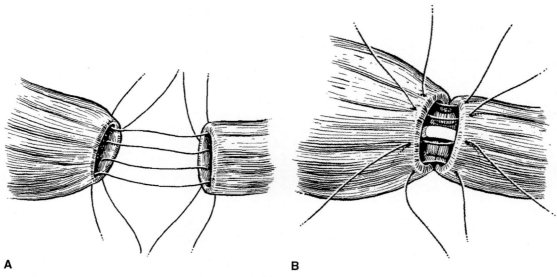

FIGURE 103-8. Esophageal anastomosis. **A:** Posterior sutures placed. **B:** Nasogastric tube is passed and anterior sutures complete the anastomosis.

fully mobilize the esophagus from the abdomen. If these maneuvers fail to bring the esophageal ends together, a primary gastric pull up is performed. On occasion, babies with EA are born with premature lungs and ventilation becomes difficult. The premature lungs require increased peak inspiratory pressures to adequately ventilate. This may result in a large portion of each mechanical breath going down the fistula rather than to the lungs because the air will travel the path of least resistance. This can be a difficult problem to manage. Attempts can be made to place

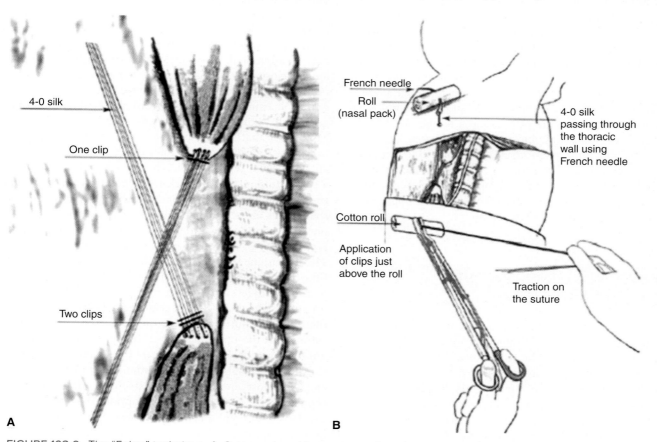

FIGURE 103-9. The "Foker" technique. **A:** Sutures placed in upper pouch and distal esophagus. Metal clips are placed to track the position of the esophageal ends using plain x-ray. **B:** Sutures are brought out the back and traction is used over time to lengthen the two segments of the esophagus.

the tip of the endotracheal tube past the fistula opening. This can rarely be sustained as a solution because of the mobility of the endotracheal tube and the close relationship of the TEF and the carina. There are several other options to control this problem. Placement of a Fogarty catheter that is inflated into the fistula with rigid bronchoscopy, followed by reintubation, often temporizes the situation. However, the Fogarty often inadvertently slips out of position causing this method to fail. Another option is to place a gastrostomy tube and put the end of the tube to underwater seal, thus increasing the resistance of the fistula tract and allowing more air into the lungs. At the time of gastrostomy tube placement, a Rumel tourniquet may be placed around the gastroesophageal junction and brought out the upper abdomen. This can be used to intermittently occlude the esophagus again forcing air into the mainstem bronchi rather than down the fistula. A more long-term solution is to divide the fistula through a right posterolateral thoracotomy. This should improve the respiratory status of the baby. If the anesthesiologist can then easily ventilate and oxygenate, the definitive repair can be done. If the baby does not improve after the fistula is divided, the distal esophagus should be stretched cranially and tacked to the prevertebral fascia with permanent sutures and the chest closed. This allows a definitive repair later when the baby has grown and the respiratory issues have resolved (Table 103-1).

● POSTOPERATIVE MANAGEMENT

In the postoperative period, the baby is nursed with the head of the bed elevated and meticulous care is taken to keep the oropharynx suctioned of saliva to prevent aspiration and pneumonia. Some surgeons will feed enterally through the tube across the anastomosis into the stomach. A contrast study of the esophagus is performed about 1 week after the operation to look for a leak. If no leak is present, the tube is removed, feeds are begun, and the chest tube is removed if no formula or saliva is seen draining. If there is a leak, large or small, the baby remains on antibiotics, the chest tube remains in place, and the study is repeated 1 week later until no leak is seen. These postoperative leaks seal with time. In addition to a leak, four more complications should be anticipated: stricture formation, gastroesophageal reflux, tracheomalacia, and recurrence of the TEF.

Stricture formation is common occurring in up to 40% of repairs. The stricture is almost always at the anastomosis, although rarely a primary cartilaginous esophageal stricture may be present in the distal esophagus in association with a TEF. Strictures are initially dilated with balloon dilator, or tapered bougie dilators that can be used over a guidewire (Savory dilators) or passed blindly (Maloney dilators). A child with a stricture that fails to stay open after serial dilation should be evaluated for gastroesophageal reflux

Table 103-1 Tracheoesophageal Fistula

Key Technical Steps

1. Confirm anatomy with plain films, pouchogram, and/or bronchoscopy.
2. Right posterolateral muscle sparing thoracotomy—use left-sided approach if aortic arch is located on the right side.
3. Retropleural dissection to posterior mediastinum.
4. Identify and divide the TEF.
5. Dissect the upper pouch looking for a proximal fistula, and avoid injury to the membranous trachea and recurrent laryngeal nerves.
6. If extra length is required, fully mobilize the upper pouch, mobilize the distal esophagus, open the esophageal hiatus, and consider upper then lower esophageal myotomies.
7. Perform an interrupted esophagoesophagotomy.
8. Place a chest tube.

Potential Pitfalls

- Ensure proper identification of the distal esophagus—the aorta has been entered thinking the TEF was being divided.
- Keep the dissection of the upper pouch on the thick esophageal wall to avoid injury to the membranous trachea and recurrent laryngeal nerves.
- Mobilize as little of the distal esophagus as necessary. Excessive mobilization may leave the proximal area ischemic, due to the segmental blood supply, resulting in a difficult postoperative stricture.
- Avoid tension, as much as possible, on the anastomosis.
- Always remember the worst native esophagus is better than an esophageal replacement. So do everything you can to bring the two ends of the esophagus together.

disease, as the stricture will not resolve until the reflux is adequately managed.

Gastroesophageal reflux occurs very commonly in this patient population, up to 70% of the time. Reflux is initially managed medically with a proton pump inhibitor with or without the addition of an H2 blocker. If medical management fails, a fundoplication may be necessary. Care must be taken when fashioning a fundoplication in these children. The distal portion of the esophagus in TEF patients does not peristalse well, and a fundoplication can lead to difficulties with dysphasia. Most pediatric surgeons will use a "floppy" Nissen fundoplication in these patients, although some prefer a partial wrap. Occasionally, these children will have a relatively short esophagus due to the initial repair and require a Collis-Nissen fundoplication to gain adequate length.

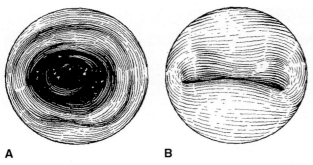

FIGURE 103-10. Bronchoscopic view of tracheomalacia. **A:** Open trachea during inspiration. **B:** The "fish mouth" collapse of the trachea during expiration.

Tracheomalacia can mimic gastroesophageal reflux disease in this patient population and occurs in up to 20% of babies born with TEF. Tracheomalacia occurs due to weakening of the tracheal cartilage resulting in "fishmouthing" of the trachea with expiration as seen on bronchoscopic view in Figure 103-10. Rigid bronchoscopy with the baby spontaneously breathing will diagnose tracheomalacia. Most babies will grow out of the malacia, but those with severe tracheomalacia require an aortopexy to stent open the trachea as seen in Figure 103-11. Recurrent TEFs occur in up to 10% of repairs. If suspected in children with respiratory issues around feeds or frequent pneumonias, it can be diagnosed with an esophagram or using a combination of rigid bronchoscopy and esophagoscopy. The best contrast study to identify a recurrence is a prone pullback esophagram where the study is done with the child lying prone allowing gravity to reveal the connection between the trachea and the esophagus. The use of rigid bronchoscopy and esophagoscopy will sometimes identify a recurrent fistula, but they are often difficult to pick up. In those difficult cases, placing methylene blue into the trachea and ventilating allows the dye to pass through the fistula if present into the esophagus where the blue dye can be seen with esophagoscopy. A recurrent fistula can be approached initially endoscopically. The fistula is identified; the mucosa is removed as best as possible

mechanically or with argon beam coagulation, and then, an adhesive is placed bronchoscopically to occlude the fistula. If this fails, an open procedure is required to separate the trachea and esophagus, repair the fistula, and place viable tissue between the suture lines. Usually, a flap of pericardium works well to prevent future recurrences.

Survival is excellent in near-term infants without cardiac anomalies. However, prematurity and the presence of a significant cardiac defect reduce the expected survival. Infants weighing >1,500 g at birth without major congenital cardiac anomalies have a 97% survival rate. If the infant is either born <1,500 g or has a major cardiac anomaly, the survival rate decreases to 59%. Infants who weigh <1,500 g at birth and have a major cardiac abnormality have only a 22% chance of survival.

Case Conclusion

On the second day of life, the baby underwent successful repair of the EA and TEF. The contrast study at 1 week showed no leak. Feeds were initiated and tolerated well, and he was discharged home. During the transition from formula to baby food, he developed some vomiting and dysphasia. A stricture was identified at the area of the anastomosis that underwent serial dilation and remained open. Other than having a "hot dog" that was underchewed get caught at the anastomotic site at age 3 requiring upper endoscopy and retrieval, he has done well and is taking all of his nutrition by mouth and thriving.

TAKE HOME POINTS

- EA and/or TEF is identified at birth with emesis and failure to pass a nasogastric tube.
- Plain film confirms EA with the tube in the proximal pouch and presence of a distal TEF when there is air seen in the abdomen.
- Evaluation involves excluding associated anomalies including chromosomal and VACTERL anomalies, identifying

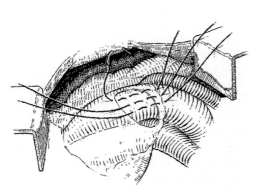
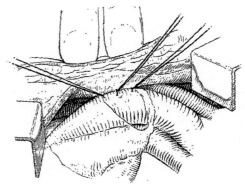

FIGURE 103-11. Aortopexy involves suturing the adventitia of the aorta to the sternum. This stents open the trachea in the babies with severe tracheomalacia.

the location of the aortic arch, and delineating the anatomy of the trachea, the esophagus, and their connections.

- Repair involves a right muscle-sparing posterolateral thoracotomy using a retropleural approach.
- Identification of the fistula and creation of an esophageal anastomosis with minimal tension provide the technical challenge.
- The anastomosis is studied at 1 week and allowed to heal on its own if a leak is identified. The leak should be retropleural and drained adequately with the chest tube.
- Postoperative complications include anastomotic leaks, strictures, gastroesophageal reflux, tracheomalacia, and recurrent TEFs.

SUGGESTED READINGS

Bruch SW, Hirschl RB, Coran AG. The diagnosis and management of recurrent tracheoesophageal fistulas. *J Pediatr Surg.* 2010;45:337-340.

Harmon CM, Coran AG. Congenital anomalies of the esophagus. In: Grosfeld JL, O'Neil JA Jr, Coran AG, et al., eds. *Pediatric Surgery.* 6th ed. Philadelphia, PA: Mosby Elsevier; 2006:1051-1081.

MacKinlay GA. Esophageal atresia surgery in the 21st century. *Semin Pediatr Surg.* 2009;18:20-22.

Spitz L, Bax NM. Esophageal atresia with and without tracheoesophageal fistula. In: Spitz L, Coran AG, eds. *Operative Pediatric Surgery.* 6th ed. London, UK: Hodder Arnold; 2006:109-120.

Skin and Soft Tissue

Melanoma

104

DANIELLE K. DEPERALTA AND VERNON K. SONDAK

Based on the previous edition chapter "Melanoma" by
Sebastian G. De La Fuente, Timothy W. McCardle, and Vernon K. Sondak

Presentation

A 37-year-old woman noted a pigmented lesion on her left arm approximately 3 months ago. She sought the attention of a dermatologist who performed a shave biopsy. Pathology was consistent with cutaneous melanoma. Breslow depth measured 1.1 mm, Clark level IV without evidence of ulceration. The tumor mitotic rate was less than 1 mitosis/mm^2. Peripheral and deep margins were involved. Physical examination reveals a healing biopsy site without residual pigmentation and no palpable lymphadenopathy.

● EPIDEMIOLOGY

Approximately 91,270 new cases of invasive melanoma and 87,290 cases of melanoma in situ are predicted to be diagnosed in 2018 in the United States. The worldwide incidence of melanoma is steadily increasing. Melanoma is 10 times more common in Caucasians than in African Americans. The mean age at diagnosis is 55 years old, and the most common primary sites are on the extremities of women and the trunk of men. Currently, melanoma accounts for approximately 5% of all skin cancer cases but is responsible for most skin cancer-related deaths, with 9,320 deaths predicted for 2018.

Even though the causes of melanoma are not fully understood, it is well established that exposure to sunlight, specifically ultraviolet (UV) radiation, is a significant risk factor. While sunburns are primarily due to UV-B (280 to 320 nm) radiation, UV-A radiation has been shown to induce mutations in various cell lines and is also considered a carcinogen. The highest-risk population includes individuals with fair skin who burn easily with sun exposure. Additional risk factors for melanoma are shown in Table 104-1.

● WORKUP

The initial evaluation of patients presenting with suspicious pigmented skin lesions should include a complete history and physical examination focusing on the characteristics of the lesion as well as the status of the regional lymph nodes. Suspicious pigmented lesions are those presenting with geometric asymmetry, irregular borders, a variety of colors within the same lesion, diameter larger than 6 mm, or changes over time (evolution) (Table 104-2) (Figure 104-1). Melanoma typically arises de novo within normal skin, but it can also arise in a pre-existing nevus. A previously stable mole that increases in size, becomes raised, or darkens in color is worrisome. The presence of pruritus, bleeding, or ulceration should also raise concern. It is important to emphasize that not all melanomas are visibly pigmented. Amelanotic melanoma lacks the classic dark or multicolored appearance, which can lead to a delay in recognition.

Suspicious skin lesions should be biopsied to establish a definitive diagnosis. The standard surgical dogma is that excisional biopsy with 1 to 2 mm margins of normal skin extending down to subcutaneous fat is preferred. However, excisional biopsy is sometimes undesirable due to the size of the lesion or its anatomic location (e.g., face, ears, digits, palm, etc.). Furthermore, it may not be routinely performed by some dermatologists, who represent the primary source of referral for these patients. Shave biopsy is a common method of diagnosis and has been shown to be reliable and accurate in the majority of cases. Ideally, the biopsy should include enough of the underlying dermis to allow determination of the depth of the lesion. Incisional or punch biopsies may also be considered for large lesions that cannot be easily removed with excisional or shave biopsy (Figure 104-2). Blood tests or imaging studies are generally not necessary in patients with clinically localized melanoma without signs or symptoms of metastatic disease. They may, however, be necessary to assess the patient's overall medical status or suitability for general anesthesia.

Table 104-1	Risk Factors for Melanoma

- Fair skin
- Red or blond hair, blue or green eyes
- Presence of many moles/dysplastic moles
- UV light exposure (especially blistering sunburns in childhood, tanning beds)
- Personal history of melanoma or nonmelanoma skin cancer
- Family history of melanoma
- Immunosuppression

Table 104-2	The ABCDEs of Melanoma Recognition

A. Asymmetry
B. Border irregularity
C. Color variation
D. Diameter > 6 mm
E. Evolution (change in lesion)

● DIAGNOSIS AND TREATMENT

Staging of melanoma is based on clinical and pathologic features and is determined according to the TNM classification system, which was updated for 2018 (Table 104-3). Clinical staging is based on the initial primary tumor biopsy, complete physical examination, and nodal FNA, which is performed in select cases. Pathologic staging includes the results of definitive surgical procedures such as wide excision, sentinel lymph node biopsy (SLNB), and radical lymphadenectomy. Patients with clinical stage I and II melanoma have localized disease, without clinical or radiographic evidence of regional or distant metastases. Clinical stage III patients harbor regional nodal or intralymphatic metastases, manifesting as enlarged lymph nodes, satellite lesions, and/or in-transit disease. Patients with clinical stage IV disease have distant metastasis. Pathologic stages I and II comprise patients with no histologic evidence of nodal involvement after undergoing sentinel lymph node biopsy. Pathologic stage III patients have histologic evidence of metastatic disease in regional lymph nodes or intralymphatic sites.

The T component of the TNM system addresses the primary tumor and is determined by the Breslow thickness, as well as the presence or absence of ulceration (Figure 104-3). Mitotic count should still be reported, but it has been eliminated as a component of the TNM staging in the 8th edition of the American Joint Committee on Cancer (AJCC) staging system. In the

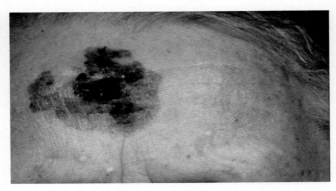

FIGURE 104-2. Forehead melanoma diagnosed with punch biopsy.

case presented above, the patient has a nonulcerated 1.1-mm melanoma, and therefore, her tumor is classified as T2a.

Other histopathologic features have prognostic implications and should be routinely described on the pathology report. These include the presence or absence of regression, microsatellitosis, vertical growth phase, angiolymphatic invasion, perineural invasion, and tumor-infiltrating lymphocytes (Table 104-4) (Figure 104-4).

● SURGICAL APPROACH

The surgical approach to primary cutaneous melanoma is radical wide excision of skin and subcutaneous tissue down to overlying fascia with a radial margin measured from the edges of the biopsy scar or any residual pigmentation (Table 104-5). The excision margin is determined by the depth and location of the primary tumor (Table 104-6). Wide excision alone (i.e., without an accompanying lymph node biopsy or dissection) can often be performed under local anesthesia, with intravenous sedation if necessary. The resected specimen is oriented and sent for permanent pathologic examination. In most cases, the resulting defect can be closed primarily, but a skin graft or myocutaneous flap coverage may be needed for large excisions or in tight areas such as the scalp, shin, or foot.

The most common first site of metastatic disease is the lymph node basin (or sometimes basins) draining the primary tumor site. Furthermore, the status of the regional nodal basin is the most important prognostic indicator in patients with clinically localized melanoma. Before the development of SLNB, many patients with primary tumor depth of 1.5 mm or greater were subjected to elective lymph node dissection for both therapeutic and staging purposes. However, the observation that elective lymphadenectomy did not provide survival benefit and was associated with significant morbidity, including lymphedema, wound infection, and nerve injury, led to the popularization of lymphatic mapping and SLNB in the 1990s. The MSLT-1 trial validated SLNB as a safe and reliable technique for axillary staging. Current guidelines recommend SLNB for patients with clinically node-negative melanoma greater than 1 mm

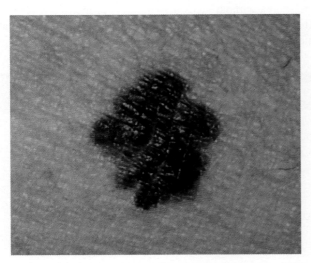

FIGURE 104-1. Melanoma presenting with asymmetry, irregular borders, and a variety of colors.

Table 104-3 | 8th Edition AJCC Staging Classification

Primary Tumor (T)

TX: primary tumor cannot be assessed
T0: no evidence of primary tumor
Tis: melanoma in situ
T1: melanomas 1.0 mm^a or less with ulceration status unknown or unspecified
  T1a: melanomas 0.1–0.7 mm or less in thickness without ulceration
  T1b: melanomas 0.8–1.0 mm with or without ulceration or 0.1–0.7 mm with ulceration
T2: melanomas 1.1–2.0 mm with ulceration status unknown or unspecified
  T2a: melanomas 1.1–2.0 mm without ulceration
  T2b: melanomas 1.1–2.0 mm with ulceration
T3: melanomas 2.1–4.0 mm with ulceration status unknown or unspecified
  T3a: melanomas 2.1–4.0 mm without ulceration
  T3b: melanomas 2.1–4.0 mm with ulceration
T4: melanomas >4.0 mm with ulceration status unknown or unspecified
  T4a: melanomas >4.0 mm without ulceration
  T4b: melanomas >4.0 mm with ulceration

Regional Lymph Node (N) and In-Transit, Satellite, and/or Microsatellite Metastases

NX: nodes cannot be assessed
N0: no regional lymph node disease
N1a: one clinically occult tumor-containing node without in-transit, satellite, and/or microsatellite metastases
N1b: one clinically detected tumor-containing node without in-transit, satellite, and/or microsatellite metastases
N1c: no regional lymph node disease with in-transit, satellite, and/or microsatellite metastases
N2a: 2 or 3 clinically occult tumor-containing nodes (i.e., detected by SLNB) without in-transit, satellite, and/or microsatellite metastases
N2b: 2 or 3 tumor-containing nodes at least one of which was clinically detected without in-transit, satellite, and/or microsatellite metastases
N2c: one clinically occult or clinically detected tumor-containing node with in-transit, satellite, and/or microsatellite metastases
N3a: 4 or more clinically occult tumor-containing nodes (i.e., detected by SLNB) without in-transit, satellite, and/or microsatellite metastases
N3b: 4 or more tumor-containing nodes, at least 1 of which clinically detected, or presence of any number of matted nodes without in-transit, satellite, and/or microsatellite metastases
N3c: 2 or more clinically occult or clinically detected tumor-containing nodes and/or presence of any number of matted nodes with in-transit, satellite, and/or microsatellite metastases

Distant Metastasis (M)

M0: no evidence of distant metastasis
M1a: metastases to skin, soft tissue, or distant lymph nodes with LDH not recorded or specified
  M1a(0): LDH normal
  M1a(1): LDH elevated
M1b: metastases to lungs with LDH not recorded or specified
  M1b(0): LDH normal
  M1b(1): LDH elevated
M1c: distant metastasis to non-CNS visceral sites with or without M1a or M1b sites of disease
  M1c(0): LDH normal
  M1c(1): LDH elevated
M1d: distant metastasis to CNS with or without M1a, M1b, or M1c sites of disease
  M1d(0): LDH normal
  M1d(1): LDH elevated

(Continued)

Table 104-3	8th Edition AJCC Staging Classification (*Continued*)

Clinical Staging

Stage	T	N	M
0	Tis	N0	M0
IA	T1a	N0	M0
IB	T1b	N0	M0
IB	T2a	N0	M0
IIA	T2b	N0	M0
IIA	T3a	N0	M0
IIB	T3b	N0	M0
IIB	T4a	N0	M0
IIC	T4b	N0	M0
III	Any T	≥N1	M0
IV	Any T	Any N	M1

Pathologic Staging

Stage	T	N	M
0	Tis	N0	M0
IA	T1a	N0	M0
IA	T1b	N0	M0
IB	T2a	N0	M0
IIA	T2b	N0	M0
IIA	T3a	N0	M0
IIB	T3b	N0	M0
IIB	T4a	N0	M0
IIC	T4b	N0	M0
IIIA	T1a/b–T2a	N1a or N2a	M0
IIIB	T0	N1b, N1c	M0
IIIB	T1a/b–T2a	N1b/c or N2b	M0
IIIB	T2b/T3a	N1a–N2b	M0
IIIC	T0	N2b, N2c, N3b, or N3c	M0
IIIC	T1a–T3a	N2c or N3a/b/c	M0
IIIC	T3b–T4a	Any N ≥N1	M0
IIIC	T4b	N1a–N2c	M0
IIID	T4b	N3a/b/c	M0
IV	Any T	Any N	M1

[a]Melanoma thickness should be reported to the nearest tenth of a millimeter. It may be measured to the nearest hundredth of a millimeter, but should be rounded to the nearest tenth of a millimeter for reporting purposes.

Modified from Amin MB, et al., eds. *AJCC Cancer Staging Manual Eighth Edition*. 2017.

in thickness. SLNB is not recommended for patients with primary tumor thickness <0.8 mm. There is still some debate regarding optimal management of patients with tumor thickness 0.8 to 1.0 mm. Current guidelines recommend that SLNB be offered to patients with primary tumor thickness 0.8 to 1.0 mm with evidence of ulceration and considered in patients without evidence of ulceration. It is our practice to routinely recommend SLNB for patients with melanoma ≥0.8 mm, regardless of ulceration. Thus, for the patient described in the Presentation, we would recommend radical wide excision with 1 to 2 cm margins, lymphatic mapping, and SLNB.

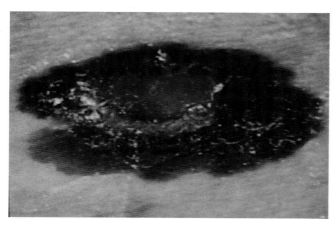

FIGURE 104-3. Melanoma, Clark level IV with a Breslow depth of 6 mm presenting with an area of ulceration in the center of the lesion.

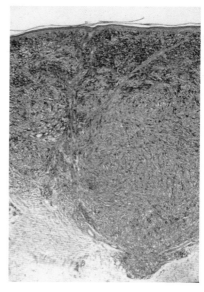

FIGURE 104-4. Dense brown melanin pigmentation in a melanoma with a nodular growth pattern.

Table 104-4	Histopathologic Factors that should be Documented on Pathology Report and their Effect on Prognosis (if any)

Histopathologic Factor	Impact on Prognosis
Tumor thickness	• Thickness ≤1 mm has best prognosis • Thickness >4 mm has worst prognosis
Ulceration	• Presence of ulceration has a worse prognosis
Growth phase	• Radial growth phase has better prognosis • Vertical growth phase has worse prognosis
Mitotic rate	• High mitotic rate has worse prognosis
Angiolymphatic invasion	• Worse prognosis
Perineural invasion	• Increased local recurrence
Regression	• No clear impact on prognosis, though remains controversial
Tumor-infiltrating lymphocytes	• Presence associated with improved prognosis
Solar elastosis	• No clear impact on prognosis
Satellitosis	• Microscopic or gross satellitosis has worse prognosis similar to nodal metastasis

Sentinel lymph node biopsy involves preoperative radionuclide lymphoscintigraphy and intraoperative injection of isosulfan blue dye. Preoperative lymphoscintigraphy, utilizing intradermally injected tracers such as ^{99m}Tc-sulfur colloid, permits determination of the lymphatic drainage patterns and allows identification of those basins at risk for melanoma metastasis (Figure 104-5A). A useful technique that combines single photon emission computed tomography with computed tomography (SPECT/CT) for localization of sentinel nodes provides considerably more anatomic detail than conventional lymphoscintigraphy. We find this particularly useful when drainage is to the neck, as the exact location of the SLN and its relationship with crucial neurovascular structures is more clearly delineated (Figure 104-5B and C).

Patients are typically injected 1 to 2 hours prior to the operation, allowing enough time for the tracer to travel to the basin of interest. The sentinel lymph node is identified intraoperatively with the aid of a handheld gamma probe. Additionally, intradermal administration of 0.5 to 1 mL of isosulfan blue dye (Lymphazurin 1%) around the intact tumor or biopsy site immediately preceding the surgical incision facilitates localization of the SLN during surgery. The combination of dye and radiolabeled colloid solution allows the surgeon to identify the SLN in more than 98% of cases. It is preferable to orient the incision for an SLNB based on the incision that would be required for a completion lymph node dissection. Removed nodes are carefully evaluated using hematoxylin and eosin staining and immunohistochemistry techniques with antibodies to one or more melanoma marker epitopes such as S100, HMB45, and MART-1/Melan-A. Intraoperative node evaluation with frozen section is unreliable for melanoma and typically not recommended. Complications of SLNB include hematoma, wound infection, seroma, and nerve injury, although serious adverse effects are very uncommon.

Table 104-5	Melanoma Surgery

Key Technical Steps

Radical Wide Excision

1. Minimum margins are measured from biopsy site/residual tumor and an elliptical skin incision created[a]
2. Dissection carried down to deep fascia
3. Wound closed in layers

Sentinel Lymph Node Biopsy

1. Patient reports to nuclear medicine for intradermal injection of ^{99m}technetium sulfur colloid to biopsy/tumor site
2. Lymphoscintigraphy defines drainage pattern
3. In the OR, the gamma probe used to confirm location of sentinel node(s)
4. Isosulfan blue dye is injected around the biopsy/tumor site
5. Targeted dissection using the gamma probe and visualization of blue dye
6. Nodal excision is complete once only background signal detected by probe without any residual visible blue or suspicious nodes
7. Sentinel nodes sent to pathology for paraffin embedding, step sectioning, and additional analysis with immunohistochemical stains

Potential Pitfalls

- Failure to anticipate need for skin graft or complex closure
- Neurovascular injury during dissection
- Failure to orient sentinel node biopsy incision to facilitate future completion node dissection
- Intraoperative frozen section should generally not be performed

[a]If not amenable to primary closure, a circular excision can be performed encompassing the minimum margins.

Table 104-6	Recommended Surgical Margins for Invasive Melanoma based on Prospective Randomized Trials

Tumor Thickness	Margin Recommendation
Melanoma in situ	0.5 cm commonly recommended, though not proven
<1.0 mm	1.0 cm
1.0–2.0 mm	1.0–2.0 cm depending on ability to achieve primary closure
>2.0 mm	2.0 cm

● SPECIAL INTRAOPERATIVE CONSIDERATIONS

If the patient will need a skin graft for coverage and an SLNB is to be performed, we commonly harvest a full-thickness skin graft from the SLNB incision site. This avoids the need for a third incision at the donor site. In patients with a tattoo adjacent to a primary melanoma, it is common for the carbon pigment from the tattoo to discolor the nodes. For this reason, it is sometimes helpful to avoid the use of blue dye so that there is no confusion when identifying the sentinel nodes. Occasionally, grossly abnormal and/or enlarged nodes are identified during SLNB. In these rare cases, it may be helpful to send the suspicious lymph node for intraoperative touch-prep analysis. Frozen section is generally not appropriate because it renders the sectioned areas of the node unusable for future immunohistochemistry.

Presentation Continued

The patient detailed above underwent radical wide excision and SLNB. Three SLNs were identified and removed. Final pathology report states that there was residual melanoma in the specimen, depth 1.2 mm, completely excised. SLNB was positive. Specifically, 2 of 3 nodes contained small foci of metastatic melanoma without evidence of extracapsular extension. Immunohistochemistry performed on the tumor-containing lymph nodes identified presence of the BRAF V600E mutation. After careful discussion she decided to be followed with nodal ultrasound and not to pursue CLND. She was referred to medical oncology to discuss adjuvant therapy options for resected stage III melanoma. The decision was made not to pursue adjuvant therapy. After 7 years, she continues to follow with her surgeon and is recurrence free.

● STAGING AND ADDITIONAL TREATMENT

The use of routine blood work and imaging studies for patients with clinical stage I or II disease is of low yield and not indicated. Given the pathologic findings above, the patient is staged as T2aN2a, Stage IIIA. Additional staging is indicated for patients with stage III or IV disease with CT or positron emission tomography (PET) scans. PET is sensitive for metastatic melanoma deposits as small as 5 to 10 mm in size but is nonspecific. The use of PET/CT fusion provides improved anatomic definition but does not eliminate false-positive results, which are still common. Brain magnetic resonance imaging (MRI) is recommended whenever patients have neurologic symptoms or distant metastases and is considered routinely for palpable stage III disease prior to surgery.

In patients with a positive SLN, overall 5-year survival is approximately 60% versus greater than 80% in patients with node-negative disease. The next step is to counsel the patient

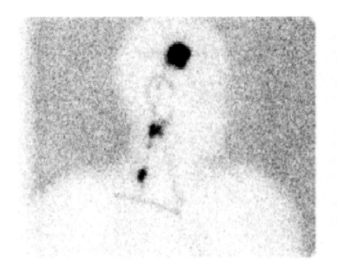

RT LAT Pix:2.4mm 99m Technetium

A

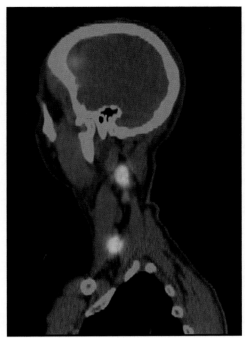

B

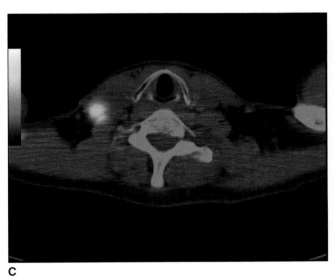

C

FIGURE 104-5. **A:** Conventional planar lymphoscintigraphy in a patient with a 2.1-mm nonulcerated melanoma of the temporal scalp. Images are taken after injecting ^{99m}technetium–sulfur colloid intradermally into the primary melanoma site. Note the anatomical landmarks defined on the scan by the technologist (ear, sternocleidomastoid muscle, and clavicle) for orientation purposes. **B:** Sagittal image from 3D SPECT/CT lymphoscintigraphy of the same patient as in A, demonstrating uptake in upper and lower cervical lymph nodes and more clearly demonstrating the relationship of the nodes to the ear, sternocleidomastoid muscle, and clavicle. **C:** Axial image from 3D SPECT/CT lymphoscintigraphy of the same patient as in A and B, showing the relationship of the upper sentinel lymph node to the undersurface of the sternocleidomastoid muscle.

regarding completion lymph node dissection (CLND), which has traditionally been the standard of care approach outside of a clinical trial, versus active nodal surveillance. Approximately, 75 to 80% of patients who undergo CLND have no additional nodal metastasis identified on final pathology, and many clinicians have questioned whether this additional operation is necessary. This was addressed by two randomized clinical trials: the German DeCOG trial and the multinational MSLT-2 trial, which both randomized melanoma patients with a positive SLNB to CLND versus nodal observation with ultrasound. In both trials, there was no difference in melanoma-specific survival between the two arms, but in the larger MSLT-2 trial, 5-year disease-free survival was

improved in patients who underwent CLND (61% vs. 57%). The CLND also afforded significant prognostic information. Lymphedema was reported in 24% of patients in the CLND group versus 6% in the observation group. Accordingly, we recommend a balanced discussion with the patient about the risks and benefits of CLND versus observation with nodal ultrasound prior to formulating a treatment plan.

In addition, the patient will need to decide whether to pursue adjuvant systemic therapy or observation. For patients with a positive SLNB, the decision to proceed with adjuvant therapy can be challenging given the treatment duration and associated toxicity of available agents. Two new options for patients with resected stage III melanoma were approved by the FDA in 2017. Immunotherapy with the programmed death 1 (PD1) inhibitor nivolumab is an option for the majority of patients and has been shown to increase recurrence-free survival by ~10% when compared with ipilimumab. Targeted therapy with combination BRAF/MEK inhibitors (dabrafenib plus trametinib) is another option that was shown to improve recurrence-free survival by 19% compared with placebo in patients whose melanoma has a BRAF mutation. Older options, including ipilimumab and interferon-alfa are now less clinically relevant in the adjuvant setting. Pembrolizumab is an another anti-PD1 agent that was recently demonstrated to improve recurrence-free survival by 14% compared with placebo. This will likely result in FDA approval of pembrolizumab for resected stage III melanoma.

● FOLLOW-UP

Controversy exists among clinicians regarding the frequency and duration of postoperative surveillance in patients with melanoma. One reasonable approach is to follow patients every 3 to 6 months for the first 2 to 3 years and annually thereafter. This schedule is influenced by a variety of factors such as the stage of the primary melanoma, number of lymph nodes involved, any prior history of melanoma, the presence of multiple atypical moles, or a family history of the disease. Patients with positive SLNB who do not undergo CLND should be followed with nodal ultrasound. Our practice is to perform ultrasound of the affected nodal basin every 4 months for 2-3 years, then every 6 months. After 5 years, ultrasound is performed annually until they are 10 years out from SLNB. We also perform annual PET-CT scans in these patients.

The main goal of surveillance is identification of new primary or recurrent disease at an early stage that would allow potential curative resection. Skin cancer education, including potential deleterious effects of sun exposure and the need for appropriate protection such as sun avoidance, protective clothing, and broad-spectrum sunscreens, should be promoted among melanoma patients and their families. Routine self–skin examination and assessment of lymph node basins are of great value, since most patients with recurrent melanoma find the disease themselves.

TAKE HOME POINTS

- Early recognition and treatment of cutaneous melanoma is associated with more favorable outcomes.
- Primary tumor thickness and histopathologic ulceration are important prognostic indicators, especially for early-stage melanoma.

- The most important prognostic factor for clinically localized melanoma is the status of the sentinel lymph node(s) draining the primary site. The optimal approach for the sentinel node-positive basin remains uncertain. CLND or nodal surveillance are both valid options.
- Current adjuvant therapy options for patients with resected stage III melanoma include observation, nivolumab or combination dabrafenib and trametinib (for patients with BRAF-mutated melanoma). Pembrolizumab is another option likely to be approved by the FDA this year. IFNα, pegylated IFNα, and ipilimumab are older options that are now less commonly used because of their side effect profiles.
- Postoperative surveillance for early-stage melanoma relies mostly on physical examination, with imaging studies performed when metastatic disease is suspected. Surveillance imaging for later-stage melanoma is commonly employed but has never been proven to be useful.

SUGGESTED READINGS

DePeralta DK, Hoang M, Tanabe KK. Approaches to regional nodes in patients with melanoma. *J Clin Oncol.* 2014;32:881-885.

Eggermont AMM, Blank CU, Mandala M, et al. Adjuvant pembrolizumab versus placebo in resected stage III melanoma. *New Engl J Med.* 2018;378:1789-1801.

Faries M, Cochran A, Andtbacka R, et al. Completion dissection vs. observation for melanoma sentinel node metastasis. *N Engl J Med.* 2017;376:2211-2222.

Han DH, Yu D, Zhao X, et al. Sentinel node biopsy is indicated for thin melanomas >0.76 mm. *Ann Surg Oncol.* 2012;19:3335-3342.

Lieter U, Stadler R, Mauch C, et al. Complete lymph node dissection versus no dissection in patients with sentinel lymph node biopsy proven melanoma (DeCOG-SLT): a multicenter, randomized, phase 3 trial. *Lancet Oncol.* 2016;17:757-767.

Long GV, Hauschild A, Santinami M, et al. Adjuvant dabrafenib plus trametinib in stage III BRAF-mutated melanoma. *N Engl J Med.* 2017;377:1813-1823.

McMasters KM, Egger ME, Edwards MJ, et al. Final results of the Sunbelt Melanoma Trial: a multi-institutional prospective randomized phase III study evaluating the role of adjuvant high-dose interferon alfa-2b and completion lymph node dissection for patients staged by sentinel lymph node biopsy. *J Clin Oncol.* 2016;34:1079-1086.

Morton DL, Cochran AJ, Thompson JF, et al. Final trial report of sentinel-node biopsy versus nodal observation in melanoma. *N Engl J Med.* 2014;370:599-609.

Schadendorf D, Fisher DE, Garbe C, et al. Melanoma. *Nat Rev Dis Primers.* 2015;1:15003.

Weber J, Mandala M, Del Vecchio M, et al. Adjuvant nivolumab versus ipilimumab in resected stage III or IV melanoma. *N Engl J Med.* 2017;377:1824-1835.

Zager JS, Hochwald SN, Marzban SS, et al. Shave biopsy is a safe and accurate method for the initial evaluation of melanoma. *J Am Coll Surg.* 2011;212:454-460.

Melanoma Presenting with Regional Lymph Node Involvement

WILLIAM R. BURNS AND MICHAEL S. SABEL

105

Based on the previous edition chapter "Melanoma Presenting with Regional Lymph Node Involvement" by Michael S. Sabel

Presentation

A 45-year-old man presented to his dermatologist after noticing a suspicious lesion on his right thigh. An excisional biopsy performed in the office demonstrated a 1.8-mm superficial spreading melanoma with ulceration. The patient now presents to your office for surgical management. On physical examination, there is a well-healed longitudinal scar on the right thigh and a palpable 2-cm, mobile, firm lymph node in the right groin.

Presentation Continued

FNA of the palpable node confirms the presence of metastatic melanoma.

● WORKUP

Unfortunately, once melanoma has spread to the lymph nodes, there is a steep drop-off in survival. Nonetheless, node-positive melanoma remains a potentially curable disease, and an aggressive surgical approach is warranted. Patients, such as this one, with biopsy proven nodal metastasis, should undergo additional evaluation for distant metastasis followed by wide local excision of the primary tumor and complete lymph node dissection if there is no radiologic evidence of distant metastasis.

A metastatic workup should be performed to evaluate any patients presenting with clinical stage III melanoma. An important part of this workup is a detailed history and physical examination. The history should include a thorough review of symptoms, focusing on symptoms consistent with metastatic disease, including any neurologic symptoms from possible brain metastases. In addition to the history and physical examination, all patients with clinically evident stage III disease should undergo staging studies. Current recommendations are for cross-sectional imaging (either a computed tomography [CT] scan of the chest/abdomen/pelvis or a whole-body positron emission tomography [PET]/CT scan). Given the propensity of melanoma to metastasize to the brain, magnetic resonance imaging (MRI) of the brain may also be considered, especially in patients with neurologic symptoms.

Several retrospective studies have suggested that these studies can lead to a change in surgical management in 15% to 35% of cases. For patients, such as the present one, with palpable inguinal adenopathy, a CT scan of the abdomen and the pelvis not only may evaluate for intra-abdominal metastasis but can also identify enlarged pelvic lymph nodes that might convert an inguinal node dissection to an inguinal–iliac dissection. It is important to note that with both CT scans and PET scans, false-positive findings are common; histologic

● DIFFERENTIAL DIAGNOSIS

All patients diagnosed with invasive melanoma should undergo a thorough physical examination, paying particular attention to the regional lymph node basins. Approximately 5% of patients will present with clinically apparent regional lymph node involvement at the time of diagnosis. Still others develop palpable lymphadenopathy months or years after excision of a primary melanoma, while occasional patients present with nodal metastasis in the absence of a detectable primary tumor (*occult primary melanoma*). Regional lymph nodes may become enlarged due to infection, inflammation, or reactive hyperplasia, particularly after an excisional biopsy of the primary tumor has been performed. However, any palpable nodes that are larger than 1 to 1.5 cm in size, hard, or fixed to adjacent structures must be considered suspicious for lymph node metastasis. In most cases, metastatic nodal involvement can be verified with a fine-needle aspiration (FNA) biopsy. Complications of an excisional biopsy (including seroma, infection, and scarring) can interfere with the performance of a subsequent lymph node dissection, so this should be reserved only for cases in which the percutaneous biopsy is negative or indeterminate; in this uncommon scenario, it can be helpful to perform excisional lymph node biopsy in combination with sentinel lymph node biopsy. When an excisional biopsy is performed, it is critical to orient the surgical incision so that it can be readily reexcised during the complete lymph node dissection if the node proves to be involved with tumor.

confirmation of an abnormal lesion should be obtained whenever feasible before concluding a patient has stage IV disease and abandoning a potentially curable surgical approach.

In some cases, the physical exam and/or staging studies may suggest that the regional disease is unresectable or borderline resectable, most often secondary to involvement of neurovascular structures. In these cases, preoperative systemic therapy should be strongly considered. Several new systemic agents have recently been approved for the treatment of unresectable stage III or stage IV melanoma. One promising approach is blockade of the immune checkpoints cytotoxic T-lymphocyte antigen-4 (CTLA-4) and programmed cell death-1 receptor (PD-1) with monoclonal antibodies to augment T-cell function. The anti-CTLA-4 antibody (ipilimumab) and anti-PD-1 antibodies (pembrolizumab and nivolumab) have led to impressive antitumor immune responses in clinical trials. Patients with a mutation in the BRAF gene, a component of a mitogen-activated protein (MAP) kinase pathway that is mutated in 50% of melanoma patients, also have the option of targeted therapies against BRAF (vemurafenib or dabrafenib) or the downstream target MEK (trametinib); these medications, which are often given in combination, can lead to dramatic clinical responses. Patients with clinically evident nodal disease, particularly if they do not seem resectable, should undergo testing of the biopsy specimen for the presence of a BRAF mutation. While treatment with either immunotherapy or targeted therapy can shrink regional disease and convert patients to potential candidates for surgery, close communication between the medical oncologist and surgeon is essential, as the proper timing of surgery is critical. Patients who stop responding, particularly with the targeted therapies, can quickly recur or progress, closing that operative window.

Presentation Continued

The patient is asymptomatic and physical examination shows no evidence of metastatic disease. A serum LDH level and CT scan of the chest, abdomen, and pelvis show no areas suspicious for metastatic disease, no involvement of neurovascular structures and no enlarged pelvic lymph nodes. The enlarged inguinal lymph node was visualized (Figure 105-1).

● SURGICAL APPROACH

The goal of a complete lymph node dissection is removal of all nodal and lymphovascular tissue within the nodal basin while preserving critical neurovascular structures (i.e., major blood vessels and motor nerves). Minor blood vessels and sensory nerves are often removed with the specimen in an attempt to reduce the risk of local recurrence. In cases where tumor invades these structures, however, complete resection of the tumor en bloc with the involved structure should be considered even if vascular reconstruction is necessary or an

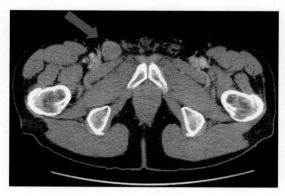

FIGURE 105-1. Contrast-enhanced CT scan demonstrates an enlarged right inguinal lymph node (*arrow*) without invasion of the adjacent femoral vessels.

acceptable postoperative motor deficit is anticipated. Closed-suction drains are frequently used to reduce the rates of postoperative seroma.

For patients with palpable disease in the axilla, a complete axillary lymph node dissection should include levels I, II, and III to provide the best regional control. In a very thin person, anterior retraction of the pectoralis major and minor muscle may allow for adequate dissection of the level III nodes. However, in many individuals, it may be necessary to divide the pectoralis minor. To do so, the pectoralis major is retracted anteriorly, and the fascia on either side of the tendon of the pectoralis minor is incised. With a finger behind the muscle to protect the axillary artery and vein, the insertion of the pectoralis minor is divided with electrocautery.

For patients with palpable disease in the groin, the extent of lymphadenectomy ("superficial" vs. "superficial and deep") is controversial. Some surgeons advocate complete superficial and deep inguinal lymph node dissections in all patients with palpable adenopathy. Others reserve deep dissection to those patients with a positive Cloquet's node or three or more involved nodes. Still others only perform deep groin dissections when there is radiographic evidence of pelvic adenopathy. If a deep groin dissection is to be performed together with a superficial dissection, this can be accomplished through one skin incision by obliquely dividing the external and internal oblique muscles to expose the pelvic retroperitoneum or alternatively by dividing the inguinal ligament. Dividing the ligament is particularly useful in cases of extensive disease low in the pelvis along the distal external iliac vessels. Although it is simpler to divide the ligament over the femoral vessels, wound healing may be improved if the inguinal ligament is detached from the anterior superior iliac spine (Table 105-1).

Case Conclusion

The patient undergoes a wide excision of the melanoma with 2-cm margins and a superficial and deep inguinal lymph node dissection. Three of eleven inguinal nodes and zero of five deep nodes are positive for lymph node metastases. There is no evidence of extracapsular extension.

Table 105-1	Superficial and Deep Inguinal Lymph Node Dissection

Key Technical Steps

1. The patient is positioned supine with the leg flexed and externally rotated in the frog-leg position.
2. An oblique, slightly S-shaped incision is created starting medial to the anterior superior iliac spine and coursing to a point 1–2 cm below the apex of the femoral triangle. An ellipse of skin over the palpable mass is included in the resection.
3. Progressively thicker flaps are raised laterally to the sartorius muscle, medially to the adductor longus and superiorly to a line from the pubic tubercle to the anterior superior iliac spine.
4. The lymph node–bearing tissue is then excised from over the femoral nerve, artery, and vein and off of the external oblique aponeurosis.
5. A deep dissection can be performed by creating a separate incision in the external oblique aponeurosis or by dividing the inguinal ligament.
6. The peritoneum and ureter are retracted medially to expose the iliac fossa. The iliac nodes are dissected off the common and external iliac vessels. The obturator nodes are dissected off the posterior surface of the external iliac vein.
7. After closure over a deep drain, the sartorius is mobilized and transposed to sit over the exposed femoral vessels.
8. A superficial drain is placed and the incision is closed.

Potential Pitfalls

- Injury to the spermatic cord structures or the contents of an unexpected hernia.
- Injury to the femoral or iliac neurovascular structures.
- Injury to the ureter.
- Bleeding from the obturator and iliac veins.

● POSTOPERATIVE MANAGEMENT

After a complete node dissection, there is a risk of recurrence in and around the dissected bed. The risk of regional recurrence increases with the size and number of involved nodes, and the presence of extracapsular extension. Some have advocated the use of adjuvant radiation to the dissected nodal basin. A prospective randomized trial demonstrated that radiation to the basin after radical lymph node dissection does decrease regional recurrence rates, although this does not appear to impact overall survival. Therefore, it is reasonable to consider postoperative radiation in patients with extracapsular extension, multiple involved lymph nodes (>2 cervical or axillary nodes or >3 inguinal nodes), or large nodes (>3 cm in the neck or axilla or >4 cm in the groin),

but the risks and benefits of adjuvant radiation must be carefully weighed. Given the higher risk of recurrence and lower morbidity of radiation after a neck dissection, the threshold for adjuvant radiation for cervical metastases is lower. On the other hand, adjuvant radiation after an inguinal node dissection is associated with significant morbidity and should be reserved for patients with a very high risk of relapse.

Patients with clinically evident regional metastases are also at a high risk of distant metastases, and most patients in this situation will ultimately die of their disease. Therefore, adjuvant therapy should be considered. For many years, high-dose interferon alpha-2b (HDI) was the only option for adjuvant therapy. However, the benefits were controversial, treatment took 1 year to complete, and there are considerable side effects. More recently, we have seen the systemic agents that proved effective in unresectable stage III or stage IV disease show efficacy in the adjuvant setting. The anti-CTLA-4 antibody ipilimumab was FDA approved in the adjuvant setting after a prospective randomized trial demonstrated an improvement in overall survival compared with placebo. The two anti-PD-1 antibodies, nivolumab and pembrolizumab, target PD-1, a T-cell receptor that binds to PD-L1 on tumor cells, inhibiting the immune system from attacking the tumor. Blocking this interaction also leads to increased T-cell activity, and both have been shown to improve recurrence-free survival compared to placebo. All of the checkpoint inhibitors carry a risk of potentially dangerous autoimmune complications, including colitis and endocrinopathies. However, in a direct comparison with ipilimumab, nivolumab was shown to be associated with better outcomes and was better tolerated by patients. Alternatively, for those patients harboring a BRAF V600 driver mutation in the MAP-kinase pathway, targeted therapy is another option. In the adjuvant setting, a combination of BRAF inhibition (dabrafenib) and MEK inhibition (trametinib) was associated with improved relapse-free and overall survival compared with placebo. Based on the available data, all patients with clinically evident nodal disease s/p resection should have a balanced discussion concerning the potential risks and benefits of adjuvant therapy. However, there remain many unanswered questions regarding adjuvant therapy, so participation in clinical trials is strongly encouraged for patients whenever possible.

TAKE HOME POINTS

- Approximately 5% of melanoma patients will present with clinically involved regional nodes.
- FNA of suspicious nodes is recommended to document regional involvement. Excisional biopsy can interfere with the subsequent node dissection.
- Workup should include a thorough history and physical examination and staging, which can be accomplished by CT or PET/CT.
- Patients with unresectable or borderline resectable regional disease should be considered for systemic therapy. The tumor should be tested for the presence of a BRAF gene

mutation. Close coordination with the medical oncologist is necessary for optimal timing of surgery after neoadjuvant systemic treatment.

- Patients with resectable disease and no definitive evidence of distant disease should undergo complete lymph node dissection. In the axilla, this typically involves levels I, II, and III. In the groin, some surgeons routinely perform a superficial and deep dissection, while other surgeons limit the deep dissection to patients with evidence of iliac or pelvic disease.
- Adjuvant radiation to the regional basin may be considered for patients at high risk of regional recurrence (multiple nodes, extracapsular extension); however, the risks (lymphedema, wound complications) must be carefully weighed against the benefits (decreased regional recurrence, no improvement in overall survival).
- All stage III melanoma patients should be referred to a medical oncologist for consideration of adjuvant therapy with either immunotherapy or targeted therapy. Patients should be encouraged to participate in on-going clinical trials.

SUGGESTED READINGS

Eggermont AM, Chiarion-Sileni V, Grob JJ, et al. Prolonged survival in stage III melanoma with ipilimumab adjuvant therapy. *N Engl J Med.* 2016;375(19):1845-1855.

Henderson MA, Burmeister BH, Ainslie J, et al. Adjuvant lymph-node field radiotherapy versus observation only in patients with melanoma at high risk of further lymph-node field relapse after lymphadenectomy (ANZMTG 01.02/TROG 02.01): 6-year follow-up of a phase 3, randomised controlled trial. *Lancet Oncol.* 2015;16(9):1049-1060.

Kirkwood JM, Manola J, Ibrahim J, et al. Eastern cooperative oncology group. A pooled analysis of eastern cooperative oncology group and intergroup trials of adjuvant high-dose interferon for melanoma. *Clin Cancer Res.* 2004;10(5):1670-1677.

National Comprehensive Cancer Network. Melanoma (Version 1.2017). https://www.nccn.org/professionals/physician_gls/pdf/melanoma.pdf. Accessed March 1, 2017.

Rodriguez Rivera AM, Alabbas H, Ramjaun A, Meguerditchian AN. Value of positron emission tomography scan in stage III cutaneous melanoma: a systematic review and meta-analysis. *Surg Oncol.* 2014;23(1):11-16.

Merkel Cell Carcinoma

WILLIAM R. BURNS AND MICHAEL S. SABEL

106

Based on the previous edition chapter "Merkel Cell Carcinoma" by Michael S. Sabel

Presentation

A 63-year-old male with history of liver transplantation presented with an enlarging red nodule on his left forearm. He initially noticed it 3 months ago but recently observed rapid growth to 3 cm in size. An excisional biopsy was performed under local anesthesia, and he was referred to your office for further evaluation and management.

● DIFFERENTIAL DIAGNOSIS

Rapid enlargement or change in a skin lesion is worrisome for a neoplastic process, although infectious and inflammatory processes should also be considered. In terms of skin cancer, basal cell carcinoma and squamous cell carcinoma are the two most prevalent. Both are associated with the chronic immunosuppression of organ transplantation, but squamous cell carcinoma is more commonly reported and is more frequently found to have high-risk features in this population. One must also consider more aggressive cancers such as melanoma, lymphoma, sarcoma, metastatic carcinoma, and Merkel cell carcinoma (MCC). Although rare, MCC often presents as a rapidly enlarging lesion and is found to be more aggressive in immunosuppressed patients. Other pathologies (such as lipoma, keratoacanthoma, epidermal cyst, pyogenic granuloma, Kaposi sarcoma, actinic keratosis, and other rarer skin lesions) should also be considered.

MCC is a rare but aggressive skin cancer. Also referred to as *neuroendocrine carcinoma of the skin* or *small cell carcinoma of the skin*, it is characterized by the presence of small blue cells on pathologic evaluation. Based on Surveillance, Epidemiology, and End Results (SEER) data, there are >1,500 new cases in the United States each year for an annual incidence of 0.79 per 100,000. MCC is most common among older individuals, with an average age at diagnosis of 69 years; only 5% of patients are younger than the age of 50. Patients with MCC typically present with an intracutaneous nodule or plaque that has grown rapidly over the preceding weeks or months. It can be flesh-colored, red, or purple. While it sometimes ulcerates, the overlying skin is frequently intact. They are most commonly found on sun-exposed areas, with approximately 50% on the face and neck, 40% on the extremities, and 10% on the trunk. Up to 80% of MCC are related to the Merkel cell polyomavirus,

whereas the remaining 20% are commonly associated with damage from ultraviolet radiation and carry a high mutational burden.

Presentation Continued

On physical examination, there is a healing biopsy site on the left forearm, which was closed with a purse-string suture (Figure 106-1). There is surrounding erythema and subtle nodularity at the periphery. There is also a palpable left axillary mass, but no other lymphadenopathy was identified. Pathologic evaluation of the biopsy identified MCC, measuring at least 11 mm in thickness with tumor extending to the deep and peripheral margins; there was no ulceration, but the mitotic rate was 61/mm^2 and lymphovascular invasion was present.

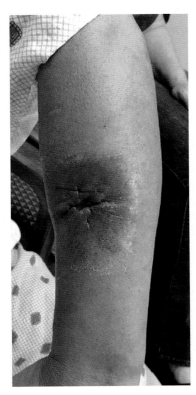

FIGURE 106-1. A 63-year-old male presents after excisional biopsy of a rapidly enlarging nodule on his left forearm.

● WORKUP

As with any patient noting a new cutaneous or subcutaneous lesion, a thorough history and physical examination is warranted. The history should include a review of pertinent risk factors, such as rapid growth or change in appearance, exposure to ultraviolet radiation, personal history of skin cancer or skin disorders, prior biopsies or ablative skin procedures, and relevant family history. The physical examination must include a complete skin and lymph node evaluation. This initial assessment will help narrow the differential diagnosis, but suspicious lesions require biopsy and pathologic evaluation to establish a diagnosis. Ideally, this is performed with an excisional biopsy, although shave biopsies of small lesions are often performed. For large pigmented lesions, a punch biopsy of the most abnormal area can also be useful.

MCC is rarely suspected at the time of presentation, but recognition of certain clinical features should increase the suspicion of MCC. The acronym *AEIOU* can help remind providers of these features: *A*symptomatic patients (lack of tenderness), *E*xpanding rapidly (significant growth in ≤3 months), *I*mmunosuppression (HIV infection, solid organ transplantation, chronic lymphocytic leukemia, etc.), *O*lder age (>50 years), and *U*ltraviolet-exposed sites on a person with a fair skin. It is estimated that up to 90% of patients with MCC have at least three of these findings.

Microscopically, MCC arises in the dermis and frequently extends into the subcutaneous fat. The tumor is composed of small blue cells with round to oval, hyperchromatic nuclei and minimal cytoplasm. There are three variants: intermediate (the most common), small cell, and trabecular. The small cell variant is identical to other small cell carcinomas and must be distinguished from metastatic small cell carcinoma. This may be accomplished through immunohistochemistry. Merkel cell tumors express CAM 5.2 and cytokeratin (CK) 20. CK7 and thyroid transcription factor-1 (TTF-1), which is typically found on bronchial small cell carcinomas, are absent on MCC. The intermediate type can often be confused for melanoma or lymphoma. MCC is invariably negative for S-100 and leukocyte common antigen, which distinguishes it from these.

Approximately 70% of patients with MCC present with localized disease, whereas 25% have clinical evidence of regional lymphadenopathy, and 5% present have distant metastases at presentation. MCC typically metastasizes to the regional lymph nodes, skin, lung, brain, bone, and liver. Patients with clinically involved lymph nodes or symptoms suggestive of distant metastases should have a computed tomography (CT) scan of the chest, abdomen, and pelvis. Positron emission tomography (PET) is also used for staging in high-risk patients. A CT scan of the chest should also be considered in patients with the small cell variant to exclude the presence of a lung mass suspicious for small cell lung cancer. Otherwise, for patients who have clinically localized disease, a chest radiograph alone is reasonable. The use of routine imaging studies in asymptomatic patients with clinically localized MCC is associated with a low rate of detecting true disease and a high false-positive rate, generating additional tests or biopsies and increasing patient anxiety without impacting overall survival.

Presentation Continued

Image-guided biopsy of the left axillary mass confirms MCC, and a PET-CT scan confirms axillary disease without evidence of distant metastasis (Figure 106-2).

● DIAGNOSIS AND TREATMENT

Similar to other rare or complex cancers, treatment options for patients with MCC are best decided in a multidisciplinary setting. Although initial treatment is usually surgical, patients should undergo appropriate staging evaluation and consideration of adjuvant therapy. Because of the high rate of local recurrence, margins of 2 to 3 cm have historically been recommended. However, low local recurrence rates have been reported after margin-negative excisions with more narrow margins. For lesions <2 cm in greatest dimension, a 1-cm margin is typically adequate. For lesions ≥2 cm,

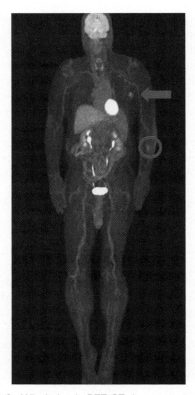

FIGURE 106-2. Whole body PET-CT demonstrates abnormal FDG uptake in the left forearm at the primary tumor biopsy site (*red circle*) and in the left axilla (*red arrow*). Other anatomic sites of FDG avidity are physiologic, and there is no evidence of distant metastatic disease.

a 2-cm margin is recommended when feasible. For patients with MCC in cosmetically sensitive areas, where even a 1-cm margin would be difficult, Mohs micrographic surgery has been reported to have comparable local control rates.

All patients with localized MCC should undergo sentinel lymph node (SLN) biopsy in conjunction with wide excision. Approximately 20% to 30% of clinically node-negative MCC patients are SLN positive, and the lymph node status is the most consistent predictor of survival. Because MCCs have a histologic appearance of small cell, approximately the size of a lymphocyte, they can be extremely difficult to detect within the lymph nodes using standard hematoxylin and eosin (H&E) staining alone. Therefore, immunohistochemical analysis of the sentinel nodes, in particular with anti-CK20, is essential. For patients having Mohs surgery, it may be preferable to perform the Mohs surgery after the patient has undergone SLN biopsy.

Presentation Continued

Wide local excision of the primary tumor site with a skin graft to close the acquired soft tissue defect and left axillary lymphadenectomy was recommended.

● SURGICAL APPROACH

Preoperative planning is critical to determine whether the primary tumor excision site is amenable to primary closure (Table 106-1). If not, reconstruction with either a skin graft or a rotational flap should be considered. The likelihood of postoperative radiation to the primary site should be taken into account when deciding the optimal method for reconstruction. Prior to surgery, the patient should also undergo lymphoscintigraphy (Table 106-1). This procedure is typically performed by an experienced radiologist in nuclear medicine, at which time a radioactive technetium (Tc-99m) sulfur colloid is injected into the dermis adjacent to the primary tumor or biopsy scar. The lymphoscintigram provides a "road map" for the surgeon to localize the SLNs that drain from the area of interest.

In the operating room, blue dye (e.g., isosulfan blue or methylene blue) is injected intradermally around the lesion (Table 106-1). In cases where proximity of the primary tumor may impact the ability to find the SLN (often termed "shine through"), the wide excision should be performed first (Table 106-1). A 1- to 2-cm margin, depending on the size of the primary tumor, is measured around the tumor (or scar from prior biopsy). If primary closure is feasible, an ellipse is drawn around the lesion to facilitate closure; a length to width ratio of 3.5:1 works well for the extremity. The skin and subcutaneous tissues should be completely excised down to the level of the muscle fascia (Table 106-1). After excision, skin flaps are elevated to allow primary wound closure (Table 106-1). However, if primary wound closure is not likely, then either a donor site for a split-thickness skin graft is prepped out or a rotational flap is marked out preoperatively. If there is any concern regarding margin status, it may be preferable to perform delayed reconstruction. This can be accomplished with standard wound dressings, a negative-pressure wound system, or a biologic wound matrix product. Once the final pathology results are known, the patient can then return to the operating room for a skin graft or rotational flap if negative margins have been attained (Table 106-1).

When excision is performed prior to SLN biopsy, all gowns, gloves, and instruments should be changed to avoid tumor contamination from the primary site to the regional nodal basin (Table 106-1). The SLN biopsy is performed through a small incision centered over the area of maximal radioactivity, such that the incision can be excised if complete lymph node dissection (CLND) is indicated in the future. Lymph nodes are considered to be SLNs if they are "hot" (i.e., possess Tc-99m), "blue" (i.e., possess blue dye), or "abnormal" (e.g., firm, enlarged, pigmented, etc.) on visual inspection and/or manual palpation. Nonsentinel lymph nodes, including those with <10% of the maximal radioactive counts, should not be removed. Despite the use of preoperative lymphoscintigraphy, intraoperative localization of an SLN can be challenging. In the rare scenario when a "hot" or "blue" lymph node cannot be identified after careful exploration of the nodal basin, a CLND is not mandatory. It is reasonable to abort the SLN biopsy procedure, obtain postoperative imaging, and discuss alternative strategies with the patient (likely with input from a multidisciplinary tumor board). More commonly, however, an SLN biopsy procedure may be required in multiple nodal basins based on the lymphatic drainage pattern of the primary tumor.

Table 106-1 Merkel Cell Carcinoma

Key Technical Steps

1. Preoperative planning for primary closure vs. skin graft or rotational flap.
2. Preoperative injection of Tc-99m colloid sulfur and lymphoscintigram and intraoperative injection of blue dye.
3. Wide excision first, if necessary, to minimize impact of "shine through" on SLN biopsy.
4. Measure adequate margins around the lesion (or scar) and excise down to include the fascia.
5. Undermine skin flaps for primary closure or rotational flap; otherwise, perform skin graft. Consider temporary graft if margin status is a concern.
6. Change position (if necessary), gowns, gloves, and instruments for performance of the SLN biopsy.

Potential Pitfalls

- Unable to close the primary tumor excision site.
- Inadequate margin for primary tumor excision.
- Inability to identify SLN.

Nonetheless, excisional biopsy of inaccessible second-order nodes (e.g., pelvic or internal mammary) is not typically recommended. For patients found to have a positive SLN, additional imaging should be considered to assess for distant disease; in the absence of distant metastasis, CLND or adjuvant radiation is typically recommended. For patients who have clinically involved lymph nodes and no evidence of distant metastasis, CLND should be performed at the time of primary tumor excision.

● SPECIAL INTRAOPERATIVE CONSIDERATIONS

There are several intraoperative clinical findings that can alter the planned surgery. Common "pitfalls" (difficulty with closure of the primary tumor site, suspicion that the margins of excision will be inadequate, and inability to locate an SLN) have already been discussed (Table 106-1). Another challenging scenario worth reviewing is when the surgeon encounters a tumor that directly invades an important neurovascular structure (e.g., long thoracic or thoracodorsal nerve, axillary or femoral vein, etc.). This almost always occurs in the context of bulky nodal disease. The ability to achieve a margin-negative resection and the expected morbidity of the procedure should be carefully considered. It is reasonable to sacrifice the long thoracic or thoracodorsal nerve, if needed, to excise all gross disease. Likewise, focal involvement of the axillary or femoral vein can be amenable to resection if only a small portion of the vein wall (or even a short segment of the vein) needs to be excised and the surgeon is comfortable performing venous reconstruction safely. Otherwise, it is best to preserve the key neurovascular structure and treat any residual disease with adjuvant radiation.

● POSTOPERATIVE MANAGEMENT

MCC is a radiosensitive tumor and radiation therapy is often part of the treatment algorithm. Adjuvant radiation is critical if surgical margins are positive or relatively close. For small primary tumors (<2 cm) in which clear margins are obtained, radiation offers toxicity but little clinical benefit. For primary tumors ≥2 cm, however, radiation should be strongly considered even if surgical margins are clear. Radiation can also be used for the regional nodal basin. For patients with low tumor burden in a positive SLN, adjuvant radiation may be considered as an alternative to CLND (although CLND is preferred at some centers). Adjuvant radiation after CLND is not necessary for patients with micrometastasis. This combination of CLND and radiation, however, is considered for patients with extensive lymph node disease or extracapsular extension. In these situations, the benefits of reducing regional recurrence must be weighed against the increased morbidity of surgery and radiation (i.e., lymphedema).

Although MCC is generally considered a chemosensitive tumor, adjuvant chemotherapy is the least studied treatment modality for MCC and currently has no established role in the treatment of regional disease. As such, systemic chemotherapy is only indicated for patients with unresectable regional disease or with distant metastatic disease. Conventional chemotherapy, most commonly platinum-based regimens (often with etoposide), can result in short-term clinical benefit. Unfortunately, chemotherapy is often toxic and rarely achieves durable responses. Immunotherapy, however, may be a better option for patients with advanced MCC. Recent clinical trials evaluating the efficacy of monoclonal antibodies inhibiting the programmed cell death receptor 1 (PD-1)/ programmed cell death ligand 1 (PD-L1) immune checkpoint, for example, have been promising. Additional studies are underway to better define the role of immunotherapy in the treatment of MCC.

Case Conclusion

He tolerated the procedure well. Pathology noted residual MCC extending to a new thickness of 12 mm in the left forearm with all margins negative. In the left axillary contents, MCC was found to involve 19 of 23 lymph nodes. His skin graft and axillary incision healed well, and the surgical drain was removed as the output decreased. His case was again discussed in multidisciplinary tumor conference with a consensus that he should undergo adjuvant radiation to the primary tumor site and regional nodal basin.

TAKE HOME POINTS

- MCC is a rare, but highly aggressive, cutaneous malignancy that is more common among elderly and immunosuppressed patients.
- Workup, including immunohistochemical staining of the biopsy, is needed to differentiate from amelanotic melanoma, lymphoma cutis, metastatic carcinoid, and metastatic small cell lung cancer.
- MCC can be treated with surgery, radiation, chemotherapy, and immunotherapy, so a multidisciplinary approach is strongly recommended.
- Local disease is treated with wide excision to achieve clear margins and often followed by adjuvant radiation.
- Clinically node-negative patients should undergo SLN biopsy in addition to wide excision. Patients with positive SLN typically undergo CLND, although radiation to the involved basin may also be considered.
- CLND followed by radiation should be considered for patients with extensive lymph node involvement or extracapsular extension.
- Chemotherapy and immunotherapy are options for patients with advanced MCC.

SUGGESTED READINGS

Becker JC. Merkel cell carcinoma. *Ann Oncol.* 2010;21(suppl 7): vii81-vii85.

Bichakjian CK, Lowe L, Lao CD, et al. Merkel cell carcinoma: critical review with guidelines for multidisciplinary management. *Cancer.* 2007;110(1):1-12.

Bichakjian CK, Olencki T, Alam M, et al. National comprehensive cancer network. Merkel cell carcinoma, version 1.2014. *J Natl Compr Canc Netw.* 2014;12(3):410-424.

Cassler NM, Merrill D, Bichakjian CK, Brownell I. Merkel cell carcinoma therapeutic update. *Curr Treat Options Oncol.* 2016;17(7):36.

Clarke CA, Robbins HA, Tatalovich Z, et al. Risk of Merkel cell carcinoma after solid organ transplantation. *J Natl Cancer Inst.* 2015;107(2):1-9.

Fitzgerald TL, Dennis S, Kachare SD, Vohra NA, Wong JH, Zervos EE. Dramatic increase in the incidence and mortality from Merkel cell carcinoma in the United States. *Am Surg.* 2015;81(8):802-806.

Heath M, Jaimes N, Lemos B, et al. Clinical characteristics of Merkel cell carcinoma at diagnosis in 195 patients: the AEIOU features. *J Am Acad Dermatol.* 2008;58(3):375.

Iyer JG, Storer BE, Paulson KG, et al. Relationships among primary tumor size, number of involved nodes, and survival for 8044 cases of Merkel cell carcinoma. *J Am Acad Dermatol.* 2014;70(4):637-643.

Nghiem PT, Bhatia S, Lipson EJ, et al. PD-1 Blockade with Pembrolizumab in Advanced Merkel-Cell Carcinoma. *N Engl J Med.* 2016;374(26):2542-2552.

Zager JS, Messina JL, Glass LF, Sondak VK. Unanswered questions in the management of stage I-III Merkel cell carcinoma. *J Natl Compr Canc Netw.* 2014;12(3):425-431.

Nonmelanoma Skin Cancer

107

ANASTASIA DIMICK

Based on the previous edition chapter "Nonmelanoma Skin Cancer" by Anastasia Dimick

Presentation

A 65-year-old white male presents with a slowly enlarging, tender 1.5-cm hyperkeratotic erythematous nodule on his left forearm. The patient first noticed the lesion about 3 months ago. He has severe photodamage (atrophic skin with numerous lentigines and senile purpura). Because of his occupation as a farmer, he has a chronic history of significant sun exposure. Previous medical history is significant for actinic keratoses (precancerous skin lesions for squamous cell carcinoma) on the face and hands, which have been treated with liquid nitrogen or cryotherapy (Figure 107-1). Family history is significant for melanoma in his father.

● DIFFERENTIAL DIAGNOSIS

In this clinical context, the most likely diagnosis is squamous cell carcinoma of the skin (Figure 107-2). Other diagnostic possibilities include basal cell carcinoma (Figure 107-3), basosquamous cell carcinoma, and melanoma. Clinical features of this lesion that point to squamous cell carcinoma are the erythematous color, the presence of hyperkeratosis or rough crusty skin, and tenderness. Melanomas can be hyperkeratotic in rare instances and sore or pruritic but are typically dark brown or black and asymptomatic. There is an uncommon variant of melanoma called amelanotic, which lacks pigment on clinical exam. These lesions may have a clinical appearance similar to basal cell carcinomas, which are usually pearly pink with telangiectatic vessels. The diagnosis of amelanotic melanoma is virtually always made on histopathologic grounds. Basosquamous cell carcinomas have clinical features of both basal cell carcinomas and squamous cell carcinomas.

● WORKUP

The patient underwent a cutaneous biopsy in the outpatient clinic. Pathology was consistent with well-differentiated squamous cell carcinoma.

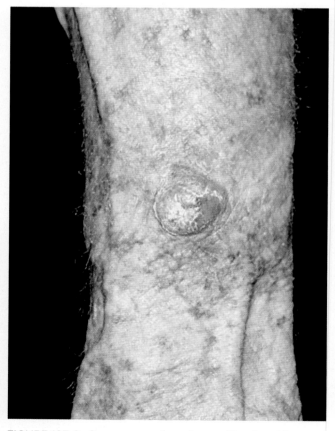

FIGURE 107-2. Squamous cell carcinoma. (Reprinted from Goodheart HP. *Goodheart's Photoguide of Common Skin Disorders*. 2nd ed. Philadelphia, PA: Lippincott Williams & Wilkins; 2003, with permission)

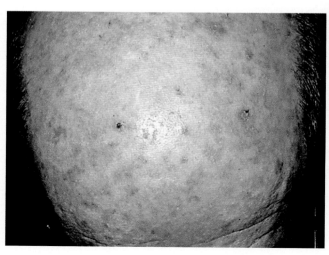

FIGURE 107-1 Actinic keratoses.

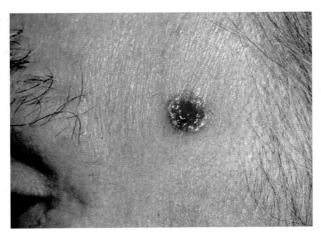

FIGURE 107-3. Basal cell carcinoma. (Reprinted from Goodheart HP. *Goodheart's Photoguide of Common Skin Disorders*. 2nd ed. Philadelphia, PA: Lippincott Williams & Wilkins; 2003, with permission).

● DISCUSSION

Squamous cell carcinoma is the second most common type of skin cancer in the United States. Basal cell carcinoma is the most common type of skin cancer in the United States. Together, these nonmelanoma skin cancers account for over 3 million cases per year. The vast majority of these cancers are caused by ultraviolet light exposure. As the population ages, the incidence is expected to increase. Risk factors for developing skin cancer include previous history of skin cancer, family history of skin cancer, fair skin (Fitzpatrick I [always burns, never tans] and Fitzpatrick II [usually burns, tans with difficulty]), severe sunburn history, excessive occupational or avocational sun exposure, and immunosuppressed state. Patients who have undergone organ transplantation have a significantly higher risk of developing skin cancer, particularly squamous cell carcinoma. Candidates for organ transplantation should receive pretransplant counseling on skin cancer prevention and a complete skin examination to identify and treat any precancerous growths, such as actinic keratoses, and cancerous lesions. Squamous cell carcinomas may also arise in burn scars, chronic ulcers, previously irradiated sites, and certain inflammatory conditions of the skin such as discoid lupus erythematosus or genital lichen sclerosus et atrophicus. Although less common than squamous cell carcinomas induced by ultraviolet radiation, these squamous cell carcinomas tend to have a more malignant course.

● DIAGNOSIS AND TREATMENT

The diagnosis of skin cancer is confirmed with a skin biopsy. There are two main histopathologic subtypes of squamous cell carcinoma: well differentiated and poorly differentiated. In general, the prognostic outcome for well-differentiated squamous cell carcinomas is good, while poorly differentiated squamous cell carcinomas tend to behave aggressively and are more likely to metastasize. In addition, other features associated with increased metastatic potential are tumor diameter greater than 2 cm and tumor depth greater than 2 mm. The overall metastatic rate of solar-induced squamous cell carcinoma is <5%. Squamous cell carcinomas of the scalp, ears, and lips have a higher metastatic rate of approximately 10% to 15%. Other squamous cell carcinomas, which behave more aggressively, are those with histologic evidence of perineural invasion. Adjuvant radiation therapy should be considered to lower the risk of metastases of squamous cell carcinomas with perineural invasion.

The mainstay of treatment for squamous cell carcinoma is excision with histopathologic confirmation of clear or negative margins. Unlike melanoma, there are no standardized excisional margins for squamous cell carcinoma. Adequate excisional margins typically range from 4 to 10 mm. Another treatment modality is Mohs micrographic surgery. Mohs micrographic surgery should be considered for squamous cell carcinomas on the face, especially those involving the H zone (temple, midface, perioral, periorbital, and periauricular regions) and neoplasms on the trunk and the extremities, which are larger than 2 cm. Mohs micrographic surgery usually results in the lowest risk of recurrence. Recurrent squamous cell carcinomas should be referred for Mohs micrographic surgery.

Treatment of basal cell carcinoma is similar to squamous cell carcinoma. In addition, electrodesiccation and curettage is an acceptable therapeutic option for small (<2 cm) basal cell carcinomas with nonaggressive histopathologic subtypes on the trunk and extremities. There are different histopathologic subtypes of basal cell carcinomas including superficial, nodular, micronodular, infiltrative, and morpheaform. Micronodular, infiltrative, and morpheaform are considered to be the aggressive growth patterns because they are more likely to recur after treatment because of ill-defined borders. Mohs micrographic surgery is the preferred therapeutic option for these basal cell carcinomas.

After successfully treating the squamous cell carcinoma, further follow-up is warranted. The patient should undergo a complete skin and lymph node examination to ensure that there are no other concerning lesions or lymphadenopathy. In addition, the patient should receive counseling on the importance of performing monthly self-skin examinations and practicing sun safety techniques such as avoiding the sun between the hours of 11 AM and 4 PM, wearing sun protective clothing, and applying a broad-spectrum sunscreen with an SPF of 30 or higher.

TAKE HOME POINTS

- Squamous cell carcinoma is the second most common type of skin cancer in the United States.
- The vast majority of these cancers are caused by ultraviolet light exposure.
- The mainstay of treatment for squamous cell carcinoma is excision with histopathologic confirmation of clear or negative margins.
- After successfully treating the squamous cell carcinoma, further follow-up is warranted. The patient should undergo a complete skin and lymph node examination to ensure that there are no other concerning lesions or lymphadenopathy.

Extremity Mass (Sarcoma)

WILLIAM R. BURNS AND ALFRED E. CHANG

Based on the previous edition chapter "Extremity Mass (Sarcoma)" by Timothy L. Frankel and Alfred E. Chang

Presentation

A 77-year-old man presents to his primary care physician with a right thigh mass. He originally noted a "lump" in this area and was treated with a course of antibiotics for presumptive lymphadenitis. Although the mass seemed to decrease in size, it soon enlarged again. An ultrasound demonstrated a 4.6-cm complex hypoechoic mass with vascular flow. He was referred to your office for further evaluation and management.

● DIFFERENTIAL DIAGNOSIS

An extremity mass can arise from a wide range of pathology, including congenital, traumatic, infectious, inflammatory, and neoplastic processes. Many of the nonneoplastic etiologies are straightforward to diagnose, but some mimic a tumor or disguise an underlying tumor. As such, traumatic injuries and infectious processes that do not fully resolve warrant careful reevaluation. Trauma, for example, can expose a previously unidentified malignancy; in very rare circumstance, trauma may even contribute to tumor growth. Likewise, an expanding soft tissue tumor may be hard to distinguish from a hematoma or abscess. When there is uncertainty, diagnostic imaging can be very helpful to assess for an underlying soft tissue tumor.

Benign soft tissue lesions (e.g., epidermoid cysts, neurofibromas, lipomas, etc.) are frequently encountered by primary care physicians and general surgeons. A careful history and physical examination is sufficient to diagnose most of these lesions. However, a small subset of patients with suspected benign soft tissue tumors actually have malignant soft tissue tumors. Fortunately, several risk factors have been identified to aid clinicians. Lesions that are >5 cm in diameter, increasing in size, located deep to the fascia, recurrent after prior excision, or causing pain are more likely to be sarcomas. Therefore, patients with these high-risk clinical findings may benefit from early referral to a sarcoma center.

Extremity sarcomas must also be differentiated from other malignancies, such as lymphoma, melanoma, and other metastatic solid tumors. Again, a thorough history and physical examination are important to expedite the evaluation. Patients with genetic syndromes (e.g., Li-Fraumeni, neurofibromatosis, hereditary retinoblastoma, etc.), exposure to chemical carcinogens, or prior radiation therapy are at increased risk for extremity sarcomas. This is also true for patients with tumors that are large, fixed to adjacent structures, located deep to the superficial fascia, or causing symptoms. While laboratory testing is not particularly helpful in the evaluation of extremity sarcomas, diagnostic imaging is very important. Suspicious lesions should be biopsied with tissue submitted for pathologic evaluation.

Sarcomas are a broad group of mesenchymal tumors, which are named according to their tissue of origin. While sarcomas have been classified into over 100 different histologic subtypes, extremity sarcomas are more broadly grouped as either bone sarcomas or soft tissue sarcomas (STS). This distinction between sarcomas of the bone versus soft tissue (i.e., fat, muscle, nerve, blood vessel, and connective tissue) is critical—not only in selecting the preferred treatment algorithm but also in identifying the appropriate subspecialty surgeon. Bone sarcomas include osteosarcoma, chondrosarcoma, Ewing sarcoma, giant cell tumor, chordoma, and undifferentiated pleomorphic sarcoma of the bone; patients with bone sarcomas most often undergo surgery by an orthopedic oncologist. STS include undifferentiated/unclassified soft tissue sarcoma, liposarcoma, leiomyosarcoma, synovial sarcoma, malignant peripheral nerve sheath tumor, rhabdomyosarcoma, fibrosarcoma, angiosarcoma, epithelioid sarcoma, clear cell sarcoma, and alveolar sarcoma of soft part, among others. STS comprise the majority of malignant extremity masses, and these patients should be evaluated by an experienced surgical oncologist or orthopedic oncologist. The most common types of extremity STS encountered in the United States are detailed below.

- Undifferentiated/unclassified soft tissue sarcoma is the subset of STS that lacks specific differentiation and cannot be otherwise classified. This designation has replaced malignant fibrous histiocytoma (MFH), as advances in pathologic evaluation have led to reclassification of many sarcomas previously labeled as MFH. There are several variants of undifferentiated/unclassified soft tissue sarcoma (i.e., pleomorphic, round cell, and spindle cell), but all are high-grade sarcomas.
- Liposarcomas are derived from adipocytes and make up 15% of STS. There are several subtypes, including well-differentiated, myxoid/round cell, dedifferentiated, and pleomorphic variants. Well-differentiated liposarcomas are

often referred to as atypical lipomatous tumors. Treatment is dependent on the subtype, so review by an experienced pathologist is crucial to ensure an appropriate plan of care.

- Leiomyosarcoma is the third most common STS and represents malignant growth of smooth muscle cells. They may occur throughout the body but are commonly found where smooth muscle cell density is highest, such as the uterus.
- Rhabdomyosarcomas are rarely seen in adults but represent the most common pediatric soft tissue tumor. They arise from skeletal muscle progenitor cells and demonstrate rapid growth and metastatic potential. Rhabdomyosarcomas can be divided into embryonal or alveolar subtypes based on their histology.
- Synovial sarcoma is a type of STS that can occur throughout the body and whose histologic features resemble those of synovial cells. There are two subtypes: monophasic (largely comprised of spindle cells) and biphasic (composed of both spindle and epithelial cells). These demonstrate an aggressive behavior.
- Angiosarcomas occur most often on the scalp or the face in the eighth and the ninth decades of life. Risk factors include old age, prior exposure to ionizing radiation, and chronic lymphedema. The latter is an important cause of morbidity following axillary or inguinal lymphadenectomy and has likely contributed to a rise in the incidence of this STS.

Presentation Continued

He denies a history of ionizing radiation, exposure to carcinogens, and family history of sarcoma. On physical examination, there is a 5-cm mass in the proximal right thigh. The lesion is nontender and immobile. There are no other masses or enlarged lymph nodes present. A number of pigmented cutaneous lesions are noted; however, none are particularly worrisome for malignancy.

● WORKUP

As stated earlier, a thorough history and physical examination is important in differentiating a benign soft tissue lesion from a malignant tumor of the extremity. The history should include a review of pertinent risk factors and assessment of how the mass has changed over time and/or impacts function of the extremity. Lesions that exhibit stability over many years and do not elicit symptoms can often be observed closely or excised if warranted. Those lesions with a suspicion of malignancy should be evaluated with diagnostic imaging. Magnetic resonance imaging (MRI) is the primary modality for evaluating extremity sarcomas. STS tend to be heterogeneous masses with enhancement on T2-weighted images, whereas benign lesions appear similar to surrounding tissues. MRI also provides measurement of tumor size, delineation of muscle compartments, and proximity to surrounding structures. When MRI is unavailable or contraindicated, a computed tomography (CT) scan can be useful.

Whichever imaging modality is used, the characteristics of an extremity mass are informative. Those suspicious for malignancy should be biopsied with tissue submitted for pathologic evaluation. For most STS, core needle biopsy is the preferred method, as the volume of tissue and retention of architecture allows for greater diagnostic certainty. When a lesion is difficult to palpate or is in close proximity to vital structures, an image-guided percutaneous needle biopsy should be considered. The access point should directly overly the lesion of interest, such that the needle tract can be easily removed with the specimen during operative extirpation. When a core needle biopsy is not possible, fine needle aspiration (FNA) may be attempted. However, FNA only provides a small amount of tissue for cytopathology, and diagnostic uncertainty (histologic subtype, tumor grade, etc.) may persist. Therefore, FNA is more often used to document local recurrence or metastasis.

Surgical biopsies are reserved for cases in which a percutaneous needle biopsy is not feasible or is unable to establish a diagnosis. Depending on the size of the lesion, it may be completely removed (lesions <3 cm) or a small wedge may be sampled (lesions >3 cm) for pathologic analysis. It is critical to orient the incision along the longitudinal axis of the limb, so as to avoid compromising a subsequent surgical procedure. In addition, meticulous hemostasis is important, as a postoperative hematoma may dissect through adjacent tissue planes; this jeopardizes a subsequent surgical procedure and has the potential to disseminate tumor cells into the hematoma cavity. Ideally, the biopsy should be performed by a surgeon trained in the management of STS, who will ultimately perform the definitive operation.

Once the diagnosis of biopsy-proven STS in made, the imaging and histologic findings are used in staging. Important characteristics used in staging of STS include size (<5 cm vs. >5 cm), tumor grade (low vs. high), and metastatic disease (absent vs. present). In addition to imaging of the extremity, patients should undergo a high-resolution CT scan of the chest to evaluate for pulmonary metastasis. Other imaging studies should also be considered, as directed by symptoms, exam findings, and histologic subtype. Lymph node metastasis, for example, is very uncommon (<5% of STS) but can be seen in specific histologic subtypes (e.g., epithelioid sarcoma and clear cell sarcoma). Thorough evaluation of the regional nodal basin in these high-risk patients may identify "occult" metastatic disease. Metastasis to regional lymph nodes is associated with poor prognosis, but not as poor as metastasis to distant sites.

Presentation Continued

MRI scan confirms the mass to be 4.5 cm in size and abutting the femoral vein (Figure 108-1). An image-guided core needle biopsy of the mass is performed. Pathologic analysis reveals a high-grade leiomyosarcoma. A CT scan of the chest does not identify any pulmonary metastasis. The case is reviewed at multidisciplinary tumor board.

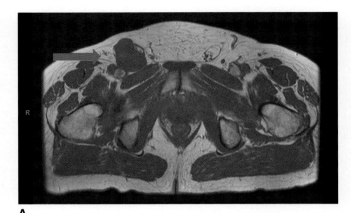

A

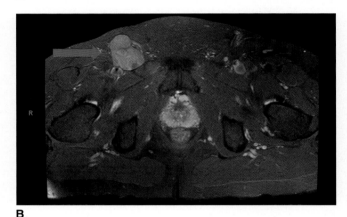

B

FIGURE 108-1. MRI study with T1-weighted sequence (**A**) and T2-weighted sequence (**B**) demonstrates a right thigh mass (*arrow*) abutting the femoral vein.

● DIAGNOSIS AND TREATMENT

The treatment of STS depends on tumor size, histologic subtype, feasibility of complete resection, and anticipated postoperative functional deficits. Whenever possible, cases should be discussed in a multidisciplinary tumor board, where diagnostic imaging and pathology can be reviewed to formulate a comprehensive treatment plan with input from medical oncologists, surgeons, and radiation oncologists. Referral to a high-volume sarcoma center should also be considered. In general, patients with small, low-grade STS are good candidates for wide excision. When negative margins are achieved, most patients do not need additional therapy. However, patients with positive margins should be considered for additional surgery to achieve negative margins or adjuvant radiation when there is concern for microscopic residual disease along critical anatomic structures (i.e., bone, major blood vessel, or major motor nerve). Patients with large (>5 cm) or high-grade STS, on the other hand, should be considered for multimodality therapy. Certain STS subtypes may benefit from systemic chemotherapy, whereas most are treated with a combination of surgical resection and radiation therapy.

The goal of operative intervention should be complete removal of the tumor to microscopically negative margins while preserving physiologic function of the extremity. Prior to 1980, however, amputation was the standard surgical approach for extremity sarcomas. Marginal resection of the tumor (i.e., removing the tumor along its capsule) was associated with up to an 80% risk of local recurrence. While wide excision of the tumor (i.e., removing the tumor with a rim of normal tissue) was better, this approach was still associated with unsatisfactorily high rates of local recurrence. Hence, radical surgery with either amputation of the joint proximal to the tumor or resection of the entire muscle compartment adjacent to the tumor was preferred; this approach was morbid but dramatically reduced local recurrence rates to well below 20%. In order to decrease morbidity and maintain low rates of local recurrence, several institutions advocated for wide excision plus adjuvant treatment. In a landmark study by Rosenberg and colleagues, patients with extremity STS were randomized to either limb-sparing surgery (i.e., wide excision with radiation therapy) or amputation. Despite only identifying local recurrences in patients undergoing limb-sparing surgery, there was no difference in overall survival between the two groups. These findings changed the approach to extremity STS, such that amputation is now reserved for those patients in whom definitive surgery would render the extremity nonfunctional.

In the last 35 years, groups have reported low rates of local recurrence in patients undergoing limb-sparing surgery plus radiation for extremity STS. The decision to administer radiation before or after surgery, however, remains controversial. Potential benefits of preoperative radiotherapy are a reduction in tumor size (which may allow for less radical surgery) and a decrease in late effects of radiation. However, this approach is also associated with an increased risk of surgical wound complications, especially in patients who are obese and/or diabetic. For patients with large, high-grade STS, there may be a role for neoadjuvant chemoradiotherapy. While specific treatment regimens vary across institutions, the two main approaches are concurrent chemoradiotherapy with single-agent chemotherapy (e.g., doxorubicin, gemcitabine, etc.) or sequential radiotherapy with multiagent chemotherapy (e.g., doxorubicin/cisplatin, doxorubicin/ifosfamide, epirubicin/ifosfamide, etc.). Clinical trials to better determine the optimal regimen are ongoing.

Presentation Continued

The patient undergoes radical resection en bloc with the overlying skin, subcutaneous tissues, muscle fascia, and segment of the femoral vein (Figure 108-2). Immediate pathologic evaluation is performed and the vascular margins are found to be negative. The femoral vein is reconstructed with an interposed segment of internal jugular vein. The sartorius muscle is transposed to cover the vessels and the soft tissues are closed in multiple layers over a surgical drain.

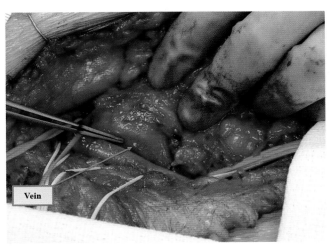

FIGURE 108-2. Intraoperative findings demonstrate a right thigh mass involving the anterior wall of the femoral vein (*arrow*), which was removed en bloc with the tumor specimen. The femoral vein was reconstructed with interposed internal jugular vein. The femoral artery was uninvolved.

● SURGICAL APPROACH

The surgical approach to STS is complete resection of the tumor en bloc with an adequate margin of adjacent soft tissue. As a general guideline, surgeons should strive for margins that include at least 1 cm of normal tissue or an intact facial layer around the tumor. This may be challenging for tumors adjacent to critical neurovascular structures, where a narrower margin is necessary to preserve function of the extremity. These patients are often recommended to have preoperative radiotherapy, as local recurrence rates remain very low even with margins as close as 1 mm. Surgeons should also consider the possibility of complex reconstruction when preoperative radiotherapy is used or when a large soft tissue defect is anticipated. In these cases, the operation should be coordinated with a plastic surgeon in the event a complex rotational flap or free tissue transfer is needed.

Just as with surgical biopsies, the incision should be oriented along the longitudinal axis of the extremity. This decreases tension on the skin closure and facilitates reoperation if a positive margin is found on final pathology. When complex reconstruction is planned, the surgical incision may be modified as long as the oncologic principles of the operation are not compromised. Prior to incision, it is important to identify (or estimate) the extent of the mass, so as to plan for complete resection with a margin of uninvolved tissue around the tumor. If fascial planes are encountered, these should be included in the resection. Nerves and arteries, on the other hand, should be preserved when they are important for limb function. If the tumor encases a vessel, en bloc resection with reconstruction can be considered. For tumors abutting bone, the involved periosteum should be removed, but the cortical bone should be left intact.

Once the specimen is resected, it should be oriented by the surgeon and taken to pathology for careful processing. If gross inspection identifies an area of concern (i.e., margin that is positive or close), additional tissue should be removed. Frozen section analysis may also help with intraoperative assessment of surgical margins; however, this pathologic interpretation can be difficult. Following initial assessment of the specimen, it is important that the entire periphery is inked to facilitate precise interpretation of the margins on final pathology.

After the resection has been completed, metallic clips should be placed along the borders of the surgical site. This helps planning if the patient requires additional surgery or adjuvant radiation. Once hemostasis is confirmed, the skin and soft tissues are reapproximated, or more complex reconstruction (rotational flap or free tissue transfer) may also be performed. Closed-suction drains can reduce the rates of postoperative seroma, but the drain sites should be placed such that they are within the radiation field. Depending on the extent of surgery, patients typically require brief hospitalization and evaluation by a physical and/or occupational therapist.

● SPECIAL INTRAOPERATIVE CONSIDERATIONS

Unexpected intraoperative findings can alter the planned surgery. In addition to the common "pitfalls" (orientation of incision, extent of resection, need for reconstruction) already discussed (Table 108-1), surgeons also face the challenge of intraoperative assessment of tumor margins. When more radical resection would result in additional morbidity, frozen section analysis can be helpful to assess the completeness of resection. However, frozen section analysis can be challenging and time-consuming. Therefore, it may be best to await final pathologic assessment of the tumor margins prior to soft tissue closure when complex reconstruction is necessary. In the event of a positive margin, this allows for additional surgery while maintaining reconstructive options. In this challenging scenario, the surgical site can be left open using either a vacuum-assisted closure device or a biosynthetic matrix. Once the pathologic review is complete, definitive reconstruction can then be performed.

● POSTOPERATIVE MANAGEMENT

In the weeks following surgery, patients often continue to have activity restrictions. As the surgical site heals, however, patients should increase their physical activity. Additional work with a physical and/or occupational therapist may be helpful to improve upon any lingering deficits. Surgical drains should be removed when the output is minimal.

The final pathology should be reviewed in a multidisciplinary tumor board, where plans for adjuvant therapy

Table 108-1	Extremity Mass (Sarcoma)

Key Technical Steps

1. Preoperative MRI assesses tumor size and proximity to surrounding structures, and core needle biopsy determines histologic subtype and pathologic grade. Review case in multidisciplinary tumor board (or refer to sarcoma center) to determine optimal multimodality therapy.
2. Surgical incision is oriented along the longitudinal axis of the extremity, unless this compromises options for complex soft tissue reconstruction.
3. STS is completely removed en bloc with a margin of uninvolved soft tissue and adjacent fascial layers.
4. Nerves and vessels critical to limb function are preserved. Segment of a vessel encased by tumor, however, can be removed when vascular reconstruction is feasible.
5. Orient the pathologic specimen and assess the margin of resection. Consider delayed reconstruction if margin status is uncertain.
6. Place metallic clips within the surgical site as markers for adjuvant radiation.
7. Close the skin and subcutaneous tissues over surgical drains, when needed. Consider physical and/or occupational therapy evaluation following surgery.

Potential Pitfalls

- Circumferential scar from surgical biopsy or prior resection requires more radical soft tissue resection.
- Intraoperative assessment of the tumor margins is challenging.
- Need for complex reconstruction to close the surgical site.

and ongoing surveillance are finalized. When radiotherapy is recommended, it may be started as early as 4 to 6 weeks after surgery. Once treatment is complete, patients should be transitioned to active surveillance, as early recognition of local recurrence and/or distant metastasis may lead to expedited therapy with improved outcomes. Patients with STS should be seen every 3 to 6 months for the first 2 to 3 years. The majority of recurrences are detected in this time frame. Depending on the risk of local recurrence and distant metastasis, periodic imaging (MRI scan of the extremity and CT scan of the chest) should be performed in asymptomatic patients. If there is no evidence of recurrence, the follow-up interval should be increased to every 6 months and then annually after 5 years. The risk of disease recurrence after 10 years is quite low, and most providers would consider stopping routine imaging at that point.

If patients develop a local recurrence, a complete clinical assessment should be performed. Patients without distant metastasis should be considered for aggressive treatment, such as re-resection or amputation. When adjuvant radiotherapy was not part of the initial treatment, it can be used to improve local control. Patient who previously received radiotherapy should also be considered for additional radiation; however, the treatment plan may be less effective. Despite aggressive local control, overall survival is largely determined by distant metastasis. In general, patients with distant metastatic disease are considered for systemic therapy. This is especially true for those with disseminated disease. Those with a solitary site (or limited extent) of metastasis, on the other hand, should be considered for additional surgery. Several studies have reported long-term disease control and survival for patients undergoing metastasectomy for extremity STS.

Case Conclusion

He tolerates the procedure well. Final pathologic analysis identifies a high-grade leiomyosarcoma (grade 2/3) measuring 5 cm in greatest dimension. All margins are negative. Twelve lymph nodes are evaluated without evidence of metastasis. His surgical drain is removed at a routine postoperative visit. He is then referred for consideration of adjuvant radiotherapy.

TAKE HOME POINTS

- STS are a broad group of mesenchymal tumors derived from fat, muscle, nerve, blood vessel, and connective tissue.
- Patients with an extremity mass suspicious for STS should undergo imaging and biopsy. These cases should be discussed in a multidisciplinary tumor board (or referred to a sarcoma center) to ensure patients receive optimal treatment.
- Small, low-grade STS can be treated with surgical resection, but large or high-grade STS should be considered for multimodality therapy. Neoadjuvant radiation may allow for less radical surgery and minimize late effects of radiation but is associated with increased surgical complication rates. Large, high-grade STS may benefit from neoadjuvant chemoradiation.
- Amputation should be avoided if a functional extremity can be maintained. When complex soft tissue reconstruction is likely, operations should be coordinated with a plastic surgeon.
- STS should be completely removed en bloc with a margin of uninvolved soft tissue and adjacent fascial layers. Critical nerves and vessels should be preserved, when possible.
- Active surveillance is recommended to aid detection of asymptomatic local recurrence and distant metastasis. Patients with local recurrence should be considered for additional surgery (with or without radiation), whereas patients with disseminated metastatic disease should be considered for systemic therapy. Surgery should also be considered for patients with limited metastatic disease.

SUGGESTED READINGS

Cormier JN, Patel SR, Herzog CE, et al. Concurrent ifosfamide-based chemotherapy and irradiation. Analysis of treatment-related toxicity in 43 patients with sarcoma. *Cancer.* 2001;92(6): 1550-1555.

Davis AM, O'Sullivan B, Turcotte R, et al. Late radiation morbidity following randomization to preoperative versus postoperative radiotherapy in extremity soft tissue sarcoma. *Radiother Oncol.* 2005;75(1):48-53.

ESMO/European Sarcoma Network Working Group. Soft tissue and visceral sarcomas: ESMO Clinical Practice Guidelines for diagnosis, treatment and follow-up. *Ann Oncol.* 2014;25(3):iii102-iii112.

Kraybill WG, Harris J, Spiro IJ, et al. Long-term results of a phase 2 study of neoadjuvant chemotherapy and radiotherapy in the management of high-risk, high-grade, soft tissue sarcomas of the extremities and body wall: Radiation Therapy Oncology Group Trial 9514. *Cancer.* 2010;116(19):4613-4621.

National Comprehensive Cancer Network. Soft Tissue Sarcoma (Version 2.2017). https://www.nccn.org/professionals/physician_gls/pdf/sarcoma.pdf. Accessed March 1, 2017.

O'Sullivan B, Davis AM, Turcotte R, et al. Preoperative versus postoperative radiotherapy in soft-tissue sarcoma of the limbs: a randomised trial. *Lancet.* 2002;359(9325):2235-2241.

Pisters PW, Pollock RE, Lewis VO, et al. Long-term results of prospective trial of surgery alone with selective use of radiation for patients with T1 extremity and trunk soft tissue sarcomas. *Ann Surg.* 2007;246:675-681.

Rosenberg SA, Tepper J, Glatstein E, et al. The treatment of soft-tissue sarcomas of the extremities: prospective randomized evaluations of (1) limb-sparing surgery plus radiation therapy compared with amputation and (2) the role of adjuvant chemotherapy. *Ann Surg.* 1982;196(3):305-315.

Wang D, Zhang Q, Eisenberg BL, et al. Significant reduction of late toxicities in patients with extremity sarcoma treated with image-guided radiation therapy to a reduced target volume: results of radiation therapy oncology group RTOG-0630 trial. *J Clin Oncol.* 2015;33:2231-2238.

Yang JC, Chang AE, Baker AR, et al. Randomized prospective study of the benefit of adjuvant radiation therapy in the treatment of soft tissue sarcomas of the extremity. *J Clin Oncol.* 1998;16(1):197-203.

Retroperitoneal Sarcoma

109

CHRISTINA V. ANGELES AND SANDRA L. WONG

Based on the previous edition chapter "Retroperitoneal Sarcoma" by Chandu Vemuri and Sandra L. Wong

Presentation

A 60-year-old woman status post left hip replacement presents after her physical therapist palpated a mass in her abdomen. On examination, she has a nontender mass in her right abdomen and right lower extremity edema. She reports feeling well other than a sensation of pressure in her abdomen. She is active and has not noticed any weight loss or fatigue.

● DIAGNOSIS

Patients with retroperitoneal sarcoma typically present with nonspecific symptoms and will often have an abdominal mass on physical examination. Some symptoms are specific to mass effect on nearby structures. Because of the location and the propensity of these tumors to push nearby organs and not invade them, diagnosis is often delayed. The majority of patients have tumors that are larger than 10 cm in size at time of initial evaluation. Retroperitoneal masses are usually malignant and about one-third of these masses are

sarcomas. The differential diagnosis also includes germ cell tumors, primary neoplasm from retroperitoneal solid organs (e.g., pancreas, duodenum, adrenal, and kidney), lymphoma, and metastatic lesions.

Occasionally, the mass is appreciated as an incidental finding on cross-sectional imaging performed for other reasons, but otherwise a CT scan of the abdomen and the pelvis with oral and IV contrast is the preferred initial radiographic evaluation. Complete workup involves a detailed history and physical examination, including assessment of diffuse lymphadenopathy, scrotal exam, and serum laboratory studies, to selectively evaluate excessive endocrine hormone production, and elevated germ cell tumor markers (e.g., alpha-fetoprotein [AFP], beta-human chorionic gonadotropin [β-hCG], and lactate dehydrogenase).

In this patient, physical examination was only remarkable for a large palpable abdominal mass and mild right lower extremity edema. CT scan of the abdomen and pelvis was significant for a massive retroperitoneal mass extending from the hepatic hilum to the pelvis and displacing the right kidney, right colon, small bowel, duodenum, and pancreas to the left (Figure 109-1). There was also compression on the

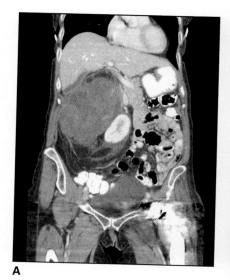
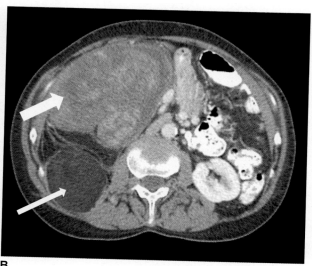

A   **B**

FIGURE 109-1. See case presentation. **A:** Retroperitoneal sarcoma occupying the majority of the right abdominal cavity is demonstrated on coronal view from the index CT scan. Note displacement of the intra-abdominal contents medially and encasement of the right kidney. **B:** Selected axial view of the liposarcoma demonstrating a homogeneous fatty appearance of the well-differentiated component (*thin arrow*) and more enhancement in the dedifferentiated component (*thick arrow*). Note displacement of the bowel into the left abdomen.

right iliac vessels, explaining her lower extremity swelling. The radiologic appearance was consistent with liposarcoma given the fatty appearance along with some solid components. A CT-guided core needle biopsy confirmed a high-grade dedifferentiated liposarcoma. CT scan of the chest did not demonstrate any evidence of pulmonary metastasis. Laboratory values were normal, including a creatinine of 0.7 mg/dL. She was referred for surgical evaluation.

● DISCUSSION

Presenting symptoms can include vague abdominal or back pain and weight loss, as well as symptoms specific to location of the tumor, such as early satiety if there is mass effect on the stomach or venous obstruction with resultant swelling of the lower extremity from a pelvic tumor. Biopsy of suspicious masses can be performed preoperatively to establish a diagnosis. Biopsy, with a core needle biopsy approach if possible, is mandatory if there is a question about the diagnosis, if there is consideration for neoadjuvant treatment, or if the tumor is felt to be unresectable.

Imaging should be directed to preparation for surgical resection. Magnetic resonance imaging (MRI) is an alternate modality that is sufficient, but not necessary, for these patients. Workup should also include evaluation of metastatic disease, most commonly to lungs or liver. Plain chest radiographs can be used to evaluate for pulmonary metastasis, but CT should be performed if any abnormalities are seen or if the sarcoma is considered a high risk for metastasis. Positron emission tomography scans do not have a defined role in assessment of retroperitoneal sarcoma.

● EVALUATION AND TREATMENT

The cornerstone of treatment for localized disease is complete surgical resection. This patient was felt to have a resectable retroperitoneal sarcoma and this was recommended. Resection should include involved intra-abdominal/retroperitoneal structures with anastomoses and reconstruction as appropriate. Sarcomas with critical vascular involvement, peritoneal implants, involvement at the root of the mesentery, or spinal cord involvement are usually considered unresectable. Incomplete resections with microscopically positive margins lead to an increased risk of local recurrence, which represents a common form of treatment failure. Great care must be taken to ensure complete resection without capsular intrusion during the index operation. Repeat resection for recurrent disease is recommended, especially if interval surveillance is able to detect early recurrences. Unfortunately, recurrent disease often predicts further recurrences, which often become increasingly more aggressive in terms of tumor biology and more technically difficult to resect with successive operations. The chance of achieving complete resection decreases with each subsequent recurrence.

Sarcomas are relatively uncommon neoplasms derived from mesenchymal cells, with an estimate of fewer than 14,000 new cases of soft tissue sarcoma in the United States each year. Only 10% to 15% of these cases will be of retroperitoneal origin. Overall, patients with retroperitoneal sarcoma have a worse disease-free survival than other sarcoma sites. More than 50 different histologic subtypes have been described, but the most commonly seen retroperitoneal sarcomas are liposarcoma or leiomyosarcoma. Prognosis is largely dictated by the ability to achieve complete surgical resection, and median survival for patients who undergo complete resection is 60 months compared to 24 months for those undergoing incomplete resection. Other factors associated with decreased survival include high histologic grade, large tumor size, and older patient age.

Multimodality treatment approaches, including systemic chemotherapy and radiation therapy, merit consideration since resection alone has unsatisfactory outcomes in high-risk tumors. There are good data to support the use of radiation in conjunction with limb-sparing procedures for extremity sarcomas. However, radiation to the retroperitoneum is complicated by dose-limiting toxicity to abdominal viscera, which are uniquely radiosensitive, and by very large treatment fields. Preoperative radiation approaches have been considered to improve rates of local control and reduce recurrences. When the sarcoma is in situ, bowel and other structures are displaced and out of the intended radiation field, allowing for more effective use of radiation. It is unlikely that radiation would change the size of the tumor or change the scope and/or extent of the planned operation. Many small series have demonstrated the safety and feasibility of radiation for selected patients with high-risk retroperitoneal sarcomas, and studies using standard external beam radiation therapy, brachytherapy approaches, or intraoperative electron beam radiotherapy approaches are ongoing to evaluate their efficacy in disease outcomes. The use of systemic chemotherapy for most histologic subtypes of retroperitoneal

Table 109-1	**Resection of Retroperitoneal Sarcoma**

Key Technical Steps

1. Midline laparotomy.
2. Thorough exploration to verify resectability.
3. Complete exposure of sarcoma and surrounding structures.
4. Resection of mass with en bloc resection of contiguous organs and vessels as needed.
5. Placement of metal clips in resection bed.
6. Reconstruction (bowel, major vessels) as needed.
7. Abdominal closure.

Potential Pitfalls

- Inadequate preoperative imaging to determine involvement of major intra-abdominal structures.
- Inadequate exposure of vessels for vascular control in a field with limited exposure due to the size of tumor.
- Rupture of tumor.

sarcoma remains controversial. Response rates are relatively low, and there is no demonstrated improvement in overall or disease-specific survival with either neoadjuvant or adjuvant chemotherapy regimens. Some commonly used cytotoxic agents include doxorubicin and ifosfamide, and increasingly gemcitabine and docetaxel. These are mostly used in patients with metastasis or unresectable disease. There is limited experience with combined chemoradiation treatments.

● SURGICAL APPROACH AND SPECIAL INTRAOPERATIVE CONSIDERATIONS

Retroperitoneal sarcomas, by definition, can originate from mesenchymal tissues throughout the retroperitoneum. Hepatic sarcomas, intra-abdominal desmoid tumors (desmoid fibromatosis), and gastrointestinal stromal tumors should be considered separately since these tumors have different presentations and management strategies. Because the location and extent of retroperitoneal sarcomas vary greatly, the surgical approach must be tailored to each patient.

A midline incision is most commonly used for access since standard laparotomy provides excellent exposure of viscera, vascular structures, and the retroperitoneum (Table 109-1). Upon entering the abdomen, thorough evaluation is made to ensure that the mass is resectable. Often, mobilization of intra-abdominal structures is necessary for this assessment. Once this decision has been made to proceed,

further dissection should be carried out in a manner to best visualize the entirety of the mass and ensure ability to obtain vascular control if necessary during the course of dissection. Structures such as bowel, mesentery, ureters, and major vessels should not be divided until resection is known to be possible. Preoperative placement of ureteral stents is recommended to decrease ureteral injury since normal anatomical landmarks are often displaced. Tumors with critical vascular involvement, peritoneal implants, involvement at the root of the mesentery, or spinal cord involvement are usually unresectable; debulking procedures are usually not considered.

Exposure in the retroperitoneum is often limited by large tumors. With the insidious growth pattern of sarcomas, contiguous structures may have to be resected en bloc to assure complete removal of tumor. Resection of colon, small bowel, kidney, adrenal gland, and inferior vena cava (IVC) must often be considered as part of the procedure depending on the location and growth pattern of the sarcoma. En bloc nephrectomy is necessary in many cases, yet the renal parenchyma is rarely invaded and the kidney can be preserved by doing a capsulectomy if the sarcoma is not encased or involve the hilum. Bowel resection is often necessary because of the extent of involvement of the mesentery/mesocolon.

Once the tumor is resected, metal clips should be placed in the resection bed to allow for later identification of the anatomic limits of the tumor. Necessary reconstructive procedures are performed at this time (Figure 109-2). Bowel anastomoses are usually performed without incident. Major

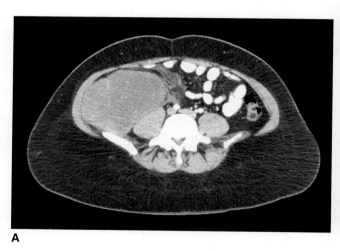
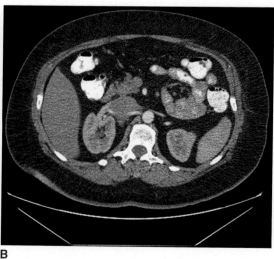

A **B**

FIGURE 109-2. Selected other case of retroperitoneal sarcomas. **A:** This is a 24-year-old woman who presented with right-sided abdominal and back pain, which continued to worsen over 2 years. She was treated for musculoskeletal pain until she presented to the ER with new right hip pain, with numbness and tingling in her right thigh. A CT of the abdomen and pelvis was done, which showed a resectable 15-cm heterogeneous mass in the right retroperitoneum displacing the right kidney and involving the psoas and colon. Preoperative biopsy identified a high-grade rhabdomyosarcoma. CT chest imaging was negative for metastasis. She underwent ureteral stent placement to help with interoperative identification of the ureter. The mass was resected en bloc with the right colon and psoas muscle. She had a primary colon anastomosis. Postoperatively, her right thigh symptoms resolved. She received adjuvant chemotherapy but experienced a recurrence with diffuse bony metastasis 1 year later. **B:** This is a 55-year-old woman who presented with worsening right-sided back pain. After many sessions with physical therapy and a chiropractor, she underwent evaluation with a thoracic/lumbar spine MRI. After finding a retroperitoneal mass, she underwent a CT of the abdomen and the pelvis, which demonstrated a mass involving the right renal vessels and the IVC. She underwent segmental resection of the IVC with en bloc right nephrectomy. The IVC was reconstructed using an interposition tube graft, and the kidney was autotransplanted after the uninvolved kidney was dissected free from the involved portions of the renal vein and artery.

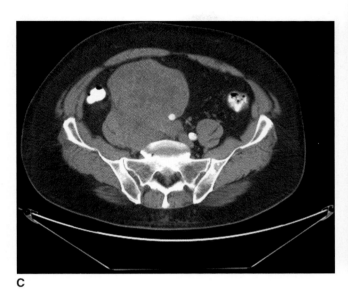
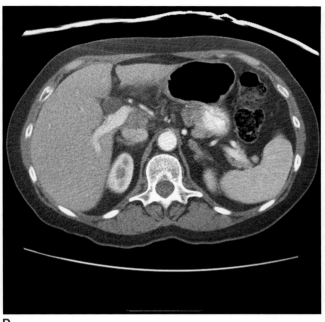

C   D

FIGURE 109-2. (*Continued*) **C:** This is a 66-year-old man with a high-grade leiomyosarcoma of the right retroperitoneum/pelvis discovered after an episode of abdominal pain. He was also noted to have right lower-extremity edema, likely due to venous compression. On CT scan, encasement of the right iliac vessels and suspected involvement of the right ureter are noted. He underwent resection of the sarcoma with en bloc resection of the right ureter, right common and external iliac artery and vein with end-to-end ureteral reconstruction (Boari flap), and vascular reconstruction of the vessels with prosthetic grafts. **D:** This is a 66-year-old woman with biopsy-proven leiomyosarcoma incidentally found during a laparoscopic cholecystectomy. The 3-cm mass is noted to straddle the portal vein and the IVC. Because of the extent of vascular involvement, this sarcoma was deemed unresectable. The patient was relatively asymptomatic and declined palliative treatment. She developed liver metastases 2 years after initial diagnosis.

vascular reconstruction techniques have been described, including primary repair or use of prosthetic graft replacements, though ligation of many vessels is generally well tolerated. Because the risk of nodal metastasis is virtually nonexistent, lymphadenectomy is unnecessary. The abdomen is closed in the standard fashion. Drains are rarely needed.

● POSTOPERATIVE MANAGEMENT

Immediate postoperative management of these patients is dictated by the extent of resection, noting that postoperative ileus is common with long procedures or if there was extensive displacement of bowel by the sarcoma.

The long-term care of these patients requires surveillance with physical exam and imaging every 3 to 6 months for the first 2 to 3 years and then annually thereafter. Interval of surveillance may vary based on the expected risk of recurrence (dependent on completeness of surgical resection and histopathologic features) and underlying performance status of

the patient. Recurrences are difficult to detect without expert review of cross-sectional imaging. It is important to be aware that well-differentiated liposarcoma may take on the appearance of "dirty fat" on cross-sectional imaging, so it can be easily missed on standard review (Figure 109-3A). Follow-up should also include chest imaging for detection of metastatic disease.

Case Conclusion

This patient underwent resection of a 4 kg, 36 × 29 × 11 cm dedifferentiated liposarcoma in a background of well-differentiated liposarcoma with en bloc kidney and adrenal resection due to encasement. The iliac vein was compressed by the tumor, yet a plane of dissection between the tumor and the iliac vessels allowed preservation of vascular structures. Her postoperative course was uncomplicated, and she had complete resolution of her lower extremity swelling.

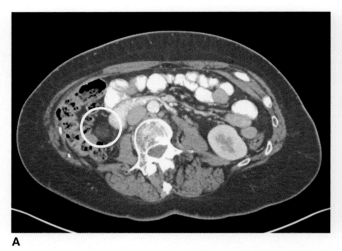

A

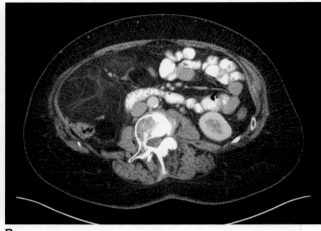

B

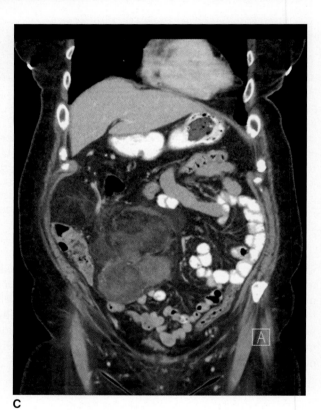

C

FIGURE 109-3. Select case of recurrent retroperitoneal sarcoma. This is a 59-year-old woman with a history of well-differentiated/dedifferentiated retroperitoneal liposarcoma diagnosed at age 40. She underwent radical resection of the sarcoma en bloc with right nephrectomy with negative margins at the time of initial diagnosis. She underwent prolonged surveillance over a 10-year period, during which her CT scans showed no evidence of recurrence or distant disease. Then, she presented with early satiety and abdominal discomfort. **A:** CT of the abdomen and pelvis performed 10 years postresection with an area of fat stranding noted on retrospective review of her imaging. **B,C:** CT of the abdomen and pelvis at time of symptoms 16 years postresection showed two main heterogeneous, solid masses along with an extensive lipomatous mass along the right retroperitoneum, extending from the posterior-lateral aspect of the liver to the pelvis. She had no evidence of distant metastasis. She underwent her second surgical resection, which included the tumor with en bloc right colon, inferior liver edge, posterior retroperitoneal soft tissue, and partial right diaphragm. There was dense scar tissue along the IVC, which required meticulous dissection.

TAKE HOME POINTS

- Differential diagnosis must also include germ cell tumors, primary neoplasm from retroperitoneal solid organs (e.g., pancreas, duodenum, adrenal, and kidney), lymphoma, and metastatic lesions.
- Preoperative imaging studies should include a CT scan of the abdomen/pelvis to assess extent of disease as well as resectability and chest imaging to evaluate for the presence of pulmonary metastases.
- The cornerstone of treatment is complete surgical resection. En bloc resection of contiguous structures may be necessary.

- Recurrence rates are relatively high. Patients should be followed closely with cross-sectional imaging and clinical evaluation.

SUGGESTED READINGS

Hollenbeck ST, Grobmyer SR, Kent KC, et al. Surgical treatment and outcome of patients with primary inferior vena cava leiomyosarcoma. *J Am Coll Surg.* 2003;197:575-579.

Jaques DP, Coit DG, Hajdu SI, et al. Management of primary and recurrent soft tissue sarcoma of the retroperitoneum. *Ann Surg.* 1990;212:51-59.

Karakousis CP. Refinements of surgical technique in soft tissue sarcomas. *J Surg Oncol.* 2010;101:730-738.

Kirane A, Crago AM. The importance of surgical margins in retroperitoneal sarcoma. *J Surg Oncol.* 2016;113:270-276.

Park JO, Qin LX, Prete FP, et al. Predicting outcome by growth rate of locally recurrent retroperitoneal liposarcoma; the one centimeter per month rule. *Ann Surg.* 2009;250:977-982.

Raut CP, Pisters PW. Retroperitoneal sarcomas: combined-modality treatment approaches. *J Surg Oncol.* 2006;94:81-87.

Siegel RL, Miller KD, Jemal A. Cancer statistics, 2016. *CA Cancer J Clin.* 2016;66(1):7-30.

Singer S, Antonescu CR, Riedel E, Brennan MF. Histologic subtype and margin of resection predict pattern of recurrence and survival for retroperitoneal liposarcoma. *Ann Surg.* 2003;238:358-370.

Trauma

Hemostatic Resuscitation

110

KEVIN B. WISE AND BRYAN A. COTTON

Presentation

A 51-year-old man presents by ground transportation after being struck by a vehicle at high speed while riding a bicycle. Bystanders telephoned Emergency Medical Services who arrived on the scene and found him interactive and complaining of pelvic pain. On arrival to the hospital, a trauma activation was called for tachycardia and hypotension. His primary survey was intact. He had a systolic blood pressure of 70/40 mmHg and a pulse of 125 bpm. His Glasgow Coma Scale (GCS) score was 15. Secondary survey revealed foreshortening of his left lower extremity.

● DIFFERENTIAL DIAGNOSIS

In contrast with penetrating trauma with often identifiable trajectories, blunt traumatic mechanisms such as a motor vehicle collision or automobile versus pedestrian have the potential to cause injuries anywhere in the body, often without external manifestation. Closed head injuries are common and may not be immediately apparent as many patients can arrive with a normal or near-normal GCS score despite significant traumatic brain injury. Scalp lacerations can also occur and have the potential for massive blood loss. Skull fractures may be present, yet only a minority of patients have classic physical exam findings such as Battle sign or raccoon eyes. Patients may suffer cervical spine injuries, necessitating cervical collar placement until such injury has been ruled out. Blunt trauma can cause direct trauma to the neck, for example from seatbelts, and indirect trauma from hyperextension or hyperflexion. With heightened awareness and increased scanning computed tomography angiogram (CTA) usage, blunt cerebrovascular injuries are increasingly recognized and diagnosed. These injuries are usually asymptomatic until neurologic signs develop secondary to stroke. Laryngotracheal injuries are also possible and often present with signs such as subcutaneous emphysema, dyspnea, hemoptysis, and hoarseness.

In the trunk, blunt injuries in the chest can cause myriad injuries including rib fractures, sternal fracture, pneumothorax, hemothorax, lung contusion, blunt cardiac injury, aortic injury, and esophageal injury. Workup during primary survey should identify life-threatening conditions such as tension pneumothorax, cardiac tamponade, and massive hemothorax. Chest x-ray and secondary survey may identify other injuries. Within the peritoneum, no organ is spared. Solid organs such as the liver, spleen, and kidney are frequently injured. Hollow viscus injuries can be present on admission but occult with signs and symptoms developing later if there is not a low index of suspicion for imaging signs such as free intraperitoneal fluid without associated solid organ injury or a subtle amount of free air. The extremities are frequently injured as well. As they are not commonly included on axial imaging, a thorough physical exam to screen for bony or vascular injury is a necessity.

● WORKUP

Evaluation and management of the injured patient are carried out in a standardized manner. The purpose of this is to quickly identify and treat life-threatening conditions. In severely injured patients, assessment and resuscitation are performed concurrently. Assessment begins with confirming a secure airway with maintenance of cervical spine precautions in patients with suspicious mechanisms of injury. If the patient's airway is compromised or the patient is unconscious (GCS ≤ 8), endotracheal intubation is indicated. Breathing and ventilation are confirmed with inspection of the chest for breath rise and auscultation. Circulation is assessed by palpation for a pulse in a major artery. External bleeding is controlled with direct pressure or a tourniquet if in an extremity is the source. The patient's level of consciousness is assessed with the GCS, and the pupils are evaluated for size and reactivity. Clothing is removed to achieve complete exposure of the patient. Particularly critical to the penetrating trauma patient is brief assessment of ventral wounds (including those involving hair-bearing areas, within skin folds, and within the axilla) and a full logroll to check for wounds on the back.

Focused assessment for the sonography of trauma (FAST) is then performed to screen for pericardial effusion and intraperitoneal bleeding. Ideally, blood is drawn, and intravenous access is obtained in parallel with the primary survey. In addition to routine laboratory studies, blood is sent for ABO typing and antibody screening, as well as coagulation assessment. A chest x-ray is then obtained. If there has been hemodynamic instability, a pelvis x-ray is indicated to assess for pelvic fracture.

A secondary survey is performed including a head to toe examination, ensuring the patient is rolled with full inspection of the back. If there is no indication for immediate operative intervention—such as hemodynamic instability with positive FAST exam, immediate return of a large volume of blood from chest tube placement, or ongoing elevated chest tube output—advanced imaging is the next priority.

Presentation Continued

The hospital's massive transfusion protocol (MTP) was activated on arrival, given a positive Assessment of Blood Consumption (ABC) score. His FAST examination was negative. The patient's chest x-ray showed no traumatic injuries. Pelvic x-ray (Figure 110-1) showed pubic diastasis, and a binder was placed with satisfactory reduction. He received five units of red blood cells (RBCs) and five units of plasma in the trauma bay for hypotension. His MTP cooler also arrived with one unit of apheresis platelets that were transfused immediately. He responded appropriately with improved blood pressure of 98/45 and heart rate to 105. The patient was taken to CT, which was remarkable for a pelvic hematoma with active extravasation (Figure 110-2). Following this, the patient was transported to Interventional Radiology where an aortogram and pelvic angiogram were obtained, but no embolization was performed as no active arterial bleeding was identified. Cystogram performed immediately after revealed an extraperitoneal bladder injury. He had a complex both column acetabular fracture, bilateral iliac wing fracture, and left inferior pubic ramus fracture. He was then admitted to the shock trauma intensive care unit.

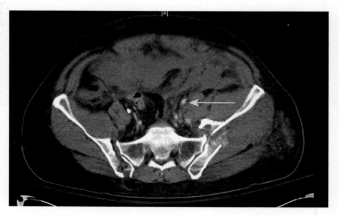

FIGURE 110-2. Axial cut of a contrasted CT scan of the pelvis demonstrating active arterial extravasation (*arrow*), pelvic hematoma, and complex pelvic fractures.

● DISCUSSION

"Injection of a fluid that will increase blood pressure has dangers in itself … if the pressure is raised before the surgeon is ready to check any bleeding that might take place, blood that is sorely needed may be lost."

Worldwide, the leading cause of death in patients under the age of 45 is injury. Exsanguination and shock secondary to hemorrhage are the cause of a significant proportion of these deaths, representing up to 40% of civilian patients. This figure rises to 80% of deaths in the military setting. Moreover, hemorrhage is responsible for half of all deaths in the first 24 hours and 80% of those dying in the operating room.

The approach to resuscitation of the bleeding patient has changed significantly over the last decade, ultimately culminating in the concept of damage control resuscitation. Originally developed by the United States Navy to describe methods to salvage a damaged, sinking ship without restoration to full working order, the term "damage control" has been adopted by trauma surgeons to describe the approach to management of the injured, hemorrhaging patient. Rather than saving a sinking ship, the goal of damage control resuscitation and surgery is to prevent or reduce the deranged physiology injured patients develop. It can be thought of as consisting of the concepts of hemostatic resuscitation and damage control surgery—early hemorrhage control with the minimum amount of operating room time required to achieve surgical hemostasis and control contamination. Definitive repair is delayed until the patient's physiology has normalized.

The goal of hemostatic (damage control) resuscitation is to treat and further prevent the disturbances in physiology of trauma patients. These are the result of the injury itself, the subsequent deficiencies in tissue perfusion, and the often-poor resuscitation techniques that follow. To achieve this end, trauma surgeons employ the three tenets of permissive hypotension, crystalloid fluid restriction, and resuscitation with blood products approximating whole blood (Figure 110-3). Broadly, hemostatic resuscitation aims to treat and prevent development of the lethal triad: hypothermia, coagulopathy, and acidosis.

Hypothermia in trauma is multifactorial, but mostly iatrogenic. Shock causes decreased metabolic activity, while prolonged exposure in the hospital setting leads to increased thermic losses through the environment. Administration of nonwarmed crystalloid intravenous fluids, frequently occurring in both the prehospital setting and trauma bay, further lowers core temperature of the injured patient. Coagulopathy is the most grievous sequela of hypothermia. It appears to occur chiefly due to decreased platelet function and clotting

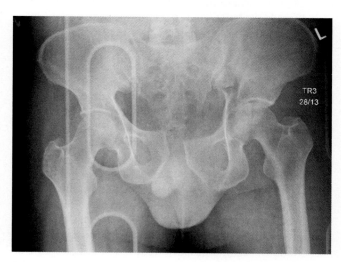

FIGURE 110-1. Anterior–posterior plain film of the pelvis demonstrating pubic diastasis and multiple pelvic fractures.

Three Tenets of Hemostatic (Damage Control) Resuscitation
1. Transfusion of blood products in ratios approximating whole blood
2. Minimization of crystalloids for resuscitation
3. Permissive hypotension until achievement of hemostasis

FIGURE 110-3. Tenets of hemostatic (damage control) resuscitation strategy.

factor activity. Reductions in platelet efficacy also result from hypothermia-induced platelet sequestration in both the liver and spleen. As with any chemical reaction, coagulation occurs slower at lower temperatures due to reduced enzyme kinetics. At a temperature of 35°C, factors XI and XII function at only 65%.

Coagulopathy contributes significantly to the morbidity and mortality of trauma. Crystalloid-based resuscitation causes a dilutional coagulopathy and is known to worsen the lethal triad. Upon arrival to the trauma center, at least 25% of injured patients have trauma-induced coagulopathy, which is associated with increased bleeding and poorer prognosis. Trauma-induced coagulopathy is worsened by inflammation and acidosis, which are often the result of tissue hypoperfusion and direct tissue injury from trauma. One such mechanism is the release of numerous anticoagulant factors, such as protein C, from ischemic cells. A consumptive coagulopathy then ensues as bleeding continues, and platelet and clotting factor stores are depleted. The severity of the coagulopathy is directly proportional to the severity of the injury. Treatment with plasma should begin with any evidence of hypotension and before laboratory confirmation of coagulopathy has returned.

Acidosis is present in many patients suffering from trauma. It is important that surgeons recognize this and address acidosis in their resuscitation strategy given that mortality rates exceed 25% when trauma patients develop a base deficit >8. The sequelae of acidosis are widespread and impact multiple organ systems. Acidosis with a pH < 7.2 decreases cardiac contractility, cardiac output, and liver and kidney perfusion. It causes vasodilation and increases the risk for cardiac arrhythmias. As pH decreases further, clotting factor activity is significantly impacted. At a pH of 7.0, factor VII activity decreases by 90%. The activity of factors II, V, and X suffer a similar impact secondary to acidosis. At a pH of <7.1, prothrombin time (PT) and partial thromboplastin time (PTT) can double. Efforts to treat this acidosis-related coagulopathy with intravenous bicarbonate are not helpful as the cause of the acidosis is not addressed; this can have the opposite of the intended effect and result in patient harm with increased carbon dioxide production. Plasma, on the other hand, is one of the most powerful acid–base buffers available. Additionally, plasma has volume expanding and endothelial stabilizing properties; all of these properties can help to reverse or attenuate coagulopathy and acidosis.

The dangers of resuscitation to normal or near-normal blood pressures have been recognized for a long time. It was thought early on that many exsanguinating patients will become hemostatic without resuscitation as they become progressively hypotensive. However, this hemostasis is disrupted by the increased blood pressure from aggressive crystalloid resuscitation. Some of these patients may fall into the category known as "transient responders." Their pathophysiology is now better understood to be a vicious feedback loop wherein crystalloid administration raises the blood pressure briefly but also causes hemodilution from coagulation factor dilution, causing increased bleeding and recurrent hypotension. This in turn prompts further fluid administration, worsening coagulopathy, and causing further hypotension. This feedback loop is hence known as the "bloody vicious cycle."

This cycle was recognized in the 1980s, and animal studies were designed to investigate this phenomenon. One of the earliest studies was conducted in a swine model. An aortotomy was performed in pigs. Three groups were resuscitated to different mean arterial blood pressure (MAP) goals. The pigs that received no resuscitation and maintained a MAP of 40 mmHg had the lowest mortality. Similar findings were replicated in rat and sheep studies. In 1994, the International Resuscitation Research Conference recommended human research in hypotensive fluid resuscitation as "attempting to normalize blood pressure seems to be counterproductive."

Evaluating the tenets of both hypotensive resuscitation and minimizing crystalloids, Bickell and colleagues built on preclinical data by conducting a study in Houston in which patients were randomized to receive prehospital fluid resuscitation (crystalloids) versus none in patients presenting with hypotension (blood pressure ≤90 mmHg) who had sustained penetrating torso injuries. The randomization resuscitation strategies were continued until the patient entered the operating room. Once patients entered the operating room, the randomized therapy was discontinued, and patients received standard of care at the time—aggressive crystalloid resuscitation. Patients who received delayed resuscitation had lower mortality compared to those who received immediate fluid resuscitation. Survivors had lower rates of postoperative complications if they received delayed resuscitation as well. The study was limited, however, as it was a single-center study that only included penetrating trauma patients.

Investigators from the Resuscitation Outcomes Consortium further investigated these two damage control resuscitation principles by randomizing patients in the prehospital setting to a systolic blood pressure of 70 mmHg or 110 mmHg. The study group was randomized to maintain a systolic blood pressure of 70 mmHg, to receive no initial fluids, and to receive boluses of 250 mL to maintain blood pressure goal. The control group (110 mmHg) received 2 L initially and additional fluid to maintain the blood pressure target. Each resuscitation protocol was maintained until hemorrhage control or 2 hours after hospital arrival. Among blunt trauma patients, 24-hour mortality was significantly lower in the study arm (3%) compared to that observed in the control group (18%), with an adjusted odds ratio of 0.17. Consistent with previous work, this study demonstrated that lower fluid volumes can be administered without worsening mortality, and, when delivered along with permissive hypotension, could improve survival.

Hemostatic resuscitation goes a step beyond simply limiting crystalloid-based resuscitation. Its goal is to actively prevent and preemptively treat the developing trauma-induced coagulopathy. As such, the American College of Surgeons Trauma Quality Improvement Program recommends a 1:1:1 ratio of plasma–platelets–RBCs in an attempt to approximate whole blood. These products are most often delivered through an institution's MTP, until laboratory data on the patient's coagulopathy is available from viscoelastic testing (thrombelastography, TEG, or thromboelastometry, TEM). In addition to the higher ratio of plasma, a higher ratio of transfused platelets–RBC is independently associated with survival.

The Pragmatic, Randomized Optimal Platelet and Plasma Ratios (PROPPR) trial randomized patients predicted to require a massive transfusion to receive plasma, platelets, and RBCs in a 1:1:1 or a 1:1:2 ratio. While 24-hour and 30-day mortality were not significantly different between the groups, outcomes of importance to the trauma patient did show a significant difference. Specifically, bleeding-related mortality was lower, and achievement of hemostasis was higher in the 1:1:1 group. In addition, there was no difference in complication rates between the two groups despite a significantly

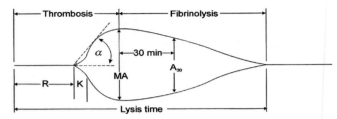

FIGURE 110-4. Standard thrombelastography (TEG) tracing.

larger volume of blood transfused to the 1:1:1 group. This is significant as critics of the high ratio approach cite transfusion-related complications such as acute lung injury as reason to minimize plasma-rich blood product transfusions.

While diagnostic shortcomings of PT, PTT, and serum fibrinogen levels in accurately characterizing coagulopathy can be met with empiric MTP-directed resuscitation, technology exists that can produce data about the entirety of the coagulation cascade including fibrinolysis. Recent interest in viscoelastic testing lies in their ability to diagnose and better characterizing the nature of coagulopathy in bleeding, injured patients. They differ from traditional laboratory measures of coagulation in that their tracings generate data about each point in the coagulation cascade (Figure 110-4). Rapid interpretation of their tracings allows directed transfusion to treat the exact component of coagulation that is deficient and responsible for the clinical coagulopathy (Table 110-1). This directed approach allows for fewer blood products to be administered to adequately treat a hemorrhaging patient, potentially decreasing transfusion-related complications. Much of the historical data on TEG usage are from the cardiac surgery literature. However, recent

Table 110-1	Normal Rapid TEG (r-TEG) Values, Their Associated Step in Coagulation, and Management Recommendations for Abnormal Values		
r-TEG Value (Normal Values)	**Definition**	**Interpretation**	**Management**
ACT > 128 s (86–118 s)	Time from start of assay to initiation of clot	Prolonged with factor deficiency or severe hemodilution	Transfuse plasma
r-value > 1.1 min (0–1.0 min)	Time between beginning of assay and initial clot formation	Prolonged with factor deficiency or severe hemodilution	Transfuse plasma
k-time > 2.5 min (1.0–2.0 min)	Time needed to reach 20 mm clot strength	Increased with hypofibrinogenemia or platelet dysfunction	Transfuse plasma Add cryoprecipitate if angle also abnormal
α-Angle < 60° (66°–82°)	Rate or acceleration of clot formation	Decreased with hypofibrinogenemia or platelet dysfunction	Transfuse cryoprecipitate Add platelets if mA is also abnormal
mA < 55 mm (54–72 mm)	Contribution of platelet function and platelet–fibrin interaction	Decreased with platelet dysfunction and/or hypofibrinogenemia	Transfuse platelets Add cryoprecipitate if angle also abnormal
Lys-30% > 3% (0%–7.5%)	Amplitude reduction 30 min after achieving mA (degree of fibrinolysis)	Increased with accelerated fibrinolysis	Tranexamic acid (TXA) or aminocaproic acid

investigations have validated its use in the care of the injured patient, demonstrating it can safely replace PT and PTT, predict blood transfusion requirement in trauma patients, and identify hypercoagulable patients who are at risk for VTE. A recent randomized trial from Denver Health Medical Center supports this. The study demonstrated that bleeding patients who were transfused using a TEG-based strategy (compared to international normalized ratio, [INR] platelet count, and fibrinogen levels) had improved 28-day survival and less overall transfusions of plasma and platelets.

Tranexamic acid (TXA) is a useful adjunct in management of a bleeding trauma patient. TXA is an antifibrinolytic agent that works by inhibiting the conversion of plasminogen to plasmin. A large, international randomized trial (Clinical Randomisation of an Antifibrinolytic in Significant Haemorrhage-2, CRASH-2) noted an improvement in mortality in injured patients who receive TXA, specifically in those with penetrating mechanism, an initial systolic blood pressure less than 75 mmHg, and receiving the agent within the first 3 hours of injury. Despite these results, widespread adoption of TXA in the United States has yet to occur. Much of this lack of acceptance is likely attributable to flaws in the methodology of the study, primary inclusion of third world and developing countries, and the applicability of the results to North American trauma centers (already incorporating the principles of hemostatic resuscitation). Most of those enrolled in CRASH-2 were treated in centers with limited availability of blood products and outside of mature trauma systems. Furthermore, fewer than half of patients underwent an operation of any type and only half of the patients in the trial received a blood transfusion of any quantity. Given the concerns over proper use of TXA, the two indications for its use in bleeding patients include hyperfibrinolysis demonstrated on TEG/TEM and in patients who are in hemorrhagic shock with a systolic blood pressure <75 mmHg and base deficit >5 as part of a MTP.

The principles of hemostatic resuscitation are namely to prevent the lethal triad before it develops. This is best achieved by limiting crystalloid resuscitation volume and preemptive correction of a patient's coagulopathy before it develops with a balanced blood product resuscitation utilizing a ratio targeting 1:1:1 plasma–platelets–RBCs. Permissive hypotension is an evidence-based resuscitation strategy allowing surgeons to use a lower goal blood pressure during workup and treatment of an injured patient until hemorrhage is controlled to decrease the risk of rebleeding. Together, these interventions have been shown to decrease the mortality of the bleeding, injured trauma patient.

Case Conclusion

This patient remains stable after admission to the shock trauma ICU and appropriate resuscitation. He then undergoes open reduction and internal fixation of his both column acetabular fracture, pubic symphysis disruption, and percutaneous screw fixation of an iliac fracture. Due to the hardware contamination risk from the extraperitoneal bladder injury, synchronous bladder repair is also performed. Foley catheter drainage is continued for 10 days postoperatively, and a postoperative cystogram prior to removal is negative. The patient is discharged home on postoperative day 12.

SUGGESTED READINGS

Bogert JN, Harvin JA, Cotton BA. Damage control resuscitation. *J Intensive Care Med.* 2016;31:177-186.

Burman S, Cotton BA. Trauma patients at risk for massive transfusion: the role of scoring systems and the impact of early identification on patient outcomes. *Expert Rev Hematol.* 2012;5:211-218.

Cannon WB. The preventive treatment of wound shock. *JAMA.* 1918;70:618-621.

Feinman M, Cotton BA, Haut ER. Optimal fluid resuscitation in trauma: type, timing, and total. *Curr Opin Crit Care.* 2014;20:366-372.

Holcomb JB, Tilley BC, Baraniuk S, et al. Transfusion of plasma, platelets, and red blood cells in a 1:1:1 vs a 1:1:2 ratio and mortality in patients with severe trauma: the PROPPR randomized clinical trial. *JAMA.* 2015;313:471-482.

Moore EE, Chin TL, Chapman MC, et al. Plasma first in the field for postinjury hemorrhagic shock. *Shock.* 2014;41(1):35-38.

Nunez TC, Cotton BA. Transfusion therapy in hemorrhagic shock. *Curr Opin Crit Care.* 2009;15:536-541.

Young PP, Cotton BA. A window of opportunity: the aggressive use of plasma in early resuscitation. *Transfusion.* 2011;51(9):1880-1882.

Emergency Department Thoracotomy

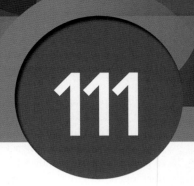

STEPHANIE SEA AND KENJI INABA

Presentation

A 19-year-old male presents to the emergency department (ED) with a single stab wound to the left parasternal chest. Emergency Medical Services (EMS) reported vitals en route are BP 80/palpable, HR 136, RR 24, and O2 saturation 90% on a nonrebreather mask. Upon arrival to the hospital, he was noted to lose vital signs, and chest compressions were started immediately by EMS.

● DIFFERENTIAL DIAGNOSIS

A trauma patient with a witnessed cardiac arrest after a penetrating thoracic injury is potentially salvageable and requires immediate intervention. The trauma team must be available on arrival for any patient at risk of traumatic arrest because rapid intervention is critical for survival. Pericardial tamponade, tension pneumothorax, massive hemorrhage, and injuries to other vital structures need to be rapidly diagnosed and aggressively treated concurrently with emergency department thoracotomy (EDT) and cardiac resuscitation.

● WORKUP

It is essential to have the trauma team activated and present in the ED before the patient arrives. Working together with emergency medicine and nursing to formulate a plan of action and to ensure proper set up of instruments prior to patient arrival can aid in a faster and more effective response, with less chance of harm to all responders.

It is key to remember that in this setting, the diagnostic workup should be minimized, and one must quickly move to treatment of the patient. Multiple diagnostic and therapeutic procedures need to be performed simultaneously when a trauma patient is about to have arrest or has arrested. Basic Advanced Trauma Life Support (ATLS) principles still apply; therefore, securing an airway, achieving vascular access, and continuing cardiopulmonary resuscitation (CPR) will be occurring concurrently. Initial laboratory tests can be drawn. A type and cross, in particular, can be valuable if the patient survives. Focused assessment with sonography for trauma (FAST) may be utilized to rapidly evaluate for the presence of cardiac motion or tamponade.

● DIAGNOSIS AND TREATMENT

Knowing the mechanism of injury and when the vital signs were lost can be valuable in deciding whether or not to perform an EDT. Patients with penetrating thoracic wounds, especially those with penetrating cardiac injury and tamponade, have the highest chance of survival. Intact signs of life are also a positive predictor of survival. However, those who arrest after blunt trauma will do poorly regardless of the degree of intervention. Currently, there is no clear data in the pediatric population as to the effectiveness of EDT.

Understanding which patients will benefit most from an EDT is critical when deciding whether or not to perform an EDT. The Eastern Association for the Surgery of Trauma (EAST) guidelines strongly recommend EDT for any patient who presents pulseless with signs of life after penetrating thoracic injury. They conditionally recommend EDT for those who present pulseless with or without signs of life after penetrating extrathoracic injury, present without signs of life after penetrating thoracic injury, or are pulseless with signs of life after blunt injury. The Western Trauma Association makes recommendations based on the duration of CPR and injury. They recommend performing an EDT in blunt trauma patients when prehospital CPR has not exceeded 10 minutes without a response or in penetrating torso trauma patients when prehospital CPR has not exceeded 15 minutes. EDT should also be considered futile when the patient's presenting rhythm is asystole and there is no pericardial tamponade. Ultrasound has been demonstrated to have a high sensitivity for the detection of survivors using these criteria, thereby making it an effective tool for discriminating potential survivors from nonsurvivors.

At our institution, an aggressive approach to the arrested patient is taken, and it is our practice to perform EDT on all arrested, penetrating injury patients and most blunt injury patients. If there was prolonged downtime, it is at the trauma surgeon's discretion not to perform the EDT. A comprehensive evaluation of EDT outcomes by Rhee demonstrated an overall survival rate of 7.4% with normal neurologic outcomes noted in 92.4% of surviving patients. Survival rates for penetrating injuries were 8.8% and 1.4% for blunt injuries. The primary factors associated with survival were the mechanism of injury, location of major injury, and the presence or absence of signs of life. Organ donation is also a tangible outcome of EDT, and the impact on society of rescuing

650

a potential organ donor must be considered in evaluating the outcomes associated with this intervention. Ultimately, rapid decision-making is critical to ensure maximum benefit after an EDT.

● SURGICAL APPROACH

It is essential that the trauma team be prepared prior to the patient's arrival. All providers should be protected with standard personal protective equipment. The role of each team member should be predetermined. This includes ensuring that the EDT tray is open and all necessary instruments are present. A second tray should be ready in case a concurrent right thoracotomy is required. Keeping the tray simple and including only the essential instruments are helpful. A scalpel; functioning Finochietto retractor; two Duval Lung Forceps; two vascular clamps (one for the hilum and one for the aorta); one long Russian forceps; four hemostats; one bone cutter; one pair of long, heavy curved scissors; and several 2-0 polypropylene sutures on a large, tapered needle are ideal. Proper lighting, an internal cardiac defibrillator, a large Foley catheter, and medications such as epinephrine and sodium bicarbonate should be readily available (Figure 111-1).

All staff assisting in the procedure should wear personal protective gear, including hat, mask with face shield, gown, and sterile gloves. Patient positioning is also important to aid in a successful EDT. Place the patient's left arm above the head or abducted at 90°. Skin preparation should be omitted as it causes the skin to be slippery and can cause injury to the provider. Draping is not required as it is time-consuming, obstructs a clear view of the anatomy, and can inhibit other procedures from occurring.

Key steps are as follows:

1. A left lateral thoracotomy incision is performed using a scalpel though the fourth or fifth intercostal space above the rib, starting at the left parasternal border and ending at the table. This will be in the inframammary fold in females and at or just below the nipple in males (Figure 111-2).

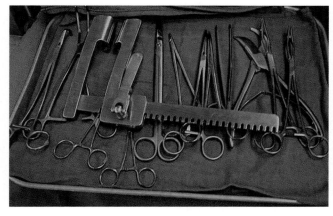

FIGURE 111-1. Instruments included in the emergency department thoracotomy tray.

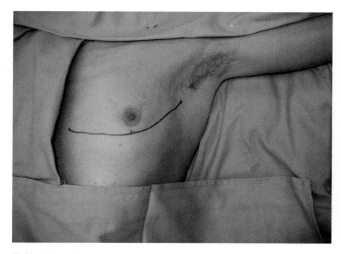

FIGURE 111-2. Skin incision for a left lateral thoracotomy.

2. Once through the skin, divide the subcutaneous tissue and both pectoralis major and minor muscles. Use large scissors to divide the remaining intercostal muscles just superior to the rib to avoid damage to the neurovascular bundle.
3. Insert the Finochietto retractor, with the crossbar closest to the bed, and spread the ribs maximally.
4. Using Duval clamps, retract the left lower lobe toward the patient's head and laterally to improve exposure of the heart and mediastinal structures (Figure 111-3).
5. Open the pericardium longitudinally to release any tamponade, avoiding the phrenic nerve.
6. At this point, assessment of any cardiac injuries can be performed and any injuries can be temporized (Figure 111-4).
7. Evaluate the lung, and if there is hilar bleeding, cross-clamping should be performed.

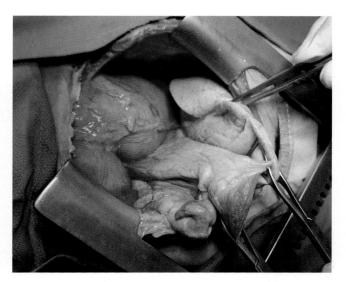

FIGURE 111-3. A left lateral thoracotomy incision with a Finochietto retractor in place—the Duvall lung clamps are on the left upper and lower lobes of the lung.

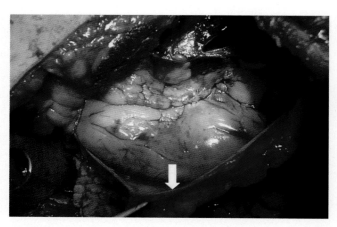

FIGURE 111-4. The *arrow* is pointing to the pericardium, which has been opened to evaluate for hemopericardium and to gain access to the heart.

8. Aortic cross-clamping is accomplished by incising the inferior pulmonary ligament. A small incision using scissors is made in the mediastinal pleura. Blunt dissection is then used to identify the aorta and encircle it. Only a small window is required, to avoid tearing the aorta or its branches. A vascular clamp is applied, avoiding injury to the esophagus.

9. A right chest tube should be placed concurrently. A clamshell incision should be performed if there is a massive right hemothorax. Scissors or a bone cutter can be used to cross the sternum. In survivors, the internal mammary arteries will need to be ligated (Figure 111-5).

Potential pitfalls:

1. Poor placement, or inadequate length, of the initial incision can make the procedure difficult.
2. Placing the Finochietto retractor with the crossbar toward the patient's midline can make extending to a clamshell incision difficult.

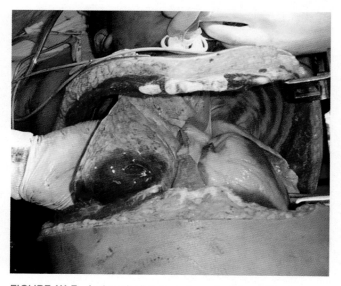

FIGURE 111-5. A clamshell thoracotomy incision with a contusion to the right lung.

3. This is a fast-paced, high-stress procedure with multiple concurrent steps requiring sharp instruments. The potential for provider injury is high.

● SPECIAL INTRAOPERATIVE CONSIDERATIONS

Upon entry into the chest cavity, if there is a cardiac injury, the immediate goal is temporary hemorrhage control followed by repair. Depending on the size of the injury, finger compression can be used to stop the bleeding. For small wounds, which make up the majority of patients who ultimately will survive, digital control is best. A Foley catheter may also provide temporary bleeding control once inserted and inflated in the wound. For larger injuries, especially on the more compliant atrial wall, a vascular clamp may be used. The wound can then be repaired with figure-of-eight, horizontal mattress sutures or a running stitch using 2-0 polypropylene suture. Of note, pledgets can be used; however, they are often time-consuming and unnecessary. They should be used sparingly and only for injuries secondary to a destructive gunshot wound where there will be tension on the suture line. Skin staples are also an alternative for emergent repair of a cardiac laceration. These can be effective in controlling bleeding in the trauma bay until definitive repair is achieved in the operating room.

Injuries in close proximity to a major coronary vessel can be difficult to manage, and care must be taken to avoid ligating these structures. Horizontal mattress sutures placed under the vessel are ideal. Repair of an injury to the coronary vessels can be attempted with interrupted sutures; however, distal injures should be ligated (Figure 111-6).

Posterior cardiac injuries may cause arrhythmias or cardiac arrest while the heart is being lifted. Exposure can be difficult. Sequentially placed laparotomy pads can be used behind the heart for elevation, or a Duval clamp at the apex of the heart can be used to elevate the heart. This should be done slowly and in close communication with anesthesia.

Hilar injuries can be temporized with digital compression or use of a vascular clamp across the hilum. While we do not perform this, an alternative that has been described is the hilar twist. This is performed by incising the inferior pulmonary ligament and twisting the entire lung 180° around the hilum.

If cardiac motion is lost, cardiac massage should be performed using both hands compressing the heart from the apex to the base. Care should be taken not to perforate the heart. Epinephrine 1 mg boluses can be injected directly into the left ventricle using an 18- or 16-gauge needle. Sodium bicarbonate in 50 mEq boluses can also be used. The use of internal cardiac defibrillation may be necessary as it is not uncommon to see return of cardiac activity as ventricular fibrillation. The cardiac paddles are placed directly on the heart in both the anterior and posterior position, and 50 J is used for defibrillation. Warm intravenous fluids poured directly on the heart can be useful in maintaining a normothermic state of the myocardium.

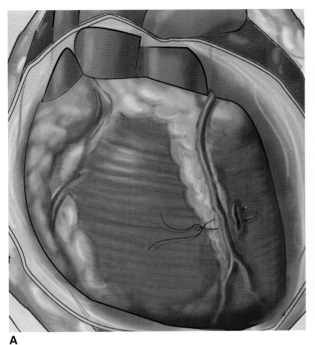
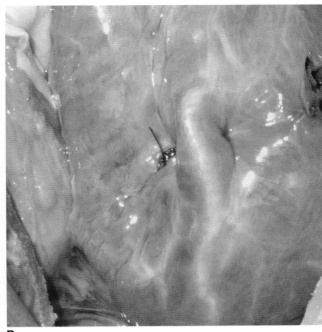

A   **B**

FIGURE 111-6. **A,B:** Schematic and actual repair of a cardiac injury near a coronary vessel using a horizontal mattress suture placed under the vessel.

● POSTOPERATIVE MANAGEMENT

The immediate goal of EDT is to achieve spontaneous cardiac motion that is organized and sufficient to perfuse the coronaries and the brain. If this occurs, the patient should be transferred directly to the operating room for definitive management. Often, after obvious control of bleeding, cross-clamping, and cardiac massage, there is still no return of spontaneous circulation. It is essential that the entire team is in agreement that all possible options have been exhausted and that the resuscitation should be terminated.

One should maintain a high level of suspicion for valvular or septal injury after the patient survives a penetrating cardiac injury. While the goal of the EDT is to control any bleeding and restart the heart, postoperative echocardiogram is routinely performed as a significant number of survivors will be identified as having an additional injury that requires intervention or monitoring.

TAKE HOME POINTS

- Rapid diagnosis and intervention are key with trauma patients arriving in cardiac arrest or in imminent cardiac arrest.
- Isolated, penetrating thoracic injuries, especially injuries to the heart with tamponade, have the highest rates of success after EDT. However, survival rates are still extremely low.
- Proper preparation, positioning, and incision will aid in a quicker and smoother EDT.

- Multiple procedures (such as intubation, vascular access, and right chest tube placement) should be performed simultaneously.
- EDT allows for decompression of a cardiac tamponade, identification and control of intrathoracic bleeding, aortic cross-clamping, cardiac massage, and defibrillation.

SUGGESTED READINGS

Burew CC, Moore EE, Moore FA, et al. Western Trauma Association critical decision in trauma: resuscitative thoracotomy. *J Trauma Acute Care Surg.* 2012;73:1359-1363.

Demetriades D, Zakaluzny S, ed. Emergency room resuscitative thoracotomy. In: Demetriades D, Inaba K, Velmahos G, eds. *Atlas of Surgical Techniques in Trauma.* Cambridge: Cambridge University Press; 2015:18-27.

Inaba K, Chouliaras K, Zakaluzny S, et al. FAST ultrasound examination as a predictor of outcomes after resuscitative thoracotomy: a prospective evaluation. *Ann Surg.* 2015;263:512-518.

Moore EE, Knudson MM, Burlew CC, et al. Defining the limits of resuscitative emergency department thoracotomy: a contemporary Western Trauma Association perspective. *J Trauma.* 2011;70:334-339.

Rhee PM, Acosta J, Bridgeman A, et al. Survival after emergency department thoracotomy: review of published data from the past 25 years. *J Am Coll Surg.* 2000;190:288-298.

Schnuriger B, Inaba K, Branco BC, et al. Organ donation: an important outcome after resuscitative thoracotomy. *J Am Coll Surg.* 2010;211:450-455.

Schnuriger B, Talving P, Inaba K, et al. Biochemical profile and outcomes in trauma patients subjected to open cardiopulmonary resuscitation: a prospective observational pilot study. *World J Surg.* 2012;36:1772-1778.

Seamon MJ, Haut ER, Van Arendonk K, et al. An evidence-based approach to patient selection for emergency department thoracotomy: a practice management guideline from the Eastern Association for the Surgery of Trauma. *J Trauma Acute Care Surg.* 2015;79:159-73.

Tang AL, Inaba K, Branco BC, et al. Postdischarge complications after penetrating cardiac injury: a survivable injury with a high postdischarge complication rate. *Arch Surg.* 2011;146:1061-1066.

Penetrating Chest Injury

112

JEFFREY J. SKUBIC AND ADIL H. HAIDER

Based on the previous edition chapter "Penetrating Chest Injury" by Albert Chi and Adil H. Haider

Presentation

A 22-year-old male presents to the emergency room with multiple stab wounds to the head, back, and left upper arm. Emergency medical services (EMS) vitals are BP 100/P, HR 104, RR 26, and O_2 saturation 97% on room air. Physical examination on arrival reveals that the patient is speaking but has diminished breath sounds on the right side; abdomen is soft; he has 2+ symmetric pulses distally; and he is moving all four extremities. He complains of chest pain and increasing shortness of breath. Initial emergency department (ED) vitals are BP 77/56, HR 126, and O_2 saturation of 96% on 100% nonrebreather mask.

● DIFFERENTIAL DIAGNOSIS

When managing unstable patients with penetrating chest injuries, trauma teams must rapidly and accurately intervene with potential life-saving procedures. Airway, breathing, and circulation must be priorities in working up the hypotensive trauma patient with an undetermined underlying cause. Three diagnoses must be considered that need immediate intervention: (1) pericardial tamponade, (2) tension pneumothorax, and (3) ongoing blood loss (e.g., hemorrhage from great vessels, pulmonary hilum, lung parenchyma, or intercostal artery). As interventions and surgical approach are very specific for each of these processes, quick assessment and judgment are necessary.

● WORKUP

In the unstable patient, surgeons must rely on clinical suspicion and physical exam findings (i.e., breath sounds absent or present, muffled or distant heart sounds) for the diagnosis of life-threatening injuries. For example, chest tube thoracostomy tube placement or needle decompression for suspected tension pneumothorax should not be delayed for confirmatory imaging. However, diagnostic adjuncts that can be performed quickly may be useful. In the case of suspected cardiac tamponade, a quick Focused Assessment Sonography for Trauma (FAST) pericardial view can determine the presence of fluid surrounding the heart. *A clinical*

caution: even with a negative pericardial window on FAST, a cardiac injury can still be present if the pericardial wound communicates with the thorax, decompressing into the chest. In the stable patient, portable upright anterior posterior chest x-ray should be performed with FAST. Computed tomography can be considered for stable patients after primary survey is performed.

● DISCUSSION

In this patient, with a penetrating wound to the chest, decreased breath sounds on the side of injury, and hypotension, a tension pneumothorax should be assumed. Immediate steps to decompress this must be undertaken.

Chest Needle Decompression

A simple pneumothorax is the most common thoracic injury after penetrating chest trauma and frequently results from an injury to the lung parenchyma. Without an adequate vent for decompression, increased intrathoracic pressure may result in kinking of the vena cava, decreased venous return to the heart, and cardiovascular collapse. In the prehospital setting, needle decompression is frequently performed on injured patients with a suspected tension pneumothorax. A decompressive needle and catheter can be inserted rapidly as a temporizing measure until a formal tube thoracostomy can be performed, although it is not without risk. It can be quite difficult to diagnose a pneumothorax in a moving ambulance.

Key Steps

1. Locate the second intercostal space and the midclavicular line.
2. Prepare site with chlorhexidine solution or an alcohol swab.
3. Make a puncture with 14-G catheter or angiocatheter from central line kit if additional length is needed secondary to body habitus.
4. Advance until rush of air is encountered and remove needle while stabilizing catheter.
5. Place a one-way valve if available.
6. Perform formal tube thoracostomy.

Pitfalls

1. Fourteen-gauge catheter length is 1¼ inches, and many patients' chest walls may require greater length to enter the chest cavity.
2. Chest needle decompression may cause additional injury to lung parenchyma causing a fatal air embolism or hematoma. There have even been reports of resultant hilar vessel injury.

Thoracostomy Tube

Drainage of the pleural space by means of a chest tube is the commonest intervention in thoracic trauma (85% of chest injuries receive tube thoracostomy), and it provides definitive treatment in the majority of cases. While a relatively simple procedure, it carries a significant complication rate, reported as between 2% and 10%. While many of these complications are relatively minor, some require operative intervention, and deaths still occur (e.g., from laceration of neurovascular bundle in inferior surface of ribs).

A chest tube is indicated to drain the contents of the pleural space. Usually this will be air or blood but may include other fluids such as chyle or gastric/esophageal contents. Chest tube insertion is also appropriate to prevent the development of a pleural collection, such as after a thoracotomy or to prevent a tension pneumothorax in the ventilated patient with rib fractures.

Absolute Indications

- Pneumothorax (*tension, open, or simple*)
- *Hemothorax*
- Traumatic arrest (bilateral)

Relative Indications

- Rib fractures and positive pressure ventilation
- Profound hypoxia/hypotension and penetrating chest injury
- Profound hypoxia/hypotension and unilateral signs to a hemithorax

Key Steps

1. Place the patient's ipsilateral arm over head to maximize exposure.
2. Don mask, gown and gloves; prep and drape area of insertion, if time allows.
3. Select site for insertion: midaxillary line, between fourth and fifth ribs at the level of the nipple in males and inframammary crease in females.
4. Infiltrate insertion site with local anesthetic, make a 3- to 4-cm incision through skin and subcutaneous tissues between the fourth and fifth ribs, parallel to the rib margins.
5. Use a Kelly clamp to push through the pleura and open the jaws widely, again parallel to the direction of the ribs.
6. Insert finger through your incision and into the thoracic cavity. Make sure you are feeling lung (or empty space) and not liver or spleen.
7. Grasp end of 28 to 36 french chest tube with the Kelly forceps (convex angle toward ribs), and insert chest tube through the hole made in the pleura.
8. After tube has entered thoracic cavity, remove clamp, and manually advance the tube posteriorly and toward the apex of the thoracic cavity avoiding the major fissure as you advance.
9. Connect chest tube to pleurovac and place to wall suction.
10. Suture in place with a nonabsorbable suture and place an occlusive dressing.

● PITFALLS

- Must confirm intrathoracic location with manual palpation of lung parenchyma. An incision placed too low can inadvertently place thoracostomy tubes intra-abdominal and not intrathoracic.
- Estimation of blood loss on initial insertion of chest tube. Placement of an additional clamp at the distal end of the chest tube during insertion decreases the amount of spillage and aids in the measurement of estimated blood loss.
- Be careful of potential injury to the chest tube inserter from rib fractures—double gloving is recommended.

Diagnosis and Recommendations

The indications for thoracotomy after traumatic injury typically include persistent shock, arrest at presentation, and ongoing thoracic hemorrhage. Operative intervention due to ongoing hemorrhage is most commonly performed after 1,500 mL of blood output on initial chest tube insertion or continued hourly blood loss of 250 mL or more for 3 consecutive hours after tube thoracostomy. Evidence of gastric contents could also represent an esophageal injury, and massive air leak from chest tube could suggest a bronchial tracheal injury.

Emergent thoracotomy is performed by an anterolateral approach as this provides the most rapid access to the heart and mediastinum. However, if there is time for operative planning, then the incision that provides the best exposure for the suspected injuries should be used.

Anterolateral Thoracotomy

Key Steps to Thoracotomy

1. Place patient in supine position with arms extended.
2. Place double-lumen endotracheal tube by anesthesia if time and stability allow; for injuries to the left chest, the endotracheal tube can be advanced in the right mainstem bronchus keeping the left lung collapsed.

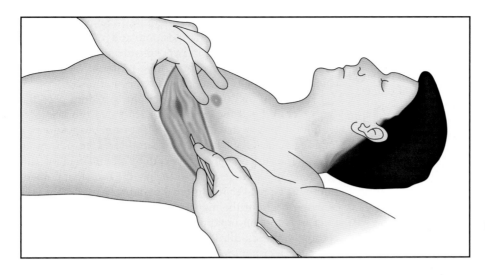

FIGURE 112-1. The emergent left anterolateral thoracotomy incision should follow the intercostal space.

3. Make the incision in the fourth intercostal space starting at the sternal border to the midaxillary line.
4. Anatomic landmarks of the fourth intercostal space are just below the nipple in males and the inframammary fold in females.
5. Enter the chest with three bold strokes of the knife: the first divides the skin and the subcutaneous tissue, the second is through the pectoralis anteriorly and serratus laterally, and the third is through the intercostal muscles entering the pleural space (Figure 112-1).

Pitfalls

- Exposure of certain structures is not always optimal with this standard thoracotomy incision.
- If the Finecetto/rib retractor is placed with the bar/spin mechanism toward the sternum, then it may obstruct extension of the incision across the sternum (clamshell thoracotomy) if required.

Resuscitative Thoracotomy

The best survival results with this procedure are seen in patients who undergo ED thoracotomy for thoracic stab injuries with isolated cardiac stab wounds and arrive with signs of life in the ED. Factors such as mechanism of injury, location of major injury, and signs of life should be taken into account when deciding whether to perform resuscitative thoracotomy in the ED.

Accepted Indications

- Penetrating thoracic injury
  - Traumatic arrest with previously witnessed cardiac activity (prehospital or inhospital)
  - Unresponsive hypotension (BP < 70 mm Hg)
- Blunt thoracic injury
  - Unresponsive hypotension (BP < 70 mm Hg)
  - Rapid exsanguination from chest tube (>1,500 mL)

Relative Indications

- Penetrating thoracic injury
  - Traumatic arrest without previously witnessed cardiac activity
- Penetrating nonthoracic injury
  - Traumatic arrest with previously witnessed cardiac activity (prehospital or inhospital)
- Blunt thoracic injuries
  - Traumatic arrest with previously witnessed cardiac activity (prehospital or inhospital)

Additional Steps to ED Thoracotomy

1. Create a window and using the Mayo scissors cut along the intercostals avoiding the neurovascular bundle on the inferior portion of the rib cage.
2. Place rib spreader into the incision with the handle toward the axilla and open to expose the workspace.
3. Mobilize the lung by cutting the inferior pulmonary ligament.
4. Manually palpate posterior ribs and palpate the spine; the thoracic aorta should be the first tubular structure encountered.
5. To cross-clamp the aorta, open the parietal pleural and place a vascular clamp across. If a nasogastric tube (NGT) is present, the NGT can be used to identify the esophagus.
6. If cardiac tamponade or a cardiac injury is suspected, open the pericardium.
7. To open the pericardium, pinch the left lateral aspect with your finger or clamp anterior to the phrenic nerve and open widely parallel to the nerve sliding scissors along the pericardium.

Pitfalls

- Injury to the aorta, the intercostal arteries, or the esophagus during aortic clamping
- Injury to the phrenic nerve when opening the pericardium

● OTHER THORACOTOMY APPROACHES

The choice of thoracic incision (Figure 112-2) for trauma repair is based on the anatomic location of injury and physiologic status. There are many incisions available for thoracic trauma. These include anterolateral thoracotomy, transsternal anterolateral "clamshell" thoracotomy, posterolateral thoracotomy, "book incision" (anterolateral thoracotomy, partial upper sternotomy to a supraclavicular extension), and median sternotomy.

The left anterolateral thoracotomy is the utility incision for resuscitation under circumstances of acute deterioration or cardiac arrest. This incision allows exposure for opening the pericardium, open cardiac massage, clamping of the descending thoracic aorta, and treatment of a large percentage of cardiac and left lung injuries.

A *left posterolateral thoracotomy* allows much greater exposure to the left hilum, including the hilar pulmonary artery, vein, and bronchus. It is also ideal exposure for the descending aorta.

A *right posterolateral thoracotomy* is indicated for right hilar injuries and also gives excellent exposure of the thoracic portion of the esophagus.

Posterolateral thoracotomy requires the patient to be repositioned in the lateral position and may exacerbate hemodynamic instability in hypovolemic patients. It is particularly well suited for approaching posterior lung parenchymal lacerations and intercostal vessel injuries.

The "book" or "trap door" incision is seldom used but can be considered for exposure of left-sided thoracic outlet injuries. It has the advantage of providing exposure of a long segment of the left common carotid and left subclavian artery. The anterolateral thoracotomy component of this incision can be made above or below the breast, and attention must be paid to the internal mammary artery. The current approach for the management of left subclavian artery injuries is to gain proximal control via anterolateral thoracotomy in the left third interspace combined with a separate clavicular incision for definitive repair.

The standard median sternotomy incision provides excellent exposure to the heart and proximal great vessels, including the ascending aorta, innominate artery, and left common carotid artery. It is recommended primarily for anticipated isolated anterior cardiac injuries where there is no need to repair injuries to other organ systems. Further exposure can be obtained with extension into either the supraclavicular area or the neck.

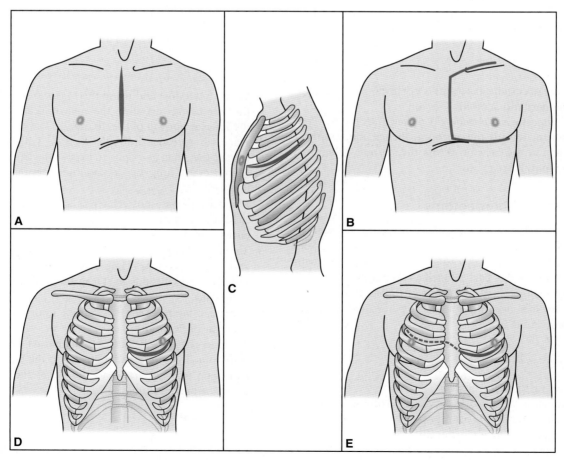

FIGURE 112-2. Thoracic incisions for trauma include (**A**) median sternotomy, (**B**) book thoracotomy, (**C**) posterolateral thoracotomy, (**D**) anterolateral thoracotomy, and (**E**) extension of an anterolateral thoracotomy across the sternum.

A clamshell thoracotomy provides almost complete exposure to both thoracic cavities. In general, the indication for performing a clamshell thoracotomy is when access is needed to both sides of the chest. For example:

- To improve exposure and access to the heart (especially right-sided structures) following a left anterolateral thoracotomy performed for profound hypotension or traumatic arrest
- To provide access to the right chest in transmediastinal injuries or multiple penetrating injury to both the left and the right chest
- To allow cardiac massage following a right-sided thoracotomy

The only part of the thoracic cavity that is not easily reached through a clamshell incision is the very superior mediastinal vessels. If there is an injury here, the sternum can be split to provide wide exposure to this area.

Resuscitative Endovascular Balloon Occlusion of the Aorta (REBOA)

REBOA has been used to improve central perfusion to the brain and heart since it was first reported during the Korean War era. With the advance of endovascular technology, it has been increasing in popularity as an alternative to resuscitative thoracotomy and aortic clamping, which are associated with high morbidity.

Indications

- Penetrating abdominal or pelvic trauma
  - Unresponsive hypotension (BP < 80 mm Hg)
- Blunt trauma patients
  - Suspected hemorrhagic source in the abdomen or pelvis.
  - Unresponsive hypotension (BP < 80 mm Hg)

Contraindications

- Aortic injury
- Mediastinal injury
- Axillary injury

Key Steps to REBOA

1. Obtain femoral artery access and insert a 5 Fr to 8 Fr sheath over a wire either percutaneously via ultrasound (or fluoroscopic) guidance or cut down.
2. Insert a large compliant balloon through your sheath and position in aortic zone 1 (left subclavian artery to celiac artery) for a suspected abdominal and/or pelvic hemorrhagic source. Position the balloon in aortic zone 3 (lowest renal artery to aortic bifurcation) for a suspected pelvic hemorrhagic source (Figure 112-3).

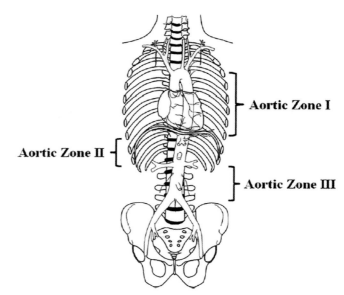

FIGURE 112-3. REBOA Zones: Zone I extends from the origin of the left subclavian artery to the celiac artery, zone II celiac to lowest renal artery, and zone III from lowest renal artery to the aortic bifurcation. Zone I is recommended for abdominal hemorrhage, while zone III is recommended for pelvic hemorrhage. Zone II is not recommended for balloon inflation.

3. Inflate the balloon with a 1/2 mixture of sterile saline and contrast under fluoroscopy. Secure your balloon in place and have an assistant continuously monitor the wire, balloon, and sheath.
4. Deflate the balloon slowly when aortic occlusion is no longer needed.
5. Remove the sheath and close the arteriotomy with either a cut down technique or percutaneous closure device.

Pitfalls

- Examine the chest radiograph before REBOA placement. A suspected aortic or mediastinal injury is a contraindication to REBOA as it may cause increased hemorrhage.
- Deflate the balloon slowly during removal. Intermittent reinflation may be needed while hemodynamics are still improving.
- Morbidity related to arterial catheter insertion includes dissection, stenosis, and perforation.

● INTRAOPERATIVE MANAGEMENT OF SPECIFIC INJURIES

Pulmonary Tractotomy for Penetrating Lung Injury

1. Once the hemithorax is entered, control of the pulmonary hilum can be accomplished with finger occlusion or

a clamp. The purpose is to prevent passage of air into the systemic circulation as well as hemostatic control.

2. Place a lung clamp on either side of the tract created by the knife or the bullet.
3. Insert a gastrointestinal anastomosis stapler through the entrance and exit wound of the lung.
4. Fire the stapling device to fully expose the injury tract.
5. Directly ligate bleeding vessels or exposed bronchi with 3-0 Vicryl figure-eight sutures.

Pitfalls

- Large unsealed areas of the lung may cause persistent blowing air leaks leading to an unplanned reoperation.

Intercostal Bleeding

1. Identify the area of injury.
2. Place a circumferential suture around the rib with an absorbable suture and large needle from within the chest cavity.
3. If necessary, a straight needle may be used to place a suture around the rib and skin and then back into the pleural cavity to get control of the vessels. These sutures can typically be removed after 48 hours.
4. Both ends of the intercostal artery must be ligated.

Pitfalls

- Including the neurovascular bundle may cause rib pain

Massive Pulmonary Hilar Bleed

1. Attempt to control bleeding with manual pressure, hemostatic suture, or rapid resection of the bleeding segment.
2. If hilar clamping is the only option, hold ventilation to allow manual grasping of the hilum with your nondominant hand.
3. Place Satinsky clamp around the entire hilum.
4. If unable to place clamp, twist the lung to rapidly control the hilum without a clamp.

Pitfalls

- Phrenic nerve injury during clamping.
- Hilar clamping is not well tolerated by patients in shock.

Pneumonectomy: Due to the substantial alterations in cardiopulmonary physiology, outcomes after traumatic pneumonectomy are very poor. Thus, this procedure should be reserved only for patients where lung salvage is not possible. That being said, the decision to proceed with this highly morbid procedure should be taken quickly and decisively as delaying this usually results in mortality.

Case Conclusion

Based on EMS reports, a chest x-ray plate was present on the ED stretcher upon arrival of the patient, and an x-ray was shot even before the automated blood pressure was measured. As hypotension was noted along with decreased breath sounds on the side of injury, the ED staff immediately performed needle decompression resulting in a rush of air and immediate improvement of blood pressure and ability to breath. The digital x-ray in Figure 112-4 appeared on the screen after needle thoracostomy and demonstrates the large tension pneumothorax prior to decompression. Note how the mediastinal structures have been shifted into the left chest. A right chest tube was then placed, which drained approximately 2 L of frank blood on insertion. This prompted emergent transfer of the patient to the operating room for a right-sided posterolateral thoracotomy. Upon exploration, a posterior intercostal artery laceration due to the stab wound was found, but no pulmonary injury was noted. The intercostal artery was ligated with large sutures placed around the rib. Two chest tubes were placed intraoperatively and managed expectantly. The importance of rapid operative intervention can be gauged from the fact that the patient's initial pH on arterial blood gas was 7.09. Intraoperatively, the patient was resuscitated with a 1:1:1 ratio of packed red blood cells, fresh frozen plasma, and platelets. By the end of the case and with reversal of hemorrhagic shock, the patient's arterial pH had normalized to 7.32. The patient was discharged home on postoperative day 4 without complications.

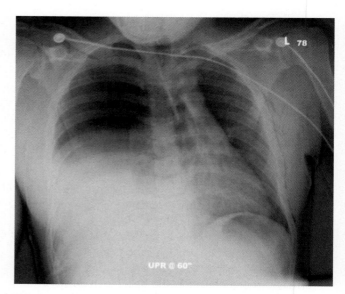

FIGURE 112-4. Chest x-ray prior to needle thoracostomy, which demonstrates a large tension pneumothorax.

TAKE HOME POINTS

- In patients with altered hemodynamics after penetrating chest injury, immediate action directed at reversing the most likely cause of instability must be taken.
- Negative FAST exam does not rule out a pericardial violation or a cardiac injury.
- Most patients with penetrating injury (up to 75%) are simply managed with a tube thoracostomy.
- If 1,500 mL of blood drains out of chest tube immediately, then the patient most likely needs an operative intervention.
- In the operating room, choice of incision is dictated by suspicion of injured structures.

SUGGESTED READINGS

Mattox KL, Wall MJ Jr, LeMaire SA. Injury to the thoracic great vessels. In: More EE, Feliciano DV, Mattox KL, eds. *Trauma*. 5th ed. New York, NY: McGraw-Hill; 2004:571-581.

Rhee PM, Acosta J, Bridgeman A, et al. Survival after emergency department thoracotomy: review of published data from the past 25 years. *J Am Coll Surg*. 2000;190:288-298.

Stannard A, Eliason JL, Rasmussen TE. Resuscitative endovascular balloon occlusion of the aorta (REBOA) as an adjunct for hemorrhagic shock. *J Trauma*. 2011;71:1869-1872.

Wall MJ, Hirshberg A, Mattox KL. Pulmonary tractotomy with selective vascular ligation for penetrating injuries to the lung. *Am J Surg*. 1994;168:665-669.

Wall MJ Jr, Soltero E, Mattox KL. Penetrating trauma. In: Pearson FG, Cooper JD, Deslauruers J, et al., eds. *Thoracic Surgery*. 2nd ed. New York, NY: Churchill Livingstone; 2002:1858-1863.

Stab Wound to the Neck

113

ANTHONY J. LEWIS AND JASON L. SPERRY

Based on the previous edition chapter "Stab Wound to the Neck"
by Gina M.S. Howell and Jason L. Sperry

Presentation

Emergency Medical Services (EMS) providers bring a 33-year-old female involved in an altercation to the emergency department, reporting a single laceration in the anterior neck. Providers on scene noted the assailant to be wielding a small pocket knife. On admission, she is normotensive, protecting her airway, has no signs or symptoms of respiratory difficulty, and is neurologically intact. She reports left neck pain. Focused neck examination reveals a single 2-cm wound anterior to the sternocleidomastoid (SCM) muscle at the level of the thyroid cartilage. There is a small, pulsatile hematoma with an associated bruit, and a moderate amount of crepitus on palpation. Plain films demonstrate subcutaneous emphysema, no tracheal deviation, and no pneumothorax.

● DIFFERENTIAL DIAGNOSIS

Penetrating trauma in the cervical region can result in significant morbidity and mortality, as it is a relatively unprotected area with a high density of vital structures. Specific injury patterns depend upon the anatomic level of injury (Table 113-1). In this case, the differential diagnosis of potential injuries is broad. This patient has a Zone II injury, placing her at risk for damage to the carotid and vertebral arteries, jugular veins, vagus nerve, larynx, trachea, esophagus, and spinal cord.

● WORKUP

The initial evaluation of every trauma patient should adhere to the principles of Advanced Trauma Life Support, beginning with rapid assessment of the airway as the chief priority in the primary survey. Oral-tracheal intubation by a skilled practitioner is the preferred method of airway control if needed; however, surgical airway creation may be needed if other intubation attempts are unsuccessful. The focused physical examination that follows should assess for signs and symptoms of significant vascular and aerodigestive tract injury (Table 113-2). "Hard" signs mandating immediate operative exploration without the need for additional diagnostic workup include shock/hypotension, active hemorrhage, expanding or pulsatile hematoma, neurologic deficit, significant subcutaneous emphysema, respiratory distress/airway compromise, or air leaking through the

Table 113-1 Anatomic Zones of the Neck and Associated Injuries

Zone	Landmarks	Important Structures
I	Clavicle—cricoid cartilage	Great vessels, proximal carotid artery, vertebral artery, lung, trachea, esophagus, thoracic duct, spinal cord, cervical nerve trunks
II	Cricoid cartilage—angle of mandible	Carotid artery and branches, jugular veins, vertebral artery, larynx, trachea, esophagus, vagus nerve, spinal cord
III	Angle of mandible—skull base	Distal internal carotid artery, vertebral artery, jugular veins, pharynx, salivary glands, cranial nerves

Table 113-2 Clinical Signs and Symptoms of Significant Injury

Vascular	Respiratory	Digestive
Hemodynamic instability[a]	Airway compromise[a]	Hematemesis
Pulsatile hematoma[a]	Air bubbling from neck wound[a]	Odynophagia
Expanding hematoma[a]	Significant subcutaneous emphysema[a]	Dysphagia
Active hemorrhage[a]	Hemoptysis	Subcutaneous emphysema
Neurologic deficit[a]	Dysphonia	
Bruit	Tracheal tenderness	
Pulse deficit	Dyspnea	

[a]Indicates hard sign of injury mandating operative exploration.

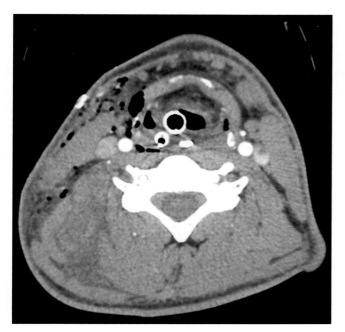

FIGURE 113-1. CTA of the neck. CTA is the initial diagnostic study of choice in the evaluation of penetrating neck wounds that do not require immediate exploration. This image demonstrates subcutaneous emphysema concerning for injury to the aerodigestive tract.

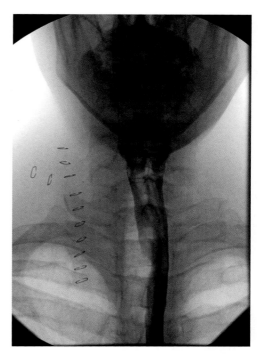

FIGURE 113-2. Barium contrast esophagogram. Clinical exam alone is unreliable in excluding esophageal injury. Formal evaluation with barium esophagogram and/or esophagoscopy is recommended to minimize the consequences of missed injury or delay in diagnosis. This image demonstrates a normal study without evidence of contrast extravasation.

neck wound. Plain chest and cervical radiographs are typically taken for all patients during this initial assessment primarily to evaluate for serious injuries (e.g., pneumothorax, hemothorax, tracheal deviation) requiring expeditious treatment.

In stable patients with wounds that penetrate the platysma but who do not need immediate exploration based upon the previously listed "hard" signs, further radiographic and endoscopic evaluation is usually recommended to evaluate for surgically significant injuries. Though practice patterns vary among institutions, computed tomography (CT) has become the backbone of modern trauma evaluation and is often used as the initial diagnostic study. The addition of intravenous contrast (computed tomographic angiography [CTA]) makes this modality even more useful for determination of injury track and proximity to vital structures, and it is the preferred method over conventional arteriography and duplex ultrasonography for the detection of vascular injuries (Figure 113-1). In addition to performing a CT, it is also prudent to formally evaluate the esophagus with barium contrast esophagography (Figure 113-2) or esophagoscopy, with many centers utilizing both techniques on a routine basis to increase sensitivity. Suspicion of laryngotracheal injury warrants laryngoscopy and bronchoscopy.

DIAGNOSIS AND TREATMENT

This patient has a penetrating wound in Zone II. She likely has a significant vascular injury based on the finding of a pulsatile hematoma and associated bruit. In addition, she may also have an injury to her aerodigestive tract as evidenced by subcutaneous emphysema on clinical and radiographic

examination. She is not unstable and does not require emergent intubation, but she does have "hard" signs of injury and therefore should go immediately to the operating room for exploration. Cervical immobilization is unnecessary due to the extremely low likelihood of unstable spine fracture in this setting, and can actually be harmful by interfering with serial neck examination and potential life-saving maneuvers.

DISCUSSION

It is universally accepted that all patients with hemodynamic instability or "hard" signs of injury require emergent operation without the need for additional diagnostic workup. There is variability, however, in the management of patients who do not fall into this category. The era of mandatory exploration for every penetrating neck wound and its high associated nontherapeutic exploration rate has certainly passed but may still serve as the most appropriate strategy in situations where immediate radiologic and endoscopic capabilities are not readily available. Selective operative management, on the other hand, relies upon serial observation and ancillary studies to effectively diagnose or rule out injuries requiring surgical intervention. There is a negligible rate of missed injury with this approach and is the strategy advocated by most, particularly for injuries that may involve Zones I and III because of the difficulty in examining and exposing these areas. Simple observation alone should be exercised with caution even in asymptomatic patients with no

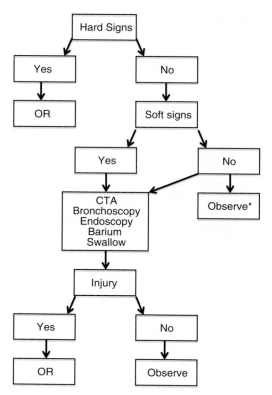

FIGURE 113-3. Suggested management algorithm for Zone II penetrating injuries. *Observation alone should be exercised with caution, as some injuries may be clinically occult at the time of presentation.

signs of significant injury, as some injuries (e.g., esophageal) are often clinically occult at the time of presentation. Delays in the diagnosis of esophageal injuries are associated with significantly worse morbidity and mortality. Although guidelines have typically recommended specific management plans based upon the anatomic zone of injury in the neck, more recent data suggest that external zone of injury does not always correlate well with the actual internal injury pattern observed.

Table 113-3	Zone II Neck Exploration

Key Technical Steps

1. Perform a neck incision along anterior border of SCM muscle.
2. Open carotid sheath and divide facial and middle thyroid veins to expose carotid artery.
3. If carotid artery injury is present, obtain proximal and distal control before definitive repair.
4. Inspect internal jugular vein and attempt primary repair if necessary.
5. Mobilize esophagus and place Penrose drain to rotate circumferentially.
6. Palpate and visualize larynx and trachea.
7. Perform esophagoscopy and/or bronchoscopy.

Potential Pitfalls

- Vagus or recurrent laryngeal nerve injury.
- Missed esophageal injury.
- Difficulty obtaining proximal or distal control of carotid artery.

A suggested management algorithm for penetrating neck injuries independent of anatomic zone is depicted in Figure 113-3.

● SURGICAL APPROACH

A standard Zone II neck exploration is performed under general anesthesia with the patient positioned supine on the operating room table with arms tucked, neck extended, and head rotated to the contralateral side (Table 113-3). A vertical neck incision along the anterior border of the SCM muscle is routinely utilized (Figure 113-4). Once the dissection is carried through skin, subcutaneous tissue, and platysma, posterolateral retraction of the SCM provides exposure to all vital structures.

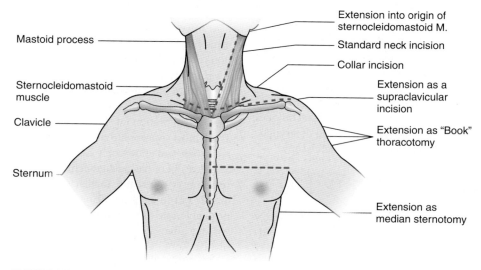

FIGURE 113-4. Incisions for exposure of penetrating neck injuries.

Unless there is another obvious injury requiring immediate attention, the vascular structures are typically explored first by opening the carotid sheath. Division of the middle thyroid and facial veins will facilitate complete visualization of the carotid artery, which lies deep and medial to the internal jugular vein. Attention is then turned to the aerodigestive tract with care taken not to injure the recurrent laryngeal nerve, which lies in the tracheoesophageal groove. Mobilization of the esophagus is accomplished by dissecting in the posterior areolar plane and then encircling the esophagus with a Penrose drain to facilitate rotation and circumferential inspection. The larynx and trachea should be visualized and palpated for signs of injury. This may require mobilization of the thyroid and/or division of strap muscles. Intraoperative esophagoscopy and bronchoscopy are often utilized to supplement direct open examination and minimize the incidence of missed injuries.

● MANAGEMENT OF COMMON ZONE II INJURIES

Vascular Injury

It is currently recommended that all common and internal carotid artery injuries should be repaired, even in patients presenting with significant neurologic deficits, as early revascularization has consistently been associated with improvement or stabilization of neurologic symptoms. Proximal and distal control of the common, external, and internal carotid arteries must be obtained before definitive repair. If exposure is less than ideal, vascular control can be accomplished with a Fogarty balloon catheter. Prior to clamping, consideration should be given to heparinization provided there are no contraindications. Shunting is usually unnecessary in the typical young trauma patient but should be employed if there is suspicion for cerebral malperfusion or evidence of poor back bleeding.

Sharp penetrating weapons typically result in relatively clean injuries that are amenable to primary repair with minimal debridement. Arteriorrhaphy can be accomplished with interrupted 6-0 polypropylene sutures. If the laceration is circumferential, an end–end repair may be performed. If the injury is near the bifurcation of the common carotid into its internal and external branches, a patch angioplasty will help minimize the development of stenosis. Large perforations or defects are unlikely from this mechanism, but if present are treated with segmental resection and interposition graft. Saphenous vein conduit is preferred for this purpose due to superior long-term patency compared with polytetrafluoroethylene.

Whenever possible, internal jugular vein injuries should be repaired. However, if the patient is unstable or simple repair is not feasible, this vessel can be ligated unilaterally with minimal morbidity. Similarly, the external carotid artery may be safely ligated secondary to extensive collateral circulation. Due to difficult access, bleeding from the vertebral vessels is best managed by temporary control of hemorrhage in the operating room using bone wax compression or insertion of a Fogarty balloon catheter, followed by immediate transfer to the arteriography suite for embolization.

Esophageal Injury

Expeditious diagnosis is critical in limiting the morbidity and mortality associated with esophageal injuries. If detected within the first 12 to 24 hours, the vast majority of full-thickness stab wound injuries can be repaired primarily in a two-layer fashion.

The area should be widely drained, and a local muscle flap should be placed to buttress the suture line, particularly if there is a concomitant tracheal or vascular injury. In the event of the latter, it is preferable to place drains via a contralateral neck incision to avoid the catastrophic consequences associated with blowout of a fresh carotid repair. Severely destructive injuries requiring esophageal exclusion with gastrostomy and jejunostomy are extremely rare. After any repair, a barium swallow should be performed between postoperative days 5 and 7 before initiating oral intake.

Tracheal Injury

Most penetrating tracheal injuries that occur as the result of stab wounds occur without significant tissue loss and can be repaired primarily. This can be accomplished in a single layer utilizing 3-0 absorbable sutures in an interrupted fashion. Again, interposition of well-vascularized tissue (omohyoid or SCM muscle) is essential to minimize risk of fistula formation. Concomitant tracheostomy is not routinely indicated to protect a tracheal repair. If performed, tracheostomy should be placed one ring distal to the injury and should be limited to severe crush injuries, major laryngeal injuries, tears that traverse >1/3 of the circumference, or when prolonged postoperative ventilatory support is anticipated. Early extubation is safe and recommended.

● SPECIAL INTRAOPERATIVE CONSIDERATIONS

It is not uncommon to find injuries that traverse more than one zone, requiring additional access incisions. Unfortunately, this is not always known beforehand in the patient who proceeds directly to the operating room without the benefit of preoperative diagnostic imaging. Zone I injuries may necessitate a median sternotomy, a supraclavicular incision with resection of the head of the clavicle, or a combined "trapdoor" approach involving the addition of an anterolateral thoracotomy. Zone III injuries are notoriously difficult to expose, requiring cephalad extension of a standard vertical Zone II incision with possible disarticulation or partial resection of the mandible and in some instances limited craniotomy. Commonly utilized surgical incisions are illustrated in Figure 113-4. In the event that adequate exposure and hemorrhage control cannot be obtained via the described approaches, consideration should be given to attempts at endovascular treatment of challenging Zone I and III injuries. Treatment in Zone II is usually feasible via standard open operative approaches, and evidence for routine use of endovascular therapy in this anatomic region is limited.

● POSTOPERATIVE MANAGEMENT

Patients will typically be monitored in the intensive care unit during the immediate postoperative period where frequent neurologic assessment and hemodynamic monitoring can be performed. Early postoperative complications related specifically to neck exploration can include hemorrhage, recurrent laryngeal nerve injury, and esophageal leak. Unilateral recurrent laryngeal nerve injury will produce hoarseness and require formal evaluation by an otolaryngologist with laryngoscopy. Postoperative hemorrhage can be rapidly fatal if not recognized promptly. The confined space of the neck can result in airway compromise if bleeding is not controlled. Fortunately, leak in the cervical esophagus typically results in localized abscess amenable to drainage, whereas leak involving the thoracoabdominal esophagus can result in fulminant mediastinitis, which is often fatal.

Case Conclusion

The patient undergoes standard central neck exploration. After evacuation of a moderate-sized hematoma, you find a clean-based laceration of her internal carotid artery and internal jugular vein, both of which are amenable to primary repair. You also find a small anterior tracheal tear, which is also repaired primarily. The esophagus is visualized externally and internally with flexible endoscopy, and there is no evidence of injury. The patient is extubated immediately after the operation and taken to the intensive care unit for monitoring. A barium swallow performed on postoperative day 1 confirmed no evidence of esophageal injury, and an oral diet is begun. The patient is discharged home on postoperative day 5.

TAKE HOME POINTS

- Assessment and management of the airway is the top initial priority.
- Hemodynamic instability or "hard" signs of injury require immediate surgical exploration.
- CT angiography is highly sensitive and specific in the diagnosis of injury in the stable patient.
- Esophageal injuries are often clinically occult at presentation, and early diagnosis is important to minimize associated morbidity and mortality.
- All common and internal carotid injuries should be repaired.
- In the setting of multiple repairs, well-vascularized flaps should be utilized to protect suture lines.
- Endovascular therapy may be a helpful adjunct in difficult anatomic regions.

SUGGESTED READINGS

Demetriades D, Theodorou D, Cornwall E, et al. Evaluation of penetrating injuries of the neck: prospective study of 223 patients. *World J Surg.* 1997;21:41-47.

Inaba K, Branco BC, Menaker J, et al. Evaluation of multidetector computed tomography for penetrating neck injury: a prospective multicenter study. *J Trauma Acute Care Surg.* 2012;72: 576-583.

Low GM, Inaba K, Chouliaras K, et al. The use of anatomic 'zones' of the neck in the assessment of penetrating neck injury. *Am Surg.* 2014;80:970-974.

Sperry JL, Moore EE, Coimbra R, et al. Western Trauma Association critical decisions in trauma: penetrating neck trauma. *J Trauma Acute Care Surg.* 2013;75:936-940.

Tisherman SA, Bokhari F, Collier B, et al. Clinical practice guideline: penetrating zone II neck trauma. *J Trauma.* 2008;64: 1392-1405.

Burns

JAMES M. CROSS, TODD F. HUZAR, AND TONYA GEORGE

Based on the previous edition chapter "Burns" by Jeffrey S. Guy

114

Presentation

A 40 year-old man was trapped inside a burning house and subsequently discovered in the hallway of his house near the front door. After being extricated from the house, he was intubated by the paramedics for a suspected inhalation injury. On examination in the emergency department, he was found to have approximately 50% total body surface area (TBSA) burn, with burns on his lower extremities, abdomen, chest, and upper extremities. He had 3rd degree burns on his chest, hands, and anterior surface of his thighs. He had a Glasgow Coma Scale score of 3T. His initial chest x-ray revealed the endotracheal tube in good position and was otherwise unremarkable. His initial arterial blood gas had a pH of 7.19, pCO$_2$ of 35, PaO$_2$ of 245, base excess of −11, and a carboxyhemoglobin of 22. The rest of his laboratory values were unremarkable. His initial weight was 85 kg.

● DIFFERENTIAL DIAGNOSIS

The differential diagnosis in this burn patient is limited to the size and type of burn as well as the presence or absence of an inhalation injury. Once the presence of an inhalation injury is identified, there is a further differential of the type and extent of the inhalation injury as well as the presence of particular toxic substances such as carbon monoxide and cyanide.

● DIAGNOSIS AND TREATMENT

Due to the requirements for specialized care, patients with large burns are often transferred to a burn center. Treatment of these patients often requires multidisciplinary expertise such as specialty-trained burn surgeons, plastic surgeons, dieticians, and physical and occupational therapists; the coordinated care of these patients is beyond the scope of this chapter. However, a typical large burn patient will be presented, and three of the most significant components of the care of this patient will be discussed: the initial resuscitation, treatment of the inhalation injury, and the basics of wound care.

Resuscitation

Burn patients lose fluid as an ongoing process, and therefore the fluid resuscitation must be a dynamic intervention based on the patient's response. There are a number of formulae in the literature, which are used as a guide for resuscitation. Each of these has its own benefits and possible complications. One of the currently most recommended formulae is the Consensus formula. It, like all resuscitation guidelines, is based on the size of the burn and the size of the patient. The fluid resuscitation in the first 24 hours is 2 mL/%TBSA/kg. The fluid recommended is Lactated Ringers; the %TBSA is the percent of the body that is burned with second or third degree burns; and kg is the weight of the patient in kilograms. There has been a concerted effort to limit the volume of resuscitation because it has been noted that within the last 10 to 20 years, patients have been receiving increasing volumes of fluid. This has led to significant complications such as pulmonary edema, abdominal compartment syndrome, and death. This increasing fluid resuscitation has been termed fluid creep.

Since this patient has a 50% TBSA burn and weighs 85 kg, his estimated fluid requirement for the first 24 hours would be 8,500 mL (50 × 85 × 2). Approximately half of the fluid is required in the first 8 hours, so the initial infusion rate would be 531.25 mL per hour, which for convenience sake, would be ordered to start at 550 mL per hour. Once that rate has started, the actual infusion rate would be changed based on how the patient responds. The patient should make between 30 and 50 mL of urine an hour. If the patient makes >50 mL per hour, the resuscitation fluid is decreased by 10% to 20%. If the urine output is below 30 mL per hour, then the fluid is titrated up by 10% to 20%.

The use of colloid in burn resuscitation is still controversial, and a comprehensive review of the evidence is beyond the scope of this chapter. The use of colloid early in resuscitation has been shown to decrease the overall amount of fluid required but has not been shown to decrease mortality rate.

Inhalation Injury

Inhalation injury can be defined in many ways but one of the more common definitions is "damage to the airways, lung parenchyma, and any associated systemic toxicity caused by inhalation of super-heated gases, particulate matter, and other by-products of combustion (Cancio, 2003)." Inhalation injury is rather complex because the damage sustained can affect any part of the tracheal–bronchial tree, which has been classified into three, distinct anatomical insults: (1) upper airways (i.e., nasopharynx to the vocal cords); (2) lower airways (below the vocal cords to the alveoli); and (3) systemic toxicity due to inhaled toxic gases. Inhalation injury has been shown to have a significant effect on morbidity and mortality both alone and in combination with thermal injury. Therefore, it is imperative to rapidly diagnose the presence of inhalation injury and associated systemic toxicity due to inhaled toxins and to manage them appropriately.

Besides the injury to the airways, the two main clinically relevant toxic gases that may contribute to morbidity and mortality associated with inhalation injury are carbon monoxide (CO) and cyanide (CN), since they can affect hemoglobin's ability to carry oxygen and utilize oxygen at the cellular level, which can lead to hypoxia and death.

The diagnosis of inhalation injury often requires a combination of history taking, physical examination, and diagnostic findings (i.e., laboratory data and bronchoscopy). Risk factors associated with inhalation injury include entrapment in a closed space fire, proximity to the fire, duration of smoke exposure, loss of consciousness, and extent of cutaneous burns. Physical examination is an important part of the workup for inhalation injury; however, exam findings such as facial burns, singed nasal or facial hair, and even carbonaceous sputum may be misleading and do not truly indicate an inhalation injury. All patients with a suspected inhalation injury should have an arterial blood gas with CO-oximetry sent at the time of evaluation to identify evidence of acidosis, hypoxia, and the presence of carbon monoxide. Regardless of what the physical exam and laboratory findings show, the gold standard for evaluating and diagnosing inhalation injury is fiberoptic bronchoscopy. In patients with inhalation injury, fiberoptic bronchoscopy may demonstrate the presence of particulate matter (i.e., soot), airway casts, and mucosal injury such as edema, erythema, ulceration, and sloughing.

The diagnosis of CO and CN poisoning is often more difficult to make since the symptoms associated with acute poisoning are often vague and nonspecific. Therefore, a patient with severe headaches, visual disturbance, syncope, and impending cardiovascular collapse should be suspected of either acute CO and/or CN poisoning. The only true way to diagnose either acute CO or CN poisoning is through laboratory studies. CO levels can be determined with CO-oximetry, which is able to measure level of carboxyhemoglobin, oxyhemoglobin, and methemoglobin levels from either an arterial or venous blood sample. The levels of carboxyhemoglobin may dictate the method of treatment. On the other hand, the diagnosis of CN poisoning is much more difficult because there is no rapid assay to measure CN levels. Current technology requires many hours for the test to be performed, and the measured level may not reflect the patient's current clinical condition.

All patients with a suspected inhalation injury must undergo rapid assessment of their airways and simultaneously be placed on 100% humidified oxygen via nonrebreather/facemask. In cases when patients present with hypoxia, cyanosis, hoarseness, stridor, significant facial, or pharyngeal edema, their airway should be secured by intubation (oro- or nasotracheal) or a surgical airway. Once the patient's airway is secured, the patient should undergo bronchoscopy that is diagnostic and potentially therapeutic for patients with significant airway debris and cast formation. Often these patients require serial bronchoscopy to evaluate their airways and to remove residual airway debris and bronchial casts. Ventilator management of patients with inhalation injury can be difficult because there is no universally accepted ventilator mode. Most clinicians will manage these patients with lung protective strategies such as low tidal volume ventilation (6 to 8 mL/kg), high positive end-expiratory pressures, permissive hypercapnia, and other maneuvers aimed at lung protection and recruitment. However, one of the issues with conventional ventilation is the inability to clear sloughed bronchial mucosa and/or bronchial casts, which can lead to airway obstruction, V/Q mismatching, increased incidence of pneumonia, and ventilator-induced lung injury. High-frequency percussive ventilation (HFPV) is a nonconventional mode of ventilation that is capable of improving clearance of airway debris and casts, decreasing ventilator-induced lung injury in the form of barotrauma, and decreasing the incidence of pulmonary infections. HFPV is a time cycle, pressure-regulated ventilator mode that combines standard pressure control breaths (10 to 30 breaths per min) superimposed on pulse, high-frequency breaths (400 to 800 breaths per min). HFPV provides a percussive element to remove obstructing airway debris and casts. This has been used successfully in many patients with inhalation injury; however, it cannot reverse the effects of inhalation injury. HFPV is often used in conjunction with inhaled agents such as bronchodilators (i.e., albuterol), mucolytic agents (i.e., *N*-acetylcysteine), inhaled anticoagulants (i.e., heparin), and 3% hypertonic saline, which work in concert to keep the airways open, prevent cast formation, and keep the airways hydrated.

CO and CN poisoning may be a concern in hypoxic patients that have sustained an inhalation injury. CO poisoning if not treated appropriately has been associated with persistent and delayed neurologic sequelae, as well as myocardial and cellular injury. For this reason, all patients with suspected CO poisoning should be placed on 100% FiO_2, whether on the ventilator or via facemask. The rationale for treating CO poisoning with 100% FiO_2 is that oxygen at this concentration shortens the half-life of carboxyhemoglobin (COHb) to 45 minutes. The COHb levels should be monitored until they are <5%. Some advocate the use of hyperbaric oxygen therapy in patients with CO poisoning because it reduces the half-life of COHb to 20 minutes; however, there are not enough data at this time to support its widespread use. CN poisoning can be rapidly lethal if not treated promptly, but since there is no

Inhalation Injury Management

Admission Evaluation

❑   ABG

❑   Co-oximetry

❑   Hydroxycobalamin (if ↑ lactate, persistent acidosis, or unexplained hypoxemia)

❑   Bronchoscopy (within 1 hour): grade injury, obtain pictures

❑   Intubate if:

    ❑   GCS < 8

    ❑   CO ≥ 20%

    ❑   BSA burns ≥ 30%

Mechanical Ventilation

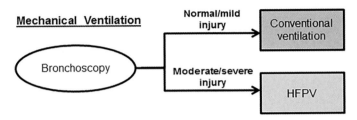

❑   Nebulized Heparin (10,000 units) and Albuterol q4h +/- nebulized *N*-acetylcysteine (3 mL of 20%)

HFPV (VDR) basic settings:
- PIP 22
- Pulse frequency (high rate) 500–550
- Sinusoidal rate (low rate) 10–12
- I:E of 1:1
- Oscillatory PEEP 5
- Demand PEEP 5
- FiO$_2$ to keep SaO$_2$ > 90%
- Convection Rise (off)

Other therapies to be considered:
- Hyperbaric oxygen therapy for CO >20%
- Serial or repeat bronchoscopy

FIGURE 114-1. Inhalation injury management.

rapid test to determine its presence in patients with inhalation injury, the clinician must treat the patient based upon clinical suspicion. The treatment of choice is IV hydroxocobalamin, which binds to hydrogen cyanide molecules forming cyanocobalamin, which is a nontoxic molecule and easily excreted in the urine. Hydroxocobalamin has been shown to be safe and effective in treating suspected cyanide poisoning in patient with inhalation injury; however, it may lead to red/pink discoloration of the skin and urine, which may affect certain laboratory studies (Figure 114-1).

Wound Care

Topical care of the burn wound is dependent on the depth of the burn. First-degree burns, which are limited to the epidermis only, require only moisturizer and symptomatic pain treatment. A second-degree burn, which involves the epidermis and varying thicknesses of the dermis, can be treated with a variety of topical therapies, and is often dependent on the practitioner's experience or preference. There are several topical treatments from which to choose. These include polysporin (bacitracin/neomycin/polymixin), mafenide acetate, oat beta glucan, collagenase, and silver sulfadiazine, to name

a few. Each of these has their own strengths and weaknesses. However, the most commonly used one has been silver sulfadiazine. Its future use may be limited by increasing bacterial resistance, and a recent Cochrane report showing that the use of silver sulfadiazine may be associated with an increased incidence of burn wound infection.

Third-degree burns, which involve the epidermis and all of the dermis, require operative treatment, since a third-degree burn will not heal normally. Prior to excision, these burns should be treated with a topical antimicrobial like those listed above. If the burn is quite large, there are a number of silver-impregnated dressings, which may prove useful and less labor intensive than topical ointments. The treatment of choice for third-degree burns is excision of all nonviable tissue and autografting to close the wounds. The larger the wound, the more imperative it is to remove the burn tissue as early as possible. It is well established that early excision and grafting improves all aspects of the care of the burn patient. Our practice is to take a patient with burns > 30% TBSA burn to the operating room within 24 hours.

For the patient in this case, we would use a large blade, such as a Watson blade (Figure 114-2), to excise large areas of burn on his arms, trunk, and legs and use a smaller blade,

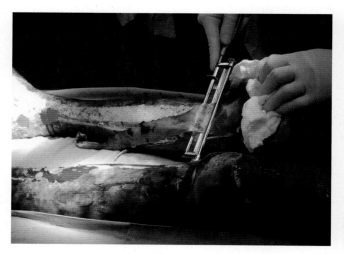

FIGURE 114-2. Excision of a burn with a Watson blade.

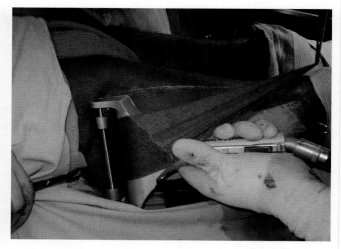

FIGURE 114-3. Harvesting of skin using a pneumatically driven dermatome.

such as the Weck blade, to excise the smaller areas on the hands and feet. If the burns are very deep and large, a fascial excision may be beneficial. To perform a fascial excision, one uses electrocautery to excise the burn down to the underlying fascia. The benefits of doing a fascial excision is that it is usually quicker and there is less blood loss. The downside is that it is cosmetically disfiguring and can lead to significant problems with distal edema in the nonburned skin (Table 114-1).

Once the burn is excised, hemostasis must be obtained for the skin grafts to be viable postoperatively. We use laparotomy pads soaked in epinephrine/saline. Topical thrombin may also be beneficial. Electrocautery may be needed to cauterize the larger bleeding vessels. Most excised burns can be covered with a split-thickness autograft. If the burn is particularly large and there are limited donor sites, the excised burn wound may be covered by either cadaveric skin or xenograft. This may be a good option if the patient has been in the operating room for an extended period of time, is cold, coagulopathic, or otherwise unstable. If the bed is adequately prepared and the patient is stable, then a split-thickness autograft is harvested to cover the excised burn. We use a

pneumatically driven dermatome to harvest the skin graft (Figure 114-3). Depending on the need, the skin graft can be used as a sheet graft, but in a large burn, such as in this case, the skin graft is meshed (Figure 114-4). There are a number of different meshers that are available. The type of mesher used depends on the size of the burn and the body part to be covered. Meshing allows fluid and blood to pass through the skin graft without collecting underneath. Formation of a hematoma or seroma formation under a skin graft will lead to the loss of the skin graft. Meshing also allows the skin graft to be expanded to cover a larger area, this is especially useful in larger burns. The downside of meshing the skin is the cosmetic outcome; meshed skin grafts do not look as good as nonmeshed, or sheet grafts.

Affixing the skin graft in place is of paramount importance. Any movement or shearing of the skin graft can lead to early skin graft loss and the need to regraft the area. There are a number of ways of affixing the graft in place. Staples are commonly used. The placement of skin staples is easy and

Table 114-1	Operative Excision of Burns

Key Technical Steps

1. Schedule early excision within 24 hours for patients with burns >30% TBSA.
2. Use a large blade (Watson) to excise areas on arms, trunk, and legs and a small blade (Weck) for areas on the hands and feet.
3. Use electrocautery to perform excision down to the underlying fascia for deep and large burns.
4. Obtain hemostasis of the burn excision site using a combination of laparotomy pads soaked in epinephrine/saline, topical thrombin, and electrocautery.
5. Consider cadaveric skin or xenograft in unstable patients or those with limited donor sites.

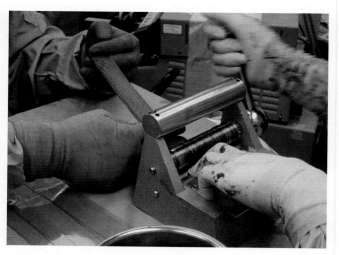

FIGURE 114-4. Meshing of the skin graft.

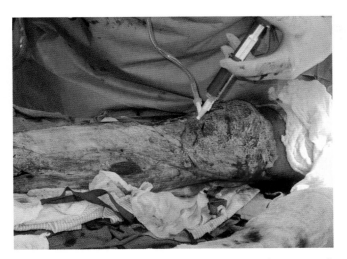

FIGURE 114-5. Application of fibrin glue prior to placement of a split-thickness skin graft.

rapid in the operating room. Postoperatively, they can be painful to remove, sometimes requiring high doses of pain medicine, or even conscious sedation. There is also the problem of the staples getting buried under the skin graft only to cause discomfort weeks to months later and difficulty in removing the buried staple. Suturing, with either absorbable or nonabsorbable suture, is also a common practice. This is more time-consuming, and may require removal postoperatively. Fibrin sealants, or fibrin glues, are becoming increasingly popular method of affixing skin grafts in place (Figure 114-5). The advantages of using a fibrin glue includes decreased operative time, improved graft take, faster mobilization after surgery, and nothing to remove postoperatively. At the end of the excision and grafting, the skin grafts are dressed with a moist nonadherent dressing and then covered with bulky absorbent dressings. If the skin graft crosses

Table 114-2	Skin Grafting

Key Technical Steps

1. Choose the appropriate type of skin graft (full-thickness vs. split-thickness) based on the location and size of the excised burn.
2. For large burns, consider meshing of a split-thickness skin graft to prevent underlying seroma or hematoma.
3. Affix the graft using one of a variety of methods: staples, sutures, or fibrin glue.
4. Dress the wound with a moist nonadherent dressing and then cover it with bulky absorbent dressings.
5. If the skin graft crosses a joint, place a splint to immobilize the area.
6. Keep the skin graft immobilized for 48 h, then start range of motion exercises.

Table 114-3	Skin Grafting

Potential Pitfalls

- Delay in excision of large burns
- Inadequate preparation of the wound bed prior to skin grafting (i.e., failure to remove all necrotic tissue)
- Inadequate hemostasis of the wound bed
- Formation of a hematoma or seroma under a graft
- Inadequate fixation of the skin graft leading to shearing and graft loss
- Failure to immobilize the graft in the immediate postoperative period
- Failure to address metabolic derangements
- Inadequate protein and calorie intake and malnutrition

a joint, a splint is placed to immobilize the area. We usually keep the skin graft immobilized for 48 hours, then start range of motion exercises.

Successful skin graft "take" is dependent on a number of factors. These include adequate operative preparation: removal of all necrotic tissue and hemostasis and properly affixing the graft in place and immobilization of the graft to prevent shearing. It is also of equal importance that the patient's metabolic derangements have been addressed. The patient with a large burn is going to be very hypermetabolic and prone to becoming malnourished. The patient must have adequate protein and caloric intake and good glycemic control. Besides supply adequate enteral nutrition, there are several adjuncts, which are beneficial. An in-depth discussion of the nutritional support of the burn patient is beyond the scope of this chapter, but the use of insulin, beta-blockers, and anabolic steroids, such as oxandrolone, have been shown to improve outcome in the severely burn patient (Table 114-2).

In summary, the patient with a large burn and inhalation injury is a particularly difficult clinical scenario. The patient requires immediate fluid resuscitation individualized to the patient's response. Inhalation needs to be diagnosed early and treatment with oxygen, intubation, bronchoscopy, and advanced ventilator management can positively impact on outcome. Finally, addressing the burn injury with topical treatment is important to prevent infection and early excision and grafting improves morbidity and mortality (Table 114-3).

TAKE HOME POINTS

- Fluid loss is an ongoing process and needs to be replaced dynamically.
- Urine output should guide resuscitation.
- There should be a high index of suspicion for inhalation injury in the right clinical scenario.
- Early excision of the full-thickness burn is a key for improved outcome.

SUGGESTED READINGS

Cancio LC, Howard PA, McManus AT, et al. Thermal injury. In: Argenta LC, eds. *Basic Science for Surgeons: A Review*. 1st ed. London, UK: WB Saunders; 2003:405-432.

Chung KK, Wolfe SE, Cancio LC, et al. Resuscitation of severely burned military casualties: fluid begets more fluid. *J Trauma*. 2009;67(2):231-237.

Huzar TF, Cross JM. Critical care management of the severely burned patient. In PR Roberts, SR Todd, eds. *SCCM Adult Comprehensive Critical Care Textbook*. Mount Prospect, IL: SCCM publishing; 2012:695-717.

Saffle JR. Fluid creep and over-resuscitation. *Crit Care Clin*. 2016;32(4):587-598.

Storm-Versloot MN, Vos CG, Ubbink DT, Vermeulen H. Topical silver for preventing wound infection. *Cochrane Database Syst Rev*. 2010;17(3):CD006478. doi:10.1002/14651858.CD006478.pub2.

Walker PF, Buehner MF, Wood LA, et al. Diagnosis and management of inhalation injury: an updated review. *Crit Care*. 2015;19:351.

Wolfe SE, Edelman LS, Kemalyan N, et al. Effects of oxandrolone on outcome measures in the severely burns: a multicenter prospective randomized double-blind trial. *J Burn Care Res*. 2006;27(2):131-139.

Blunt Abdominal Trauma from Motor Vehicle Crash

115

CARLA KOHOYDA-INGLIS AND STEWART C. WANG

Based on the previous edition chapter "Blunt Abdominal Trauma from Motor Vehicle Crash" by Carla Kohoyda-Inglis and Stewart C. Wang

Presentation

A 32-year-old man with no significant past medical history presents as the unrestrained driver of an older, mid-sized, 4-door sedan involved in a severe head-on motor vehicle crash with a large tree (Figure 115-1). Bystanders found the man unresponsive and pulled him from the vehicle. On arrival of emergency responders, the man was responsive only to painful stimuli, had labored respirations, and was bleeding from the mouth. Emergency medical services (EMS) also found a large amount of damage to the steering wheel and 13 inches of intrusion in the toepan area (Figure 115-2).

● DIFFERENTIAL DIAGNOSIS

Care of injured patients begins with assessment at the scene by emergency responders to get the right patient to the right place in the right period of time, so that they can receive definitive treatment. This patient met Field Triage Decision Scheme Step 1 (Physiologic) criteria with decreased level of consciousness (Glasgow Coma Scale, GCS ≤ 13) and was appropriately transported to a high-level trauma center. Passenger compartment intrusion >12 inches at the occupant site or 18 inches anywhere in the vehicle is associated with a high risk of severe (Injury Severity Score, ISS >15) injury to that occupant and a Step 3 (Mechanism of Injury) criterion for field triage of injured patients.

Unlike penetrating trauma, blunt trauma such as motor vehicle crashes may cause internal injuries in multiple body compartments with little external evidence. Initial evaluation (primary survey) of the patient in the emergency room focuses on quickly identifying and treating life-treating injuries that affect **A**irway, **B**reathing, **C**irculation, **D**isability (neurologic) (Table 115-1).

On primary survey, he was awake and alert, but complaining of right lower chest and right upper abdominal pain. His vital signs were BP 110/80, RR 12, HR 95, and T36.7. Physical examination revealed decreased breath sounds in the right chest and tenderness on palpation on the right lower chest wall and right upper abdomen without peritoneal signs. FAST (Focused Abdominal Sonography for Trauma) ultrasound exam showed fluid at the right hepatorenal fossa with right kidney irregularity. Portable CXR showed fluid in the right chest; pelvis XR was normal. A chest tube was placed for the right hemothorax with 900 cc initial output and slow subsequent output.

● WORKUP

In the absence of indication for immediate surgical exploration (e.g., hemodynamic instability with positive FAST or high chest tube output), 3-dimensional imaging to detect occult internal injuries from blunt trauma is the next priority. CT scans in this patient showed (1) a large complex liver

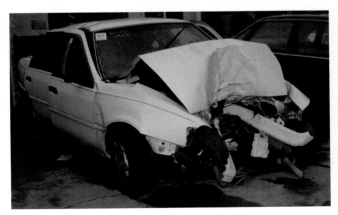

FIGURE 115-1. Vehicle damage from frontal crash into large tree.

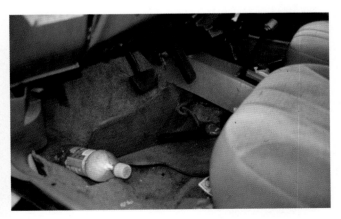

FIGURE 115-2. Interior damage with >12 inches of toepan intrusion into the driver's space. This meets Step 3 (Mechanism of Injury) criteria for field triage and is associated with significant risk of severe injury.

Table 115-1	Primary Survey of the Injured Patient
A	Airway with cervical spine protection
B	Breathing and ventilation
C	Circulation with hemorrhage control
D	Disability (neurologic evaluation)
E	Exposure/environmental control

laceration extending completely through the medial segment of the left lobe and into the lateral segment of the left lobe and the right lobe (Figure 115-3A). (2) Poorly perfused right kidney, narrowing of the right renal artery with extravasation of intravenously administered contrast material from the right renal artery and a large right perinephric hematoma (Figure 115-3B).

● INITIAL MANAGEMENT

Surgical management of the multiply injured patient involves the principles of quick stabilization and resuscitation followed by prioritized treatment of individual injuries. With control of the airway and ability to ventilate the patient, the highest priority is to control hemorrhage, especially arterial bleeding. The presence of active contrast extravasation (arterial bleeding) from the right kidney on abdominal CT mandates immediate intervention. Experience over the past few decades has shown that many solid abdominal organ injuries can be managed without open abdominal exploration and also that hemorrhage control with interventional radiologic techniques provides better organ salvage rates than open operations, which frequently result in organ removal (e.g., nephrectomy, splenectomy) rather than repair to control bleeding. Since there were no immediate hard indications for open

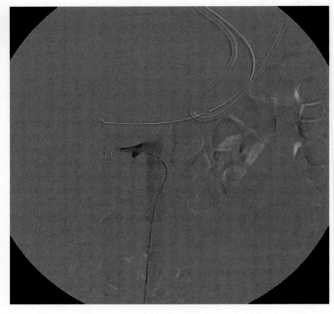

FIGURE 115-4. Bleeding from the right renal artery was controlled after placement of 5 and 8 mm coils.

exploration (hemodynamic instability, hollow organ injury, penetrating mechanism), this patient underwent radiologically guided embolization of the right kidney and liver with successful control of the bleeding (Figures 115-4 and 115-5). The patient was then admitted to the ICU for supportive care.

While hemorrhage control is paramount as indication for surgical intervention in the initial postinjury period, the sequelae of organ injury in the days following may also require intervention. It is also important to reassess the patient for injuries missed during the initial assessment. Bile leak is common following large liver injuries and must be controlled (washout and drain placement, often laparoscopic) to avoid bile peritonitis. A HIDA scan is a sensitive test for bile

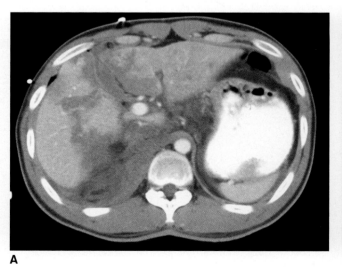
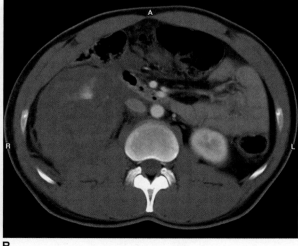

FIGURE 115-3. CT scan images from the patient in the scenario demonstrating **(A)** large complex liver laceration and **(B)** large perinephric hematoma with contrast extravasation.

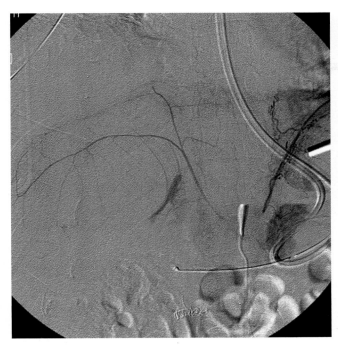

FIGURE 115-5. Extravasation from a descending branch of the right hepatic artery. This was subsequently controlled with injection of Gelfoam.

leakage. In this patient, screening HIDA scan on postinjury day 3 showed bile extravasation from the liver with drainage into the right chest tube via the pleural cavity. A clinical diagnosis of right diaphragmatic injury was made. Right-sided diaphragm injuries from blunt trauma are much less common than injuries to the left side. Small isolated right diaphragm injuries may not require operative repair since they are much less likely to develop complications such as organ herniation due to the large liver buttressing it underneath. However, due to the interval development of increased liver elevation on chest x-ray as well as the complication of bile leak into the pleural cavity, operative repair was indicated in this case.

● OPERATIVE MANAGEMENT

The patient was explored through a midline abdominal incision. The liver was found to be partially herniated into the right chest (Figure 115-6). In order to safely reduce the fractured liver back into the abdominal cavity, the midline abdominal incision was extended into the right chest (thoracoabdominal incision) to allow the liver to be pushed down from above. The large diaphragm tear was easily repaired with pledgeted sutures (Figure 115-7). The thin, pliable nature of the diaphragm can result in significant disorientation of torn edges and optimal repair is facilitated by alignment of the edges with tags, stay sutures, or clamps during the repair. The right pleural cavity was irrigated and drainage maintained with a chest tube. Source control and drainage is an important surgical principle when tissues have been damaged and contents contaminate body cavities. The gallbladder was found to be partially avulsed in the line of the liver

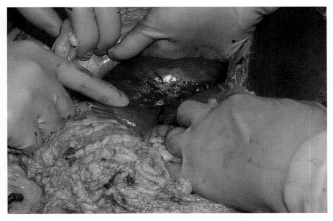

FIGURE 115-6. Large liver laceration found on abdominal exploration.

laceration and was resected. Multiple drains were placed to drain the leak from bile ducts too small to control individually. The abdominal cavity volume was insufficient to allow primary fascial closure following the reduction of the liver due to the intestinal swelling induced by injury and operation. Closure of the fascia with resultant increased abdominal compartment pressures would have compromised renal as well as pulmonary function in this patient with significant injuries to both of those organ systems and also increased the chances for incisional dehiscence. The fascia was bridged with a temporary dressing and closed at a subsequent operation. Temporary closure techniques (e.b. V.A.C., ABThera) have simplified the management of complex trauma patients requiring abdominal operations for damage control.

● KEY POINTS

- The ABCDs take top priority: Airway, Breathing, Circulation, Disability.
- Indications for urgent laparotomy following blunt trauma include the following:
  - Hemoperitoneum in the setting of hemodynamic instability
  - Perforation of hollow viscus or peritonitis

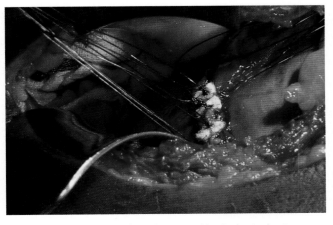

FIGURE 115-7. Repair of diaphragm with pledgeted sutures.

- At urgent laparotomy, the primary objective is damage control of bleeding and peritoneal soilage. It is better to do a partial operation for damage control than to complete a large complex operation on a sick, unstable, multiply injured patients.
- Most solid organ injuries can be managed without open operation; advances in 3D medical imaging and interventional radiologic techniques have markedly decreased the need for open abdominal exploration.
- Not all clinically important injuries will be immediately diagnosable, even with extensive 3D scanning. Follow-up evaluations and a high index of suspicion are essential.

SUGGESTED READINGS

Demetriades D, Velmahos GC, ed. Indications for and techniques of laparotomy. In: David Feliciano, Kenneth Mattox, Ernest Moore, eds. *Trauma*. 6th ed. New York: McGraw-Hill Professional; 2007.

Franklin GA, Casós SR. Current advances in the surgical approach to abdominal trauma. *Injury*. 2006;37(12):1143-1156.

Lee JC, Peitzman AB. Damage-control laparotomy. *Curr Opin Crit Care*. 2006;12(4):346-350.

Sasser SM, Hunt RC, Sullivent EE, et al. Guidelines for field triage of injured patients. Recommendations of the National Expert Panel on Field Triage. *MMWR Recomm Rep*. 2009;58(RR-1):1-35.

Damage Control Laparotomy

116

MITCHELL J. GEORGE AND JOHN A. HARVIN

Presentation

A 21-year-old male with no known past medical history presents to the emergency department after a gunshot wound to the abdomen. He is complaining of abdominal pain. His first vital signs show him to be hypotensive and tachycardic. Physical examination reveals an intact airway, equal bilateral breath sounds, and a single wound to the anterior abdominal wall next to the umbilicus.

X-rays of the torso reveal a single projectile in the right hemipelvis. Focused abdominal sonography for trauma (FAST) shows fluid in the abdomen. The institution's massive transfusion protocol is activated. The patient is taken emergently to the operating room for laparotomy.

Upon entering the abdomen, a large amount of bright red blood is encountered. The hemoperitoneum is evacuated, and continued bleeding is observed from the aortic bifurcation. Given that it appears arterial, the supraceliac aorta is compressed against the spine. A right medial visceral rotation (mobilizing the right colon and small bowel mesentery off the retroperitoneum) is performed. Bleeding is controlled with manual compression of the retroperitoneum, while distal control is obtained by clamping the common iliac arteries. With supraceliac aortic compression still present as proximal control, the hematoma is entered and a destructive aortic injury is identified at the aortic bifurcation. A clamp is placed proximal to the injury, and supraceliac aortic compression is released.

● SURGICAL APPROACH

Decision to Perform Damage Control

The goal of a damage control laparotomy (DCL) is to prevent the irreversible spiral toward death that occurs when patients develop the "lethal triad": hypothermia (temperature <35°C), acidosis (pH < 7.2), and coagulopathy. The decision to perform damage control should be made as early as possible so that these metabolic derangements are avoided. While many have suggested certain predictive lab values, vital signs, and transfusion thresholds as indications for DCL, none have been validated in a high-quality study. This decision is highly dependent on surgeon judgment. The potential metrics to suggest the need for DCL are listed in Table 116-1.

Table 116-1	Parameters Guiding Patient Selection for DCL

Potential Metrics to Suggest Need for DCL

Injury Patterns
- Abdominal vascular injury with ≥2 visceral injuries
- Major inaccessible venous injury
- Bleeding requiring packing

Physiologic Parameters
- Hypothermia (Temperature < 35°C)
- Acidosis (pH < 7.20 or base excess < -14)
- Sustained Hypotension (SBP < 70 mm Hg)
- Coagulopathy (nonmechanical bleeding)
- Estimated blood loss > 5 L
- Tactical DCL

While the surgeon is certainly focused on the operative task at hand, she/he must also be aware of the patient's overall transfusion requirements, temperature, and intraoperative blood gas values. Communication with the anesthesiologist is critical.

All efforts should be made to minimize iatrogenic contributions to physiologic failure. Such efforts include active warming of the patient and transfusion of warmed blood products to prevent hypothermia. High ratios of red blood cells, fresh frozen plasma, and platelets with minimal crystalloid and colloid should be given to prevent or reverse coagulopathy. After decision to proceed with damage control, the two mandatory goals of the operation are (1) hemorrhage control and (2) contamination control (Figure 116-1).

Damage Control Laparotomy

The principle of permissive hypotension should be employed until hemorrhage control is obtained. Multiple randomized clinical trials have shown improved mortality and decreased overall transfusion volumes when patients are resuscitated only to a mean arterial pressure (MAP) of 50 mm Hg or systolic blood pressure of 70 mm Hg. Once hemorrhage has been controlled, patients can then be resuscitated to normal blood pressure or another end point of resuscitation (e.g., urine output, pH, base excess). Again, a high ratio (1:1:1) of red blood cells, fresh frozen plasma, and platelets is the preferred resuscitative strategy. Crystalloid and colloid should be avoided.

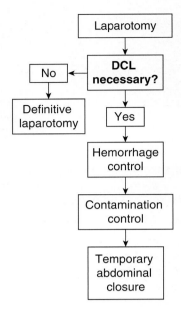

FIGURE 116-1. Decision tree for DCL and sequence of surgical approach.

The abdomen should be entered sharply through a xipho-pubic incision through the linea alba. Upon entering the peritoneum, the hemoperitoneum is manually removed using laparotomy pads and a closed suction device. Using a hand-held retractor, the abdominal cavity is quickly surveyed while evacuating the hemoperitoneum. Any quadrant that is found to have continued bleeding is packed with laparotomy pads. To improve exposure superiorly over the liver and to prevent tearing of the liver during retraction, the falciform ligament is clamped, divided, and tied off. Venous bleeding can be initially controlled with abdominal packing. If bleeding persists after packing, arterial injury should be suspected. If arterial bleeding is suspected, the supraceliac aorta can be temporarily compressed against the spine with an instrument (Table 116-2).

Hemorrhage Control

Common areas of hemorrhage include solid organs and intra-abdominal or retroperitoneal vascular structures. Liver lacerations with complete capsular disruption can be explored and bleeding structures ligated or coagulated. A Pringle maneuver (compression of the porta hepatis) can help decrease bleeding from the liver wound and to differentiate venous from arterial bleeding as arterial bleeding should cease or decrease with the porta occluded. Hepatotomy and exploration of liver lacerations should be avoided in a patient on the brink of the lethal triad. The vast majority of liver injuries that cannot be controlled with suture ligation and coagulation can be controlled with packing. If arterial bleeding is suspected, postoperative hepatic angiography is indicated prior to return to the operating room for reexploration.

Bleeding from the spleen can often be treated with direct suture repair and topical hemostatic agents. Alternatively, the spleen can be mobilized and wrapped in a sheet of

Table 116-2	Trauma Laparotomy

Key Technical Steps

1. Table selection: fluoroscopic capable
2. Patient positioning: supine in cruciform position
3. Preparation and drape: chin to knees
4. Incision: Xipho-pubic
5. Two options for packing:
   - Pack all 4 quadrants, then remove packs starting from area that does not appear to be bleeding
   - Evacuate hemoperitoneum from all four quadrants and pack only those that are bleeding
6. Digital or clamp occlusion of arterial bleeding sources for initial control
7. Reassessment of patient physiologic status with anesthesia team

Potential Pitfalls

- Placement of EKG leads or monitoring equipment in anterior or lateral on chest invading the operative field
- Allowing drapes or linens to lay over side rails of operating room bed precluding fast and easy placement of self-retaining retractor
- Extension of incision below umbilicus if large pelvic hematoma is known
- Failure to communicate with anesthesia team regarding timing of arterial clamping

polyglactin mesh to tamponade bleeding. In coagulopathic patients, ongoing bleeding from major splenic injuries is to be expected, and splenectomy should be performed.

The kidney is a more infrequent cause of massive bleeding given its confinement within Gerota's fascia. Nonetheless, ongoing renal bleeding in a hemodynamically unstable patient is an indication for renal exploration. A vertical incision is made in Gerota's fascia, and the kidney is delivered into the operative field. Again, suture ligation or coagulation can be attempted to stop bleeding. In the damage control situation, if bleeding can be stopped, complex nephrorrhaphy should be delayed until the reexploration. Ongoing bleeding from the kidney despite these measures should result in prompt nephrectomy.

In the damage control situation, the majority of intra-abdominal and retroperitoneal arterial injuries should be shunted. Temporary intravascular shunting has been used extensively in military and civilian settings. Shunts can be fashioned from chest tubes, nasogastric tubes, or commercially produced vascular shunts. Once the appropriate size has been selected, the shunt is flushed with saline, inserted proximally and distally, and secured to the proximal and distal artery with silk ties. Heparinization postoperatively is not necessary, and the shunt can be left in for 48 hours. Removal of the shunt and definitive repair is performed at the reexploration.

The internal iliac artery, inferior mesenteric artery, and celiac axis can be safely ligated. The remainder of the major intra-abdominal and retroperitoneal arteries should be salvaged. Injury to the aortic bifurcation may require rapid repair with a bifurcated Dacron graft given the difficulty shunting this injury.

The iliac veins and infrarenal inferior vena cava can be ligated if repair is time-consuming or associated with massive blood loss. The suprarenal inferior vena cava and portal vein should be repaired whenever possible given the high mortality associated with ligating such injuries. An excellent option for venous injuries is to shunt them as well. They may be repaired in a delayed fashion which will allow for better outflow for the affected extremity or organ.

Massively transfused, acidotic patients with aortic and/or iliac artery or vein injuries should be considered for prophylactic four compartment fasciotomy of the affected limb (or both). If fasciotomy is not performed, compartments should be closely monitored in the intensive care unit (Table 116-3).

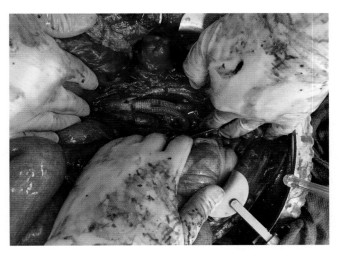

FIGURE 116-2. Dacron graft in place of obliterated aortic bifurcation with proximal and distal anastomotic sites visible.

Presentation Continued

At the time of hemorrhage control, the patient has received 44 units of packed red blood cells, 44 units of plasma, 42 units of platelets, and 20 units of cryoprecipitate. He has no evidence of coagulopathy but is hypothermic (temperature 34°C) and acidotic (pH 7.25). Given this, we choose to perform a DCL.

A shunt is desired but can not be fashioned given the aortic bifurcation injury. So, a bifurcated Dacron graft is quickly sewn proximally and distally and flow is reestablished to the lower extremities (Figure 116-2).

Contamination Control

After control of hemorrhage, hollow viscus injuries are quickly addressed to limit contamination of the peritoneal cavity. Uncontrolled leakage of stool, bile, pancreatic fluid, or urine will cause major morbidity and must be controlled during the initial damage control operation. Inspection of both hemidiaphragms for injury at this time is crucial—concurrent bowel,

biliary, bladder, or ureteral injury risks contamination of the chest cavity. If a full-thickness diaphragm laceration is found, perform warm saline lavage through the perforation and drainage by tube thoracostomy. The diaphragm is repaired with nonabsorbable suture. The bowel should be systematically inspected in a rapid fashion, starting proximally and moving distally. Small injuries of the stomach, small bowel, or colon with viable edges can be closed temporarily. Areas sustaining major damage should be resected with the expectation that intestinal continuity will be restored at a following operation. Leaving blind loops of bowel in the damage control situation is safe for up to 72 hours. Placement of feeding tubes should be deferred until the definitive operation is performed.

Pancreatic or biliary injury is challenging given the proximity of multiple vital structures. For severe pancreatic injury distal to the superior mesenteric vein, distal pancreatectomy is acceptable during the initial operation. Severe pancreatic injury proximal to the superior mesenteric vein or severe injury to the ampullary region may require pancreaticoduodenectomy. Pancreaticoduodenectomy following trauma is decreasing in incidence as some advocate for drainage alone of these injuries. The need for pancreaticoduodenectomy is largely driven by the status of the duodenum and ampulla of Vater.

Damage to the urinary bladder can be quickly closed in two layers with absorbable suture and drained with a Foley catheter. Ureteral injuries take longer to repair and can be temporarily ligated or externally drained and repaired in a delayed fashion (Table 116-4).

Table 116-3	Hemorrhage Control and Potential Pitfalls

Key Technical Steps

1. Packing can control the vast majority of liver hemorrhage.
2. For penetrating trauma through the retroperitoneum, medial and lateral visceral rotations are required for adequate exploration.
3. Proximal and distal control should be obtained prior to exploring retroperitoneal hematomas.

Potential Pitfalls

- Attempted salvage of bleeding solid organs such as the spleen or kidney should not be performed in acidotic, hypothermic, or coagulopathic patients.

Presentation Continued

Once hemorrhage is controlled, thorough exploration of the remainder of the abdomen reveals multiple destructive small bowel injuries and a right colon injury. The injured areas of small bowel are resected in one segment, and a right hemicolectomy is performed. The patient is left in discontinuity.

Table 116-4	GI Contamination Control and Potential Pitfalls

Key Technical Steps

1. Inspect both hemidiaphragms for lacerations
2. Run the bowel quickly and systematically
3. Close simple injuries to the stomach, duodenum, and small bowel in a single layer
4. Resect all nonviable segments of bowel
5. Inspect the pancreas for injury; drain injured areas
6. Repair simple bladder injuries and divert ureteral injuries with external drainage

Potential Pitfalls

- Attempted definitive repair of bowel, pancreatic, or biliary injury should not be performed in a coagulopathic, acidotic, or hypothermic patient

Temporary Abdominal Closure

Temporary abdominal closure is a prerequisite prior to transfer to the ICU. Multiple methods and devices exist to serve this purpose. The simplest is skin-only closure with towel clips; however, this obstructs postoperative imaging. Suture closure of skin only has been performed; however, this places the massively resuscitated patient at higher risk of abdominal compartment syndrome (ACS). Commonly, temporary closure of the abdominal cavity with negative pressure drainage is being employed. Negative pressure dressings allows active drainage of the peritoneal cavity and encourage early fascial closure. Bowel or abdominal wall edema due to resuscitation and capillary leakage is allowed to expand with this closure, discouraging intra-abdominal hypertension or its progression to ACS.

Presentation Continued

The rest of the abdomen is without injury. The patient's abdomen is temporarily closed with a negative pressure vacuum device. Bilateral four compartment fasciotomies are performed, and the patient is transferred to the ICU.

● POSTOPERATIVE MANAGEMENT

Resuscitation continues on arrival of the patient to the ICU. Physiologic and biochemical derangement caused by the original injury is compounded by the stress of surgery, heat loss from an open abdominal cavity, and bleeding during the operation. Efforts of resuscitation should focus on reversing the lethal triad of hypothermia, coagulopathy, and acidosis. We continue high ratios of red blood cells, plasma, and platelets well into the ICU phase of care until the patient is fully resuscitated and the lethal triad reversed. The patient should be covered with warm blankets and IV fluids, or blood products should be warmed before administration.

Coagulation panels should be resent upon arrival to the ICU and corrected with appropriate blood products. The blood bank should be made aware of the patient with fresh blood product in the room at all times until the patient returns to the OR. The trend of a patient's acidosis is more indicative than its magnitude at this stage, and a rising lactic acid should be presumed as worsening delivery of oxygen to organs and peripheral tissues, prompting search for missed injury or continued intra-abdominal hemorrhage.

These patients are at risk for postoperative ACS, which is defined as pathologically elevated intra-abdominal pressure associated with organ dysfunction. Bladder pressure should be monitored as the patient's resuscitation continues. A diagnosis of ACS should prompt swift return to the operating room.

● SECOND LOOK SURGERY

The patient should be approaching physiologic normality prior to returning to the OR. This includes correction of hypothermia, absence of coagulopathy, and stoppage of vasopressors. The goal of the first reexploration is to evaluate for further abdominal injury, restore intestinal continuity, and close the abdominal fascia.

Case Conclusion

The patient is taken back to the OR the next day for a second look. The entire abdomen is inspected and no further injury is found, and the patient is hemostatic. There are no other bowel injuries noted. An ileostomy is matured to restore intestinal continuity, and the fascia is closed.

TAKE HOME POINTS

- The decision to pursue damage control management is multifactorial and determined by mechanism of injury, injury pattern, and degree of physiologic derangement.
- The vicious cycle of hypothermia, acidosis, and coagulopathy can be prevented or reversed by quick control of surgical bleeding and administration of balanced blood products.
- Discussion between the anesthesia and operating teams is paramount during the entirety of the operation.
- Vascular injuries should not be repaired in coagulopathic patients. These should be either ligated if appropriate or shunted with delayed repair.
- Visceral injury requires closure or resection to limit the burden of peritoneal contamination.
- Second look surgery should focus on identifying any further injury and restoring intestinal continuity.

SUGGESTED READINGS

Johnson JW. Evolution in damage control for exsanguinating penetrating abdominal injury. *J Trauma.* 2001;51(2):269-271.

Lamb CM, et al. Damage control surgery in the era of damage control resuscitation. *Br J Anaesth.* 2014;113(2):242-249.

Rotondo MF, et al. 'Damage Control': an approach for improved survival in exsanguinating penetrating abdominal injury. *J Trauma.* 1993;35(3):375-382.

Stone HH, et al. Management of major coagulopathy with onset during laparotomy. *Ann Surg.* 1983;197(5):532-535.

Voiglio EJ, et al. Abbreviated laparotomy or damage control laparotomy: why, when and how to do it? *J Visc Surg.* 2016;153:13-24.

The Abdominal Compartment Syndrome and Management of the Open Abdomen

117

CLAY COTHREN BURLEW

Presentation

A 57-year-old man is admitted to the surgical intensive care unit (ICU) after being ejected during a rollover motor vehicle collision. He has a history of hypertension, coronary artery disease, and a prior deep venous thrombosis requiring warfarin therapy. His postinjury diagnoses include bilateral rib fractures with hemopneumothoraces, a grade 3 liver injury, and bilateral femur fractures. Over the next 24 hours, he requires intubation and has bilateral chest tubes placed. His femur fractures are placed in skeletal traction at the bedside. He receives 8 L of crystalloid, 10 units of fresh frozen plasma, and 6 units of packed red blood cells during his resuscitation. On morning rounds, his blood pressure is 80/50 mm Hg and heart rate is 100 bpm. On further evaluation, his urine output has been less than 10 cc/hr for the past 4 hours, and his peak airway pressure is 50 cm H_2O. His hemoglobin has been stable for the past 8 hours with his coagulation status normalized; his serum creatinine is 1.06 g/dL. Chest film shows no residual pneumothorax, and his hemothoraces have been evacuated. His bladder pressure is 25 cm H_2O. Abdominal ultrasound evaluation for oliguric renal failure reveals no hydronephrosis and scant ascites.

DIFFERENTIAL DIAGNOSIS

In any critically ill patient, there are many etiologies that can cause cardiopulmonary embarrassment and a low urine output. In this trauma patient, sources such as hypovolemic/hemorrhagic and cardiogenic shock should be ruled out. The patient's total volume status, trend in hemoglobin values, and signs of ongoing hemorrhage should be determined. Additionally, a chest film will rule out hemopneumothoraces, and a cardiac ultrasound can evaluate cardiac filling and rule out cardiac tamponade. The cardiac ultrasound, echocardiography, transesophageal Doppler, or noninvasive cardiac evaluation (i.e., FloTrac) can identify primary cardiac failure with low cardiac output. Urine electrolytes and a history of

agents that could cause renal failure may help differentiate acute renal failure from oliguria that associated with abdominal compartment syndrome (ACS). Regardless, a diagnosis of intra-abdominal hypertension (IAH) and accompanying ACS has to remain in one's differential in the at-risk patient.

ACS may be due to either intra-abdominal injury or disease processes (primary) or due to large volume resuscitation (secondary) or a combination of these. In secondary ACS, massive resuscitation utilizing crystalloid and blood products results in bowel edema, retroperitoneal edema, and often ascites. ACS can be an elusive diagnosis if not considered by the intensivist, and an evaluation of shock in any critically ill patient should include an evaluation for IAH. This patient is at risk for ACS due to both his intra-abdominal injury and his large volume resuscitation.

WORKUP

Clinical evaluation rather than imaging is central to the diagnosis of ACS which is typified by the combination of IAH plus end-organ derangements. Specific clinical indices that should herald the diagnosis of ACS include decreased urine output, increased pulmonary pressures, increased peak airway pressures, decreased cardiac preload, significant cardiac dysfunction, and elevated intracranial pressure. As noted previously, these end-organ variables can be seen in a variety of shock states and with specific injury patterns. Therefore, central to the diagnosis of ACS is the identification of IAH.

Physical examination is not overtly helpful in the diagnosis of IAH. Patients may have abdominal distension, but clinical exam appears to be reliable only about 40% of the time. IAH is determined by measuring the patient's bladder pressure. The bladder acts as a passive reservoir and hence transmits intra-abdominal pressure. The patient's bladder pressure is measured after instilling 25 to 50 cc of saline via a three-way Foley catheter with the drainage tube clamped. One should interpret the bladder pressure in patients with external compression on the bladder (such as pelvic packing for hemorrhage), those with bladder rupture, marked adhesive disease, or a neurogenic bladder with caution; these patients may not have bladder pressure measurements that are reflective of the intra-abdominal pressure. IAH is defined as a bladder pressure >12 mm Hg. In general, intra-abdominal pressures over 20 cm H_2O become worrisome, but it is the combination of IAH with end-organ derangements that determines intervention. ACS is a late event in the spectrum of IAH; therefore, monitoring at-risk patients allows one to identify IAH and intervene in an attempt to prevent the sequelae of ACS.

DIAGNOSIS AND TREATMENT

With a bladder pressure of 25 cm H_2O and evidence of end-organ derangements (low urine output, elevated airway pressures, and hypotension), this patient has ACS. Emergent decompression is indicated. If the patient had evidence of a significant intra-abdominal fluid component (i.e., ascites evident on bedside ultrasound), initial decompression with a percutaneous drain and repeat measurement of the bladder pressure is a reasonable first step. Removing a significant amount of ascites can drop the abdominal pressure enough to obviate the need for a decompressive laparotomy. For this patient, however, decompression via midline laparotomy is indicated. The laparotomy allows egress of ascites and blood and the edematous bowel protrudes from the abdominal cavity (Figure 117-1); the intra-abdominal pressure drops to zero, and rapid correction of the patient's cardiopulmonary embarrassment is typical.

SURGICAL APPROACH

Decompressive laparotomy is performed via a midline incision. Although this is typically and optimally performed in the operating room, for patients too unstable to transport, it

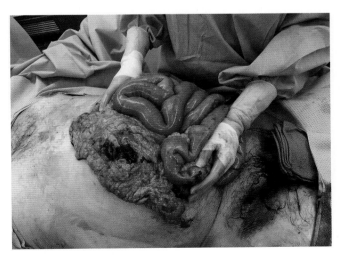

FIGURE 117-1. Decompressive midline laparotomy allows egress of bowel, ascites, and blood from the abdominal cavity.

Table 117-1	Temporary Abdominal Coverage

Key Technical Steps

1. Fenestrate the 1010 Steri-Drape
2. Place the drape over the bowel and circumferentially under the fascia of the laparotomy incision
3. Place 2 JP drains along the fascial edges
4. Run the JP drain tubing cephalad from the laparotomy opening
5. Cover everything with an occlusive Ioban dressing
6. Place the drains to wall suction

Potential Pitfalls

- If there is a lack of visceral coverage, two Steri-Drapes may be necessary
- JP drains exiting inferiorly may not afford a sealed/closed suction system; drains should exit superiorly
- Pulling the Ioban tightly across the open abdomen may result in recurrent ACS as the bowel swells from ongoing resuscitation; leaving some expansion room is critical
- Covering the 1010 Steri-Drape with either a towel of laparotomy pad prior to Ioban placement prevents visualization of the viscera; early ischemia or bleeding can be missed

can be performed in the ICU. In fact, bedside laparotomy for secondary ACS requires minimal equipment: scalpel, suction, cautery, and temporary closure dressings.

Following decompression, coverage of the eviscerated bowel while controlling the ascitic effluent from the abdomen is necessary. Our preferred option for temporary coverage of the abdominal viscera for open abdomen patients utilizes a 1010 Steri-Drape (3M Health Care, St. Paul, MN), 2 Jackson-Pratt drains, and a large Ioban (3M Health Care, St. Paul, MN) (Table 117-1). Small holes are cut in the plastic 1010 Steri-Drape with a scalpel to allow fluid to pass through the drape; the holes should be small slits in the plastic to prevent the Ioban from sticking to the underlying bowel. The plastic drape is placed to cover the entirety of the bowel and is then tucked under the fascia circumferentially (Figure 117-2A). Occasionally, two Steri-Drapes must be used in an overlapping manner to cover all of the viscera. Two Jackson-Pratt (JP) drains are placed along the fascial edges with the tubing running cephalad; these drains will control any ascitic fluid that is generated during the patient's ongoing resuscitation (Figure 117-2B and C). The large Ioban then covers the 1010 drape, drains, and adjacent abdominal wall as an occlusive and sterile seal (Figure 117-2D). The advantages of this temporary coverage include rapid execution, effective decompression while controlling effluent, direct visualization of the bowel, and fluoroscopic compatibility.

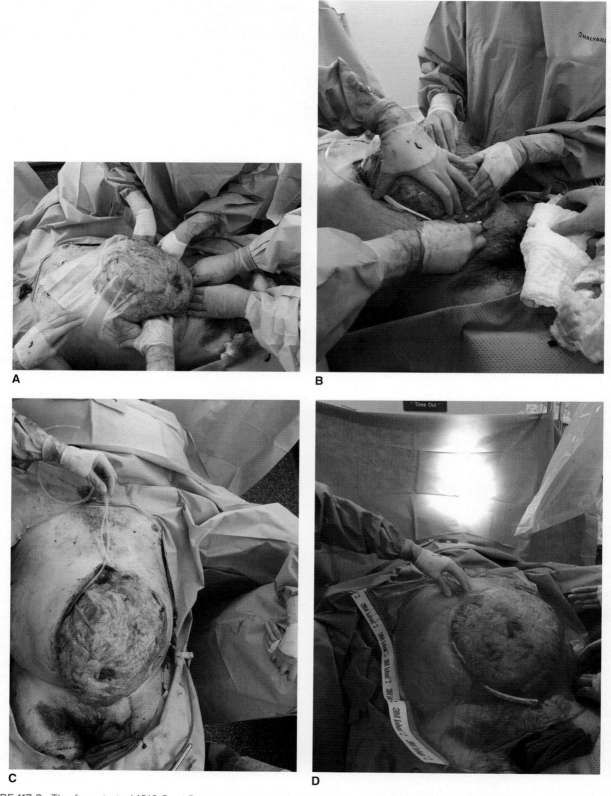

FIGURE 117-2. The fenestrated 1010 Steri-Drape covers the bowel and is tucked under the fascia circumferentially **(A)**. Two Jackson-Pratt drains are placed along the fascial edges with the tubing running cephalad to control the resuscitation-associated ascitic fluid **(B,C)**. A Large Ioban provides a sterile seal over the plastic drape, drains, and adjacent abdominal wall **(D)**.

Another option for temporary coverage is a vacuum-assisted closure device or negative pressure wound therapy (NPWT) system; one must ensure that recurrent ACS does not occur due to suction-related pressure on the abdominal contents. Additionally, while NPWT is critical to the management of patients with an open abdomen past the initial 24 to 48 hours, early use of these devices is not necessary.

Regardless of temporary closure technique, one has to ensure that recurrent ACS does not occur; a patient can develop ACS despite an open abdomen. Leaving some "expansion space" in the temporary covering is critical as the bowel will likely continue to swell with ongoing resuscitation. To ensure the patient does not have recurrent ACS, bladder pressures are monitored in those with hemodynamic instability or low urine output.

Following ICU management of the open abdomen patient (see Postoperative Management section), the patient is returned to the operating room for attempts of fascial closure. Primary closure of the native fascia is the goal at the first return to the operating room; the majority of patients have this accomplished at repeat laparotomy. One may wish to monitor airway pressures during the fascial closure to ensure recurrent IAH and ACS are not impending.

If abdominal fascial closure is not possible at second laparotomy, there are several options for management. Sequential fascial closure techniques are commonly used and employ three key components: (1) fascial tension toward the midline to prevent lateral retraction, (2) vacuum-assisted reduction of abdominal viscera with control of abdominal effluent, and (3) repeated attempts at further fascial closure every 24 to 48 hours. Options to provide midline traction of the fascia, and hence prevent loss of the abdominal domain, include simple sutures (over the top of the sponges used in the vacuum-assisted closure) or commercially available bridging devices.

Our preferred approach in Denver is closure sequentially performed with the combination of a Wound Vac™ and constant fascial tension with sutures (Figure 117-3A and B). Patients are returned to the operating room every 2 days for fascial closure with interrupted sutures and replacement of the sponges until fascial approximation is accomplished.

Other options for bowel coverage include prosthetic placement (mesh or biologics) with closure of the subcutaneous tissue and skin over the top to prevent desiccation and evisceration should the prosthetic fail. Closing only the skin and subcutaneous tissue over the exposed viscera with a planned hernia is always an option. In patients with retraction of the skin and fascia, who have an exposed visceral block, skin graft placement directly onto the granulating intestines can provide successful coverage. Component separation for abdominal wall reconstruction is performed 9 to 12 months later once the skin graft has separated from the underlying bowel.

● POSTOPERATIVE MANAGEMENT

The postoperative care of the open abdomen patient is not markedly different from the care of any critically ill patient. Patients should have appropriate resuscitation, normalization of adverse physiology including hypothermia and coagulopathy, and proactive management to prevent complications (e.g., lung protective ventilation strategies, insulin therapy for stress-induced hyperglycemia, and treatment of adrenal suppression). The postoperative issues that are unique in this population, however, include careful fluid administration, enteral nutrition support, and management of abdominal injuries. Fluid administration in the first 24 postoperative hours must balance cardiac

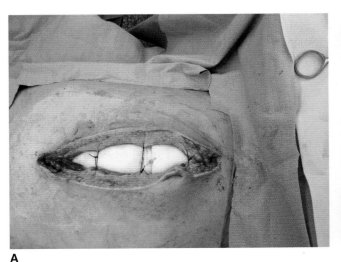
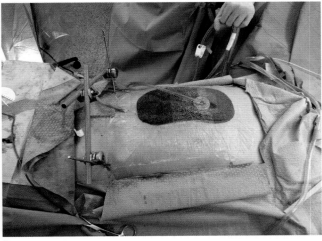

A   **B**

FIGURE 117-3. The Denver sequential fascial closure technique utilizes a white wound VAC sponge over the viscera, no. 1 PDS sutures over the sponge to prevent lateral retraction of the fascia **(A)**, and a black sponge over this as a "sponge sandwich" for vacuum-assisted reduction of abdominal viscera and control of abdominal effluent **(B)**.

performance (often fluid-responsive) versus the generation of visceral and retroperitoneal edema (necessarily fluid restrictive). While the use of colloid is appealing in open abdomen patients, the evidence to date does not support its use. Damage control resuscitation, typically initiated in the trauma bay and continued in the operating room, should not be abandoned during postoperative care in the ICU; higher plasma to red cell ratios is associated with fascial closure rates.

Although the protruding viscera of the open abdomen patient may cause hesitancy in the initiation of enteral nutrition, several studies support starting tube feeds in this trauma population. Enteral nutrition in the patient with an open abdomen is not only feasible, but it has been shown to be associated with an increase in successful fascial closure, a decrease in complications, and a decrease in mortality. Once the patient's deranged physiology is corrected, enteral nutrition should be considered if the bowel is in continuity.

For patients with significant visceral edema, direct peritoneal resuscitation (DPR) can be a useful adjunct. In this technique, a 19-Fr round Blake drain is placed in a dependent portion of the abdomen and is used to infuse hypertonic dialysate. The dialysate flushes through the abdominal contents and is removed via the two JP drains located just under the temporary abdominal closure covering (i.e., the 1010 Steri-Drape and Ioban closure). The 2.5% peritoneal dialysis solution is infused at a rate of 1.5 mL/kg/h, which causes the edematous bowel to shrink over the ensuing 24 to 48 hours. Of note, standard wound VAC sponges, especially the white sponge, do not allow egress of the dialysate from the abdomen; the accumulated fluid can recreate ACS. Therefore, the temporary closure with the 1010 Drape and Ioban should be used when DPR is performed.

The complications observed in patients following open abdomen management are similar to those of any patient undergoing an exploratory laparotomy: abscess, anastomotic leak, and enterocutaneous (EC) fistula. In general, these complications are treated using the similar approaches. Management of the complication is similar. Occasionally, the abscess or anastomotic leak is identified while the abdomen is still open; this permits earlier drainage and may facilitate diversion.

The enteroatmospheric (EA) fistula is a complication that is unique to the open abdomen. These occur in the small minority of patients who do not attain fascial closure despite repeated techniques and are left with a "frozen abdomen." If the soft tissue can be mobilized to cover the opening, the fistula tract can be intubated and an enterocutaneous fistula (ECF) promoted. This (ECF) may ultimately heal, but the coverage also prevents further breakdown of adjacent bowel and numerous sites of EA fistulas. Other management options for EA fistulas include "patching" the bowel opening with a biologic (acellular dermal matrix, flexible silica gel lamellar, or cadaveric skin) and using fibrin glue as an additional sealant. Control of the contamination from the EA fistula is often the most problematic; use of a "floating stoma" and incorporation of NPWT appear to have some success in management.

Case Conclusion

ACS is diagnosed in our patient and he undergoes a midline laparotomy. Following decompression, his airway pressures normalize, his urine output increases, and his hemodynamics improve. He is managed with DPR utilizing the 1010 Steri-Drape and Ioban temporary closure technique. Enteral nutrition is instituted on postoperative day 1 via his nasogastric tube. He is returned to the operating room on postoperative day 2; partial fascial closure is accomplished, DPR is halted, and NPWT with fascial retention sutures are placed in the remaining open portion of the fascia. Sequential fascial closure is performed at laparotomy 3 and 4 on postoperative days 4 and 6, with final closure on day 6. Intramedullary nails of bilateral femur fractures are performed on hospital day 3, and his chest tubes are removed on hospital day 5. Following his inpatient stay, he is transferred to an acute rehabilitation facility for further care. At 1 year following injury, he is ambulatory and has no evidence of abdominal wall hernia.

TAKE HOME POINTS

- ACS may be due to either intra-abdominal injury or disease processes (primary) or due to large volume resuscitation (secondary) or a combination of these.
- Secondary ACS is typified by marked bowel edema, retroperitoneal edema, and resuscitation-associated ascites.
- An evaluation of shock in any critically ill patient should include an evaluation for IAH and ACS.
- ACS is defined as the combination of IAH plus end-organ derangements: decreased urine output, increased pulmonary pressures, increased peak airway pressures, decreased cardiac preload, significant cardiac dysfunction, and elevated intracranial pressure.
- Physical examination may not diagnose ACS. IAH is determined by measuring the patient's bladder pressure.
- Emergent decompression is indicated for ACS.
- The optimal temporary coverage for the open abdomen includes rapid execution, effective decompression while controlling effluent, direct visualization of the bowel, and fluoroscopic compatibility.
- Patients can develop ACS despite an already open abdomen.
- If abdominal fascial closure is not possible at second laparotomy, sequential fascial closure techniques are commonly used and employ three key components: (1) fascial tension toward the midline to prevent lateral retraction, (2) vacuum-assisted reduction of abdominal viscera with control of abdominal effluent, and (3) repeated attempts at further fascial closure every 24 to 48 hours.

SUGGESTED READINGS

Balogh ZJ, Lumsdaine W, Moore EE, Moore FA. Postinjury abdominal compartment syndrome: from recognition to prevention. *Lancet.* 2014;384(9952):1466-1475.

Burlew CC, Moore EE, Cuschieri J, et al. Who should we feed? A western trauma association multi-institutional study of enteral nutrition in the open abdomen after injury. *J Trauma Acute Care Surg.* 2012;73:1380-1388.

Burlew CC, Moore EE, Johnson JL, et al. 100% fascial approximation can be achieved in the post-injury open abdomen. *J Trauma.* 2012;72:235-241.

Dennis A, Vizinas TA, Joseph K, et al. Not so fast to skin graft: transabdominal wall traction closes most "domain loss" abdomens in the acute setting. *J Trauma Acute Care Surg.* 2013;74(6):1486-1492.

Haddock C, Konkin DE, Blair NP. Management of the open abdomen with the abdominal reapproximation anchor dynamic fascial closure system. *Am J Surg.* 2013;205(5):528-533.

Joseph B, Zangbar B, Pandit V, et al. The conjoint effect of reduced crystalloid administration and decreased damage-control laparotomy use in the development of abdominal compartment syndrome. *J Trauma Acute Care Surg.* 2014;76(2):457-461.

Kirkpatrick AW, Roberts DJ, De Waele J, et al. Intra-abdominal hypertension and the abdominal compartment syndrome: updated consensus definitions and clinical practice guidelines from the world society of the abdominal compartment syndrome. *Intensive Care Med.* 2013;39(7):1190-1206.

Regli A, De Keulenaer B, De Laet I, et al. Fluid therapy and perfusional considerations during resuscitation in critically ill patients with intra-abdominal hypertension. *Anaesthesiol Intensive Ther.* 2015;47(1):45-53.

Roberts DJ, Zygun DA, Grendar J, et al. Negative-pressure wound therapy for critically ill adults with open abdominal wounds: a systematic review. *J Trauma Acute Care Surg.* 2012;73(3):629-639.

Weaver JL, Smith JW. Direct peritoneal resuscitation: a review. *Int J Surg.* 2015;(S1743-9191):1224-1228.

118

Complex Liver Injury

JEREMY L. WARD AND CARLOS H. PALACIO

Presentation

A 24-year-old man presents to the emergency department via emergency medical services (EMS) after a fall from approximately 30 feet. On arrival, he opens his eyes spontaneously, follows commands, and is oriented. He has bilateral and equal breath sounds and palpable peripheral pulses. His initial vital signs include systolic blood pressure (SBP) of 110 mm Hg, heart rate (HR) of 89, respiratory rate of 26, and oxygen saturation of 98%. He has right upper quadrant tenderness associated with a large contusion of the right upper quadrant and flank. Chest x-ray is negative. Pelvic x-ray demonstrated a right pelvic fracture. A focused assessment with sonography for trauma (FAST) demonstrates fluid in the right upper quadrant.

● DIFFERENTIAL DIAGNOSIS

Blunt injuries, including those resulting from a fall, involve the transfer of force to the thorax, abdomen, pelvis, head, spine, and extremities. In these cases, the initial differential diagnosis for potential injuries is exceptionally broad. Mechanism of injury can assist in the initial triage and risk stratification. In this case, a fall from 30 feet is associated with significant injuries and mortality, as a 48-foot fall is associated with 50% of mortality. The initial evaluation of a blunt trauma patient should follow the Advanced Trauma Life Support protocol, with primary survey, secondary survey, and adjunct tests such as chest x-ray, pelvis x-ray, and FAST. The purpose of the primary survey is to focus on those diagnoses which are acutely life threatening. The secondary survey allows for a more detailed examination of the patient and leads to clues as to additional diagnoses.

With this patient, the primary and secondary surveys, x-rays, and FAST have ruled out significant hemothorax, pneumothorax, and pericardial effusion. The differential diagnosis, especially considering the finding of fluid on FAST, should include solid organ and hollow viscus injury, and given the pelvic fracture on x-ray, extraperitoneal hemorrhage should be suspected.

● WORKUP

As the initial evaluation progresses through the primary and secondary surveys, chest x-ray, pelvic x-ray, and FAST exam, the clinician should actively plan for the next steps in evaluation and management. Acute life-threatening injuries should be addressed with urgency, and endotracheal intubation, insertion of chest tubes, application of pelvic binders, or transfusion of blood may be warranted. On initial evaluation, patients with peritonitis should proceed to the operating room (OR) for laparotomy. Additionally, patients with hypotension and a positive FAST should proceed to the OR for control of intra-abdominal hemorrhage. In the setting of a hypotensive patient with a negative FAST, retroperitoneal or pelvic hemorrhage should be suspected. Patients who are hemodynamically stable with mechanism of injury suspicious for intra-abdominal or pelvic injury should be emergently evaluated with computed tomography (CT).

This patient has blunt abdominal injury and is hemodynamically stable and without peritonitis. He has multiple indications to pursue CT of the abdomen and pelvis, including the mechanism of injury, free fluid in the abdomen on FAST, and pelvic fracture on plain radiograph.

Presentation Continued

The patient is taken for CT scan. During CT, he remains hemodynamically stable. Imaging reveals a grade IV liver laceration without active extravasation of intravascular contrast (Figure 118-1).

● DIAGNOSIS AND TREATMENT

After diagnosis of blunt liver injury, it is important to note certain characteristics of the injury to determine the optimal management. First, the grade of the injury must be determined. Second, the injury must be comprehensively evaluated for extravasation of intravenous contrast. The American Association for the Surgery of Trauma Organ Injury Scale is the most widely utilized system for injury stratification. For liver injury, the scale covers grades I to VI (Table 118-1). This grading system is highly predictive for the need of operative interventions and the development of complications related to the injury. In patients with low-grade (I to III) injury without contrast extravasation, the need for operative intervention is exceptionally unlikely. These injuries are safely managed nonoperatively, and the global management strategy of patients with low-grade liver injuries should largely be based upon the associated injuries. Hemodynamically stable

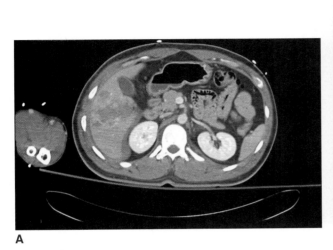
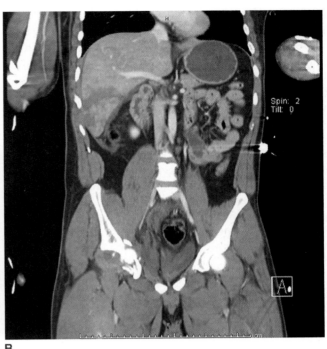

A

B

FIGURE 118-1. **A,B:** CT images. Axial and coronal images of high-grade injury without extravasation.

Table 118-1	Grading of Liver Injuries
Grade	**Injury Description**
I	
Hematoma	Subcapsular, nonexpanding, < 10% surface area
Laceration	Capsular tear, nonbleeding, < 1-cm deep parenchymal disruption
II	
Hematoma	Subcapsular, nonexpanding, hematoma 10%–50%; intraparenchymal, nonexpanding, < 2 cm in diameter
Laceration	<3 cm parenchymal depth, < 10 cm in length
III	
Hematoma	Subcapsular, > 50% of surface area or expanding; ruptured subcapsular hematoma with active bleeding; intraparenchymal hematoma > 2cm
Laceration	>3 cm parenchymal depth
IV	
Hematoma	Ruptured central hematoma
Laceration	Parenchymal destruction, involving 25%–75% of hepatic lobe
V	
Laceration	Parenchymal destruction of > 75% of hepatic lobe
Vascular	Juxtahepatic venous injury (retrohepatic inferior vena cava/major hepatic veins)
VI	
Vascular	Hepatic avulsion

Reprinted from Moore EE, Shackford SR, Patcher HI, et al. Organ injury scaling: spleen, liver and kidney. *J Trauma.* 1989; 29(12):1664-1666, with permission.

patients without peritonitis who have high-grade injuries (IV to V) can also be safely managed nonoperatively. High-grade injuries, however, do observe a failure rate of 5% to 10%, and most injuries requiring surgical intervention are high grade. Hemodynamic instability due to hemorrhage is the most common cause of failure. As such, patients with high-grade injuries should be admitted to an intensive care unit (ICU) for close monitoring and serial hemoglobin assessments.

The presence of extravasation of contrast on CT is of important significance. This finding is also associated with failure of nonoperative management. In hemodynamically stable patients with extravasation on CT, angiography and selective embolization are indicated. This adjunct to nonoperative management can reduce the failure rate and need for surgical intervention. Angiography is only indicated in cases where extravasation is visualized on CT, regardless of the grade of injury.

In this case, the patient is hemodynamically stable and without peritonitis. He has a high-grade liver injury, but he is a candidate for nonoperative management and meets criteria for ICU admission.

Presentation Continued

The patient is admitted to the ICU. Five hours later, he develops peritoneal signs, hypotension (SBP 89), and tachycardia (HR 110). Transfusion is initiated and the patient is transported to the OR for immediate laparotomy. In the OR, large volume of hemoperitoneum is evacuated. The liver is circumferentially packed, which controls the hemorrhage. The abdominal viscera are systematically evaluated for additional injuries and none are identified. A temporary abdominal closure is applied with a negative pressure dressing and the patient is transferred to the ICU.

● SURGICAL APPROACH

Although nonoperative management is the cornerstone of therapy for liver injury, the surgeon must have a thorough understanding of the anatomy of the liver and the algorithms and techniques utilized for surgical management of liver injuries (Table 118-2). Liver injuries resulting in hemorrhagic shock are rare and frequently high grade. The combination of a high-grade injury with the patient's hemodynamic instability can create an environment of significant stress for the inexperienced surgeon. Given the rarity of the need for operative intervention, surgeons should maintain familiarity with the surgical algorithms and techniques for managing complex liver injuries. The initial step in surgical management is placement of perihepatic packing. Initially, packing is sequentially placed throughout the abdomen in all four quadrants as the hemoperitoneum is evacuated and the patient resuscitated. The initial packing is then sequentially removed and the liver injury is evaluated. If the liver injury is found to be the cause of hemorrhage, carefully planned

Table 118-2	Operative Management of Liver Injury

Key Technical Steps

1. Laparotomy for trauma—midline incision, evacuation of hemoperitoneum, packing of four quadrants
2. Sequential removal of packing after resuscitation
3. Evaluation of the extent of liver injury
4. Bimanual compression of liver to control hemorrhage
5. Circumferential packing of the liver to achieve tamponade; if hemorrhage is controlled, perform temporary abdominal closure after completion of abdominal exploration
6. Planned removal of packing at 48 h
7. Pringle maneuver when packing does not control hemorrhage
8. Direct vessel ligation to control bleeding; may require mobilization, finger fracture, or stapled hepatotomy to expose the injury
9. Possible resection to expose or remove injury
10. Suspicion for injury to hepatic vein or retrohepatic vena cava when Pringle maneuver does not control bleeding
11. Preplanned strategies for addressing recurrent hemorrhage, bile leak, or devitalized tissue at take back for removal of perihepatic packing

Potential Pitfalls

- Excessive perihepatic packing can obstruct venous return
- Placement of packing into the injury will cause further parenchymal disruption and exacerbate hemorrhage
- Deep liver sutures can injure intrahepatic structures; avoid in central locations
- Injury to the common bile duct can result from Pringle maneuver; use appropriate clamp or vessel loop
- Additional unnecessary surgical interventions on the liver can result in additional avoidable hemorrhage; if perihepatic packing achieves control of hemorrhage, this should be considered definitive

circumferential liver packing should be pursued. The goal of the liver packing is to return the liver parenchyma to its anatomic position and tamponade any bleeding. Liver packing should not be placed into the laceration, but rather, folded dry laparotomy pads should be positioned around the surface of the liver, beginning posteriorly and progressing anteriorly, such that the injured parenchyma is reapposed and tamponade applied (Figure 118-2). Care must be taken to not apply excessive packing, as venous return from the infrahepatic vena cava can become obstructed resulting in hemodynamic instability. Most commonly, this simple maneuver will control the hemorrhage. In cases where hemorrhage is controlled with packing, this maneuver should be considered definitive. A temporary abdominal closure should be

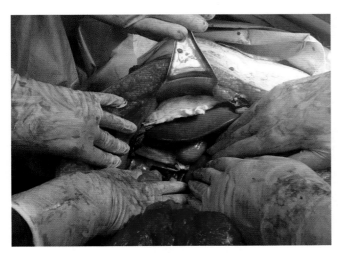

FIGURE 118-2. Perihepatic packing. Folded laparotomy pads placed circumferentially around the injured liver.

applied, and the patient should be transported to the ICU for additional resuscitation and correction of metabolic derangements. At this point, CT of the injury (if not previously obtained) or angiography may be useful, as selective embolization may be of benefit. The patient is returned to the OR 48 hours later and the packs are removed. The liver injury is usually hemostatic; however, the surgeon must be prepared to pursue additional hepatic interventions.

When packing fails to control hemorrhage or when significant hemorrhage is encountered with the planned removal of packing, additional surgical maneuvers are required (Table 118-2). The first step to immediately control the hemorrhage is bimanual compression (or repacking the liver). When compressive techniques are insufficient, or when an alternative method is required to address the injury, a Pringle maneuver should be applied. This is achieved by first opening the gastrohepatic ligament, avoiding injury to any accessory of the left hepatic artery that may be present.

Opening this ligament will allow control of the vascular inflow of the liver by placing a Rummel tourniquet around or vascular clamp across the hepatoduodenal ligament containing the porta hepatis (Figure 118-3). If this maneuver controls the hemorrhage, the source is either a branch of portal vein or a branch of hepatic artery, or both. Surgical control of the hemorrhage with direct vessel ligation should then be pursued. This involves exploration of the liver injury, visualization of the bleeding vessels, and suture ligation. This may require mobilization of the right or left liver. Thus, the trauma surgeon must be knowledgeable in the anatomy of the liver, its attachments, and its standard and aberrant vascular inflow and outflow. Mobilization of the liver will frequently allow better hemorrhage control with bimanual compression and improve exposure for exploration and vessel ligation. For deeper vascular injuries, the finger fracture technique may be employed with ligation and division of sequentially deeper intraparenchymal structures until the source of hemorrhage is identified. The trauma surgeon should be familiar with the use of cutting linear staplers in liver surgery. These can quickly accomplish hepatotomy and exposure of the bleeding vessels for direct vessel ligation. Although early literature regarding liver resection for trauma was fraught with high mortality, more recent literature suggests improved and acceptable safety of liver resection for trauma. For some injuries, the stapler can be used for nonanatomic resection of the injured liver. This resection can expose the injured vessels for ligation or remove the source of hemorrhage with the specimen. The trauma surgeon should be prepared to utilize whichever techniques will allow for simplest and most expedient control of bleeding. In some cases, this will be direct vessel ligation, with or without hepatotomy. In other cases, this may be resection.

The most challenging cases in liver trauma arise when hemorrhage cannot be controlled with packing or a Pringle maneuver. In these cases, a juxtahepatic venous injury should be presumed (hepatic vein or retrohepatic cava),

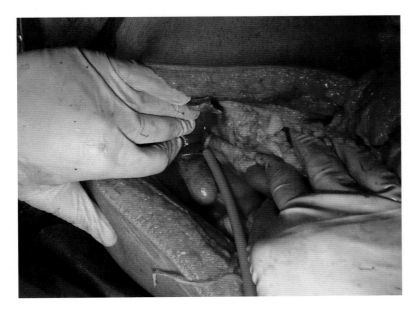

FIGURE 118-3. Pringle maneuver. A Rummel tourniquet is placed around the porta hepatis utilizing a vessel loop.

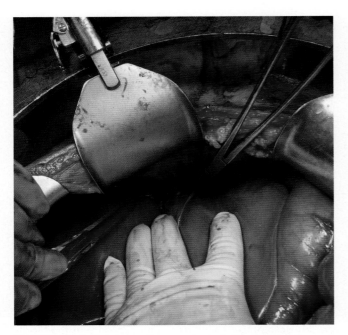

FIGURE 118-4. Total hepatic vascular isolation. For total vascular isolation, vascular control of the porta hepatis (Pringle), suprahepatic vena cava, and suprarenal infrahepatic vena cava must be achieved. Intra-abdominal control of suprahepatic vena cava with vascular clamp is shown.

and total hepatic vascular isolation should be considered (Figure 118-4). To achieve this, the inferior vena cava should be controlled immediately cephalad to the right renal vein. This will control inflow to the retrohepatic cava. If not already done, the falciform ligament should be taken down and the triangular ligament opened. This will expose the hepatic veins and the suprahepatic cava. Mobilization of the left liver from the diaphragm will allow additional exposure of the suprahepatic cava, which can then be controlled below the diaphragm. Alternatively, a phrenotomy can be made with the heavy curved scissors, beginning near the xiphoid and progressing posteriorly slightly to the patient's right toward the hepatic veins. Mediastinal transdiaphragmatic control of the suprahepatic inferior vena cava can then be quickly achieved in an extrapericardial or intrapericardial manner, and sternotomy can be avoided. Once total hepatic vascular isolation has been achieved, the surgeon should expeditiously continue with completing the mobilization of the right liver, which was begun with opening the triangular ligament. Complete mobilization of the right liver will then expose the retrohepatic portion of the inferior vena cava. Care must be taken to identify and control any accessory hepatic veins. These are generally multiple and small, draining from the liver directly to the IVC. Occasionally, robust accessory right hepatic veins are encountered. Due to the presence of adrenal and dorsal veins, which have not been controlled, the surgeon should be prepared for ongoing hemorrhage from the IVC during this process (despite total hepatic vascular isolation). Once the injury is identified, vascular control of the injury can often be improved

to reduce the ongoing hemorrhage. Venovenous bypass can be considered in cases where complex repair of the IVC is required. This allows decompression of the portal system, decompression of the IVC, and maintenance of venous return. The IVC can then be repaired in a manner to prevent stenosis if possible. Native vein (left internal jugular), bovine pericardium, or synthetic material (e.g., polytetrafluoroethylene, PTFE) can be used for patch repair of the IVC. Due to the difficulty in obtaining control of hemorrhage, exposure of the injury, and complexity of repair, mortality for retrohepatic caval injuries remains high.

On planned relaparotomy for removal of perihepatic packing, evaluation of the liver should be undertaken. Bile leakage, necrosis, and devitalized liver may require surgical intervention. Whenever possible, bile leaks should be addressed at this time. If it is not possible to find the source of the bile leak, the patient should be closed with drains in place and proceed to early endoscopic retrograde cholangiopancreatography (ERCP) with sphincterotomy and placement of stent. Devitalized liver should be debrided. Appropriate management of necrosis is controversial, but it should be noted as a risk factor for subsequent morbidity.

Presentation Continued

In the ICU, the patient remains stable with no hemodynamic or laboratory evidence of bleeding. At 48 hours, the patient returns to the OR for planned relaparotomy and removal of perihepatic packing. On removal of the laparotomy pads, there is significant bile staining on the pads, there is significant necrosis of segment VI, and hemorrhage from the injury ensues. The hemorrhage is controlled with bimanual compression. A Rummel tourniquet is placed around the porta hepatis but is not tightened. The right lobe is fully mobilized exposing the injured liver. A cholecystectomy is performed, the Pringle is applied, and a nonanatomic resection of the injured liver is completed with cutting linear staplers. The argon beam coagulator and topical cellulose hemostatic agents are used to control parenchymal bleeding from the liver edge. A closed suction drain is then positioned and the abdomen is then sutured closed.

● SPECIAL INTRAOPERATIVE CONSIDERATIONS

In some cases, parenchymal sutures can be used to control liver bleeding. Traditionally, heavy chromic sutures are used on large blunt needles. Care should be taken to avoid using these sutures for deep or central injuries due to the importance of the structures located there. Omental packs can also be used in liver injuries, generally in combination with sutures. For penetrating injuries, a tamponade of the injury tract can be achieved with balloon or Sengstaken-Blakemore tube. Topical hemostatic agents and devices can also be useful, such as cellulose agents, bipolar sealers, or argon beam coagulators. However, the most useful adjunct is generally the addition of an experienced set of hands, and assistance should be sought early for complex injuries.

● POSTOPERATIVE MANAGEMENT

Complications of liver injury are observed with increasing frequency in association with increasing grade. The surgeon should be vigilant in evaluating the patient for the development of a complication. Early infectious complications include infected necrosis and abscess formation. Early signs of infection should prompt CT imaging, especially in patients with known necrosis or those who underwent angiography and embolization. A combination of antibiotics and percutaneous drainage is usually sufficient; however, some patients may require operative drainage or resection. Biliary complications include biloma formation and bile leaks. While small bilomas may resolve spontaneously, most will require percutaneous drainage with or without ERCP and stent placement. Complete liver failure is rare and devastating, and transplant has been used in some of these cases. Patients who present in a delayed manner with acute upper gastrointestinal hemorrhage should be suspected of having hemobilia, especially in the setting of jaundice or right upper quadrant pain. While endoscopy may provide a diagnosis, in the setting of hemobilia, it is frequently nondiagnostic and always nontherapeutic. Angiography is the diagnostic modality of choice and embolization the intervention of choice.

Outpatient management generally involves avoidance of contact sports or activities with high risk of reinjury, such as horseback riding. The duration of activity restrictions is controversial as is the need for repeat imaging.

Case Conclusion

The patient progressed without incident. He was extubated 1 day after closure and was discharged home shortly thereafter. His drain was removed in the clinic.

TAKE HOME POINTS

- Patients with blunt abdominal trauma who present with peritonitis should undergo emergent laparotomy.
- Patient with blunt abdominal trauma who present with hypotension and positive FAST should undergo emergent laparotomy.

- Patients with penetrating abdominal injury who present with peritonitis or hypotension should undergo emergent laparotomy.
- Hemodynamically stable patients without peritonitis who have blunt liver injury can safely be managed nonoperatively regardless of the grade of injury.
- Patients with extravasation of intravenous contrast on CT should undergo hepatic angiography with selective embolization.
- Patients with high-grade injuries are more likely to fail nonoperative management or have complications.
- After perihepatic packing to control hemorrhage, consider CT or angiography to assess for intrahepatic vascular injury amenable to embolization.
- Complications of liver injury include hemorrhage, bile leak or biloma, necrosis, infection and abscess, and hemobilia.

SUGGESTED READINGS

Kozar RA, Feliciano DV, Moore EE, Moore FA, Cocanour CS, West MA, et al. Western Trauma Association/critical decisions in trauma: operative management of adult blunt hepatic trauma. *J Trauma.* 2011;71(1):1-5.

Kozar RA, Moore FA, Cothren CC, Moore EE, Sena M, Bulger EM, et al. Risk factors for hepatic morbidity following nonoperative management: multicenter study. *Arch Surg.* 2006;141(5):451-458.

Kozar RA, Moore FA, Moore EE, West M, Cocanour CS, Davis J, et al. Western Trauma Association critical decisions in trauma: nonoperative management of adult blunt hepatic trauma. *J Trauma.* 2009;67(6):1144-1148.

Kutcher ME, Weis JJ, Siada SS, Kaups KL, Kozar RA, Wawrose RA, et al. The role of computed tomographic scan in ongoing triage of operative hepatic trauma: a Western Trauma Association multicenter retrospective study. *J Trauma Acute Care Surg.* 2015;79(6):951-956.

Pachter HL, Spencer FC, Hofstetter SR, Coppa GF. Experience with the finger fracture technique to achieve intra-hepatic hemostasis in 75 patients with severe injuries of the liver. *Ann Surg.* 1983;197(6):771-778.

Peitzman AB, Marsh JW. Advanced operative techniques in the management of complex liver injury. *J Trauma Acute Care Surg.* 2012;73(3):765-770.

Polanco P, Leon S, Pineda J, Puyana JC, Ochoa JB, Alarcon L, et al. Hepatic resection in the management of complex injury to the liver. *J Trauma.* 2008;65(6):1264-1269.

Stassen NA, Bhullar I, Cheng JD, Crandall M, Friese R, Guillamondegui O, et al. Nonoperative management of blunt hepatic injury: an Eastern Association for the surgery of trauma practice management guideline. *J Trauma Acute Care Surg.* 2012;73(5 suppl 4):S288-S293.

Duodenal Injury

BENJAMIN DAVID CARR AND MARK R. HEMMILA

Based on the previous edition chapter "Duodenal Injury" by Filip Bednar and Mark R. Hemmila

Presentation

A 22-year-old man is brought to the hospital by emergency medical services after being stabbed during a domestic dispute. He arrives in the emergency room (ER) with a kitchen knife protruding out of his abdomen in the right upper quadrant. By report, the knife has a blade at least 10-inches long. The knife blade is now buried in his abdominal wall up to the handle. His initial systolic blood pressure (SBP) is 80 mm Hg.

● DIFFERENTIAL DIAGNOSIS

This patient has a penetrating mechanism of injury with possible traumatic injuries to the abdomen, retroperitoneum, and chest region. Vital structures and injuries that could prove rapidly lethal include pericardial tamponade, tension pneumothorax, and arterial or venous blood vessel laceration. It is imperative to consider and evaluate for these injuries during the initial assessment in the trauma bay.

● WORKUP

The primary survey focuses on airway, breathing, circulation, neurologic deficit, and exposure using the Advanced Trauma Life Support protocol. This patient may or may not require endotracheal intubation in the ER. He should have large-bore intravenous access established but not receive significant crystalloid fluid administration until operative intervention is underway. A focused assessment with sonography for trauma (FAST) exam quickly evaluates the patient's pericardial space for evidence of pericardial fluid and/or tamponade. A flat-plate chest radiograph will reveal the presence of a hemothorax or pneumothorax requiring chest tube placement. It is important to logroll this patient, examining for additional evidence of injury. If time permits, a blood sample should be obtained for blood type and crossmatch. Type-specific or O negative blood products should be available for immediate administration, if necessary.

Presentation Continued

In the present case, FAST exam is negative for pericardial blood but positive for a fluid stripe between the liver and the kidney in the right upper quadrant of the abdomen. Chest x-ray shows no hemothorax or pneumothorax. Given the mechanism of injury and fascial penetration, this patient has a clear indication for immediate operative exploration.

His ER workup should be expeditious and ideally last <10 minutes. The knife should be left in place and prepped into the operative field. The surgeon should be prepared to explore for injuries to the liver, biliary system, duodenum, inferior vena cava (IVC), right kidney, stomach, small bowel, colon, and vascular system in retroperitoneal zones 1 (central abdomen) and 2 (flank).

● TREATMENT

A generous midline laparotomy is the standard approach for a trauma patient in this circumstance (Table 119-1). The patient should be surgically prepped and draped from the sternal notch to the groin. One leg should be prepped and draped into the field from the groin to the knee. Endotracheal intubation, if not already performed, should occur just prior to skin incision. Blood products must be available. Entry into the abdomen should be accomplished quickly and safely, using a scalpel with limited passes to divide the skin, subcutaneous tissue, and fascia. Next, the peritoneum is sharply divided over the length of the incision both cephalad and caudad with heavy scissors. An examination of the position of the knife blade, trajectory, and injuries is quickly made prior to removing the knife. All four quadrants should be rapidly packed off with laparotomy sponges and the small bowel eviscerated toward the midline. Once all four quadrants are packed, a careful exploration and systematic control of significant acute hemorrhage are performed one quadrant at a time. If time permits, allowing the anesthesia team to catch up with blood product administration prior to starting the exploration can be helpful to the patient. The most likely vascular structures to be injured under these circumstances include the intrahepatic vasculature, the portal triad, IVC,

Table 119-1	Duodenal Injury Repair

Key Technical Steps

1. Midline laparotomy from the xiphoid to the pubic symphysis.
2. Rapid packing of all four quadrants.
3. Careful exploration and hemostasis by quadrants.
4. Mobilization of the hepatic flexure medially.
5. Kocher and/or Cattell-Braasch maneuvers to fully expose the entire duodenum.
6. Damage control vs. definitive repair.
7. External drainage of suture lines and provision of feeding access.
8. Possible delayed closure and second-look laparotomy once stable to reassess bowel viability and exploration for other occult injuries.

Potential Pitfalls

- Failure to control acute hemorrhage from vascular structures surrounding the duodenum prior to duodenal assessment.
- Decision between damage control approach and definitive repair based on the patient's status and other injuries.
- Protection of the right ureter and kidney during medial visceral rotation.
- Avoidance of iatrogenic vascular and pancreatic injuries during the duodenal mobilization and assessment.
- Failure to plan for pancreatic or duodenal leak.

right renal pedicle, celiac axis, superior mesenteric vessels, aorta, and the pancreaticoduodenal complex of blood vessels.

Duodenal Exposure

Once initial hemostasis has been obtained and the patient has been adequately resuscitated, a systematic exploration of the abdominal viscera is performed. In this case, the surgeon has to have a high suspicion for duodenal and pancreatic injuries along with the other abdominal viscera in the area of the penetration. Exposure of the duodenal loop and pancreatic head is achieved using a combination of the Kocher and the Cattell-Braasch maneuvers (Figure 119-1). The surgeon may also elect to divide the ligament of Treitz to further expose the fourth portion of the duodenum and the duodenojejunal junction. To begin the exposure, the retroperitoneal attachments of the hepatic flexure of the colon and the gastrocolic ligament are initially divided to gain access to the lateral aspect of the second portion of the duodenum. A Kocher maneuver is performed by incising the peritoneum lateral to the duodenal C-loop and then mobilizing the duodenum and the pancreatic head medially. This will allow visualization of the majority of the first, second, and a portion of the third section of the duodenum.

The Cattell-Braasch maneuver is a full right to medial visceral rotation including the right colon and small bowel. To perform this maneuver, the white line of Toldt is incised lateral to the right colon, and the right colon and cecum are mobilized medially. Attention must be given to identify and protect the right ureter in the process. This maneuver allows the surgeon access to the base of the bowel mesentery, which is also mobilized from the right lower quadrant to the

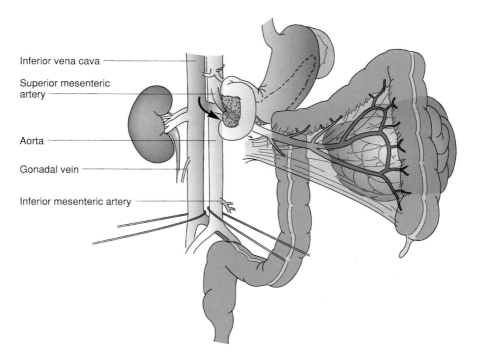

Inferior vena cava

Superior mesenteric artery

Aorta

Gonadal vein

Inferior mesenteric artery

FIGURE 119-1. The Cattell-Braasch and Kocher maneuvers allow rotation of the right colon and the small intestine completely away from the right retroperitoneum, allowing exposure of the duodenum and the pancreatic head, as well as the vascular structures and kidney. (Reprinted from Mulholland MW, Lillemoe KD, Doherty GM, Maier RV, Upchurch GR. *Greenfield's Surgery.* 4th ed. Philadelphia, PA: Lippincott Williams & Wilkins; 2006, with permission.)

ligament of Treitz. This exercise will further expose the third and the fourth portions of the duodenum with additional mobilization provided by division of the ligament of Treitz itself. Once the full medial visceral rotation is performed, the surgeon also has access to all of the right-sided retroperitoneal organs and vascular structures including the IVC, right renal complex, and the superior mesenteric blood vessels.

Injury Assessment and Repair

With full exposure and the patient stabilized, the surgeon has to assess the degree of duodenal injury before selecting the proper repair or damage control approach. Duodenal injuries are graded (Table 119-2), and it is important to ascertain the location of the laceration in relation to the other nearby anatomic structures. A crucial maneuver is to assess whether the duodenal papilla is involved as this will determine whether a simple or a complex repair is required. If uncertainty exists, a cholecystectomy and an on-table cholangiogram can be performed to assess the common bile duct. Passing a balloon catheter ("biliary Fogarty") or a similar small catheter through the cystic duct stump following cholecystectomy and feeding, it distally can prove to be a simple maneuver to identify the relationship of the ampulla to the area of injury.

Options for repair of a duodenal laceration include simple primary closure with or without debridement, simple repair and drainage with pyloric exclusion, Roux-en-Y duodenojejunostomy, duodenal diverticularization (antrectomy, oversewing of the duodenum, and loop gastrojejunostomy), and a full pancreaticoduodenectomy for massive injuries of the pancreaticoduodenal complex. In general, the simplest repair that gets the job done and an operation that will "fail well" is preferred. Performance of a Whipple procedure for trauma should be the option of last resort and is best conducted in stages. All of these repairs should have

consideration given to supplementation of the repair with buttressing of vulnerable suture lines and strategic placement of external drainage devices. Drainage of the pancreas and attention to provision of feeding access for the patient in the form of a nasojejunal tube, gastrojejunostomy tube, or a distal feeding jejunostomy are imperative.

Most simple duodenal injuries are closed primarily without tension using a single- or double-layer closure technique in a transverse fashion to avoid narrowing the bowel lumen. Suture lines may be buttressed with an omental flap or a serosal flap by oversewing with a loop/limb of the jejunum. Another option for more extensive lacerations or perforations of the duodenum, which cannot be closed primarily, is to create a Roux limb of the jejunum and use it to repair the luminal defect by constructing a duodenojejunostomy in a side-to-side fashion. Pyloric exclusion can offer protection of a fresh suture line and temporarily redirect gastric outflow (Figure 119-2). To create pyloric exclusion, a distal longitudinal gastrostomy is made on the anterior surface of the stomach. The pyloric ring is grasped with an Allis clamp, pulled into the stomach, and the pyloric opening oversewn with a running 2-0 or 3-0 Prolene suture. Another option is to staple the pylorus shut with a thoracoabdominal (TA) stapler. A draining loop gastrojejunostomy is then fashioned. More complex repairs such as duodenal diverticularization (biliary and pancreatic diversion from the affected duodenum) have become less favored with the more frequent use of a pyloric exclusion approach. Complex type III duodenal injuries (>50% of the duodenal circumference or more than a simple perforation) will require selection of a more complex repair, and this may be best accomplished at a second operation.

Decompression of a duodenal repair with an antegrade or a retrograde duodenostomy tube can reduce the rate of fistula formation. Most simple lacerations of the duodenum can be repaired primarily, and decompression and pyloric exclusion

Table 119-2	AAST Grading of Duodenal Injuries
Grade	**Injury Description**
I	Intramural hematoma—involving a single portion of the duodenum Laceration—partial thickness, no perforation
II	Intramural hematoma—involving more than one portion of the duodenum Laceration—disruption of <50% of the circumference
III	Laceration—disruption of 50%–75% of the circumference of D2 Laceration—disruption of 50%–100% of the circumference of D1, D3, D4
IV	Laceration—disruption of >75% of the circumference of D2 Laceration—involvement of the ampulla or the distal common bile duct
V	Laceration—massive disruption of the pancreaticoduodenal complex Vascular—devascularization of the duodenum

Advance one grade for multiple injuries up to grade III. D1, first portion of the duodenum; D2, second portion of the duodenum; D3, third portion of the duodenum; D4, fourth portion of the duodenum.

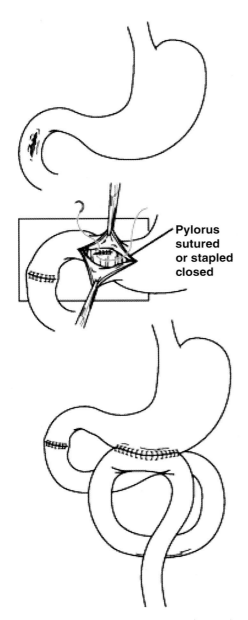

Pylorus sutured or stapled closed

FIGURE 119-2. The pyloric exclusion procedure: primary repair of the duodenal injury, protective closure of the pylorus, and gastrojejunostomy to re-establish enteric continuity.

are often not necessary. There has been a recent trend in the literature suggesting that pyloric exclusion is associated with greater morbidity. However, the patients who receive pyloric exclusion also have more associated pancreatic injuries and a higher rate of grade IV or V injuries. No prospective randomized trials are available to answer this question definitively.

The most important goal in selecting any repair or drainage procedure of the duodenum lies in understanding of not only how it will work but often in how it will affect the patient if it fails. The second key aim is to be constantly aware of the overall state of the patient. If the patient is moving toward the lethal triad of hypothermia, acidosis, and coagulopathy, damage control will become the primary goal with reconstructions reserved for a later operation.

● SPECIAL INTRAOPERATIVE CONSIDERATIONS

Isolated injury to the duodenum is rare, and injury to the duodenum is typically associated with injuries to other vital structures in the area. The surgeon may encounter severe hemorrhage from portal structures, the aorta, the IVC, the superior mesenteric or celiac vessels, or the renal vessels. Exsanguination from any of these is the most rapid mode of death from this type of injury. During the Kocher and Cattell-Braasch maneuvers, the surgeon must be ready to obtain control of vascular structures in the area. Frank bleeding or a large hematoma should warrant the surgeon in taking appropriate steps to gain proximal and distal vascular control prior to further exploration. The Pringle maneuver or clamping of the hepatic pedicle will provide control of portal and hepatic hemorrhage. The superior mesenteric and pancreaticoduodenal vessels may be controlled by manual occlusion of the supraceliac aorta and compression of the pancreaticoduodenal complex with tightly rolled laparotomy sponges after the Kocher and Cattell-Braasch maneuvers. Right renal hilum injuries may be exposed by mobilizing the kidney out of Gerota's fascia. Full aortic clamping may be necessary depending on the extent and location of the vascular injury. Walking the clamps to isolate just the area of injury once vascular control has been achieved will lessen the ischemic burden. IVC injuries may be repaired primarily, if properly visualized. In these scenarios, more definitive duodenal or pancreatic repair will often have to be delayed to a later time, and simple drainage with temporizing measures will suffice for initial control of the area. Resuscitation, stabilization, and avoidance of the lethal triad of hypothermia, acidosis, and coagulopathy are important.

● POSTOPERATIVE MANAGEMENT

Patients are typically admitted to the intensive care unit (ICU) after an initial trauma laparotomy and stabilization. Critical care goals include proper resuscitation and warming of the patient with reversal of any significant coagulopathy. Monitoring for ongoing hemorrhage is essential. Many patients will be admitted with an open abdomen secondary to perioperative resuscitation and massive visceral swelling. Management of the open abdomen requires care, diligence, and constant attention to avoid an enterocutaneous fistula. If the abdomen is open, the surgeon should plan for re-exploration within the next 12 to 48 hours based on the patient's response to resuscitation. Tube feeding may begin within 24 to 48 hours of injury, provided the patient has stabilized and a repair of the injury has been performed. However, the majority of patients with duodenal injury may have enteral feeding intolerance lasting weeks after injury.

Postoperative complications after a duodenal injury include duodenal narrowing, duodenal leak with attendant abscess formation, and occult injury to other surrounding viscera, most notably the pancreas or biliary tree. Useful diagnostic studies to evaluate for these complications may include upper gastrointestinal contrast studies, computerized tomography (CT) scan, endoscopic retrograde cholangiopancreatography (ERCP), magnetic resonance cholangiopancreatography (MRCP), and hepatobiliary iminodiacetic acid (HIDA) scans. Long-term duodenal narrowing with functional obstruction will most likely require a definitive operative repair with duodenorrhaphy, Roux-en-Y duodenojejunal reconstruction, or gastrojejunostomy. Duodenal leaks are a common occurrence despite adequate vascularity and buttressing of the repair. Drainage of suture lines will allow for the formation of a stable fistula tract. Duodenal fistulas will often close spontaneously, and a definitive repair or fistula closure operation should be delayed until the patient has fully recovered from his acute injuries. The presence of distal feeding access in the form of a feeding jejunostomy or a nasojejunal tube is absolutely necessary and should be considered as part of the initial operation, if allowed by the patient status. Pancreatitis can lead to dehiscence of suture lines. Vascular repairs near the pancreas should utilize native tissue rather than prosthetic graft material whenever possible. Protecting the repair with tissue coverage from omentum is extremely wise. Pancreatic duct or biliary tract injuries may require stents or drainage tube placement involving endoscopic or radiologic techniques in addition to operative interventions as necessary.

Case Conclusion

On operative exploration, the injured man was found to have a lateral laceration of the second portion of his duodenum without associated vascular injuries. The duodenal defect was repaired primarily in two layers. In performing the repair, the duodenum was closed in a transverse direction and the suture line covered by omentum. The site was also drained externally using a closed suction drain. Despite these precautions, the patient did develop a duodenal leak, which was well controlled with the closed suction drain. Enteral nutrition was provided via a nasojejunal tube placed at the time of operation. By 6 weeks after his initial operation, his duodenal leak had resolved and he was tolerating oral intake.

TAKE HOME POINTS

- Duodenal injuries are frequently associated with injuries to other surrounding viscera and vascular structures.
- Proper exposure to assess the duodenal injury is essential and is achieved with a combination of the Kocher and Cattell-Braasch maneuvers.
- Definitive repair or damage control measures are performed based on the overall patient status and the extent of the duodenal injury.
- External drainage of all duodenal repair suture lines is recommended.
- Feeding access must be obtained to provide the patient with the necessary nutrition for proper recovery. This feeding access should be capable of functioning even if the duodenal repair fails.
- A high suspicion must be maintained postoperatively for duodenal repair breakdown, leak, and abscess formation.

SUGGESTED READINGS

Carrillo EH, Richardson JD, Miller FB. Evolution in the management of duodenal injuries. *J Trauma.* 1996;40:1037-1045.

Dickerson RN, Voss JR, Schroeppel TJ, et al. Feasibility of jejunal enteral nutrition for patients with severe duodenal injuries. *Nutrition.* 2016;32:309-314.

Ivatury RR, Nassoura ZE, Simon RJ, et al. Complex duodenal injuries. *Surg Clin North Am.* 1996;76:797-812.

Malhotra A, Biffl WL, Moore EE, et al. Western Trauma Association critical decisions in trauma: Diagnosis and management of duodenal injuries. *J Trauma Acute Care Surg.* 2015;79:1096-1101.

Schroeppel TJ, Saleem K, Sharpe JP, et al. Penetrating duodenal trauma: a 19-year experience. *J Trauma Acute Care Surg.* 2016; 80:461-465.

Seamon MJ, Pieri PG, Fisher CA, et al. A ten-year retrospective review: does pyloric exclusion improve clinical outcome after penetrating duodenal and combined pancreaticoduodenal injuries? *J Trauma.* 2007;62:829-833.

Snyder WH, Weigelt JA, Watkins WL, et al. The surgical management of duodenal trauma: precepts based on a review of 247 cases. *Arch Surg.* 1980;115:422-429.

Stovall RT, Peltz E, Jurkovich GJ. Duodenal and pancreatic trauma. In: Ashley SW, Cance WG, Chen H, et al., eds. *Scientific American Surgery.* Hamilton, ON: Decker Intellectual Properties Inc.; 2016.

Velmahos GC, Constantinou C, Kasotakis G. Safety of repair for severe duodenal injuries. *World J Surg.* 2008;32:7-12.

Weigelt JA. Duodenal injuries. *Surg Clin North Am.* 1990;70: 529-539.

Pancreatic and Duodenal Trauma

120

BROOKE C. BREDBECK AND CARLTON C. BARNETT JR.

Presentation

A 22-year-old female was kicked in the epigastrium by a horse and transported to the nearest emergency department. She reports falling back after the blow without hitting her head and denies loss of consciousness. She complains only of epigastric pain. Her heart rate is 110 bpm. A large supraumbilical contusion is visualized with no other abnormalities noted. Abdominal and chest x-rays are negative for rib fractures or free air, and lung fields are clear. Focused abdominal sonography for trauma (FAST) is negative for free fluid or cardiac tamponade.

● DIFFERENTIAL DIAGNOSIS

This patient presents with blunt trauma to the epigastrium. Therefore, any organs or vessels residing in this region are vulnerable to injury. These include the stomach, duodenum, pancreas, transverse colon, liver, spleen, and vessels associated with these structures. Additionally, the force of impact poses risk for skeletal fracture in the vertebral column and ribs.

● WORKUP/DIAGNOSIS

The majority of early deaths due to blunt abdominal trauma are due to exsanguinating hemorrhage. Therefore, initial workup should proceed under advanced trauma life support (ATLS) guidelines, with careful monitoring of vital signs for evidence of hemorrhagic shock and investigation for sources of bleeding. If the patient is hemodynamically unstable or free intra-abdominal fluid is present, immediate exploratory laparotomy is indicated. Perforated viscus also mandates laparotomy and may present with subdiaphragmatic free air; however, this may be missed on initial abdominal x-ray particularly if the patient is supine.

Though it is a useful diagnostic modality for intraperitoneal fluid collections, FAST is unreliable in diagnosing retroperitoneal fluid. Therefore, when examining patients with epigastric trauma, indicators of hemodynamic instability should prompt definitive operative management even in the face of a negative FAST or x-ray.

In the hemodynamically stable patient with a negative initial workup, computed tomography (CT) with intravenous

contrast aids in the diagnosis of retroperitoneal injury. CT has approximately 80% sensitivity and specificity for identifying a pancreatic or duodenal injury, which may manifest as hypoattenuation or comminution of pancreatic and duodenal structures. Extraluminal gas, fat stranding, and fluid collecting in the retroperitoneum are additional signs that suggest pancreatic or duodenal disruption (Figure 120-1).

Presentation Continued

CT shows circumferential wall thickening of a portion of the duodenum and extraluminal gas and a linear region of nonenhancement near the head of the pancreas.

● TREATMENT

Nonsurgical management of low-grade duodenal and pancreatic injuries is appropriate. Minor hematomas in either the duodenum or pancreas do not require surgical intervention,

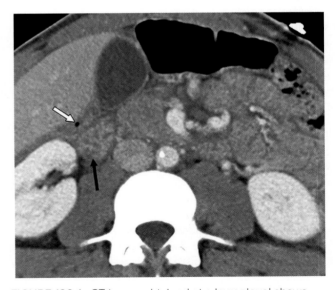

FIGURE 120-1. CT image obtained at a lower level shows thickening of the duodenal wall in the descending part (*black arrow*). Adjacent to the duodenum is a small collection of extraluminal air (*white arrow*), which indicates a small grade II laceration of the wall. (Reprinted from Linsenmaier U, Wirth S, et al. Diagnosis and classification of pancreatic and duodenal injuries in emergency radiology. *Radiographics*. 2008;28:1591-1602, with permission.)

and laparotomy for such isolated findings only puts the patient at risk of operative complications (immediate and long-term bowel obstruction and hernia). Structurally or functionally disruptive injuries require operative intervention. Examples include transection of the main pancreatic duct, full laceration of the duodenal lumen, or duodenal hematoma causing outlet obstruction.

SURGICAL APPROACH

If surgery is performed to investigate suspected duodenal or pancreatic trauma, a methodical exposure of all surrounding structures should also be performed. Therefore, the surgeon should begin with a midline laparotomy incision to ensure adequate exposure. A generous Cattell-Braasch maneuver or right medial visceral rotation will allow superior visualization of the head, neck, and a significant portion of the body of the pancreas as well as the third portion of the duodenum. The Cattell-Braasch maneuver frees the terminal ileum and identifies the ligament of Treitz. Subsequently, a Kocher maneuver can be accomplished by incising the peritoneum at the right edge of the duodenum and reflecting the duodenum and pancreas to the left. The dissection should extend to the level of the aorta and allows for visualization of the pancreatic head and duodenal C-loop. Further dissection through the fascia exposes more distal aspects of the duodenum as well as the common bile duct. Complete inspection of the pancreas is finalized by incision of the gastrocolic ligament to access the remainder of the lesser sac.

Once all injuries have been identified, the surgeon must consider the patient's current condition (e.g., extent and severity of injuries, hemodynamic status, and prognosis) to guide intraoperative management. For example, if the patient is severely injured with a poor prognosis, damage control laparotomy may be preferable to definitive repair. If the patient is otherwise minimally injured and there are few easily reparable injuries, definitive repair is more reasonable.

In a patient with low-grade duodenal injuries (grades I and II), primary repair with monofilament in the direction of the pattern of injury is preferred. Though transverse repair does provide the benefit of preventing luminal narrowing, tension-free repair in these cases is of pre-eminent importance. In intermediate or high-grade injuries, removal of portions of the duodenum or primary repair with pyloric exclusion should be considered. Pancreatic injuries are managed based on the probability that main ductal disruption is present. If main ductal disruption is unlikely, injuries may be managed by simple closed suction drainage; otherwise, they ought to be managed by resection of the affected portion. Resection in distal pancreatic injuries is accomplished by distal pancreatectomy, usually by stapling. Proximal resection in cases of pancreatic head injuries is more complex. A duodenum-preserving pancreatic head resection may be indicated in cases of pancreatic head injury without duodenal devascularization, while a pancreaticoduodenectomy may be necessary if severe duodenal compromise is suspected. Partial pancreatectomy performed to salvage the pancreatic tail requires pancreaticojejunostomy for diversion of pancreatic enzymes; this procedure has an added benefit of decreasing the likelihood of pancreatic insufficiency and the need for splenectomy.

SPECIAL INTRAOPERATIVE CONSIDERATIONS

Likelihood of main pancreatic ductal disruption is judged intraoperatively by visual inspection, but can be aided by advanced imaging modalities like intraoperative pancreatogram.

POSTOPERATIVE MANAGEMENT

Late diagnosis of pancreatic ductal injury may be catastrophic because it can lead to highly morbid infectious complications. Therefore, if ductal injury has not been definitively ruled out before or during surgery, magnetic resonance cholangiopancreatography (MRCP) or even endoscopic retrograde cholangiopancreatography (ERCP) in the very early postoperative period is recommended. Additionally, trending serum amylase/lipase levels can direct early therapy. If amylase/lipase increases rather than stabilizing or decreasing, it may indicate persistent pancreatic fistula or occult duodenal perforation.

Common postoperative complications include pancreatic fistula, duodenal fistula and/or stricture, duodenal outlet obstruction from expanding hematoma, pancreatic pseudocyst, pancreatitis, intra-abdominal abscess, and pancreatic insufficiency. Some complications, such as low-output pancreatic fistula, can be managed conservatively. Others, such as duodenal fistula/stricture and abscess, may require imaging either to investigate the severity of the problem or to guide further management. Prevention and aggressive treatment of infection in the postoperative period is paramount. Abscesses should be drained to achieve source control and patients should begin with broad-spectrum antibiotic therapy, which can be narrowed as cultures and sensitivities become available.

Providing adequate nutrition optimizes the patient's wound healing and immune system; in some patients, nutritional support via feeding jejunostomy is therefore recommended (Table 120-1).

Case Conclusion

The patient was managed nonoperatively given the low-grade duodenal and pancreatic injury found on CT. Because a pancreatic laceration was visualized, MRCP was performed on the first postoperative day to rule out injury to the main pancreatic duct. Serum amylase and lipase trended down after initial injury, and the patient was discharged in good condition the next day.

Table 120-1	Pancreatic and Duodenal Trauma

Key Technical Steps

1. Obtain exposure to the pancreas, duodenum, and surrounding structures starting with a generous Cattell-Braasch maneuver or right medial visceral rotation.
2. Perform a Kocher maneuver to reflect the duodenum and pancreatic head to the left.
3. Obtain access to the lesser sac through the gastrocolic ligament.
4. Carefully assess the head, body, and tail of the pancreas for injury.
5. Subsequent surgical decision-making should be based on the grade and location of the injury and overall injury status and prognosis.
6. Consider intraoperative pancreatography in a stable patient if unable to assess if there is a main pancreatic ductal disruption. Alternatively, a postoperative MRCP or ERCP can be performed.
7. Consider placement of a nasojejunal or surgical jejunostomy tube.

Potential Pitfalls

- Inadequate exposure and evaluation for pancreatic or duodenal injury.
- Failure to evaluate the pancreatic duct resulting in a delayed diagnosis of ductal disruption.
- Risk of tension resulting in a leak or luminal narrowing resulting in a stricture after primary repair of a duodenal injury.
- Need for splenectomy during distal pancreatic resection.
- Delay in diagnosis and/or treatment of postoperative complications such as fistula or abscess.

TAKE HOME POINTS

- Pancreatic and duodenal traumas are causes of high morbidity and mortality at two different time points in management: (1) immediately after injury due to massive exsanguination and (2) late morbidity/mortality due to delayed (missed) diagnosis of injury, normally presenting with systemic inflammatory response syndrome and eventual infectious complications. Therefore, early diagnosis of pancreatic and duodenal injuries is essential in preventing catastrophic postoperative sepsis and abscess formation.
- Regardless of the individual injury patterns, the surgeon should be mindful that severely injured patients may benefit from damage control operations rather than immediate definitive repair.
- Generally, repair or selective removal of damaged tissue is preferred in settings of pancreatic and duodenal trauma. Complex, timely operations with high morbidity, such as the pancreaticoduodenectomy, should be reserved only for cases of severe devascularization or similarly severe injury patterns.

SUGGESTED READINGS

Biffl WL. Duodenum and pancreas. In: Mattox KL, Moore EE, Feliciano DV, eds. *Trauma*. 7th ed. New York, NY: McGraw-Hill; 2012.

Bredbeck BC, Moore EE, Barnett CB. Duodenum preserving pancreatic head resection (Beger procedure) for pancreatic trauma. *J Trauma Acute Care Surg*. 2015;78(3):649-651.

Cruvinel NJ, Pereira BM, Ribeiro MA, Rizoli S, Fraga GP, Rezende-Neto JB. Is there a role for pyloric exclusion after severe duodenal trauma? *Rev Col Bras Cir*. 2014;41(3):228-231.

Malhotra A, Biffl WL, Moore EE, et al. Western trauma association critical decisions in trauma: diagnosis and management of duodenal injuries. *J Trauma*. 2014;79(6):1096-1101.

Melamud K, LeBedis CA, Soto JA. Imaging of pancreatic and duodenal trauma. *Radiol Clin North Am*. 2015;53:757-771.

Moore FA, Feliciano DV, Andrassy RJ, et al. Early enteral feeding, compared with parenteral, reduces postoperative septic complications. The results of a meta-analysis. *Ann Surg*. 1992;216(2):172-183.

Rogers SJ, Cello JP, Schecter WP. Endoscopic retrograde cholangio-pancreatography in patients with pancreatic trauma. *J Trauma*. 2010;68:538-544.

Pelvic Fracture

121

OLIVER L. GUNTER JR. AND H. ANDREW HOPPER

Based on the previous edition chapter "Pelvic Fracture" by Avi Bhavaraju and Oliver L. Gunter

Presentation

A 22 year-old is on a motorcycle group ride when he crashes his motorcycle on the highway. He is helmeted. He is thrown approximately 30 feet. The patient is found unconscious by emergency medical services (EMS). He is hypotensive with systolic blood pressure in the 80s. He responds to a 1 L normal saline (NS) fluid bolus by EMS, and systolic blood pressure is now 100 mm Hg.

Upon arrival to the trauma bay, he is awake but confused. He is tachycardic with heart rate in the 140s. Systolic blood pressure is back in the 80s. He is given 2 units of uncrossmatched O positive blood. He is complaining of lower abdominal pain and significant bilateral hip pain.

● DIFFERENTIAL DIAGNOSIS

This is a case of undifferentiated shock due to blunt trauma. The differential diagnosis of undifferentiated shock in trauma includes the following: hemorrhage (i.e., from the thorax, abdomen, pelvis, retroperitoneum, extremity or long bone, or external), tension pneumothorax, cardiac tamponade, spinal cord injury, or myocardial ischemia or arrhythmia.

● WORKUP

In accordance with the Advanced Trauma Life Support (ATLS) guidelines, the immediate priorities in this patient are to secure the airway and assess breathing and circulation (ABCs). History and physical examination, when available, may alert the provider to the possibility of a pelvic fracture, as in this case scenario. Patients may complain of pelvic, hip, lower abdomen, or lower back pain. Often, this pain can be worsened by position or lower extremity movement. Furthermore, the patient should be assessed for pelvic ring instability. This is best performed by applying gentle pressure from the lateral aspect of each iliac wing with both hands. Also, providers should examine the lower extremities for abnormal rotation of shortening as this can often be a clue to a fracture or dislocation. Blood at the urethral meatus may indicate bladder or urethral disruption, which occurs with high frequency in association with pelvis fractures. Digital rectal exam should be performed to asses for gross blood, high-riding prostate, and rectal tone.

Important laboratory tests include type and screen, complete blood count, electrolytes, coagulation studies, and resuscitation markers (blood gas, lactate, and base deficit).

Chest and pelvis films in the trauma bay can help direct resuscitation and treatment plans. Focused Assessment with Sonography for Trauma (FAST) is useful in evaluating for hemoperitoneum, especially in blunt trauma. All of these modalities can be performed during the initial trauma resuscitation, are quick and minimally invasive, and can provide useful information regarding the potential source of hemorrhage. If a patient is hemodynamically stable, then computerized tomography (CT) should be performed. It is an invaluable diagnostic tool for evaluating multisystem trauma patients. The addition of intravenous contrast makes CT a rapid and sensitive imaging modality to evaluate sources of hemorrhage. Extravasation of contrast in proximity to pelvic fractures may indicate active bleeding that requires further management.

Presentation Continued

The patient in the scenario undergoes a chest x-ray with no acute findings (Figure 121-1). Pelvis x-ray shows widening of the pubic symphysis (Figure 121-2). There is diastasis of the right sacroiliac (SI) joint.

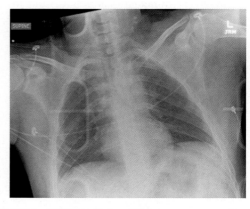

FIGURE 121-1. AP CXR obtained in the emergency department.

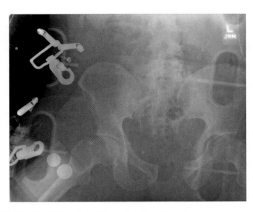

FIGURE 121-2. AP pelvis film obtained in the emergency department.

DIAGNOSIS AND TREATMENT

Once a pelvic fracture has been diagnosed on an antero-posterior pelvis radiograph, additional imaging may further characterize the fracture pattern and identify other associated injuries. Pelvic inlet and outlet views show fractures of the pelvic ring, while oblique projections better demonstrate acetabular injuries. CT imaging of the pelvis with reconstructed views are useful for operative planning and can identify even occult fractures with high sensitivity.

Pelvic fractures may be classified into five categories based on mechanism and predominant force vectors:

1. Anteroposterior compression (APC) injuries
2. Lateral compression (LC) injuries
3. Vertical shear (VS) injuries
4. Combined mechanical injuries (CMIs)
5. Acetabular fractures (AFs)

Grading is from one to three in the order of increasing severity of ligamentous and bony injuries. Those with significant ligamentous disruption and diastasis are often referred to as "open-book" fractures.

While lower-grade injuries may be managed nonoperatively with weight-bearing restriction, more severe injuries require surgical stabilization.

CT scan with IV contrast is a useful imaging modality for patients with multiple injuries. Contrast extravasation indicates active hemorrhage and demonstrates pelvic or retroperitoneal hematomas. Most pelvis fracture–related bleeding will tamponade and cease spontaneously; severe injuries may require arteriography and embolization to control hemorrhage.

Disruption of the pelvic ring increases the pelvic volume. In the setting of pelvic fracture–related bleeding, patients may benefit from closed reduction to reduce the pelvic volume and tamponade of ongoing hemorrhage. This is achieved with external fixation devices, with commercially available pelvic binders, or with a sheet tightly wrapped around the pelvis.

Presentation Continued

The patient was resuscitated according to ATLS guidelines. He stabilized after transfusion of 2 units of blood in the trauma bay. A pelvic binder was placed in order to collapse the pelvic volume and attempt to minimize further bleeding. Initial FAST was positive for fluid in the pelvis. He subsequently underwent CT imaging. A large volume of contrast-enhanced urine was identified within the peritoneum on delayed images compatible with intraperitoneal bladder rupture (Figure 121-3). An "open-book" pelvic fracture was confirmed, and three-dimensional reconstruction was performed to aid in operative planning (Figure 121-4).

SURGICAL APPROACH

The initial management of a patient with pelvic injuries should begin with a thorough assessment according to ATLS guidelines. Mechanism of injury and physiologic state determine the subsequent course. For hemodynamically stable patients, the initial management is weight-bearing restriction and formal orthopedic evaluation.

Hemodynamically unstable patients must be evaluated and managed systematically. Patients in shock must have the source of hemorrhage identified and controlled in the midst of ongoing resuscitation. Adequacy of resuscitation should be monitored simultaneously. Life-threatening injuries should be addressed in the order of severity as they are identified.

Although pelvic injuries can be associated with significant hemorrhage, associated injuries are common and must be evaluated. Screening radiographs can rule out intrathoracic or pelvic injuries. If a pelvic fracture is found, external reduction of the pelvic ring is a useful temporizing maneuver to minimize ongoing bleeding. Abdominal ultrasound can expeditiously identify patients that require immediate

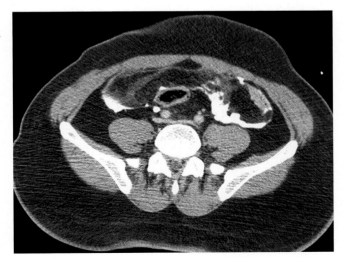

FIGURE 121-3. Axial CT image showing extravasation of contrast from the bladder.

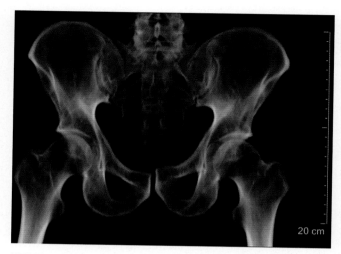

FIGURE 121-4. 3D reconstruction of open-book pelvic fracture.

Table 121-1   Pelvic Fracture

Key Technical Steps
1. Determine if the patient is hemodynamically stable
2. Identify and control sources of bleeding
3. Obtain initial diagnostic studies (chest x-ray, pelvic x-ray, FAST) in the trauma bay
4. Begin resuscitation with blood products if indicated
5. Reduce pelvic volume to tamponade bleeding (bedsheet, pelvic binder, or ex-fix)
6. Obtain CT to define facture pattern and to identify associated abdominal/thoracic injuries
7. Perform angioembolization for contrast extravasation or continued/recurrent pelvic hemorrhage

Potential Pitfalls
- Difficulty in determining initial management strategy (i.e., exploratory laparotomy vs. angiography with possible embolization) in hemodynamically unstable patients with a + FAST and a pelvic fracture
- Danger of releasing tamponade and worsening of bleeding during laparotomy in patients with a pelvic hematoma
- Bleeding from an uncontrolled pelvic source—quick intervention with ongoing resuscitation is required until bleeding is stopped
- Underrecognition of shock from pelvic hemorrhage

laparotomy. Evaluation and splinting of long bone injuries minimize fracture-related bleeding. Lacerations with significant external hemorrhage can be controlled with external pressure or a tourniquet. If the patient can be stabilized, further imaging may be indicated. CT imaging of the brain, spine, and torso is an invaluable tool (particularly in the setting of polytrauma) with the addition of IV contrast to rule out solid organ injury and bleeding.

Significant pelvic hemorrhage can be difficult or impossible to control, primarily because of anatomic inaccessibility of the injured vessels. Although external reduction combined with either intra- or extraperitoneal packing may be utilized, arteriography with embolization can selectively embolize individual vessels. This method is preferable to nonselective operative ligation of one or both internal iliac arteries. An aortogram with bilateral iliac runoff, followed by selective angiography of both internal and external iliac systems, is the initial approach taken. If contrast extravasation is seen, selective embolization with coils or foam should be performed. Strong consideration should be given to embolizing vessels that have evidence of vessel spasm or an abrupt cutoff since these usually represent signs of injury. This approach is successful in upwards of 80% to 90% of patients. It is essential to continue the resuscitation throughout the hemorrhage control process until appropriate endpoints are met to prevent the lethal combination of hypothermia, coagulopathy, and acidosis. Recurrent instability may require reassessment and repeat angiography to assess for rebleeding. Inability to control pelvic hemorrhage by means of external reduction, pelvic packing, angioembolization, or operative ligation is associated with high mortality (Table 121-1).

● SPECIAL INTRAOPERATIVE CONSIDERATIONS

Patients with pelvic fractures undergoing laparotomy require special consideration, as the technique utilized may differ from the standard laparotomy for trauma. If an external compression device is present, exposure can be severely limited, and great care must be taken when deciding to remove this device as the patient may hemorrhage from reexpansion of the pelvic volume. If possible, the standard laparotomy incision should be limited to a supraumbilical incision, as extending the incision below the semilunar line may lead to further hemorrhage by increasing anterior extension of a pelvic hematoma. Limiting the laparotomy incision will also aid in the preperitoneal packing of the pelvis, as this requires a separate lower incision. Damage control techniques for rapid control of hemorrhage followed by temporizing measures with delayed reconstruction should be considered for patients who are severely physiologically compromised.

Intraoperative control of pelvic bleeding is technically challenging and often ineffective. Ligation of the hypogastric arteries is one technique to control pelvic arterial bleeding, but this technique may be complicated by difficult exposure and distorted anatomy in the face of an extensive retroperitoneal hematoma. Venous pelvic bleeding usually arises from cancellous bone or the sacral venous plexus, is diffuse in nature, and is difficult or impossible to control with ligation. This type of pelvic bleeding is best controlled by tamponade. Management of pelvic bleeding during laparotomy is done by tightly packing the pelvis via an intraperitoneal approach in combination with temporary abdominal closure. Postoperatively, the patient may need to be managed with angiography and embolization if there is continued hemorrhage. Once stabilized, the patient can be returned to the operating room for re-exploration. At this time, the pelvic packing can be removed, bowel continuity can be restored, and any additional injuries can be addressed. Definitive closure follows traditional principles of damage control laparotomy. At this point, stabilization of the pelvis fracture, either internal or external, may be considered in conjunction with orthopedics.

Open pelvic fractures deserve special consideration. An open pelvis fracture involves direct communication between a fracture fragment and the rectum, vagina, or skin of the perineum or groin. While open pelvis fractures only account for 2% to 4% of all pelvis fractures, the mortality of this injury has been estimated at 45% and can acutely result from uncontrolled bleeding from the fracture site because the wound is open to the environment and receives no internal tamponade. Initial management should focus on control of acute hemorrhage and wound management. Associated regional injuries are common and may include injuries to the bladder, urethra, vagina, and anorectum, which may increase the risk of infection and complexity of subsequent reconstruction. Consideration should be given to fecal and urinary diversion to reduce the risk of pelvic sepsis and to facilitate operative repair of the fractures.

● POSTOPERATIVE MANAGEMENT

Postoperative management of pelvic fractures involves a multifaceted approach to patient care. They key elements to consider are weight-bearing status, deep venous thrombosis (EVT) prophylaxis, monitoring for postoperative complications, and long-term follow-up. Postoperative weight-bearing status is highly variable, but most unstable pelvis fractures require several weeks of lower extremity non–weight bearing.

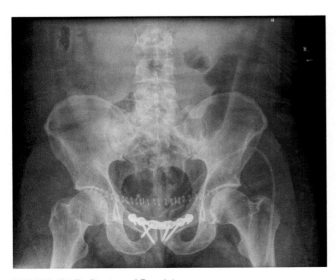

FIGURE 121-5. Post-op AP pelvis.

The incidence of DVT in patients with pelvic trauma is reported to be as high as 60%. Routine DVT prophylaxis is recommended. DVT prophylaxis may be mechanical (ambulation, sequential compression devices) or chemical (e.g., low molecular weight heparin, Coumadin).

Sciatic or lumbosacral nerve injury can be seen after severe pelvic fracture (10%–15% incidence). In zone 3 sacral fractures, rates of nerve injury can be as high as 50%. Nonunions and malunions also occur. Pain and pelvic or limb deformity are the most common complaints from patients. Females may have higher rates of urinary symptoms, cephalopelvic disproportion, and gynecologic pain. The bladder is injured in approximately 3.4% and the urethra in 1% of patients with pelvic trauma.

Case Conclusion

As the CT scan revealed an intraperitoneal bladder rupture, the patient was urgently taken to the operating room. Exploratory laparotomy was performed. A defect in the dome of the bladder was identified. The trigone of the bladder was examined and found to be without injury. There was no injury to the ureters or the urethral opening. The bladder laceration was closed in two layers. Watertight closure was ensured by instilling 200 mL of normal saline into the bladder. A Foley catheter was placed. Once the abdomen was closed, the case was turned over to the orthopedic surgeons. The patient underwent open reduction and internal fixation of pelvic fracture with a plate and closed treatment of right SI joint diastasis (Figure 121-5). The patient was normalized over the next few days. He was discharged from the hospital to a rehabilitation facility for further physical therapy.

TAKE HOME POINTS

- Pelvic fractures may be classified into five categories based on mechanism and predominant force vectors: lateral compression (grades I to III), anter (grades I to III), vertical shear, combined mechanism, and acetabular fractures. Grading is from one to three in the order of increasing severity of ligamentous and bony injuries.
- Workup of pelvic fractures may include x-rays (i.e., anterior and posterior, inlet and outlet, oblique, and Judet views). CT of the abdomen and pelvis should be obtained with IV contrast to evaluate for concomitant intra-abdominal injuries. Noncontrast scans with thin cuts and reconstructed views can be used for determining management strategy.
- Initial workup should follow ATLS guidelines.
- Because of a high rate of concurrent truncal injuries, patients with pelvic fractures require a full trauma workup and evaluation.
- Angioembolization should be considered in patients with the following: contrast extravasation on CT, uncontrolled

pelvic hemorrhage identified intraoperatively, or recurrent pelvic hemorrhage.

- Orthopedic management pearls:
  - Temporary pelvic stabilization for hemodynamically unstable patients can be achieved using a bedsheet, pelvic binder, or external fixator.
  - Patients should be referred to an orthopedic surgeon for definitive repair, which may require transfer if no qualified orthopedic surgeon is available.
  - DVT prophylaxis should be initiated early.
  - Weight bearing should be limited as necessary.

SUGGESTED READINGS

Bjurlin MA, Fantus RJ, Mellett MM, Goble SM. Genitourinary injuries in pelvic fracture morbidity and mortality using the National Trauma Data Bank. *J Trauma.* 2009;67:1033.

Burgess AR, Eastridge BJ, Young JW. Pelvic ring disruptions: effective classification system and treatment protocols. *J Trauma.* 1990;30(7):848-856.

Cannada LK, Taylor RM, Reddix R, et al. The Jones-Powell Classification of open pelvic fractures: a multicenter study evaluating mortality rates. *J Trauma Acute Care Surg.* 2013;74:901.

Dalal SA, Burgess AR, Siegel JH, et al. Pelvic fracture in multiple trauma: classification by mechanism is key to pattern of organ injury, resuscitative requirements, and outcome. *J Trauma.* 1989;29(7):981-1000.

Davis JW, et al. Western trauma association critical decisions in trauma: management of pelvic fracture with hemodynamic instability. *J Trauma.* 2008;65:1012-1015.

Denis F, Davis S, Comfort T. Sacral fractures: an important problem. Retrospective analysis of 236 cases. *Clin Orthop Relat Res.* 1988;227:267.

Dente CJ, Feliciano DV, Rozycki GS, et al. The outcome of open pelvic fractures in the modern era. *Am J Surg.* 2005;190:830.

Geerts WH, Code KJ, Jay RM, et al. A prospective study of venous thromboembolism after major trauma. *N Engl J Med.* 1994;331:1601-1606.

Grotz MR, Allami MK, Harwood P, et al. Open pelvic fractures: epidemiology, current concepts of management and outcome. *Injury.* 2005;36:1.

Guillamondegui OD, et al. Pelvis fractures. In: Cameron J, ed. *Current Surgical Therapy.* 8th ed. Philadelphia, PA: Mosby Elsevier Science; 2004.

Hauschild O, Strohm PC, Culemann U, et al. Mortality in patients with pelvic fractures: results from the German pelvic injury register. *J Trauma.* 2008;64:449.

Weis EB Jr. Subtle neurological injuries in pelvic fractures. *J Trauma.* 1984;24:983

Yoshihara H, Yoneoka D. Demographic epidemiology of unstable pelvic fracture in the United States from 2000 to 2009: trends and in hospital mortality. *J Trauma Acute Care Surg.* 2014;76:380.

Critical Care

Airway Emergency

122

SAMUEL A. SCHECHTMAN, DEREK T. WOODRUM, AND DAVID W. HEALY

Based on the previous edition chapter "Airway Emergency"
by Derek T. Woodrum and David W. Healy

Presentation

A 25-year-old male is brought to the emergency department as a level I trauma after being thrown from a snowmobile. At the scene, emergency responders placed the patient in a cervical collar and administered high-flow oxygen via face mask. In the emergency department, his pulse oximetry saturation is 92%, and he has partially obstructed (snoring, noisy) breathing. Due to hypotension and a focused abdominal sonogram positive for free fluid, he is taken directly to the operating room for an exploratory laparotomy. Intravenous and intra-arterial accesses are already in place.

After removing the anterior portion of the cervical spine collar, a rapid sequence induction of anesthesia and direct laryngoscopy are performed in the operating room with manual in-line cervical stabilization and cricoid pressure. The laryngoscopist is unable to visualize the vocal cords or pass an endotracheal tube into the trachea. The saturations begin to fall into the 80s.

● DISCUSSION

An airway emergency is one of the most critical, time-sensitive situations encountered by surgeons and anesthesiologists. Surgeons will likely be involved in several cases involving airway management during their careers. This example case occurred in the operating room in a "controlled" setting. Yet, smaller hospitals may not have in-hospital 24-hour anesthesia services, and emergency airway management may fall to the surgical team. Even when a full complement of help is available, the surgical team may be the first responder to an airway emergency on rounds, in the trauma bay, or at off-site locations such as radiology suites or burn debridement rooms. Finally, the surgical team will occasionally be called upon for obtaining a surgical airway in the operating room in settings of trauma and/or impossible ventilation and intubation.

The purpose of this chapter is to highlight salient points when approaching an airway emergency. It is crucial that the physician has a previously thought-out and well-understood approach to airway management. We discuss pre-induction airway evaluation, rapid sequence induction for standard intubation, and subsequent approaches when intubation is unsuccessful. Surgical airway management is also reviewed in the setting of cannot intubate and cannot oxygenate scenarios.

● DIFFERENTIAL DIAGNOSIS

This patient's hypoxia is likely caused by several factors including hypoventilation from partial airway obstruction, depressed mental status, and opioid administration. Other factors to consider include pulmonary contusion, aspiration, pneumothorax or hemothorax associated with rib fractures, depressed cardiac output from cardiac contusion, tamponade, and/or aortic dissection. In the setting of trauma and suspected craniofacial injuries, laryngotracheal trauma must be considered.

● WORKUP

In an airway emergency, there is limited time for additional workup. A pre-existing chest radiograph can diagnose pneumothorax, hemothorax, or widened mediastinum—but the main focus should be on the airway exam. The goal in an urgent situation is to maintain oxygenation while simultaneously identifying predictors of difficult ventilation and intubation. This risk stratification will help guide immediate and subsequent airway management. If a patient is hypoxemic with little or no ventilatory effort, the airway should be supported by chin lift with or without an oral pharyngeal airway as oxygen is applied.

The airway exam is performed to specifically aid in the prediction of three situations: difficult mask ventilation, difficult intubation, and difficult surgical airway access. Table 122-1 lists risk factors for difficulty with each of these three techniques. The ability to mask ventilate is extremely important in maintaining gas exchange and life. It may be continued for some time if intubation is unsuccessful. Figure 122-1 illustrates the Mallampati scoring system, which describes how much of the oropharynx can be visualized. A Class III (no visualization of the uvula but the soft palate can be seen) or Class IV (the soft palate cannot be visualized)

Table 122-1	Risk Factors for Difficult Mask Ventilation, Difficult Intubation, and Difficult Cricothyrotomy		
Difficult Mask Ventilation	**Difficult Intubation**	**Difficult Cricothyrotomy**
Mallampati 3 or 4	Mallampati 3 or 4	Prior surgery to the neck
Obesity	Limited extension	Hematoma or infection
Sleep apnea	Cervical collar	Obesity and limited access (e.g. flexion scoliosis)
Presence of beard	Hospital bed	Radiation
Prior neck radiation	Limited mandibular protrusion	Tumors (including thyroid goiter)

Mallampati score alerts to the likelihood of *both* difficult mask ventilation and intubation with direct laryngoscopy. With this, alternative airway devices and airway expert consultation should be obtained immediately.

The recommended brief airway exam in the emergency setting includes assessment of mouth opening, Mallampati class, and mandibular protrusion (ability to extend the lower teeth anterior to the upper teeth). The presence or absence of teeth and facial hair is noted, and neck mobility—particularly extension—is assessed if the patient has a cleared cervical spine. Additionally, any prior anesthetic and/or airway history should be reviewed if readily available.

In the setting of suspected laryngotracheal trauma, otolaryngology consultation, flexible fiber-optic laryngoscopy, and computed tomography (CT) images are valuable diagnostic tools. Yet, in an emergent setting or without the presence of an otolaryngologist, these tools are unlikely to be available. If laryngotracheal trauma is suspected, attempting oral or nasal endotracheal intubation should be avoided, as this can result in further injury including complete laryngotracheal separation and subsequent asphyxiation. Management of these injuries is beyond the scope of this chapter, but a surgical airway is the indicated strategy for securing the airway with known or suspected laryngotracheal trauma.

● RAPID SEQUENCE INDUCTION

After the airway exam is completed and urgent calls for assistance are made, preoxygenation is performed prior to induction of anesthesia. This is best carried out utilizing a non-rebreathing mask with a collapsible air reservoir. In a patient breathing spontaneously, an Ambu® (Copenhagen, Denmark) bag is not ideal for preoxygenation as it is difficult to draw oxygen from the self-expanding bag. If the airway is partially obstructed but respiratory effort is present, a jaw thrust/chin lift maneuver should be performed. After preoxygenation and application of cricoid pressure, general anesthesia should be induced to optimize intubating conditions. Table 122-2 lists the common emergency induction agents and muscle relaxants. The comparative advantages and disadvantages are outside the scope of this chapter, but etomidate is used frequently for its maintenance of hemodynamic stability on induction.

Ketamine can be used for induction of anesthesia while maintaining respiratory effort and spontaneous ventilation. This agent can also serve to maintain hemodynamic stability with induction. The use of ketamine does induce central stimulation of the sympathetic nervous system, leading to adverse effects in trauma patients including increased intracranial pressure, pulmonary artery pressure, and myocardial work. Therefore, it is best avoided in patients with coronary artery disease, uncontrolled hypertension, congestive heart failure, arterial aneurysms, and increased intracranial pressure.

The use of succinylcholine or rocuronium in the doses listed will provide optimal intubating conditions within 60 seconds. Contraindications to succinylcholine are listed below. Due to these contraindications, rocuronium is frequently used in rapid sequence induction of anesthesia. It will provide approximately 30 to 45 minutes of muscle relaxation. Now, many institutions have the availability of sugammadex, a reversal agent for neuromuscular blockade. If immediate reversal of rocuronium is required, a dose of 16 mg/kg of sugammadex can be administered.

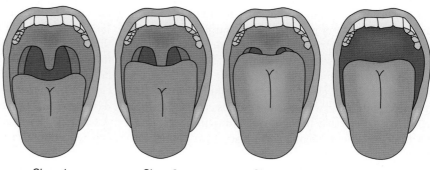

FIGURE 122-1. Mallampati score.　　Class 1　　　　Class 2　　　　Class 3　　　　Class 4

Table 122-2	Common Emergency Induction Agents and Muscle Relaxants

Induction Agent	Dose
Etomidate	0.2–0.3 mg/kg IV
Sodium thiopental	3–5 mg/kg IV
Propofol	2–3 mg/kg IV
Ketamine	1–2 mg/kg IV
Muscle Relaxant	**Dose**
Succinylcholine	1–1.5 mg/kg IV
Rocuronium	0.6–1.2 mg/kg IV

Succinylcholine is a widely used and relatively safe muscle relaxant, but the potential complications should be known. Any provider administering it *must* be familiar with the absolute contraindications and avoid its use in patients with burns (having occurred beyond 24 hours), hyperkalemia, upper motor neuron lesions, neuromuscular disorders, and a personal or family history of malignant hyperthermia.

● UNABLE TO VENTILATE

In this chapter's case scenario, intubation was not successful after rapid sequence induction and direct laryngoscopy. In this situation, a well–thought-out backup plan must be readily instituted. Figure 122-2 illustrates a flow diagram on how to manage an unsuccessful intubation. It is a modification of the American Society of Anesthesiologists Difficult Airway Algorithm, focusing on the goals of maintaining gas exchange and oxygen saturation as the airway is managed. Key points are noted in the text following the flowchart.

1. If the initial intubation attempt is unsuccessful, the pulse oximetry reading should be noted while optimizing intubation conditions for subsequent attempts. If the saturation is already dropping below 90%, *further intubation attempts should not be made.*
2. Oxygenation and ventilation with bag–mask should be attempted immediately while calling for surgical airway supplies and preparing for a surgical airway. A surgical airway is not the next step, but parallel preparations should be made.
3. If bag–mask ventilation is successful, the patient is "re"preoxygenated before subsequent attempts are made at intubation utilizing alternate airway techniques by an airway expert familiar with these alternatives.
4. If bag–mask ventilation is unsuccessful, a laryngeal mask airway (LMA) should be placed. If LMA placement is successful and ventilation through the LMA is adequate, an airway expert may then consider trans-LMA intubating techniques.

5. If LMA placement is unsuccessful, or inadequate at providing effective oxygenation, a surgical airway should be promptly established (see below).

Of critical importance is the immediate call for help from experienced providers if the initial attempt at intubation is unsuccessful. The goal is oxygenation and gas exchange, and this should be accomplished with bag–mask ventilation if intubation is unsuccessful. We recommend against the use of advanced alternative airway devices (videolaryngoscopes, intubating supraglottic airways, fiberoptic intubations, etc.) by inexperienced providers. Just as an anesthesiologist is unlikely to safely perform an appendectomy (even after observing the procedure hundreds of times), it is unlikely that a surgical team member will be successful in using unfamiliar and advanced airway devices in a critical situation. The strong focus should remain on oxygen delivery and airway patency—this is the reason for LMA placement if intubation and bag–mask ventilation are unsuccessful. The reported incidence of difficult bag–mask ventilation combined with difficult laryngoscopy is estimated to be 0.40%.

● SURGICAL APPROACH

If intubation is unsuccessful, and mask ventilation and LMA placement are inadequate to permit additional attempts by alternate airway methods, a surgical airway through emergency front of neck access should be performed without delay. Recent literature from the Difficult Airway Society supports performing a scalpel cricothyrotomy (Figure 122-3, Table 122-3). The Difficult Airway Society advises that this is the fastest and most reliable approach to securing the airway in cannot intubate and cannot oxygenate circumstances. However, cannula techniques have also been supported, as study in human cadavers has shown higher first attempt success rates with cannula techniques. Still, oxygenation through cannulas can only be achieved by using high pressure sources (less likely to be readily available), risking barotrauma. Other techniques such as use of the Melker Emergency Cricothyrotomy Catheter Sets® (Cook Medical, Bloomington, IN) often involve additional equipment with more complex steps, potentially lengthening the time to secure an airway in a situation where seconds matter. Still, the wire-guided technique utilizing a Melker cricothyrotomy kit is often widely available.

The Difficult Airway Society supports that regardless of the chosen front of neck access technique, it should be done by well-trained personnel. The chosen technique should be easy to perform emergently based upon available equipment and provider familiarity. During any attempt at a surgical approach, efforts should continue at rescue oxygenation through the upper airway (supraglottic airway device, nasal insufflation, tightly fitting face mask).

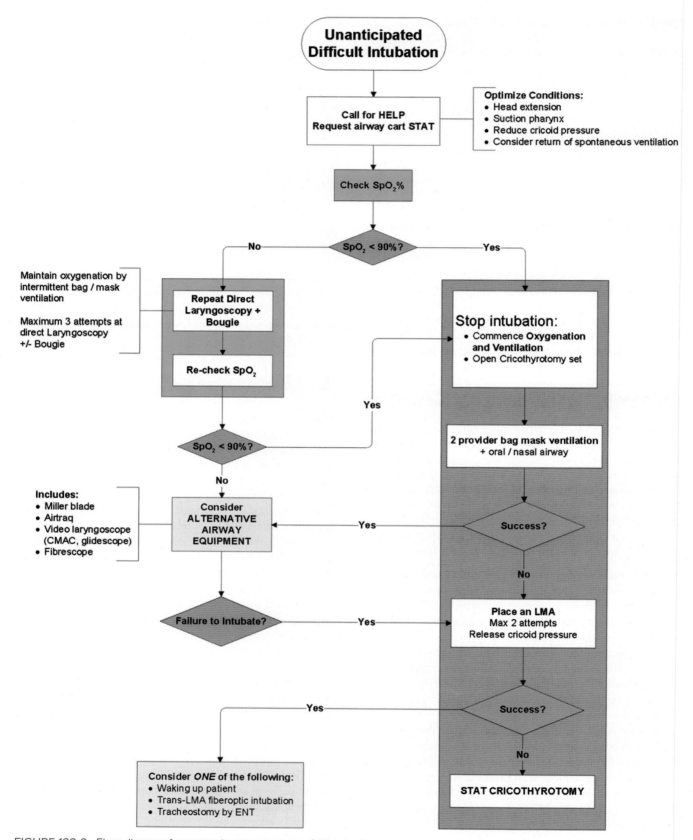

FIGURE 122-2. Flow diagram for managing an unsuccessful intubation.

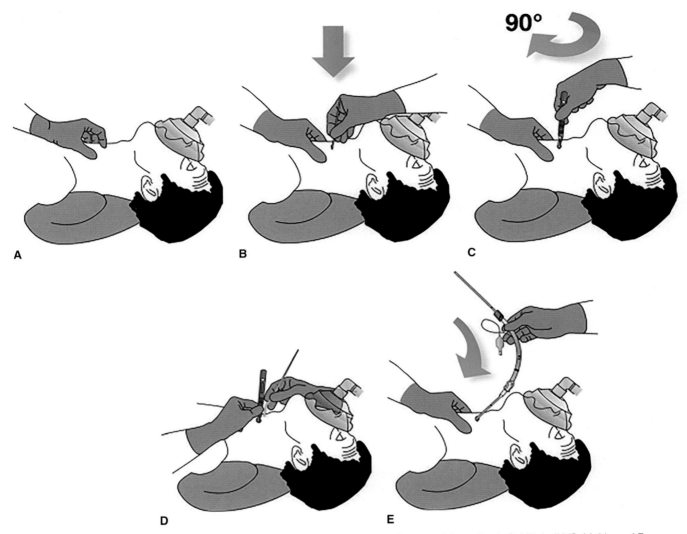

FIGURE 122-3. Difficult Airway Society scalpel cricothyrotomy technique. (Reprinted from Frerk C, Mitchell VS, McNarry AF, et al. Difficult Airway Society 2015 guidelines for management of unanticipated difficult intubation in adults. *Br J Anaesth.* 2015;115(6):827-848, with permission.)

● POSTOPERATIVE MANAGEMENT

After establishing a definitive airway—that is, a cuffed tube in the trachea—placement is confirmed by listening for bilateral breath sounds and checking for return of end-tidal CO_2. The latter is accomplished either by observing color change on an in-line device or by return of CO_2 to a gas analyzer on an anesthesia machine. However, blood must be flowing to the lungs in order for CO_2 delivery to take place. In the setting of very low cardiac output (exsanguination, massive myocardial infarction [MI], or pulmonary embolus) or in cardiac arrest without cardiopulmonary resuscitation, CO_2 will not be detected even if the airway is correctly positioned. Pulse oximetry and arterial blood gas sampling are used in an adjunctive manner. A chest x-ray (CXR) should be ordered to confirm position and to check for adequate inflation of all lung lobes (an emergency operation should not be delayed for a CXR, of course).

TAKE HOME POINTS

- Immediate consultation with an airway management expert gives the greatest chance for successful outcome in emergency airway management.
- Rapid sequence induction followed by direct laryngoscopy (accompanied by manual in-line cervical stabilization if cervical spine stability is uncertain) is the current standard of care.
- An understanding of the failed airway algorithm (memorized!) is crucial for logical, safe, and sequential handling of the emergency airway.
- Alternative airway devices beyond a standard LMA require previous experience for successful placement. Their use is not recommended in an emergency without prior familiarity.

Table 122-3   Surgical Scalpel Cricothyrotomy

Equipment

1. Scalpel with a number 10 blade.
2. Bougie with coude (angled) tip.
3. Tube, cuffed, size 6.0 mm.

Key Technical Steps

1. Place a shoulder roll to optimize position—neck extension (do not extend neck in cervical spine injury)
2. Continue attempts at rescue oxygenation via upper airway
3. Stand on patient's left side if right-handed
4. Use thumb, index, and middle fingers to identify laryngeal anatomy
5. Stabilize larynx using the left hand
6. Use left index finger to identify cricothyroid membrane
7. Hold scalpel in the right hand and make a transverse stab incision through the skin and cricothyroid membrane with the cutting edge of the blade facing you
8. Keep scalpel perpendicular to the skin and turn it through 90° so that the sharp edge points caudally
9. Swap hands, hold scalpel with the left hand
10. Maintain gentle traction pulling scalpel toward you laterally with the left hand keeping the scalpel handle vertical to the skin
11. Pick up the bougie with your right hand
12. Holding the shaft of the bougie parallel to the floor at a right angle to the trachea, slide the angled "coude" tip down the side of the scalpel blade furthest from you into the trachea
13. Rotate and align the bougie with the patient's trachea and advance up to 10–15 cm
14. Remove scalpel
15. Stabilize trachea and tension skin with the left hand
16. Railroad a lubricated 6.0-mm cuffed tracheal tube over the bougie
17. Rotate the tube as it is advanced
18. Remove the bougie
19. Inflate the cuff and confirm ventilation with capnography
20. Secure the tube

Potential Pitfalls

- Trauma to lateral vascular structures or wrong level incision if a transverse incision is used. These are two reasons for vertical midline incision in the emergency setting.
- False passage of tracheostomy tube.

SUGGESTED READINGS

Apfelbaum JL, Hagberg CA, Caplan RA, et al. Practice guidelines for management of the difficult airway: an updated report by the American Society of Anesthesiologists Task Force on Management of the Difficult Airway. *Anesthesiology.* 2013;118(2):251-270.

Bell RB, Verschueren DS, Dierks EJ. Management of laryngeal trauma. *Oral Maxillofac Surg Clin North Am.* 2008;20:415-430.

Cook TM, Woodall N, Frerk C, et al. Major complications of airway management in the UK: results of the Fourth National Audit Project of the Royal College of Anaesthetists and the Difficult Airway Society. Part 1: anaesthesia. *Br J Anaesth.* 2011;106(5):632-642.

Frerk C, Mitchell VS, McNarry AF, et al. Difficult Airway Society 2015 guidelines for management of unanticipated difficult intubation in adults. *Br J Anaesth.* 2015;115(6):827-848.

Heard AMB. *Percutaneous Emergency Oxygenation in the Can't Intubate, Can't Oxygenate Scenario*; 2013.

Hung O, Murphy M. Context sensitive airway management. *Anesth Analg.* 2010;110(4):982-983.

Kheterpal S, Han R, Tremper KK, et al. Incidence and predictors of difficult and impossible mask ventilation. *Anesthesiology.* 2006;105(5):885-891.

Kheterpal S, Healy D, Aziz MF, et al. Incidence, predictors, and outcome of difficult mask ventilation with combined with difficult laryngoscopy: a report from the multicenter perioperative outcomes group. *Anesthesiology.* 2013;119(6):1360-1369.

Melker JS, Gabrielli A. Melker cricothyrotomy kit: an alternative to the surgical technique. *Ann Otol Rhinol Laryngol.* 2005;114(7):525-528.

Verschueren DS, Bell RB, Bagheri SC, et al. Management of laryngotracheal injuries associated with craniomaxillofacial trauma. *J Oral Maxillofac Surg.* 2006;64:203-214.

Cardiovascular Failure

JOSEPH FERNANDEZ-MOURE, JEREMY CANNON, AND LEWIS J. KAPLAN

123

Presentation

A 54-year-old man (90 kg) has undergone an emergency ruptured abdominal aortic aneurysm repair and is cared for in your intensive care unit (ICU). An estimated blood loss (EBL) of 2.2 L was replaced with 2.6 L lactated Ringer's, 4 units packed red blood cells (PRBCs), 4 units fresh frozen plasma (FFP), and 1 unit of apheresis platelets. His abdomen was closed. Hemodynamics are supported with low-dose epinephrine at 0.05 mcg/kg/min. He remains mechanically ventilated and sedated on assist control (AC)/volume control ventilation. In the early morning, there is a change in hemodynamics to HR 122 bpm, RR 12, BP 88/48 mm Hg, SpO_2 88%, and his ABG is 7.21/58/56; hemoglobin is stable at 9.7 gm%. The patient now requires an increase in epinephrine to 0.12 mcg/kg/min to address a falling mean arterial pressure (MAP).

● DIFFERENTIAL DIAGNOSIS

Given the plethora of diagnoses that may explain these findings, it is easiest to group them into discrete categories as follows:

1. *Disordered Compartment Pressure–Volume Relationships*
   These include intra-abdominal hypertension (IAH) and the abdominal compartment syndrome (ACS), tension pneumothorax, tension hemothorax, and pericardial tamponade.
2. *Disorders of Intravascular Volume*
   The chief disorder here is postoperative hemorrhage, but capillary leak, infection-related vasodilatation, and septic shock may create a plasma volume deficit as well. While this is early in the postoperative time course for infection to be present, an iatrogenic colon perforation or necrotizing soft tissue infection of the surgical site should be considered. Finally, individual genetics may craft a more robust than anticipated inflammatory cascade leading to this presentation.
3. *Disorders of Intravascular Flow Including Vascular Tone*
   Flow-related issues are primarily related to compartment pressure impeded venous return as above or pulmonary embolism. Reduced tone is most commonly related to

sepsis sequelae such as septic shock, while increased tone is related to hypertension and its related sequelae such as hypertensive urgency or emergency, neither of which is likely in this scenario. There are other scenarios where excessive hypertension may lead to reduced cardiac output in those with cardiomyopathy such that end-organ failure results, but these events are less likely outside of the heart failure population.

4. *Disorders of Cardiac Mechanics*
   Primary myocardial failure from acute myocardial infarction heads the differential in this category. Reduced flow from the new onset of an atrial dysrhythmia (more common) or ventricular dysrhythmia (less common) should be specifically sought. An isolated troponin leak without an associated mechanical defect noted on echocardiographic evaluation would not result in this presentation. Indeed, a troponin leak is a frequent event in this patient population and has been reported in up to 55% of patients undergoing emergency open repair; rates after endovascular repair range from 4% to 12%.

● WORKUP

In general, workup of the four different but somewhat related groups of differential diagnoses occurs in parallel rather than in series. IAH or the ACS should be specifically evaluated using bladder pressure; physical examination is notoriously lacking in fidelity to rule these conditions in or out. A lab profile to include hemoglobin concentration should be sent, ideally using point-of-care testing for rapid turn around even as a clinical lab specimen is sent for confirmation in addition to other profiles including creatine kinase–muscle/brain (CK-MB) and troponin-I assessment; an ECG is ideal to evaluate for injury or infarction patterns as well. Coagulopathy assessment using standard measures such as prothrombin time (PT), international normalized ratio (INR), activated partial thromboplastin time (aPTT), fibrinogen, and thromboelastography (if available) is similarly appropriate.

In addition, a rapid bedside assessment of hemoglobin should be made by evaluating the patient's conjunctivae and nail beds for paleness or pallor. While peripheral temperature assessment will disclose evidence of poor perfusion, it will not define the etiology. Instead, additional objective data are important to ascertain. A portable CXR is the key in evaluating for space-occupying lesions within the pleural space as well as a change in the cardiac silhouette. While awaiting the portable chest radiograph, ultrasonography may be performed to assess cardiac chamber size, global contractility, pericardial space–occupying lesions, and inferior vena cava (IVC) diameter and collapse as well as the presence or absence of pleural space–occupying lesions including gas or fluid. These assessments may be loosely grouped as "ICU ultrasound" as they interrogate for ICU relevant abnormalities that will inform either additional testing or therapeutic undertakings. Abnormalities noted on ICU cardiac ultrasound should be followed with a formal cardiac echocardiography to evaluate detailed cardiac structure and function. The ICU cardiac ultrasound does not serve as a substitute for an echocardiographic technician obtained and cardiologist interpreted organ-based ultrasound assessment.

● DIAGNOSIS AND TREATMENT

In this patient, the intra-abdominal pressure (IAP) was mildly elevated (IAP = 16 mm Hg), the conjunctivae remained fairly pink, and the CXR indicated a well-positioned oral endotracheal tube and no change in the cardiac silhouette with the exception of full pulmonary hila; no pneumothorax was identified, the central venous catheter was in good position, and both costophrenic angles were blunted. The ICU ultrasound, on the other hand, was quite abnormal with regard to global performance and chamber size leading to an emergency echocardiogram. The IVC was dilated at 4.2 cm and did not collapse with respiratory change. The right ventricle (RV) was mildly dilated, and the left ventricle (LV) was full and hypokinetic with septal bowing from right to left. The left atrium was dilated with an atrial diameter of 3.8 cm; pulmonary artery (PA) pressures were estimated to be elevated. The ECG demonstrated atrial fibrillation and suggested myocardial injury with T-wave inversions in V_2 and V_4 ST segments with R-wave progression failure consistent with anterior infarction; troponin-t was elevated at 2.8.

Standard treatment for acute myocardial infarction includes venodilatation, afterload reduction, supplemental oxygen, anticoagulation, beta-blockade for arrhythmia prevention and rate-related work reduction, and for specific patients, therapy for arterial occlusion (percutaneous coronary intervention [PCI] or fibrinolysis). This is followed by antiplatelet agents, continued afterload reduction, and statin therapy. For inpatients, a time metric from ischemia recognition to PCI time of ≤90 minutes is the standard of care; this parallels the "door to balloon" metric for those presenting to the emergency department.

Presentation Continued

Emergency cardiology consultation leads to rapid transport to the catheterization lab for intervention. Concomitantly, dobutamine is started in place of epinephrine for inotropic support as well as vasodilatation in light of the dilated ventricles and evidence of increased PA pressures by echocardiography. Cardiac catheterization leads to percutaneous transluminal coronary angioplasty (PTCA) and drug-eluting stent placement in the left anterior descending (LAD) and circumflex arteries but is complicated by progressively challenging ventilation marked by failure of CO_2 clearance as well as hypoxemia with a P/F ratio < 100. Progressive hypotension that is unresponsive to high-dose dobutamine and epinephrine is evaluated with an echocardiogram that shows global hypokinesis and full chamber sizes. The patient is evaluated for temporary support using extracorporeal membrane oxygenation (ECMO) to allow myocardial and pulmonary recovery.

● SURGICAL APPROACH

Surgical Decision-Making

The key elements involved in this decision are severity of illness, reversibility of the underlying disorder, bleeding risk, and anatomic access suitability as well as the absence of conditions that are incompatible with recovery and survival. Combined postintervention cardiac and secondary pulmonary failure that is not manageable with conventional techniques may be temporized with ECMO to allow recovery. Since both cardiac and pulmonary support is required, this patent is most suitable for venoarterial (VA) ECMO instead of venovenous (VV) ECMO in which native pump function without mechanical assistance is required. Intra-aortic balloon pumping alone would not be sufficient for this patient as pulmonary support is also required (Figure 123-1).

Key Technical Steps

It is essential to have excellent familiarity with all of the devices you intend to use, as well as to have the essential supplies for a back-up plan if your original one encounters difficulties requiring a plan change. Identify and mark the sites of cannulation for venous drainage and arterial inflow. Either the right atrium or the IVC may be used for venous drainage, and the common femoral artery is used for arterial inflow access due to its ease of cannulation. Another option for arterial inflow is a chimney graft to the right subclavian artery, which is particularly attractive in this patient with recent aortic surgery and a need to perfuse the aortic arch. Consider evaluating the intended site with ultrasonography to measure vessel diameter as an aid in cannula selection and to ensure that there is no venous clot or heavily calcified

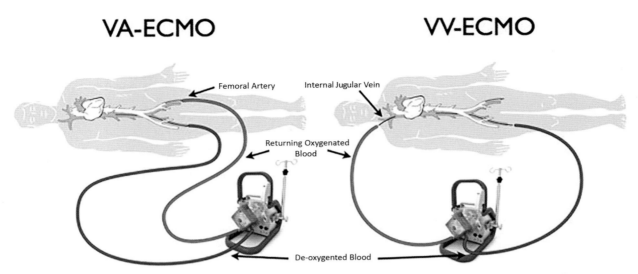

VA-ECMO

VV-ECMO

Femoral Artery

Internal Jugular Vein

Returning Oxygenated Blood

De-oxygented Blood

FIGURE 123-1. Schematic of venoarterial versus venovenous ECMO. (From Cove ME, MacLaren G. Clinical review: MCS for cardiogenic shock complicating acute myocardial infarction. *Crit Care.* 2010;14:235; originally published by BioMed Central with permission from MAQUET GmbH & Co. KG.)

arterial plaque that would drive alternate site selection. Consider concomitant placement of an antegrade femoral cannula to also direct a portion of the inflow down the limb to avoid ipsilateral limb ischemia based upon luminal partial occlusion by the main cannula, especially in those with preexisting evidence of peripheral arterial disease.

Preparation and sterile draping is required as is full barrier protection for team members in the room given arterial access using large-bore cannulae and arterial pressure. Anticoagulation using unfractionated heparin is given prior to cannulation to minimize both local and device thrombosis. Cannulation proceeds using Seldinger's technique most commonly and should employ the largest cannula that may be accommodated by the patient's vascular anatomy. The cannulae should be well secured

to avoid malpositioning or even dislodgement during routine ICU care. The cannula are attached to the primed ECMO circuit using a careful heparin flush technique to avoid the introduction of air bubbles into the circulation.

It is essential to monitor LV function after starting VA-ECMO using arterial waveform pulsatility as well as multiply repeated echocardiographic interrogations as LV function may acutely deteriorate. Diuresis for reduction of total body salt and water is commonly need in ECMO recipients regardless of modality and should be specifically considered. Ongoing monitoring of anticoagulation is similarly required to reduce clotting potential and thromboembolism. Continued vigilance for extremity ischemia distal to the site of arterial access is similarly important to monitor (Figure 123-2 and Table 123-1).

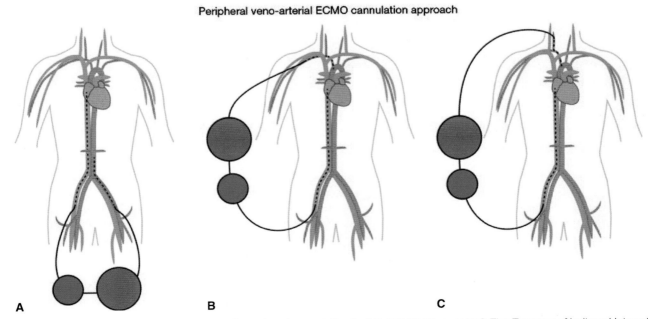

Peripheral veno-arterial ECMO cannulation approach

A   **B**   **C**

FIGURE 123-2. **A-C:** Common alternate sites of peripheral cannulation for VA-ECMO. (Copyright © The Trustees of Indiana University.)

Table 123-1	Veno-Arterial ECMO

Key Technical Steps

1. Determination of cannulation sites
2. Evaluation of cannula size
3. Anticoagulation
4. Seldinger's technique insertion of cannulae
5. Durable securing of cannulae
6. Connection to circuit
7. Evaluation of LV function
8. Adjustment to maintenance mechanical ventilation
9. Consideration of reduction of total body salt and water

Potential Pitfalls

- Vessel injury
- Cannula malposition
- Limb ischemia

Presentation Continued

Maintenance ventilation is initiated at a low rate (as oxygenation and CO_2 clearance is principally circuit driven) limiting peak airway pressure to <20 cm H_2O pressure to avoid biotrauma and reducing FIO_2 to <0.5. Common settings may include AC 6 to 10/pressure control = 20/40% FiO_2/+10 positive end-expiratory pressure (PEEP), but others may serve equally well and may be individualized to the underlying pulmonary process; given the light sedation, often used, an inhalation:exhalation (I:E) ratio driven approach may be better tolerated by those who are awake instead of a fixed inspiratory time approach.

● SPECIAL INTRAOPERATIVE CONSIDERATIONS

Patients with heavily calcified femoral vessels and those with femoral-based arterial reconstructions generally need an alternate arterial inflow site. The right common carotid artery, axillary artery, or the subclavian artery may be used as alternate access sites. A selective advantage of the subclavian site is that it also facilitates ambulation, which may be problematic when the carotid site is instead selected when this technique is used for pulmonary transplant patients who need VA-ECMO. The benefit in this patient is staying out of the groin as well as perfusing the aortic arch.

● POSTOPERATIVE MANAGEMENT

Titration goals once the VA-ECMO circuit is employed broadly include a $SaO_2 > 90\%$, a venous O_2 saturation (venous line sampled) approximately 75% of the arterial saturation

(parallels the normal A-Vo_2 difference), and age and comorbidity appropriate indices of adequate tissue perfusion including an appropriate MAP and lactate. Continuous evaluation for suitability for weaning should be undertaken to enable as rapid as possible transition back to native cardiac function driven circulation and nonpump managed oxygenation and CO_2 clearance.

Major complications of ECMO in general include bleeding (most common complication), limb ischemia, thromboembolism, vascular injury, and heparin-induced thrombocytopenia. There are additionally specific VA-ECMO complications that include:

1. Coronary artery hypoxemia due to reduced oxygen in the blood that fills the LV compared to the richly oxygenated blood that perfuses the viscera and lower extremities when using femoral cannulation
2. Cerebral hypoxemia
3. Pulmonary edema and parenchymal hemorrhage that is associated with left atrial or ventricular distension in the setting of poorly preserved LV function
4. Cardiac or aortic thrombosis in the setting of impaired LV outflow when retrograde aortic filling occurs via a femoral artery cannulation site
5. Neurologic injury that includes a range of toxic–metabolic encephalopathy to stroke, which is difficult to parse between elements unique to VA-ECMO as compared to those related to the underlying condition that necessitated ECMO as a rescue strategy

Case Conclusion

After 10 days, the patient's LV function has improved as has the PaO₂ and PaCO₂ triggering two successful trials of discontinuation of VA-ECMO. Accordingly, cannulae are removed, and the arterial site is compressed for 30 minutes. Consider ultrasound evaluation of the site after manual compression has been completed. Alternative approaches include using a closure device as well.

TAKE HOME POINTS

- ECMO is a rescue strategy that may support only pulmonary function or combined cardiac and pulmonary function.
- ECMO modality selection is essential as it drives cannulation site selection.
- Anticoagulation is required for ECMO and also underpins the most common complication, bleeding.
- Frequent echocardiographic interrogation of LV function is essential in VA-ECMO management and titration.
- VA-ECMO has a unique spectrum of complications compared to VV-ECMO.
- Ultrasound is an invaluable tool in all phases of the course of ECMO patient management.

- Optimal management of ECMO patients (initiation, titration, and weaning) requires a dedicated and trained team, and a dedicated and well-equipped center.

SUGGESTED READINGS

Biscotti M, Bachetta M. The "sport model": extracorporeal membrane oxygenation using the subclavian artery. *Ann Thorac Surg.* 2014;98(4):1487-1489.

Cannon JW, Gutsche JT, Brodie D. Optimal strategies for severe acute respiratory distress syndrome. *Crit Care Clin.* 2017;33(2):259-275.

Pellegrino V, Hockings LE, Davies A. Veno-arterial extracorporeal membrane oxygenation for adult cardiovascular failure. *Curr Opin Crit Care.* 2014:20(5):484-492; doi:10.1097/MCC.0000000000000141.

Posluszny J, Rycus PT, Bartlett RH, et al.; on behalf of the ELSO Member Centers. Outcome of adult respiratory failure patients receiving prolonged (≥14 days) ECMO. *Ann Surg.* 2016;263(3):573-581; doi:10.1097/SLA.0000000000001176.

Smith M, Vukomanovic A, Brodie D, Thiagarajan R, Rycus P, Buscher H. Duration of veno-arterial extracorporeal life support (VA ECMO) and outcome: an analysis of the Extracorporeal Life Support Organization (ELSO) registry. *Crit Care.* 2017;21:45. https://doi.org/10.1186/s13054-017-1633-1.

Terri S, Andrew G, Amandeep S, et al. Veno-arterial extracorporeal membrane oxygenation (VA-ECMO) for emergency cardiac support. *J Crit Care.* 2018;44:31-38. https://doi.org/10.1016/j.jcrc.2017.10.011.

Thiagarajan RR, Barbaro RP, Rycus PT, et al.; on behalf of the ELSO Member Centers. Extracorporeal life support organization registry international report 2016. *ASAIO J.* 2017;63(1):60-67; doi:10.1097/MAT.0000000000000475.

Acute Kidney Injury (Acute Renal Failure)

ANNA TYSON AND ANTHONY CHARLES

124

Based on the previous edition chapter "Acute Renal Failure" by April E. Mendoza and Anthony G. Charles

Presentation

A 63-year-old man presents to the emergency room complaining of acute-onset abdominal pain. He described the pain as initially located in the left lower quadrant but now generalized. He has developed nausea and vomiting. His last bowel movement was a day prior to presentation. He admits to fever and chills and has been diaphoretic. He denies prior episodes of similar abdominal pain.

His past medical history is significant for non-insulin-dependent diabetes mellitus for over 10 years controlled with metformin and essential hypertension managed with an angiotensin converting enzyme (ACE) inhibitor. His past surgical history is significant for an appendectomy 45 years ago. He has never undergone a screening colonoscopy. He has no known allergies.

His vitals revealed a temperature of 100°F, pulse rate of 120 per minute, respiratory rate of 32, and a blood pressure of 90/53. Physical exam showed an obese man, in acute painful distress. He has no jugular venous distension and his chest exam was unremarkable. Abdominal examination revealed generalized abdominal tenderness with rebound and guarding. The remainder of the exam revealed warm extremities with brisk capillary refill and no evidence of edema. Abdominal computed tomography (CT) with intravenous (IV) contrast shows free air and free fluid in the abdomen with significant inflammation around the sigmoid colon.

He is taken to the operating room for exploratory laparotomy, which confirms perforated sigmoid diverticulitis with extensive abdominal soilage. He undergoes a sigmoid colectomy and Hartman's procedure. The following morning, he remains mechanically ventilated. His vitals have remained stable; however, he has become oliguric with a urine output of only 15 mL per hour.

● DIFFERENTIAL DIAGNOSIS

Acute kidney injury (AKI) (previously acute renal failure) describes a spectrum of renal dysfunction, reflecting serum creatinine, glomerular filtration rate (GFR), and urine output. Unlike chronic kidney disease, AKI develops over hours to days. Recent consensus defines AKI as an increase in serum creatinine ≥0.3 mg/dL in 48 hours, an increase ≥1.5 times the baseline creatinine in 7 days, or a decrease in urine output to <3 mL/kg over 6 hours. AKI can also be characterized by the RIFLE criteria, which consists of five categories of renal dysfunction: risk, injury, failure, loss, and end-stage renal disease (Table 124-1).

AKI can be oliguric or nonoliguric. Nonoliguric renal failure is often reversible but may develop into oliguric failure without prompt recognition and treatment. Oliguria is defined as urine output <400 mL per day, <16.6 mL per hour, or <0.5 mL/kg/h in adults (<1.0 mL/kg/h in children weighing <10 kg). Anuria is defined as urine output <50 mL per day.

Early identification and treatment of AKI are crucial to prevent further progression of renal injury. In general, the etiology of AKI is organized into three groups: prerenal, renal, and postrenal (Table 124-2). Although this categorization is a useful guide to diagnosing AKI, physicians must remember that a patient's renal dysfunction may be multifactorial.

Table 124-1	The RIFLE Criteria
Risk	1.5-fold increase in serum creatinine[a] GFR decrease by 25% Urine output <0.5 mL/kg/h for 6 hours
Injury	Twofold increase in serum creatinine GFR decrease by 50% Urine output <0.5 mL/kg/h for 12 hours
Failure	Threefold increase in serum creatinine GFR decrease by 75% Urine output <0.5 mL/kg/h for 24 hours or anuria for 12 hours
Loss	Complete loss of kidney function (need for RRT) for more than 4 wk
ESRD	Complete loss of kidney function (e.g., need for RRT) for more than 3 mo

[a]Creatinine may not be elevated early in AKI despite reduced GFR as there may not have been enough time for creatinine to accumulate.

720

Table 124-2	Etiologies of Acute Kidney Injury		
Prerenal		**Renal**	**Postrenal**
• Hypovolemia • Mechanical ventilation • Abdominal compartment syndrome • Cardiomyopathy • Heart failure • Aortic stenosis • Dissecting aortic aneurysm • Malignant hypertension • Acutely decompensated liver disease with portal hypertension • Drugs that alter renal blood flow (NSAIDs, ACEIs, ARB)s		• Profound shock • Severe sepsis • Multiorgan failure • Myoglobinuria • Acute interstitial nephritis • Hypersensitivity reactions • DIC • TTP/HUS • Scleroderma • Nephrotoxic drugs (aminoglycosides, amphotericin, cisplatin) • Other nephrotoxins (ethylene glycol, CIAKI)	• Papillary necrosis • Retroperitoneal mass • Urethral stricture • Prostatic hypertrophy • Ureteral injury • Hematoma compressing the renal pelvis or ureter • Malignancy of the bladder, ureter, intestine, or uterus • Neurologic disorder causing urinary retention

Prerenal

Prerenal causes of AKI describe processes that decrease renal blood flow. The most common cause of renal hypoperfusion in the postoperative setting is hypovolemia, whether due to blood loss or volume depletion. Hypovolemia secondary to third spacing, and insensible fluid loss should be high on the differential as a cause of this patient's oliguria owing to his peritonitis and emergent laparotomy. However, other causes of renal hypoperfusion should be entertained.

Medications such as nonsteroidal anti-inflammatory drugs (NSAIDs), ACE inhibitors, and angiotensin receptor blockers may alter renal blood flow and exacerbate AKI. Consider holding these medications in the postoperative patient with AKI. Redistributive shock, such as cardiogenic or septic shock, particularly in patients with a long-standing history of diabetes and hypertension may result in poor renal perfusion. Abdominal compartment syndrome with evidence of increased bladder pressures, hypotension, and increased peak inspiratory pressures on the ventilator must also be considered.

Prerenal disorders account for 20% to 40% of cases of AKI in intensive care unit (ICU) patients. The AKI in these patients can often be corrected by treating the underlying condition, but persistent hypoperfusion of the kidney may lead to acute tubular necrosis (ATN).

Renal

Renal causes of acute renal dysfunction describe diseases of the renal parenchyma, namely, intrinsic glomerular disease (nephritic or nephrotic), ATN, or acute interstitial nephritis (AIN). Glomerular disease may be primary (idiopathic) or secondary (due to a paraneoplastic syndrome, medication, or other systemic diseases). ATN is the most common intrinsic renal disorder and accounts for 40% to 50% of

AKI in ICU patients. The etiology of ATN is numerous, but potential causes in the surgical patient include ischemia and nephrotoxins such as myoglobin and hemoglobin, contrast-induced acute kidney injury (CIAKI), antibiotics (aminoglycosides, cephalosporins, sulfonamides, vancomycin), and anesthetic agents (methoxyflurane, enflurane). AIN is often drug induced (due to certain antibiotics, nonsteroidal anti-inflammatory drugs or NSAIDs, antiepileptics, or diuretics).

Postrenal

Postrenal causes of renal dysfunction are uncommon (10%) and can often be identified by physical examination. Removing or replacing the urinary catheter can usually diagnose an enlarged prostate or a clogged catheter. Physical examination can identify a full bladder, or a bladder scan can be used in the case of obese patients. Direct ureteral injury has an incidence of 1% to 2% during abdominal surgery. Injuries include ligation, transection, devascularization, and partial laceration of the ureter. Though rare, bilateral ureteral injury will present with significant acute renal dysfunction.

Presentation Continued

The patient is extubated the following morning and is awake but confused. Physical examination reveals normal heart and chest sounds. His abdomen is mildly distended and generalized edema is present. He denies pain except for tenderness at the incision site on palpation. His central venous pressure (CVP) ranges from 4 to 6 cm H_2O. His current blood pressure recordings have been between 100 to 110 mm Hg systolic and 50 to 80 mm Hg diastolic. Review of the chart shows a preoperative creatinine of 1.5 mg/dL with a postoperative creatinine now at 3.2 mg/dL.

● WORKUP

The initial diagnostic evaluation for acute renal dysfunction should start with a review of the patient's history and a physical examination. In particular, check to see if the patient has a history of pre-existing renal disease, as this carries a higher risk of developing postoperative acute renal failure. Adjunctive invasive monitoring, urinary catheterization, trends in urine and serum chemistry (sodium, potassium, urea, and creatinine), urine microscopy, and ancillary tests such as bladder and renal ultrasonography play an additional role in identifying and categorizing the cause of renal dysfunction and subsequent renal failure.

Examination

Assessing the neurologic function, perfusion status, and signs of volume overload gives the clinician a better idea of the cause, severity, and progression of renal dysfunction. This patient has signs of volume overload as evidenced by peripheral edema. His abdomen is mildly distended, but not tense, which points away from abdominal compartment syndrome. Neither rectal nor stomal exam reveals melena, frank blood, or evidence of prostate enlargement. The bladder is not palpable. His catheter was flushed to ensure no obvious obstruction in the tubing. Physical exam findings important in the diagnosis of AKI are described in Table 124-3.

Laboratory and Ancillary Testing

New-onset oliguria should prompt a workup to distinguish between prerenal and renal causes of oliguria. This should include checking serum and urine electrolytes, urinalysis, and urine microscopy. Common findings on urine microscopy are listed in Table 124-4.

The addition of urine electrolytes is imperative in the workup of new-onset renal dysfunction. Sodium reabsorption increases in the setting of renal hypoperfusion (in an attempt by the kidneys to preserve circulating volume). As such, urine sodium is usually decreased (<20 mEq/L) in patients with prerenal renal failure. In contrast, patients with intrinsic renal disease lose the ability to concentrate urine, resulting in high levels of urine sodium (>40 mEq/L). However, one must remember that in patients with pre-existing renal insufficiency, patients on certain diuretics, and elderly patients, urine sodium may be falsely elevated, and a high urine sodium level in these patients does not rule out a prerenal cause of their oliguria. Liver cirrhosis and other medical problems also affect the excretion of sodium. Urea and nitrogen by-products remain relatively constant and should be considered in these circumstances (Table 124-5).

Calculating the fractional excretion of sodium (FENa) is a useful adjunct to the interpretation of urine electrolytes. FENa represents the ratio of sodium clearance to creatinine clearance by the kidneys. FENa < 1% is associated with prerenal conditions (the kidney preserves the ability to filter sodium and concentrate urine), while FENa > 2% is associated with renal injury (the kidney loses the ability to maximally concentrate urine). In the setting of furosemide and bumetanide use, calculating the

Table 124-3 Physical Exam and Possible Indications of AKI

Physical Exam	Possible Indications
Vitals signs	
Temperature	Possible infection
Blood pressure	Hypertension: nephrotic syndrome, malignant hypertension Hypotension: hypovolemia, redistributive shock
Heart rate	Tachycardia: shock, arrhythmias Bradycardia: inadequate renal perfusion
Weight loss/gain	Fluid overload (edema) or hypovolemia
Mouth	Dehydration
Neck	Distended jugular veins: fluid overload possibly of cardiac origin Collapsed jugular veins: hypovolemia
Chest	Pulmonary crackles/rales: fluid overload New murmurs/rubs: heart failure, endocarditis, pericarditis
Abdomen	Bladder fullness, masses: genitourinary obstruction
Rectum	Enlarged prostate
Skin	Rash: interstitial nephritis, drug rash Blue toes: atheroembolic events

Table 124-4 Common Urinalysis and Urine Microscopy Findings and Possible Indications

Laboratory Finding	Possible Indication
Muddy brown/granular casts	ATN
Epithelial cell casts	ATN
Red cell casts	Vasculitis, glomerulonephritis
Sterile pyuria	Interstitial nephritis
Proteinuria	Glomerular disease
Uniform, round RBC[a]	Extrarenal bleeding
Dysmorphic RBC	Glomerular disease

[a]RBC, red blood cell.

Table 124-5	Key Lab Findings of Prerenal and Renal Causes of AKI	
Laboratory Test	**Prerenal Findings**	**Renal Findings**
BUN to creatinine ratio	>20:1	10–20:1
Urine specific gravity	>1.020	1.010–1.020
Urine sediment	Hyaline casts	Granular/epithelial casts
Urine sodium	>20 mEq/L	>40 mEq/L
FeNa percent	<1%	>2%
FeUrea percent	<35%	>35%
Urine osmolality	<350 mOsmol/kg	>500 mOsmol/kg

fractional excretion of urea (FEUrea) may be more appropriate and accurate (Table 124-6).

Cardiac dysfunction remains a potential cause of oliguria. In critically ill patients, EKG, cardiac enzymes, echocardiography, chest radiograph, and serum chemistry panel should be considered. Renal ultrasonography can be useful if the initial workup does not identify the diagnosis. This is a fast, noninvasive method to evaluate obstructive causes of renal failure and identify signs of chronic disease.

Invasive Monitoring

Hypovolemia is the most common cause of postoperative oliguria and must be identified and corrected rapidly. Patients with new-onset oliguria should have indwelling urinary catheters placed to accurately measure urine output during the workup and initial treatment of renal failure. Central venous and arterial catheters and/or pulse contour

Table 124-6	Important Formulas
Creatinine Clearance (Men)
CL_{Cr} (mL/min) $= \dfrac{(140-age) \times weight\ (kg)}{72 \times serum\ creatinine\ (mg/dL)}$
Creatinine Clearance (Women)
CL_{Cr} (mL/min) $= 0.85 \times CL_{Cr}$ for men
Fractional Excretion of Sodium (FENa)
$\dfrac{Urine[Na] \times Plasma[Cr]}{Plasma[Na] \times Urine[Cr]} \times 100$
Fractional Excretion of Urea (FEUrea)
$\dfrac{Urine[Urea] \times Plasma[Cr]}{Plasma[Urea] \times Urine[Cr]} \times 100$

continuous cardiac output (PiCCO) monitors provide useful hemodynamic measurements to assess the patient's volume status and perfusion. Low CVP may indicate hypovolemia. Similarly, low central venous oxyhemoglobin saturation ($ScvO_2$) may indicate low cardiac output, either from low preload or cardiac dysfunction.

Renal biopsy is rarely indicated in the acute setting. This invasive test is reserved for cases when all tests and workup have remained unrevealing and the condition continues without improvement. That being said, renal biopsy may be useful for the evaluation of acute glomerulonephritis or vasculitis or isolated hematuria with proteinuria.

Presentation Continued

The patient's urine output has continually decreased now with a total of 50 mL of urine in 24 hours, although he has received several liters of fluid. He is 15 L positive and now has crackles bilaterally on chest exam with increasing extremity edema. His CVP is elevated at 15. Cardiac enzymes and BNP (brain natriuretic peptide) are within normal limits, and he has had no EKG changes consistent with evolving heart disease. His creatinine has climbed to 6 mg/dL from his baseline of 1.5 mg/dL. His BUN (blood urea nitrogen) is approaching 70 mg/dL, and his ABG (arterial blood gas) reveals a pH of 7.25. A urinalysis shows epithelial cell casts. Renal replacement therapy (RRT) is now considered the next best step in his management.

● DIAGNOSIS AND TREATMENT

The patient is diagnosed with AKI secondary to ATN. Underresuscitation in the face of sepsis, emergent surgery, and third spacing likely resulted in his renal dysfunction and ischemic injury that further evolved into ATN. Underlying renal insufficiency made him especially susceptible to this injury.

Early identification and supportive measures are the only treatment options and must be initiated rapidly to prevent/reduce further injury. Once supportive measures prove futile and renal dysfunction continues, RRT should be initiated.

Fluid Resuscitation

Administering a fluid challenge remains the gold standard for initial management of AKI. Lactated Ringers and other potassium-containing solutions should be avoided to prevent hyperkalemia. In general, a fluid challenge of 1 to 3 L crystalloid is recommended, although fluid resuscitation should be targeted to physiologic endpoints, such as CVP, mean arterial pressure (MAP), and urine output. Overly aggressive resuscitation can lead to pulmonary congestion and worsening of respiratory function. Colloid solutions are more expensive and offer no benefit over crystalloids for initial resuscitation. Low-dose dopamine (2 µg/kg/min) has no proven benefit in acute oliguric renal failure.

Diuretics

For patients with AKI in the setting of fluid overload, judicious use of diuretics may be indicated. Loop diuretics are preferred as first-line therapy, beginning with 40 to 80 mg of IV furosemide. If the patient does not respond within 30 to 60 minutes, the dose may be doubled. If the patient still does not respond, clinicians may consider adding a thiazide diuretic. However, patients that remain unresponsive to a short trial of diuretics should progress to RRT.

Renal Replacement Therapy (RRT)

Patients with persistently worsening renal function despite supportive measures should be evaluated for RRT. Specific indications for RRT are described in Table 124-7. Hyperkalemia and metabolic acidosis are two of the most common acute indications for RRT. If these imbalances are mild, and the underlying AKI is reversible, physicians can attempt pharmacologic management of the hyperkalemia or metabolic acidosis. Severe imbalances, especially in the setting of fluid overload, are best managed by RRT.

Several options for RRT exist, the two most common being hemodialysis and hemofiltration. Hemodialysis removes solutes from the blood by diffusion by the use of a concentration gradient. This method allows for rapid clearance of solutes, permitting intermittent hemodialysis. However, hemodialysis also results in significant fluid shifts during treatment sessions, increasing the risk for hypotension. Hemofiltration, on the other hand, clears solutes by the use of a pressure gradient. This process is slower than hemodialysis and has less risk of hypotension but must be performed continuously. Removal of solutes is more gradual and physiologic, making it a better choice for many ICU patients who cannot tolerate large fluid or electrolyte shifts.

Table 124-7	Indications for Renal Replacement Therapy
Acidosis refractory to medical therapy (pH < 7.1)	
Acute, severe electrolyte changes (commonly hyperkalemia)	
Intoxications (methanol, ethanol)	
Volume overload	
Uremia—any of the below symptoms or findings:	
Encephalopathy	
Severe azotemia (BUN > 100 mg/dL)	
Significant bleeding	
Uremic pericarditis	

PROGNOSIS

Most patients with AKI recover renal function; however, they may not return to their pre-injury baseline. Even mild degrees of AKI in the setting of nonoliguric renal failure are associated with increased morbidity and mortality. The RIFLE criteria are associated with worse prognosis. Compared to patients without AKI, relative risk for mortality increases by 2.4 (CI 1.94 to 2.97) for risk, 4.15 (CI 3.14 to 5.48) for injury, and 6.37 (CI 5.14 to 7.9) for failure categories.

CLINICAL APPROACH TO ACUTE RENAL DYSFUNCTION

Adequate perioperative resuscitation is crucial for preventing renal dysfunction. Invasive monitoring may prove a helpful adjunct in surgical patients with AKI. Mortality is increased in this subset of critically ill patients.

Key clinical components:

1. Examine the patient.
2. Ensure proper perioperative resuscitation; minimize exposure to nephrotoxins; monitor fluid balance.
3. Employ the trends in serum and urine chemistry to help confirm the diagnosis and guide therapeutic endpoints.
4. Consider adjunctive monitoring such as echocardiogram prior to invasive monitoring.
5. Consider the need for RRT if patient meets criteria.

Figure 124-1 describes the initial workup and management of patients with clinical findings consistent with AKI.

Pitfalls in management include:

1. Failure to examine the patient and review pre-existing comorbidities
2. Indiscriminate use of diuretics in the face of hypotension and underresuscitation
3. Prolonged use of diuretics when patient meets criteria for dialysis
4. Ignoring respiratory status in acute renal failure
5. Misinterpreting information gathered from invasive monitoring

Case Conclusion

The patient was started on RRT. His pre-existing comorbidities made him susceptible to acute renal dysfunction and ultimately renal loss when his clinical course was complicated by hypotension and sepsis. The patient required dialysis for 6 weeks and eventually regained renal function. His favorable outcome is likely a result of proper resuscitation and the appropriate use of RRT.

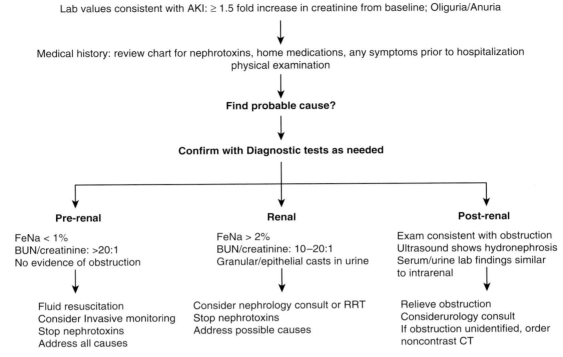

Lab values consistent with AKI: ≥ 1.5 fold increase in creatinine from baseline; Oliguria/Anuria

Medical history: review chart for nephrotoxins, home medications, any symptoms prior to hospitalization physical examination

Find probable cause?

Confirm with Diagnostic tests as needed

Pre-renal

FeNa < 1%
BUN/creatinine: >20:1
No evidence of obstruction

Fluid resuscitation
Consider Invasive monitoring
Stop nephrotoxins
Address all causes

Renal

FeNa > 2%
BUN/creatinine: 10–20:1
Granular/epithelial casts in urine

Consider nephrology consult or RRT
Stop nephrotoxins
Address possible causes

Post-renal

Exam consistent with obstruction
Ultrasound shows hydronephrosis
Serum/urine lab findings similar
to intrarenal

Relieve obstruction
Considerurology consult
If obstruction unidentified, order
noncontrast CT

FIGURE 124-1. Diagnostic workup and evaluation of a patient with oliguria.

TAKE HOME POINTS

- Use baseline chemistries to assess renal function.
- Ensure adequate perioperative resuscitation.
- Surgical patients must be assumed to have a prerenal cause until proven otherwise.
- All types of redistributive shock are also prerenal causes of AKI and renal failure.
- Be cognizant of comorbidities.
- Avoid nephrotoxic medications, such as aminoglycosides, IV contrast, etc.
- Diuretics may be utilized only after correction of hypovolemia.
- Use of diuretics does not alter the course of renal failure.
- Consider RRT when patient meets criteria.
- Renal failure is associated with increased mortality in surgical patients.

SUGGESTED READINGS

Bellomo R, Ronco C, Kellum JA, et al. Acute renal failure-definition, outcome measures, animal models, fluid therapy and information technology needs: the Second International Consensus Conference of the Acute Dialysis Quality Initiative (ADQI) Group. *Crit Care.* 2004;8:204-212.

Diskin CJ, Stokes TJ, Dansby LM, et al. The comparative benefits of the fractional excretion of urea and sodium in various azotemic oliguric states. *Nephron Clin Pract.* 2010;114:145-150.

Fatehi P, Hsu C. Evaluation of acute kidney injury (acute renal failure) among hospitalized patients. In: Palevsky PM, Sheridan AM, eds. *UpToDate.* 2016. https://www.uptodate.com/contents/evaluation-of-acute-kidney-injury-among-hospitalized-adult-patients

Marino PL.Oliguria and acute renal failure. In: *The ICU Book.* 4th ed. Philadelphia, PA: Lippincott Williams & Wilkins; 2013.

Mullin RJ. Acute renal failure. In: Cameron JL, eds. *Current Surgical Therapy.* Philadelphia, PA: Mosby; 2008;1200-1206.

Okusa MD, Rosner MH. Overview of the management of acute kidney injury (acute renal failure). In: Palevsky PM, Sheridan AM, eds. *UpToDate.* 2016.

Patschan D, Müller GA. Acute kidney injury. *J Inj Violence Res.* 2015;7(1):19-26.

Stafford RE, Cairns BA, Meyer AA. Renal failure. In: Souba WW, Fink MP, Jurkouch GS, et al., eds. *ACS Surgery: Principles and Practice.* New York, NY: WebMD Professional Publishing; 2006: 1408-1412.

Thomas ME, Blaine C, Dawnay A, et al. The definition of acute kidney injury and its use in practice. *Kidney Int.* 2015;87:62-73.

Adrenal Insufficiency

125

KAZUHIDE MATSUSHIMA AND HEIDI L. FRANKEL

Based on the previous edition chapter "Adrenal Insufficiency" by Steven R. Allen and Heidi L. Frankel

Presentation

A 67-year-old female sustained multiple injuries in a motor vehicle crash 7 days ago. These injuries included a subarachnoid hemorrhage and bilateral lower extremity fractures, necessitating several days of ventilator support. Over the past 24 hours, she has required reintubation (using rapid sequence methodology employing etomidate and succinylcholine) for increasing respiratory difficulty and has developed progressive tachycardia and hypotension despite adequate fluid administration.

Her past medical history is significant for chronic liver disease secondary to hepatitis C, chronic obstructive pulmonary disease (COPD), hypertension, diabetes, and rheumatoid arthritis for which she takes 15 mg of prednisone daily.

● DIFFERENTIAL DIAGNOSIS

A broad differential diagnosis is pertinent to identify and treat all potential etiologies leading to her hemodynamic instability. Due to the patient's intubation and underlying pulmonary disease, ventilator-associated pneumonia leading to sepsis and septic shock must be considered. Other pulmonary causes, such as a pulmonary embolism (PE), may also contribute to this clinical picture. Additionally, with her age and multiple comorbidities, an acute cardiac event, such as a myocardial infarction (MI), is possible. Her orthopedic injuries also predispose her to fat emboli. Finally, adrenal insufficiency (AI) must be considered as she was intubated with etomidate, which has been found to cause AI, although less likely after a bolus dose, and her chronic use of steroids. Other etiologies of AI should also be considered in critically ill patients.

Presentation Continued

On physical exam, she is an obese woman who appears her stated age. She is arousable but does not consistently follow commands.

Her vital signs demonstrate a temperature of 38.6°C, a regular heart rate of 130/min, and blood pressure of 85/40 mmHg on continuous norepinephrine administration. Her respiratory rate is 25/min on the ventilator with a FiO₂ of 0.6, and positive end-expiratory pressure (PEEP) of 7.5 cmH₂O. Her current oxygen saturation is 92%. Her current central venous pressure is 10 mmHg, and her urine output is only 10 mL per hour. She has received three 1 L boluses of crystalloid with no improvement in hemodynamic status. On further workup, blood cultures were consistently negative. Her white blood count was within normal limits of 11,000 mm³ and hemoglobin was stable at 9.7 g/dL. The electrolyte panel demonstrated sodium of 131 mmol/L and potassium of 5.3 mmol/L. Liver function tests revealed mildly elevated transaminases with total bilirubin of 2.1 mg/dL. The CT scan of the chest was negative for a PE, and her echocardiogram demonstrated an ejection fraction of 65% with no obvious wall motion abnormalities. Cardiac enzymes were not elevated.

● DIAGNOSIS AND TREATMENT

In the face of hemodynamic instability unresponsive to fluid resuscitation and dependent on vasopressors and having ruled out other etiologies including sepsis, PE, and acute MI, AI is the one likely diagnosis that remains. AI seems relevant in light of her chronic steroid use and severe stress from injury. Further, AI is common in patients with acute and chronic liver disease. Other signs that suggest the diagnosis of AI include persistent, unexplained fever, weakness, and the inability to wean the ventilator support as well as hyponatremia and hyperkalemia. Other tests that may point toward the diagnosis of AI include mild eosinophilia with mean eosinophil counts of 3.5% versus 0.9% in those with normal adrenal function. These laboratory abnormalities are, however, more likely in the face of chronic AI.

Adrenal function may be assessed by several tests although none are considered to be extremely reliable. The random cortisol level is most helpful. Cortisol is normally secreted in a diurnal cycle. However, this diurnal variation is often lost in the critically ill patient. Thus, cortisol may be assayed at any time in the critically ill patient. Within the literature, many values have been proposed as the appropriate minimum value (range, 10 to 34 µg/dL); however, many would agree that a random cortisol over 18 is a normal response to stress. The results of random cortisol level should be carefully interpreted in patients with certain disorders that are related to cortisol-binding globulin excess or deficiency including chronic liver disease or obesity. Furthermore, cortisol level can be inaccurate in patients on chronic glucocorticoid supplementation. While the adreno-corticotropic hormone (ACTH) stimulation test may also be diagnostic and has been used over the decades, the use of the ACTH stimulation test should not be used to determine the indication for treatment with glucocorticoid. This test is conducted by administering 250 µg of ACTH (cosyntropin) either intravenously or intramuscularly. Cortisol levels are measured before and then 30 and 60 minutes after administration of the cosyntropin. This test may be performed at any time of the day. The "delta 9" may be helpful in making the diagnosis of AI. In a multicenter, randomized trial, Annane demonstrated that those patients who showed a change in baseline cortisol levels by ≤9 µg/dL at 30 or 60 minutes during the ACTH stimulation test had lower mortality rates if they received corticosteroids. This test is thought to demonstrate adrenal reserve in the face of critical illness or sepsis but does not assess the integrity of the hypothalamic–pituitary–adrenal axis. It is also argued that those patients who are maximally stressed may be effectively secreting the maximum amount of cortisol. Therefore, while it may be sufficient, the delta value may not be very high and may be <9 µg/dL. The utility of the delta 9 may be limited for this reason. More important, the multicenter CORTICUS trial did not report outcome differences between responders and nonresponders to a stimulation test. Thus, the use of a cosyntropin stimulation test of cortisol to define AI has fallen out of favor. Free cortisol may also be helpful in identifying AI. More than 90% of cortisol is bound to proteins including cortisol-binding globulin and albumin. Experts would agree that the biologically active portion of cortisol is that which is free, or not bound to proteins. Delayed test results make this test impractical in critically ill patients. More work must

be done to assess the true utility of this test and to develop a more clinically relevant diagnostic aid.

Other tests exist but should not be utilized in the critically ill population and include the insulin tolerance test and metyrapone test. The insulin tolerance test may lead to profound hypoglycemia, while the metyrapone test may exacerbate an adrenal crisis.

Finally, the diagnosis of acute AI in the patient with liver failure is a difficult one. Much literature relies on use of an ACTH stimulation test; however, it is not evident that the delta 9 strategy is any more valid in this patient population than it is overall.

Presentation Continued

Since the differential diagnosis had been narrowed to include AI without any other obvious cause of the hemodynamic instability, a random cortisol level was drawn and found to be 8 mg/dL. Given strong suspicion in the setting of hemodynamic instability, it was determined that the patient should be treated for AI.

● TREATMENT OF AI

AI may be separated into AI in those who regularly take exogenous corticosteroids for other medical problems such as rheumatoid arthritis or asthma, also known as secondary AI and acute AI. Faced with the effects of AI, one must appropriately supplement the patient with corticosteroids (Table 125-1). For those on chronic steroids in the face of stress from critical illness, one should consider increasing the dose of corticosteroids. How long one should supply the elevated dose or whether an elevated dose is even required is not well described in the literature.

Hydrocortisone is the corticosteroid of choice as both prednisone and cortisone require hydroxylation to obtain the active compound of prednisolone and cortisol, respectively. One must consider the replacement of mineralocorticoids

Table 125-1	Corticosteroid Equivalents		
Corticosteroid	**Glucocorticoid Potency**	**Mineralocorticoid Potency**	**Equivalent Dosage (Glucocorticoid Potency, mg)**
Cortisone	0.8	1.0	25
Hydrocortisone	1.0	1.0	20
Prednisolone	4	0.8	5
Methylprednisolone	5	0.5	4
Triamcinolone	5	0	4
Fludrocortisone	10	12.5	NA
Dexamethasone	25	0	0.75

as well in AI. This is not necessary if hydrocortisone is used due to the combined activity of both glucocorticoids and mineralocorticoids. However, the major protocol difference between two large trials that had discordant results in patients with septic shock was that the "positive" trial also included use of a mineralocorticoid in addition to administration of hydrocortisone.

The administration of hydrocortisone (150 to 200 mg daily for 5 to 7 days) has been shown to lead to a decreased vasopressor requirement as well as improved organ dysfunction, fewer ventilator days, fewer ICU days, and most importantly lower 28-day mortality. The exact dose is controversial as many studies have demonstrated positive effects with varying dosages ranging from 50 mg every 6 hours to 100 mg of hydrocortisone every 8 hours with a treatment length of 1 to 5 days.

A 2002 study by Annane and associates demonstrated a 28-day survival benefit in patients with septic shock and AI who received both hydrocortisone and fludrocortisone with no difference in adverse events between the study group and the placebo control group. However, one must use caution as a more recent study known as the CORTICUS trial demonstrated no significant difference in mortality between patients who received hydrocortisone versus placebo. Additionally, there was no difference in patients who did not have a response to the ACTH stimulation test compared to those who did respond. While shock was reversed more quickly in those who received hydrocortisone, there was no survival benefit. A recent meta-analysis by Annane confirmed these results. It remains unknown whether the administration of fludrocortisone (high mineralocorticoid potency) in addition to hydrocortisone is associated with survival benefit in the treatment of patients with AI.

Finally, literature is not conclusive that steroid administration in those with AI in the face of liver failure will result in improved outcomes.

Case Conclusion

The patient was treated with 50 mg of hydrocortisone every 6 hours for 5 days. Within several hours of her first dose of steroids, her hemodynamic status stabilized and the pressor support was weaned without incident, and she was subsequently extubated. She was transitioned from hydrocortisone to oral prednisone as her condition improved, and she was able to take medications by mouth. She was later discharged from the intensive care unit in stable condition on her home dose of prednisone.

TAKE HOME POINTS

- AI may present with subtle signs that mimic other clinical etiologies including sepsis, pulmonary embolus, and acute MI.
- One must establish a broad differential diagnosis in order appropriately rule out each of the life-threatening entities.

- Clinical signs may include hypotension, tachycardia, and fever as well as weakness and an inability to wean the patient from the ventilator.
- Laboratory studies that may point toward AI include hyponatremia and hyperkalemia as well as a mild eosinophilia, although these are more common in those with chronic AI.
- The diagnosis of AI may be made by a random cortisol level. The use of an ACTH stimulation test is usually not required. The treatment of AI should be not delayed while laboratory results are pending, particularly in patients with septic shock.
- Treatment with hydrocortisone at a dose of 50 to 100 mg every 6 to 8 hours is considered the preferred standard. The length of the treatment course is dependent on the patient's clinical response.

SUGGESTED READINGS

Annane D, et al. Corticosteroids in the treatment of severe sepsis and septic shock in adults: a systematic review. *JAMA.* 2009;301:2362-2375.

Annane D, et al. Effect of treatment with low doses of hydrocortisone and fludrocortisone on mortality in patients with septic shock. *JAMA.* 2002;288:862-871.

Annetta M, et al. Use of corticosteroids in critically ill septic patients: a review of mechanisms of adrenal insufficiency in sepsis and treatment. *Curr Drug Targets.* 2009;10:887-894.

Cooper MS, Stewart PM. Adrenal insufficiency in critical illness. *J Intensive Care Med.* 2007;22:348-362.

Cooper MS, Stewart PM. Corticosteroid insufficiency in acutely ill patients. *N Engl J Med.* 2003;348:727-734.

Edwin SB, Walker PL. Controversies surrounding the use of etomidate for rapid sequence intubation in patients with suspected sepsis. *Ann Pharmacother.* 2010;44:1307-1313.

Fede G, et al. Adrenocortical dysfunction in liver disease: a systematic review. *Hepatology.* 2012;55:1282-1291.

Grossman AB. Clinical review#: the diagnosis and management of central hypoadrenalism. *J Clin Endocrinol Metab.* 2010;95:4855-4863.

Hamrahian A. Adrenal function in critically ill patients: how to test? When to treat? *Cleve Clin J Med.* 2005;72:427-432.

Johnson KL, Rn CR. The hypothalamic-pituitary-adrenal axis in critical illness. *AACN Clin Issues.* 2006;17:39-49.

Marik PE, Gayowski T, Starzl TE; Hepatic Cortisol Research and Adrenal Pathophysiology Study Group. The hepatoadrenal syndrome: a common yet unrecognized clinical condition. *Crit Care Med.* 2005;33:1254-1259.

Marik PE, et al. Recommendations for the diagnosis and management of corticosteroid insufficiency in critically ill adult patients: consensus statements from an international task force by the American College of Critical Care Medicine. *Crit Care Med.* 2008;36:1937-1949.

Nylen ES, Muller B. Endocrine changes in critical illness. *J Intensive Care Med.* 2004;19:67-82.

Rivers EP, et al. Adrenal insufficiency in high-risk surgical ICU patients. *Chest.* 2001;119:889-896.

Sprung CL, et al. Hydrocortisone therapy for patients with septic shock. *N Engl J Med.* 2008;358:111-124.

Trifan A, et al. Update on adrenal insufficiency in patients with liver cirrhosis. *World J Gastroenterol.* 2013;19:445-456.

Acute Respiratory Distress Syndrome (ARDS)

126

LILLIAN S. KAO

Based on the previous edition chapter "Acute Respiratory Distress Syndrome (ARDS)" by Pauline K. Park, Krishnan Raghavendran, and Lena M. Napolitano

Presentation

A 65-year-old female underwent an urgent left hemicolectomy for a partially obstructing colon cancer. She has multiple comorbidities including coronary artery disease, hypertension, and chronic renal failure requiring hemodialysis. On postoperative day 5, she develops fever, abdominal pain, and leukocytosis. Abdominal radiographs confirm extensive pneumoperitoneum. Emergent laparotomy confirms anastomotic disruption. Resection of the anastomosis with end colostomy and Hartman's procedure is performed. The patient develops worsening severe hypoxemia in the operating room, with a PaO$_2$ of 85 mm Hg on FiO$_2$ 1.0. She is maintained intubated and mechanically ventilated and is admitted to the surgical intensive care unit (ICU) postoperatively.

● DIFFERENTIAL DIAGNOSIS

The differential diagnosis in surgical patients with severe hypoxemia and acute respiratory failure includes bacterial pneumonia and cardiogenic or noncardiogenic pulmonary edema. This patient could have heart failure leading to pulmonary edema or volume overload related to her chronic renal failure. If the hypoxemia is of sudden onset, then aspiration pneumonitis or pulmonary embolus should be considered. In this patient with an anastomotic disruption, acute respiratory distress syndrome (ARDS) should be at the top of the list. ARDS is a syndrome defined by (1) the presence of bilateral pulmonary infiltrates of acute onset within 1 week of a known clinical insult; (2) PaO$_2$:FiO$_2$ (P/F) ratio of ≤300; and (3) respiratory failure not fully explained by volume overload. It is important to establish a definitive diagnosis in patients with severe hypoxemia, as definitive treatment strategies must be aligned with the diagnosis.

● WORKUP

The workup for ARDS includes diagnostic imaging and laboratory tests to exclude the other potential diagnoses of the acute hypoxemic respiratory failure. ARDS is ultimately a clinical diagnosis, excluding other etiologies of severe hypoxemia. ARDS-associated mortality rates remain high, at approximately 40%, and therefore an early diagnosis is critical to initiation of optimal management.

Chest Radiograph

This patient had a normal chest radiograph preoperatively and developed bilateral infiltrates with the development of abdominal sepsis (Figure 126-1). The bilateral opacities are not explained fully by pleural effusions, lobar or lung collapse, or nodules.

Transthoracic Echocardiography

This diagnostic test is used to evaluate for cardiogenic pulmonary edema. This patient's echocardiogram demonstrated a hyperdynamic state with an estimated ejection fraction of 70% and no evidence of left ventricular dysfunction, left atrial hypertension, or valvular disease. This is consistent with her diagnosis of abdominal sepsis and does not confirm a diagnosis of heart failure. There is no evidence of right heart strain or right ventricular dysfunction that may be present in patients with pulmonary embolus.

Laboratory Tests

Arterial blood gas confirms hypoxemia, PaO$_2$ of 85 mm Hg on FiO$_2$ 1.0, which confirms a P/F ratio of 85 which is ≤300 mm Hg. No other specific laboratory tests confirm a diagnosis of ARDS.

Cultures

Respiratory cultures should be obtained to evaluate for possible bacterial or aspiration pneumonia as the etiology of the patient's acute respiratory failure. Since the patient is intubated, use of bronchoscopy or mini bronchoalveolar lavage to obtain quantitative bacteriology is preferred. Additionally, in a patient with suspected ARDS associated with sepsis, cultures (i.e., blood and intra-abdominal) may help guide treatment of the underlying etiology once source control has been obtained.

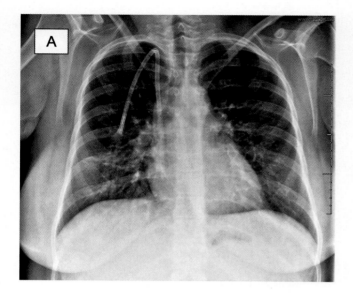

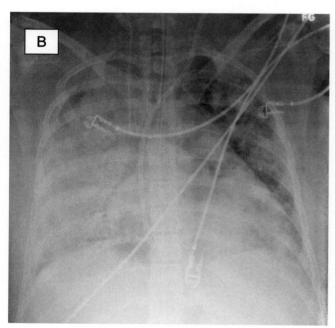

FIGURE 126-1. Preoperative chest radiograph (**A**) and on ICU admission (**B**).

Electrocardiogram

Electrocardiogram (EKG) reveals sinus tachycardia with no conduction abnormalities. In patients with pulmonary embolus or acute cor pulmonale, a right heart strain pattern may be present. EKG is also helpful to evaluate for possible acute myocardial infarction.

Chest Computed Tomography Scan

Computed tomographic (CT) pulmonary angiography is used to diagnose pulmonary embolism and may also be useful in identification of effusion, pneumothorax, or posterior dependent atelectasis that can help to guide treatment strategies. Some patients with severe hypoxemia will not be stable for transport for CT imaging. Four (4)-extremity venous duplex scan may be considered to evaluate for extremity venous thrombosis, which would warrant initiation of systemic anticoagulation. However, presence of a venous thrombosis is not diagnostic of pulmonary embolism as the etiology of the severe hypoxemia.

● DIAGNOSIS

This patient has severe ARDS. The timing of the onset of hypoxemic respiratory failure is acute, or within 7 days of a clinical insult (in this case, abdominal sepsis from an anastomotic leak), which is consistent with ARDS. Additionally, the patient has bilateral infiltrates on chest radiograph, hypoxemia (P/F ≤ 300 mm Hg), and no evidence of cardiogenic pulmonary edema.

The original ARDS criteria were created at the 1994 American-European Consensus Conference (AECC) and differentiated between acute lung injury (ALI) and ARDS based on the P/F ratio. ALI was defined as a P/F ratio of 200 to 300 mm Hg and ARDS was defined as a P/F ratio of ≤200 mm Hg. Furthermore, the AECC definition did not require a minimum positive end-expiratory pressure (PEEP). In 2012, the Berlin definition of ARDS was published. The new definition included a criterion addressing the specific timing of the respiratory onset in relation to a known trigger (1 week). Additionally, using the Berlin definition, ALI no longer exists and ARDS is stratified into mild, moderate, and severe based on P/F ratio (Table 126-1). A minimum PEEP or CPAP of 5 cm H$_2$O is required for mild ARDS, and a minimum PEEP of 5 cm H$_2$O is required to diagnose moderate or severe ARDS. The Berlin criteria also modified the AECC criterion for the absence of left atrial hypertension; pulmonary edema may be present but should not fully explain the hypoxemic respiratory failure. In the absence of a known ARDS risk factor, objective assessment (e.g., echocardiography) is recommended to exclude the presence of hydrostatic edema.

The Berlin criteria addressed some of the criticisms of the AECC definition and resulted in a slight improvement in the prediction of mortality. Nonetheless, ARDS remains a clinical diagnosis and requires the clinician to recognize the constellation of clinical features.

● PATHOPHYSIOLOGY

ARDS is characterized by diffuse alveolar damage and hyaline membranes representing epithelial injury and increased permeability of the endothelium and epithelium. This results in the accumulation of protein- and neutrophil-rich pulmonary edema in the lung interstitium and in the distal airways. Additional mechanisms impair the removal of pulmonary edema fluid and inflammatory cells from the lung (Figure 126-2).

Table 126-1	The Berlin Definition of ARDS

	Acute Respiratory Distress Syndrome
Timing	Within 1 week of a known clinical insult or new or worsening respiratory symptoms
Risk factor	Objective assessment (i.e., echocardiography) required to exclude hydrostatic edema if no risk factor present
Chest imaging	Bilateral opacities—not fully explained by effusions, lobar or lung collapse, or nodules
Oxygenation Mild Moderate Severe	200 mm Hg < P_aO_2/FiO_2 ≤ 300 mm Hg with PEEP or CPAP ≥ 5 cm H_2O 100 mm Hg < P_aO_2/FiO_2 ≤ 200 mm Hg with PEEP ≥ 5 cm H_2O P_aO_2/FiO_2 ≤ 100 mm Hg with PEEP ≥ 5 cm H_2O
Left atrial hypertension	No requirement for measuring pulmonary arterial wedge pressure or of excluding left atrial hypertension Respiratory failure not fully explained by cardiac failure or fluid overload

● TREATMENT

Treatment of the Cause

The first priority in management of ARDS is treatment of the underlying cause or precipitating event. In this patient, treatment of the abdominal sepsis is required, including broad-spectrum empiric antibiotics, surgical source control, resuscitation, and cardiorespiratory support.

Respiratory Support with Mechanical Ventilation

LUNG PROTECTIVE VENTILATION

Recommendations regarding the use of specific ventilation strategies have been published by in a joint clinical practice guideline endorsed by the American Thoracic Society, European Society of Intensive Care Medicine, and the Society of Critical Care Medicine. The goal of mechanical ventilation is to increase oxygenation while minimizing the risk of further lung injury, known as ventilator-induced lung injury. Low tidal volume (6 mL/kg) ventilation, adjusted to maintain plateau pressures (Pplat) </= 30 cm H_2O is associated with a significant reduction in mortality (Table 126-2) and is the standard ventilator management of ARDS across all strata of severity. This strategy allows for permissive hypercapnia. With the development of the National Institutes of Health (NIH)-sponsored ARDS Clinical Trials Network, large well-controlled trials of ARDS therapies have been completed. Thus far, the only mechanical ventilation strategy found to improve survival rates is lung protective ventilation using low tidal volumes.

In the ARDS patient with persistent hypoxemia, additional strategies including recruitment maneuvers (RM), "open lung" ventilation with higher PEEP, and mechanical ventilation with higher mean airway pressures (airway pressure release ventilation or high-frequency oscillatory ventilation, HFOV) may be considered. However, these strategies are either only conditionally recommended (RMs and higher PEEP) or strongly recommended against (HFOV).

HIGHER PEEP

There is no consensus regarding the optimal strategy for setting PEEP. While higher PEEP may have benefits related to improved alveolar recruitment and oxygenation, it also has theoretical risks of barotrauma, increased dead space, and increased pulmonary vascular resistance. Synthesis of data from randomized trials is challenging due to variations in strategies for delivering higher PEEP. For example, a recent trial evaluating RM in addition to titration of PEEP versus low PEEP resulted in patients in the experimental group having worse outcomes.

Prone Positioning

The clinical practice guideline recommends prone positioning for more than 12 hours per day in adult patients with severe ARDS. Proposed benefits of prone positioning include improved ventilation-perfusion matching, increased alveolar recruitment, and increased end-expiratory lung volume. This translates to improved oxygenation in 70% to 80% of patients with ARDS; maximal improvements are seen in the most hypoxemic patients. Based on subgroup

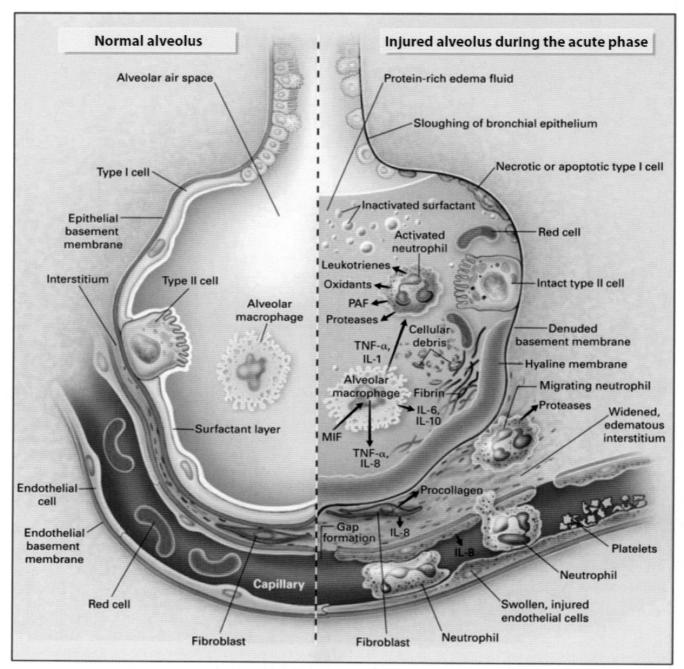

FIGURE 126-2. The normal alveolus and the injured alveolus in the acute phase of acute lung injury and the acute respiratory distress syndrome. In the acute phase of the syndrome, there is sloughing of both the bronchial and alveolar epithelial cells; protein-rich hyaline membranes form on the denuded basement membrane. Neutrophils adhere to the injured capillary endothelium and marginate through the interstitium into the air space, which is filled with protein-rich edema fluid. In the air space, alveolar macrophages secrete cytokines; interleukin (IL)-1, -6, -8, and -10; and tumor necrosis factor-α (TNF-α), which act locally to stimulate chemotaxis and activate neutrophils. IL-1 can also stimulate the production of extracellular matrix by fibroblasts. Neutrophils can release oxidants, proteases, leukotrienes, and other proinflammatory molecules such as platelet-activating factor (PAF). A number of anti-inflammatory mediators are also present in the alveolar milieu including IL-1 receptor antagonist, soluble TNF receptor, autoantibodies against IL-8, and cytokines such as IL-10 and -11 (not shown). The influx of protein-rich edema fluid into the alveolus leads to the inactivation of surfactant. MIF, macrophage-inhibitory factor. (Adapted from the Massachusetts Medical Society, with permission.)

Table 126-2   Low Tidal Volume Ventilation Strategy from ARDS Network (www.ardsnet.org)

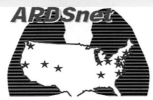

NIH NHLBI ARDS Clinical Network
Mechanical Ventilation Protocol Summary

INCLUSION CRITERIA: Acute onset of
1. $PaO_2/FiO_2 \leq 300$ (corrected for altitude)
2. Bilateral (patchy, diffuse, or homogeneous) infiltrates consistent with pulmonary edema
3. No clinical evidence of left atrial hypertension

PART I: VENTILATOR SETUP AND ADJUSTMENT
1. Calculate predicted body weight (PBW)
   Males = 50 + 2.3 [height (inches) - 60]
   Females = 45.5 + 2.3 [height (inches) -60]
2. Select any ventilator mode
3. Set ventilator settings to achieve initial V_T = 8 ml/kg PBW
4. Reduce V_T by 1 ml/kg at intervals $\leq$ 2 hours until V_T = 6ml/kg PBW.
5. Set initial rate to approximate baseline minute ventilation (not > 35 bpm).
6. Adjust V_T and RR to achieve pH and plateau pressure goals below.

OXYGENATION GOAL: PaO_2 55-80 mmHg or SpO_2 88-95%
Use a minimum PEEP of 5 cm H_2O. Consider use of incremental FiO_2/PEEP combinations such as shown below (not required) to achieve goal.

Lower PEEP/higher FiO2

FiO_2	0.3	0.4	0.4	0.5	0.5	0.6	0.7	0.7
PEEP	5	5	8	8	10	10	10	12

FiO_2	0.7	0.8	0.9	0.9	0.9	1.0
PEEP	14	14	14	16	18	18-24

Higher PEEP/lower FiO2

FiO_2	0.3	0.3	0.3	0.3	0.3	0.4	0.4	0.5
PEEP	5	8	10	12	14	14	16	16

FiO_2	0.5	0.5-0.8	0.8	0.9	1.0	1.0
PEEP	18	20	22	22	22	24

PLATEAU PRESSURE GOAL: $\leq$ 30 cm H_2O
Check Pplat (0.5 second inspiratory pause), at least q 4h and after each change in PEEP or V_T.
If Pplat > 30 cm H_2O: decrease V_T by 1ml/kg steps (minimum = 4 ml/kg).
If Pplat < 25 cm H_2O and V_T< 6 ml/kg, increase V_T by 1 ml/kg until Pplat > 25 cm H_2O or V_T = 6 ml/kg.
If Pplat < 30 and breath stacking or dys-synchrony occurs: may increase V_T in 1ml/kg increments to 7 or 8 ml/kg if Pplat remains $\leq$ 30 cm H_2O.

pH GOAL: 7.30-7.45
Acidosis Management: (pH < 7.30)
  If pH 7.15-7.30: Increase RR until pH > 7.30 or $PaCO_2$ < 25 (Maximum set RR = 35).

If pH < 7.15: Increase RR to 35.
  If pH remains < 7.15, V_T may be increased in 1 ml/kg steps until pH > 7.15 (Pplat target of 30 may be exceeded).
  May give $NaHCO_3$
Alkalosis Management: (pH > 7.45) Decrease vent rate if possible.

I: E RATIO GOAL: Recommend that duration of inspiration be $\leq$ duration of expiration.

---

analyses of multiple randomized trials and an individual patient data meta-analysis, prone positioning improves mortality in patients receiving it more than 12 hours per day and in patients with severe ARDS. Complications include a higher rate of endotracheal tube obstruction and pressure ulcers.

High-Frequency Oscillatory Ventilation

High-Frequency Oscillatory Ventilation (HFOV) aims to limit volutrauma by delivering very small tidal volumes while simultaneously limiting trauma due to atelectasis by using higher mean airway pressures. However, randomized trials have failed to demonstrate improved mortality, and at least one large multicenter randomized trial reported increased harm. Thus, the clinical practice guideline recommends strongly against the use of HFOV in patients with moderate to severe ARDS. The use of HFOV in patients with refractory severe hypoxemia due to ARDS remains unclear.

Recruitment Maneuvers

Recruitment maneuvers (RMs) attempt to increase the amount of aerated lung to improve gas exchange. RMs are performed by sustained inflation with continuous positive airway pressure (i.e., 30 cm H_2O PEEP for 30 seconds) or controlled ventilation at increased airway pressure. RM can improve oxygenation, but may also result in transient adverse events (hypotension, hypoxemia) or pneumothorax, and have not been shown to improve survival. The clinical practice guideline provides only a conditional recommendation for RMs in patients with moderate or severe ARDS given the low to moderate quality of evidence.

Extracorporeal Membrane Oxygenation

Venovenous extracorporeal membrane oxygenation (ECMO) is the most common strategy employed in patients with severe ARDS unresponsive to other management strategies, with a 50% survival rate reported in 1,473 adults with ARDS treated with ECMO from the Extracorporeal Life Support Organization (ELSO). The CESAR trial was a multicenter trial performed in the United Kingdom that randomized 180 patients to conventional mechanical ventilation versus ECMO and demonstrated that ARDS management with a standardized algorithm including ECMO in an expert center resulted in improved 6-month outcome (death or severe disability at 6 months, 63% vs. 47%; RR, 0.69; 95% CI, 0.05 to 0.97; $P = 0.03$). But compliance with a low tidal volume ventilation strategy was not mandated in the control cohort. The clinical practice guidelines provide no recommendation for or against its use due to the lack of sufficient evidence.

Subsequent to publication of the clinical practice guidelines, the ECMO to Rescue Lung Injury in Severe ARDS (EOLIA) trial was published. In an international, randomized trial, 249 patients were randomized to a strategy of early ECMO versus conventional mechanical ventilation with ECMO permitted as rescue. The trial was stopped early for futility; the 60-day mortality was not significantly lower with early ECMO, however 28% of the conventional ventilation patients crossed over to ECMO and the secondary outcome of mortality + crossover was significantly higher. Interpretation of this result is controversial.

Therapies Targeted at the Lung Injury

The use of a fluid-conservative strategy after patients with ARDS are no longer in shock was associated with improved oxygenation and a significant reduction in the duration of mechanical ventilation, and no difference in 60-day mortality or nonpulmonary organ failures. Therefore, conservative volume management and titrated diuretic administration (furosemide [Lasix], bumetanide [Bumex]) with either intermittent administration or continuous infusion can be considered. In patients with nonuniform infiltrates, positioning the patient with the good lung down can improve oxygenation by improving perfusion to the more aerated portion of the lung.

Supportive Therapies

Patients with ARDS require adequate sedation and analgesia, usually administered by IV continuous infusion titrated to effect. In critically ill patients with ARDS with a P/F ratio <150 mm Hg, early administration of a neuromuscular blocking agent (cisatracurium) for 48 hours improved the adjusted 90-day survival and increased the time off the ventilator without increasing muscle weakness. Neuromuscular blockade may be required in these severe cases, but prolonged neuromuscular blockade has been associated with myopathy and neuropathy in critically ill patients. Measures to reduce ventilator-associated pneumonia (VAP) are instituted, as ARDS patients can require prolonged mechanical ventilation and are at high risk for VAP. Early mobilization and physical therapy to reduce ICU-acquired weakness is an important component of care. All ARDS patients require nutritional support, and enteral nutrition is preferred as it is associated with decreased infectious complications in ICU patients. In some, but not all studies, administration of a specialized enteral nutrition formula (with omega-3 fatty acids [eicosapentaenoic acid, gamma-linolenic acid] and antioxidants) was associated with improved outcomes (reduced mortality, increased ventilator-free and ICU-free days, reduced organ failure and improved oxygenation).

● ADJUNCTIVE PHARMACOLOGIC THERAPIES

Pharmacologic therapies include inhaled nitric oxide and inhaled prostacyclin.

Inhaled Nitric Oxide

Inhaled nitric oxide (INO) is a selective pulmonary vasodilator that improves oxygenation by increasing blood flow in ventilated areas to improve ventilation/perfusion matching. A meta-analysis of 12 trials and 1,237 patients confirmed that INO significantly increased oxygenation that persisted through day 4 of treatment, but no significant effect of INO on hospital mortality was identified.

Inhaled Prostacyclin and Other Vasodilatory Prostaglandins

Prostacyclin is a selective pulmonary vasodilator and inhibitor of platelet aggregation. When aerosolized, its vasodilatory action improves ventilation/perfusion matching in the lung, resulting in improved oxygenation and no effect on systemic arterial blood pressure. Inhaled iloprost is a more stable analog of prostacyclin and is approved by the FDA for pulmonary hypertension, and can be used instead of INO in ARDS patients with severe hypoxemia to improve oxygenation.

● SPECIAL CONSIDERATIONS

Complications in ARDS patients are common. Clinicians must pay careful attention to early recognition of potential complications, particularly pneumothorax and VAP. The latter is a common risk factor for development of ARDS, and almost 60% of patients with ARDS from other risk factors can develop VAP. Evaluation for other common infectious complications (central line–associated bloodstream infection, catheter-associated urinary tract infection) in ICU patients should be considered if fever and/or leukocytosis develop during the ICU stay.

● FOLLOW-UP

It has been documented that ARDS patients who survive have significant functional impairments during initial recovery, but most achieve near-normal lung function at 1 year, which persists without deterioration at 5 years. The major disability in these patients is a combination of exercise limitation, physical and psychological sequelae, and decreased physical quality of life. ARDS patients should have follow-up to assess the recovery of their pulmonary function. Chest radiograph, pulmonary function tests, and chest CT imaging are all considered dependent on the patient's clinical condition at follow-up.

Case Conclusion

This patient with sepsis-associated ARDS was treated with low tidal volume ventilation, conservative fluid administration, prone positioning, and sepsis management. She required 12 days of mechanical ventilation and was successfully weaned and extubated. Quantitative lower respiratory tract cultures obtained by bronchoalveolar lavage were negative for bacterial pathogens. She completed a course of systemic antibiotics for treatment of abdominal sepsis due to secondary peritonitis. She did not require supplemental oxygen on discharge home. Arterial blood gas confirmed adequate oxygenation on room air.

TAKE HOME POINTS

- The Berlin definition of ARDS includes timing within 1 week of a clinical insult, the acute onset of bilateral infiltrates, $PaO_2/FiO_2 \leq 300$ mm Hg (with PEEP ≥ 5 cm H_2O across all strata or CPAP ≥ 5 cm H_2O for mild), and inability to fully explain the hypoxemia based on cardiac failure or volume overload.
- ARDS can be caused by both direct (pulmonary) and indirect (nonpulmonary) etiologies.
- Any patient with the acute onset of bilateral pulmonary infiltrates and severe hypoxemia in the setting of risk factors such as trauma and sepsis should be evaluated for ARDS.
- ARDS-associated mortality rates remain high, at approximately 40%, and therefore an early diagnosis is critical to initiation of optimal management.
- Low tidal volume (6 mL/kg) ventilation is associated with decreased mortality in ARDS.

- A fluid-conservative management strategy, supplemented with targeted diuretic administration, is associated with improved ICU outcomes in ARDS.
- Evidence-based clinical practice guidelines exist regarding mechanical ventilation in patients with ARDS.

SUGGESTED READINGS

Brower RG, Matthay MA, Morris A, et al. Ventilation with lower tidal volumes as compared with traditional tidal volumes for acute lung injury and the acute respiratory distress syndrome. *N Engl J Med.* 2000;342(18):1301-1308.

Combes A, Hajage G, Capellier A, et al. for the EOLIA Trial Group, REVA and ECMONet. Extracorporeal Membrane Oxygenation for Severe Acute Respiratory Distress Syndrome. *N Engl J Med.* 2018;378:1965-1975, DOI: 10.1056/NEJMoa1800385

Fan E, Del Sorbo L, Goligher EC, et al. An official American Thoracic Society/European Society of Intensive Care Medicine/Society of Critical Care Medicine Practical Guideline: mechanical ventilation in adult patients with acute respiratory distress syndrome. *Am J Respir Crit Care Med.* 2017;195(9):1253-1263.

Herridge MS, Tansey CM, Matte A, et al. Canadian critical care trials group. Functional disability 5 years after acute respiratory distress syndrome. *N Engl J Med.* 2011;364:1293-1304.

Napolitano LM, Park PK, Raghavendran K, et al. Nonventilatory strategies for patients with life-threatening 2009 H1N1 influenza and severe respiratory failure. *Crit Care Med.* 2010;38(4):e74-e90.

Papazian L, Forel JM, Gacouin A, et al. ACURASYS study investigators. Neuromuscular blockers in early acute respiratory distress syndrome. *N Engl J Med.* 2010;363(12):1107-1116.

Peek GJ, Mugford M, Tiruvoipati R, et al, CESAR trial collaboration. Efficacy and economic assessment of conventional ventilator support versus extracorporeal membrane oxygenation for severe adult respiratory failure (CESAR): a multicenter randomized controlled trial. *Lancet.* 2009;374:1351-1363.

Pipeling MR, Fan E. Therapies for refractory hypoxemia in acute respiratory distress syndrome. *JAMA.* 2010;304(22):2521-2527.

Raghavendran K, Napolitano LM. ALI and ARDS: advances and challenges. *Crit Care Clin.* 2011;27:xiii-xiv.

Stewart RM, Park PK, Hunt JP, et al. NHLBI ARDS Clinical Trials Network. Less is more: improved outcomes in surgical patients with conservative fluid administration and central venous catheter monitoring. *J Am Coll Surg.* 2009;208(5):725-735.

The ARDS Definition Task Force. Acute respiratory distress syndrome: the Berlin definition. *JAMA.* 2012;307(23):2526-2533.

Wiedemann HP, Wheeler AP, Bernard GR, et al. Comparison of two fluid-management strategies in acute lung injury. *N Engl J Med.* 2006;354:2564-2575.

Ventilator-Associated Pneumonia

127

KUNJAN S. BHAKTA AND KRISHNAN RAGHAVENDRAN

Based on the previous edition chapter "Ventilator-associated Pneumonia" by Krishnan Raghavendran

Presentation

A 28-year-old male was involved in a motor vehicular accident travelling at 60 miles per hour. He sustained a significant traumatic brain injury (Glasgow Coma Scale of 8), was intubated at site, and transported to the ED. Subsequent workup revealed multiple cerebral contusions with no midline shift, infiltrates in the base of the right lung zones, mild hypoxia, and a femur fracture. He was then admitted to the ICU and was managed with supportive care including monitoring of intracranial pressure, mechanical ventilation, early nutrition, and appropriate prophylaxis for prevention of venous thromboembolism and stress-related mucosal disease. On the 4th day following trauma, he mounted a febrile response to 101°F, had a new onset infiltrate in the right upper lobe, and developed a leukocytosis.

● DIFFERENTIAL DIAGNOSIS

Presence of fever, leukocytosis, and a new infiltrate in a patient who has been endotracheally intubated and mechanically ventilated should raise a strong suspicion for ventilator-associated pneumonia (VAP). The patient at the time of initial presentation had evidence of hypoxia with an infiltrate in the lung and this should raise the possibility of aspiration-induced lung injury. Aspiration-induced pneumonitis may manifest signs similar to infection but a major aspiration event is unlikely at a point where the patient has been intubated with a cuffed tube. However, aspiration pneumonitis is a risk factor for development of aspiration pneumonia. Isolated pulmonary contusion without any other evidence of thoracic trauma is unlikely and is not likely to manifest fever and leukocytosis. Pulmonary infarctions secondary to pulmonary embolism should also be considered in the differential diagnosis. Finally, acute development of a dense infiltrate in the right upper lobe should also raise the possibility of migration of the endotracheal tube down the right main stem bronchus with resultant occlusion of the right upper lobe bronchus and subsequent collapse. However, a collapse is not associated with fever or leukocytosis.

● WORKUP

This patient underwent a bronchoscopy and quantitative bacteriology from the bronchoalveolar lavage. A Gram stain from the lavage was additionally obtained. Patient at this time had a febrile episode with a temperature of 39°C and white count of 16,000/μL. A chest x-ray showed evidence of a dense right upper lobe infiltrate. The tip of the endotracheal tube was visualized at 4 cm above the carina.

● DISCUSSION

VAP, defined as a pulmonary infection occurring after at least 48 hours of ventilation, is the leading cause of death in the ICU, with estimated prevalence rates of 10% to 65% and mortality rates of 25% to 60%. The incidence of VAP using the latest data from the National Healthcare Safety Network demonstrates an incidence of 0-5.8/1,000 ventilator days. VAP remains a major cause of mortality and morbidity in the critically ill patient. Despite significant advances that have been made in recent years to reduce the incidence of VAP in most ICUs, it still is considered the major cause of mortality and increased economic burden associated with the intubated/mechanically ventilated patient. The crucial aspect in the management lies with the ability to accurately diagnose and to promptly treat VAP.

● DIAGNOSIS AND TREATMENT OF VAP

Diagnosis of VAP remains a major challenge in the care of the critically ill. Though this is a controversial subject, there are areas that are generally agreed upon and are in use in most ICUs in the country. VAP is considered only if the patient has been intubated for at least 48 hours and most ICUs follow the Centers for Disease Control (CDC) criteria of fever, leukocytosis or leukopenia, and new-onset infiltrate. However, the incidence of VAP has been grossly underreported. In an attempt to improve surveillance across ICUs, the CDC has introduced new definitions (see Table 127-1). This algorithm is to be primarily used for surveillance and for future reporting, but it is currently not intended to be used for clinical

736

Table 127-1	CDC Surveillance Algorithm for Ventilator-Associated Events

Patient has a baseline period of stability or improvement on the ventilator, defined by ≥ 2 calendar days of stable or decreasing daily minimum*
FiO_2 or PEEP values. The baseline period is defined as the 2 calendar days immediately preceding the first day of increased daily minimum PEEP or FiO_2.

*Daily minimum defined by lowest value of FiO_2 or PEEP during a calendar day that is maintained for > 1 hour.

After a period of stability or improvement on the ventilator, the patient has at least one of the following indicators of worsening oxygenation:
1) Increase in daily minimum* FiO_2 of ≥ 0.20 (20 points) over the daily minimum FiO_2 of the first day in the baseline period, sustained for ≥ 2 calendar days.
2) Increase in daily minimum* PEEP values of ≥ 3 cm H_2O over the daily minimum PEEP of the first day in the baseline period,+ sustained for ≥ 2 calendar days.

*Daily minimum defined by lowest value of FiO_2 or PEEP during a calendar day that is maintained for > 1 hour.

+Daily minimum PEEP values of 0-5 cm H_2O are considered equivalent for the purposes of VAE surveillance.

Ventilator-Associated Condition (VAC)

On or after calendar day 3 of mechanical ventilation and within 2 calendar days before or after the onset of worsening oxygenation, the patient meets <u>both</u> of the following criteria:
1) Temperature > 38 °C or < 36°C, **OR** white blood cell count ≥ 12,000 cells/mm³ or ≤ 4,000 cells/mm³.
AND
2) A new antimicrobial agent(s) (see Appendix for eligible antimicrobial agents) is started, and is continued for ≥ 4 calendar days.

Infection-related Ventilator-Associated Complication (IVAC)

On or after calendar day 3 of mechanical ventilation and within 2 calendar days before or after the onset of worsening oxygenation, ONE of the following criteria is met **(taking into account organism exclusions specified in the protocol):**
1) Criterion 1: Positive culture of one of the following specimens, meeting quantitative or semiquantitative thresholds as outlined in protocol, <u>without</u> requirement for purulent respiratory secretions:
   - Endotracheal aspirate, ≥10⁵ CFU/mL or corresponding semiquantitative result
   - Bronchoalveolar lavage, ≥10⁴ CFU/mL or corresponding semiquantitative result
   - Lung tissue, ≥ 10⁴ CFU/g or corresponding semiquantitative result
   - Protected specimen brush, ≥10³ CFU/mL or corresponding semiquantitative result
2) Criterion 2: Purulent respiratory secretions (defined as secretions from the lungs, bronchi, or trachea that contain ≥ 25 neutrophils and ≤10 squamous epithelial cells per low power field [lpf, ×100])' **PLUS** organism identified from one of the following specimens (to include qualitative culture, or quantitative/semiquantitative culture without sufficient growth to meet criterion #1):
   - Sputum
   - Endotracheal aspirate
   - Bronchoalveolar lavage
   - Lung tissue
   - Protected specimen brush

' If the laboratory reports semiquantitative results, those results must correspond to the above quantitative thresholds. See additional instructions for using the purulent respiratory secretions criterion in the VAE Protocol.

(Continued)

Table 127-1	CDC Surveillance Algorithm for Ventilator-Associated Events (*Continued*)

3) Criterion 3: One of the following positive tests:
- Organism identified from pleural fluid (where specimen was obtained during thoracentesis or initial placement of chest tube and NOT from an indwelling chest tube)
- Lung histopathology defined as: 1) abscess formation or foci of consolidation with intense neutrophil accumulation in bronchioles and alveoli; 2) evidence of lung parenchyma invasion by fungi (hyphae, pseudohyphae or yeast forms); 3) evidence of infection with the viral pathogens listed below based on results of immunohistochemical assays, cytology, or microscopy performed on lung tissue
- Diagnostic test for *Legionella* species
- Diagnostic test on respiratory secretions for influenza virus, respiratory syncytial virus, adenovirus, parainfluenza virus, rhinovirus, human metapneumovirus

Possible Ventilator-Associated Pneumonia (PVAP)

Source: Ventilator-Associated Event (VAE) Protocol. January 2018. Centers for Disease Control and Prevention. Available at: http://www.cdc.gov/nhsn/pdfs/pscmanual/10-vae_final.pdf

management. In theory, these newer criteria will identify other ventilator-associated conditions such as acute respiratory distress syndrome (ARDS), atelectasis, and pulmonary edema, which are all clinical conditions that contribute to mortality but that are also preventable.

Once the clinical suspicion of VAP is entertained, a bacteriologic workup is then initiated. Determination of specific bacteriology and early initiation of appropriate broad-spectrum antibiotics remain the cornerstone of diagnosis and treatment of VAP. Sputum Gram stains or cultures are considered inappropriate as they are neither sensitive nor specific. The specimen used for quantitative bacteriology should be obtained either through a bronchoscope or by the use of a coaxial catheter that is inserted blindly through the endotracheal tube. The latter approach

called the mini-BAL does not involve a bronchoscope, and the diagnostic yield is considered similar to that from conventional bronchoscopy. Additionally, some ICUs use a protective brush inserted via a bronchoscope to obtain direct cultures from the affected area of the lung. The brush is then retrieved and directly plated onto the culture media. Significance is attributed to observed bacterial burden of more than 10^4 CFU/mL.

Regardless of the diagnostic modality used to ascertain the specific bacteriology, appropriate broad-spectrum antibiotic therapy should be initiated as soon as the cultures are obtained. Treatment regimens should be based on local antibiograms. Appropriate antibiotics should cover *Staphylococcus aureus, Pseudomonas aeruginosa*, and other Gram-negative bacilli (see Table 127-2). Coverage for methicillin-resistant *Staphylococcus aureus* (MRSA) using vancomycin or linezolid should be used in units where the known resistant rates are >10% to 20% or if the resistance rate is unknown. Two antipseudomonal antibiotics from two differing classes should be used for certain risk factors (see Table 127-3) and in ICUS where >10% of Gram-negative isolates are resistant to the antibiotic being considered for monotherapy.

Table 127-2	Bacteriology of Isolated Organisms from VAP Reported to the National Healthcare Safety Network, 2009–2010

Organism	No. (%) of pathogens
Staphylococcus aureus (MSSA and MRSA)	2,043 (24.1)
Pseudomonas aeruginosa	1,408 (16.6)
Kleibsiella sp	854 (10.1)
Enterobacter	727 (8.6)
Acinetobacter baumannii	557 (6.6)
Escherichia coli	504 (5.9)
Serratia spp.	386 (4.6)

Table 127-3	Risk Factors for Multidrug-Resistant Pathogens and MRSA

Prior intravenous antibiotic use within 90 d
Septic shock at time of VAP
ARDS preceding VAP
Five or more days of hospitalization prior to the occurrence of VAP
Acute renal replacement therapy prior to VAP onset

Table 127-4   Measures to Prevent VAP

- Avoidance of endotracheal intubation
  - Use noninvasive positive pressure ventilation when possible
- Minimize sedation
  - Avoid benzodiazepines
  - Daily and paired spontaneous awakening and breathing trials
- Provide early exercise and mobility
- Use of endotracheal tubes with subglottic drainage ports in patients expected to intubate >48 h
- Avoid unnecessary manipulation/changes of the ventilatory circuit
- Elevate head of bed
- Oral care with chlorhexidine
- Hand washing/disinfection

● PREVENTION OF VAP

With the introduction of VAP bundle and recent understanding of the pathogenesis of VAP, major strides have been taken in recent years in the institution of prevention strategies for VAP. A detailed list of various methodologies used to prevent VAP and items included in the VAP bundle are provided in Table 127-4.

Case Conclusion

The patient was diagnosed with VAP on the 4th day following trauma. Because of the high incidence of MRSA in this ICU, the patient was started on vancomycin and cefepime. The quantitative cultures were consistent with 10^5 *Klebsiella pneumoniae*. The vancomycin was discontinued, and the cefepime was deescalated to ceftriaxone. Antibiotics were continued for a total of 8 days at which time the white count and fever had subsided. The ventriculostomy catheters were removed on the 6th day following trauma and patient continued to improve clinically. He was extubated on the 9th posttrauma day and was subsequently transferred to an adult rehabilitation facility.

TAKE HOME POINTS

- One of the most common nosocomial infections and a significant cause of mortality and morbidity in the critically ill.

- The risk of VAP is cumulative and its incidence increases with the duration of mechanical ventilation.
- The diagnosis of VAP remains an ongoing challenge. Current standards involve a combination of clinical criteria and quantitative bacteriology of the lower respiratory tract. Newer criteria are now in use for surveillance and reporting but are not intended for clinical use.
- It is important to obtain quantitative bacteriology prior to initiation of antibiotics.
- The initiation of antibiotics should be prompt, broad spectrum and also depend on available microbiograms of the individual ICU.
- As important as it is to initiate early and appropriate broad-spectrum antibiotics, it is equally important to deescalate or discontinue the antibiotics once the quantitative cultures are finalized.
- The duration of treatment varies and generally ranges from 8 to 14 days.
- Prevention of VAP is most effective when multiple risk factors are addressed. Formal protocols such as adoption of VAP bundle have been very effective in reducing the overall incidence of VAP.

SUGGESTED READINGS

CDC. Ventilator Associated Event Protocol. January 2018. Available at: http://www.cdc.gov/nhsn/pdfs/pscmanual/10-vae_final.pdf

Chastre J, Fagon JY. Ventilator-associated pneumonia. *Am J Respir Crit Care Med.* 2002;165(7):867-903.

Guidelines for the management of adults with hospital-acquired, ventilator-associated, and healthcare-associated pneumonia. *Am J Respir Crit Care Med.* 2005;171(4):388-416.

Iregui M, Ward S, Sherman G, et al. Clinical importance of delays in the initiation of appropriate antibiotic treatment for ventilator-associated pneumonia. *Chest.* 2002;122(1):262-268.

Kalil AC, et al. Management of adults with hospital-acquired and ventilator-associated pneumonia: 2016 clinical practice guidelines by the infectious diseases society of America and the American thoracic society. *Clin Infect Dis.* 2016;63(5):575-578.

Kollef MH. Prevention of hospital-associated pneumonia and ventilator-associated pneumonia. *Crit Care Med.* 2004;32(6):1396-1405.

Raghavendran K, Mylotte JM, Scannepeico F. Nursing home-associated pneumonia, hospital-acquired pneumonia and ventilator-associated pneumonia (VAP): the contribution of dental biofilms and periodontal inflammation. *Periodontol 2000.* 2007; 44:164-177.

Raghavendran K, Wang J, Bellber C, et al. Predictive value of sputum gram stain for the determination of appropriate antibiotic therapy for VAP. *J Trauma.* 2007;62(6):1377-1383.

Sievert DM, et al. Antimicrobial-resistant pathogens associated with healthcare- associated infections: summary of data reported to the National Healthcare Safety Network at the Centers for Disease Control and Prevention, 2009–2010. *Infect Control Hosp Epidemiol.* 2013;34(1):1-14.

Sepsis and Septic Shock

128

LISA M. KODADEK AND PAMELA A. LIPSETT

Based on the previous edition chapter "Septic Shock" by Pamela A. Lipsett

Presentation

A 68-year-old man presents to the emergency department with severe acute abdominal pain located in his left lower quadrant for the past 2 days. He reports a fever of 101°F, diarrhea 4 days ago, and now constipation for the past day. He has not vomited, but he has been nauseated and unable to tolerate solid foods or liquids. He has made little urine in the past day. He reports a history of acute diverticulitis requiring two previous hospitalizations in the past year and hypertension controlled with medication. He is unable to give a more complete history because of increasing confusion. His vital signs reveal an elevated temperature of 39°C, a pulse of 128, a respiratory rate of 32, and a blood pressure of 74/38 mm Hg. His oxygen saturation is 90% on 60% FIO_2 face mask. His examination demonstrates an acutely ill-appearing man in pain and respiratory distress. He is mildly confused but without focal neurologic findings. He is tachypneic with rapid shallow respiratory efforts but clear lungs. His cardiac examination is normal aside from hypotension and tachycardia. His extremities are cool. His abdominal examination reveals a distended abdomen that is rigid and painful to palpation both generally and especially in the left lower quadrant where there is a suggestion of fullness.

DIFFERENTIAL DIAGNOSIS

The patient is presenting in shock and the shock is most likely related to the abdominal pain. Differential diagnoses may include perforated viscus with intra-abdominal contamination as well as other causes of peritonitis. In this age group, the most common etiologies of a rigid abdomen and shock are related to diverticulitis, perforated ulcer, perforated malignancy of the gastrointestinal tract, or even appendicitis. A history of diverticulitis makes this diagnosis most likely, but a broad differential must be considered.

Shock is defined as inadequate tissue perfusion and may be classified based on underlying etiology (Table 128-1). With a history of poor oral intake and diarrhea, this patient may be dehydrated, but it is unlikely his depressed blood pressure is due entirely to hypovolemia. Furthermore, his diastolic pressure is quite low and suggestive of vasodilation consistent

with distributive shock rather than vasoconstriction as often seen in hypovolemic shock. Cardiac and noncardiac causes of shock should be considered, but investigation should not delay resuscitation. Further studies should be obtained to identify the etiology of shock.

WORKUP

Laboratory evaluation demonstrates an elevated white blood cell (WBC) count of 24,000/mm³, hemoglobin of 15.0 g/dL, and a depressed platelet count of 100,000/cu mm. Electrolytes reveal sodium of 142 mEq/L, potassium of 3.4 mEq/L, chloride of 100 mEq/L, bicarbonate of 20 mEq/L, glucose of 180 mg/dL, blood urea nitrogen of 48 mg/dL, and serum creatinine of 1.8 mg/dL. Lactate is elevated to 4.9 mmol/L. An arterial blood gas reveals pH of 7.30, $PaCO_2$ of 30 mm Hg, and PaO_2 of 60 mm Hg. A plain chest radiograph shows clear lungs and a modest respiratory effort. A plain abdominal radiograph is fairly unremarkable. A computed tomography (CT) scan without contrast demonstrates an inflammatory mass in the sigmoid colon with pericolonic fluid extending into the pelvis and a small amount of localized free air adjacent to the colon. An electrocardiogram shows sinus tachycardia without any other acute changes.

DIAGNOSIS AND TREATMENT

Sepsis is defined as life-threatening organ dysfunction caused by a dysregulated host response to infection. Septic shock is a subset of sepsis in which underlying circulatory and cellular/metabolic abnormalities are profound enough to substantially increase mortality. The 2016 Sepsis-3 guidelines provide an approach for identifying and diagnosing patients with sepsis and septic shock. Patients with suspected infection should be assessed using a quick SOFA (qSOFA) score consisting of three clinical criteria easily assessed at the bedside: altered mentation, systolic blood pressure (SBP) of 100 mm Hg or less, and respiratory rate (RR) of 22 per minute or greater. In the case presentation, the patient meets all three of the qSOFA criteria (confusion, RR 32, SBP 74 mm Hg). In cases where a patient meets 2 or more of the qSOFA criteria, the Sequential [Sepsis-Related] Organ Failure Assessment

740

Table 128-1   Differential Diagnosis of Shock

Hypovolemic Shock	Extracardiac Obstructive Shock	Cardiogenic Shock	Distributive Shock

Hemorrhagic
  Gastrointestinal
  Trauma
	Elevated Intrathoracic Pressure
	  Positive-pressure ventilation
	  Tension pneumothorax
		Arrhythmias	*Anaphylaxis*
			
			Burns

Nonhemorrhagic
  Burns
  Dehydration
  Diarrhea
  Polyuria
    Diuretic use
    Diabetes insipidus
  Vomiting
	Extrinsic Vascular Compression
	  Mediastinal tumors
	Pericarditis
		Mechanical
		  Valvular regurgitation
		  Valvular stenosis
		  Ventricular aneurysm
		  Ventricular septal defects
			Endocrine
			  Myxedema coma
			  Adrenal insufficiency

Third-Space Losses
  Ascites
  Peritonitis
	Vascular Flow Obstruction
	  Acute pulmonary hypertension
	  Air embolism
	  Aortic dissection
	  Pericardial tamponade
	  Pulmonary embolism
	  Tumors
		Myocardial Infarction
		  Cardiomyopathy
		  Intrinsic depression
		  Myocarditis
		  Pharmacologic
		    Beta blockers
		    Calcium channel blockers
			Infection/Inflammation
			  Pancreatitis
			  Sepsis
			Snake bite
			Trauma
			  Spinal cord injury

(SOFA) score should then be applied to assess for organ dysfunction and evidence of sepsis (Table 128-2).

SOFA variables include PaO_2/FIO_2, Glasgow Coma Scale, mean arterial pressure (MAP), administration of vasopressors, serum creatinine or urine output, bilirubin, and platelet count. The patient in the case presentation clearly has evidence of organ dysfunction with a SOFA score of ≥2 points since he demonstrates abnormalities of his respiratory, central nervous, cardiovascular, renal, and hematologic systems. An acute change in total SOFA score ≥2 points consequent to the infection is diagnostic for sepsis. Septic shock is diagnosed when clinical criteria for sepsis are met and the patient exhibits persistent hypotension requiring vasopressors to maintain MAP ≥65 mm Hg and a serum lactate level >2 mmol/L despite adequate volume resuscitation. In the case scenario, the patient's hypotension (if persistent and requiring vasopressors after volume resuscitation), in addition to the lactate of 4.9 mmol/L, is diagnostic of septic shock.

Treatment of sepsis and septic shock requires early diagnosis, source control of the underlying infection, timely antibiotic administration, and effective resuscitation. The patient should be approached with therapies consistent with guidelines provided by the Surviving Sepsis Campaign (SSC). Given the respiratory compromise apparent at presentation, immediate attention should focus on supporting the patient's respiratory effort with additional oxygen (100% face mask). He is likely to require intubation and mechanical ventilation to decrease the work of breathing and to improve his oxygenation.

The SSC guidelines currently recommend initial quantitative resuscitation of patients with sepsis-induced tissue hypoperfusion (Table 128-3). Sepsis-induced tissue hypoperfusion may be defined as hypotension persisting after the initial fluid challenge of 30 mL/kg or a blood lactate concentration ≥4 mmol/L. The specific goals of resuscitation to be attained during the first 6 hours after recognition of sepsis are central venous pressure (CVP) of 8 to 12 mm Hg, MAP of ≥65 mm Hg, urine output of ≥0.5 mL/kg/h, central venous oxygen saturation ($ScvO_2$) of 70% or mixed venous oxygen saturation (SvO_2) of 65%, and normalization of lactate. Crystalloids are the initial fluid of choice in the resuscitation of patients with sepsis and septic shock. Albumin may be used in adjunct for fluid resuscitation of patients who require substantial amounts of resuscitation fluids. Normalization of lactate was added as a resuscitation goal in the 2012 SSC guidelines. This new guideline was based on two multicenter randomized controlled trials (EMShockNet and LACTATE) that used lactate normalization both as a single target for resuscitation and in combination with normalization of $ScvO_2$. There is evidence that normalization of lactate by 20% or more per 2 hours for the patient's first 8 hours in the ICU is associated with decreased mortality.

With respect to control of infection and treatment, blood cultures should be obtained before administration of combination of broad-spectrum antibiotics if possible, but more importantly, antibiotics should be administered within 1 hour of recognition of sepsis or septic shock. For the patient in the case scenario, expected pathogens include enteric gram-negative bacteria, facultative aerobic gram-positive organisms, and anaerobes. Resistant pathogens are unlikely to be present in the patient described but should be

Table 128-2   Sequential [Sepsis-Related] Organ Failure Assessment (SOFA) Score[a]

	Score				
System	0	1	2	3	4
Respiration					
PaO₂/FIO₂, mm Hg (kPa)	≥400 (53.3)	<400 (53.3)	<300 (40)	<200 (26.7) with respiratory support	<100 (13.3) with respiratory support
Coagulation					
Platelets, × 10³/μL	≥150	<150	<100	<50	<20
Liver					
Bilirubin, mg/dL (μmol/L)	<1.2 (20)	1.2–1.9 (20–32)	2.0–5.9 (33–101)	6.0–11.9 (102–204)	>12.0 (204)
Cardiovascular	MAP ≥ 70 mm Hg	MAP < 70 mm Hg	Dopamine <5 or dobutamine (any dose)[b]	Dopamine 5.1–15 or epinephrine ≤0.1 or norepinephrine ≤0.1[a]	Dopamine >15 or epinephrine >0.1 or norepinephrine >0.1[b]
Central Nervous System					
Glasgow Coma Scale[c]	15	13–14	10–12	6–9	<6
Renal					
Creatinine, mg/dL (μmol/L)	<1.2 (110)	1.2–1.9 (110–170)	2.0–3.4 (171–299)	3.5–4.9 (300–440)	>5.0 (440)
Urine output, mL/d				<500	<200

[a]Organ dysfunction can be identified as an acute change in total SOFA score ≥2 points consequent to infection. The baseline SOFA score can be assumed to be zero in patients not known to have pre-existing organ dysfunction.

[b]Catecholamine doses are given as μg/kg/min for at least 1 hour.

[c]Glasgow Coma Scale ranges from 3 to 15; higher score indicates better neurologic function.

PaO₂/FIO₂, ratio of arterial oxygen partial pressure to fractional inspired oxygen; mm Hg, millimeters mercury; kPa, kilopascal; MAP, mean arterial blood pressure.

a consideration for patients with recent hospitalization or those who develop septic shock in the hospital.

Vasopressors may be used in conjunction with appropriate fluid resuscitation to maintain a MAP ≥ 65 mm Hg. Norepinephrine is the first choice for vasopressor administration; epinephrine may be added or potentially substituted for norepinephrine when an additional agent is necessary. Vasopressin is not recommended as the first choice for a single initial vasopressor, but it may be added to norepinephrine to raise the MAP or decrease the amount of norepinephrine required. Dopamine may be used as an alternative to norepinephrine in selected patients with low risk of tachyarrhythmia and bradycardia. A trial of dobutamine may be appropriate if there is evidence for myocardial dysfunction, but when used alone for sepsis, it will almost certainly lower blood pressure.

Current SSC guidelines do not support routine use of blood transfusions for septic patients. In the absence of myocardial ischemia, severe hypoxemia, hemorrhage, or ischemic heart disease, red blood cell transfusion should only be administered if the hemoglobin level is <7.0 g/dL. The appropriate target hemoglobin concentration is 7.0 g/dL to 9.0 g/dL.

Once the patient has been adequately resuscitated, a specific anatomical diagnosis of infection should be sought. If intervention is warranted to obtain source control through surgical drainage or other intervention, this should be completed within 12 hours of recognition. The description of the CT scan in the case scenario suggests that this patient has Hinchey Stage III disease (Table 128-4) and an intervention will be required. While open surgery has classically been applied to the treatment of complicated diverticulitis, percutaneous treatment followed by one-staged repair has been reported with increasing

Table 128-3	Surviving Sepsis Campaign Bundles

To be completed within 3 hours:

1. Measure lactate level
2. Obtain blood cultures prior to administration of antibiotics
3. Administer broad-spectrum antibiotics
4. Administer 30 mL/kg crystalloid for hypotension or lactate ≥4 mmol/L

To be completed within 6 hours:

5. Apply vasopressors (for hypotension that does not respond to initial fluid resuscitation) to maintain arterial pressure (MAP) ≥ 65 mm Hg
6. In the event of persistent arterial hypotension despite volume resuscitation (septic shock) or initial lactate ≥4 mmol/L (36 mg/dL):
   - Measure central venous pressure (CVP)[a]
   - Measure central venous oxygen saturation (ScvO$_2$)[a]
7. Remeasure lactate if initial lactate was elevated[a]

[a]Targets for quantitative resuscitation included in the guidelines are CVP of ≥8 mm Hg, ScvO$_2$ of ≥70%, and normalization of lactate.

Adapted from Dellinger RP, Levy MM, Rhodes A, et al. Surviving sepsis campaign: international guidelines for management of severe sepsis and septic shock. *Crit Care Med.* 2013;41(2):580-637.

success. An exhaustive review of diverticulitis management is beyond the intended scope of this chapter.

SPECIAL CONSIDERATIONS

It is important to note that the 2012 SSC recommendations are still based in large part on a landmark 2001 study by Rivers et al., which demonstrated decreased mortality for patients with sepsis who were treated with an early goal-directed therapy (EGDT) protocol. Subsequent studies, including ProCESS (Protocolized Care for Early Septic Shock), ProMISe (Protocolized Management in Sepsis), and ARISE (Australasian Resuscitation in Sepsis Evaluation), have failed to replicate the mortality benefit seen in the initial EGDT study. A 2015 systematic review and meta-analysis by Angus et al. pooled 5 randomized clinical trials and determined there was no difference in mortality between EGDT and usual care; EGDT was associated with increased utilization of resources including ICU care and vasopressors. Sepsis and septic shock represent an area of active and prodigious research investigation, and evidence-based guidelines will continue to reflect advances in knowledge. Guidelines from the SSC, updated every 4 years, will continue to reflect the most recent literature, and clinicians must update their practices to ensure optimization of patient outcomes and appropriate use and allocation of resources.

The quantitative SSC resuscitation goals represent current best practice, but these should not be considered gold standard. For example, MAP interpretation may be difficult in patients with chronic hypertension. While central and mixed venous oxygen saturations are helpful to assess the difference between oxygen delivery and consumption, these lab values are typically obtained via invasive monitors. CVP is not an accurate determination of volume status, particularly in mechanically ventilated patients or those with increased abdominal pressure or pre-existing decreased ventricular compliance. Other methods, such as the pulse pressure variation, the passive leg raise test, and bedside ultrasound examination, can assess intravascular volume status without necessitating placement of a central venous catheter.

POSTOPERATIVE MANAGEMENT

Once source control has been obtained, ongoing support in the ICU is necessary following the intervention until organ dysfunction has resolved. While the exact duration of

Table 128-4	Hinchey Stages for Diverticulitis	
Stage	**Definition**	**Treatment**
Stage I	Small (<4 cm) confined pericolonic or mesenteric abscess	Antibiotics, nothing by mouth/clear liquids
Stage II	Large pericolonic abscess (>4 cm) often extending to the pelvis	Antibiotics, nothing by mouth, percutaneous drainage followed by elective one-staged procedure with controlled infection
Stage III	Rupture of a pericolonic abscess causing purulent peritonitis	As above if sepsis is controlled; otherwise, perform laparotomy if sepsis continues. Resection of involved colon and reanastamosis, with or without diversion. A laparoscopic approach may be feasible
Stage IV	Free rupture of an inflamed diverticulum causing feculent peritonitis	As above with exploratory laparotomy in most cases, possible one- or two-staged procedure Classic three-staged procedure largely abandoned

antibiotics will depend on the source and degree of source control, most infections can be treated with antibiotics for 14 days or less. Recent studies suggest that patients with intra-abdominal infection can be treated with 4 days of antibiotics following source control. Antibiotic requirement beyond a 14-day time frame suggests inadequate source control or complication.

Case Conclusion

The patient was intubated and received 14 L of crystalloids in addition to norepinephrine to support intravascular volume and blood pressure. Following blood cultures, piperacillin–tazobactam was administered within 1 hour of his presentation. His urine output improved from 5 to 10 mL per hour to 35 mL per hour before he went to interventional radiology for percutaneous drainage of his pelvic abscess. Within 4 hours of drainage, his norepinephrine requirement abated. His ventilatory requirement continued for 3 days, but following a spontaneous breathing trial on day 4, he was successfully extubated and liberated from mechanical ventilation. He began to spontaneously diurese on day 2.5 and was assisted with diuretics to remove the fluid he had gained while in shock. He was transferred to the ward for rehabilitation on day 5 after presenting in septic shock.

TAKE HOME POINTS

- Sepsis is defined as life-threatening organ dysfunction caused by a dysregulated host response to infection.
- Septic shock is a subset of sepsis in which underlying circulatory and cellular/metabolic abnormalities are profound enough to substantially increase mortality.
- Sepsis and septic shock are emergencies requiring early diagnosis, source control, timely antibiotic administration, and effective resuscitation.
- The Surviving Sepsis Campaign (SSC) guidelines provide evidence-based treatment strategies and are updated every 4 years based on current literature.

- Initial resuscitation for sepsis and septic shock should precede any attempt at source control beyond antibiotic administration.
- Recent studies suggest antibiotics may be administered for shorter periods after source control.

SUGGESTED READINGS

Angus DC, Barnato AE, Bell D, et al. A systematic review and meta-analysis of early goal-directed therapy for septic shock: the ARISE, ProCESS and ProMISe Investigators. *Intensive Care Med.* 2015;41(9):1549-1560.

ARISE Investigators and ANZICS Clinical Trials Group. Goal-directed resuscitation for patients with early septic shock. *N Engl J Med.* 2014;371:1496-1506.

Dellinger RP, Levy MM, Rhodes A, et al. Surviving sepsis campaign: international guidelines for management of severe sepsis and septic shock. *Crit Care Med.* 2013;41(2):580-637.

Jansen TC, van Bommel J, Schoonderbeek FJ, et al. LACTATE study group: early lactate-guided therapy in intensive care unit patients: a multicenter, open-label, randomized controlled trial. *Am J Respir Crit Care Med.* 2010;182:752-761.

Jones AE, Shapiro NI, Trzeciak S, et al. Emergency Medicine Shock Research Network (EMShockNet) investigators: lactate clearance vs central venous oxygen saturation goals of early sepsis therapy: a randomized clinical trial. *JAMA.* 2010;303:739-746.

Mouncey PR, Osborn TM, Power GS; The ProMISe Trial Investigators. Trial of early, goal-directed resuscitation for septic shock. *N Engl J Med.* 2015;372:1301-1311.

Rivers E, Nguyen B, Havstad S, et al. Early goal-directed therapy in the treatment of severe sepsis and septic shock. *N Engl J Med.* 2001;345(19):1368-1377.

Sawyer RG, Claridge JA, Nathens AB, et al. Trial of short-course antimicrobial therapy for intraabdominal infection. *N Engl J Med.* 2015;372(21):1996-2005.

Shankar-Hari M, Phillips GS, Levy ML, et al. Developing a new definition and assessing new clinical criteria for septic shock for the third international consensus definitions for sepsis and septic shock (sepsis-3). *JAMA.* 2016;315(8):775-787.

Singer M, Deutschman CS, Seymour CW, et al. The third international consensus definitions for sepsis and septic shock (sepsis-3). *JAMA.* 2016;315(8):801-810.

Yealy DM, Kellum JA, Huang DT, et al.; The ProCESS Investigators. A randomized trial of protocol-based care for early septic shock. *N Engl J Med.* 2014;370(18):1683-1693.

Abdominal Compartment Syndrome

ASHLEY D. MEAGHER AND HEATHER LEIGH EVANS

Based on the previous edition chapter "Abdominal Compartment Syndrome" by Rebecca Plevin and Heather L. Evans

Presentation

A 62-year-old man presents to the hospital with severe back pain and hypotension and is diagnosed with a ruptured abdominal aortic aneurysm. He is emergently taken to the operating room where he undergoes successful placement of an endovascular stent graft. The patient receives 12 units of packed red blood cells, 12 units of fresh frozen plasma, and 2 units of platelets intraoperatively and is admitted to the ICU for further resuscitation and mechanical ventilator support. In the next 6 hours, the patient develops progressive hypoxemic respiratory failure with increasing peak airway pressures, hypotension unresponsive to further blood product resuscitation, oliguria, and rising creatinine. On physical exam, his abdomen is distended and tense to palpation.

DIFFERENTIAL DIAGNOSIS

While creating the differential diagnosis of abdominal distension and multisystem organ failure (MSOF) in the critically ill patient, the clinician must first rule out life-threatening causes. In this patient who is persistently hypotensive despite massive blood product transfusion, the immediate concern is continued bleeding. Endovascular repair can be complicated by stent migration, endoleak, or iatrogenic injury at the cannulation site.

Emergency surgical procedures repair with prolonged hypotension increases the risk of bowel ischemia, which may result in worsening clinical picture of refractory shock, as well as abdominal distension. Whole blood lactate should be evaluated, and if elevated, suspicion for ischemia should be high.

Large retroperitoneal hemorrhage, with massive blood product transfusion, can lead to the development of intra-abdominal hypertension (IAH) and abdominal compartment syndrome (ACS), which present as increasing abdominal distension, elevated intra-abdominal pressures, and new-onset organ failure.

Bowel obstruction is possible given the patient's abdominal distension. Physical exam would help elucidate inciting factors such as an abdominal wall hernia or scars suggestive of prior abdominal surgery. In the absence of these factors or other chronic medical conditions, bowel obstruction in this clinical setting is unlikely. Abdominal distension is a frequent first sign of Ogilvie's syndrome (acute colonic pseudo-obstruction), but it does not typically present this early in the hospital course. Similarly, toxic megacolon from *Clostridium difficile* colitis must also be ruled out. This bacterial infection can lead to massive bowel wall edema and ileus, which would explain the patient's progressive abdominal distension and septic symptoms. *Clostridium difficile* is less likely in a newly hospitalized patient, but as there is no background information about his prior health and antibiotic history, colitis must remain on the differential to avoid missing a catastrophic complication such as bowel perforation. This infection should be placed higher on the differential if the patient had received antibiotics recently, had a recent hospitalization, transferred from a long-term health care facility, or has a significant leukocytosis (>18,000/μL), even in the absence of diarrhea.

Ileus is common following critical illness and massive resuscitation. It is typically self-limited and improves with time. Ongoing shock and fluid resuscitation could prolong the duration of an ileus. However, ileus alone would not cause the constellation of hypotension, oliguria, and hypoxemia. The clinician must consider that a systemic inflammatory response such as transfusion-related acute lung injury (TRALI) or adult respiratory distress syndrome (ARDS) may develop as a consequence of the initial episode of shock and resuscitation or due to a secondary insult postoperatively. In addition to MSOF, each of these conditions can cause ileus due to release of inflammatory mediators and result in abdominal distension.

DIAGNOSIS

The first step in working up this patient is to perform physical examination and obtain laboratory studies, specifically a complete blood count (CBC) to evaluate for a sudden drop in hemoglobin and hematocrit and a whole blood lactate level. Significant hematocrit decrease would indicate ongoing hemorrhage, either from the aneurysm or an iatrogenic vascular injury from the femoral cannulation. Any indication of ongoing hemorrhage would necessitate return to the operating room for hemorrhage control.

Evaluation for IAH or ACS should be done by measuring intra-abdominal pressure, which is generally performed via bladder manometry using the Foley catheter for transduction. Serial measurement of abdominal girth can provide objective evidence of increasing distension.

In the absence of immediate indications for operative intervention, imaging studies may be useful. Plain radiographs of the abdomen to look for free air or the presence of pneumatosis intestinalis would indicate bowel perforation or ischemia. Bedside ultrasound can be used to evaluate for volume status, collapsible inferior vena cava (IVC), and the presence of free fluid in the abdomen, as well as hematoma at the cannulation sites. Of course, if the patient were stable enough, a computed tomography (CT) scan would provide important information about the patient's vessels to rule out hemorrhage or if there is pneumatosis intestinalis.

Given his shock and MSOF, sepsis is within the differential, so the patient must be optimized from a medical standpoint while the clinician searches for an infectious source. Central venous access should be obtained, if not already present, and resuscitation escalated, with resuscitation endpoints according to the Surviving Sepsis Campaign guidelines. Specimens should be obtained for culture to rule in infectious sources and eventually guide microbial therapy, but broad-spectrum antibiotics should be initiated without delay if sepsis is high on the differential.

There are a number of possible explanations for the sudden increase in peak airway pressures. If central venous access was placed, iatrogenic pneumothorax must be ruled out by chest x-ray (CXR), and the patency of the endotracheal tube and large bronchi must be evaluated for airway obstruction with airway secretions. The patient's decreased urine output should be investigated by checking the position of the Foley catheter and ruling out catheter obstruction. Obtaining urine electrolytes and calculating the fractional excretion of sodium (FeNa) would be useful to evaluate for acute tubular necrosis as a potential cause of early oliguric renal failure.

Presentation Continued

As part of his workup, CBC reveals a hemoglobin of 9.5 g/dL (slightly increased from one obtained 4 hours ago) and a serum lactate of 3 mmol/L (which is rising from 2.5 mmol/L 4 hours prior). Peak airway pressures on the ventilator are >50 mm Hg, and CXR does not demonstrate a pneumothorax or evidence of lobar collapse. The patient's urine output remains <5 mL per hour. On bedside ultrasound, the patient had a significant amount of free intra-abdominal fluid, as well as a collapsed IVC. The bladder pressure, initially 12 mm Hg on arrival to the ICU, is now 23 mm Hg.

Based on this workup, the patient has ACS, but unrecognized bowel ischemia cannot be ruled out entirely. Diagnostic paracentesis (and possible therapeutic) is one option at this point, but due to the concern for significant bowel edema, exploratory laparotomy and decompression of the abdomen are deemed the more appropriate next step.

● DISCUSSION

The standard intra-abdominal pressure (IAP) is 5 to 7 mm Hg in critically ill adults; IAH is defined as sustained IAP ≥ 12 mm Hg. ACS is defined as sustained IAP > 20 mm Hg that is associated with new organ dysfunction/failure. IAH also involves elevated IAP but does not result in organ dysfunction. IAH is graded based on the degree of hypertension (Table 129-1). Risk factors for ACS include massive fluid resuscitation and tissue edema, abdominal surgery, ileus, sepsis, and hemorrhage (Table 129-2). ACS is therefore most often found in the most critically ill of ICU patients.

The types of ACS are differentiated by their respective causes. Primary ACS occurs after injury, or disease of the abdominopelvic organs leads to increased IAP, such as with hemorrhage from a large liver laceration or a ruptured abdominal aortic aneurysm. Secondary ACS results from factors external to the abdominal compartment. ACS following massive fluid resuscitation and resulting bowel edema is a classic example of secondary ACS. IAH can be broken down into hyperacute, acute, subacute, and chronic based on the length of time over which the condition develops (seconds, hours, days, and months to years, respectively). Hyperacute IAH is usually the result of physiologic processes such as sneezing or Valsalva. Chronic IAH occurs in pregnancy, liver failure, ascites, and intra-abdominal tumor. These subtypes, of course, do not always require intervention. Even morbid obesity may be associated with a chronic elevation of the baseline IAP. In order to be considered diagnostic for ACS, the elevated IAP pressure must be sustained and associated with a new pathologic process in one or more organ systems.

Measurement of IAP is the gold standard for diagnosing ACS using modifications of the Kron's technique, whereby bladder pressure is measured using a urinary catheter (Table 129-3). There are several commercially available products for measuring bladder pressures. "Homemade" devices to measure bladder pressure can also be assembled, but it is important to remember that these devices may produce less reliable results, increased risk of urinary tract infection, and require added expertise and time to obtain data.

CT scan can provide useful clues to the diagnosis. Intrahepatic IVC narrowing may occur as a result of abdominal pressure preventing adequate filling. Bowel walls may appear thickened secondary to edema, and the diaphragms may appear elevated. The patient may have a

Table 129-1	Grading System for Intra-abdominal Hypertension
Grade I: IAP 12–15 mm Hg	
Grade II: IAP 16–20 mm Hg	
Grade III: IAP 21–25 mm Hg	
Grade IV: IAP ≥ 25 mm Hg	

testinal, and neurologic dysfunction. These conditions are associated with increased ICU length of stay and morbidity, and IAH/ACS are independent predictors of mortality in critically ill ICU patients. ACS and IAH are much less common with the advent of crystalloid-sparing resuscitation strategies. Massive transfusion with blood products in hemorrhage and the judicious use of pressors in sepsis have resulted in decreasing incidence of ACS. However, it is vital for a clinician to recognize ACS when it occurs and act expeditiously.

● TREATMENT

Treatment of IAH (Table 129-4) is targeted at preventing progression to ACS, notably improving abdominal wall compliance or intra-abdominal space. There are a few nonoperative techniques that can be attempted, in the correct clinical situation. Large-volume paracentesis of pancreatic ascites, for example, removes the driver of bowel edema, as well as creates "space" for the edematous bowel. However, the clinician must be cognizant of the edematous bowel to avoid perforation while performing paracentesis. This should be accomplished using ultrasound-guided or CT-guided techniques. Nasogastric decompression, use of vasopressors in balance with judicious fluid resuscitation, and dialysis for fluid removal may contribute to an overall effort to reduce IAP.

Table 129-2 Risk Factors for IAH or ACS

Diminished Abdominal Wall Compliance
Abdominal surgery
Major trauma
Major burns
Prone positioning
Increased Intra-abdominal Contents
Gastroparesis/gastric distension
Ileus
Colonic pseudo-obstruction
Volvulus
Capillary Leak/Fluid Resuscitation
Acidosis
Damage control laparotomy
Hypothermia
Sepsis
Miscellaneous
Mechanical ventilation
Obesity

"round belly sign," defined as an anteroposterior:transverse ratio >0.8 when measured at the level where the left renal vein crosses the aorta. Ascites may be seen, as in the case of severe pancreatitis. Frequently, these patients are not stable enough for safe transport to radiology for CT scan, and bedside point-of-care ultrasound has emerged as a promising technology for evaluation of free fluid as well as IVC compression.

ACS is clinically significant because it increases risk of developing respiratory, cardiovascular, renal, gastroin-

Table 129-3 The Modified Kron's Technique for Measuring Bladder Pressure

Measuring Bladder Pressure
1. Insert an 18-gauge IV catheter into the culture port of the Foley catheter; remove needle.
2. Attach IV catheter to pressure tubing.
3. Attach tubing to 1-L NS, 60-mL Luer Lock Syringe, and disposable pressure transducer.
4. Position patient supine and zero transducer at the midaxillary line.
5. Inject 25 mL saline into the urinary bladder and clamp Foley catheter distal to the culture port.
6. Measure bladder pressure at end expiration.

Table 129-4 Nonoperative Management of Increased IAH

Decrease mass effect	Evacuate intraluminal contents: NGT, colonic decompression, minimize enteral nutrition, prokinetic agents
	Remove space-occupying lesions: surgical debridement/excision, percutaneous drainage of fluid collections
	Optimize fluid status: avoid excessive IVF, target daily fluid balance net even to negative 3 L, diuresis, hemofiltration
	Optimize tissue perfusion: keep APP ≥60 mm Hg with judicious IVF, vasoactive medications
Increase abdominal wall compliance	Provide adequate sedation/analgesia, position the patient in reverse Trendelenburg/elevate head of bed, remove constrictive abdominal dressings, administer pharmacologic paralysis

Deep sedation with temporary neuromuscular blockade may be used to increase abdominal wall compliance, if the IAH is thought to be reversible or if surgical intervention should be avoided in a patient with severe medical comorbidities, such as severe cirrhosis.

● SURGICAL APPROACH

When a patient develops ACS with MSOF, surgical decompression should be performed. The overall goal is to decrease IAP, allowing for increased visceral perfusion. There is no consensus among experts regarding an IAP value that requires surgical intervention. Rather, surgery is necessary when there is evidence of end-organ dysfunction despite optimal medical therapy. Delaying decompression leads to further tissue ischemia, organ failure, and increased mortality.

Surgical treatment consists of decompressive laparotomy (Table 129-5). In general, the edematous bowel readily releases from the abdomen, and any ascites or hemorrhage should be evacuated. Fascial reapproximation is typically not possible without causing recurrence of ACS, and the abdomen is left open with a temporary abdominal closure (TAC). This also facilitates a second look operation once the patient is stabilized to assess for any ongoing intra-abdominal pathology, such as bowel ischemia.

There are various methods for the placement of a TAC following decompressive laparotomy including prosthetic mesh; Bogota bag, which is a sterilized plastic bag such as a 3-L intravenous fluid bag; vacuum packing (often used in damage control laparotomy following trauma, see Table 129-5);

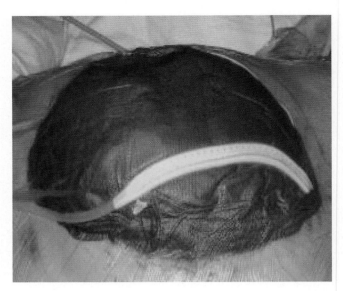

FIGURE 129-1. Vacuum-packed abdomen.

and negative pressure systems such as vacuum-assisted closure devices. In addition to decreasing the risk of further ACS and allowing access to the abdomen if needed, vacuum packs and negative pressure devices have the additional benefit of removing abdominal transudate (Figure 129-1). However, care must be taken with wound vacuums to apply the devices correctly in order to minimize the risk of enterocutaneous fistula formation.

● POSTOPERATIVE MANAGEMENT

Patients are still at risk for ACS after surgical decompression. Even with vacuum packs or negative pressure system, recurrent ACS is possible, particularly if massive fluid resuscitation continues. It is thought that these systems do not always allow for necessary expansion of intra-abdominal volume during postoperative resuscitation and reactive tissue edema.

Because patients remain at risk for ACS following decompressive laparotomy, postoperative care focuses on decreasing IAP by the same methods described above. Bladder pressures should be monitored postoperatively, and the clinician must remain vigilant for further signs of organ dysfunction that could indicate a repeat episode of ACS. Repeat ACS episodes are an indication for return to the operating room and reopening of the laparotomy.

Patients who undergo laparotomy for ACS need eventual abdominal closure. However, prolonged hospitalization with an open abdomen/vacuum pack often leads to tissue contraction and loss of domain, which makes it difficult or impossible to close the abdomen in a one-stage procedure. Early fascial closure should be attempted, as soon as the bowel edema has resolved, to decrease risk of fistula and hernia formation. Even so, these patients may require mesh to augment fascial closure, skin grafting to achieve complete soft tissue coverage, and finally component separation to maintain long-term abdominal wall integrity.

Table 129-5	Creating an Abdominal Vacuum Pack

Key Technical Steps

1. Incise ~1-in slits in a variety of locations on a large plastic drape.
2. If possible, drape the exposed bowel with omentum.
3. Lay the drape flat in a subfascial position, taking care to cover all abdominal contents and to pack the drape into the paracolic gutters.
4. Cover drape with sterile gauze.
5. Place two flat Jackson-Pratt drains on top of the gauze.
6. Cover the wound with sterile towels and an iodine impregnated polyurethane drape (3M Ioban; 3M Healthcare, St. Paul, Minnesota) and place drains to low continuous suction.

Potential Pitfalls

- Use care on entering the abdomen given the high potential for enterotomy due to significant bowel edema.
- Ensure complete coverage of the bowels when placing TAC to decrease risk of fistula formation.

Case Conclusion

The patient is taken to the operating room and undergoes decompressive laparotomy. A large retroperitoneal hematoma is encountered and small ascites, but the patient's intestines are boggy and edematous. A vacuum pack is placed intraoperatively, and the patient returns to the ICU for hemodynamic monitoring including bladder pressure measurements every 4 hours. Over the course of the next 12 hours, the patient's hemodynamics stabilize and kidneys begin to function. He is taken back to the operating room for second look procedure, at which time no intestinal necrosis is found. His bowels are still too edematous to fully close the fascia. Over the following weeks, the patient's fascia is closed in a staged manner. Renal function continues to improve, and he is successfully extubated. He is discharged to a skilled nursing facility with wound vacuum in place over his midline soft tissue defect, which heals over the course of several months.

TAKE HOME POINTS

- ACS affects multiple organ systems. It is important to rule out other causes of injury to each affected organ system.
- IAH: sustained pathologic IAP ≥12 mm Hg. ACS: sustained pathologic IAP >20 mm Hg accompanied by new organ dysfunction/failure.
- The modified Kron's technique is the gold standard for measuring IAP, whereby the intracystic pressure is measured after injecting 25 mL of saline into the urinary bladder.
- IAH may be treated nonoperatively by evacuating intraluminal contents, increasing abdominal compliance, optimizing fluid status, and optimizing tissue perfusion.
- Surgical decompression is necessary when signs of organ dysfunction emerge despite best nonoperative management.
- TAC is advocated in order to decrease the risk of subsequent ACS episodes and facilitate second looks.
- Bladder pressures should be measured even after decompressive laparotomy because compartment syndrome can occur even with TAC.

- Enterocutaneous fistulae are a known complication of temporary negative pressure dressings.
- Early or at least same-stay attempts at fascial closure should be performed.

SUGGESTED READINGS

Acosta S, Wanhainen A, Björck M. Temporary abdominal closure after abdominal aortic aneurysm repair: a systematic review of contemporary observational studies. *Eur J Vasc Endovasc Surg.* 2016;51(3):371-378.

Al-Bahrani AZ, et al. A prospective evaluation of CT features predictive of intra-abdominal hypertension and abdominal compartment syndrome in critically ill surgical patients. *Clin Radiol* 2006;62:676-682.

Balogh ZJ, Lumsdaine W, Moore EE, Moore FA. Postinjury abdominal compartment syndrome: from recognition to prevention. *Lancet.* 2014;384(9952):1466-1475.

Cheatham ML. Nonoperative management of intraabdominal hypertension and abdominal compartment syndrome. *World J Surg.* 2009;33(6):1116-1122.

Kirkpatrick AW, Roberts DJ, De Waele J, et al. Intra-abdominal hypertension and the abdominal compartment syndrome: updated consensus definitions and clinical practice guidelines from the World Society of the Abdominal Compartment Syndrome. *Intensive Care Med.* 2013;39:1190.

Kron IL, Harman PK, Nolan SP. The measurement of intra-abdominal pressure as a criterion for abdominal re-exploration. *Ann Surg.* 1984;199(1):28-30.

Malbrain ML, et al. Prevalence of intra-abdominal hypertension in critically ill patients: a multicentre epidemiological study. *Intensive Care Med.* 2004;30(5):822-829.

Reintam A, et al. Primary and secondary intra-abdominal hypertension—different impact on ICU outcome. *Intensive Care Med.* 2008;34(9):1624-1631.

Seternes A, Rekstad LC, Mo S, et al. Open abdomen treated with negative pressure wound therapy: indications, management and survival, *World J Surg.* 2017;41(1):152-161.

Sugrue M, Buhkari Y. Intra-abdominal pressure and abdominal compartment syndrome in acute general surgery. *World J Surg.* 2009;33(6):1123-1127.

van Brunschot S, Schut AJ, Bouwense SA, et al. Dutch pancreatitis study group. abdominal compartment syndrome in acute pancreatitis: a systematic review. *Pancreas.* 2014;43(5):665-674.

Nutritional Support in the Critically Ill Patient

130

KYLE J. VAN ARENDONK AND ELLIOTT R. HAUT

Based on the previous edition chapter "Nutritional Support in the Critically Ill
Surgery Patient" by Kyle J. Van Arendonk and Elliott R. Haut

Presentation

J.B. is a 35-year-old multisystem trauma victim injured in a high-speed motorcycle crash. After undergoing embolization for bleeding secondary to his open book pelvic fracture, he developed abdominal compartment syndrome requiring decompressive laparotomy. The operation revealed multiple liver lacerations and a small bowel perforation that was resected and primarily anastomosed. Over the next several days, he experienced a significant systemic inflammatory response and multiple organ dysfunction requiring the use of vasopressors and mechanical ventilation.

The above patient suffering from major multisystem trauma is a common scenario managed by the surgical critical care team. One of the many challenges facing the team is finding a way to provide nutrition through the long intensive care unit (ICU) course that likely will ensue.

● WORKUP

Calculating Nutritional Requirements

Energy requirements vary based on the clinical scenario, but a general estimate is 25 to 30 kcal/kg/d. Higher energy requirements can be seen in patients with burns, sepsis, and multisystem trauma. Energy requirements can also be calculated using published predictive equations such as the Harris-Benedict equation (Table 130-1), which gives a measure of resting energy expenditure (REE) that can then be adjusted by an activity or stress factor to calculate total daily energy expenditure (Table 130-2). Finally, indirect calorimetry can also be used. Indirect calorimetry uses a "metabolic cart" to measure the amount of oxygen consumed and carbon dioxide eliminated in order to calculate a patient's actual (as opposed to predicted) REE. In order to maintain accuracy, indirect calorimetry is typically limited to patients who are on mechanical ventilation and who are at a relatively steady state.

Carbohydrates, protein, and fat provide 4, 4, and 9 kcal/g, respectively. Ethanol provides 7 kcal/g. In clinical settings, dextrose, with an energy content of 3.4 kcal/kg, should typically be used rather than carbohydrate for calculations

(Table 130-3). For parenteral nutrition, 10% and 20% lipid solutions contain 1.1 and 2 kcal/mL, respectively. In the ICU setting, infusions of propofol also provide significant calories that must be considered (1.1 kcal/mL) (Table 130-1). In general, approximately 60% of calories should come from carbohydrate, 25% to 30% from fat, and 10% to 15% from protein. Protein seems to be the nutrient most important for wound healing, immune function, and preventing the loss of lean body mass. Critically ill patients are therefore often given additional protein based upon either simple equations (estimating 1 to 2 g/kg/d of protein need) or by calculating their actual nitrogen balance (see below).

● TREATMENT

The first two issues that must be addressed are when to begin nutrition and via what route that nutrition should be provided.

Table 130-1	Useful Formulas
Harris-Benedict Equation (kcal/24 h) for Estimating Resting Energy Expenditure (REE)	REE (men) = 66.5 + (13.8 × weight in kg) + (5 × height in cm) − (6.8 × age) REE (women) = 655 + (9.6 × weight in kg) + (1.8 × height in cm) − (4.7 × age)
Caloric Content of Nutrients/Infusions	Carbohydrate: 4 kcal/g Dextrose: 3.4 kcal/g Protein: 4 kcal/g Fat: 9 kcal/g Ethanol: 7 kcal/g Propofol: 1.1 kcal/mL 10% Lipid Solution: 1.1 kcal/mL 20% Lipid Solution: 2 kcal/mL
Nitrogen Balance	Nitrogen balance = (protein intake ÷ 6.25) − (UUN + 4)
Respiratory Quotient (RQ)	Carbohydrate: 1.0 Protein: 0.8 Fat: 0.7 Underfeeding: <0.7 Overfeeding: >1.0

Table 130-2	Approximate Stress Factor Multipliers for REE	
Elective Surgery	1.2
Multisystem Trauma	1.3–1.5
Sepsis	1.5–1.8
Burns	1.5–2.0

Timing

The benefits of early enteral nutrition in the critically ill and injured patients have been well established. Ideally, enteral nutrition should be initiated within the first 24 to 48 hours following ICU admission. Early provision of enteral nutrition can dampen the inflammatory response and is associated with lower mortality, decreased morbidity, and improved outcomes.

Enteral Versus Parenteral Route

The enteral route is preferred over the parenteral route whenever possible because of both the benefits of enteral nutrition and the risks associated with parenteral nutrition. Enteral

Table 130-3	Sample Calculations
	Goal: provide 70 kg patient with 25 kcal/kg/d and 1.0 g protein/kg/d 70 kg × 25 kcal/kg/d = 1,750 kcal/d 70 kg × 1.0 g protein/kg/d = 70 g protein/d
Tube Feeds	Chosen tube feed contains 1.5 kcal/mL and 0.06 g protein/mL 1,750 Kcal/d ÷ 1.5 kcal/mL = 1,167 mL/d 1,167 mL ÷ 24 h = 49 mL/h 1,167 mL × 0.06 g protein/mL = 70 g protein The tube feeds can be run continuously at 49 mL/h, which will provide 25 kcal/kg d and 1.0 g protein/kg/d
CPN	Chosen CPN solution contains 70 g amino acids and 285 g dextrose in 1,000 mL and will be added to 250 mL of 20% lipid emulsion Total volume = 1,250 mL 1,250 mL ÷ 24 h = 52 mL/h 70 g amino acid × 4 kcal/g = 280 kcal 285 g dextrose × 3.4 kcal/g = 969 kcal 250 mL × 2 kcal/mL = 500 kcal Total kcal/d = 1,749 1,749 kcal/d ÷ 70 kg = 25 kcal/kg/d The CPN can be run continuously at 52 mL/h, which will provide 25 kcal/kg and 1.0 g protein/kg/d

nutrition has been shown to stimulate the production of secretory immunoglobulin A, preserve upper respiratory tract immunity, maintain the intestinal brush border, preserve gut-associated lymphoid tissue, and prevent the translocation of bacteria across the intestinal wall, all leading to a decrease in infectious complications in surgical ICU patients.

Enteral nutrition also avoids the many risks inherent to parenteral nutrition, including mechanical complications of central venous access placement (i.e., pneumothorax, hemothorax, arterial puncture, etc.), line sepsis, electrolyte disturbances, and liver dysfunction. With the use of parenteral nutrition, gut disuse leads to mucosal atrophy, bacterial overgrowth, diminished blood flow, and decreased gut immunity, all of which may lead to increased translocation of bacteria across the intestinal wall.

● ROUTES FOR ENTERAL NUTRITION

Enteral feeds can be provided through several routes. Gastric feeds can be provided via an orogastric or nasogastric tube or via a gastrostomy tube, placed either surgically, endoscopically (percutaneous endoscopic gastrostomy [PEG] tube), or percutaneously via interventional radiology. Postpyloric feeds can be given via a nasoduodenal or nasojejunal tube, a surgical jejunostomy tube, or a PEG tube with a jejunal extension (PEG-J).

Bedside placement of nasoduodenal tubes can be time-consuming and at times difficult. The critical care teams and surgical teams should plan ahead whenever possible and have a nasoduodenal tube placed intraoperatively under direct manipulation in patients undergoing laparotomy who are expected to need enteral nutritional access. When a nasoduodenal feeding tube is placed in the ICU, a two-step procedure should be utilized to avoid inadvertent bronchial placement and the potential complications that can result (Figures 130-1 and 130-2). Newer devices with more advanced technologies now exist. The Kangaroo™ feeding tube, which has a 3-mm camera within it, can provide real-time imaging guidance that may facilitate correct anatomic tube placement in the ICU in a more safe and expeditious manner. The Cortrak™ tube placement system uses an electromagnetic transmitter on the tube, which can be sensed and followed outside the patient via a special receiving unit. After proper placement is confirmed, taking the small amount of extra time to secure the tube to the nose (i.e., via a commercial device such as the AMT bridle™) can increase the likelihood that the enteral tube stays in position through periods of patient agitation and patient repositioning.

No evidence exists for a mortality benefit with postpyloric feeds rather than gastric feeds. However, postpyloric feeds may decrease the risk of regurgitation, aspiration, and pneumonia. Given the higher risk of aspiration with gastric feeds, many providers suggest that critically ill patients at high risk of aspiration should preferentially be fed via a postpyloric route, especially if showing any signs of intolerance

1. Prior to placement, estimate the length of tube needed to extend just below the patient's carina (typically about 30 cm).

2. With the stylet in, insert the tube to the measured length and obtain a chest x-ray to confirm that the tube is midline rather than extending laterally (towards the lung) into either bronchi (Figure 130-2A).

3. After midline position is confirmed, advance the tube with the stylet to the desired position.

4. Obtain an abdominal x-ray to confirm successful positioning (Figure 130-2B).

5. Reposition as needed.

6. When correct placement is confirmed, fasten the tube securely and remove the stylet.

7. Begin tube feeds.

FIGURE 130-1. Two-step procedure for nasoduodenal feeding tube placement.

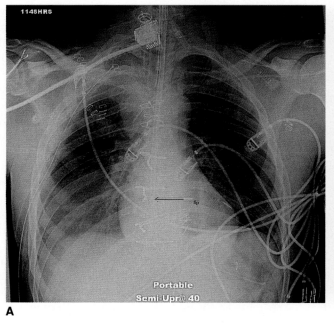
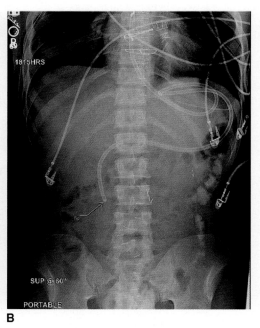

A   B

FIGURE 130-2. Radiographs showing **(A)** initial insertion of the feeding tube into the distal esophagus to confirm midline positioning beyond the carina and **(B)** advancement of the feeding tube into a postpyloric position.

to gastric feeds. However, gastric feeds can still be used safely in the majority of patients and are often the suggested first-line treatment.

Monitoring of Enteral Feeding

Tolerance of enteral feeding should primarily be assessed via a through physical examination and clinical assessment, with the absence of nausea, vomiting, and abdominal distention and the passage of flatus and stool acting as reliable signs of adequate tolerance. Another way to monitor the tolerance of gastric feeds is to measure gastric residual volumes, which can be checked approximately every 6 hours and are considered acceptable when less than approximately 200 to 300 cc (exact values vary by institution). However, gastric residuals poorly predict the risk of aspiration and pneumonia and therefore are frequently being abandoned as a routine part of patient care. In centers where gastric residuals are still routinely measured, repeated high gastric residuals may be used to encourage the transition to postpyloric feeding, but repeatedly holding tube feeds when gastric residuals are high in the absence of any clinical signs of feeding intolerance is discouraged.

A common problem in the ICU patient receiving enteral feeds is the frequent stopping of enteral feeds for frequent, often daily, trips to the operating room or to diagnostic testing. Tube feeds at an hourly goal rate cannot provide full nutrition when they are routinely infusing for only a small portion of each 24-hour period. If these patients are already intubated or have a tracheostomy in place, the need for anesthesia induction for intubation is precluded, and tube feeds can therefore safely be left running during these periods in order to maximize nutritional support. In the case of postpyloric feeding, the risk of aspiration even when induction of anesthesia is required is exceedingly low. Nutrition should therefore be continued during procedures or diagnostic testing whenever possible. Some centers also use a nurse-driven protocol, which allows the nurse to adjust the tube feed hourly rate to achieve a 24-hour total goal volume.

Enteral Nutrition in Specific Patient Populations

Clinical scenarios do exist in which enteral nutrition must be avoided. For example, bowel perforation, bowel obstruction, and discontinuity of the gastrointestinal tract (i.e., damage control surgery) preclude enteral feeding. However, research is showing the number of these conditions is fewer than previously thought. In cases of acute pancreatitis, enterocutaneous fistulae, and the open abdomen, enteral nutrition has historically been held, but now has been shown to be safe and even beneficial.

For acute pancreatitis, increasing evidence shows that early enteral nutrition improves outcomes. Gastric and jejunal feeds may even provide similar benefit, contrary to intuition that would suggest that gastric feeds would stimulate the pancreas and worsen the inflammatory response. For proximal enterocutaneous fistulae, enteral feeds can be provided

distal to the fistula. For more distal fistulae, proximal enteral feeds can be given, and the length of small bowel present prior to the fistula will determine if enteral nutrition will be adequate. In these cases, as well as in cases of short gut syndrome, the addition of "supplemental" parenteral nutrition may be necessary to achieve total caloric needs.

Historically, enteral nutrition has also been delayed for several days until bowel function has returned (as marked by presence of bowel sounds, passage of flatus, bowel movements, etc.) after any gastrointestinal surgery. However, increasing evidence shows that early enteral feeding in postoperative patients is not only safe but also beneficial in accelerating the return of bowel function after surgery. In addition, within the ICU population in particular, some level of gastrointestinal dysfunction is very common. The typical signs marking return of bowel function are not necessarily reliable, and enteral nutrition should not be delayed based simply upon the lack of bowel sounds or passage of flatus and stool.

Finally, enteral nutrition should be avoided in patients with significant hemodynamic instability. In patients requiring vasopressor support or large-volume fluid or blood product resuscitation, enteral nutrition is typically withheld until the patient is more hemodynamically stable and fully resuscitated. Although ischemic bowel is a rare complication of enteral nutrition, theoretically enteral nutrition may require an increase in splanchnic blood flow requirement that cannot be supported in low cardiac output states. For this reason, hemodynamic instability has been considered a contraindication to early enteral feeding. However, enteral support can be provided to patients on stable low doses of vasopressors while watching carefully for any signs of intolerance.

● ROLE OF PARENTERAL NUTRITION

When early enteral nutrition is *not* possible, decision-making depends on the patient's nutritional status prior to admission to the ICU. No nutritional support is necessary for the first seven days in previously healthy patients without evidence of malnutrition, after which parenteral nutrition should then be initiated. However, if patients have evidence of malnutrition prior to the episode of critical illness, parenteral nutrition should be initiated as soon as possible. In these high-risk patients, initial hypocaloric dosing of their parenteral nutrition (≤20 kcal/kg/d or 80% of energy requirements) may provide significant benefits, after which parenteral nutrition can be increased to meet full energy requirements once the patients have stabilized. Parenteral nutrition can generally be stopped once enteral nutrition has begun and is able to provide a majority (>60%) of the patient's energy requirements.

Parenteral nutrition can also be used to supplement enteral support in cases in which enteral support cannot meet a patient's full caloric requirements after approximately seven days. Maintaining at least a portion of patients' nutritional support via the enteral route is important, as even "trickle" or "trophic" feeds (usually considered 10 to 30 cc/h of tube feeds) may be beneficial in maintaining the intestinal brush border and preventing mucosal atrophy.

Parenteral nutrition requires adequate venous access. Peripheral parenteral nutrition (PPN) is a lower osmolality solution that can safely be given through a peripheral vein, although it is only rarely able to provide full nutritional support. PPN is often used as a bridge until full enteral support can be achieved or adequate venous access is obtained for central parenteral nutrition (CPN). CPN consists of a high osmolality solution that can provide full nutrition but must be given through a central venous line.

Several approaches can help decrease line sepsis when using parenteral nutrition. Lines should be placed in a standardized fashion using a checklist to ensure adherence to best practices for sterility. A single-lumen peripherally inserted central catheter (PICC) or a single-lumen central line is preferred over the use of any multiple-lumen catheters because of the lower risk of line sepsis. The subclavian vein is preferred (vs. internal jugular or femoral) given its lower rate of infection. The central line should be a new line inserted with a fresh stick rather than changed over a guide wire at a pre-existing central line site. Ideally, the central line should be limited to provision of parenteral nutrition ("dedicated") without any other use (i.e., blood draws or medication administration). Tunneled lines should be considered when an extended period of parenteral nutrition is expected.

Presentation Continued

After a long course in the SICU, J.B. was slowly weaning from mechanical ventilation. His prealbumin was measured to be 25 (normal range 18 to 38). His nitrogen balance was calculated to be positive. A metabolic cart was completed, and his respiratory quotient (RQ) was 1.1. His tube feeds were adjusted appropriately. His glycemic control, initially maintained with an insulin drip, was converted to a subcutaneous regimen.

● MONITORING ADEQUACY OF NUTRITIONAL SUPPORT

The concept of nitrogen balance is based on the balance between anabolism and catabolism. Providing nutritional support to the critically ill patient is meant to shift this balance to the anabolic state so that the patient's protein need not be utilized for gluconeogenesis (catabolism). The ideal state of positive nitrogen balance is then a greater intake of nitrogen than excretion of nitrogen, while a negative nitrogen balance is to be avoided. Nitrogen balance is calculated by subtracting total nitrogen losses (urine, stool, insensible losses) from nitrogen intake (Table 130-1). Nitrogen intake is calculated based on 6.25 g of protein containing 1 g of nitrogen, while nitrogen losses are estimated by measuring a 24-hour urine urea nitrogen (UUN) and adding an estimate of stool and insensible losses.

Adequacy of nutrition can also be estimated using the respiratory quotient (RQ), which is calculated via indirect calorimetry. The RQ is the ratio of carbon dioxide produced to oxygen consumed. Each of the major nutrients has a unique RQ: protein (RQ = 0.8), fat (RQ = 0.7), and carbohydrates (RQ = 1.0). Pure carbohydrate metabolism therefore has an RQ of 1.0, while pure fat oxidation has an RQ of 0.7. The ideal RQ on an individual patient is approximately 0.8. An RQ under 0.7 represents underfeeding with resulting lipolysis and ketosis. An RQ over 1.0 represents overfeeding (Table 130-1).

Reassessment of the adequacy of nutritional support in meeting requirements should be done at regular intervals. In addition to indirect calorimetry and the other methods mentioned, a number of laboratory values also serve as markers of adequate nutrition. Albumin and transferrin levels have half-lives of approximately 20 and 10 days and so do not serve as ideal markers of changes made in the short-term. Prealbumin is a more useful marker with its shorter half-life of about 2 days. Retinol-binding protein is a relatively new marker with an even shorter half-life of about 12 hours. Unfortunately, each of these markers also reflects the acute phase response to critical illness and therefore may not accurately reflect nutritional status in the ICU setting.

Critically ill patients should have their glucose levels monitored closely. The optimal target range of blood glucose continues to evolve with newly emerging research and may be different for specific patient populations (i.e., cardiac surgery). One large trial showed reduced sepsis, reduced ICU length of stay, and lower hospital mortality with strict glucose control, keeping glucose levels 80 to 110 mg/dL, compared to "conventional" therapy (keeping glucose levels <200 mg/dL). However, more recently, another large trial has brought this practice into question after showing increased mortality in patients receiving strict glucose control compared to a more lenient approach (keeping glucose levels <180 mg/dL), thought to be secondary to differences in episodes of hypoglycemia. Many institutions have therefore now relaxed the upper limit of their goal range for glucose control, with target glucose ranges of 140 to 180 or 150 to 180 mg/dL frequently being used.

Overfeeding and Refeeding Syndrome

Overfeeding patients in the critical care setting should be avoided with the same vigilance that underfeeding is avoided. Overfeeding can cause harmful metabolic consequences, including hyperglycemia and hypertriglyceridemia. In addition, overfeeding can have deleterious effects on weaning from mechanical ventilation by burdening the patient with an extra load of carbon dioxide that must be expired. This diagnosis must be considered and ruled out in any patient who does not have another more obvious cause for failure to wean from mechanical ventilation.

When initiating nutritional support in the critically ill, the critical care team must avoid the risk of refeeding syndrome. This condition typically occurs when the sudden introduction of nutrition in a relatively malnourished patient stimulates the release of insulin, causing phosphate, potassium, and magnesium to shift intracellularly. The diagnosis is made when hypophosphatemia, hypokalemia, and hypomagnesemia are discovered after initiation of nutritional support in at-risk patients, such as those with prolonged malnutrition, excessive gastrointestinal losses, chronic alcohol abuse, metastatic cancer, or recent abdominal surgery, all of which lead to depletion of the above electrolytes. Refeeding syndrome can result in generalized muscle weakness and difficulty in weaning the patient from mechanical ventilation due to the depletion of adenosine triphosphate stores resulting from hypophosphatemia. The condition can be avoided by slowly reintroducing nutrition in patients at high risk of developing the syndrome.

Immunonutrition

More recently, the focus has shifted from nutritional *support* to nutritional *therapy* as a way to augment the immune system in critically ill patients. For example, a relative arginine depletion is thought to limit T-cell function and contribute to the immunosuppressed state following injury or major surgery. In addition, omega-3 fatty acids appear to have immune-modulating benefits in postoperative patients. Immune-modulating enteral feeds containing arginine and omega-3 fatty acids have shown promising results with regard to decreasing postoperative complications, especially in high-risk patients. Additional research is needed regarding the use of arginine and omega-3 fatty acids as well as other antioxidants such as selenium, vitamin C, and vitamin E, but these immune-modulating formulas appear to have a variety of clinical benefits in the critically ill.

Case Conclusion

After weaning from mechanical ventilation, J.B. was transferred from the ICU. His tube feeds were continued while he regained swallowing function with the help of speech and language pathologists. He was able to support his nutrition with an oral diet before transfer to a rehabilitation facility.

The importance of appropriate nutritional support in the critically ill cannot be overemphasized. Failure to provide adequate nutrition has been shown to increase morbidity and mortality in the ICU. Appropriate nutritional support in the critically ill limits the inflammatory response and decreases the rate of ICU complications.

TAKE HOME POINTS

- Early nutrition is beneficial in critically ill patients.
- Enteral nutrition is preferable to parenteral nutrition whenever possible.
- Consider risks of gastric versus postpyloric feeding.
- Overfeeding should be avoided as much as underfeeding.
- Use objective data (i.e., laboratory values, nitrogen balance, and indirect calorimetry) to guide changes in nutritional support.

SUGGESTED READINGS

Al-Omran M, Albalawi ZH, Tashkandi MF, Al-Ansary LA. Enteral versus parenteral nutrition for acute pancreatitis. *Cochrane Database Syst Rev.* 2010;(1):CD002837.

Chang YS, Fu HQ, Xiao YM, Liu JC. Nasogastric or nasojejunal feeding in predicted severe acute pancreatitis: a meta-analysis. *Crit Care.* 2013;17(3):R118.

Davies AR, Morrison SS, Bailey MJ, et al. A multicenter, randomized controlled trial comparing early nasojejunal with nasogastric nutrition in critical illness. *Crit Care Med.* 2012;40(8):2342-2348.

Elke G, van Zanten AR, Lemieux M, et al. Enteral versus parenteral nutrition in critically ill patients: an updated systematic review and meta-analysis of randomized controlled trials. *Crit Care.* 2016;20(1):117.

Fivez T, Kerklaan D, Mesotten D, et al. Early versus late parenteral nutrition in critically Ill children. *N Engl J Med.* 2016;374(12):1111-1122.

Investigators N-SS, Finfer S, Chittock DR, et al. Intensive versus conventional glucose control in critically ill patients. *N Engl J Med.* 2009;360(13):1283-1297.

Jiang H, Sun MW, Hefright B, Chen W, Lu CD, Zeng J. Efficacy of hypocaloric parenteral nutrition for surgical patients: a systematic review and meta-analysis. *Clin Nutr.* 2011;30(6):730-737.

Marimuthu K, Varadhan KK, Ljungqvist O, Lobo DN. A meta-analysis of the effect of combinations of immune modulating nutrients on outcome in patients undergoing major open gastrointestinal surgery. *Ann Surg.* 2012;255(6):1060-1068.

McClave SA, Taylor BE, Martindale RG, et al. Guidelines for the provision and assessment of nutrition support therapy in the adult critically Ill patient: Society of Critical Care Medicine (SCCM) and American Society for Parenteral and Enteral Nutrition (A.S.P.E.N.). *JPEN J Parenter Enteral Nutr.* 2016;40(2):159-211.

Reignier J, Mercier E, Le Gouge A, et al. Effect of not monitoring residual gastric volume on risk of ventilator-associated pneumonia in adults receiving mechanical ventilation and early enteral feeding: a randomized controlled trial. *JAMA.* 2013;309(3):249-256.

SECTION **14**

Transplant

Acute Liver Failure

131

Based on the previous edition chapter "Acute Liver Failure" by Bernard J. Dubray and Christopher D. Anderson

Presentation

A 32-year-old, 45-kg Asian female is transferred in from an outside hospital. She appears mildly jaundiced with confusion, being only oriented to person. She is tachypneic and tachycardic but not requiring any hemodynamic vasopressor support. On exam, ophthalmic evaluation is normal except for scleral icterus, the patient's chest is clear, examination of the abdomen reveals a firm palpable liver edge, there is bruising on her arms, and the patient has a tremor. According to family, the patient was otherwise healthy and well until a few weeks ago, when she began complaining of flulike symptoms and fatigue. She was treated with a course of antibiotics without success, and then began taking over-the-counter cold medications, which "didn't help no matter how much she took" as well as "a lot of different herbal medications." One day prior, she began to quickly deteriorate and became confused so her family brought her to a local emergency room. She was found to have markedly elevated liver enzymes (AST 3990 IU/L, ALT 3570 IU/L, total bilirubin 4.5 mg/dL), with acidosis on arterial blood gas (pH 7.20), and she was admitted to her local hospital, before being transferred to a tertiary center later that day as she deteriorated further.

● DIFFERENTIAL DIAGNOSIS

The patient in the case presentation has acute liver failure (ALF), known historically as fulminant hepatic failure. ALF is characterized by a rapid deterioration in liver function along with other organ dysfunction, in a patient without chronic fibrotic liver disease. ALF patients typically present with nonspecific symptoms (i.e., fatigue, malaise, anorexia) and jaundice before progressing to the hallmark symptoms of a coagulopathy and hepatic encephalopathy. As ALF progresses, multiorgan dysfunction occurs with renal failure, cardiovascular collapse, and respiratory failure. Most urgently, patients with ALF may die of cerebral edema that leads to brain death, which can occur within days of development of symptoms.

ALF occurs when a primary insult causes marked hepatocyte death, with subsequent activation of the innate immune response (monocytes, Kupffer cells). This then causes a large production of inflammatory mediators leading to a marked systemic response, resulting in liver disease with an associated overwhelming systemic inflammatory response syndrome (SIRS) and organ failure. Parallel to this, circulating monocytes become functionally impaired and less able to respond to infection, predisposing the ALF patient to sepsis, a frequent cause of death in ALF.

There are numerous causes of ALF (Table 131-1), and it is critical for management and prognosis to establish a correct diagnosis. ALF is stratified into hyperacute (<7 days), acute (7 to 28 days), and subacute (4 to 26 weeks) based on duration between jaundice/icterus and encephalopathy, and the different etiologies are associated with these stratifications. Acetaminophen-induced liver injury, and hepatitis A and E virus are typically hyperacute, hepatitis B virus (HBV) and autoimmune causes are acute, and non–acetaminophen drug–induced liver injury and Wilson's disease are common causes of a subacute presentation. Geography is also relevant in defining ALF, since in Eastern countries and the developing world, almost 95% of ALF cases are viral (hepatitis A/B/E virus), whereas Western countries have a more heterogenous picture, with acetaminophen overdose being most common, in the United Kingdom (45% of patients) and United States, compared with non–acetaminophen drug hepatotoxicity being common in Germany and France.

While rapid deterioration in liver function is the hallmark of ALF, sudden elevations of liver transaminases and bilirubin, along with coagulopathy and altered level of consciousness, can also be seen in several other disease processes. If no primary injury is present, then these other conditions must be considered in the differential diagnosis:

(a) **Acute Decompensation of Cirrhosis**—A patient may be unaware that they are cirrhotic, particularly with HBV, Willson's disease, or autoimmune disease where they may be well compensated. An acute decompensation of their cirrhosis can mimic the symptoms of ALF.

(b) **Autoimmune Hepatitis (AIH)**—Patients with AIH can develop a sudden onset of a marked jaundice and transaminitis, which can be mistaken for ALF.

(c) **Acute Alcoholic Hepatitis**—This is easily missed if alcohol abuse is not detected. Patients present with an elevated GGT that is five times the upper limit of normal, with increased WBC and no other signs of sepsis.

(d) **Preeclampsia/HEELP Syndrome/Acute Fatty Liver of Pregnancy**—This should be considered in pregnant and recently postpartum women.

Table 131-1	Etiologies of Acute Liver Failure		
ALF Etiology	**Hyperacute (<7 d)**	**Acute (<8–28 d)**	**Subacute (4–26 wk)**
Medication	Acetaminophen Halothane	Rifampin INH Phenytoin	Non–acetaminophen antibiotics Valproate
Viral infections	Hepatitis A Hepatitis E	Hepatitis B	Epstein-Barr Cytomegalovirus Varicella
Toxins	Wild mushrooms (*Amanita phalloides*)	Carbon tetrachloride Wild mushrooms	Herbal supplements (kava, ephedra)
Autoimmune	—	Autoimmune	Autoimmune
Metabolic	—	—	Wilson's disease Reyes syndrome
Vascular	—	—	Budd-Chiari

(e) **Multiorgan Dysfunction from Sepsis**—Severe sepsis can cause multiorgan dysfunction, with cholestasis causing jaundice, and a SIRS presentation that mimics ALF.

(f) **Malignant Infiltration**—A diffuse hepatic infiltration of malignant cells from lymphoma, or a rapidly progressive metastatic tumor, can lead to rapidly progressive liver failure.

(g) **Acute Ischemic Injury/Hypoxic Hepatitis**—Common in elderly patients with cardiovascular disease and congestive heart failure causing hypotension and hypoxia. It also occurs with surgical injury or trauma to the vascular inflow to the liver.

(h) **Pancreatitis**—Presents with elevated liver enzymes and bilirubin, with a SIRS response similar to ALF, but without the coagulopathy and encephalopathy.

● WORKUP

ALF can evolve rapidly, so an urgent and methodical workup should be simultaneous to patient treatment and stabilization, ensuring quick identification of diagnostic details that guide appropriate therapy. In some cases of ALF, the patient's presentation can change dramatically over the day from being awake to brain death caused by cerebral edema, so everything must be expedited. A comprehensive history from both patient and relatives is important for obtaining information about symptoms, medication frequency, and describing the interval between jaundice and encephalopathy, which is helpful for defining ALF prognosis and subtype.

The severity of the liver injury is determined by the liver enzymes (AST, ALT, GGT, alkaline phosphatase) and bilirubin. Next, an INR to assess coagulopathy, arterial ammonia, and an arterial blood gas is used to assess the prognosis and

urgency for transplantation. Finally, further labs are used to determine the etiology of the ALF, including the following:

(a) Viral serologies for HBV (HBsAg, HBcAb) along with the DNA PCR test, and serologies for hepatitis A virus (anti-HAV IgM) and hepatitis E virus (anti-HEV IgM).

(b) Other viral serologies for herpes simplex (anti-HSV IgM), varicella virus (anti-VZV IgM), and also DNA PCR test for cytomegalovirus (CMV), Epstein-Barr virus (EBV), herpes simplex virus (HSV), and parvovirus.

(c) Autoimmune markers: antinuclear antibodies (ANA), anti-smooth muscle antibodies (ASMA), antisoluble liver antigen (anti-SLA), antineutrophil cytoplasmic antibody (ANCA).

(d) Urine toxicology screen

(e) Serum acetaminophen level

(f) Serum copper level and serum ceruloplasmin level for Wilson's disease.

Diagnostic imaging has a reduced role in the initial workup for ALF, as it less helpful for diagnosis, but may aid in making therapeutic decisions. A liver duplex ultrasound assesses the patency and direction of flow of the hepatic artery and vein and portal vein, and a CT scan of the abdomen can assess liver volume and texture and also exclude other diagnoses such as pancreatitis. Nodular liver morphology consistent with underlying chronic liver disease may change the differential diagnosis as described above. The role for liver biopsy is ill defined and limited, and while it may not diagnose the cause, it can provide useful prognostic information and rule out other causes such as autoimmune hepatitis and malignant infiltration. If performed, the biopsy should be transjugular, rather percutaneous given the coagulopathy associated with ALF.

During the workup of ALF, the patient should be monitored, and general supportive measures should be initiated to maintain patient stability and prevent complications that might become contraindications for transplantation.

Presentation Continued

The history from the patient and family described flulike symptoms for several weeks; however, the confusion and jaundice only occurred in the last day. The patient had been taking many doses of OTC cold medications (likely containing acetaminophen), and with further probing, it was found that she was also taking extrastrength acetaminophen. Viral serologies and PCR were drawn and pending, autoimmune markers, serum copper, and urine toxicology were normal. Acetaminophen level was 50 mcg/mL, approximately 24 to 36 hours after the patient's last acetaminophen dose.

● DIAGNOSIS AND TREATMENT

Not all cases of ALF require transplantation, but when transplant is required, it is unique among surgical emergencies: one cannot immediately proceed to the operating room like occurs in other general surgical emergencies. The nature of transplantation involves waiting, often for several days for a suitable organ (deceased or living donor) to become available; therefore, the surgical treatment of ALF requires medical management to limit complications until that transplant can occur. The overall treatment of ALF involves a general diagnosis algorithm, along with a parallel organ medical management strategy. The general diagnosis algorithm is (a) Recognition of ALF; (b) Assessment for Immediate Transplantation; (c) Identification of Disease Etiology; (d) Potential Therapeutic Interventions; and (e) Decision on Transplantation.

(a) **Recognition of ALF**

Patients with ALF can present with nonspecific symptoms (i.e., fatigue, malaise, anorexia, abdominal pain), which may go unnoticed until jaundice evolves. The hallmark of ALF is severe liver dysfunction associated with encephalopathy and coagulopathy; however, for optimal outcome, the disease needs to be recognized as early as possible, preferably prior to these hallmark symptoms.

(b) **Assessment for Expedited Transplantation**

Some patients need an expedited move to transplantation, even prior to all diagnostic results being available. The King's College Criteria (Table 131-2) is a metric used to stratify patients based on their risk of death without transplantation, which allows prioritizing those for expedited transplantation. Those meeting the criteria should be evaluated and listed for transplantation immediately.

(c) **Identification of Disease Etiology**

There are many causes of ALF including viral, medications, autoimmune, toxic, metabolic, and vascular causes. Potential therapies exist for some etiologies such as viral hepatitis and acetaminophen overdose, making laboratory and serologic diagnosis of these etiologies vital. Autoimmune etiologies, and vascular etiologies such as Budd-Chiari, may also have potential therapeutic interventions as well, although their effectiveness is less clear. In contrast, many of the other remaining etiologies including toxic causes such as wild mushrooms or herbal supplements, and metabolic causes such as Wilson's disease, do not have therapeutic interventions, making a diagnosis critical since transplant is the only definitive therapy available.

Wild mushroom poisoning (from *Amanita phalloides*) should be suspected in patients with severe gastrointestinal symptoms such as nausea, vomiting, diarrhea, and abdominal cramping within 24 hours of mushroom ingestion. Wilson's disease, representing up to 12% of all ALF cases, occurs primarily in women, and lab tests show elevated serum and urine copper levels, a high bilirubin to alkaline phosphatase ratio, and decreased serum ceruloplasmin level. A slit-lamp ophthalmic examination can identify Kayser-Fleischer rings in 50% of Wilson's disease patients. Finally, many drugs can cause hepatotoxicity and ALF, either by binding to cytochrome system molecules, inducing oxidative stress, or causing mitochondrial or hepatocyte toxicity. The most common—and most commonly missed—drug-induced ALF is from antibiotics such as amoxicillin–clavulanate.

Table 131-2	Kings College Criteria for Liver Transplant Listing	
ALF due to Acetaminophen	**ALF due to Other Causes**

• pH <7.3 after resuscitation
  or
• Lactate >3 mmol/L
  or
• All of the following 3 criteria
  • Encephalopathy >grade III
  • Cr >3.4
  • INR >6.5
	• INR >6.5
	  or
	• Any 3 of the following criteria
	  • Indeterminate and drug induced
	  • Age >40 y or <10 y
	  • INR >3.5
	  • Interval jaundice–encephalopathy >7 d
	  • Bilirubin >17.5

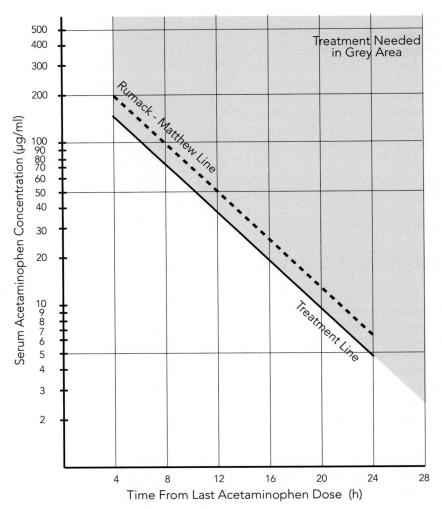

FIGURE 131-1. Rumack-Matthew nomogram.

(d) Potential Therapeutic Interventions

Several etiologies for ALF have potential therapies, which if initiated early can avoid a transplant, making early diagnosis important.

Hepatitis B Virus (HBV): The detection of HBsAg (>10,000 UI/mL) and/or HBV DNA, along with high titres of IgM HBcAb, implicates HBV. In ALF, the typical innate immune response against HBV does not occur, and instead, cytotoxic CD8 T cells destroy hepatocytes after recognizing hepatitis B core antigen on the hepatocyte cell surface. Immediate treatment with the antiviral therapy entecavir improves survival from 20% to more than 80%.

Acetaminophen: Need for treatment is calculated by the Rumack-Matthew nomogram (Figure 131-1), based on both the acetaminophen plasma concentration, and the time postingestion, using the antidote treatment *N*-acetylcysteine (NAC). NAC replenishes the liver stores of glutathione, which is depleted by excess acetaminophen metabolites; if given early (<24 hours) before there is too much liver damage, NAC can reverse the ALF.

Budd-Chiari: ALF from Budd-Chiari is uncommon and presents with right upper quadrant pain, edema/fluid retention, and a striking hepatomegaly—a clinical picture, which helps distinguish it from other ALF where the liver is small. Therapeutic options can be effective on rare occasions, including anticoagulation and transjugular intrahepatic portocaval shunting (TIPS).

Autoimmune Causes: When positive auto antibodies (+ANA, +ASMA, +ANCA, + anti-SLA) are detected at ≥1:40 titer, or if a liver biopsy suggests an autoimmune etiology, a potential therapy is high-dose corticosteroids. There is debate, however, as a recent multicenter study showed no survival benefit with steroids, and even a potential reduced survival in the sickest patients treated with steroids.

Other Viruses: Although they are rare causes of ALF, both HSV and VZV can be treated with acyclovir antiviral therapy, and CMV can be treated with ganciclovir antiviral therapy.

(e) Decision on Transplantation

For patients with ALF having either liver injury so severe on presentation to require transplantation, those with potentially reversible injury unresponsive to therapy, or those with disease etiologies without potential therapy who eventually progressed to where liver recovery is unlikely—liver transplantation is the only remaining therapeutic option to prevent death. The other part of the decision for transplantation, however, is identifying who is not a candidate for transplantation. The only absolute contraindication to transplantation in ALF is unrecoverable brain injury from increased intracranial pressure (ICP) due to cerebral edema. Relative contraindications include bacteremia (a common complication impacting 30% of ALF patients), hemodynamic instability requiring rising vasopressor requirements, and uncontrolled ARDS.

When addressing the general diagnosis algorithm, a concurrent organ management strategy is necessary to limit complications and potential contraindications to transplantation: (a) Neurologic Support/Cerebral Edema; (b) Renal Failure Support; (c) Hemodynamic Support; (d) Respiratory Support; (e) Nutritional Support.

(a) **Neurologic Support/Cerebral Edema**
ALF causes significant hyperammonemia, and the ammonia enters cerebral astrocytes where it is converted to osmotically active glutamine which in turn induces cerebral edema. Those at risk for cerebral edema have grade III-IV encephalopathy or serum ammonia >150 mcg/dL. Cerebral edema increases ICP, which can eventually limit cerebral blood flow. Management includes intravascular volume control with CVVHD, and general measures to reduce ICP including head of bed at 30 degrees, endotracheal intubation, avoidance of hypertension, and propofol sedation. Further strategies for ICP reduction

include hyperthermia, mannitol, and NSAID treatment (Table 131-3). Standard medical therapies to reduce serum ammonia levels (lactulose and rifaximin) may be used but do not have proven impact on survival in ALF patients.

(b) **Hemodynamic Support**
ALF patients need adequate volume resuscitation to ensure adequate cardiac output, while avoiding over resuscitation that exacerbates cerebral edema. ALF is characterized by a hyperdynamic circulation, with high cardiac output and low systemic vascular resistance, and an adequate mean arterial pressure and cerebral perfusion pressure is maintained using vasopressors such as norepinephrine and vasopressin.

(c) **Renal Failure**
Acute renal failure occurs in up to 80% of ALF patients. Management includes adequate volume resuscitation, avoidance of nephrotoxic agents, infection treatment, and renal replacement therapy with CVVHD.

(d) **Respiratory Support**
Respiratory failure and ARDS can occur with ALF. Hypercapnia, which may raise ICP, can be limited by increasing minute ventilation. The lowest level of PEEP to achieve adequate oxygenation should be used to avoid worsening cerebral edema.

(e) **Nutritional Support**
ALF is a catabolic state with 60% increased energy requirements, and four-fold increased protein catabolism

Table 131-3　Strategies for Treating Increased ICP in ALF

Strategy	Approach
Body position	• Head of bed 30 degree • Head midline, avoiding twist of neck
Analgesia/sedation	• ↓ environmental stimulation • Propofol to sedate, avoid cough or strain against ventilator
Volume/fluids	• Resuscitation with isotonic fluid ↑ MAP, ↓ lactate • Avoid volume overload that can worsen cerebral edema
Blood pressure	• Use vasopressors to increase MAP • Norepinephrine first, then add vasopressin
Oxygenation	• Goal is to maximize O_2 level • Lowest PEEP to achieve O_2 level, to avoid ↑ cerebral edema
Ventilation	• Hyperventilation may ↓ ICP acutely, as a rescue therapy • Normal ventilation once hyperosmotic agent started
Temperature	• Goal is 35–36 degree using heating/cooling blanket, antipyretics • ↑ temp causes ↑ oxidative metabolism. ↓ temp causes shivering
Osmotic pressure	• IV 3% hypertonic NS bolus to maintain Na <150 mol/L • IV 25% mannitol to maintain serum osmolality <320 mOsm/L
Dialysis ultrafiltration	• Large volume of blood product and meds cause overload • CRRT to remove excess fluid, and ↓ serum NH_3
Pharmaceutical	• Thiopental Rx: ↓ ICP, ↑ cerebral O_2, ↓ cerebral blood flow • Indomethacin Rx: ↓ ICP, caution from nephrotoxic effects

requiring at least 40 g of protein administration per day. ALF patients can develop sudden hypoglycemia, and up to half of ALF patients need glucose infusions.

Presentation Continued

Having diagnosed acetaminophen poisoning, based on the Rumack-Matthew nomogram, NAC therapy was initiated. After resuscitation, the patient's pH was 7.25, INR 6.2, and she progressed to grade IV encephalopathy, requiring intubation. Meeting Kings College Criteria, an expedited evaluation for transplantation was performed, and the patient was listed for transplant with a status 1 designation. While awaiting transplantation, measures were used to limit cerebral edema and ICP, renal support was provided using CVVHD, hypotension was managed with norepinephrine, and hypoglycemia was treated with a D10W infusion.

● SURGICAL APPROACH

With the decision to perform a liver transplant for ALF, one must consider those factors unique to ALF compared to end-stage liver disease. First, patients with ALF are often hemodynamically unstable on vasopressors, so implanting the liver via a "piggyback technique" is favored since this approach avoids vena cava clamping. Second, because ALF patients lack chronic portal hypertension, they do not have collateral veins and do not tolerate portal vein clamping as easily as those with end-stage liver disease, thus a temporary portacaval shunt can be created to decompress the portal system following hepatectomy. Third, ALF is associated with massive necrosis, and extensive manipulation of the liver during the hepatectomy can release a surge of toxic inflammatory mediators and cytokines into the systemic circulation. The standard "caval replacement technique" requires less manipulation and rotation making this approach more appropriate in patients with significant encephalopathy (assuming patient is hemodynamically stable).

(1) **Incision and Exposure**
A right-sided hockey-stick incision is performed, dividing the rectus sheath and right external oblique, internal oblique, and transversus abdominis to enter the abdomen. A self-retaining retractor is used to expose the upper abdomen and retract the intestine.

(2) **Hepatectomy—Division of Ligaments**
The falciform, right and left triangular ligaments are divided with electrocautery. The gastrohepatic ligament is divided, ligating any potential replaced left hepatic artery crossing in this plane.

(3) **Hepatectomy—Hepatoduodenal Ligament**
Approaching the hepatoduodenal ligament, the cystic duct is divided, allowing for a high division of the common hepatic duct (ligating any potential replaced right hepatic artery running posterior to the bile duct). The

various branches of the hepatic artery (classically, the right and left branch) are divided, leaving the portal vein, which is dissected free from tissue circumferentially along its length to its bifurcation.

(4) **Hepatectomy and Implantation—Caval Replacement Technique**
The lateral borders of the vena cava are dissected from the peritoneum, dividing the adrenal vein and encircling both the suprahepatic and infrahepatic vena cava. After clamping the suprahepatic vena cava with a Satinsky clamp, the infrahepatic vena cava with an angled Debakey clamp, and the portal vein with an angled clamp, the vena cava, and portal vein are divided, and the liver is removed. After placing the donor allograft into the field orthotopically, the suprahepatic vena cava of the donor is anastomosed end-to-end to the recipient suprahepatic vena cava with a 4-0 nonabsorbable monofilament suture. The liver is flushed via the portal vein with iced saline to remove preservation fluid, and the infrahepatic vena cava of the donor is anastomosed end-to-end to the recipient infrahepatic vena cava with a 4-0 nonabsorbable monofilament suture.

(5) **Hepatectomy and Implantation—Piggyback Technique (Alternate Approach)**
In the piggyback technique, the vena cava is preserved, and the liver is dissected off the vena cava by dividing all of the short hepatic veins, up to the level of the hepatic veins, which are isolated. A Satinsky clamp is applied to the hepatic veins, and an angled clamp to the portal vein, and the hepatic veins and portal vein are divided allowing removal of the liver with retention of the vena cava. A common orifice for the allograft outflow is created by dividing the bridges of the three hepatic veins. After placing the donor allograft into the field, the suprahepatic vena cava of the donor is anastomosed to the common orifice of the hepatic veins with a 4-0 nonabsorbable monofilament suture, while the liver is flushed with iced saline and the donor infrahepatic vena cava is ligated.

(6) **Portal Vein, Hepatic Artery, and Biliary Anastomosis**
Both the donor and recipient portal vein are shortened to avoid redundancy and anastomosed end-to-end using a 6-0 nonabsorbable monofilament suture. A growth factor (air knot) is placed to avoid narrowing of the portal vein. The proper hepatic artery of the donor and the proper hepatic artery of the recipients are shortened to avoid redundancy and anastomosed end-to-end with a running 7-0 nonabsorbable monofilament suture using a parachute technique. Any anomalous hepatic artery variants (replaced left or right artery) present are implanted into hepatic artery branches. The donor bile duct is shortened by dividing above the cystic duct takeoff and anastomosed end-to-end to the recipient duct with 6-0 absorbable monofilament suture.

(7) **Completion**
If desired, flows can be measured in the hepatic artery and portal vein. A nasoduodenal feeding tube is positioned in the duodenum, and the incision closed with a 1-0 absorbable monofilament suture and the skin reapproximated with clips.

Presentation Continued

Two days after listing for transplant, a potential 59-year-old donor liver became available, and a deceased-donor liver transplant was performed using a "piggyback technique" for implantation, because the patient was on perioperative vasopressor support, and CVVHD renal support. Following successful implantation, hemodynamic support requirements significantly decreased.

● SPECIAL INTRAOPERATIVE CONSIDERATIONS

Because of the unpredictable nature of transplanting a non-native organ, it is common for special intraoperative circumstances to arise that require consideration

(a) **Hepatic Artery Dissection**

If a hepatic artery dissection occurs during the hepatectomy, a donor iliac artery can be anastomosed to the infrarenal aorta to create an aortoiliac conduit to provide arterial inflow to the donor allograft.

(b) **Portal Vein Thrombosis**

While less common in ALF given the lack of portal hypertension, a portal vein thrombus can be treated with a portal vein thrombectomy or eversion thrombectomy to restore suitable portal flow. If this is not successful, a donor iliac vein can be used to create either a superior mesenteric vein jump graft, or a renoportal shunt.

(c) **Biliary Size Mismatch**

If a significant mismatch exists between the donor and recipient bile ducts that hinders an acceptable anastomosis, a Roux-en-Y hepaticojejunostomy should be performed.

Presentation Continued

Intraoperatively, during the hepatic artery isolation of the hepatectomy, an arterial dissection occurred. An aortoiliac conduit was created and used as the arterial inflow, anastomosing it end-to-end to the donor common hepatic artery with 5-0 nonabsorbable monofilament sutures. Hepatic artery flow measurements showed excellent hepatic artery flow of 850 mL/min.

● POSTOPERATIVE MANAGEMENT

Transplantation is the rare surgical procedure where the postoperative management may be more important than the operative surgery, and given the high incidence of potential complications, a successfully functioning transplant depends on managing these complications.

(a) **Bleeding**

Given the extensive operative dissection, multiple vascular anastomoses and concomitant coagulopathy, postoperative bleeding is common. The threshold should be low to reexplore in the event of significant postoperative transfusions.

(b) **Vascular Complications**

Vascular complications may compromise the allograft if it occurs soon after transplant. A duplex ultrasound is performed on postoperative day 1 to assess the vasculature, and any concerns warrant reexploration. Immediate hepatic artery stenosis or hepatic artery thrombosis (HAT) necessitates arterial reconstruction with an aortoiliac conduit. Later, hepatic artery issues can be resolved in interventional radiology with stenting. Portal vein thrombosis requires immediate portal vein thrombectomy and frequently an eventual retransplantation.

(c) **Biliary Complications**

Biliary complications are the most common complications. Both bile duct leaks and obstructions can be managed with immediate surgical revision using a Roux-en-Y hepaticojejunostomy. Later, biliary complications can be resolved in interventional radiology or via ERCP with balloon dilation and or stenting.

(d) **Infections**

Given the posttransplant immunosuppression, infections are commonplace. Infections can be related to the transplant (i.e., cholangitis, abscess) or systemic (bacteremia, viremia). Transplant-related infections are treated with drainage and antibiotics. Systemic infections are treated with antibiotic or antiviral therapy as appropriate.

Case Conclusion

The liver transplant was successful, renal function recovered, her mental status improved, allowing hospital discharge on postoperative day 10. Four weeks following discharge, the bilirubin increased to 15.2 mg/dL and imaging described a biliary obstruction at the anastomosis. Following biliary dilation, a biliary stent was placed via ERCP, and upon removal of the stent 2 months later, the biliary stricture had resolved. The patient remains clinically well 3 years posttransplant (Table 131-4).

TAKE HOME POINTS

- While severe liver dysfunction with coagulopathy and encephalopathy are the hallmark of ALF, many other conditions must be considered in the differential diagnosis.
- ALF can evolve rapidly, so the workup and evaluation must be urgent and methodical and occur simultaneously to stabilization of the patient.
- Early recognition of ALF symptoms and accurate diagnostic choices are key in identifying those patients where therapies exist to treat the cause of the acute liver failure.

Table 131-4	Deceased Donor Liver Transplant

Key Technical Steps

Recipient Hepatectomy

1. Right-sided hockey-stick incision
2. Division of 4 ligamentous attachments of liver
3. Dissection hepatoduodenal ligament elements (division of hepatic arterial branches, high ligation of common hepatic duct and isolation of portal vein)
4. Caval replacement technique—isolation and division of retrohepatic vena can
5. Piggyback technique—division of short hepatic veins with resection of liver off vena cava

Allograft Implantation

1. Caval replacement technique—anastomosis of supra— and infrahepatic vena cava
2. Piggyback technique—anastomosis of suprahepatic vena cava and infrahepatic vena cava ligation
3. Portal vein anastomosis -> allograft reperfusion
4. Hepatic artery anastomosis -> arterial reperfusion
5. Bile duct anastomosis
6. Closure of abdomen

Potential Pitfalls

- Lack of collateral veins in ALF causing increased bleeding and intestinal edema with portal clamping
- Intimal dissection of recipient hepatic artery necessitating aortoiliac conduit.
- Size mismatch of donor allograft to recipient, or size mismatch of vascular or biliary anastomosis.

- The Kings College Criteria is useful in prioritizing those patients who will require transplantation.
- A liver transplant is a technically difficult operation involving microvascular anastomoses. The surgeon must be adaptable and be able to resolve size and anatomical differences between the donor liver and the recipient.
- Posttransplant complications are common, and successful transplant outcomes depend on the posttransplant recognition and management of complications.

SUGGESTED READINGS

Bernal W, Lee WM, Wendon J, Stolze Larsen F, Williams R. Acute liver failure: a curable disease by 2024. *J Hepatol.* 2015;62:S112-S120.

Bernal W, Wendon J. Acute liver failure. *N Engl J Med.* 2013;369: 2525-2534.

Cardoso FS, Marcelino P, Bagulho L, et al. Acute liver failure: an up-to-date approach. *J Crit Care.* 2017;39:25-30.

Damm TW, Kramer DJ. The liver in critical illness. *Crit Care Clin.* 2016;32:425-438.

Detry O, De Roover A, Honore P, Meurisse M. Brain edema and intracranial hypertension in fulminant hepatic failure: pathophysiology and management. *World J Gastroenterol.* 2006;12:7405-7412.

EASL Clinical Practical Guidelines on the management of acute (fulminant) liver failure. *J Hepatol.* 2017;66:1047-1081.

Rabinowich L, Wendon J, Bernal W, et al. Clinical management of acute liver failure: results of an international multi-center survey. *World J Gastroenterol.* 2016;22:7593-7603.

Rumack BH, Matthew H. *Pediatrics.* 1975;55:871-876.

Shalimar SKA. Management in acute liver failure. *J Clin Exp Hepatol.* 2015;5:S104-S115.

Wang DW, Yin WM, Yao YM. Advances in the management of acute liver failure. *World J Gastroenterol.* 2013;19:7069-7077.

Variceal Bleeding and Portal Hypertension

132

MICHAEL J. ENGLESBE AND SETH A. WAITS

Based on the previous edition chapter "Variceal Bleeding and Portal Hypertension" by Brendan J. Boland and Andrew S. Klein

Presentation

A 63-year-old female with a history of nonalcoholic steatohepatitis (NASH) presents to the emergency room with multiple bouts of hematemesis. Her family reports that she vomited large amounts of blood several times at home. Prior to this event, she had no complaints. Her blood pressure is 70/40 and her heart rate is 118. She is awake but confused. On physical examination, she has moderate cachexia, mild scleral icterus, and splenomegaly.

● DIFFERENTIAL DIAGNOSIS

When evaluating patients with upper gastrointestinal (GI) bleeding in the setting of chronic liver disease, the clinician must have a high suspicion for bleeding esophageal varices. Most patients with decompensated liver disease (cachexia, ascites, encephalopathy, or renal dysfunction) will have evidence of esophageal varices on upper endoscopy, many of which will become clinically significant. Patients with variceal hemorrhage may present with hematemesis or melena. The bleeding is usually brisk and will not be associated with abdominal pain. Portal hypertension is the underlying cause for development of esophageal varices. The average portal vein (including splenic and superior mesenteric vein) pressure ranges between 1 and 4 mm Hg higher than the hepatic vein free pressure and not more than 6 mm Hg greater than central venous pressures. Pressures that exceed these limits define portal hypertension. More commonly, portal hypertension is used to define a constellation of symptoms related to elevated mesenteric venous pressures, including ascites, gastrointestinal bleed due to varices, and the development of mesenteric venous collaterals. Portal hypertension may be caused by liver disease in addition to prehepatic or posthepatic venous obstruction. In contrast to patients with cirrhosis of the liver, patients with noncirrhotic portal hypertension usually have only splenomegaly.

Other potential etiologies for bleeding in this patient include a Mallory-Weiss tear or severe esophagitis, though bleeding is usually less severe and these diagnoses are generally associated with pain. Consideration of peptic ulcer disease with bleeding from either the stomach or the duodenum must also be considered, as this is the most common etiology of GI bleed in patients without liver disease. A history of dyspepsia, infection with *Helicobacter pylori*, and nonsteroidal anti-inflammatory drug use are risk factors for ulcers.

● WORKUP

The management of a patient with bleeding esophageal varices is similar to that of any bleeding patient. Early intubation is critical for airway protection in patients with hematemesis and encephalopathy. Establish large bore intravenous access and initiate aggressive resuscitation with blood and blood products in the emergency department for any unstable patient. Draw a comprehensive set of labs including CBC, electrolytes, renal function, liver function, and coagulation panel. Transfuse to a goal hemoglobin level of 8 grams per deciliter and avoid overresuscitation, which can exacerbate portal hypertension and bleeding. Patients with liver disease can have complex coagulation disorders and targeted resuscitation is critical. Non–goal-directed resuscitation with fresh frozen plasma is an effort to correct the INR is misguided. Rotational thromboelastometry (ROTEM) may be helpful in guiding resuscitation.

● DIAGNOSIS AND TREATMENT

Pharmacotherapy

Infusion of vasopressin is indicated if the patient is unstable. This is a potent splanchnic vasoconstrictor and lowers portal pressures while simultaneously increasing systemic pressure. Alternatively, octreotide may be used but can exacerbate hypotension. Patients with a GI bleed and ascites are at risk of developing spontaneous bacterial peritonitis, which carries a significant mortality risk. Prophylactic antibiotics have shown benefit in several trails and should be administered prior to endoscopic therapy. Intravenous ceftriaxone, ciprofloxacin, levofloxacin, or oral norfloxacin (if appropriate) should be given.

Endoscopy

After appropriate resuscitation, the most important step in the management of a patient with hemodynamic instability and an upper GI bleed is endoscopy. This should be done in the emergency department without delay. When varices are identified, endoscopic ligation (banding) is the preferred treatment. The varix is suctioned into a channel within the endoscope and a band is deployed, strangulating the varix and causing thrombosis. If banding cannot be performed for technical reasons, endoscopic sclerotherapy with a chemical sclerosant such as sodium tetradecyl sulfate, sodium morrhuate, ethanolamine oleate, or absolute alcohol can be attempted.

Presentation Continued

The patient was aggressively resuscitated, and endoscopy was performed in the emergency department. Despite all efforts, bleeding was not able to be stopped. Interventional radiology consultation was made.

Transjugular Intrahepatic Portosystemic Shunt (TIPS)

The combination of pharmacotherapy and endoscopy successfully manage variceal bleeding in 90% of patients. A TIPS should be considered in patients with recurrent bleeds or in patients with whom pharmacotherapy and endoscopy are unsuccessful. A TIPS is placed through an endovascular approach from the internal jugular vein. A common channel is created between the hepatic vein (usually the right) and the portal vein (usually the right). This channel is established with wire access and an 8- to a 12-mm stent is deployed between these two vessels. TIPS successfully manages acute bleeding in over 80% of cases. Patency rates for TIPS have improved significantly over the past decade with the introduction of covered stents. Screening ultrasounds to check flow in the TIPS are necessary so that early intervention can be done to prevent in-stent occlusion. In most cases, a stenotic TIPS can be crossed with a guidewire and recanalized with balloon dilation or repeat stent placement. Primary-assisted patencies at 1 and 2 years are reported to be 83% and 79%, respectively, and secondary patency at 1 and 2 years are reported to be 96% and 90%. The most common complication of TIPS is new-onset or worsening encephalopathy. This can be difficult to manage. In general, the presence of encephalopathy is a contraindication to TIPS placement.

Other Techniques

In a patient with significant encephalopathy or when TIPS fails, balloon-occluded retrograde transvenous obliteration (BRTO) is a highly effective and minimally invasive treatment for isolated varices. This technique utilizes an occlusion balloon to control the blood flow and delivery of sclerosant through prominent draining veins of portosystemic shunts. With the shunt outflow occluded, the goal is to fill the variceal complex sufficiently with a sclerosing agent and obliterate the varices without refluxing into the systemic or portal circulation.

Direct balloon occlusion by a nasoenteric tube is another technique to effectively stop variceal bleeding. This is rarely done in hospitals with advanced endoscopic and interventional radiology capabilities. Although several types of tube exist, the steps for effective placement are similar. Following endotracheal intubation, the occlusion tube is inserted into the mouth and advanced into the stomach. The intragastric location of the balloon is confirmed by x-ray, and the distally located gastric balloon is inflated. Gentle traction is applied to the tube until it is lodged against the gastroesophageal junction and secured in place. The esophageal balloon is then inflated to provide occlusion of the varices. The balloon can only be left in place for relatively short period time as too much tension on the balloon can cause gastric and esophageal necrosis.

In some cases, splenic embolization can effectively manage recurrent GI bleed from portal hypertension. This is especially effective in patients with left-sided portal hypertension who are not candidates for surgical management.

● SURGICAL MANAGEMENT OF A VARICEAL BLEED OR PORTAL HYPERTENSION

Surgery is rarely necessary for patients with GI bleed or significant portal hypertension. Most importantly, patients with decompensated liver disease are unlikely to survive major surgical procedure. These patients should be considered for liver transplantation. It is rare that a patient with decompensated liver disease develops a gastrointestinal bleed that cannot be managed with the techniques detailed above.

A multidisciplinary committee should review all complex cases. Key members of this committee include advanced endoscopists, interventional radiology, hepatology, and transplantation surgery. Indications for surgery in adults are as follows:

- Patients with GI bleed who fail all other options. Most of these patients will have mesenteric venoocclusive disease.
- Severe and long-standing thrombocytopenia with non-cirrhotic portal hypertension.
- Severe and disabling abdominal pain. This is usually from massive splenomegaly. Many patients with mesenteric venoocclusive disease will have abdominal pain and no other complications; few of these patients should have surgery because their pain is unlikely to get better.
- Massive splenomegaly affecting lifestyle. The spleen crosses the abdominal midline and occupies much of the pelvis.

Operative exposure to the neck and/or groin for vein procurement is needed in many cases. An arterial line and central line should be placed in most cases. The central line will be used to assess the CVP in calculations of the

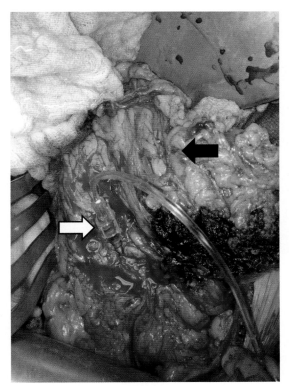

FIGURE 132-1. Measurement of mesenteric vein pressures. Select a vein that will be easy to ligate following cannulation. Cannulate the vein with an angiocatheter and measure pressures with the assistance of the anesthesia team. The *white arrow* represents the cannula in an omental branch. The *black arrow* demonstrates the omentum retracted superiorly.

portal-systemic pressure gradient. Additional tubing and anesthesia equipment will be needed for intraoperative mesenteric venous pressure measurements (Figure 132-1). All members of the operative team (surgical, nursing, and anesthesia) should be prepared for significant intraoperative bleeding, as is frequently experienced during liver transplantation or open abdominal vascular surgery. Overresuscitation will worsen this bleeding; the goal CVP during the dissection should be 5 mm Hg. This requires frequent communication between the anesthesiologists and surgeons. At our center, we prefer to enter the abdomen through a midline incision. Aggressive retraction of the costal margin will facilitate access to the short gastric veins in the upper abdomen. This is best achieved with an Omni™ or Thompson™ retractor.

The final surgical approach to manage severe portal hypertension is determined by operative findings. The surgeon must understand the patient's physiology and how to best assure long-term management of portal hypertension while accepting reasonable operative risk. Consideration must be made for future options if the current surgical procedure fails. Prosthetic graft material or cryopreserved vein should be reserved for patients in severe extremis from acute portal hypertensive complications. Surgical options include the following.

Splenectomy with Proximal Splenic Artery Ligation and Esophagogastric Devascularization

The indications for this procedure include patients with a life-threatening complication from portal hypertension and complex mesenteric venoocclusive disease or poor venous drainage of the spleen (left-sided portal hypertensive physiology) (Figure 132-2). Patients with long-standing thrombocytopenia (platelets < 35,000 per µL) and massive splenomegaly need a splenectomy. The spleen is fibrotic and will remain large (and platelet counts will remain low) following shunt surgery alone. Massive splenomegaly will make many portal hypertension surgical procedures impossible. Because of this, splenectomy is the first portion of the procedure. If there is significant portal hypertension and collaterals, preoperative splenic embolization should be done immediately prior to the procedure. If done more than a few hours before the splenectomy, the patient will have significant adverse symptoms, and the spleen will become soft and easy to injure during surgery. The size of the spleen and the severity of the portal hypertension usually favor an open procedure; however, laparoscopic splenectomy can be performed in selected instances. To complete the esophagogastric devascularization, identify any collateral vessels behind the stomach and ligate these veins with clips. Repeat portal pressure measurement should be performed after splenectomy to determine whether a shunt is needed. A shunt should be done if there

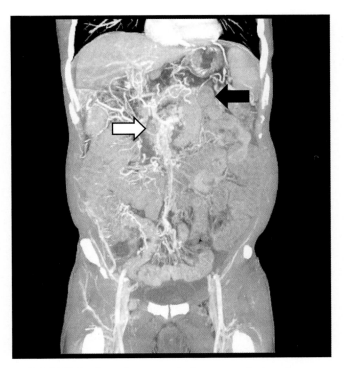

FIGURE 132-2. Complex mesenteric venoocclusive disease. These patients can usually be managed with splenectomy. The *white arrow* represents the occluded superior mesenteric vein and portal vein. The *black arrow* represents the occluded splenic vein.

is a viable target for mesenteric venous inflow and central venous outflow and a postsplenectomy mesenteric-systemic gradient of 12 mm Hg.

Proximal Splenorenal Shunt

This procedure is indicated for persistent portal hypertension following splenectomy and functions as a nonselective shunt. The confluence of the superior mesenteric vein and splenic vein should be patent with a patent splenic vein. A pressure gradient between the splenic vein and central venous system of 12 is needed to maintain shunt patency. Generous mobilization of the splenic vein is needed to this procedure. This is not always technically possible, and alternative approaches include minimal dissection of the splenic vein and use of a vein conduit or an alternative shunt procedure.

Inferior Mesenteric Vein to Left Renal Vein Shunt

The inferior mesenteric vein is too small to provide adequate inflow for a shunt in most patients. In some patients to complex mesenteric venoocclusive disease, the inferior mesenteric vein can be large and spared of chronic occlusive disease. These patients should have a splenectomy. As described above, if there is significant mesenteric venous pressure following splenectomy and there are not better inflow vessels available, the inferior mesenteric vein to left renal vein shunt is a good option.

Distal Splenorenal Shunt

Classically, a distal splenorenal shunt was not thought to be associated with postshunt encephalopathy in cirrhotic patients. More recent experience notes that encephalopathy remains common in these patients. As a result, patients with significant cirrhosis or progressive liver disease rarely benefit from this procedure. Patients with significant ascites should not have a selective shunt such as a distal splenorenal shunt as this often exacerbates this issue. In cases where a shunt is performed, follow-up imaging with ultrasound should be performed in the days after the procedure to assess patency. If shunt cannot be seen on ultrasound, a CT scan of MRI of the abdomen with mesenteric vein reconstructions may be performed (Figure 132-3).

Meso-Rex Shunt

A meso-Rex shunt restores normal physiology and has been reported to be associated with improved liver and cognitive function. It is performed by using venous conduit to shunt the superior mesenteric vein or splenic vein to the portal vein in the Rex recess. The procedure is indicated for patients with portal vein thrombosis, a patent superior mesenteric vein (or splenic vein), and intrahepatic portal veins, including the junction between the right and left lobes of the liver. Vein conduit is required for this procedure and internal jugular vein is

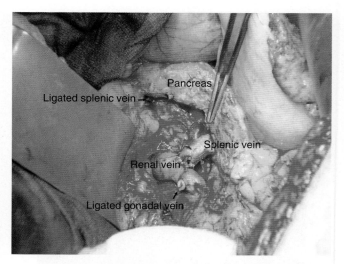

FIGURE 132-3. Distal splenorenal shunt. Anatomic labels noted in figure.

favored. The intrahepatic portal vein is not always adequate for an anastomosis. One must be prepared to do an alternative shunt procedure and do not procure conduit until the portal vein in the Rex recess is determined to be patent and suitable for anastomosis. Postoperative ultrasound should be performed to assess patency and provide a baseline.

Other Shunts

Surgery for portal hypertension requires novel approaches to unique patient problems and a willingness to change the plan during surgery depending on intraoperative findings. Numerous variations on the surgical procedures detailed above should be considered. Large collateral vessels are occasionally appropriate for shunt creation. These vessels tend to be thin walled and meticulous technique is paramount. For example, a large coronary vein can be used for anastomosis to the portal vein in the Rex recess or to the retrohepatic inferior vena cava.

● POSTOPERATIVE CARE

A typical hospitalization may be between 3 and 7 days. Avoid volume overload; it will affect shunt flow. Carefully monitor liver function. Many patients have a preoperative propensity for thrombosis; consider postoperative fractionated or unfractionated heparin. Discharge these patients on systemic anticoagulation. All splenectomy patients need a postoperative aspirin. If the platelet count goes over 300,000 per μL, inpatient and outpatient systemic anticoagulation is required for 3 months or greater. Patients do not need nasogastric tubes and diets can be advanced quickly. A surveillance abdominal ultrasound is obtained prior to discharge to verify patency of the shunt. If the shunt cannot be visualized, more advanced imaging can be considered on a case-by-case basis. Patients with preoperative ascites will need to continue diuretics for several weeks. Endoscopy to assess for stigmata of portal hypertension and follow-up imaging of the shunt should be done at scheduled intervals for several years as an outpatient. Early diagnosis and intervention by interventional radiology will facilitate long-term shunt patency.

Case Conclusion

The patient was brought to the angiography suite emergently for TIPS. A TIPS was successfully placed and the bleeding stopped. The patient developed postprocedure encephalopathy, which was medically managed with lactulose. The patient was referred for liver transplant evaluation.

TAKE HOME POINTS

- Gastroesophageal varices are the likely source of acute upper GI bleeding in patients who have a known history of cirrhosis or who have clinical stigmata of chronic liver disease.
- Aggressive resuscitation and early endoscopy (banding) are keys to accurate diagnosis.
- Octreotide and vasopressin are the preferred pharmacologic treatments for bleeding gastroesophageal varices.

- TIPS is an effective short- and long-term management of severe acute bleeding that fails endoscopy and for recurrent GI bleeds.
- Surgical management of portal hypertension should be reserved for patients who fail all medical, endoscopic, or interventional radiology approaches to care. Patients with decompensated liver disease are unlikely to benefit from surgical management and should be evaluated for liver transplantation.
- Patients with noncirrhotic portal hypertension can achieve long-term benefit from surgical shunts.

SUGGESTED READINGS

Garcia-Tsao G, Bosch J. Management of varices and variceal hemorrhage in cirrhosis. *N Engl J Med.* 2010;362(9):823–832.

Olson JC, Saeien K. Gastrointestinal issues in liver disease. *Crit Care Clin.* 2016;32(3):371-384.

Shneider BL, Bosch J, de Franchis R, et al. Portal hypertension in children: expert pediatric opinion on the report of the Baveno v Consensus Workshop on Methodology of Diagnosis and Therapy in Portal Hypertension. *Pediatr Transplant.* 2012;16(5):426-437.

Toshikuni N, Takuma Y, Tsutsumi M. Management of gastroesophageal varices in cirrhotic patients: current status and future directions. *Ann Hepatol.* 2016;15(3):314-325.

End-Stage Renal Disease (Renal Transplantation)

SUZIE S. LEE AND DEREK MOORE

Based on the previous edition chapter "End-Stage Renal Disease (Renal Transplantation)" by Leigh Anne Dageforde and Derek Moore

133

Presentation

A 56-year-old male with polycystic kidney disease and hypertension arrives at your transplant center for evaluation. His nephrologist predicts he will require dialysis in the next 4 months and recommends him for evaluation for renal transplantation.

● DIFFERENTIAL DIAGNOSIS

Causes for end-stage renal disease (ESRD) and therefore potential kidney transplant are numerous and can be grouped into several major categories including glomerulonephritis, hereditary, metabolic, toxic, multisystem disease, congenital, tumors, and chronic obstruction. Most patients have undergone a workup for their chronic kidney disease with a nephrologist and arrive to see a transplant surgeon with a diagnosis regarding the etiology of the renal failure. The first successful kidney transplant was performed between identical twins in Boston in 1954. Since then, with the advent of immunosuppression, transplants for ESRD from both living and deceased donors have increased in number to around 18,000 annually in the United States.

● WORKUP

The workup for a potential transplant candidate involves a detailed history and physical as well as appropriate laboratory studies and imaging as indicated. Key components of the history include information regarding the etiology of renal failure, the length of time on dialysis, and the amount of urine the patient makes, if any. Other pertinent past medical history includes cardiac and pulmonary disease, cancer, and infections. In addition, information about prior transplants and transfusion of blood products must be obtained due to the affect on the degree of sensitization to human leukocyte antigens (HLA) and the ease of obtaining a negative crossmatch to potential donors. The physical exam should focus on elements of the patient's anatomy that might preclude them from safe transplantation, especially severe peripheral vascular disease or prior deep vein thrombosis (DVT) that might manifest as diminished femoral and pedal pulses or lower extremity swelling.

Testing for all potential transplant candidates involves both evaluation for safety of the operative procedure and assessment for risk factors, such as active infection or malignancy, associated with adverse outcomes in the setting of immunosuppression. Laboratory studies include complete blood count, comprehensive metabolic panel, coagulation panel, HLA typing, and viral serologies (HBV, HCV, HIV, CMV). Additionally, all patients should have a chest radiograph, EKG, and tuberculosis skin test. All transplant candidates undergo psychosocial evaluation to screen for characteristics that may be associated with medication or postoperative care noncompliance. Other testing is primarily related to recommended screening exams based on patient age and gender: colonoscopy for all patients >50 years old, Pap smear if female without prior hysterectomy, mammogram if female over 40 years old, and PSA if male over 50 years old. If the patient has not made urine for over 5 years, a voiding cystourethrogram may be considered to assure adequate bladder volume for anastomosis of the donor ureter. Some centers perform a CT scan on all patients on dialysis more than 5 years to evaluate for renal cell carcinoma. For a history of systemic lupus erythematous or DVT, patients should undergo a hypercoagulable workup; for those with a history of DVT, a venous phase CT is recommended to evaluate for patency of the iliac veins. Patients with viral serology positive for hepatitis C virus are referred to a hepatologist and undergo a liver biopsy and screening for hepatocellular carcinoma.

● DIAGNOSIS AND TREATMENT

Once a patient is cleared for transplantation, investigation for potential donors ensues. The two options for donors include living (either related or unrelated) and deceased. Donors must be healthy themselves and undergo a detailed history and physical as well as any age-appropriate testing. Compatibility of donors and recipients is based on HLA/major histocompatibility complex haplotypes both type I and type II. For patients with willing living donors who are not a satisfactory match, some transplant centers are willing to arrange paired matches. Transplant candidates without living donors are placed on the list for deceased donor renal transplant.

Preoperative history and physical should include updates since the last clinic visit as well as repeat labs, chest x-ray, and EKG as some patients may be close to a year from their last clinic visit when a kidney becomes available. Patients on dialysis should have their fluid status and electrolytes evaluated for possible preoperative dialysis, although most on their routine dialysis schedule will not require it. Preoperative consent should include not only transplantation but also induction of immunosuppression, which will begin during the transplantation operation.

Immunosuppression includes two phases for transplant recipients: induction and maintenance. Induction regimens differ depending on transplant centers, but most include anti-thymocyte immunoglobulin with steroids. The maintenance phase usually includes a calcineurin inhibitor (cyclosporine or tacrolimus), mycophenolate mofetil, and prednisone, although some centers have had success with steroid avoidance protocols.

● SURGICAL APPROACH

In the operating room, a three-way Foley catheter is placed so that sterile saline can be infused to fill the bladder prior to anastomosis of the ureter. Transplanted kidneys are generally placed into the right iliac fossa with anastomosis of the renal artery and vein to the right iliac vessels unless contraindicated due to recipient anatomy, prior operation or transplantation, or known vascular disease. The right side is chosen preferentially because the right external iliac artery and vein are often more superficial than the left. In type I diabetics who may be candidates for pancreas transplantation, the kidney is placed on the left side to preserve the right for an eventual pancreas allograft. The Gibson transplant incision is a gently curving incision from the symphysis pubis to just superior and medial to the anterior superior iliac spine (ASIS). The layers of the abdominal wall are incised until the retroperitoneal space is reached. The inferior epigastric vessels are often divided. The spermatic cord is retracted medially in males; the round ligament is divided in females. The external iliac vessels are isolated with care taken to ligate all crossing lymphatics to prevent lymphocele. Proximal and distal control of the artery and vein are achieved with atraumatic vascular clamps. The donor kidney is then taken off ice, but attempts are made to keep it cold while the anastomosis is being completed. The renal artery and vein are then sewn to the external iliac artery and vein in an end-to-side fashion with fine monofilament nonabsorbable suture (Table 133-1).

After the vascular anastomoses are complete and the kidney is reperfused, attention is turned to the ureter. The three-way Foley is clamped and the bladder distended with irrigation, so it can be identified. A large-gauge needle is inserted into the presumed bladder to ensure proper identification. The detrusor muscle and the bladder mucosa are opened, and a mucosa-to-mucosa neoureterocystostomy is performed over a ureteral stent with absorbable suture. The

| Table 133-1 | Kidney Transplant Procedure |

Key Technical Steps

1. Three-way Foley with flush inserted prior to prep.
2. Right (or left if anatomic limitation to right) gently curving or "hockey stick"–shaped incision from 2 fingerbreadths superior to the syphilis pubis and 2 fingerbreadths medial to the anterior superior iliac spine.
3. Divide inferior epigastric vessels.
4. Reach retroperitoneal space and stay extraperitoneal by sweeping down the peritoneum medially.
5. Dissect external iliac vessels carefully dividing surrounding lymphatics to gain proximal and distal control.
6. Donor renal artery and vein are sewn to the external iliac artery and vein in an end-to-side fashion with fine monofilament suture, followed by reperfusion of the kidney.
7. Bladder distended with fluid and detrusor muscle and bladder mucosa opened.
8. Mucosa-to-mucosa neoureterocystostomy is performed over a ureteral stent with absorbable suture.
9. Detrusor muscle of the bladder is then closed loosely with absorbable suture.
10. Anastomoses checked and hemostasis obtained.
11. Incision closed in several anatomic layers.

Potential Pitfalls

- Twisting of the donor vessels during anastomosis.
- Anastomosing the ureter to the colon or the rectum instead of the bladder.
- Multiple or short donor vessels requiring careful anastomosis.
- Living donor vessels do not have Carrel patch.
- Inadequate reperfusion of the kidney.

detrusor muscle of the bladder is then closed loosely over the neoureterocystostomy with absorbable suture. Hemostasis is achieved and the incision is closed. After closing the muscular layer over the kidney, a Doppler is used to confirm good flow to the kidney. A closed-suction drain may be left to evaluate for collection of lymph, urine, or blood, but is not required.

● POSTOPERATIVE MANAGEMENT

Postoperative management of renal transplant patients requires adequate fluid resuscitation. Patients who receive a living donor transplant will often have a large diuresis the night of the operation and may require hourly mL per mL replacement intravenous fluid based on the amount of urine output. Relative hypotension should be treated aggressively to avoid compromising renal perfusion. Mild hypertension is acceptable but systolic blood pressures > 180 mm Hg should be treated. Other postoperative orders include strict ins and outs, daily weights, morning labs including immunosuppressant levels, pain medications (avoid morphine due to active metabolite that is cleared renally), immunosuppression medications, antiviral prophylaxis, DVT prophylaxis, and Foley catheter instructions (usually left in place until postoperative day 3).

Postoperative graft function can be described as immediate, slow, or delayed. Immediate graft function is common in living donor transplants. Patients have immediate urine output and decreasing serum creatinine. Slow graft function is subjective and defined as oliguria (although not seen in those patients producing urine from their native kidneys) and a serum creatinine that does not fall initially. Delayed function describes a patient that requires dialysis in the first week posttransplant.

As with any operative intervention, complications can occur following renal transplantation (Table 133-2). Several complications can occur in the more immediate postoperative period including wound infection, seroma, and lymphocele. Wound infection occurs uncommonly in renal transplant recipients, but the risk of wound infection may be significantly increased in obese patients. Treatment consists of drainage of the infection and antibiotics. Seromas are sterile collections of fluid usually in the subcutaneous space. Symptomatic collections can be treated with aspiration, although this runs the risk of infecting the sterile collection and the fluid often reaccumulates. Serial aspirations or percutaneous drainage may be required for treatment of seromas.

Lymphoceles usually occur in the subfascial plane and are due to accumulation of lymph leakage created by the disruption of the lymphatics surrounding the iliac vessels during intraoperative dissection. Often, lymphoceles are small and asymptomatic but can be large and cause pain, swelling, ureteral obstruction, venous obstruction leading to DVTs or renal vein thrombosis, or urinary incontinence from compression of the bladder. Diagnosis is made by ultrasound and often reveals a round, septated cystic mass. Treatment is not required for small, asymptomatic lymphoceles. For

collections concerning for a urine leak, infection, or compression of the kidney, percutaneous drainage is necessary. The aspirate should be tested for creatinine to rule out urine leak. Obstructive or infected lymphoceles are managed with infusion of a sclerosing agent or surgical intervention with marsupialization externally or internally into the peritoneal cavity (see Figure 133-1 for CT image of lymphocele).

Vascular complications include bleeding, renal vein or artery thrombosis, and renal artery stenosis. Graft thrombosis occurs within the first 2 to 3 days postoperatively and may be related to surgical technique, although patients with a history of a hypercoagulable state are at higher risk. Compression of the renal hilum by a large fluid collection or hematoma can contribute to vascular thrombosis. Symptoms include oliguria (although unreliable if the patient's native kidneys were still producing urine), graft swelling, tenderness, and hematuria. Laboratory tests reveal rising serum creatinine. Evaluation is best achieved with a transplant ultrasound with Doppler, although a radioisotope nuclear medicine scan may also be used. Arterial or venous thromboses often require transplant nephrectomy. Renal artery stenosis is usually a late complication occurring 3 months to several years postoperatively. Diagnosis is made via transplant ultrasound with Doppler. Treatment is first with percutaneous angioplasty followed by surgical intervention as needed.

Urologic complications include urinary extravasation and ureteral obstruction. Urine leaks can occur at the level of the bladder, ureter, or renal calyx and presents as copious drainage through a JP drain or fluid drainage from the incision. Both drainage fluid and serum creatinine should be checked, and a Foley catheter should be placed. The fluid from a urine leak will have a creatinine that is significantly higher than the serum creatinine. If the urine leak is small, Foley catheter placement and bladder decompression may

Table 133-2	Potential Complications Following Renal Transplantation

Potential Complications

- Seroma
- Lymphocele
- Urinary extravasation
- Ureteral obstruction
- Ureteral stenosis
- Bleeding
- Renal artery or vein thrombosis
- Renal artery stenosis

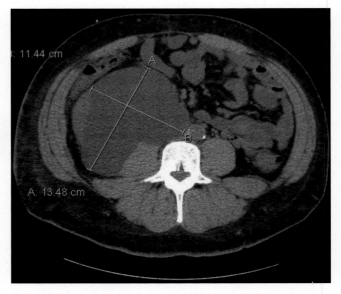

FIGURE 133-1. Right groin lymphocele following kidney transplantation.

allow the leak to seal. Large leaks require percutaneous nephrostomy tube placement and stenting if the intraoperative stent was removed or no stent was used. Some urine leaks require definitive surgical repair. Repair of the ureter should be performed over a double-J stent.

Ureteral obstruction presents with impaired graft function and oliguria. The obstruction can be secondary to compression by clots, lymphoceles, fibrosis, or ureteral stenosis. Diagnosis can be made by ultrasound that demonstrates hydroureter. A retrograde pyelogram may show the area of obstruction. Obstruction is managed surgically by evacuating the hematoma, lymphocele, or collection causing the obstruction. Similar to the treatment of urine leaks, percutaneous stent placement followed by surgical intervention may be required for ureteral stenosis.

Postoperatively in the outpatient setting, patients require labs every few days to check immunosuppressant levels as

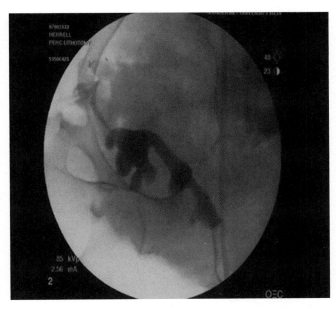

FIGURE 133-2. Nephrostogram demonstrating left-sided renal transplant with long-segment ureteral stricture and no bladder filling.

well as graft function. Transplant recipients follow up initially with the surgeon, but once all surgical issues are resolved, care often returns to the nephrologist. Nephrologists often manage long-term management of immunosuppressants and concerns for rejection.

TAKE HOME POINTS

- Transplant candidates must tolerate a large operation, have adequate anatomy for transplantation, and be healthy enough to start immunosuppression.
- Intraoperatively, tension-free, wide anastomoses are necessary.
- Careful attention to postoperative urine output and blood pressure; aggressive fluid resuscitation may be needed to replace urinary losses.
- Complications require prompt attention and management.

SUGGESTED READINGS

Greco F, Hoda MR, Alcaraz A, et al. Laparoscopic living-donor nephrectomy: analysis of the existing literature. *Eur Urol.* 2010;58(4):498-509.

Kayler L, Kang D, Molmenti E, et al. Kidney transplant ureteroneocystostomy techniques and complications: review of the literature. *Transplant Proc.* 2010;42(5):1413-1420.

Pascual J, Zamora J, Galeano C, et al. Steroid avoidance or withdrawal for kidney transplant recipients. *Cochrane Database Syst Rev.* 2009;1:CD005632.

Ponticelli C, Moia M, Montagnino G. Renal allograft thrombosis. *Nephrol Dial Transplant.* 2009;24(5):1388-1393.

Rajiah P, Lim YY, Taylor P. Renal transplant imaging and complications. *Abdom Imaging.* 2006;31(6):735-746.

Case Conclusion

Your patient receives a deceased donor kidney notable for multiple renal arteries. He tolerates the procedure well and has an uncomplicated postoperative course. Three months later, he has elevated serum creatinine, which continues to rise on serial laboratories but is otherwise asymptomatic. Transplant ultrasound demonstrates hydronephrosis. He undergoes percutaneous antegrade nephrostogram, which confirms hydronephrosis secondary to a 3-cm segment of ureteral stenosis at the anastomosis (Figure 133-2). Because of the long length of stenosis, endoscopic management such as balloon dilation or endoureterotomy is determined to be inadequate. A nephrostomy tube is left in place until the patient is scheduled for return to the operating room for ureteral reconstruction.

Ureteral stenosis is the most common major ureteric complication following renal transplant with incidence varying from 2.6% to 15%.[1] It usually presents within 3 months of transplantation and affects the distal ureter. Ischemia of the distal ureter is implicated as the main cause of ureteral stenosis, and therefore, care should be taken to not overskeletonize the ureter during the procurement and backtable preparation.

Endoscopic interventions such as balloon dilation or short-term stents are more successful for shorter segments of disease and within 3 months of transplant.[2]

There are multiple options for reconstruction including reimplantation to the bladder, Psoas hitch, Boari flap, and ureteroureterostomy. As with any anastomosis, the goal is a tension-free reconstruction. Mobilization of the bladder reinforced with a Psoas hitch may eliminate tension and allow reimplantation. If the ureter is too short, the bladder can be elongated with Boari flap to meet the ureter. Another option is to reimplant the donor ureter into native ureter.[3]

REFERENCES FOR CLINICAL SCENARIO

1. He B, Bremner A, Han Y. Classification of ureteral stenosis and associated strategy for treatment after kidney transplant. *Exp Clin Transplant*. 2013;11(2):122-127.

2. Giessing M. Transplant ureter stricture following renal transplantation: surgical options. *Transplant Proc*. 2011;43(1):383-386.

3. Pike TW, Pandanaboyana S, et al. Ureteric reconstruction for the management of transplant ureteric stricture: a decade of experience from a single centre. *Transpl Int*. 2015;28(5):529-534.

SECTION 15

Head and Neck

15

Head and Neck

134

Melanoma of the Head and Neck

HAROLD HEAH AND MICHAEL E. KUPFERMAN

Based on the previous edition chapter "Melanoma of the Head and Neck" by Andrew Kroeker, Andrew Shuman, and Erin McKean

Presentation

A 76-year-old Caucasian man presents with a pigmented lesion over the malar eminence of the right cheek; he had first noticed this lesion 2 years ago. It was initially dark, round, and pea sized but has enlarged over the past 4 months. Along with the enlargement, its margins have become more irregular; the lesion has become more heterogeneous in color, with varying degrees of pigmentation. The lesion did not hurt or bleed and he did not notice any ulceration.

● WORKUP

History

At first presentation, it is essential to obtain a thorough medical history and directed physical examination. Cutaneous melanomas of the head and neck are readily visible since this part of the body is exposed, but lesions can sometimes be obscured by hair if located on the scalp or the auricles. Patients may present with a new pigmented skin lesion or a previously present nevus that has changed in appearance. Other symptoms suggestive of melanoma include pruritus, pain, bleeding, and ulceration. Pertinent history also includes:

- Significant unprotected sun exposure
- Previous sunburns
- Use of tanning beds
- Family history (first degree relative) of melanoma
- Personal history of skin malignancies
- Large number of nevi or atypical nevi (>50)

Physical Examination

When examining the suspected skin lesion, the mnemonic "ABCDE" is used:

A—Asymmetry: The shape is asymmetrical with one half appearing different from the other.
B—Border: Irregularity of borders around the lesion.
C—Color: Heterogeneity in color of the lesion.
D—Diameter: Usually >6 mm in size.
E—Evolving/evolution: On serial examinations, the lesion demonstrates change in shape, color, and increase in size over time.

Examination should encompass the draining lymph node basin of the lesion. For the head and neck, this includes examination of the parotid, suboccipital, as well as anterior and lateral neck nodal basins. If perineural invasion is suspected, gross sensation around the lesion and motor function, such as facial movements, should be evaluated. Finally, the patient should undergo a complete skin examination by a dermatologist.

The head and neck are the most common sites for mucosal melanoma. This is a rare entity that accounts for <2% of all melanomas with clinicopathologic behavior distinct from cutaneous melanomas. They occur on mucosal surfaces of the upper aerodigestive tract and genitourinary tract and behave more aggressively, conveying poorer prognosis than cutaneous melanomas. Mucosal melanomas tend to present in an advanced stage due to obscure primary sites such as within the sinonasal tract or in the nasopharynx. Presenting symptoms include epistaxis, nasal obstruction, or blood-tinged sputum, and some may also have middle ear effusions from eustachian tube obstruction. Physical examination requires thorough examination of the mucosal surfaces of the upper aerodigestive tract and includes flexible fiber-optic nasopharyngoscopy. It is also important to ascertain any prior history of cutaneous melanomas, and examination should encompass the patient's skin surfaces to rule out the possibility of the mucosal melanoma being a metastatic deposit (Figures 134-1–134-3).

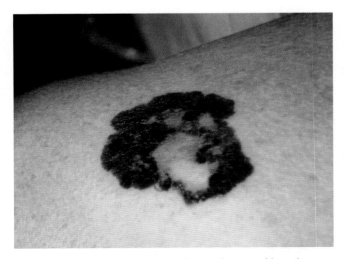

FIGURE 134-1. Superficial spreading melanoma. Note the irregular borders, color heterogeneity, and asymmetry. (Reprinted from Craft N, Fox LP, Goldsmith LA, et al. *VisualDx: Essential Adult Dermatology*. Philadelphia, PA: Wolters Kluwer; 2010, with permission.)

5-year survival by stage

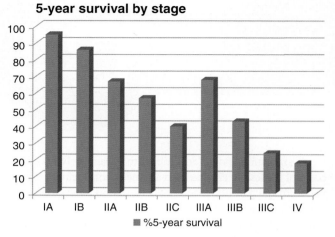

FIGURE 134-2. Cutaneous melanoma—5-year survival based on AJCC TNM stage.

Investigations and Diagnosis

All worrisome lesions should be biopsied to obtain tissue for histopathologic assessment and confirmation of diagnosis. Excisional, incisional, and punch biopsies are all reasonable options, and the choice would depend on the site and size of the lesion. An important factor to consider during the biopsy is to obtain adequate tissue depth so that the depth of invasion can be properly assessed by the pathologist. In view of this, shave biopsies are not recommended when the

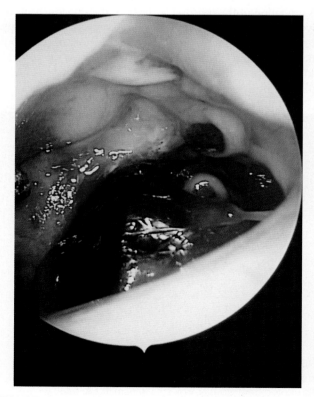

FIGURE 134-3. Mucosal melanoma on the left eustachian cushion. Patient had presented with left hearing loss from middle ear effusion.

differential diagnosis is a melanoma as the depth of invasion would often be indeterminate. When performing an excision biopsy of the lesion, a margin of 1 to 3 mm is recommended as wider margins can potentially reduce the accuracy of sentinel lymph node mapping if later indicated. As for incision and punch biopsies, they should be performed at the thickest portion of the lesion. In general, frozen section (FS) analysis is not recommended for melanocytic lesion as both depth of invasion and degree of cytologic atypia are difficult to accurately interpret with FS.

The histopathology result of the biopsy should be reported in a synoptic reporting format as developed by the College of American Pathologists (CAP) and recommended by the American Joint Committee on Cancer (AJCC). This includes the following:

- Procedure
- Anatomic site
- Histologic subtype
- Tumor thickness (Breslow thickness) and anatomic (Clark) levels
- Ulceration
- Margins
- Mitotic rate
- Vascular invasion
- Perineural invasion
- Tumor regression
- Growth patterns and phases

Upon biopsy and confirmation of melanoma, the disease should then be staged based on the eighth edition of the AJCC Cancer Staging Manual. The T stage (primary site) is determined by the Breslow depth. Lesions with ≤1.00-mm invasion are staged as T1, 1.01 to 2.00 mm as T2, 2.01 to 4.00 mm as T3, and >4.00 mm as T4. The T stages are further divided into "a" and "b," "a" being the absence of ulceration and "b" being with ulceration. Additionally, T1a lesions have <0.8-mm depth of invasion without ulceration, while T1b are categorized as having 0.8- to 1-mm depth of invasion with or without ulceration. The N status is determined by the number of involved lymph nodes, N1 being 1 node involved, N2 being 2 to 3, and N3 being ≥4 nodes. The N stage is further divided into "a," "b," and "c": "a" denotes presence of clinically occult nodes (detected by sentinel lymph node biopsy [SLNB]); "b" denotes presence of clinically detectable lymph node; "c" denotes presence of in-transit, satellite, and/or microsatellite metastases. In-transit metastasis is defined as intralymphatic tumor in the skin or subcutaneous tissue >2 cm from the primary site but not yet involving the regional nodal base. Clinically evident lymph nodes can be evaluated preoperatively with fine needle aspiration cytology (FNAC). This low-cost and minimally invasive method has been shown to be highly sensitive in diagnosing lymph node involvement. In the absence of clinically evident nodal disease, primary lesions of stages T1b and higher should undergo lymphoscintigraphy and SLNB for more accurate N-status assessment. The sentinel lymph node is defined as the first lymph node or group of nodes to which the malignant cells are most likely to metastasize from the primary site. This is performed by intradermal injection of radiotracer (such as Tc-99m tilmanocept or Tc-99m sulfur colloid) around the primary site followed by capturing of images using a scintillation camera to identify the uptake at the primary site and sentinel lymph node/s. In the head and neck with its more anatomically complex structures, a single photon emission computed tomography (SPECT) is often useful in localizing the sentinel lymph nodes.

As advanced cutaneous melanomas have a high risk of distant metastasis, a metastatic workup should be performed for Stage III and IV disease. This would include computed tomography (CT) scans of the neck, chest, abdomen, and pelvis with contrast, MRI of the brain, serum lactate dehydrogenase (LDH), and possibly fluorodeoxyglucose–positron emission tomography (FDG-PET) scans. Though costly, FDG-PET scans have been shown to be superior in detecting distant metastasis compared to conventional CT scans (Figure 134-4 and Tables 134-1 and 134-2).

● TREATMENT

Treatment of Primary Site

The treatment of primary lesion involves performing a wide local excision (WLE) with adequate margins. T1 lesions require 1-cm margins, 1- to 2-cm margins for T2, and 2-cm margins for T3-4 lesions. Frozen sections have a limited role in assessment of the margins, and a rush permanent histologic assessment should be performed instead. The incision should be perpendicular to the skin surface and beveling should be avoided. The incision extends deep to the dermis into the subcutaneous tissue layer. In the face, staying superficial to the superficial musculoaponeurotic system (SMAS) can help to avoid damage to the facial nerve branches. In cases where the tumor extends into the deeper planes, the WLE has to be extended to the appropriate depth to ensure complete. As permanent histopathologic assessment of margins usually take a few days to be return, a delayed closure method can be adopted. The wound is first dressed and only closed upon return of negative margins. Depending on the site and size of the wound, closure techniques can vary. Primary closure is the simplest technique, but if the skin defect is sizeable, various local flaps or distant free flaps can be utilized (Figure 134-5).

Treatment of Nodal Basin

Clinically N0 Disease

In the absence of clinically evident nodal disease, SLNB should be performed at the time of the WLE for any lesions staged T1b and above. The Multicenter Selective Lymphadenectomy Trial (MSLT-1) demonstrated the prognostic value of SLNB for intermediate-thickness and thick melanomas (Breslow thickness >1.00 mm) but did not demonstrate improvement in survival. In general, SLNB is not indicated for lesions with Breslow thickness ≤0.75 mm as risk factors like ulceration and high mitotic figure count are rare in such thin lesions and the risk for occult nodal metastasis is low. When performing SLNB, intradermal radiotracer injections around the primary site should be performed preoperatively to allow for uptake at the sentinel lymph node at the time of surgery. Intraoperatively, the surgeon will then use a gamma probe to identify the sentinel lymph node(s). Additional intradermal injection of a colored dye such as methylene blue or isosulfan blue at the time of surgery can also provide a visual guide to identify sentinel lymph nodes. The lymph nodes are then sent for permanent histopathology examination.

Completion neck dissection in the setting of positive micrometastasis after SLNB is useful for more accurate staging in view of possible positive micrometastases in non-sentinel lymph nodes as well as improving regional control of the nodal basin. It is, however, unclear if completion neck dissection improves survival and the results of the MSLT-2 trial should provide useful information to answer this question for head and neck melanomas.

Clinically N Positive

In the setting of positive nodal disease without evidence of distant metastasis, clearance of the lymph nodes in the nodal basin should be performed. If the positive node is within the parotid bed, the patient should have a parotidectomy as well as an appropriate neck dissection to clear the draining nodal basin.

Adjuvant Therapy

Adjuvant Radiation Therapy

Adjuvant radiation therapy to the primary site after complete resection with widely clear margins is generally not recommended except in certain situations. Desmoplastic melanoma is a subset of the disease that has a high propensity for local recurrence, and adjuvant radiation to the primary site has been shown to improve local control. Adjuvant radiation to the neck or parotid nodal basins in node-positive disease improves regional control but at the expense of increased treatment-related morbidity. Another scenario where adjuvant radiation is useful would be for mucosal melanomas. In these patients, adjuvant radiation is recommended as it has been shown to improve both locoregional control as well as survival. In cases with positive nodal disease, the neck should also be treated after appropriate neck dissection.

Adjuvant Systemic Therapy

Melanomas are generally resistant to traditional chemotherapy agents used for head and neck malignancies. However, there have been exciting developments in targeted therapy, immunotherapy, and combinations of traditional chemotherapy with interferon for use in the setting of stage III and IV melanomas. High-dose interferon by itself or in

10 min RT Cheek HEAD/NECK LYMPHOSCINTIGRAPHY 1

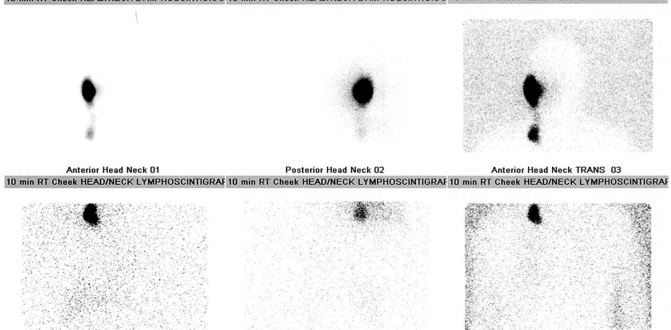

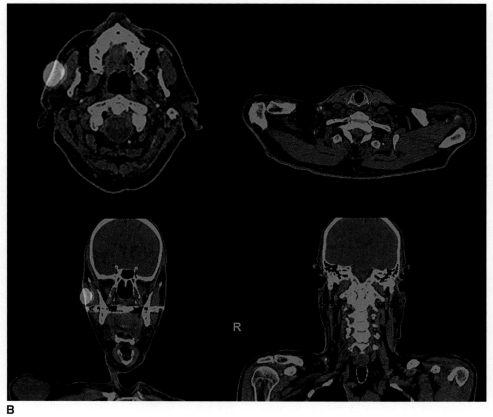

FIGURE 134-4. **A:** Preoperative lymphoscintigraphy. **B:** SPECT. Demonstrates relationship of sentinel lymph node to other structures of the head and neck.

Table 134-1	Eighth Edition AJCC TNM Cutaneous Melanoma Guide 2017	
Classification		
T	**Thickness (mm)**	**Ulceration status**
Tis	N/A	N/A
T1 T1a T1b	≤1.0 <0.8 <0.8 0.8–1.0	Without ulceration With ulceration With or without ulceration
T2 T2a T2b	>1.0–2.0	Without ulceration With ulceration
T3 T3a T3b	>2.0–4.0	Without ulceration With ulceration
T4 T4a T4b	>4.0	Without ulceration With ulceration
N	**No. of tumor-involved regional lymph nodes**	**Presence of in-transit, satellite, and/or microsatellite metastases**
N0	0	N/A
N1 N1a N1b N1c	 1 clinically occult (detected on SLNB) 1 clinically detected No regional lymph node disease	No No Yes
N2 N2a N2b N2c	 2–3 clinically occult (detected on SLNB) 2–3 clinically detected 1 clinically occult or detected	No No Yes
N3 N3a N3b N3c	 ≥4 clinically occult (detected on SLNB) ≥4 clinically detected ≥2 clinically occult or detected and/or any number of matted nodes	No No Yes
M	**Site**	**Serum LDH**
M0	No distant metastases	N/A
M1a M1a(0) M1a(1)	Distant skin, soft tissue, and/or nonregional lymph node	Normal Elevated
M1b M1b(0) M1b(1)	Lung metastases with or without M1a sites	Normal Elevated
M1c M1c(0) M1c(1)	All other non-CNS[a] visceral metastases with or without M1a or M1b sites	Normal Elevated
M1d M1d(0) M1d(1)	CNS[a] metastasis with or without M1a, M1b, or M1c sites	Normal Elevated

[a]CNS, central nervous system.

| Table 134-2 | | Eighth Edition AJCC Cutaneous Melanoma Staging 2017 | | | | | | | |

	T0	T1a	T1b	T2a	T2b	T3a	T3b	T4a	T4b
N0	N/A	IA	IA	IB	IIA	IIA	IIB	IIB	IIC
N1a	N/A	IIIA	IIIA	IIIA	IIIB	IIIB	IIIC	IIIC	IIIC
N1b	IIIB	IIIB	IIIB	IIIB	IIIB	IIIB	IIIC	IIIC	IIIC
N1c	IIIB	IIIB	IIIB	IIIB	IIIB	IIIB	IIIC	IIIC	IIIC
N2a	N/A	IIIA	IIIA	IIIA	IIIB	IIIB	IIIC	IIIC	IIIC
N2b	IIIC	IIIB	IIIB	IIIB	IIIB	IIIB	IIIC	IIIC	IIIC
N2c	IIIC	IIIC	IIIC	IIIC	IIIC	IIIC	IIIC	IIIC	IIIC
N3a	N/A	IIIC	IIIC	IIIC	IIIC	IIIC	IIIC	IIIC	IIID
N3b	IIIC	IIIC	IIIC	IIIC	IIIC	IIIC	IIIC	IIIC	IIID
N3c	IIIC	IIIC	IIIC	IIIC	IIIC	IIIC	IIIC	IIIC	IIID
M1	IV								

combination with other chemotherapy agents has been shown to improve overall survival, but this is at the expense of significant treatment toxicity. Immunotherapy in the form of cytotoxic T-lymphocyte–associated antigen (CTLA)-4 and anti–PD-1 inhibitors, such as ipilimumab and nivolumab, have also emerged as viable and effective adjuvant treatment options in the setting of advanced melanomas. They have demonstrated improved survival in patients with advanced unresectable disease and distant metastasis.

The tumor specimens should be tested for BRAF and c-KIT mutations to identify patients suitable for targeted therapy. C-KIT inhibitors like imatinib and BRAF inhibitors like vemurafenib and dabrafenib are now FDA approved for treatment of appropriate advanced melanoma patients in whom these mutations are identified.

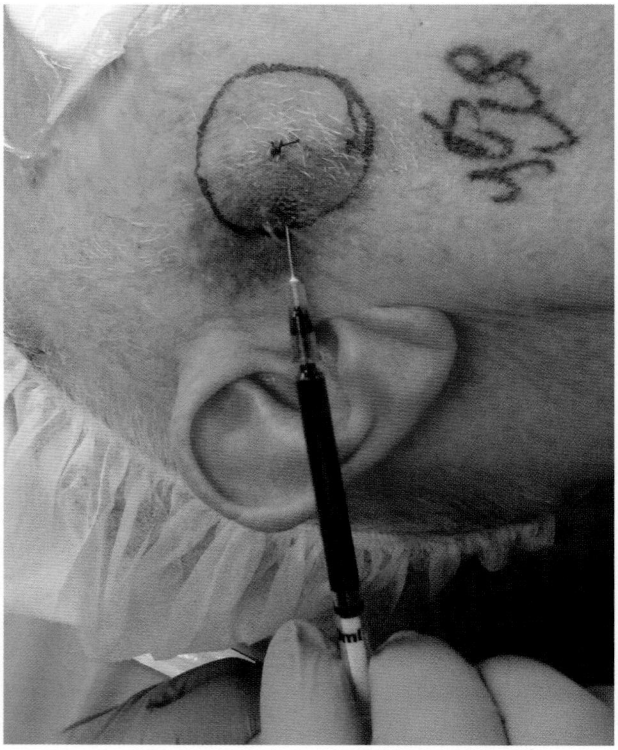

Metastatic Disease

Historically, patients with distant metastasis have poor prognosis, and treatment was generally palliative in intent. The mean 5-year survival for Stage IV disease is about 18% but varies depending on the sites of metastases and M staging (M1a, b, or c). However, with the emergence of the various systemic therapies discussed earlier, such as immunotherapy and interferon and targeted therapies, improvements in survival have been seen in this group of patients. A prospective trial using anti–PD-1 agent to treat metastatic melanoma recently reported a 5-year survival of 34%.

● DISCUSSION

The incidence of melanoma has been steadily increasing in the United States, from 14 per 100,000 in the early 1990s to about 24 per 100,000 in 2013. Paradoxically, despite this increase over the past two decades, there has not been a corresponding rise in mortality from the disease. This could be explained by the heightened public awareness of this condition, resulting in earlier diagnosis. The overall 5-year survival for melanoma is about 90% with Stage I disease accounting for >80% of new cases diagnosed. Melanoma can affect adults of various ages with people aged 55 to 74 years

FIGURE 134-5. Patient prepped for wide local excision of a left cheek melanoma and sentinel lymph node biopsy. A 2-cm margin has been drawn around the lesion, and intradermal injection of isosulfan blue around the lesion is being administered. Note the suture that had been placed to mark the site of the lesion after the initial biopsy.

accounting for about 45% of all new cases, and there are more males affected with a male-to-female ratio of 1.7:1. The head and neck are common sites for melanoma given that sun exposure is a predisposing factor, accounting for about 20% of all cutaneous melanomas. The anatomical sites that are most sun exposed are also the most common sites of the disease, namely, the face, scalp, auricle, and neck.

There are several histologic subtypes of melanomas described, and those found in the head and neck includes (1) superficial spreading melanoma, (2) nodular melanoma, (3) lentigo maligna melanoma, (4) desmoplastic melanoma, and (5) mucosal melanoma. The most common types are the superficial spreading and nodular melanomas. Lentigo maligna refers to a type of melanoma in situ and is a precursor to lentigo maligna melanoma. Though not yet exhibiting invasion, lentigo maligna should be excised, but smaller margins of 0.5 cm are adequate. Subtype of melanoma is part of the synoptic histopathology report but has less significance in terms of prognosis compared to Breslow depth, ulceration, and mitotic figure count.

Surgery is still the treatment of choice for resectable, melanomas, and clear margins should be the aim of the surgeon. This can sometimes pose a challenge in the head and neck, given the proximity to structures like the eye and facial nerve. The surgeon may be tempted to sacrifice on margins to preserve skin for closure or to avoid creating anesthetically unpleasant surgical defect, but one has to bear in mind that the aim is for negative margins in order to achieve long-term locoregional control and survival. As such, it is vital for the surgeon to engage the patient in the operative planning so that they can be onboard with the overall treatment plan and outcomes.

● SURVEILLANCE

The goal of surveillance is to detect recurrent disease early and initiate treatment in a timely manner to allow for improved oncologic outcomes. These patients are also 5 to 6 times more likely to develop new skin primaries than the general population. The new primaries can occur anywhere but more commonly affect the same site as the initial primary lesion. All melanoma patients should undergo regular screening of their skin by a dermatologist at 6- to 12-month intervals.

The frequency of surveillance visits depends on the stage of the disease. For stage IA to IIA disease, patients should be followed up at 6- to 12-month intervals for the first 5 years and annually thereafter. At each review, they should have a thorough history taken and a targeted physical examination. No imaging investigations are necessary unless clinically indicated by relevant signs or symptoms detected during the visit. For stage IIB to IV disease, these patients require closer surveillance with visits every 3 to 6 months for the first 2 years and then 3 to 12 months thereafter. Imaging investigations should be done every 3 to 12 months for the first

2 years to screen for asymptomatic recurrent or metastatic disease and then only as clinically indicated thereafter.

Patients with melanoma in situ should undergo yearly skin surveillance as they are also at increased risk of skin malignancies, including invasive melanoma.

Case Conclusion

The patient was seen in postoperative follow-up to discuss the final pathology and staging. The Breslow depth was 2.95 mm with clear margins, and the sentinel lymph node was negative. His disease was staged as T3aN0M0 (Stage IIA) after pathology review; no adjuvant therapy was recommended. His wound defect was subsequently closed with a local rotation-advancement flap. He has been scheduled for routine follow-up in 3 months time.

TAKE HOME POINTS

- Surgery is the primary treatment modality for melanoma.
- Sentinel lymph node biopsy should be performed for intermediate-thickness and thick melanomas.
- Though the surgeon should keep preservation of aesthetics in mind, this should be secondary to oncologically sound surgery, and proper discussion with the patient is vital to achieve outcomes that are acceptable by both.
- Appropriate histopathologic and clinical staging is necessary for both risk stratification and selection of appropriate treatment modalities.

SUGGESTED READINGS

Agrawal S, Kane JM 3rd, Ballo MT. The benefits of adjuvant radiation therapy after therapeutic lymphadenectomy for clinically advanced, high-risk lymph node-metastatic melanoma. *Cancer.* 2009;115:5836-5844.

Andtbacka RH, Gershenwald JE. Role of sentinel lymph node biopsy in patients with thin melanoma. *J Natl Compr Canc Netw.* 2009;308-317.

Balch CM, Soong SJ, Smith T, et al. Long-term results of a prospective surgical trial comparing 2 cm vs. 4 cm excision margins for 740 patients with 1–4 mm melanomas. *Ann Surg Oncol.* 2001;8:101-108.

Balch CM, Soong SJ, Gershenwaldt JE, et al. Prognostic factors analysis of 17,600 melanoma patients: validation of the American Joint Committee on Cancer melanoma staging system. *J Clin Oncol.* 2001;19:3622-3634.

Balch CM, Gershenwald JE, et al. Final version of 2009 AJCC melanoma staging and classification. *J Clin Oncol.* 2009;27:6199-6206.

Bamboat ZM, Konstantinidis IT, Coit DG, et al. Observation after a positive sentinel lymph node biopsy in patients with melanoma. *Ann Surg Oncol.* 2014;21:3117-3123.

Byers RM. Treatment of the neck in melanoma. *Otolaryngol Clin North Am.* 1998;31:833-839.

Chang AE, Karnell LH, Menck HR. The national cancer database report on cutaneous and noncutaneous melanoma: a summary of 84,836 cases from the past decade. *Cancer.* 1998;83:1664-1678.

Flaherty KT, Puzanov I, et al. Inhibition of mutated, activated BRAF in metastatic melanoma. *N Engl J Med.* 2010;363:809-819.

Hodi FS, O'Day SJ, et al. Improved survival with ipilimumab in patients with metastatic melanoma. *N Engl J Med.* 2010;363:711-723.

Kirkwood JM, Ibrahim JG, Sosman JA, et al. High-dose interferon alfa-2b significantly prolongs relapse-free and overall survival compared with the GM2-KLH/QS-21 vaccine in patients with resected stage IIB-III melanoma: results of Intergroup Trial E1694/S9512/C509801. *J Clin Oncol.* 2001;19:2370-2380.

Larkin J, Chiarion-Sileni V, Gonzalez R, et al. Combined nivolumab and ipilimumab or monotherapy in untreated melanoma. *N Engl J Med.* 2015;373:23-34.

Morton DL, Thompson JF, Faries MB, et al. Final trial report of sentinel-node biopsy versus nodal observation in melanoma. *N Engl J Med.* 2014;370:599-609.

Moreno MA, Roberts DB, Kupferman ME. Mucosal melanoma of the nose and paranasal sinuses, a contemporary experience from the M.D. Anderson Cancer Center. *Cancer.* 2010;116:2215-2223.

Pasquali S, Mocellin S, Campana LG, et al. Early (sentinel lymph node biopsy-guided) versus delayed lymphadenectomy in melanoma patients with lymph node metastases: a personal experience and literature meta-analysis. *Cancer.* 2010;116:1201-1209.

Rigel DS, Friedman RJ, Kopf AW, et al. ABCDE—an evolving concept in the early detection of melanoma. *Arch Dermatol.* 2005;141:1032-1034.

Schmalbach CE, Nussenbaum B, et al. Reliability of sentinel lymph node mapping with biopsy for head and neck cutaneous melanoma. *Arch Otolaryngol Head Neck Surg.* 2003;129:61-65.

Schmalbach CE, Johnson TM, Bradford CR. The management of head and neck melanoma. *Curr Probl Surg.* 2006;43:781-835.

Surveillance, Epidemiology and End Results. (2016). Available at: http://seer.cancer.gov.

Wagner M, Morris CG. Mucosal melanoma of the head and neck. *Am J Clin Oncol.* 2008;31:43-48.

Yamamoto M, Fisher KJ, Wong JY, et al. Sentinel lymph node biopsy is indicated for patients with thick clinically node-negative melanoma. *Cancer.* 2015;121:1628-1636.

Head and Neck Cancer

ZHEN GOOI AND CAROLE FAKHRY

135

Based on the previous edition chapter "Head and Neck Cancer" by Matthew Spector and Erin McKean

Presentation

A 68-year-old gentleman presents to the emergency room with complaints of hoarseness and pain with swallowing that has been getting worse over the past 2 months. His past medical history is significant for chronic kidney disease and insulin-dependent diabetes mellitus. He has an extensive smoking history of at least 30 pack years.

On initial examination in the emergency room, he has marked inspiratory stridor and he is drooling. He is tachypneic and is currently saturating at 91% on 10 L via face mask. His voice has a rough quality to it. Palpation of his neck reveals subtle bulge in the region of his left thyroid lamina.

● DIFFERENTIAL DIAGNOSIS

- Malignancy is at the top of the list of differential diagnoses. Potential cancers that are known to occur in the larynx include squamous cell carcinoma (SCC), verrucous carcinoma, adenocarcinoma, neuroendocrine carcinoma, sarcoma, and lymphoma. In a patient with an extensive smoking history and the clinical findings as described above, SCC is at the top of the differential. Squamous cell carcinoma is also the most common malignancy affecting the mucosa of the head and neck region. While less likely in this scenario, other causes of airway obstruction include:
  - Inflammatory/infectious—epiglottitis secondary to bacterial infection and Ludwig's angina
  - Benign lesions—vocal cord papilloma, hemorrhagic polyp, and laryngocele
  - Allergic reactions causing angioedema

● WORKUP

Given the concern that the patient has an airway obstruction, a flexible fiber-optic scope exam is a useful adjunctive procedure that can quickly identify the location and extent of upper airway obstruction. In this case, it shows an ulcerative friable mass occupying almost his entire glottis. The immediate concern in this patient's presentation is that of impending airway compromise. He will require his airway to be secured with the safest procedure. Options to secure the airway include oral or nasal intubation or a tracheostomy. In this case, the most expedient manner to achieve this will be an awake tracheostomy. This allows the patient to retain his capacity to breathe during the operation and avoids the scenario of not being able to intubate or mask ventilate the patient following induction of general anesthesia. For an awake tracheostomy, local anesthesia is infiltrated into the skin and subcutaneous tissues of the midline neck below the cricoid cartilage. After the neck is prepped and draped, a 3-cm vertical skin incision is made in the midline below the inferior border of the cricoid cartilage. Dissection is carried out to identify the avascular plane of the midline raphe between the sternohyoid and sternothyroid neck muscles. Any overlying thyroid isthmus tissue is divided to reach the trachea. The inferior border of the cricoid cartilage is identified, and a cricoid hook is used to provide superior retraction of the laryngotracheal complex. A tracheotomy is made in between the first and second tracheal rings. The "high" location of this tracheostomy is performed in anticipation of possible definitive surgical resection that will require incorporation of the superior tracheal rings as a resection margin during laryngectomy.

The alternative is to perform an awake transoral/transnasal intubation, preferably with the assistance of fiber-optic scopes in the hands of doctors who have experience and competency with management of the difficult airway. This comprises of pretreatment of the nasal cavity with nasal decongestant and topical anesthetic also applied to the base of the tongue and posterior pharyngeal wall. For both of these strategies, it is imperative to discuss with anesthesia team the intubation plan and alternatives of securing the airway in the event of a failed intubation attempt. After securing airway, attention turns to the diagnostic evaluation. Once his airway is secured, the patient can be safely induced, and under general anesthesia, a direct laryngoscopy should be performed to assess for the exact sites of involvement of his laryngeal mass as well as biopsy of the mass. In this patient's case, he is shown to have a bulky ulcerative lesion centered on the left true vocal cord, extending to the anterior commissure and the anterior half of the contralateral vocal cord. Superiorly, the cancer involves the entire false vocal cord. There is no involvement of the subglottis, pyriform sinuses, or postcricoid region. Biopsy of this mass reveals keratinizing squamous cell carcinoma.

Computed tomography (CT) of the neck with contrast enables for characterization of any extralaryngeal spread of the cancer that may not be appreciated on direct laryngoscopy, as well as the presence of neck nodal metastasis. Additionally, for staging purposes, CT scan of the chest with contrast is also recommended. Evaluation of the chest is important for anyone with an advanced laryngeal malignancy and for patients with extensive smoking history who are at increased risk for a second primary tumor. In this patient's case, the cancer is shown to invade through the left lamina of the thyroid cartilage. There is no suspicious cervical lymphadenopathy. The CT of the chest shows extensive emphysematous changes.

● DIAGNOSIS AND TREATMENT

Based on the information obtained from clinical examination and radiologic imaging, this patient is staged as a Stage IV, T4aN0M0 laryngeal squamous cell carcinoma. Squamous cell carcinoma is the most common malignancy affecting the head and neck region with an estimated incidence of 13,000 cases in the United States and 4,000 deaths being attributable to it. The larynx is comprised of three subsites—the supraglottic larynx is represented by the area above the true vocal folds and includes the laryngeal surface of the epiglottis, false vocal cords, aryepiglottic folds, and arytenoids. The glottis is comprised of the true vocal folds, while the subglottis is the area below the true vocal folds up to the inferior border of the cricoid. The staging for glottic cancer involves assessment of anatomical extent and vocal fold function. T1 glottic cancers are limited to the vocal cord, while T2 cancers extend to either the supraglottis or subglottis or cause impaired vocal cord mobility. Glottic cancers causing either vocal cord fixation, invasion into the paraglottic space, or inner cortex of the thyroid cartilage are classified as T3. T4a cancers invade through the outer cortex of the thyroid cartilage and/or structures beyond the larynx such as the trachea, strap muscles, thyroid, or esophagus. T4b cancers invade into either the prevertebral space or mediastinal structures or encase the carotid artery. Figure 135-1 shows pathways for spread of a primary cancer involving the glottis.

Treatment options for patients with advanced laryngeal cancer are divided into two main categories, surgical and nonsurgical. Surgical management of advanced laryngeal cancer in principle involves a total laryngectomy. In a select number of patients, a partial laryngectomy that preserves some components of the laryngeal apparatus may be possible; however, this is usually restricted to patients with limited involvement of their cancer to one or two laryngeal subsites. Primary nonsurgical management involves concurrent chemoradiation, with the preferred chemotherapeutic agent being cisplatin and radiation therapy usually being administered over the course of 7 weeks to a total dose of 70 Gy to the primary site and 44 to 50 Gy to sites of intermediate risk. There is evidence to show that an up-front surgical approach involving a total laryngectomy is superior to concurrent chemoradiation for stage T4a cancers.

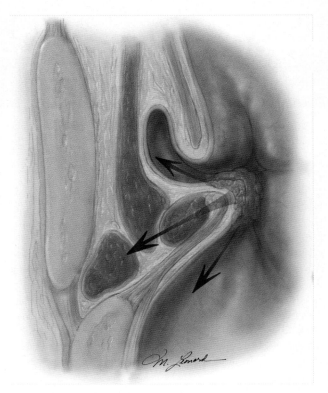

FIGURE 135-1. Pathways for spread for a primary cancer involving the glottis with *arrows* from top to bottom representing supraglottic, paraglottic, and subglottic spread. (Reprinted from Myers J, Hanna E. *Cancer of the Head and Neck.* 5th ed. Philadelphia, PA: Wolters Kluwer; 2016, with permission).

● SURGICAL APPROACH

As alluded to earlier, surgical management of this patient's advanced laryngeal cancer will involve a total laryngectomy. Additionally, a left hemithyroidectomy will also be performed due to the extralaryngeal extension of the cancer through the left thyroid cartilage lamina. Bilateral elective neck dissections are carried out in this patient because of his advanced stage, extralaryngeal extension, and involvement of the contralateral glottis. These features increase the risk of occult nodal metastasis to around 20%. The nodal stations at risk in advanced glottis cancer are levels II to IV and VI.

At the start of surgery, his tracheostomy tube is exchanged for a flexible endotracheal tube to allow for ease of access to the neck. A curvilinear skin incision is designed, extending across a natural skin crease of the neck from the posterior border of one sternocleidomastoid muscle to the other. The inferior aspect of this incision incorporates the prior tracheostomy stoma. Skin incision is made and carried down to the layer below the platysma muscle, dividing it in the process. Subplatysmal skin flaps are raised superiorly to the level just above the hyoid bone to expose the suprahyoid muscles and inferiorly to the clavicle.

The right neck dissection is started. The inferior border of the submandibular gland is skeletonized, followed by identification of the anterior and the posterior bellies of the digastric muscle. The hypoglossal nerve is identified deep to the digastric muscle and traced posteriorly toward its intersection point with the internal jugular vein close to the skull base. This allows for freeing up of the lymph node packet overlying the digastric muscle and carotid sheath in level II, marking the superior limit of the neck dissection. Following this, the fascia overlying the anterior border of the sternocleidomastoid muscle is divided in a broad-based fashion from levels II through IV. This allows the lymph node packet to be progressively separated from its attachments to the sternocleidomastoid muscle as dissection proceeds in a posterior–medial direction with lateral retraction of the sternocleidomastoid muscle. During this process, the omohyoid muscle is divided in level III. At the superior portion of level II, using the transverse process of C1 and posterior belly of the digastric muscle as landmarks, the spinal accessory nerve is identified and traced superiorly toward its intersection point with the internal jugular vein close to the skull base and inferiorly at its entry point into the sternocleidomastoid muscle. The posterior border of the sternocleidomastoid muscle marks the posterior limit of the neck dissection. The inferior attachments of the lymph node packet at the level of the clavicle are divided, marking the inferior limit of the dissection. Next, the lymph node packet is then freed off the floor of the neck, using the cervical nerve rootlets as landmarks for the medial limit of the dissection. Dissection at this point processes from a posterior to anterior fashion, elevating the lymph node packet off the carotid sheath contents, taking care to preserve the internal jugular vein, vagus nerve, and carotid artery. The entire neck dissection lymph node packet is left attached to the strap muscles marking the anterior limit of the neck dissection. This process is repeated on for the left neck. Figure 135-2 shows the completed right

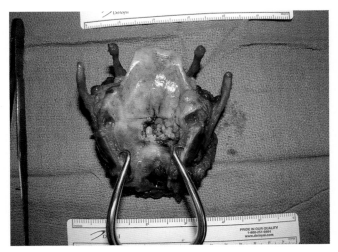

FIGURE 135-2. Total laryngectomy specimen with posterior cricoid cartilage showing a transglottic cancer with preepiglottic and paraglottic space spread (not belonging to this patient). (Reprinted from Myers J, Hanna E. *Cancer of the Head and Neck.* 5th ed. Philadelphia, PA: Wolters Kluwer; 2016, with permission).

neck dissection wound bed following removal of the lymph node bearing tissue.

Following completion of the neck dissection, attention is turned toward performing the laryngectomy. Superiorly, the suprahyoid muscles are divided from their attachment points at the superior edge of the body and greater cornu of the hyoid bone. Care is taken to stay close to the hyoid bone during this step to avoid injury to the hypoglossal nerve. Inferiorly, the strap muscles are dived at their attachment points to the sternum. Next, the lateral border of the left thyroid lobe is identified. The superior and inferior thyroid vascular pedicles are identified and divided as close to the lateral edge of the thyroid lobe as possible. The thyroid isthmus is divided, and the right thyroid lobe is reflected off the laryngotracheal complex, while the left thyroid lobe together with the left level VI lymph node packet is kept attached to the eventual laryngectomy specimen. Next, the lateral borders of the laryngectomy specimen are delineated by dividing the overlying constrictor muscles at the lateral borders of the thyroid lamina. Pirifrom sinus mucosa is elevated bluntly of the inner aspect of the thyroid lamina, taking care not to inadvertently enter the pharynx during this step. Attention is then turned toward performing the tracheal incision to separate the trachea from the laryngeal complex. The tracheotomy is made between the third and fourth tracheal rings anteriorly, with the tracheal incisions then beveling obliquely superiorly for 2 tracheal rings in order to create a wider laryngectomy stoma. This opening, with a short anterior wall and long lateral and wide posterior walls, becomes the new laryngectomy stoma and is temporarily prevented from retracting into the mediastinum by placement of 1 to 2 stay sutures to the inferior neck skin flap. The avascular plane between the trachea and esophagus is identified, and dissection is carried superiorly to the level just inferior to the postcricoid mucosa. Once the superior, inferior, and lateral borders of the eventual laryngectomy specimen have been identified and dissected free, the next step is to complete the pharyngeal mucosal incisions. The pharynx is entered superiorly through the preepiglottic space. Identification of the epiglottis and its subsequent retraction in an anterior inferior direction allow for clear visualization of the intraluminal laryngeal contents. The mucosal cuts are completed taking care to incorporate a margin around the laryngeal cancer and sparing as much normal-appearing piriform sinus mucosa as possible. A cricopharyngeal myotomy is then performed, and a nasogastric tube is placed into the patient's nostril and advanced into the stomach through the esophageal inlet. Hemostasis is secured in the laryngectomy and neck dissection wound bed, and the neck is copiously irrigated with saline. Figure 135-3 shows a representative total laryngectomy specimen.

The neopharynx is then reconstructed by bringing together the remaining pharyngeal mucosa with the residual tongue base tissue in a transverse fashion over the nasogastric tube. First, a single 3-0 Vicryl suture is used to bring together the midline inferior pharyngeal mucosa to the midline tongue base, dividing the pharyngeal defect into

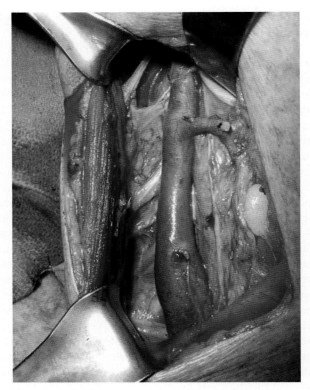

FIGURE 135-3. Right neck following selective neck dissection of levels II to IV showing preservation of spinal accessory nerve, internal jugular vein, and sternocleidomastoid muscle. (Reprinted from Myers J, Hanna E. *Cancer of the Head and Neck.* 5th ed. Philadelphia, PA: Wolters Kluwer; 2016, with permission).

2 halves. Subsequently, interrupted sutures are then placed to approximate the mucosa of the pharynx with the mucosal layer and muscular layer of the tongue base from a lateral to medial fashion, taking care to invert the mucosal edges. The mucosal closure is reinforced by bringing together an additional layer of overlying fascia with interrupted sutures along the length of the pharyngeal closure. A leak test is performed by insufflating diluted hydrogen peroxide through the oral cavity and into the oropharynx, and any areas of leakage are reinforced.

The medial attachments of the sternocleidomastoid muscle to the clavicle are divided on each side for 2 cm, allowing for the stoma to be situated more superficially once it is matured. Maturation of the stoma is then performed. Using 2-0 Prolene sutures sewn in interrupted half-mattress fashion, the submucosal layer of the tracheal rings is approximated to the inferior neck skin flap, and the posterior membranous trachea is approximated to the superior neck skin flap. Two 15-Fr flat Blake drains are placed, one on either side of the neck, to drain the neck dissection bed deep to the sternocleidomastoid muscle. The neck is then closed in a multilayered fashion, with interrupted 3-0 Vicryl sutures for the platysma layer, 4-0 Vicryl for the subdermal layer, and staples for the skin.

● SPECIAL INTRAOPERATIVE CONSIDERATIONS

Gross extranodal extension of cancer into the sternocleidomastoid muscle, internal jugular vein, or spinal accessory nerve will necessitate sacrifice of these structures. Preoperative examination with direct laryngoscopy enables planning for where the eventual entry into the pharynx can be made for mucosal incisions. In the event that there is gross extension of cancer involving the epiglottis, entry into the pharynx can be made in either the postcricoid mucosa inferiorly or the piriform sinus mucosa opposite to the side of the main cancer bulk laterally. Extension of cancer to involve a major portion of the piriform sinus mucosa or posterior pharyngeal wall will necessitate sacrifice of these structures. In the event of an inadequate amount of mucosa available for reconstruction of the pharynx, regional flaps such as the pectoralis major myocutaneous flap or free tissue transfer from the radial forearm or anterolateral thigh can be used.

In patients who are deemed suitable candidates by speech and language pathologists without a history of radiation to the neck, a tracheoesophageal puncture can be created at the time of surgery for eventual placement of a voice prosthesis 7 to 10 days after surgery. The tracheoesophageal puncture is performed 1 cm below the superior edge of the laryngectomy stoma before creation of the neopharynx. A red rubber catheter is used to stent the opening, also allowing for temporary feeding in the postoperative period while the suture line of the neopharynx reconstruction is allowed to heal.

● POSTOPERATIVE MANAGEMENT

Broad-spectrum antibiotics are administered for a further 24 hours. Feeding via the nasogastric tube can be initiated after 24 hours postoperatively, in the absence of ongoing nausea/emesis. The patient's head of bed is kept elevated. Meticulous care of the new laryngectomy stoma is performed, which involves humidification, removal of crusting, and suctioning of secretions, in order to avoid any mucous plugging. Close attention should be paid to the contents of the closed suction drain bulbs for salivary discharge, which are indicative of pharyngeal leak. In the absence of any salivary content within the drain bulbs, a leak test with the patient swallowing some water-soluble contrast material can be performed at day 5 to 7 postoperatively. A soft diet can be commenced after if this test is negative for any anastomotic leak. The neck drains may be removed after if the output is <20 mL over a time period of 24 hours.

Neck staples may be removed after 7 days and stomal sutures at 2 weeks. If a tracheoesophageal puncture was performed at the time of surgery, a voice prosthesis is inserted in place of the red rubber catheter at 10 days. Formal training on the use of their voice prosthesis is carried out at 3 weeks. In the meantime, the patient may phonate using an electrolarynx device. Rehabilitation after neck dissections involves the patient performing range of motion shoulder exercises. Depending on final pathologic staging of this patient's cancer, adjuvant radiation will be administered for features of T3/T4 staging, N2/N3 nodal disease, and perineural/lymphovascular invasion. Adjuvant chemoradiation is indicated for features of extracapsular nodal extension and positive margins (Table 135-1).

Table 135-1 Total Laryngectomy

Key Technical Steps

1. Apron neck incision and raising of subplatysmal flaps
2. Completion of neck dissections if indicated
3. Superior dissection limit—separating suprahyoid musculature off the hyoid bone
4. Perform ipsilateral hemithyroidectomy if indicated
5. Divide superior constrictor muscle at the lateral edges of the thyroid lamina
6. Inferiorly, divide strap muscles from sternal attachments
7. Perform tracheotomy and bevel tracheal incisions superiorly and identify tracheoesophageal plane
8. Entry into pharynx via either preepiglottic space (superior), piriform sinus (lateral), or postcricoid (inferior)
9. Perform mucosal incisions sparing uninvolved piriform sinus mucosa
10. Cricopharyngeal myotomy
11. Reconstruction of the pharynx
12. Maturation of laryngectomy stoma
13. Closure of the neck

Potential Pitfalls

- Failure to accurately stage laryngeal cancer preoperatively
- Injury to hypoglossal nerve during dissection in the region of the hyoid bone
- Inadvertent transection into tumor at time of pharyngeal entry because of failure to recognize site and extent of involvement
- Inadequate sparing of piriform sinus mucosa precluding primary pharyngeal reconstruction
- Failure to invert mucosa during pharyngeal reconstruction predisposing to anastomotic leak
- Not beveling tracheal incisions, leading to a narrowed laryngectomy stoma

TAKE HOME POINTS

- An awake tracheostomy is the preferred method to secure a patient's airway in the scenario of an obstructive laryngeal mass with respiratory compromise.
- Accurate staging of advanced laryngeal cancer requires a combination of intraoperative examination of the larynx, CT scan with contrast of the chest and neck.
- Advanced laryngeal cancer with gross extralaryngeal extension is best treated with an up-front surgical approach involving a total laryngectomy. Elective neck dissections should be performed at the time of laryngectomy to address occult nodal metastatic disease.
- Following an up-front surgical management of laryngeal cancer, patients should receive adjuvant radiation or chemoradiation for high-risk disease features.

SUGGESTED READINGS

Bernier J, Dmoenge C, Ozsahin M, et al. Postoperative irradiation with or without concomitant chemotherapy for locally advanced head and neck cancer. N Engl J Med. 2004;350 (19):1945-1952.

Deschler DG, Moore MG, Smith RV. Quick reference Guide to TNM Staging of Head and Neck Cancer and Neck Dissection Classification. 4th ed. Available at: www.entnet.org/sites/default/files/neckdissection_quickrefguide_highresFINAL.pdf.

Forastiere AA, Zhang Q, Weber RS, et al. Long term results of RTOG 91–11: a comparison of three nonsurgical treatment strategies to preserve the larynx in patients with locally advanced larynx cancer. J Clin Oncol. 2013;31(7):845-852.

Grover S, Swisher-McClure S, Mitra N, et al. Total laryngectomy versus larynx preservation for T4a larynx cancer: patterns of care and survival outcomes. Int J Radiat Oncol Biol Phys. 2015;92(3):594-601.

National Comprehensive Cancer Network. Head and neck cancer (version 1.2016). Available at: https://www.nccn.org/professionals/physician_gls/pdf/head-and-neck.pdf. Accessed September 10, 2016.

INDEX